Anaesthesia for Children

To Margaret McClelland
and John Stocks

Anaesthesia for Children
WITH A SECTION ON INTENSIVE CARE

T.C.K. BROWN
MBChB, MD (Melb), FANZCA, FRCA
Director of Anaesthesia,
Royal Children's Hospital,
Melbourne

G.C. FISK
MA, BM, BCh, FANZCA
Formerly Director of Paediatric Anaesthesia,
Prince of Wales Hospital, Sydney; and
Senior Lecturer, School of Paediatrics,
University of New South Wales

FOREWORD BY
GORDON H. BUSH
MA, DM, FRCA, DA
Emeritus Consultant in Paediatric Anaesthesia,
Royal Liverpool Children's Hospitals,
Liverpool, UK

SECOND EDITION

OXFORD
BLACKWELL SCIENTIFIC PUBLICATIONS
LONDON EDINBURGH BOSTON
MELBOURNE PARIS BERLIN VIENNA

© 1979, 1992 by
Blackwell Scientific Publications
Editorial Offices:
Osney Mead, Oxford OX2 OEL
25 John Street, London WC1N 2BL
23 Ainslie Place, Edinburgh EH3 6AJ
238 Main Street, Cambridge
     Massachusetts 02142, USA
54 University Street, Carlton
     Victoria 3053, Australia

Other Editorial Offices:
Librairie Arnette SA
2, rue Casimir-Delavigne
75006 Paris
France

Blackwell Wissenschafts-Verlag
Meinekestrasse 4
D-1000 Berlin 15
Germany

Blackwell MZV
Feldgasse 13
A-1238 Wien
Austria

First published 1979
German edition 1985
Second edition 1992

Set by Setrite Typesetters, Hong Kong
Printed and bound in Great Britain by
William Clowes Ltd, Beccles and London

DISTRIBUTORS

Marston Book Services Ltd
PO Box 87
Oxford OX2 ODT
(*Orders*: Tel: 0865 791155
          Fax: 0865 791927
          Telex: 837515)

USA
Blackwell Scientific Publications, Inc.
238 Main Street
Cambridge, MA 02142
(*Orders*: Tel: 800 759-6102
          617 225-0401)

Canada
Times Mirror Professional Publishing, Ltd
5240 Finch Avenue East
Scarborough, Ontario M1S 5A2
(*Orders*: Tel: 800 268-4178
          416 298-1588)

Australia
Blackwell Scientific Publications
(Australia) Pty Ltd
54 University Street
Carlton, Victoria 3053
(*Orders*: Tel: 03 347-0300)

A catalogue record for this book is
available from the British Library

ISBN 0-632-03023-2

Contents

Contributors

The following either wrote the chapters or contributed to the chapters indicated in brackets:

ROD WESTHORPE (Deputy Director) [3, 4, 21, Appendix 5]
ROBERT EYRES [13, 24]
IAN MCKENZIE [2, 25]
STEPHEN ROBINSON [8, 10]
BARBARA MAIN [17]
JILL ROBERTSON [17]
PETER LAUSSEN [1, 26]
MARY DWYER [3, 10]
All of the Department of Anaesthetics, Royal Children's Hospital, Melbourne

FRANK SHANN (Director) [29, 37]
ROBERT HENNING [13, 24]
JAMES TIBBALLS (Deputy Director) [31, 35]
WARWICK BUTT [37]
All of the Intensive Care Unit, Royal Children's Hospital, Melbourne

ALAN DUNCAN (Director) [9, 32, 33]
PAUL SWAN [36]
All of the Intensive Care Unit, Princess Margaret Hospital for Children, Perth, Western Australia

DILIP PAWAR (Delhi) [8]
OLLI MERETOJA (Helsinki) [2]
BRIAN ANDERSON (Auckland, New Zealand) [25]
JUDY KERMODE (Perth, WA) [25]
ITALO ZAMUDIO (Chile) [27]
Anaesthetists who contributed while working at Royal Children's Hospital, Melbourne

RON WALL [Appendices 1, 2]
Biomedical Engineer, Royal Children's Hospital, Melbourne

JULIE JONES [5]
Psychiatrist, Royal Children's Hospital, Melbourne

ROGER HALL [18]
Dental Surgeon

LARRY MCNICOL [11 Liver transplantation]
Anaesthetist, Austin Hospital, Melbourne

STEPHEN HORTON [Appendix 3]
RICHARD MULLALY [Appendix 3]
Perfusionists, Royal Children's Hospital, Melbourne

TOM KARL [Appendix 4]
Cardiac Surgeon, Royal Children's Hospital, Melbourne

Other contributors

Physicians: L. LANDAU [25], N. CAMPBELL [1], K. WATERS [25], J. COURT [25], G. WARNE [25], P.D. PHELAN [1], P. SLY [1], H. POWELL [1], M. SOUTH [1]

Surgeons: A. AULDIST [12], S. BEASLEY [11], K. STOKES [11], R. DICKENS [19], G. HARLEY [16], D. WALLACE [14], J. KEOGH [20], E. GUAZO [14], R. BERKOWITZ [15]

Anaesthetists: G. WOTHERSPOON (Sydney) [28], J. GILLIES [16]

Foreword

It was my privilege to write the foreword to the first edition of this important addition to the world literature on paediatric anaesthesia, and I am most grateful for the added pleasure and honour of performing this task for the second edition. The fact that a second edition is now required some 12 years later is testimony not only to the continuing popularity of this book, but also to the advances that have been made in this specialty in the intervening years. It is also a tribute to the significant contribution that has been made to paediatric anaesthesia by our colleagues in Australia. The editors and all those involved in writing and producing this new textbook are to be congratulated on their immense dedication and sheer hard work.

The contents of this new edition have naturally undergone extensive revision to incorporate advances in new drugs, techniques, equipment and concepts to reflect modern standards and practice. These changes have occurred in all chapters but, in particular, major rewriting has taken place in the sections on pharmacology, plastic surgery (to incorporate the important work now being performed in craniofacial surgery), and of course in cardiac surgery, where such tremendous progress has been made in the diagnosis, evaluation and correction of congenital cardiac anomalies.

The extended role of the paediatric anaesthetist to cover areas of concern outside the operating theatre suite, whilst being developed more than 10 years ago, is now fully recognized, and this is reflected in the important addition of a new chapter on pain and its management.

This aspect of anaesthetic practice has largely been neglected, partly because of the tremendous workload of the anaesthetist within the theatre complex itself, and the lack of suitable staffing levels. Thankfully the approach to postoperative and other painful situations is now recognized, and requires radical solutions world-wide. With the advent of new techniques now available, the next few years will undoubtedly see a more humane and successful resolution of this common problem.

The other areas in which the paediatric anaesthetist has been in great demand are, of course, in all aspects of intensive care and resuscitation. The editors have therefore most properly extended this part of the book to include circulatory failure and shock, cardiac arrest, neurological emergencies and new developments in supportive therapy. These chapters indicate the current approach to these challenges. The recognition of the need for a dedicated and full-time involvement in this highly specialized and time-consuming branch of medicine has long been recognized in paediatric hospitals in Australia. The resultant expertise and experience are acknowledged throughout the world.

I feel entirely confident that this second edition will achieve the same success as the first. It will continue the excellent traditions of anaesthesia for children which were established by the pioneers of the field in Australia. It was, after all, an appreciation that inspired the production of this book in the first place.

Gordon H. Bush

Preface

Much progress has been made in paediatric anaesthesia since the following case was reported at the Anaesthetic Section of the British Medical Association (Australia Branch) over 60 years ago. 'Problems were encountered keeping a clear airway with an open ether anaesthetic during a harelip repair by an orthopaedic surgeon. The pathologist reported the death as being due to an overdose of ether, but the anaesthetist described looking into the mouth and seeing bubbles rising through a pool of blood in the pharynx and expressed his own conviction that the baby drowned in his own blood. He went on to plead for small tubes and endotracheal anaesthesia in such cases, the advantages of which had been so clearly demonstrated recently by Magill.'

Although tragedies still occur, they are less frequent because training in the principles and practice of anaesthesia for children has improved, and has been available to more anaesthetists. Programmes of training need careful planning. It must be recognized that adequately supervised practical training should be backed up by theoretical teaching and active involvement with medical and surgical colleagues in assessing and managing patients outside the operating theatre. Exposure of trainees to these programmes can stimulate enquiring minds to suggest new ideas and developments, as can involvement in research. In a well-planned teaching department both teachers and trainees can help to raise the standards of care still further.

It is evident that paediatric anaesthesia has taken great strides forward since the first edition of this book in 1979. Many new books have appeared, major paediatric anaesthetic meetings and courses have been held throughout the world and the literature in the field has increased so much that a specialist journal, *Paediatric Anaesthesia*, is being launched.

The importance of individual patients, as they develop from birth to adolescence through rapid stages of maturation, has been emphasized. As they grow, their responses to stress, separation from parents and exposure to strangers in unfamiliar surroundings also change.

Anaesthetists need to understand these reactions and the ways in which they can make hospitalization, anaesthesia and surgery more pleasant and less psychologically stressful. Smooth induction, an operation without complications and comfortable recovery are the goals to be achieved. Our patients can respond to and be reassured by kindly handling, and should not just be quietened with sedatives. Anaesthetists should work together with other medical, nursing and ancillary staff to create an environment where the child does not feel threatened or neglected. Parents are also important because they have anxieties that can be allayed by an understanding anaesthetist. Anxious parents transmit anxiety to their child, so it is helpful to everybody to reassure the parents. The chapter on 'The Child in Hospital' should help readers to gain a better understanding of their young patients. Its inclusion in the first edition brought many favourable comments and it is notable that in recent years the handling of children and their parents has been a subject of great interest to paediatric anaesthetists.

Children requiring surgery sometimes have syndromes or associated diseases which are significant in their overall anaesthetic management. Increased experience and greater awareness and understanding of these problems are reflected in the expansion of Chapter 25 on medical conditions.

The section on intensive care has been expanded, reflecting the marked increase in the importance of this field, and the developments that have accompanied it.

Many people have helped in the preparation of this edition, most of whom work or have worked at the Royal Children's Hospital. We hope that the presentation of their combined knowledge and experience has been distilled into a clear, concise and comprehensive source of practical ideas and useful information for paediatric anaesthetists. We hope it will help many anaesthetists in training and those who care for children in their anaesthetic practice, and ultimately benefit our patients.

T.C.K.B.

G.C.F.

Acknowledgements

The preparation of this second edition has involved many contributors who have prepared chapters or parts thereof, or have given constructive comments on other sections. Each chapter has thus had the input of at least three, and often more, experienced paediatric anaesthetists. They are all individually acknowledged in the list of contributors, with an indication of the chapters they wrote either wholly or in part.

We owe very special thanks to Cathy Taylor, our secretary, who typed the manuscript, and without whose help our task would have been much more arduous.

Our wives, Janet and Flora, and our families deserve a special vote of thanks for their tolerance and support, and for all they gave up to allow us to accomplish this task.

The Educational Resource Centre's team of photographers and artists under Gigi Nieuwenhuis and Cornell Papov have been a great help in preparing the illustrations.

We would also thank the staff of Blackwell Scientific Publications, in particular Mr Peter Saugman and Mr Mark Robertson, for their encouragement and help.

Many illustrations were previously published in *Anaesthesia and Intensive Care* and we thank the Editor for permission to reproduce these.

T.C.K.B.

G.C.F.

An Appreciation: The Development of Paediatric Anaesthesia in Australia

Margaret McClelland and John Stocks, to whom this book is dedicated, had a strong influence on paediatric anaesthesia in Australia.

Dr Margaret McClelland

Dr Margaret McClelland was born at Berriwillock, Victoria, in 1905. She qualified in medicine at Melbourne University, and subsequently worked at Queen Victoria Hospital, Melbourne, the Coast Hospital and the Royal Alexandra Hospital for Children in Sydney before going to London in 1936. She spent 10 years there, mainly at the Central Middlesex Hospital, where she undertook her anaesthetic training. In 1943 she helped to elucidate the adverse interaction between trichlorethylene and soda lime.

One day she was shocked to see a child screaming and struggling on his way to theatre; she thought 'there must be a better way than this' and determined there and then to devote her anaesthetic career to improving the lot of children undergoing surgery. There is no doubt that she succeeded.

In 1946 she returned to Melbourne and soon had a busy anaesthetic practice, being one of the original members of the Melbourne Anaesthetic Group, the first such group in Melbourne. By 1947 she was sought after as an anaesthetist for neonatal surgery. She was the first anaesthetist in Melbourne to use muscle relaxants for infants. Gradually her involvement at the Royal Children's Hospital increased until she was appointed half-time Anaesthetist in charge, and then in 1956 she became full-time Director of Anaesthesia. She was actively involved in research and the development of the Animal Research Laboratory at the hospital, particularly in relation to hypothermia and cardiac surgery, which was then in its infancy. In association with Mr Harry Adams of C.I.G. she developed equipment specially for use with infants and children. Death associated with anaesthesia was of special interest and concern to her and through her efforts in raising the standard of paediatric anaesthesia she has contributed to a great reduction in childhood

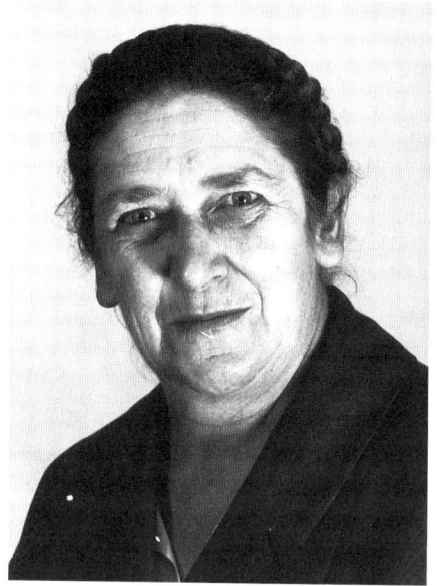

Dr Margaret McClelland

mortality in our community. Her dictum was that 'death due to anaesthesia is usually due to carelessness or ignorance'.

She was one of Australia's leading anaesthetists and a foundation fellow of the Australian Faculty of Anaesthetists, as well as an honorary FFARCS (Eng). She examined in the final FFARACS examinations, was President of the Australian Society of Anaesthetists in 1964, and in 1967 was honoured by the Faculty of Anaesthetics with the Orton Medal for distinguished services to anaesthesia. In 1970 she was made an honorary Fellow. She became an officer of the Order of the British Empire in 1975. Her many interests included current affairs, ornithology and geology. In her latter years her activities were limited by physical disability. She died in 1990.

Dr John Stocks

Dr John Stocks was born in Young, New South Wales, and graduated from Sydney University. During these early years he was Sydney University and New South Wales country chess champion.

In 1959 he appeared as a quiet man on the Melbourne anaesthetic scene, preceded by a reference that indicated his dedication: 'given a problem he would work at it until he had it mastered'. He completed his training at the Royal Children's Hospital and St Vincent's Hospital, and returned to become assistant to the Director of Anaesthesia at the Royal Children's Hospital in 1961. In 1963, with Ian McDonald, he introduced postoperative respiratory support and prolonged nasotracheal intubation for infants. This led to the development of the Intensive Care Unit in the hospital. He became recognized internationally for this work. His dedication to the care of sick children won him the respect of his colleagues and it was acknowledged by many paediatric surgeons that their advances were largely due to the improved postoperative intensive care that he had developed. In 1969 he became Director of Intensive Care, and in 1970 he became Director of Anaesthesia as well when Dr McClelland retired. He was a quiet, rather shy person whose tremendous knowledge was most effectively imparted through his Paediatric Anaesthetic Notes which were widely used all over Australia and New Zealand, and even reached as far as Canada, Scotland and Scandinavia. It was his intention to expand his notes into a book, but he was struck down by complications of an illness which he had bravely endured since his school-

days. After a long illness borne with immense fortitude, he died on 11 March 1974 aged 43 years, leaving his wife Lois and two children. The tribute from his department sums him up: 'A humble, diligent, quiet doctor, who led by example and served sick children with unsurpassed devotion.'

We undertook to write the first edition of this book in place of the one John Stocks had intended to write, and many who contributed to it in a variety of ways were colleagues and friends of his. It had been his intention to dedicate his book to Margaret McClelland and we feel that it is fitting to dedicate it to both of these outstanding paediatric anaesthetists.

Other early contributors to paediatric anaesthesia in Australia

We have outlined the contributions of Drs Margaret McClelland and John Stocks to the development of paediatric anaesthesia in Melbourne. Several others made significant contributions: Dr Ian McDonald, well known in Australia as a cricketer, became the first registrar with anaesthetic duties at the Children's Hospital, in 1951. He later became assistant to the Director of Anaesthesia. He played a leading part in paediatric anaesthesia in Melbourne. He helped to develop paediatric anaesthetic equipment and was co-author, with John Stocks, of one of the earliest papers on prolonged nasotracheal intubation. Dr L.G. Morton joined the sessional staff immediately after the war. In 1949 W.H.J. Cole became a sessional anaesthetist. His contribution to anaesthesia has been largely through the clinical study of a large number of anaesthetic drugs, and at the age of 52 he received an MSc for his researches. Dr Helene Wood made a substantial contribution to patient care of children, both in anaesthesia and in intensive care, during the decade from 1965. In 1970 she became deputy director of anaesthesia and was acting director for some time while John Stocks was ill.

The first specialist paediatric anaesthetist in Sydney was Dr A.D. Morgan who was appointed to the Royal Alexandra Hospital for Children in 1940. He presented a paper on 'Anaesthesia in Children' at the BMA Congress in Brisbane in 1949. Dr Charles Sara became honorary anaesthetist in 1948. He was influential in establishing intubation for plastic and neurosurgery, in the development of respiratory resuscitation of the newborn and in promoting the importance of temperature and humidification in paediatric anaesthesia. In 1955 Dr Verlie Lines

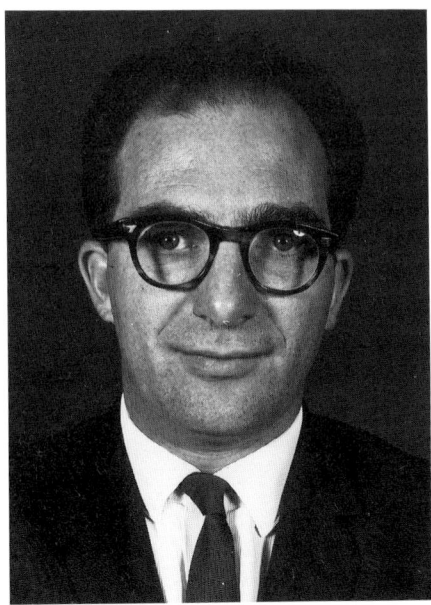

Dr John Stocks

became the first full-time staff anaesthetist, and in 1959 Dr George Lomaz became the first full-time Director of Anaesthesia.

Dr Gilbert Brown gave most of the difficult anaesthetics for children in Adelaide before the war. He was a founder member and the first President of the Australian Society of Anaesthetists. Dr Mary Burnell, later Dean of the Faculty of Anaesthetists, was the person most responsible for the development of paediatric anaesthesia in South Australia during World War II. She was instrumental in the appointment of a full-time director (Dr W. Gunner) at the Adelaide Children's Hospital and the establishment of the Department of Anaesthetics. Soon afterwards, Dr Tom Allen took over and in 1965, with Dr Ian Steven who succeeded him as Director, published another of the earliest papers on prolonged nasotracheal intubation.

The first recorded anaesthetic used at Princess Margaret Children's Hospital in Perth was chloroform, for an intussusception, on 12 July 1909. Rectal anaesthesia had a vogue there in the 1920s and ethyl chloride was introduced in 1922. The first recorded intubation was performed by Dr Mayerhofer in 1926. It became common practice for some years to intubate children for tonsillectomy, but then it was abandoned until relatively recently. Dr Gilbert Troup, one of the founders of the Australian Society of Anaesthetists and the Faculty of Anaesthetists, undoubtedly contributed to the development of paediatric anaesthesia there. He was associated with the hospital from 1922 and was honorary anaesthetist from 1930 to 1947. Dr Douglas Wilson was part-time Honorary Director of Anaesthesia from 1947 to 1956 and remained an honorary anaesthetist until 1963. He is regarded as the real pioneer of paediatric anaesthesia in Western Australia. He made most of his own equipment, including some special endotracheal tubes, a humidifier, pulse meters and extensions for intravenous needles. He carried out nearly all the neonatal anaesthesia in Perth for several years.

In 1960, Dr Nerida Dilworth was appointed the first full-time Director of Anaesthesia. Later she became a member of the Board of the Faculty of Anaesthetists. Soon afterwards, Dr Peter Brine, who later became President of the Australian Society of Anaesthetists, joined the visiting staff.

Dr Tess Brophy (Crammond) was largely responsible for improving the standard of paediatric anaesthesia in Brisbane after she returned from overseas in 1957. She became a member of the Board and later Dean of the Faculty of Anaesthetists, and also the first Professor of Anaesthesia in Queensland.

Dr Jackson Rees from Liverpool, who was the Australian Society of Anaesthetists' overseas visitor in 1963, provided a great stimulus to further developments in paediatric anaesthesia.

Anaesthesia for children in Australia has benefited from the presence of long established children's hospitals in most of the major cities, and from the many leading anaesthetists in the country who have had a particular interest in children.

1: Anatomy and Physiology

INTRODUCTION

The neonate differs in many ways from the fully developed adult. The changes that occur in the neonatal period (the first 28 days of life) and during infancy (1−12 months) are continuous and significant. In anaesthesia these lead to gradually changing responses to environmental factors (e.g. susceptibility to temperature change), to drugs and to procedures carried out by anaesthetists and surgeons. The rate of change varies with age, tending to be more rapid in the neonatal period, and in different organs.

An important difference is the relatively greater (2−2.5 times) surface area/body weight ratio of the neonate compared with older children and adults. When comparing measurements of physiological function between neonates and adults, the relationship to surface area or to body weight is used. Measurements such as metabolic rate or oxygen consumption will be similar when related to surface area, but are doubled when related to weight. Resting oxygen consumption is 6−8 ml/kg/min in the neonate, 5−6 ml/kg/min in infants and 3−4 ml/kg/min in adults. The increased oxygen consumption per kg implies increases in other functions that determine oxygen and carbon dioxide transport, such as pulmonary ventilation and cardiac output. The cardiac output is mainly achieved by a more rapid heart rate.

The greater surface area contributes to thermal instability in neonates due to increased heat loss.

Appreciation of the variations in anatomy and physiology during development from infancy to maturity provides the basis for good patient care. Changes in the airway, cardiovascular, respiratory and central nervous systems, fluid and electrolyte status and temperature maintenance are of particular importance to the anaesthetist. A knowledge of fetal physiology is needed to understand changes at birth and features persisting in premature infants that have anaesthetic implications.

ANATOMICAL DIFFERENCES OF SIGNIFICANCE TO THE ANAESTHETIST

Relative body proportions

The body proportions differ. The head is relatively much larger and the limbs smaller in the neonate and infant. During anaesthesia, there can be significant heat loss from the large head if it is exposed. During resuscitation in burns cases variations in the percentage of surface area of the head and limbs are taken into consideration (see Fig. 20.1).

Nervous system

The brain is relatively larger in newborns and infants, and receives a greater proportion of cardiac output, than in adults.

In humans there is a spurt in brain growth from the last quarter of pregnancy through the first 2 years, by which age the brain has reached over 80% of its adult mass. This brain growth spurt does not occur at the same stage of development in other species. The cholesterol content of the brain is used as an index of myelination. It increases at a slightly lower rate than brain mass during the first 2 years.

The thickness of the myelin sheath has been used to assess gestational age because it is independent of pathological influences such as toxaemia, maternal diabetes, hypoxia or brain damage. Slower nerve conduction and easier access to the brain of certain drugs, including barbiturates and morphine, is associated with incomplete myelination (see Chapter 2).

The water content of the brain decreases from about 92% during the latter half of fetal life to about 82% by the end of the first year, but most of this decrease occurs by the second or third month of postnatal life.

The spinal cord reaches the coccyx in the 12-week fetus, gradually ending more proximally due to more rapid growth of the vertebral column. It terminates at the lower border of L3 at birth and at the L1−L2 interspace in adults. This is of significance during lumbar puncture, which should therefore be performed through the L4−L5 or L5−S1 spaces in infants. The lower end of the dura is usually at the level of S2 but there is some variation, and if it is lower there is an increased hazard of dural puncture with caudal injections (see Fig. 22.3).

The depth of the epidural space and nerves below the skin is obviously less in infants. The epidural space is about 1−1.5 mm/kg beneath the skin. The location of nerves using fascia and aponeuroses to gauge depth may be difficult in neonates, as these layers are thinner and not easily felt (see Chapter 22).

Neuromuscular junction

By the end of the first trimester, motor nerve fibres have made contact with the peripheral muscles but it is not until 26−28 weeks that the motor nerve endings differentiate to form end plates, and this process is still incomplete at term, particularly in the limbs. After high frequency repetitive stimuli, the action potential amplitude declines more rapidly and the neonatal motor end plate takes longer to recover than that of older infants. Less acetylcholine is available within the neuromuscular junction. This means there is a lower margin of safety when administering muscle relaxants (see Chapter 2).

Airway

The differences in the anatomy of the airway are important in laryngoscopy and intubation. The epiglottis is longer and usually U-shaped (Fig. 1.1). The larynx is situated at a higher level opposite C3−4 vertebrae in the neonate and descends during the first 3 years and again at puberty to its final position opposite C6. The descent of the larynx as the child grows is shown in Fig. 1.2 [1].

The length of the trachea correlates better with weight ($r = 0.72$) than with age, but varies from 3.2 to 7 cm in babies under 6 kg (Fig. 1.3) [2]. The angle at which the bronchi branch from the trachea is similar to that in adults − 30° on the right and 47° on the left (Fig. 1.4).

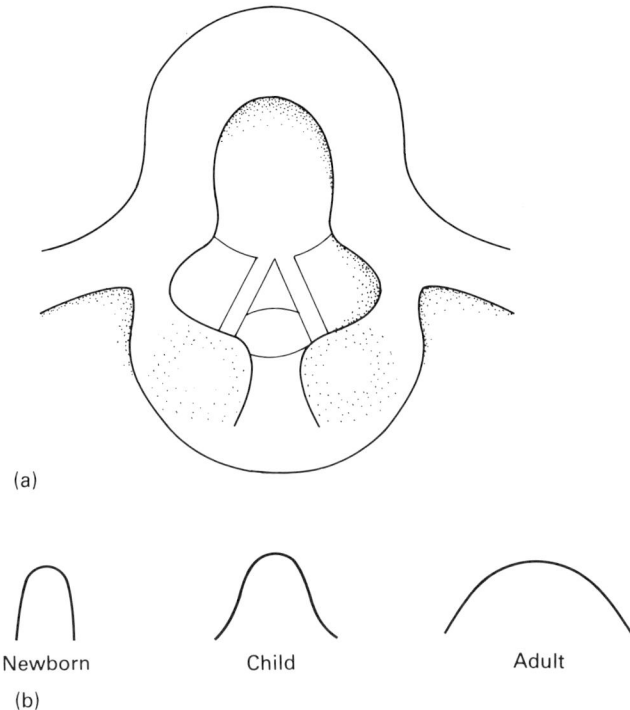

(a)

Newborn   Child   Adult

(b)

Fig. 1.1 The epiglottis is relatively larger and more U-shaped in the neonate.

The angle of the mandible is 140° compared to 120° in the young adult.

The large head should be stabilized and does not need to be raised on a pillow to improve visualization of the larynx. Because the larynx is situated relatively higher in the neck there are fewer intervertebral joints above the larynx that can be flexed to alter the angle of view. For this reason and because of the anterior inclination of the larynx it is useful to press the larynx backwards to bring it into view (see Chapter 7).

As the narrowest part of the larynx before puberty is the cricoid ring, an uncuffed tube should be used. There should be a small leak when pressure is applied. The end of the tube should be mid-trachea (about 2 cm below the vocal cords in a full-term infant) to avoid bronchial intubation, especially when the neck is flexed, or accidental extubation if the neck is extended. The right main bronchus is more likely to be intubated than the left because the tip of the bevel of the tube is on the right and the bronchial angle is less. After puberty when the cricoid enlarges, the narrowest part of the larynx is at the vocal cord level. This is an irregular shape and a cuffed tube is needed.

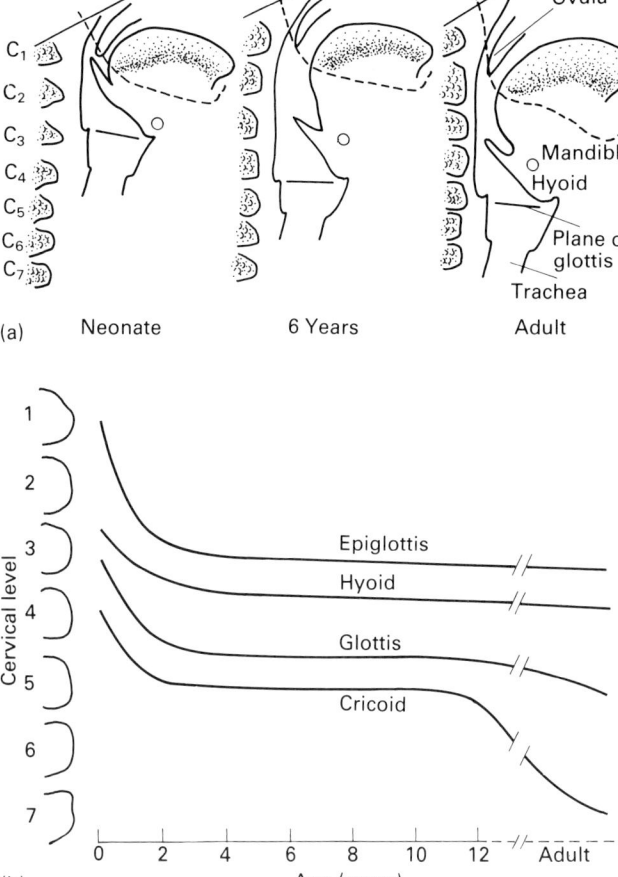

Fig. 1.2 (a) This shows the relative position of the larynx in relation to the cervical vertebra during growth. (b) This shows graphically the levels of the various components of the larynx at different ages. (Redrawn from R.N. Westhorpe [1].)

The same size of tube that will pass through the cricoid ring comfortably in an infant or small child will fit through the nose for nasal intubation, but for adults a smaller tube is needed.

Airway abnormalities occur in newborns. These include obstruction by subglottic and tracheal stenosis, and laryngeal clefts and webs. Functional obstruction results from infantile larynx (laryngomalacia), vocal cord palsy, and tracheomalacia. The infantile larynx has a prominent omega-shaped epiglottis, which, with the arytenoid cartilages, collapses inwards during inspiration, causing stridor (see Fig. 15.6). This is not usually a threat to life. In tracheomalacia, the tracheal rings may be inadequate or compressed by other structures, resulting in obstruction during expiration. Intubation may be needed to maintain the airway (see Chapter 33).

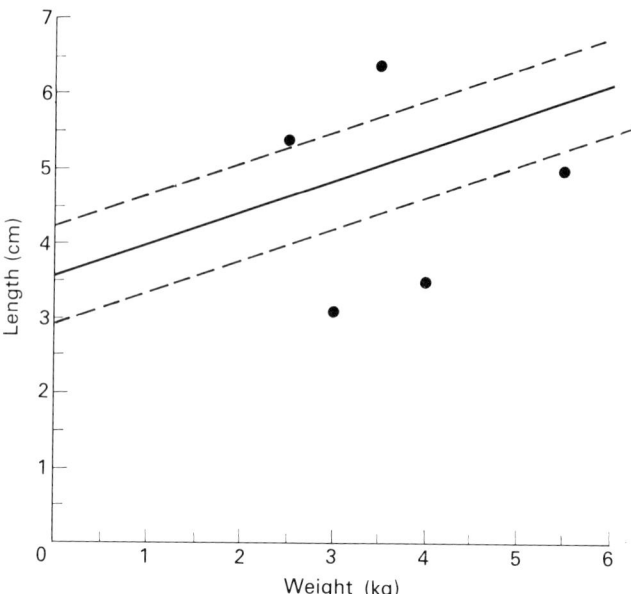

Fig. 1.3 Tracheal length in relation to weight. Patients falling outside the normal range are indicated so that the widest individual variation can be appreciated. (Derived from A. Meursing [2].)

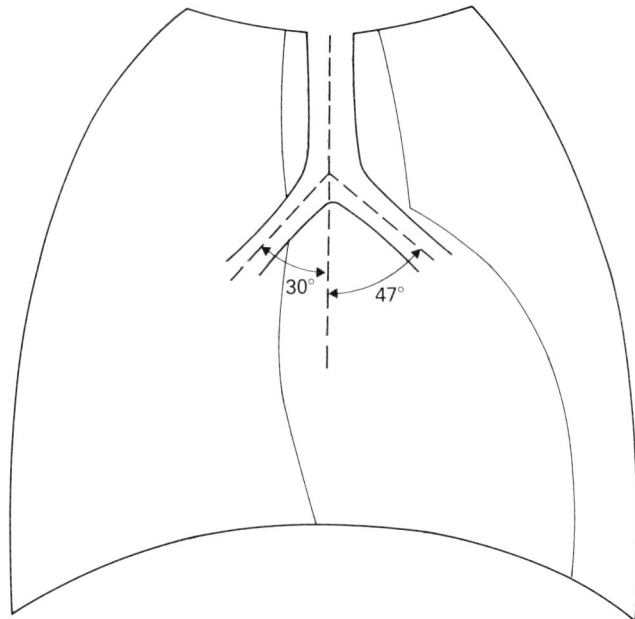

Fig. 1.4 Bronchial angles in neonates (mean of 40 measurements) illustrating how the measurements were made on neonatal chest X-rays. (T.C.K. Brown.)

RESPIRATORY SYSTEM

Introduction

Measurements of respiratory function have only been made in newborn infants in the last 40 years [3] and studies in infants beyond the neonatal period are more recent [4, 5]. Lack of co-operation makes these measurements difficult in infants and small children. If gently handled, newborn infants who have been fed will remain asleep even during complex measurements. This has allowed many studies to be made under basal conditions. Older infants have proved much more difficult to investigate and some form of sedation has always been necessary. This has limited the number and, to some extent, the value of respiratory investigations undertaken in babies beyond the neonatal period. Measurements of respiratory mechanics, lung volumes and gas exchange are readily performed in paediatric and neonatal intensive care units and during anaesthesia, but it is difficult to relate the measurements made in these abnormal situations to normal breathing.

Anatomy of the lungs and chest

Some knowledge of the differences in structure of the lung between the neonate and adult is essential to compare pulmonary function at different ages.

By the 16th week of fetal life the bronchial tree has developed. The number of airways proximal to the alveolar ducts does not increase significantly from birth to adult life [6], but there is substantial growth of the alveolar portion of the lung, with an increase in the number and surface area of alveolar ducts and alveolar sacs. There is uncertainty about the number of alveoli present at birth, but a reasonable estimate is 20 million. The maximum increase in number occurs before the age of 8 years, by which time there are about 370 million. The alveoli are very shallow at birth, with a surface area of $0.4 \, mm^2$. After birth, the alveoli increase in depth but they do not reach the average adult size of about $1 \, mm^2$ until adolescence. Thus growth in lung volume in the early years of life is mainly due to an increase in the number of alveoli, whereas during adolescence it is mainly in alveolar size.

There are important differences in the structure of the bronchial walls between children and adults. Children's bronchi have more cartilage and connective tissue, and proportionally more glands in the major bronchi, and there is less muscle, particularly in the smaller bronchioles. Small airway obstruction is thus more commonly due to inflammation and oedema in infants, and to muscle spasm in older patients.

The average diameter of the trachea in the newborn infant is 6 mm in comparison to 14 mm in the adult. Therefore any oedema from inflammation or the use of an inappropriately large endotracheal tube may cause significant airway obstruction in the infant.

The shape of the chest wall in neonates and infants influences lung volume and the mechanics of breathing. The ribs are more horizontal so that anteroposterior expansion is limited, while the lack of the bucket-handle movement of the ribs limits transverse expansion of the chest in inspiration. Consequently the diaphragm is relatively more important in ventilation in neonates and infants than in older patients.

The ribs and costal cartilages are more compliant in infants, so that sternal and rib retraction occurs more easily when negative intrathoracic pressure is increased. This is seen with airway obstruction or reduced pulmonary compliance.

In the diaphragm and intercostal muscles of infants there are fewer Type I muscle fibres, which are the slow-contracting, high-oxidative fibres adapted for sustained activity. This contributes to the early fatigue of these muscles when work of breathing is increased. Type I fibres reach the mature proportion of 55% by 8−9 months of age. In the newborn, only 25% are Type I fibres and in the premature neonate, as few as 10% [9]. Similar changes are seen in the intercostal muscles, where the proportion of Type I fibres is 65% at maturity, 46% in the neonate and 20% in the premature.

Respiratory rate

The resting respiratory rate of a newborn infant is between 30 and 40 breaths per minute; this gradually falls to the adult level of 15−16 breaths per minute by late childhood. There are two theories proposed to explain the optimal respiratory rate: one is that for a given level of alveolar ventilation there is a frequency which is least costly in terms of the work of breathing to overcome the compliance and resistance of the respiratory system; the other is that the optimal frequency for a given alveolar ventilation is the one that is least costly in terms of the average force generated by the respiratory muscles. Calculations based on both theories show that the optimal frequency for a newborn infant is between 30 and 40 breaths per minute [10]. At rest, the child's minute ventilation depends on metabolic demands and the respiratory rate is set for minimum energy expenditure. When the work of breathing increases, as in parenchymal

lung disease or airways obstruction, a much larger portion of total energy expenditure is needed to maintain adequate ventilation. In sick infants with these diseases, mechanical ventilation may be useful by reducing the work of breathing. Positive end-expiratory pressure (PEEP) or constant positive airway pressure (CPAP) may allow expiration to be completed more readily in some situations by reducing expiratory airway obstruction. This expiratory obstruction increases the time constant of expiration, and if the rate of respiration is also increased there may not be enough time for the respiratory system to return to its elastic equilibrium volume at end expiration. The result is over-expansion of the lungs. This has been called 'inadvertent PEEP'. It acts as an inspiratory load, increasing the work of breathing.

The inspiratory time constant is the time in seconds necessary for alveolar pressure to reach 63% of the total change in airway pressure during inspiration. It is dependent on compliance and resistance. In a healthy neonate, one time constant is approximately 0.12 sec and the equilibration of pressure takes five time constants, i.e. 0.6 sec. This is less than in older patients [30]. Patients with reduced compliance ('stiff lungs') have a reduced time constant and breathe more rapidly at lower tidal volumes to minimize the work of breathing. When mechanically ventilating neonates, inspiratory and expiratory times must be adjusted to allow adequate inspiration and complete expiration. Prolonged expiration may be necessary when there is airway obstruction.

Volume measurements

Tidal volume (V_T), minute volume, alveolar ventilation, dead space/tidal volume ratio (V_D/V_T), and functional residual capacity (FRC) have been measured in babies with acceptable accuracy. Other measurements such as vital capacity, total lung capacity and forced respiratory volume cannot be made because they require active patient co-operation. Volume change during crying has been recorded as representing vital capacity but this measurement has limited value.

TIDAL VOLUME AND DEAD SPACE

V_T has been measured by collecting expired gas over a timed interval and by allowing the baby to breathe to atmosphere while enclosed in a body plethysmograph. Both measurements have given similar results, but when collecting expired gas it is difficult to keep instrument dead space to a minimum. Alveolar ventilation, V_D and V_T have been estimated by analysis of carbon dioxide in mixed expired gas, end tidal gas and 'arterialized' capillary blood. Dead-space volume calculated from the Bohr equation [10] averaged about 2.2 ml/kg giving a V_D/V_T ratio of about 0.3 (see Table 1.1). Strang [11] calculated the V_D/V_T ratio by measuring the change in carbon dioxide concentration during expiration. His results were much higher than those found using the Bohr equation [$PECO_2 \times V_T = Paco_2 \times (V_T - V_D)$].

The V_D/V_T ratio is about 0.3 in both infants and adults.

Minute ventilation of 220 ml/kg and alveolar ventilation of 140 ml/kg are about twice the adult figures of 100 ml/kg and 60 ml/kg respectively, but if the alveolar ventilation is expressed in relation to surface area, the results in adults and infants are almost identical at about 2.3 l/m²/min.

The practical importance of dead space of 6−7 ml in a 3 kg newborn infant is that this can be increased considerably by apparatus dead space unless steps are taken to minimize it. Equipment such as the low dead space Rendell Baker−Soucek mask with a connecting elbow, in which the fresh gas flows directly into the mask, was designed to achieve this. Intubation also reduces dead space. If ventilation is controlled, dead space is not usually a problem because one tends to hyperventilate babies. It may be desirable to add dead space by not cutting the tube to compensate for hyperventilation.

Limited chest wall function and the reliance on the diaphragm as the main muscle of respiration mean that the tidal volume is relatively fixed during spontaneous ventilation in neonates and infants. Thus an increase in alveolar ventilation depends mainly on increasing respiratory rate. This occurs when metabolism is increased, but it may also be an early sign of impending respiratory failure.

FUNCTIONAL RESIDUAL CAPACITY

Functional residual capacity has been determined by helium dilution [12], nitrogen washout [13], and in a body plethysmograph [4, 8] with the infant lying supine. In the one study comparing nitrogen washout and plethysmographic methods in newborn infants, the plethysmograph showed a higher FRC, suggesting that there was gas trapped in the lung [13] due to airway closure during normal tidal ventilation, and that closing volume exceeds FRC in the infant. The closing volume approximates to FRC at 6 years and for the next few years it is lower than FRC. Ventilation is most effective between the ages of 10 and 20 years when Pao_2 values reach their highest levels [14].

The measurements of FRC in neonates and infants are comparable relative to size to the findings in older patients (Table 1.1). Most measurements of FRC in older children and adults are made in either the sitting or upright positions. It has been shown that FRC increases by 25−30% on changing from the supine to the erect position. Another problem is deciding the body measurement to which the lung volume should be related. FRC related to body weight measured in young adults in the supine position is similar to that found in infants.

Because closing volume exceeds FRC in neonates, they have a lower $Paco_2$ and oxygen reserve than older

Table 1.1 Lung volume measurements in infants

Age	Author	V_T (ml/kg)	V_D (ml/kg)	V_D/V_T	Minimum ventilation (ml/kg/min)	Alveolar ventilation (ml/kg/min)	FRC (ml/kg)
Newborn (0−4 weeks)	Average	6.5	2.2	0.31	220	140	25 (He dilution) 32 (body plethys.)
1−8 weeks	Howlett [7]	10.4	—	—	—	—	35.5 (body plethys.)
4−46 weeks	Phelan and Williams [4]	—	—	—	—	—	30 (body plethys.)
1−6 months	Doershuk et al. [8]	8.8	—	—	234	—	32 (body plethys.)
1−12 months	Stocks and Godfrey [5]	—	—	—	—	—	33 (body plethys.)
Adult	Comroe et al. [66]	6.6	2.2	0.3	100	60	34 (supine)

V_T = tidal volume.
V_D = dead-space volume.
FRC = functional residual capacity.

children. This, combined with an increased oxygen consumption (6–8 ml/kg/min) in the neonate, which is related to the higher basal metabolic rate, means that the neonate will become hypoxaemic more rapidly in hypoxic situations. Alveolar ventilation per kg is greater in neonates and the $\dot{V}A/FRC$ ratio is greater, being 4–5:1 (140:35) in neonates and about 2:1 (60:35) in adults. The greater alveolar ventilation offsets the fall in Pao_2 resulting from the low closing volume.

Respiratory mechanics

COMPLIANCE

Lung compliance (volume change per unit pressure change) increases during the first few hours after birth from 1.5 ml/cmH$_2$O to about 6 ml/cmH$_2$O. Lung compliance has been measured during spontaneous breathing (dynamic compliance, Cdyn) in newborns by a number of authors [15, 16] and a value between 5 and 6 ml/cmH$_2$O reported. Compliance increases with increasing lung size, so that a newborn infant has a compliance of 5 ml/cmH$_2$O, while an adult's compliance is 200 ml/cmH$_2$O. This simply means that the adult lung is larger. To allow a direct comparison of compliance between lungs of different sizes, some reference is necessary. The most useful comparison is obtained by expressing compliance in relation to FRC: this is termed specific compliance. Specific compliance is very similar in the newborn period, in later infancy, and in adults (Table 1.2). Measurement of Cdyn in the uncooperative

individual is of limited value because of the inability to control the volume history of the lungs. If the subject has been breathing at low lung volumes for some time, Cdyn will be less than after 1 or 2 large breaths. This is because some alveoli collapse at low lung volumes. Nevertheless the measurements of Cdyn do indicate that there is no great difference in the elastic properties of the lung between the newborn and the adult.

The chest wall is very compliant in the neonate and probably accounts for less than 15% of total respiratory elastance. The very soft rib cage of the infant is probably responsible for this high compliance. After infancy, the chest wall becomes more rigid and, after about the age of 1 year, there is little change in the ratio of lung to chest-wall compliance.

Because the ribs are horizontal and the rib cage of an infant is soft, it contributes little to increased intrathoracic volume during inspiration, at least in the supine position. During quiet breathing there is apparent movement of the rib cage during inspiration, but if there is airway obstruction or respiratory distress, sternal retraction occurs. Because adequate ventilation depends on diaphragmatic movement, anything that inhibits diaphragmatic descent will cause hypoventilation. Abdominal distension with gas can seriously impair inspiration, and has been known to precipitate respiratory failure in conditions such as acute viral bronchiolitis. Inflation through a face mask may introduce a large amount of gas into the stomach, but this can be avoided if ventilation is gentle. Figure 1.5 shows the changes in compliance during anaesthesia when an infant's stomach was accidentally distended with air, after deflation, and when the

Table 1.2 Measurements of respiratory mechanics in infants

Age	Authors	Cdyn (ml/cmH$_2$O)	Specific compliance (ml/cmH$_2$O/ml)	Airway resistance (cmH$_2$O/l/sec)	Pulmonary resistance (cmH$_2$O/l/sec)
Newborn (1–4 weeks)	Average	5.3	0.059	19	31
1–8 weeks	Howlett [7]	—	0.062	—	20–57
4–46 weeks	Phelan and Williams [4]	—	0.056	—	14–33
1–12 months	Doershuck et al. [8]	—	—	10–30	—
1–12 months	Stocks and Godfrey [5]	—	—	11–24	—
Adult	Marshall [20]	—	0.050	—	—
	Briscoe and DuBois [21]	—	—	—	—
	Comroe [66]	—	—	0.05–0.15	—

Cdyn = dynamic compliance.
FRC = functional residual capacity.

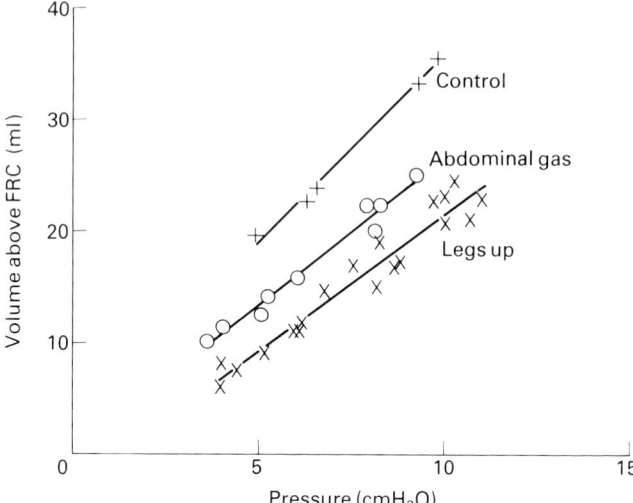

Fig. 1.5 This demonstrates the compliance changes which occurred in an infant when the stomach was accidentally distended with air (○), after it was deflated (+), and when the infant was placed in an extreme lithotomy position for surgery (×).

infant was placed in an extreme lithotomy position for surgery.

RESISTANCE TO BREATHING

Airway and pulmonary resistance have been measured in neonates [15, 16] and in infants and young children up to the age of 5 years [4, 5, 8]. Table 1.2 shows the mean values for airway and pulmonary resistance in neonates, and the individual measurements given by the authors who studied older infants. Resistance decreases with increasing lung and body size. A useful relationship has been found between the reciprocal of airways resistance and lung volume which is termed specific conductance. One of the problems in comparing measurements of resistance in infants and those in older children and adults is that the measurements in the younger subjects have usually been made during nose breathing. It has been shown that the nose contributes about 42% of the total airways resistance in newborn infants [17] and in adults up to 63% [18]. Most measurements in adults are made during mouth breathing. Overall, the measurements of airway and pulmonary resistance in infants are probably not too dissimilar to those in adults when allowance is made for the difference in lung size (see Table 1.2). The same pressure gradient is needed to overcome airway resistance during normal resting ventilation in infants as in adults [19].

Peripheral airways smaller than 2 mm in diameter contribute a very small proportion of total airway resistance in adults because their total cross-sectional area is greater than the trachea and bronchi. This is particularly important because many diseases begin in these peripheral airways and will not be detected by simple tests of airway resistance until they are well advanced. In children under the age of 6 years, peripheral airways contribute about half of the total airways resistance [22], and therefore disease narrowing the small airways is more likely to cause substantial breathing problems. This is one reason why bronchiolitis and asthma cause more frequent and serious problems in young children. Insertion of an endotracheal tube increases airways resistance and therefore the work of breathing. This does not usually produce any clinically obvious difference because energy normally consumed by spontaneous respiration is a very small proportion (3%) of total energy expenditure.

Gas exchange

VENTILATION/PERFUSION RELATIONSHIPS

Significant ventilation/perfusion (V/Q) mismatch also occurs in the newborn. In the normal adult the ventilation/perfusion ratio is 0.8–0.9 decreasing from the apex to the base of the lung when sitting upright. The alveolar-to-arterial oxygen gradient is 4–5 mmHg in the adult and the arterial-to-alveolar carbon dioxide gradient is 1–2 mmHg. In the neonate, lung expansion and changes in pulmonary blood flow occur soon after birth, but the ventilation/perfusion ratio is low — about 0.4 — due to airway closure and gas trapping. This mismatch is reflected in a lower normal oxygen tension in the neonate — 50–70 mmHg (6.7–9.3 kPa) soon after birth. In the pre-term infant the shunt is greater, and may persist longer than in full-term infants. This mismatch is further aggravated by parenchymal lung disease, as in newborn respiratory distress syndrome [23].

V/Q mismatch, high oxygen consumption and high closing volumes (see above) make neonates more likely to become hypoxaemic.

Control of breathing

CHEMORECEPTORS

Peripheral and central chemoreceptors are well developed in the neonate and transmit information about the ventilation requirements to the respiratory centre. Before birth, the fetal Pao_2 is about 30 mmHg (4 kPa) and after birth there is an immediate increase in tension to 50 mmHg (6.7 kPa), and then within a few hours to 70 mmHg (9.3 kPa). This exceeds the normal fetal oxygen tension and means that the oxygen-sensitive aortic and carotid body chemoreceptors have little influence in the control of breathing initially until they are reset to a higher oxygen tension threshold level [24]. After the chemoreceptors have been reset, a fall in oxygen tension will stimulate increased ventilation, but in neonates this is transient because they are unable to sustain the hyper-ventilatory response. Subsequently, ventilation falls towards the previous inadequate level.

The ventilatory response to carbon dioxide tension appears to be more mature. The CO_2 response curve is shifted to the left compared to the adult, which means that the chemoreceptors begin to increase ventilation at lower CO_2 levels. The response is linear until the carbon dioxide tension reaches about 60 mmHg (8 kPa), at which level it reaches a plateau.

MECHANORECEPTORS

Reflexes from the chest wall, upper airway and lung influence the respiratory centre, so that ventilation meets metabolic demands with minimal work of breathing. Most of the proprioreceptive information and reflexes arise from the chest wall muscle spindles. These are stretch-sensitive receptors detecting the forces applied to the chest wall and the workload. The larger airways have receptors that sense lung inflation and deflation, irritants of the airway mucosa, and changes resulting from alterations in the interstitial lung fluid [24]. The Hering–Breuer reflex is initiated by lung distension, terminates inspiration and prolongs expiratory time. It becomes active in infants, slowing respiration, but its role in the neonate is not clearly understood.

CENTRAL CONTROL

Although the respiratory centres respond to chemoreceptors and mechanoreceptors, periodic respiration and apnoeic episodes may occur, most commonly in premature and ex-premature babies, associated with immaturity of the central respiratory control. There is debate about the age at which the risk of these episodes ceases — between 52 and 60 weeks post gestation. They are significant if they last longer than 15 seconds and are

associated with cyanosis and bradycardia [25]. Other factors, such as general anaesthesia, hypothermia, anaemia and hypoglycaemia may be associated with apnoeic episodes. They may be symptoms of pathological conditions such as neonatal seizures, intraventricular haemorrhage and sepsis. Lung problems that decrease FRC and increase the work of breathing, such as bronchopulmonary dysplasia and atelectasis, may also contribute.

Pulmonary surfactant

Pulmonary surfactant is a complex of chemical substances present in the normal mature lung that is important in the maintenance of the physical properties of the alveoli and small airways. It alters surface tension in the alveoli during deflation, preventing atelectasis.

Surfactant is approximately 90% lipids and 10% proteins. The lipid component is mostly phospholipid, with a small amount (<10%) of neutral lipids, predominantly cholesterol. The role of the proteins and neutral lipids is poorly understood; the former are probably important in the regulation of surfactant production.

There are at least seven phospholipids associated with the surfactant complex. Of these, two appear to be the most important for surfactant function: phosphatidylcholine (PC) and phosphatidylglycerol (PG). Phosphatidylcholine, also known as lecithin, accounts for approximately 80% of the phospholipids. It is the main surface-active component, but is a solid at body temperature. Phosphatidylglycerol has little surface activity, but it enables PC to become a liquid at body temperature, so that it can spread on to the alveolar surface.

Surfactant molecules have a bipolar structure, with hydrophilic and hydrophobic ends.

Surfactant is produced by the alveolar Type-II pneumocytes, which cover approximately 2% of the alveolar surface. These cells appear in the fetal lung at around 22 weeks' gestation, but are not present, or functioning in a mature fashion, until about 34 weeks. Surfactant is synthesized in the endoplasmic reticulum and stored in granules known as lamellar bodies, from where it is secreted on to the alveolar surface. The PG is then reabsorbed, leaving the PC molecules, which have a bipolar structure, as a monolayer. The hydrophilic ends float in lung fluid and the hydrophobic ends protrude into the alveoli.

During breathing, as the alveolar surface expands and contracts, the PC molecules move apart during

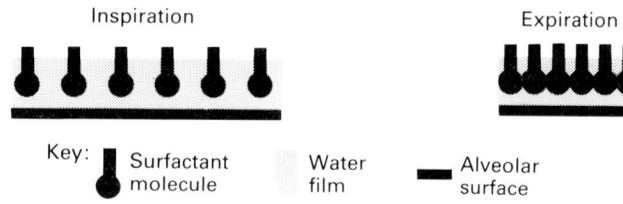

Inspiration   Expiration

Key: ▮ Surfactant   ▯ Water   ▬ Alveolar
       ● molecule   film   surface

Fig. 1.6 Surfactant molecules float in the water film coating the alveolar surface. During inspiration the molecules are spaced apart, while during expiration they become packed together. This packing results in surface solidification and prevents alveolar collapse.

inspiration and together during expiration (Fig. 1.6). Towards the end of expiration they come close together, forming a solid matrix which prevents further collapse of the alveolus. This is the mechanism by which surfactant is said to lower alveolar surface tension. Abnormalities of surfactant quantity or composition lead to alveolar collapse (atelectasis) and to difficulty in re-expansion, and so to increased work of breathing [26].

A number of conditions are associated with surfactant deficiencies. These include pre-term birth and newborn respiratory distress syndrome ('hyaline membrane disease'), pulmonary oedema, pneumonia, and the adult respiratory distress syndrome (ARDS). The first of these is due to inadequate surfactant production, and the others to disruption of surfactant function.

Attempts to improve surfactant function have only been properly investigated in newborn respiratory distress syndrome. Replacement therapy has been moderately effective in pre-term babies, with a reduction in mortality and improvement in lung function.

Clinical application

The factors outlined above indicate why the neonate and small infant are more likely than older patients to develop respiratory failure. Postoperative ventilation may be required after prolonged general anaesthesia in the premature and ex-premature infant, especially after major thoraco-abdominal surgery. Postoperative respiratory monitoring (e.g. apnoea alarm) is essential if the neonate is at risk of apnoeic episodes.

During anaesthesia with nitrous oxide and oxygen, FRC decreases. This may be due to the rapid diffusion of these gases, resulting in atelectasis. When air is used as the carrier gas for a volatile anaesthetic in neonatal anaesthesia, satisfactory oxygen saturations can be maintained without added oxygen, particularly if up to 5 cmH$_2$O PEEP is also used. The explanation is that the decrease in FRC will be minimized because nitrogen is only slowly diffusable and splints the alveoli, and the PEEP will prevent airway closure so that the air can reach the alveoli. These factors have important practical implications, particularly in neonatal anaesthesia. If alveolar collapse can be minimized, the tendency to postoperative apnoea is reduced in ex-premature infants.

A number of important points deserve comment. Infants with congenital heart disease resulting in increased pulmonary blood flow and pulmonary hypertension have decreased compliance. With manually controlled ventilation, it is possible for an anaesthetist to feel the increased compliance when a pulmonary artery is banded to reduce pulmonary blood flow. Compliance is also decreased in newborn respiratory distress syndrome. In acute viral bronchiolitis there is a marked increase in airways resistance and in FRC. The apparent change in compliance is probably due to hyperinflation secondary to airway disease. Controlled ventilation in these infants requires a slower rate than in newborn respiratory distress syndrome, with a relatively short inspiratory phase and prolonged expiration. Asthmatics have the same problem.

CARDIOVASCULAR PHYSIOLOGY

Fetal circulation

During fetal life, oxygenated blood from the placenta returns via the umbilical vein. There is a species difference in placental function, and although most data from sub-primates suggest an umbilical vein Po_2 of 30 mmHg (4.0 kPa) with an oxygen saturation of 80%, it is likely that this may be higher in the human fetus. Most of this passes directly through the liver via the ductus venosus to the inferior vena cava, which has an oxygen saturation of approximately 67%. A small portion perfuses the liver, especially the left lobe. About 60% of this blood passes directly through the foramen ovale into the left atrium while the remainder, having diverged at the crista dividens, mixes with deoxygenated blood (Po_2 18 mmHg, 2.4 kPa), with a saturation of 40%, from the head and neck via the superior vena cava and from the coronary sinus. Most of this blood passes into the right ventricle and pulmonary artery. Because pulmonary vascular resistance is high, the lungs receive only about 10% of the right ventricular output, while the remainder flows through the large ductus arteriosus into the descending aorta. This reduces the Pao_2 below the ductus to 19–20 mmHg (2.5–2.9 kPa), about 35–40% saturation, compared to the Pao_2 of 25–28 mmHg (3.3–3.7 kPa), about 60% saturation, in the ascending aorta. The heart and brain are therefore perfused with better-oxygenated blood. Most of the right ventricular output is diverted to the aorta, so that the majority of the combined ventricular output goes to the placenta and returns via the inferior vena cava. The pulmonary and bronchial veins, coronary sinus and thebesian veins contribute about 10% of the venous return.

The concept of cardiac output as defined in adults cannot be applied to the fetus. Rather, the combined ventricular output needs to be considered. In the fetal lamb, right ventricular output is about 60–65% of the total, whilst the left ventricle ejects 35–40% of the combined ventricular output. Total cardiac output increases in proportion to growth during the second half of pregnancy. Towards term, the proportion passing to the placenta falls. In the fetus, resistance to flow from the right and left ventricles is similar and so is the thickness of the walls of the ventricles and great arteries. After birth, the higher systemic resistance results in thickening of left ventricular and aortic walls.

Transition to postnatal circulation

At birth several changes occur (Fig. 1.7) [27]. There is a transition from high pulmonary artery pressure, high pulmonary vascular resistance and low systemic vascular resistance in the fetus, to the postnatal state of reduced pulmonary vascular resistance and increased systemic vascular resistance. At birth, the umbilical vessels are clamped and then close. This results in an increase in systemic vascular resistance and an increase in left ventricular end-diastolic pressure. The lungs expand, reducing pulmonary vascular resistance and right ventricular end-diastolic pressure. The increased blood flow through the lungs and increased left ventricular end-diastolic pressure lead to a rise in left atrial pressure. When this exceeds right atrial pressure, the foramen ovale functionally closes. The ductus arteriosus constricts in response to an increased Pao_2 and is functionally closed by days 2–3. Fibrous tissue grows in from mounds that develop in the ductal wall during the last 3 months of pregnancy, so that by 2 months of age the ductus becomes an avascular fibrous cord — the ligamentum arteriosum. Once the ductus arteriosus has closed, pulmonary artery

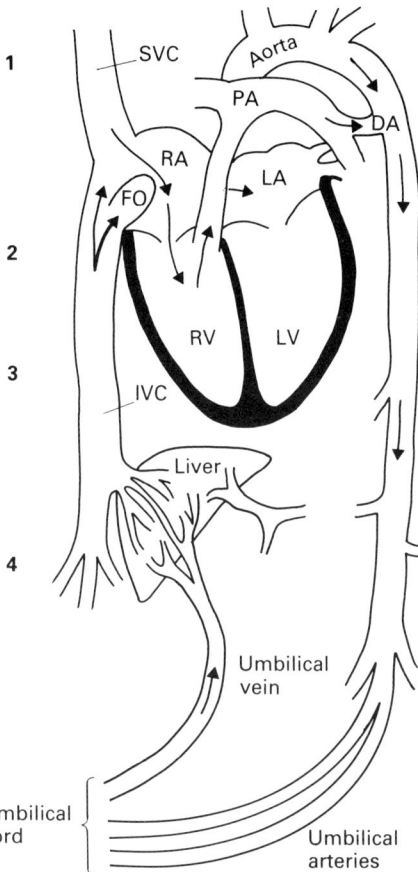

Fig. 1.7 Diagram of the fetal circulation and the circulatory changes at birth: **1** Pulmonary vessels open up as respiration begins; **2** Umbilical vessels close; **3** Foramen ovale closes when left atrial pressure exceeds right atrial pressure; **4** Ductus arteriosus closes as pulmonary artery resistance falls.

pressure falls toward adult levels within 2–3 weeks, with most of the change occurring in the first 3 days. This is due initially to a reduction in vasoconstrictor tone resulting from a rise in arterial oxygen tension, and later to a thinning of the media of the pulmonary vessels.

The fall in pulmonary vascular resistance may be delayed in infants who have congenital heart disease with left-to-right shunt. At first, the high pulmonary blood flow causes increased pulmonary artery pressure but later, if the cause is untreated, pathological changes develop in the vessel walls, causing a permanent increase in pulmonary vascular resistance that eventually reduces flow. When this pathological pulmonary hypertension has developed, surgical correction of congenital cardiac anomalies is often unsatisfactory.

When ductal blood flow is necessary to maintain life in

babies with cardiac defects, the ductus can be kept open with a prostaglandin E_1 or E_2 infusion (0.05–0.1 μg/kg/min). Alternatively, in some premature babies it may be desirable to attempt to close an open ductus. Prostaglandin synthetase inhibitors such as salicylate or indomethacin (0.2 mg/kg 6-hourly × 3 doses) may be used.

After 2–4 weeks, pulmonary vascular resistance (related to surface area) and pulmonary artery pressure (15–30:5–10 mmHg; 2.0–4.0:0.7–1.3 kPa) fall to levels which remain constant into adulthood.

Closure of the ductus arteriosus is delayed by hypoxia. In the neonate, episodes of hypoxia cause pulmonary vasoconstriction which is more marked in less mature infants. The rise in pulmonary vascular resistance leads to a fall in left atrial pressure and possibly a rise in right atrial pressure, so that the foramen ovale opens. At the same time, relaxation of the ductus tone and pulmonary vasoconstriction alters the pulmonary/systemic pressure relationships so that flow may reverse through the ductus. If there is myocardial depression as well, a fall in aortic pressure may make the situation worse. When small babies are anaesthetized, hypoxia during induction and intubation can lead to this situation, which must be avoided by meticulous technique. Cyanosis does not improve immediately when the baby is ventilated with oxygen. In conditions such as congenital diaphragmatic hernia, where cyanosis is a presenting feature, the transitional circulation may persist. It may not readily reverse with oxygen alone and may require controlled ventilation with neuromuscular blockade, sedation, correction of acidosis, haemodynamic support with inotropes and the use of vasodilators (e.g. tolazoline, nitroglycerine, prostaglandin, nitroprusside) to break the hypoxic cycle.

Postnatal development

After birth, the myocardium responds to changing haemodynamic demands. Most significant is the increased work of the left ventricle and the decrease in that of the right ventricle.

Much of the knowledge of myocardial development is based on animal studies. The newborn myocyte is smaller, more rounded and more primitive in appearance. Mitoses occur frequently, particularly in the left ventricle. Hyperplasia by myocyte replication occurs in response to an increased pressure load in the neonatal period and is complete by 3–6 months in humans. The biochemical basis of this is not known, but enzymes for cell replication, including deoxyribonucleic acid (DNA) polymerase, disappear from the myocyte in infancy.

Further postnatal ventricular growth is due to hypertrophy, with increased myocyte size and maturation in response to increasing demand.

The two ventricles grow at different rates during infancy and childhood. The left ventricle grows most rapidly early, the thickness increasing more than 50% in the first 6 months.

Biochemical changes also occur within the neonatal myocardium, especially in the sarcoplasmic reticulum. There is relatively less sarcoplasmic reticulum in the fetal myocardium than in the adult, but there is a progressive increase during development. There are significant increases in the activity of several calcium-related functions in the sarcoplasmic reticulum. These include calcium adenosine triphosphatase (ATP-ase) activity, calcium re-uptake and phospholamban concentration. The relative immaturity of sarcoplasmic reticular regulation of calcium concentration within the cytoplasm of myocytes means that the immature heart is more dependent on trans-sarcolemmal calcium flux to generate force development and relaxation than in the adult. With increasing maturity, voltage-dependent calcium channels regulating calcium entry into the cell increase in numbers, along with the increase in sarcolemmal sodium calcium exchange mechanisms [28].

Such findings are clinically important; calcium is a useful inotrope in the neonatal period and calcium channel-blocking agents administered to neonates to treat superventricular tachycardias may result in cardiovascular collapse.

Autonomic control

Cardiac parasympathetic innervation and function in the neonate are similar to those in the adult. No age-related differences in the density or distribution of cholinergic fibres have been found in animal studies.

Cardiac sympathetic function is present at birth, although significant postnatal development occurs. The myocardial content of noradrenaline increases with age, along with the concentration of myocardial enzymes associated with noradrenaline production and degradation. Sympathetic stimulation will produce both chronotropic and inotropic effects in neonates; however, the chronotropic effect predominates. While noradrenaline production within adrenergic nerves increases with age, cardiac adrenergic receptors appear to be present and fully functional at birth [29]. Circulating catecholamine levels are elevated in the newborn and help to maintain the functional response of the infant heart on the background of a relatively low vagal inhibitory tone.

Autonomic control of the circulation is incompletely developed in the newborn, with a diminished heart rate and blood-pressure response to baroreceptor stimulation. This is consistent with the lower level of sympathetic efferent neural output.

While it is often stated that newborns have a higher resting vagal tone, there is no evidence to support this statement. Rather, the bradycardic and hypotensive response seen in newborns to stimuli such as hypoxaemia and airway instrumentation reflect the functional immaturity of myocardial sympathetic innervation [30].

Heart rate

The normal heart rate in babies is much higher than in adults — 120–160 per minute in neonates (Fig. 1.8). An adequate heart rate is important in babies because their stroke volume cannot increase much and their cardiac output is therefore heart-rate dependent.

Bradycardia may occur during anaesthesia from several causes. Hypoxia from any cause is a potent cause of bradycardia in infants. Stimuli such as laryngoscopy, intubation, endotracheal suction and traction applied to eye muscles, tonsils, etc. may cause reflex bradycardia. It may also occur with the administration of certain drugs such as suxamethonium, neostigmine or halothane. The cause should be corrected and, if reflexly or drug induced, atropine may be needed.

Electrocardiogram

The ECG in the neonate is more commonly used to monitor rate and rhythm than as a diagnostic aid. In general, as infants grow, the ECG changes reflect the increasing dominance of the left ventricle as its wall thickness increases [32].

Blood pressure

Blood pressure is directly proportional to cardiac output and peripheral resistance. The neonatal blood pressure is determined by high flow and low resistance. Because blood pressure gradually increases, peripheral resist-

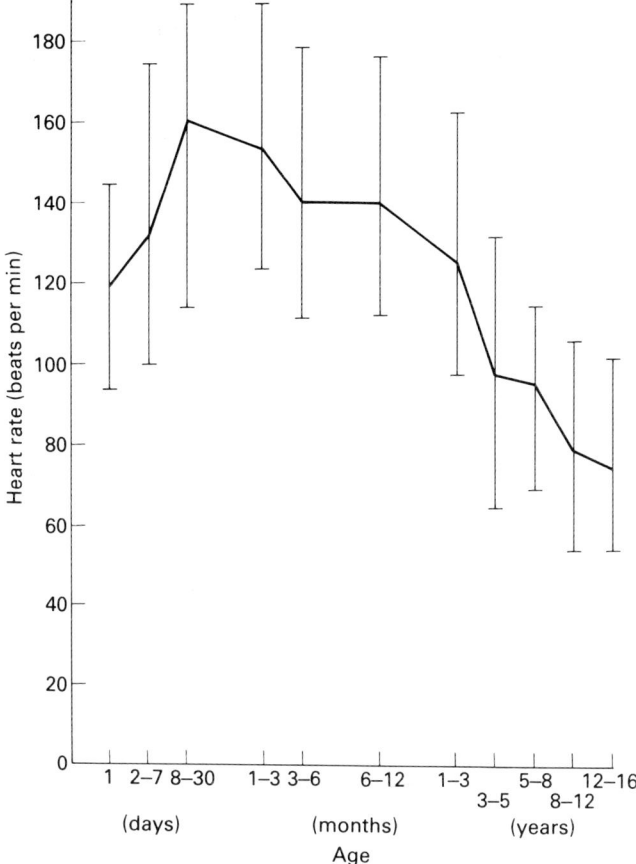

Fig. 1.8 Changes in heart rate with age (derived from figures from Shinebourne [31].)

ance must increase more rapidly than cardiac output (ml/min/kg) decreases.

Normal systolic blood pressure at birth varies between 70 and 90 mmHg and rises to about 100 mmHg by 1 year. (Fig. 1.9). In premature infants the pressures are lower. The blood pressure remains relatively constant until about 6 years of age and then gradually rises towards adult values, reaching 120 mmHg systolic at 18 years.

Cardiac output

The cardiac output in the first week of life is high, ranging from 280 to 430 ml/min/kg of body weight. During the following 6–8 weeks, cardiac output decreases in relation to body weight. At 3 weeks it has fallen to 200–300 ml/min/kg and by 8 weeks is only 150 ml/min/kg [33].

Immature myocardium develops less tension per unit area than mature muscle at any pre-load because only

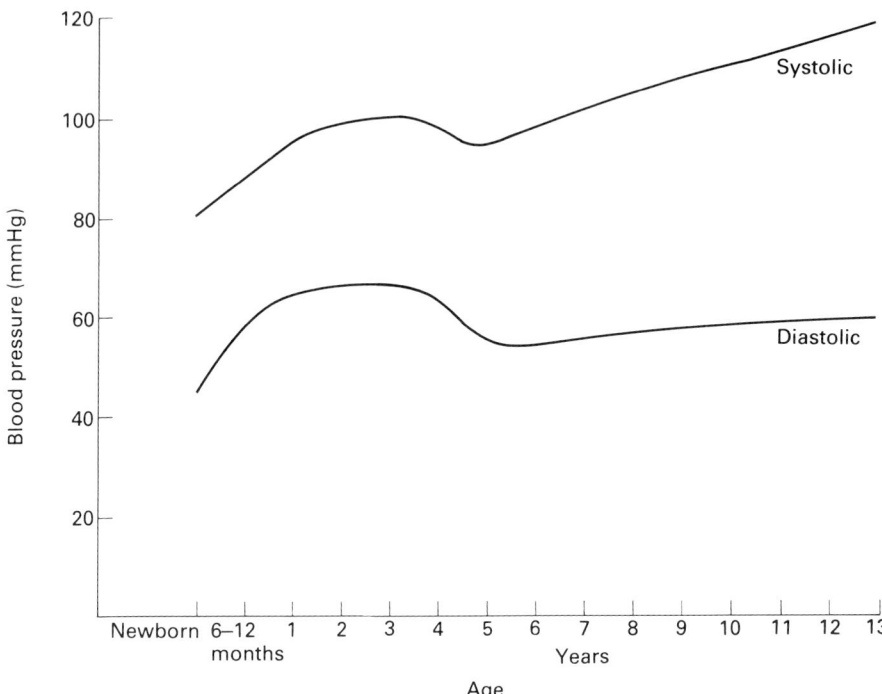

Fig. 1.9 Blood pressure changes with age (derived from figures by A.S. Nadas and D.C. Fyler (1972) [31].)

30% of the neonatal myocardium has contractile elements, compared to approximately 60% in the mature adult myocardium. Myofibril size and organization increase throughout infancy, as do the number and organization of mitochondria and sarcomeres [34].

The smaller proportion of contractile tissue is associated with reduced compliance of the ventricle [35]. This means that neonates and infants have a relatively fixed stroke volume and therefore their cardiac output is heart-rate dependent.

The cardiac index (l/min/m^2) is similar (about 4.5 ± 0.9: SD) in infants and children, implying that as surface area decreases cardiac output (l/min/kg) decreases. The ejection fraction of 0.63 in children and 0.68 in infants is also similar. The left and right ventricular end-diastolic volumes are less (about 40 ml/m^2) in infants under 1 year than in children over 2 years (about 70 ml/m^2) [36, 37].

BLOOD

Blood volume

Blood volume measured at birth is 70–90 ml/kg, depending on whether the cord is clamped immediately or not. During the first 24 hours, fluid shifts from the intra- to the extravascular space so that blood volume decreases

slightly [38]. Adult blood volume is usually estimated as 70 ml/kg and it seems that the figures of 80–100 ml/kg, previously used for neonates, are too high.

The cardiac output/blood volume ratio is higher in infants than adults, so that although the blood volume is comparable to that in older patients, the flow is relatively greater, increasing oxygen carriage.

Haemoglobin and oxygen carriage

Haemoglobin at birth ranges from 18 to 20 g/100 ml blood. The level drops steadily until 2–3 months of age, when it levels off and gradually rises again towards adult values at puberty (Fig. 1.10) [39]. Erythropoietin regulates red cell production in response to oxygen availability. It induces differentiation of the progenitor cell into red-cell precursors and stimulates the subsequent steps in red-cell maturation. The relatively hypoxic environment *in utero* is a stimulus for its presence in fetal plasma, but it disappears shortly after birth as the arterial oxygen saturation increases and oxygen carriage by the red cells improves. In both full-term and premature infants, there is a rise in plasma erythropoietin at about 3 months of age, which is reflected in an increasing reticulocyte count [39] (Fig. 1.11). Red cell survival is shorter in infants than in adults.

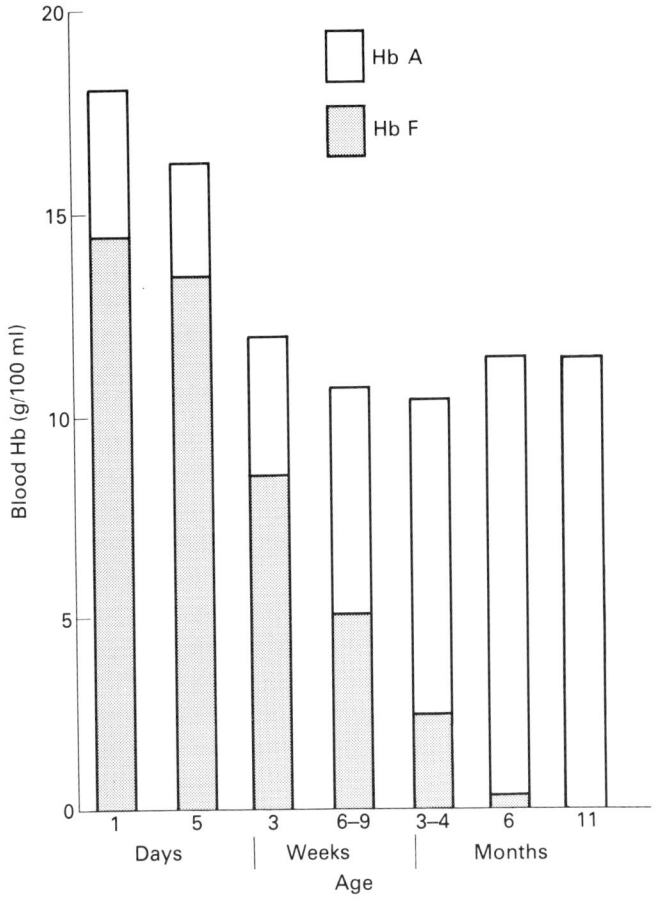

Fig. 1.10 Changes in the total and in the proportion of fetal and adult haemoglobin during the first year of life.

Fetal haemoglobin (haemoglobin F) has two alpha and two gamma chains in its molecule, in contrast to two alpha and two beta chains in adult haemoglobin. The proportion of fetal haemoglobin F is about 90–95% until 36 weeks' gestation, when the beta chains characteristic of adult haemoglobin begin to replace the gamma chains in the haemoglobin produced. At birth, haemoglobin F is still predominant (75–80%) but gradually decreases so that by 6 months only small amounts remain (Fig. 1.10).

Haemoglobin F has a greater affinity for oxygen than adult haemoglobin (haemoglobin A). This is due to a reduced binding of 2,3-diphosphoglycerate (2,3-DPG) to haemoglobin F and as 2,3-DPG and oxygen tend to compete for binding to haemoglobin, a reduction in 2,3-DPG increases the affinity for oxygen [40]. Although the actual binding site is different it has been suggested that 2,3-DPG binds mainly with the basic imidazole nitrogen of histidine in position 143 of the beta chain of

haemoglobin. In the gamma chain in haemoglobin F, histidine is replaced by the neutral amino acid serine that does not combine with the acidic 2,3-DPG. 2,3-DPG does combine with other sites on beta and gamma chains but to a much lesser extent [41].

The haemoglobin–oxygen dissociation curve is shifted to the left and P_{50} is lower than in adult haemoglobin (Fig. 1.12). The P_{50} in infants will therefore depend on the proportion of fetal haemoglobin present and the 2,3-DPG levels in the red cells.

Physiological anaemia is maximal at 3–6 months of age. It is due to lack of erythropoietin and the more rapid breakdown of red cells containing haemoglobin F. The reduced oxygen carriage is partially offset by the increasing haemoglobin A content of the cells, resulting in greater oxygen release in the tissues.

The advantage of a low P_{50} in the fetus (Fig. 1.12) is that oxygen is taken up more readily in the placenta, but it is less readily released in the tissues. This is offset by lower tissue P_{O_2} levels increasing oxygen tension gradient and by carbon dioxide uptake by the red cells facilitating oxygen release.

Iron stores and blood loss in the newborn

Most of the fetal iron stores are built up in the last trimester of pregnancy. The consequence of premature delivery is that the baby has less iron and a reduced haemoglobin level. This disadvantage continues, so that the physiological anaemia which normally occurs between 3 and 6 months is more severe (Table 1.3).

Moderate blood loss can be tolerated by a full-term infant and sufficient oxygen can be carried even if the haemoglobin drops to 10–12 g/100 ml. Because haemoglobin carries most of the iron stores, significant blood loss will result in iron-deficiency anaemia. This anaemia will be worse in prematurity and during the period of physiological anaemia. Repeated blood sampling can add to the problem. Iron supplementation or even blood transfusion may be needed.

Table 1.3 Physiological anaemia of infancy

Birth	Minimum Hb level (about 3 months)
Full-term	11.4 ± 0.9 g/100 ml
1200–2400 g	9.6 ± 1.4 g/100 ml
Below 1200 g	7.8 ± 1.4 g/100 ml

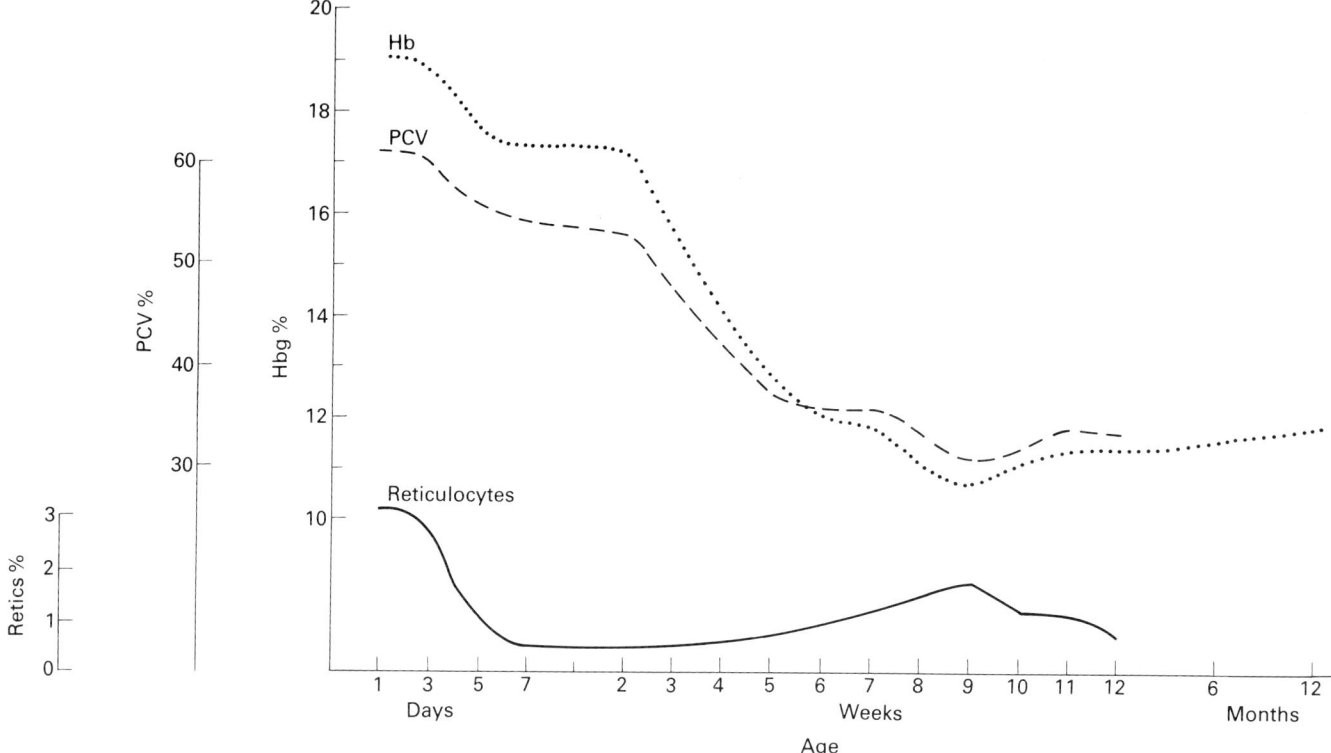

Fig. 1.11 Changes in haemoglobin, PCV and reticular sites during the first year of life (derived from figures from Y. Matoth [37]).

BODY FLUIDS

Body water may be as much as 80–85% of body weight in the premature infant, decreasing to 75% at full term and 60–65% in adults. Initially, a greater proportion is extracellular than intracellular. At about 4–6 months

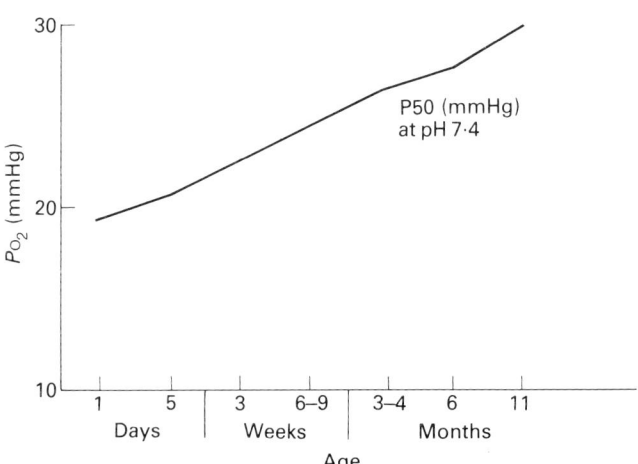

Fig. 1.12 Changes in P_{50}–Po_2 where 50% of the haemoglobin is oxygenated (at pH 7.4) during the first year of life.

after birth, the volume of the two compartments is similar and then the intracellular proportion increases and the extracellular decreases (Fig. 1.13) [42, 43]. The significance of these changes is discussed further in Chapter 2 (neonates may have a greater volume of distribution of drugs, mainly distributed in the extracellular space) and Chapter 29 (fluids and electrolytes — extracellular electrolyte losses will require more mmols to replace the deficit in neonates, e.g. chloride in pyloric stenosis).

NEONATAL RENAL PHYSIOLOGY

Introduction

The kidney is an active organ controlling body fluid volume and the excretion of water, electrolytes, drugs and other wastes. Renal function depends on renal blood flow, glomerular filtration, and tubular reabsorption and secretion. The fetus relies primarily on the placenta for its homeostasis, although the kidney does function. At birth, homeostasis is taken over by the kidneys which rapidly improve their function during the first few days,

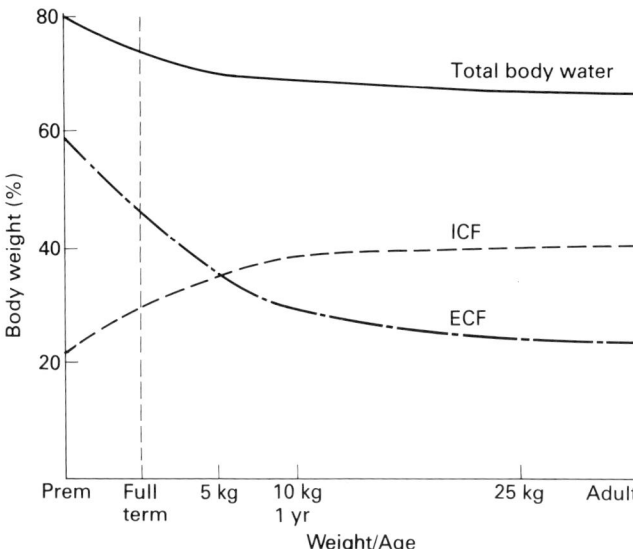

Fig. 1.13 Distribution of body water: this graph illustrates the changing ratio of intracellular to extracellular fluid during early life (figures derived from Friis Hansen and D.B. Cheek).

although development of full function relative to surface area may take up to 2 years. This rapid improvement takes place whether the infant is full term or premature, although in the latter, function is less efficient.

The main factors influencing the development of renal function are gestational age and changes from a high renal vascular resistance and low blood flow to a lower resistance and increasing blood flow.

The formation of new glomeruli ceases when the fetus reaches 2100–2500 g.

During the first few days after birth, when the stress of delivery causes a catabolic load and renal function is most immature, there is a higher level of plasma urea and creatinine than later, when most protein and electrolyte intake is used in growth, thereby decreasing the load to be excreted.

Renal blood flow

Renal blood flow depends on arterial blood pressure and renal vascular resistance. Systolic arterial pressure at birth is about 70–90 mmHg (9.3–12.0 kPa). Renal blood flow in a 3 kg infant is about 150 ml/min in the first 12 hours, increasing to 250–335 ml/min during the first week. The proportion of cardiac output supplying the kidneys is about 4–6% during the first 12 hours, 8–10% in the first week, rising to 20–25% at maturity.

A relatively greater proportion of the blood flow goes

to the medulla and juxtamedullary glomeruli in the newborn [44]. The cortex, which in adult life receives 90% of the renal blood flow, develops later. The increase in cortical blood flow as the infant develops is accompanied by a greater ability to excrete a sodium load. Renal vascular resistance rises and renal blood flow is reduced by adrenaline and noradrenaline in infants, while isoprenaline has little effect. High Pa_{O_2} levels increase renal vascular resistance.

Glomerular filtration

Formation of glomeruli ceases at about 34 weeks' gestation (2000–2400 g) but maturation of glomerular function continues for several months. The low glomerular filtration rate (GFR) in infants compared with adults, even when related to body surface area [45], is due to the low renal blood flow and perfusion pressure. Other factors are smaller filtering surface area and smaller pores in the membrane [46]. When GFR is extrapolated to an equivalent surface area to an adult, it is about 30 ± 10 (SD) ml/min/1.73 m^2 during the first 12 hours rising to 70 ± 20 ml/min by 3 months and 105 ± 20 ml/min from age 2 years to adulthood (Fig. 1.14) [47]. The reduced glomerular filtration is the limiting factor in the delayed excretion of many drugs (see Chapter 2).

Tubular function

The renal tubule consists of the proximal convoluted tubule, the loop of Henle and the distal convoluted tubule which leads into the collecting duct. These all

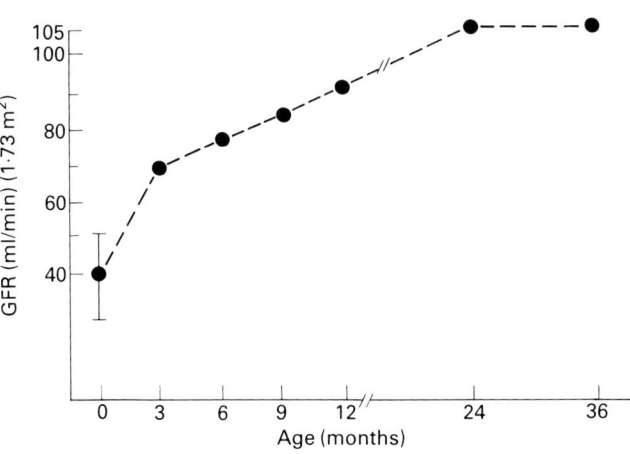

Fig. 1.14 Comparative changes in glomerular filtration rate with age using figures standardized to body surface area of 1.73 m^2.

develop at different rates, the distal nephron maturing sooner than the proximal convoluted tubule; the loop of Henle matures even later. The proximal tubule is responsible for reabsorption of most of the water (80%), glucose, amino acids and electrolytes including bicarbonate and phosphate and the secretion of ammonia.

Sodium reabsorption in the proximal tubule is generally proportional to the filtered sodium load. Under normal circumstances infants can tolerate a varied sodium intake, but under conditions of sodium loading the neonatal kidney may not be able to excrete the excess of sodium because the cortical nephrons are not fully developed [48]. There is a direct linear relationship between proximal tubular sodium and water reabsorption and the oncotic pressure in the postglomerular vessels [49]. Later, the control of sodium excretion and the handling of excess sodium improve, when the cortical nephrons develop.

Sodium reabsorption continues in the loop of Henle and in the distal tubule where aldosterone controls the final adjustment of sodium reabsorption to maintain body sodium and extracellular fluid volume.

Renin—angiotensin and aldosterone levels are high at birth and remain so during the first few months of life. The response of the target cells develops during the perinatal period: premature infants are insensitive, while the full-term newborn is responsive to aldosterone.

Water excretion by the kidney is determined by many factors. These include the length of the loop of Henle, the rate of excretion of urea and electrolytes, the osmotic pressure of the renal interstitium and the availability of and response to antidiuretic hormone (ADH or vasopressin). The latter controls the permeability of the distal nephron. Urinary dilution is deficient during the first 3—5 days of life, when urine flow rate does not respond to an acute water load. The neonate is thus at risk if too much water is given.

Maximum urine concentration in infants is about 700 mmol/l compared with 1200 mmol/l in the older child and adult. The decreased concentrating ability is probably due to there being a lower solute load in the glomerular filtrate with fewer osmotically active particles, than to immaturity of the tubules. This reflects the anabolic growth in infants after the first 2 or 3 days. Tissue growth consumes protein and electrolytes so that the urea concentration and osmotic pressure of the renal interstitium rises only slowly. The administration of urea or a high protein diet increases interstitial osmotic pressure, resulting in a marked increase in concentrating ability. During the first month, a significant increase in medullary sodium concentration occurs, which helps to increase the reabsorption of water and improve concentrating ability [50].

The circulating level of antidiuretic hormone is very high at birth and falls during the first postnatal days to adult levels, but the renal response to ADH is less in immature than mature collecting ducts.

Amino acid excretion is higher in infants under 4 months than in children over 2 years.

Acid—base balance

The kidney is important in hydrogen ion balance because it regulates bicarbonate concentration and secretes hydrogen ion, which is buffered by phosphate and ammonia in the tubular fluid.

The neonate has a low plasma pH (7.30—7.42) associated with low bicarbonate levels (18—22 mmol/l) because the maximum concentration to which the tubules can reabsorb bicarbonate (resorptive tubular maximum) is lower than in older children [51].

Other buffering mechanisms are inefficient, so that the ability to excrete acid is reduced during the first week but rapidly increases thereafter. Phosphate excretion is low in very young infants and this limits titratable acid formation and tolerance of a high phosphate intake. Plasma phosphate levels are relatively high in neonates. Ammonia excretion is limited. By 1 month of age, the kidney can respond to an ammonium chloride load.

Conclusion

The immaturity of renal function at birth places the newborn at risk when fluid or electrolyte stresses occur, but this risk decreases so that by 1 year only very severe stresses will not be compensated by the kidney. The functions of the kidney tend to develop more rapidly during the first few weeks and then maturation progresses more gradually.

It must be remembered that factors which disturb renal haemodynamics may delay kidney maturation or temporarily reduce a poorly developed function. These include hypoxia, hypotension from any cause, low cardiac output, and abnormal water or electrolyte loads.

TEMPERATURE

Skin

The skin is an important organ for the maintenance of heat, fluid and electrolyte balance and for protection against infection and the entry of toxic substances.

The epidermis is the most important barrier. It is only 2—3 cell layers thick at 28 weeks' gestation, but is fully developed by 32 weeks. After very premature birth the epidermis develops rapidly [52].

Fluid losses are greater through immature than fully developed epidermis. Pre-term infants weighing less than 1250 g may lose 40—150 ml/kg/24 h compared with 10—15 ml/kg/24 h in full-term infants [53]. Toxins may be more readily absorbed, e.g. alcohol, surface antibiotics and iodine — the latter may cause neonatal hypothyroidism [54]. Permeability to oxygen and carbon dioxide may be six times greater before 32 weeks' gestation than in full-term infants [55].

Sweat glands are formed by 25 weeks but only function after 36 weeks' gestation. Even then they are much less efficient than those of adults, even though there are six times as many glands per unit area [56].

Temperature homeostasis in the newborn

The newborn is homeothermic and within a few minutes of birth can respond to cold exposure by peripheral vasoconstriction and increased metabolism. Oxygen consumption is low at birth but rapidly rises to 7—8 ml/kg/min in the full-term infant. In premature or small-for-dates infants, this rise is more gradual and may take several days.

Infants have a greater problem in maintaining body temperature than older children or adults because their surface area to body weight ratio is 2—2.5 times greater, their skin and subcutaneous fat that insulate the body are thinner, and their total mass is smaller, so that the body heat sink is less.

Thermoregulation

The temperature-regulating centre is situated in the hypothalamus. It has receptors which respond to changes in blood temperature as small as 0.1—0.2°C, and it also receives information from temperature receptors in the skin. Skin vessel calibre is adjusted reflexly to minor variations in environmental temperature which are sensed in the skin. When the environmental temperature change is greater or body temperature is altered, heat loss is increased or decreased by changes induced by the temperature-regulating centre in the hypothalamus, including responses mediated via the vasomotor centre. The hypothalamus also regulates metabolism and the centres controlling related functions have modulating connections with the temperature-regulating centre.

In some pathological states associated with infection and pyrogens in the blood, the set point of the hypothalamus is raised and the heat-losing mechanisms are activated at higher temperatures. This explains inappropriate responses such as rigors which increase heat production even though temperature is elevated.

Heat production

Heat production is increased with activity, by shivering in response to cold and by non-shivering thermogenesis. The neonate does not usually shiver during the first few days of life unless exposed naked to low environmental temperatures (below 15°C) [57]. Their main method of heat production is by non-shivering thermogenesis, achieved by increasing the metabolic activity of brown fat. This is a specialized tissue with a high mitochondrial content, found largely in the interscapular region, but also near major blood vessels [58], in the neck, around the kidneys [59], and in the perineal and inguinal regions [60]. Brown fat has a rich sympathetic innervation which can be activated by stimulation of the ventromedial nucleus of the hypothalamus [61]. Exposure to cold increases brown fat metabolism. The local tissue temperature rises, warming the blood passing through it and thus helping to maintain body temperature. Oxygen consumption may double and this is accompanied by an increase in blood flow through the brown fat, where the oxygen uptake can be increased by over six times [62]. The blood flow may reach 25% of the cardiac output. Depletion of brown fat in infants reduces their ability to respond to cold. The metabolic response to cold is depressed by hypoxia because additional oxygen is required for the increased metabolism. Such conditions include birth asphyxia, respiratory distress syndrome, inadequate respiration associated with prematurity, hypoglycaemia and depression by sedative drugs. Beta adrenergic blocking agents also block brown fat metabolism.

Heat loss

The body loses heat by evaporation, radiation, convection and conduction (Fig. 1.15). Evaporative loss from the skin is related to the amount of sweating and also the relative humidity. It is greater when humidity is low. The newborn has six times more sweat glands per unit area than the adult, but the peak response is only one-third of the adult response [56]. In a hot environment, the only way to dissipate heat may be by evaporation and the infant may therefore become

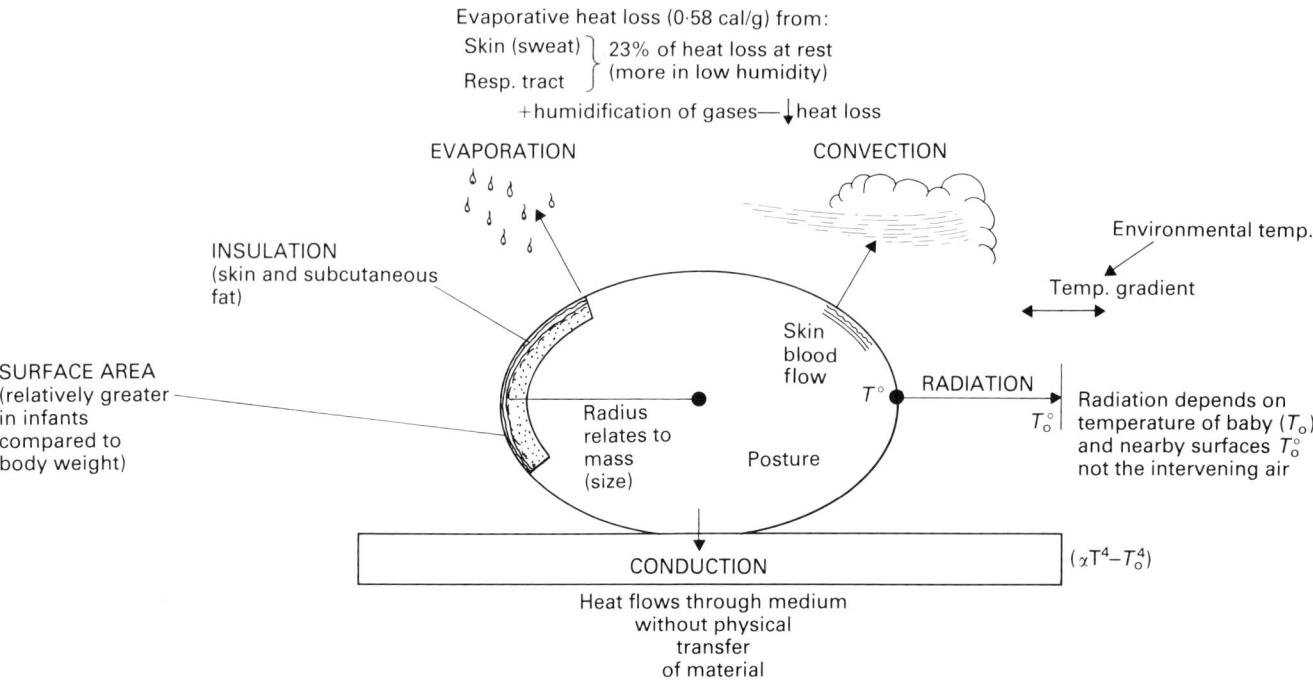

Fig. 1.15 A diagrammatic representation of the factors affecting heat loss from the body.

hyperthermic. Immature infants are in greater danger because their ability to sweat is less; before 32 weeks' gestation they do not sweat at all [63].

Respiratory heat loss is increased if the nasal re-warming mechanism is bypassed, as it is when the patient is intubated. The cooling due to breathing cold dry gases can be reduced by warming and humidifying the inspired gases.

As the environmental temperature decreases, radiant heat loss increases absolutely and in proportion to other

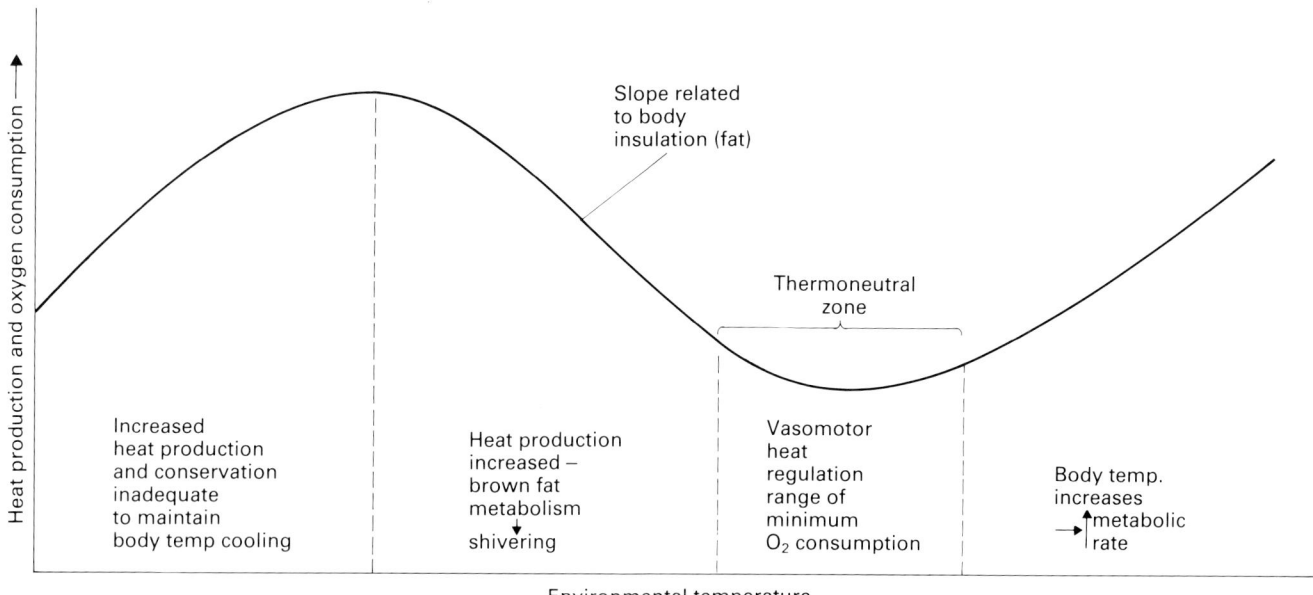

Fig. 1.16 Thermoneutral zone. A diagram illustrating the changes in heat production with environmental temperature and the factors which influence oxygen consumption and heat production.

heat-losing mechanisms [64]. Radiant heat is lost to nearby objects and is independent of the intervening air temperature. Thus air in an incubator may be close to body temperature but if the incubator is in a cold environment and its wall temperature is low there may be substantial heat loss from the infant to the incubator wall (Fig. 1.15). Significant heat loss by radiation may occur when it is cold outside, if a naked or only slightly clothed infant is placed near a closed window. Clothing reduces radiant heat loss.

Convective heat loss is the transfer of heat by movement of the surrounding air. It can be increased if there is significant air movement. Draughts should be avoided where lowering of the body temperature is not desired.

Conduction is heat transfer from molecule to molecule, for example, heat transfer from the body to the surface with which it is in contact. The use of a warming blanket under the infant will minimize these losses.

Thermoneutral environment

The thermoneutral environment is the range of environmental temperatures within which the body will maintain its temperature with minimal oxygen consumption (Fig. 1.16). The critical temperature is the point at which extra heat must be generated if the body temperature is not to fall. It is the lower end of the thermoneutral range.

The metabolic response to cold, expressed as a rise in oxygen consumption, correlates best with the difference between abdominal skin temperature and environmental temperature. In the thermoneutral range, oxygen consumption is minimal and body temperature can be controlled by variations in skin blood flow alone. Neonates, and in particular premature babies, have a narrow thermoneutral range because they have a relatively large surface area and are poorly insulated. Environmental temperatures exceeding body temperature prevent heat loss and the infant will gradually gain heat with an accompanying rise in metabolic rate. The critical temperature at which oxygen consumption begins to increase (Fig. 1.16) depends largely on maturity and age. In a draught-free environment with 50% relative humidity a full-term 3 kg baby has a lower critical temperature (about 33°C at birth, decreasing to 32°C by 2 weeks of age). In contrast, a 1 kg newborn premature infant with less subcutaneous fat and less efficient temperature regulating mechanisms will require an environmental temperature of 35.5°C to prevent increases in heat pro-

duction or losses greater than 25% of basal values [64]. Cold stress will lead to increased oxygen consumption and heat production, unless cold is extreme or the baby is sick, with impaired ability to respond to cold.

The rate of increase in oxygen consumption below the critical temperature is dependent on the temperature difference between the body and the environment and on the infant's insulation. Clothing the infant provides extra insulation from the environment and thus a temperature of 6–8°C lower will be tolerated before oxygen consumption increases more than 25% [65]. If sick babies are nursed in a thermoneutral environment, increased oxygen consumption is avoided at a time when their response to stress is impaired. The morbidity and mortality of neonates, especially the premature, has been reduced by careful attention to the environmental temperature in which they are nursed. Sick infants are often nursed under overhead heaters with servo-control from the abdominal skin.

Anaesthesia

Anaesthetic drugs depress the reflexes which maintain body temperature. Muscle relaxants prevent shivering, and anaesthetics such as halothane dilate peripheral blood vessels, thereby increasing heat loss. Blood loss leading to circulatory impairment will decrease tissue metabolism, further impairing the maintenance of body temperature. An adequate circulating blood volume should be maintained. As heat production mechanisms are depressed during anaesthesia, patients, especially babies, will tend to cool unless steps are taken to maintain body temperature. These include warming the operating theatre above the usual 20°C, keeping the infant covered when possible, placing the patient on a warming mattress, using warmed, humidified gases when the patient is intubated, and warmed solutions for preparing the operating field. Intravenous fluids and blood should also be warmed. The period at which the infant is at greatest risk is during the induction of anaesthesia, and before draping the patient for surgery. An overhead heater should be used for all infants during this period.

Consequences of cooling

If children, especially babies, cool significantly during anaesthesia, recovery may be delayed, respiration depressed and heart rate, blood pressure and cardiac output lowered. Apart from shivering, muscle activity may be diminished and the infant may be lethargic. There is then an increased danger of regurgitation and aspiration, leading to pulmonary complications. These changes are reversible on rewarming.

Signs of infection and surgical complications may be masked. Babies often do not develop an elevated temperature in response to infection.

ENERGY BALANCE IN THE FETUS AND NEWBORN

Newborn infants, especially those born prematurely, cannot tolerate periods of fasting or fluid restriction as well as older age groups. Metabolic requirements are high, especially for temperature regulation, but body reserves of carbohydrate and fat may be low or negligible.

During fetal life, metabolic requirements are less than postnatally because respiratory and muscular activity is low and the environmental temperature is constant. Throughout gestation the major energy requirement is for growth and, towards term, laying down fat and glycogen stores. Indirect measurements suggest an oxygen consumption of about $4-5$ ml/kg/min in the human fetus at term.

Glucose is the main metabolic fuel in the fetus. Most comes via the placenta from the maternal circulation, but a little may also be produced from amino acids and fats by the fetal liver. Fetal blood sugar is usually $70-80\%$ of the maternal level and fluctuates with it.

Glycogen stores are laid down throughout gestation, in the liver, myocardium and skeletal muscle, mostly in the last trimester. Thus at 33 weeks' gestation, a fetus has about 9 g of stored glycogen, and 7 weeks later at term this has increased to about 34 g.

White fat accumulates from mid-gestation but, as with glycogen, most is laid down in the last few weeks. At 28 weeks there are virtually no stores; by 34 weeks $7-8\%$ of body weight is fat, and at term, 16%.

At birth, the fetus' metabolic economy is abruptly altered. The supply of the main metabolic fuel — glucose — stops. Extra energy is immediately required for breathing, other muscular activity and digestion, but most of all for temperature maintenance. At rest, in an appropriately warm environment, oxygen consumption rises to $7-8$ ml/kg/min. With cold stress and activity it will have to rise two-to-threefold more.

Glycogen stores are mobilized rapidly in response to catecholamine release, and are usually virtually exhausted in $3-4$ hours. Despite this, blood sugar levels drop to a lowest level at about 4 hours of age, and rise only slowly to more normal levels in the succeeding days. Fat stores are rapidly mobilized, increasing plasma free fatty acid and glycerol levels, and the infant switches over to a metabolism in which the main fuel is fat rather than glucose. The enzymes of the newborn liver are less able than in older age groups to produce glucose from pyruvate or amino acids (gluconeogenesis) in the face of glycogen depletion and hypoglycaemia.

Practical implications

Premature infants are born before appreciable stores of glycogen or fat have accumulated, and therefore cannot maintain adequate blood sugar for any period of fasting. Severe hypoglycaemia can result in apnoea, convulsions and permanent brain damage. Even fasting before operation, or the period of reduced glucose supply caused by blood transfusion (glucose 3 gm/500 ml decreasing to 2.7 and 2 gm/500 ml at 1 and 2 weeks in ACD blood) can result in hypoglycaemia in the most premature infants. The inability to maintain fasting blood sugar can persist for weeks. Thus the ex-premature infant admitted for 'routine' hernia repair should not be fasted too long without intravenous glucose and fluid. Plasma glucose should be checked intraoperatively if glucose is not being given in these patients.

Small-for-dates infants resulting from uteroplacental insufficiency have the same inability to withstand fasting as premature infants, because of reduced glycogen and fat stores.

Conclusion

An understanding of the differences between neonates, infants and older children is important for the paediatric anaesthetist, so that the management of anaesthesia and maintenance of homeostasis is appropriate for the age of the patient. It also helps in the understanding of responses to the drugs.

REFERENCES

1 Westhorpe R.N. The position of the larynx in children and its relationship to the ease of intubation. *Anaesth Intens Care* 1987, **15**, 384.
2 Meursing A.E.E. Thesis. Some aspects of infant trachea. 1985.
3 Cross K.W., Oppe T.E. Respiratory rate and volume in premature infants. *J Physiol* 1952, **116**, 168.
4 Phelan P.D., Williams H.E. Ventilatory studies in healthy

infants. *Paediat Res* 1969, **3**, 435.

5 Stocks J., Godfrey S. Specific airway conductance in relation to postconceptual age in infancy. *J Appl Physiol* 1977, **43**, 144.

6 Thurlbeck W.M. Postnatal growth and development of the lung. *Am Rev Resp Dis* 1975, **111**, 803.

7 Howlett G. Lung mechanics in normal infants and infants with congenital heart disease. *Arch Dis Child* 1972, **47**, 707.

8 Doershuk C.F., Downs T.D., Matthews L.W., Lough M.D. A method of ventilatory measurements in subjects 1 month to 5 years of age. *Paediat Res* 1970, **4**, 165.

9 Keens T.G., Bryan A.C., Levison H., Yanuzzo C.D. Developmental pattern of human muscle fibre types in human ventilatory muscles. *J Appl Physiol* 1978, **44**, 909.

10 Mead J. Control of respiratory frequency. *J Appl Physiol* 1960, **15**, 325.

11 Strang L.B. Alveolar gas and anatomical dead space measurements in normal newborn infants. *Clin Sci* 1961, **21**, 107.

12 Berglund G., Karlberg P. Determination of FRC in newborn infants. *Acta Pediat* 1956, **45**, 541.

13 Nelson N.M., Prod'hom L.S., Cherry R.B., Lipsitz P.L., Smith C.A. Pulmonary function in the newborn infant: methods — ventilation and gaseous metabolism. *Pediatrics* 1963, **30**, 963.

14 Mansell A., Bryan C., Levison H. Airway closure in children. *J Appl Physiol* 1972, **33**, 771.

15 Cook C.D., Cherry R.B., O Brien D., Karlberg P., Smith C.A. Studies of respiratory physiology in the newborn infant. *J Clin Invest* 1955, **34**, 975.

16 Burnard E.D., Grattan-Smith P., Picton-Warlow C.G. Grauaug A. Pulmonary insufficiency in prematurity. *Aust Pediat J* 1965, **1**, 12.

17 Polgar G., Kong G.P. The nasal resistance of newborn infants. *J Pediat* 1965, **67**, 557.

18 Butler J. The work of breathing through the nose. *Clin Sci* 1960, **19**, 55.

19 Polgar G. Opposing forces to breathing in newborn infants. *Biol Neonat* 1967, **11**, 1.

20 Marshall R. The physical properties of the lungs in relation to the subdivisions of lung volume. *Clin Sci* 1957, **16**, 507,

21 Briscoe W.A., Dubois A.B. The relationship between airway resistance, airway conductance and lung volume in subjects of different age and body size. *J Clin Invest* 1958, **37**, 1279.

22 Hogg J.C., Williams J., Richardson J.B., Macklem P.T., Thurlbeck W.M. Age as a factor in the distribution of lower airways conductance and in the pathologic anatomy of obstructive lung disease. *New Engl J Med* 1970, **282**, 1283.

23 Krauss A.N., Soodalter J.A., Auld P.A.M. Adjustment of ventilation and perfusion in the full term and distressed neonate. *Paediatrics* 1971, **47**, 865.

24 Davis G.M., Bureau M.A. Pulmonary and chest wall mechanics in the control of respiration in the newborn. *Clin Perinatol* 1987, **14**, 551.

25 Marchal F., Bairam A. Neonatal apnoea and apnoeic syndromes. *Clin Perinatol* 1987, **14**, 509.

26 Morley C.J. Surfactant therapy in very premature babies. *Br Med Bull* 1988, **44**, 919.

27 Rudolph A.M. The changes in the circulation after birth. Their importance in congenital heart disease. *Circulation* 1970, **41**, 343.

28 Fisher D.J., Towbin J. Maturation of the heart. *Clin Perinatol* 1988, **15**, 421.

29 Friedman W.F. The intrinsic physiological properties of the developing heart. *Prog Cardiovasc Dis* 1972, **15**, 87.

30 Geis P.W., Tatooles C.J., Priola D.V., Friedman W.F. Factors influencing neurohumoral control of the heart in the newborn dog. *Am J Physiol* 1975, **228**, 1685.

31 Shinebourne E.A. Growth and development of the cardiovascular system: functional development. In: Davis J.A., Dobbing J. (Eds.) *Scientific foundations of paediatrics*, (1974) William Heineman, London, p. 208.

32 Thomaidis C., Varlamis G., Karamperis S. Comparative study of the ECG of healthy full term and premature newborns. *Acta Paediat Scand* 1988, **77**, 653.

33 Rudolph A.M. Circulatory changes during the perinatal period. *Paed Cardiol* 1983, **4**, (Supp 11), 17.

34 Friedman W.F. The intrinsic physiologic properties of the developing heart. In: Friedman W.F., Lesch M., Sonnenblick E.H. (Eds.) *Neonatal heart disease*, (1973) Grune and Stratton, New York.

35 Kirkpatrick S.E., Pitlick P.T., Naliboff J., Freidman W.F. Frank–Starling relationship as an important determinant of fetal cardiac output. *Am J Physiol* 1976, **231**, 495.

36 Graham T.P., Jarmakani J.M., Atwood G.F., Ganent R.V. Right ventricular volume determinations in children. Normal values and observations with volume and pressure overload. *Circulation* 1973, **47**, 144.

37 Graham T.P., Jamarkani J.M. Haemodynamic investigations of congenital heart disease in infancy and childhood. In: Freidman W.F., Lesch W.F., Sonnenblick F.W. (Eds.) *Neonatal heart disease*, (1973) Grune and Stratton, New York.

38 McCue C., Garner F.B., Hurt W.G., Schelen E.C., Sharpe A.R. Placental transfusion. *J Pediat* 1968, **72**, 15.

39 Matoth Y., Zaizov R., Vasarno I. Postnatal changes in some red cell parameters. *Acta Paediat Scand* 1971, **60**, 317.

40 Oski F.A., Delivoria-Papadopoulous M. The red cell, 2,3-diphosphoglycerate, and tissue oxygen release. *J Pediat* 1970, **77**, 941.

41 Oski F.A., Gottlieb A.J. The interrelationship between red blood cell metabolites, haemoglobin, and the oxygen–equilibrium curve. In: *Progress in haematology*, (1971) Vol VII. William Heinemann Medical Books, London, pp. 33–67.

42 Friis Hansen B. Body composition during growth. *Pediatrics* 1971, **47**, 264.

43 Cheek D.B. Extracellular volume: its structure and measurement and the influence of age and disease. *J Pediatr* 1961, **58**, 103.

44 Jose P.A., Slotkoff L.M., Lilienfield L.S. Calgagno P., Eisner G.M. Intrarenal blood flow distribution in the canine puppy. *Clin Res* 1970, **18**, 504.

45 Barnett H.L. Renal physiology in infants and children — method for estimation of glomerular filtration rate. *Proc Soc Exp Biol Med* 1940, **44**, 654.

46 Arturson G., Groth T., Grotte G. Human glomerular membrane porosity and filtration pressure. *Clin Sci* 1971, **40**, 137.

47 Roy L.P. Renal physiology in children. *Anaesth Intens Care* 1973, **1**, 453.

48 Fetterman G.H., Shuplock N.A., Philipp F.J., Gregg H.S. The growth and maturation of human glomeruli and proximal convolutions from term to adulthood. *Pediatrics* 1965, **35**, 601.

49 Brenner B.M., Troy J.L., Daugharty T.M., MacInnes R.M. Quantitative importance of changes in postglomerular colloid

osmotic pressure in mediating glomerular tubular balance in the rat. *J Clin Invest* 1973, **52**, 190.

50 Edelman C.M., Wolfish N.M. Dietary influence on renal maturation in premature infants. *Pediat Res* 1968, **2**, 421.

51 Edelman C.M., Rodriguez Soriano J., Boichis H., Grushkin A.B., Acosta M.I. Renal bicarbonate reabsorption and hydrogen ion excretion in normal infants. *J Clin Invest* 1967, **46**, 1309.

52 Rutter N. The immature skin. *Br Med Bull* 1988, **44**, 957.

53 Baumgart S., Engle W.D., Fox W.W., Polin R.A. Radiant warmer power and body size as determinants of insensible water loss in the critically ill neonate. *Paediat Res* 1981, **15**, 1495.

54 Coakley J.C., Francis I., Gold H., Mathur K., Connelly J.F. Transient primary hypothyroidism in the newborn. *Aust Paediat J* 1989, **25**, 25.

55 Cartlidge P.H., Rutter N. Percutaneous respiration in the newborn infant. Effect of gestation and altered ambient oxygen concentration. *Biol Neonatol* 1987, **52**, 301.

56 Foster K.G., Hey E.N., Katz G. The response of sweat glands of the newborn baby to thermal stimuli and intradermal acetylcholine. *J Physiol* 1969, **203**, 13.

57 Adamsons K., Gandy G.M., James L.S. The influence of

58 Hull D. The structure and function of brown adipose tissue. *Br Med Bull* 1966, **22**, 92.

59 Aherne W., Hull D. Brown adipose tissue and heat production in the newborn infant. *J Pathol* 1966, **91**, 223.

60 Heaton J.M. The distribution of brown adipose tissue in humans. *J Anat* 1972, **112**, 35.

61 Hall G.M., Lucke J.N. Brown fat: a thermogenic tissue of anaesthetic importance? *Br J Anaes* 1982, **54**, 907.

62 Heim T., Hull D. The blood flow and oxygen consumption of brown adipose tissue in the newborn rabbit. *J Physiol* 1966, **186**, 42.

63 Hey E.N., Katz G. Evaporative water loss in the newborn baby. *J Physiol* 1969, **200**, 605.

64 Hey E.N., Katz G. The optimal thermal environment for naked babies. *Arch Dis Child* 1970, **45**, 328.

65 Hey E.N. The relationship between environmental temperature and oxygen consumption in the newborn baby. *J Physiol* 1969, **200**, 589.

66 Comroe J.H., Foster R.E., DuBois A.B., Briscoe W.A., Carlsen E. *The Lung*, 2nd edn (1962). Year Book Publishers, Chicago.

thermal factors upon oxygen consumption of the newborn infant. *J Pediat* 1965, **66**, 495.

2: Paediatric Anaesthetic Pharmacology

GENERAL PRINCIPLES

To produce a predictable response and minimize the side effects of drugs the anaesthetist needs to know the patient's age, weight and physical status. 'Sick' children and neonates require careful titration of anaesthetic drugs, whereas older, robust patients may tolerate more rapid injection of precalculated doses of drugs.

Pattern of drug responses with development

There are several ways of comparing neonatal with adult doses. The problem is whether mg/kg, mg/m^2 or some nomogram is the most appropriate method. The choice is arbitrary and frequently depends on convenience, but the method chosen may indicate relative resistance or sensitivity. For example, on a mg/kg basis neonates are resistant to suxamethonium, but when dose is related to surface area the sensitivity is comparable to adults [1].

  Pharmacokinetic changes may produce opposing effects on initial response and duration of action. For example, 'resistance' to a loading dose due to the relatively large extracellular fluid compartment in the neonate may be followed by 'sensitivity' to subsequent doses, associated with immature metabolic and renal function slowing clearance.

At a pharmacodynamic level, membrane and receptor maturation are likely to influence the concentration of drug that will produce an effect. The picture is complicated by the fact that drug concentrations may be measured in plasma, serum or whole blood. Further, the relation of blood concentrations to tissue concentrations to which receptors are exposed depends on protein binding, pH, ionization and tissue penetration. The differences may be considerable. For a pharmacodynamic purist, biophase receptor concentrations of the drug should be compared to assess sensitivity, but in general this is impractical.

Finally, at every step there will be the usual biological variation which confounds the treating physician who attempts to 'squeeze' patients into tight protocols. Pharmacokinetic data only give a guide to the changing dose requirements with age. Despite these problems the anaesthetist should know the patient's weight and can avoid overdosage if he knows which ages and conditions are associated with sensitivity to usual mg/kg doses.

In older children, renal and hepatic clearance is more rapid than in adults, while protein binding and brain and heart function are similar to that of an adult.

The overall picture for many drugs is that compared with adults there may be a period of sensitivity in the neonate, followed by relative resistance and the need for larger doses in infants and young children, declining towards adult doses in adolescents.

PHARMACOKINETICS

The absorption, distribution and elimination of drugs vary with age.

Absorption

The rate and degree of absorption depend on the route of administration. In paediatrics, patient acceptance of the route is an important consideration. Many recent advances have depended on new methods of administration rather than on new drugs.

The intravenous route avoids problems with variability of absorption; other routes of drug administration introduce extra steps in the path of the drug to the site of action, making doses and responses more variable.

Inhalation anaesthetic agents equilibrate more rapidly to a higher tissue concentration in infants compared to adults. For example, the ratio of alveolar to inspired concentration of halothane with controlled ventilation, is about 0.55 at 3 minutes and 0.83 at 20 minutes in infants, compared with 0.4 at 3 minutes and 0.55 at 20 minutes in adults [2]. This faster equilibration results from a combination of increased alveolar ventilation (for a given Pa_{CO_2}), especially in proportion to functional residual capacity (FRC), and increased cardiac output. This correlates with the increased oxygen and CO_2 transport per kg in infants. The consequence is that despite infants having a higher minimum alveolar concentration (MAC) for halothane than adults, they will be anaesthetized more rapidly. They also develop cardiovascular side effects more rapidly.

Inhalation of nebulized solutions may evolve as a useful delivery system for other systemically active drugs. Endotracheal adrenaline and atropine have a place during resuscitation, until intravenous access is obtained.

Gastric emptying is usually the rate-limiting step for drug absorption, as access to the large surface area of the small intestine is the most important factor in gastrointestinal absorption. Gastric emptying may be delayed in patients who are sick, have suffered trauma or received opioids. These patients are also the group least in need of preoperative sedation, which is the anaesthetist's main indication for oral medication. Despite complex physicochemical interactions across membranes, the limitation on oral drug absorption in toddlers is whether or not they take it. If the child's confidence and co-operation are gained and the mixture offered is palatable, the desired drug absorption will occur. Attempting to force a child to take a drug orally may be more distressing than an injection. The 'fentanyl lollipop' is an attempt to overcome this problem.

Drugs such as thiopentone, methohexitone and paracetamol may be given rectally. Rectal pH varies between 7 and 12 [3] so that absorption is variable. Usually, large doses are used to achieve the desired effect, but this may result in prolonged action unless the excess is removed — e.g. methohexitone — once the patient is asleep [4].

Intramuscular injection, although reliable, is painful due to splitting of the muscle fibres. It may be the single worst aspect of a child's hospitalization, and if less distressing alternatives are available, they are generally preferred. Muscle blood flow is reduced in the shocked patient, causing decreased absorption. If a second dose of opioid is given because the first one was ineffective, there is a danger of overdose when the patient is resuscitated and muscle blood flow is restored. Neonatal muscle, which is only 20% of body mass (50% in the adult), receives 10% of the neonate's relatively high cardiac output (11% in the adult) [5]. This suggests that neonatal muscle receives about four times the blood flow per gram of tissue that adult muscle receives. The higher muscle blood flow explains the more rapid onset of intramuscular injections, e.g. ketamine or suxamethonium, in neonates and small children compared to adults. The intramuscular route is contraindicated in patients with coagulopathy.

Transdermal drug administration is not yet widely used in paediatric anaesthesia, except for local anaesthetic EMLA (eutectic mixture of local anaesthetics) cream. Painless, prolonged, controlled transdermal drug delivery is appealing, but very slow onset and offset times (the skin beneath a patch acting as a reservoir if the patch is removed before it is exhausted) mean that planning and monitoring these applications will be important. Scopolamine (hyoscine) and fentanyl long-acting transdermal preparations are already available.

Subcutaneously administered drugs are taken up more slowly than intramuscularly because the blood flow is less. The action of the drug can thereby be prolonged (e.g. naloxone, insulin). Subcutaneous infusions have been used for morphine in children with chronic pain, maintaining drug levels simply with infrequent injections.

Intranasal and sublingual administrations of lipid-soluble drugs (e.g. intranasal sufentanil premedication) avoid both the dermal barrier (the mucosa being an easier membrane to cross) and first-pass metabolism by the liver.

The absorption of local anaesthetics varies depending on the site of injection, being more rapid in more vascular tissue, but may be modified by the addition of vasoconstrictors and changing pH (see Local Anaesthetics below).

Distribution

Once absorbed, drugs are distributed according to tissue blood flow and solubility in that tissue. The neonate demonstrates striking differences compared to the adult. The cardiac output on a per kg basis is double that of the adult, whilst the neonate's small size reduces the circulation time.

The size of the brain in relation to the rest of the body will influence distribution and redistribution of fat-soluble drugs. In the neonate, the ratio of brain to fat and muscle tissue is about 1:3 and the brain constitutes half of the vessel-rich group of tissues. In adults, by contrast, the ratio of brain to fat and muscle tissue is about 1:30 and the brain comprises only about one quarter of the vessel-rich group of tissues. Although neonatal and adult brains have similar blood flows on a ml/100 g basis, the neonatal brain receives about one third of the neonate's high cardiac output compared with only one seventh in the adult. Thus, despite having relatively less lipid per gram than mature brain, the neonatal brain represents a substantial reservoir for lipid-soluble drugs such as general anaesthetic agents, and the potential for redistribution to muscle or fat is limited. This may be a factor in the clinical impression of a prolonged 'hangover' in neonates from anything greater than small doses of lipid-soluble general anaesthetic agents.

Unionized drugs cross the blood–brain barrier relatively easily, and therefore this ill-defined barrier is more significant in the uptake of partially ionized drugs that have a central action. In neonates, immaturity allows some substances to cross this barrier more readily. It has been shown that morphine uptake is greater in the neonatal brain [6].

Ionized drugs such as muscle relaxants tend to distribute to the extracellular space. In the neonate this represents 45% of body weight, whereas in the adult it is only about 20% [7, 8]. On this basis a larger loading dose would be expected but this is balanced by an increased sensitivity at the receptor level.

Albumin-bound drugs form an inactive reservoir in the blood. Binding is influenced by pH, the pKa of the drug and the affinity of the drug for the binding site, the latter determining which of competing drugs will be bound. Recent work suggests that some drugs bound to α_1 acid glycoprotein are accessible to tissue receptors. Plasma protein binding holds the drug in the circulation and hence reduces volume of distribution. High tissue binding, on the other hand, will increase the volume of distribution (V_D).

Neonates have lower levels of albumin. Postnatally, more sites may be occupied by endogenous substances such as bilirubin, so that there will be a larger free fraction of drugs normally bound to albumin. The most striking protein variation in neonates is due to the low level of α_1 acid glycoprotein (α_1 AGP), which slowly rises to near adult levels by about 6 months of age. This protein is a potent binder of basic drugs. Opioids and local anaesthetics, both groups with relatively narrow therapeutic indices, are bound by α_1 AGP. The role of the low levels of α_1 AGP in increasing the susceptibility of neonates to toxicity from these drugs, compared to pharmacodynamic factors, has not been defined. 'Safe' blood levels are usually quoted as total concentration (either in plasma or whole blood). Levels quoted as safe in adults, particularly for the more highly protein-bound drugs such as bupivacaine, may represent toxic levels in neonates as a result of the increased free fraction.

Elimination

Although some drugs may be excreted unchanged by the lungs, kidneys, skin or gastrointestinal tract, most are metabolized, usually by the liver, to more ionized forms, to facilitate excretion, commonly by the kidneys.

The metabolic processes involve either phase I reactions, which modify a chemical group on the drug by, for example, oxidation, reduction, hydroxylation or hydrolysis, or by phase II synthetic reactions where conjugation with glucuronide, sulphate, acetate or amino acids occurs, or both of these. The development of these processes is not uniform in neonates and alternative pathways may be used which make prediction of poor handling by the neonate difficult. Of phase I reactions in neonates, oxidation is weak but rapidly increases over days, whereas reduction is less depressed and hydrolysis appears mature. Of phase II reactions, sulphation is present early, whereas other conjugation reactions develop over months. Glucuronidation, the immaturity of which is a key factor in hyperbilirubinaemia of the newborn, develops over about 2 months. Its deficiency in neonates is the cause of chloramphenicol toxicity — 'grey baby syndrome'. In the adult it is the major metabolic route for morphine, but it has been suggested that the neonate can use sulphate conjugation as an alternative route for morphine metabolism before glucuronidation develops; this also occurs with paracetamol.

The neonatal kidney is immature. Parts of the tubule and their functions mature at different rates. They mature more rapidly in the early weeks but full maturity may not be reached until the second year (see Chapter 1).

Glomerular filtration is the rate-limiting step for the excretion of many drugs, particularly the aminoglycoside antibiotics. Because the glomerular filtration rate (GFR) changes rapidly during the early weeks, blood levels of nephrotoxic drugs such as gentamicin must be monitored so that therapeutic levels are achieved without causing toxicity.

Penicillin excretion is enhanced by tubular transport mechanisms, which can be blocked by probenecid in adults. These are immature in neonates, so the excretion is delayed. Consequently, after the initial loading dose, smaller or less frequent doses will be needed to maintain therapeutic blood levels. Tubular secretion may also assist with the excretion of conjugated drugs.

A number of drugs used in anaesthesia have a similar pattern of dosage with development, premature infants having a low requirement, which increases in full-term neonates, further between 3−12 months and then declines through childhood to adult levels, which decrease further in the elderly. This applies to non-depolarizing muscle relaxants, inhalation agents and some induction agents.

PHARMACODYNAMICS

Changes in pharmacodynamics during development are probably an important source of differences, particularly between premature and full-term neonates and adults. Information confirming this is scarce, but changes may occur at different levels.

Receptors

SPECIFIC

Specific receptor sites may change in type or number with development. In the rat, evidence for different receptor subtypes for opioid-mediated analgesia and respiratory depression [9] is based on the fact that the amount of agonist required to produce analgesia is 40 times greater in younger (less than 14 days) than older rats, while susceptibility to respiratory depression is unchanged. The developmental aspects of receptors for acetylcholine, adrenaline, dopamine, serotonin, histamine and opioids are likely to be important for anaesthetists. For example, marked bradycardia and consequent decrease in cardiac output are more likely in infants and small children than in adults, following drugs such as suxamethonium given alone.

NON-SPECIFIC

Non-specific (possibly physicochemically specific, but not necessarily stereospecific) receptor sites in the brain for volatile anaesthetic agents may be affected by membrane development. The change of the MAC of halothane in newborn rats correlates with increased brain water [10]. Decreased solubility of halothane, due to the more aqueous membranes in younger subjects, means that a higher partial pressure is required to produce the same (effective) dry weight concentration of halothane in the membrane. This correlates well with the increased MAC requirement of infants but, in premature and mature neonates the decreased MAC may possibly be due to tissue sensitivity, overriding the effect of decreased membrane solubility of the volatile agents.

Tissue responses

Increased cardiorespiratory depression due to volatile agents in neonates is likely to be due not only to kinetic factors but also to central nervous system (CNS) and cardiorespiratory immaturity.

The sympathetic nervous system is less developed in the neonate, so that drugs that activate or block sympathetic activity tend to have less effect than in the adult. Adrenergic receptors develop earlier than their central connections, so directly acting exogenous catecholamines are more effective in neonates than sympathetic activation, although the cardiac response is still less than in adults, due to myocardial immaturity (see Chapter 1).

INHALATION AGENTS

Introduction

Inhalation anaesthesia remains a widely used technique for induction in children, especially when intravenous access is difficult to establish or the child is frightened of needles. Often, if premedication has been effective, anaesthesia can be induced without disturbing the patient. Although total intravenous anaesthesia is increasingly being advocated, inhalation anaesthesia is likely to remain an important part of paediatric anaesthesia in the foreseeable future.

CHOICE AND AVAILABILITY OF INHALATION ANAESTHETIC AGENTS

Halothane is currently the most generally available inhalation agent world-wide, although its use is decreasing in litigation-conscious countries due to the rare cases of halothane hepatitis.

Enflurane is also widely used but isoflurane is becoming increasingly popular particularly in more affluent countries. It is particularly useful for neurosurgery and when induced hypotension is desired (see Chapters 14 and 24).

Methoxyflurane is no longer available, despite its very useful analgesic properties even in subanaesthetic concentrations, its potent bronchodilator effects and its relatively low toxicity in children.

Trichloroethylene is a very cheap agent, a potent analgesic and a useful alternative to nitrous oxide when a balanced anaesthetic is used. However, its manufacture for medical use has been discontinued because the production plants are outdated and it is not economically viable to replace them.

Diethyl ether, the 'safe' anaesthetic used widely for so many years, is diminishing in use largely because of its flammability. It is still used in drawover ether–air anaesthesia.

Cyclopropane, a gaseous anaesthetic, is even more flammable and is hardly used now for this reason, but was popular, especially in children, until halothane became widely accepted, because of its very rapid induction and good muscle relaxation.

Sevoflurane, a new agent introduced in Japan, is potentially useful in paediatric anaesthesia, especially for short procedures and for day surgery. It has a blood gas solubility coefficient of 0.63, which makes induction and emergence very rapid. It is readily vaporized (BP 58.5°C, saturated VP at 20°C 157 mmHg), is non-irritant to inhale and has little tendency to cause laryngeal spasm, so it is ideal for inhalation induction. MAC is 1.7 to 2.1% in adults and 2.5% in children. It is estimated to be 2.1% in infants. It has minimal effect on the cardiovascular system and is the least arrhythmogenic halogenated agent when given with adrenaline. Its disadvantages are 4–5% metabolism to inorganic fluoride and it produces trace amounts of reactive compounds with soda lime. The clinical significance of both these factors is probably minimal and the latter is non-existent if an open breathing system is used.

Desflurane is another new agent under trial, but it seems less likely to be useful in paediatric anaesthesia. Its boiling point is close to room temperature (23°C) which means it will require a special vaporizer.

THE IDEAL INHALATION AGENT

This should have a low blood gas solubility coefficient and be non-irritant to the airways so that induction and termination of anaesthesia is rapid. Other desirable features include cardiovascular stability, non-flammability, no metabolic degradation, lack of liver or kidney toxicity and minimal postoperative vomiting.

Nitrous oxide

Some of the problems of nitrous oxide have had much publicity in recent years and there are some situations where it is better avoided. It is still an important agent in paediatric anaesthesia because it is odourless, well tolerated and has a rapid onset. It hastens the onset of anaesthesia when volatile agents are added because 50–70% nitrous oxide provides 1/2 to 2/3 MAC and because of its influence on the uptake of the second agent.

Its low blood gas solubility coefficient (0.46) makes its onset and offset rapid. Although its MAC in adults is 105% it is likely that the MAC will be lower in neonates, as the MAC of other inhalation agents which have been studied is lower in the very young. It would follow that less supplementation would be needed to provide adequate anaesthesia.

The diffusion of nitrous oxide is more rapid than nitrogen. This may lead to problems within enclosed air cavities, e.g. pneumothorax, lung cyst (Chapter 12), obstructed bowel (Chapter 11) and during air embolism. (Chapter 14). Middle-ear pressure may rise if the Eustachian tube is blocked, disrupting the ossicular chain or interfering with grafts during myringoplasty (Chapter 15).

If the patient requires an increased inspired oxygen concentration (FiO_2) then the concentration of nitrous oxide must be reduced. Pulse oximetry allows fine control of the required inspired oxygen concentration.

CARDIOVASCULAR EFFECTS

The relative lack of cardiovascular depression, partly related to a stimulatory effect of N_2O on the sympathetic nervous system offsetting some intrinsic myocardial depressant effects, has been one reason for this agent's popularity. The direct depressant effect may be unmasked by interaction with other drugs such as high-dose fentanyl or midazolam.

The suggestion that pulmonary hypertension may be increased in predisposed patients (e.g. congenital heart disease with high pulmonary flow) is now considered unlikely. For open heart surgery in children, nitrous oxide is often avoided except for induction, owing to the risk of intravascular air bubbles being expanded.

RESPIRATORY EFFECTS

In neonates, airway closure occurs during normal breathing. Thus with high FiO_2 or the use of N_2O, absorption of alveolar content may produce alveolar collapse in the alveoli distal to the airway closure. This may be overcome by keeping alveoli inflated with PEEP, sighs or large tidal volumes, or N_2O may be avoided. When air is used as the carrier gas, nitrogen will tend to remain in the alveoli and splint them open because it is less soluble than N_2O (see Chapter 9).

FLAMMABILITY

Nitrous oxide can support combustion and thus is not as useful as the nitrogen in air in decreasing the risk of ignition of flammable equipment when surgical lasers are used, especially in the airway.

METABOLIC TOXICITY

Neurological and bone marrow toxicity follow prolonged use of N_2O (e.g. as intensive care sedation), due to the acute inhibition of enzyme systems related to vitamin B_{12} and folate metabolism. It may be prudent, even though adverse outcome has not yet been demonstrated, to avoid repeated or prolonged exposure to N_2O in severely ill patients (e.g. septicaemia, large burns, multi-system failure).

Medical air

The need to avoid N_2O may coincide with the need to control FiO_2, making the availability of medical air very important in paediatric centres. Atelectasis, lung toxicity and retinopathy of prematurity may be associated with a high FiO_2.

Volatile agents

The selection of a volatile agent depends on several factors:

1 Availability and cost — most hospitals have a choice of two or three agents.
2 Pharmacological properties — rate of onset and elimination (depends on blood gas solubility), analgesic properties and the effects on the cardiovascular and respiratory systems.

3 Patient factors — age, intercurrent disease, type of surgery, etc.

4 Role of the agent in the anaesthetic technique — whether it is being used as the main agent or as a supplement.

COMPARATIVE PHARMACOLOGY

The components of general anaesthesia — hypnosis, reflex suppression, analgesia and muscle relaxation — are often considered in relation to balanced anaesthesia when several drugs are used, but the contribution of each of these components in relation to the effect of each inhalational agent is rarely considered. They produce some of each effect but the only comparative measure is minimum alveolar concentration (MAC — the alveolar concentration of an agent which prevents purposeful movement in response to an incision in 50% of unpremedicated patients). It has been observed clinically that trichloroethylene, for instance, is a potent analgesic but a poor muscle relaxant which may increase relaxant requirements, whereas isoflurane and enflurane have a relatively greater effect on muscle and reduce the requirements for muscle relaxants.

MAC AND AGE

Minimum alveolar concentration varies with age, particularly in early life.

Halothane has an MAC in neonates (0–31 days) of 0.9%, increasing in infants (1–6 months) to 1.2% [11]. By 5 years the MAC of halothane has declined to 0.9%, whilst the usual 0.8% applies at 40 years, although declining further with age [12].

The MAC of isoflurane follows a similar pattern [13], and a further reduction in MAC with prematurity has been shown [14]. Isoflurane MAC for premature infants <32 weeks gestational age is 1.3%, 32–37 weeks 1.4%, term neonates (0–31 days) 1.6%, infants (1–6 months) 1.9%. This peak in MAC in young infants falls to 1.8% in older infants (6–12 months), to 1.6% for children 1–5 years of age, and 1.2 in adults (Fig. 2.1).

This pattern is likely to be common to all volatile agents but they have not all been measured. The reasons for the changes are not understood. The decreased solubility of these drugs in the more aqueous brain membranes of infants would be expected to require higher alveolar concentrations to produce the same effective membrane concentration [10], accounting for the 'resist-

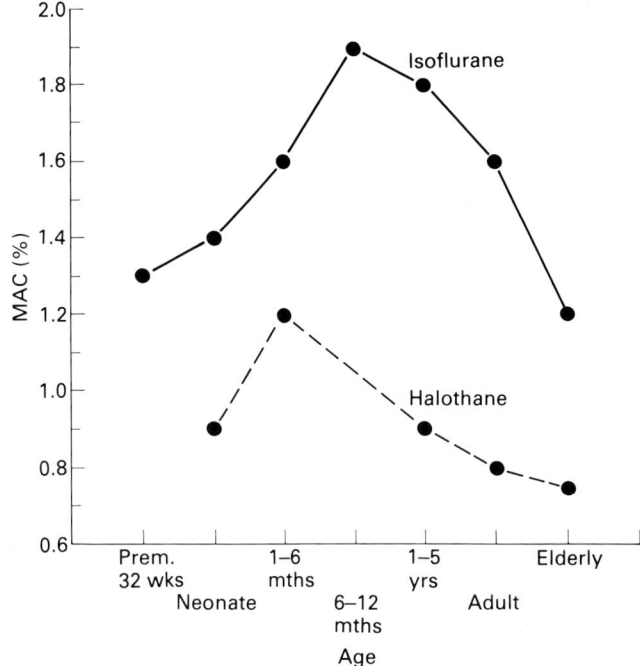

Fig. 2.1 Minimum alveolar concentration changes with age, showing that neonates and the elderly have low MAC whereas infants and young children have the highest levels.

ance' of infants. The lower requirements of premature infants may be pharmacodynamic rather than kinetic, relating to immature CNS function.

INDUCTION

Inhalation induction of anaesthesia is often used in children. The rate of induction will depend on the blood gas partition coefficient, the concentration administered and the age of the patient. If the inspired concentration can be increased rapidly without coughing or breath-holding, the alveolar concentration needed to produce anaesthesia will be reached more rapidly (referred to as overpressure). Uptake will also be increased if nitrous oxide (blood gas partition coefficient 0.47) is used as a carrier gas. In the past this effect was shown to be even more marked with ethylene (blood gas partition coefficient 0.14) which could increase the uptake of methoxyflurane (blood gas partition coefficient 12) to resemble a nitrous oxide halothane induction [15].

Induction can be induced more rapidly with halothane than isoflurane in children. Halothane has a higher blood gas partition coefficient but higher concentrations are less irritant and a smoother induction can be achieved.

Induction with isoflurane may be improved if the patient has had atropine to reduce the production of secretions.

The uptake of some anaesthetics is enhanced by the concurrent inhalation of carbon dioxide to stimulate respiration. This was a common technique with ether and may enhance isoflurane induction [16] but is hazardous with agents such as halothane where hypercarbia is associated with cardiac dysrhythmias.

An important practical consequence of the rapid induction that occurs in children with inhalational agents is the rapid onset of cardiovascular depression. The high concentrations used at induction must be lowered quickly once the child is anaesthetized. The pulse rate especially, and the blood pressure, should be monitored. If halothane in oxygen is used for induction in children over 6 months old, the MAC for endotracheal intubation (intubation without straining on the tube), is about 50% higher than the MAC [17]. Provided there is no airway obstruction, this will be achieved within 5 minutes spontaneously breathing 3.5–4% halothane in oxygen. Similar figures apply to enflurane [18].

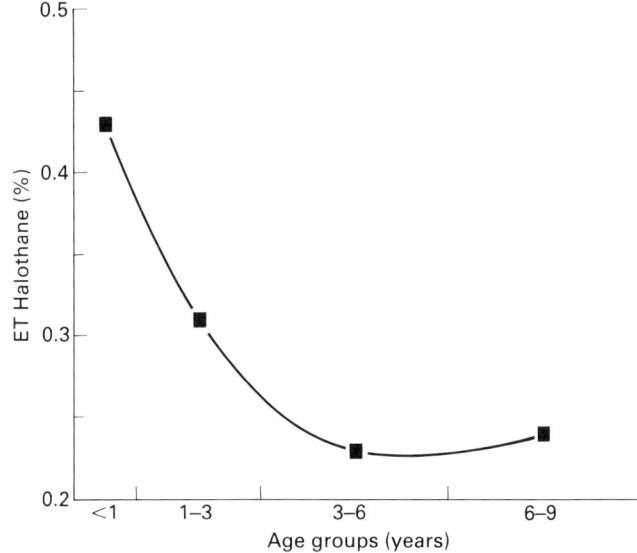

Fig. 2.2 The concentration (mean for age groups) at which infants and children awaken on emergence from halothane anaesthesia, showing that the concentration decreases with age. (P. Morris, personal communication.)

EMERGENCE

Recovery from anaesthesia is more rapid with agents with low blood gas solubility coefficients. After prolonged anaesthesia, agents with high lipid solubility are sequestered in muscle and fat and take a long time to eliminate. It has also been shown that awakening from halothane occurs at concentrations which vary with age, being higher in infants and lower when premedication or thiopentone has been used (Fig. 2.2) [19].

CARDIOVASCULAR EFFECTS

In paediatrics, neonates are the most susceptible to adverse cardiovascular effects of volatile agents. The neonatal heart is less compliant, has less muscle per gram of tissue, and the balance of autonomic innervation is different (see Chapter 1). Cardiac output is rate-dependent and sensitive to inadequate preload. Less reserve when exposed to direct myocardial depressants and increased afterload can be expected.

Marked falls in cardiac output occur with halothane and isoflurane anaesthesia (1.5 MAC) in infants and small children [20]. Halothane decreases heart rate and cardiac output more than isoflurane. Cardiac output will return to control levels for both agents if the rate is

increased with atropine. Indirect measures of contractility (ejection fraction and left ventricular end-diastolic volume) are depressed more by halothane than isoflurane. Halothane causes more direct myocardial depression than isoflurane, while the latter causes more vasodilatation. Enflurane's effects are intermediate.

Baroreceptors are active even in premature babies. In neonates their sensitivity is the same but the baroreceptors are reset during isoflurane anaesthesia so that a slower heart rate is associated with a given blood pressure [21]. Because cardiac output is rate-dependent in neonates, these baroreceptor effects can become important.

Dysrhythmias

In usual clinical concentrations, life-threatening dysrhythmias are rare. Bradycardia or tachycardia are the main forms of dysrhythmia seen with volatile agents. Ventricular fibrillation occasionally occurs. Defibrillation was required in less than 1/50 000 paediatric halothane anaesthesias [22].

Bradycardia can follow the administration of some drugs, especially suxamethonium, as well as fentanyl, vecuronium and propofol. It is more likely when two or more of these are given together in the absence of parasympathetic blocking drugs such as atropine. Manipulation of the airway, external ocular muscles and peritoneum by the surgeon or anaesthetist can cause reflex bradycardia. Halothane may potentiate these effects. Occasionally, the bradycardia may progress to asystole or ventricular fibrillation. These problems seem to be less common with enflurane and even less so with isoflurane. Prevention depends on anticipation and careful monitoring. Atropine or glycopyrrolate should be readily available or used prophylactically.

Tachycardia may be provoked by sympathetic stimulation or sympathomimetic agents combined with volatile agents, and may lead to ventricular dysrhythmia. Halothane, in particular, sensitizes the myocardium to this effect [23]. The sensitivity is reduced by the concurrent administration of lignocaine. Isoflurane has a similar, but lesser effect. Using three ventricular ectopic beats as the dysrhythmia endpoint in adults breathing 1.25 MAC halothane in oxygen, the ED50 for adrenaline when injected submucosally in the nose was 2.1 μg/kg but it increased to 3.7 μg/kg when 0.5% lignocaine was added, while with 1.25 MAC isoflurane 6.7 μg/kg adrenaline was needed. These combinations had steep dose−response curves. Enflurane had a flat curve, so that although the ED50 was 10.9 μg/kg, about 10% of patients had three ventricular ectopic beats at low doses of adrenaline [23]. Children seem more resistant to ventricular dysrhythmias caused by this interaction. Adrenaline, 10 μg/kg, seems a reasonable maximum safe dose for infiltration for children having nitrous oxide halothane relaxant anaesthesia [24]. It may need to be reduced with higher concentrations of halothane in the presence of hypercarbia and when injected into vascular areas. Care must be taken to calculate the actual adrenaline dose: 1 in 200 000 adrenaline used in local anaesthetic solutions is sufficient for local vasoconstriction and contains 5 μg/ml.

The use of topical cocaine in combination with submucosal adrenaline, especially with halothane, deserves particular attention. The cocaine produces a sympathomimetic action by blocking the re-uptake of noradrenaline, which also exaggerates the effect of adrenaline. This is true of both exogenous and endogenous adrenaline, making anxious patients especially at risk. Rare but tragic deaths from ventricular fibrillation have occurred in elective nasal surgery in teenagers, with the combination of cocaine, adrenaline and halothane. Cocaine is well absorbed transmucosally, and the maximum dose is unclear but 1 mg/kg seems safe. Solutions of 2−5% are effective. Halothane should be avoided in these cases if adrenaline is injected.

Dysrhythmias that are not a clinical problem are common. Halothane−nitrous oxide induction induced dysrhythmia in 60% of children [25], usually junctional rhythm, which resolved spontaneously. In patients with underlying cardiac valve abnormalities, ventricular hypertrophy or conduction defects, the dysrhythmia may be more serious.

RESPIRATORY EFFECTS

Volatile agents affect the depth and rate of breathing, acting directly on the respiratory centre and on peripheral neural mechanisms. They also directly affect bronchial muscle tone and the muscles of respiration. They can be irritant to the airways. Halothane has been studied more extensively in children than have the other volatile agents.

The effect of 0.5% halothane in children is to increase respiratory rate and decrease tidal volume, with little effect on minute ventilation or EtCO2. With increasing concentration, especially over 1%, tidal volume and ventilation decrease, rate and EtCO2 increase with an associated decrease in cardiac output [26]. There is a response to carbon dioxide stimulation [27]. Intercostal muscles are depressed more than the diaphragm by halothane, so that its respiratory effects are exaggerated in patients with impaired diaphragmatic function (either primary or secondary to abdominal distension) [28].

The ventilatory response to hypoxia is suppressed by as little as 0.1 MAC halothane [29] and abolished by 1.1 MAC. Patients recovering from halothane anaesthesia are therefore at increased risk from hypoxia and this risk is probably even greater in neonates. Ventilation increases to compensate for apparatus dead space under 0.5% halothane [30] but at higher concentrations respiratory depression and CO2 retention occur.

The small respiratory reserve of infants prompts most anaesthetists to control their ventilation even for short procedures. Neonates should be ventilated because respiration is depressed when breathing nitrous oxide−halothane. It is notable that after 30 days, term babies tolerate mask anaesthesia for minor surgery with this anaesthetic without marked respiratory depression when breathing spontaneously [31].

Enflurane and isoflurane also cause respiratory depression, as shown by a dose related rise in Paco$_2$, and decreased responses to hypoxia and hypercarbia, as is the case with halothane. These agents differ from halothane in that they depress respiratory rate, but they depress tidal volume less than halothane. All these agents are bronchodilators and may depress hypoxic pulmonary vasoconstriction.

INTRACRANIAL PRESSURE EFFECTS

Volatile anaesthetic agents can increase intracranial pressure by vasodilatation, thereby increasing cerebral blood volume. The vasodilatation is dose dependent and is greatest with halothane and least with isoflurane. As time passes the effect with halothane decreases. Controlled ventilation with hypocapnia may also reduce vasodilatation. Cerebrospinal fluid reabsorption (in dogs) is increased by isoflurane and decreased by halothane and enflurane [32].

Enflurane may cause fitting. This can be associated with a rise in intracranial pressure even in the paralysed patient. It is not recommended for neurosurgery.

Volatile anaesthetic agents should be avoided in patients with acute intracranial hypertension, at least until the dura is opened.

METABOLISM AND TOXICITY

Metabolites of volatile anaesthetic agents may cause organ damage. The metabolism of halothane is similar in both children and adults [33]. In adults, only 0.2% of isoflurane is excreted in the urine as metabolites, whereas 2% of enflurane, 20% of halothane and 20−50% of methoxyflurane is metabolized. A low blood gas partition coefficient will speed postoperative respiratory excretion of unchanged anaesthetic and correlate with smaller tissue stores of the drug intraoperatively, which will decrease vital organ exposure. Isoflurane has not been found to be toxic to either liver or kidneys.

Liver toxicity has been much discussed. Halothane commonly causes minor liver enzyme changes, which are of doubtful clinical significance. 'Halothane hepatitis' is a rare entity, with a much lower incidence in children than in adults. Fulminant hepatic necrosis is associated with repeated exposures, and may be accompanied by fever and eosinophilia. The pathophysiology is unknown, but may involve a halothane metabolite initiating an immune reaction. Retrospective reviews at paediatric hospitals in England and the USA of 165 000 and 200 000 halothane anaesthetics respectively [34, 35] found only three cases of apparent halothane hepatitis, all of which resolved. Lethal halothane hepatitis has occurred in childhood. One report of seven cases in children included

one death [36]. When the safety and benefits of halothane are balanced against the risk of hepatitis, it would seem that in children halothane can be used when it is warranted, although it would be sensible to use another agent if jaundice or unexplained fever has followed a recent halothane anaesthetic [37, 38]. Thousands of children have had halothane on many (up to 200) occasions without adverse effects.

Enflurane has been reported as causing hepatitis, but is believed to have an even lower incidence of this problem than halothane [39]. Isoflurane does not seem to cause liver necrosis, but methoxyflurane has been associated with hepatitis [40].

Fluorinated volatile agents are metabolized to a varying degree to produce fluoride ions. Levels of 50−80 μmol/l produced following 2.5−3 MAC hours' exposure of methoxyflurane in adults causes tubular damage and polyuric renal failure [41]. Fluoride levels of 33 μmol/l caused a 25 % reduction in maximum urine osmolality in adults [46]. The serum fluoride levels for similar exposure in children aged 7−14 years was only about half that for adults (Fig. 2.3) [42, 43] presumably due to increased fluoride uptake by bone and teeth. Children are therefore relatively protected from the renal toxicity of methoxyflurane. Pre-existing renal impairment, or the presence of other nephrotoxins (e.g. gentamicin) increase the risk of fluoride-induced polyuric renal failure [44]. Enzyme induction by other drugs may increase fluoride levels.

The other halogenated agents are metabolized to a

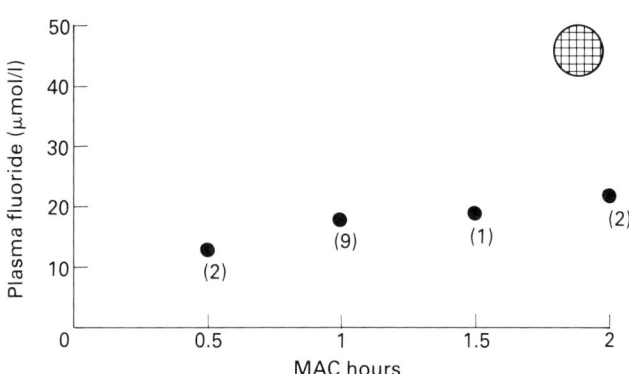

Fig. 2.3 Plasma fluoride levels following different MAC hours exposure to methoxyflurane in children aged 7−14 years. The hatched area is the approximate equivalent concentration in adults, showing that the levels are much lower in children for the same exposure. Numbers in brackets = number of patients. MAC was measured with a mass spectrometer [42].

lesser degree, so that fluoride production is unimportant [45] except after prolonged enflurane anaesthesia [46].

MUSCLE EFFECTS

The volatile agents produce varying degrees of muscle relaxation and potentiation of neuromuscular blockade, which is most marked with enflurane. Halothane in particular may cause postoperative hypertonicity and 'shivering', which increases oxygen consumption. It may also impair airway patency and chest-wall movement, making supplementary oxygen important during recovery. Abnormal responses may occur in patients with certain muscle disorders such as malignant hyperthermia (see below).

POLLUTION

Operating theatre pollution is more difficult to control in paediatric anaesthesia, where inhalation induction and open circuits are generally used. No significant effects of anaesthetic gas pollution have been demonstrated by rigorous statistical analysis, although idiosyncratic responses such as headache, dysrhythmia and liver dysfunction have been reported. Recommended maximum levels are often based on the minimum achievable under ideal conditions rather than on specific effects of higher concentrations. Paediatric anaesthetists should minimize pollution where possible. Atmospheric pollution from anaesthetics is insignificant in the overall problem of environmental pollution [47].

INTRAVENOUS INDUCTION AGENTS

Ideally, intravenous induction should be painless, rapid, non-irritant, not depressant to the cardiorespiratory system, without muscle movements or allergic responses, and short-acting without 'hangover'. The drug should be cheap and easily stored. No drug achieves all these ideals, but despite many innovations, thiopentone, first used in 1934, remains the 'standard' by which other agents are measured.

Thiopentone

Thiopentone is a barbiturate with a short action due mainly to redistribution. The high lipid solubility allows both rapid brain penetration (in association with high cerebral blood flow) and rapid redistribution (especially

to muscle with its large mass but less blood flow). The elimination half-life in children is about 6 hours compared to 12 hours in adults [48]. This is because clearance in children is twice the adult rate although the volume of distribution, protein binding and distribution phase kinetics are similar. Theoretically, this difference will reduce residual sedation in children, especially following repeated doses or infusions, but because of the dominance of redistribution with usual doses this is rarely significant clinically. The likely decreased metabolism of thiopentone in prematures and neonates has not been quantified, but protein binding has been shown to be about 10% less than in adults [49]. There is a clinical impression of more 'hangover' from thiopentone in these patients, but distribution phase differences, due to small muscle and fat compartments in relation to the CNS, are more likely than depressed metabolism to prolong thiopentone's clinical effects.

The average dose of thiopentone is about 5 mg/kg but must be modified by several factors:
1 *Age*. Recent studies have shown that neonates need a smaller induction dose (ED50 3.4 mg/kg). The ED50 increases to 6.5 mg/kg between 1 and 6 months of age and then declines to about 5.6 mg/kg between 6 and 12 months, thereafter slowly falling during childhood to about 4–5 mg/kg (Fig. 2.4) [50, 51]. Suppression of a

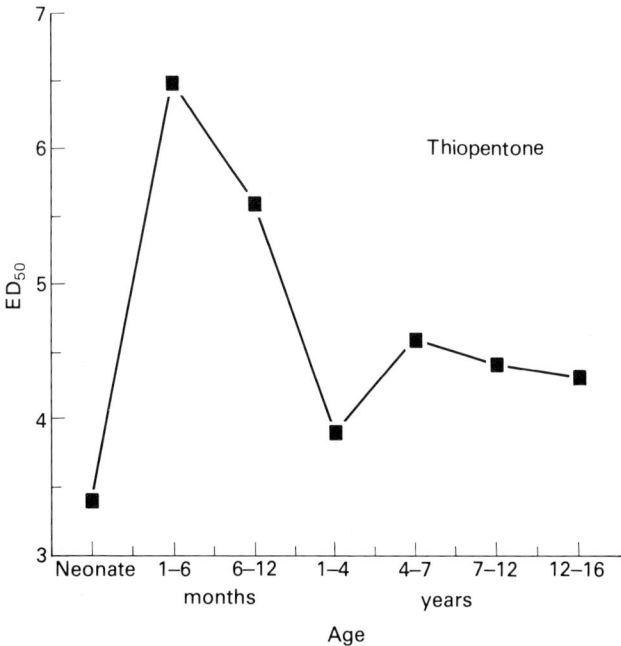

Fig. 2.4 The ED50 sleep dose of thiopentone at different ages. (Data derived from Westrin [50], and Jonmarker [51].)

painful stimulus (trapezius squeeze) required a higher dose — 7 mg/kg in infants and children from 1 month to 4 years compared with 3.7 mg/kg in adults [52]. An experimental study in puppies during the first weeks of life showed that dose requirements steadily increased from birth (Fig. 2.5). In practice, neonates need less and infants and children more thiopentone per kg for induction than adults. The neonatal dose should be tailored to the degree of development and vigour of the baby.

2 *Premedication.* Effective premedication provides sedation and decreases anxiety. Anxiety increases central arousal and sympathetic activity. The beta-adrenergic effects of this increase cardiac output, mostly to muscles, so that relatively less of the output goes to the brain and a larger dose of thiopentone is needed. ED50 was found to be 8 mg/kg in unpremedicated patients compared to 4 mg/kg in a premedicated group [53].

3 *Hypovolaemia.* Hypovolaemic patients require smaller doses of thiopentone given slowly. The blood volume is reduced and hence concentration will be increased unless the dose and rate of injection are reduced. The brain and heart receive preferential flow so that a greater proportion of cardiac output goes to those organs, leading to greater depression unless a small dose is given, otherwise precipitous hypotension may occur [54].

4 *Cardiac output.* Children with severe valvular stenosis, pericardial tamponade or cardiomyopathy may decompensate, so that cardiac output becomes inadequate unless doses are much reduced. It may be wise to use an alternative drug with less myocardial depressant action, such as fentanyl or ketamine, in such cases.

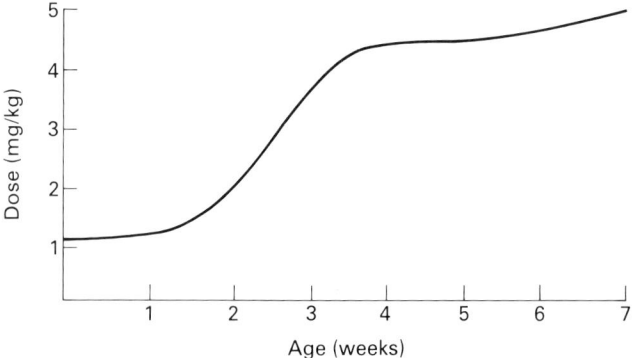

Fig. 2.5 ED50 for head drop in a litter of seven puppies following thiopentone administered at a standard rate into the external jugular vein. (Data from J. Allt Graham and T.C.K. Brown.)

Central nervous system (CNS) actions of thiopentone anaesthesia are not accompanied by analgesia at low doses. Thiopentone reduces cerebral metabolism and CO_2 production and hence decreases cerebral blood flow. This makes thiopentone a useful means of reducing intracranial pressure (ICP), in contrast to the volatile agents. Neurosurgical access and acute control of raised ICP can be assisted, but care must be taken to avoid hypotension, as cerebral perfusion pressure (ICP-MAP) may be compromised. The use of thiopentone for ICP control over several days may not improve outcome. Its suggested role as a 'cerebral protective' agent in ischaemia has not been established.

The cardiovascular response to thiopentone induction is a fall in cardiac output. This is due to direct myocardial depression, but the resultant fall in blood pressure is modified by an increase in systemic vascular resistance. In infants, the heart rate falls unless atropine is given, further depressing cardiac output. In atropine-premedicated children, the heart rate rises [55]. Neonates and children with cardiovascular compromise need careful titration for the safe use of thiopentone.

The respiratory effects of thiopentone seem to be largely secondary to CNS depression. Apnoea may result, especially in those already at increased risk, such as premature and neonatal patients and those with a history of sleep apnoea. In patients with 'difficult' or obstructed airways, in whom one may not be able to assist ventilation, the occurrence of apnoea may be catastrophic. Thiopentone should be used with great caution, if at all, in such patients.

The barbiturates are contraindicated in patients with either acute intermittent or variegate porphyria (see Pharmacogenetics below).

Anaphylactic reactions to thiopentone are rare, but when they occur they are often life threatening (see Chapter 27).

Methohexitone

Methohexitone is another short-acting barbiturate which has a shorter elimination half-life (3 hours compared with 6 hours for thiopentone) in children [56]. It is an oxybarbiturate with a methyl substitution on one $-N-$ which causes the excitatory movements sometimes seen at induction. Pain on injection and hiccoughs can occur. The usual dose is about 2 mg/kg, but the same principles apply to modifying its dose as discussed above. In some centres it is used rectally (10–15 mg/kg).

Propofol

Propofol is a phenol derivative supplied in a soya emulsion and egg phospholipid, to make an injectable emulsion. It has a rapid onset of action, with quick awakening due to redistribution and a rapid clearance from the plasma. Elimination half-life is short. It is claimed that patients awaken more rapidly and clearly after propofol than after thiopentone. This may be more obvious in adults because thiopentone is quickly redistributed in children. Reported recovery times in children have varied, showing either similar recovery times to thiopentone [57] or a reduction in recovery time of 30–50% [58–60]. Ninety minutes after an induction dose the thiopentone and propofol groups are indistinguishable. Patients receiving propofol awaken more rapidly after repeated doses or infusions.

The dose of propofol recommended for induction varies. The ED50 was found to be 2 mg/kg in premedicated children and 2.5 mg/kg in unpremedicated patients [61]. The ED90 was 3.5 mg/kg in premedicated children and over 4 mg/kg when unpremedicated [62]. This may reflect the flat dose–response curve of propofol [63] which makes the assessment of average dose more difficult. The ED50 has also been shown to be greater for infants (3.2 mg/kg) than teenagers (2.4 mg/kg) [64].

A major disadvantage of propofol is the frequency of pain on injection, especially in peripheral veins. This can be overcome by the addition of 1 mg/kg lignocaine to 3 mg/kg propofol.

Because propofol has a short duration of action and rapid clearance it has been used by infusion or repeated doses, because patients awaken rapidly when it is stopped. At present the major disadvantage of infusions is cost.

The cardiovascular effects of propofol include moderate hypotension, with a decrease or no change in heart rate. It decreases peripheral vascular resistance and probably also causes some myocardial depression. These effects are less marked in children. Propofol appears to decrease responsiveness to airway manipulation and laryngoscopy. Intubation is accompanied by less hypertension and tachycardia than following thiopentone.

It causes transient depression of respiration and, in some children, apnoea. Nausea is less common than after thiopentone. It decreases intracranial pressure but

seizure activity following its administration has been reported. If injected intra-arterially, it causes less damage than thiopentone. Propofol has been used in patients with porphyria.

Ketamine

Ketamine is a dissociative anaesthetic that blocks transmission of impulses from lower centres and the thalamus to the cortex. The activity of the vital brain-stem centres thus remain more active than with other anaesthetic agents.

Ketamine has a sympathomimetic effect. The cardiovascular effects result from central sympathetic stimulation producing a rise in heart rate and blood pressure and, in most situations, overriding of its intrinsic myocardial depressant effect. Pulmonary vascular resistance is not increased by ketamine [65]. There is a reduced tendency for cardiovascular decompensation to occur with blood loss. It increases cerebral blood flow and intracranial pressure. As a consequence, it is contraindicated when a rise in intracranial pressure is to be avoided. This is less of a problem with prematures and infants before the cranial sutures close, because there is some room for expansion of intracranial contents [66].

Ketamine's respiratory effects differ from other anaesthetic agents, causing a small, dose-related shift of the CO_2 response curve to the right. Functional residual capacity (FRC) [67], tidal volume and respiratory rate are maintained, and airway reflexes remain active. Aspiration can occur but is less likely than during conventional anaesthesia due to the preservation of laryngeal muscle tone. Laryngospasm is rare. Salivation can be a nuisance but can be prevented by an anticholinergic such as atropine or hyoscine. It is a bronchodilator.

Muscle tone is well maintained and this makes it easier to change a child's position during anaesthesia and to hold position when, for instance, bandages are applied during burn dressings.

Nystagmus, eye opening and involuntary muscle movement occur frequently.

Ketamine has analgesic properties even at low, subanaesthetic concentrations.

The main disadvantage of ketamine is the tendency to dream and hallucinate during emergence. This is more likely in people who are aware of their dreams. Although these excitatory phenomena are thought to be rare in children, they do occur but are often not recognized.

Ketamine pharmacokinetics vary in the younger age

groups. $T_{1/2}$ beta is 30 minutes at 4 years, 1 hour at 1 year and 3 hours at less than 3 months old. The clearances at these ages are 25, 35 and 12 ml/kg/min. Protein binding is only 10% in neonates and 30% in adults [68].

ADMINISTRATION

Ketamine has been given by a variety of routes but is usually injected intravenously or, in the absence of venous access, intramuscularly. An intravenous dose of 1–2 mg/kg is followed by a staring gaze as the patient gradually loses consciousness within a minute or two. An intramuscular dose of 3–4 mg/kg causes loss of consciousness within 3–4 minutes. An intravenous cannula can then be inserted for further administration. For short procedures each mg/kg given intravenously provides 4–5 minutes' anaesthesia when given alone in unpremedicated children, and 5–7 minutes if an opiate premedication has been given [69]. Usually, diazepam or midazolam is given intravenously at induction or in increments of 0.05–0.1 mg/kg for premedication (0.3 mg/kg) to suppress the undesirable hallucinations and dreams which can occur with ketamine.

Maintenance of ketamine anaesthesia can be achieved by further incremental doses or by an infusion with additional increments if necessary. When a longer anaesthetic is anticipated (over an hour), a larger initial dose of 5–6 mg/kg provides smoother maintenance and a lower dose requirement in the later stages. Contrary to the prolongation of action achieved by premedication with opiates in short cases [69], an intravenous bolus of morphine does not increase the duration of action of ketamine during long cases. Presumably the peak effect of morphine passes and the levels decline before the action of ketamine wears off.

It is difficult to achieve satisfactory anaesthesia using ketamine as a sole agent with the suggested doses in babies under 3 months and with the long $T_{1/2}$ and low clearance, large doses are undesirable. As basal anaesthesia accompanying regional blocks in infants, it should be given in small doses slowly to avoid apnoea, which has occurred when it has been given in large doses or too rapidly.

Postoperatively, children should be allowed to awaken quietly. Postoperative sleep after ketamine (with diazepam) lasts approximately as long again as the anaesthetic time. This is a disadvantage of the use of large doses for longer anaesthetics. Postoperative vomiting is less common than following conventional anaesthetics.

Midazolam

Midazolam is a benzodiazepine which has sedative, anxiolytic, amnesic and anticonvulsant effects. Unlike diazepam, it has no long-acting metabolites, is relatively short acting and is water soluble and non-irritant in solution. Strictly speaking midazolam should not be regarded as an induction agent, because of its rather slow onset time and unreliable hypnotic action, but it is effective in combination with fentanyl. The usual recommended dose is 0.3 mg/kg but some patients will not lose consciousness with even 0.6 mg/kg [70].

PHARMACOKINETICS

Midazolam is shorter acting in children than adults. V_D.ss is 1.3 l/kg. Elimination half-life of 1.2 hours in children is shorter than adults (1.5–2.5 hours) and plasma clearance of 9 ml/kg/min is greater than 6–8 ml/kg/min in young adults and 4–5 ml/kg/min in the elderly. Following intramuscular, rectal and oral administration, peak serum concentrations were at 15, 30, and 53 minutes and bioavailability was 87%, 18% and 27% respectively, following 0.15 mg/kg. The oral dose is thus about three times the intramuscular dose. When larger oral doses are given, relatively less is absorbed (15% at 3 mg/kg) [71].

The cardiovascular effects are minimal in healthy children, while apnoea can occur following rapid intravenous injection. Synergism occurs between midazolam and fentanyl, alfentanil and thiopentone [72–74]. Restlessness sometimes occurs during recovery from midazolam.

Etomidate

Etomidate has the advantage of minimal cardiovascular and respiratory depression and rapid recovery. Pain on injection is common and not reliably prevented by fentanyl or lignocaine [75]. Movement on injection occurs frequently. Suppression of steroid hormone production following prolonged infusions has resulted in its use and availability being limited.

OPIOIDS

Morphine, pethidine and papaveretum have been used for many years in children, but have usually been avoided in neonates and small infants because of the fear of respiratory depression. Babies, 12–60 hours old, have a depressed ventilatory response to CO_2 after pethidine, and more so after morphine. It has been suggested that penetration into the immature brain was easier but the immature respiratory centre may also be more susceptible to the depressant effects of these drugs [6].

Pharmacokinetic changes in the neonatal period may contribute to this sensitivity. Protein binding is decreased. Clearance of morphine [76], fentanyl [77], alfentanil [78] and sufentanil [79] is decreased in neonates but increases to adult levels within weeks. The reduced clearance prolongs the elimination half-life and, in the case of alfentanil, increased $V_D.ss$ prolongs $T_{1/2}$ beta further. Morphine and sufentanil have a decreased $V_D.ss$ in neonates despite which the $T_{1/2}$ beta is still longer than in adults.

Attitudes to analgesia in infants and children have changed. It has been recognized that the stress response can be suppressed by analgesics [80]. Fentanyl appears to be better than the older drugs to use in neonates for operative analgesia. It has been shown that even premature infants were breathing spontaneously within 2–3 hours after receiving 30–50 µg/kg [81, 82], but it is probable that these infants had developed tolerance following prolonged sedation in intensive care units. When 7.5 µg/kg fentanyl was used as the sole anaesthetic, 50% of neonates less than 1 week old had a 20% rise in heart rate or blood pressure within 30 minutes, suggesting that the dose was inadequate, while following 12.5 µg/kg no supplementation was required within 120 minutes [83]. When fentanyl was used as the sole anaesthetic in neonates, the blood levels at extubation were lower than expected from adult studies [84] but profound respiratory depression has been reported in a baby less than 3 months old with low blood levels [85]. No significant cardiovascular effects were observed in premature infants (with 30 µg/kg) [77], term neonates (10 µg/kg) [86], and infants (35 µg/kg) [87]. The muscle rigidity which may follow high doses of fentanyl can be controlled with muscle relaxants.

It would seem to be safe to use high-dose fentanyl in neonates provided facilities are available for post-operative ventilation if necessary. The doses indicated above are higher than necessary for patients who have not been on infusions. They should be reduced (under 10 µg/kg), particularly in neonates, if they are to breathe spontaneously postoperatively. Infants over 3 months old do not have increased sensitivity to fentanyl-induced respiratory depression [85].

Morphine is still a useful analgesic as it provides better sedation, lasts longer and costs less than fentanyl. It can release histamine, lowering the blood pressure (especially if given as a large i.v. bolus), and sometimes causes itching and bronchospasm. It has been used for infusions (see Chapter 8). In neonates, 5–20 (usually 10) µg/kg/hour is often used in intensive care units. These rates produce blood levels similar to those required by adults [76]. Higher infusion rates for prolonged periods in neonates have been associated with seizures [88].

All opioids cause respiratory depression and patients must be monitored carefully, particularly neonates and those with potential airways obstruction. They also cause nausea and vomiting.

The commonly used intramuscular dose of morphine is 0.2 mg/kg, and of pethidine, 1 mg/kg. The latter has antispasmodic properties and is better than morphine in asthmatics. For epidural use the more lipid-soluble drugs, pethidine and fentanyl, are shorter acting but less likely to cause respiratory depression than morphine.

Codeine 0.5 mg/kg, is a useful analgesic which can be administered orally, rectally or intramuscularly. Methadone can be given orally (90% bioavailability) or intravenously (0.3–0.4 mg/kg). It has a long duration of action.

OPIOID ANTAGONISTS

Naloxone is a specific opioid antagonist. It has a short $T_{1/2}$ beta due to a small volume of distribution and a high clearance rate. Clearance is decreased in the neonate due to slow glucuronidation. If it is used to reverse opioid-induced respiratory depression the patient must be monitored, because the opioid may have continuing effects when the action of naloxone wears off. It can be given by infusion to avoid this problem (e.g. 10 µg/kg/h or titrated to the desired effect). Doses should be titrated to reverse postoperative respiratory depression without losing the analgesic effect of the opioid. The required dose may be very small.

MUSCLE RELAXANTS

Physiological factors affecting dose

The response to muscle relaxants and the doses required change during growth from birth to adolescence. Neuromuscular transmission is immature until the age of 2 months [89, 90] and the response to tetanic nerve stimulation and the rate of muscle contraction are less than in older children. The response is more variable during the first few months, as there are many physiological changes which affect drug action occurring at this time. In general the maturation process is dependent more on the duration of extra-uterine life than on post-conceptual age.

The type of muscle fibre influences the response to muscle relaxants: type 1 fibres (slow twitch, high oxidative) are more sensitive to non-depolarizing muscle relaxants than type 2 fibres (fast twitch) [91]. The distribution of muscle fibres changes — for example, 55% of muscle fibres in the adolescent diaphragm are type 1 slow-twitch fibres compared with 26% at full term and 14% in premature infants of 30 weeks' post-conceptual age [92]. With fewer of the more sensitive type 1 fibres, the neonatal diaphragm would be expected to remain more active than peripheral muscles during neuromuscular block. It has been observed clinically that during recovery from muscle paralysis, diaphragmatic activity begins at deeper levels of peripheral neuromuscular block in neonates than in older children. These differences are clinically significant, because most dose-response studies in children have been performed on peripheral hand muscles. If the diaphragm is relatively more resistant to paralysis, the clinical dose requirement to cause respiratory paralysis will be greater [93].

Neuromuscular blocking agents are distributed in the extracellular fluid compartment, which constitutes a greater proportion of total body water during the first months of life [94–97]. The distribution volume (l/kg) decreases with age, increasing the plasma concentration

achieved. The concentration required for effect may change as the neuromuscular junction matures. The net effect of these counteracting changes depends on the muscle relaxant used, and results in slightly different age-dependent potencies. The different age-dependent durations of effect of various muscle relaxants depend on redistribution and on elimination by metabolism, renal excretion or spontaneous degradation. Recovery from atracurium is little affected by age but vecuronium is long-acting in the neonate [103]. Atracurium degradation is slower if the body temperature falls [106].

Non-depolarizing relaxants

When the doses required to produce 95% neuromuscular block (ED95) are compared in neonates, infants, children and adolescents, the requirement in children aged 3–10 years is greater than in the younger and older age groups (Table 2.1) [93]. This may be due to differences in body composition during growth. The fat compartment increases two- to threefold to its maximum of as much as 30% of body weight during the first year of life, thereafter diminishing towards puberty [7]. The muscle compartment as a proportion of body weight decreases during the first year of life and thereafter it increases two- to threefold until it reaches a maximum of 40% by the end of the active growth phase. Adults have more fat and less muscle tissue than children, therefore when a neuro-

Table 2.1 ED95 doses of neuromuscular blocking (NMB) agents in paediatric patients. Adult ED95 doses are taken from a recent review article [109] and mivacurium [120] and suxamethonium [105] data. Values are expressed as µg/kg

Ref.	NMB-agent	Anaes	Neonates <1 mth	Infants <1 yr	Children 3–10 yrs	Adolescents >12 yrs	Adults
[100]	D-tubocurarine	N_2O-O_2	–	410	500	440	480
[99]		Hal	340	290	320	–	
[100]	Alcuronium	N_2O-O_2	–	200	270	240	220
[107]	Pancuronium	N_2O-O_2	72	66	93	77	67
[98]		Hal	–	47	70	–	
[111]	Vecuronium	N_2O-O_2	48	47	81	55	43
[102]		Hal	–	–	60	45	
[110]	Atracurium	N_2O-O_2	220	230	320	300	210
[103]		N_2O-O_2	120	160	200	–	
[101]		Hal	–	170	170	180	
[104]		Hal	–	160	260	160	
[118]	Mivacurium	N_2O-O_2	–	–	110	–	80
[119]		Hal	–	–	90	–	
[123–124]	Suxamethonium	N_2O-O_2	–	730	440	270	300

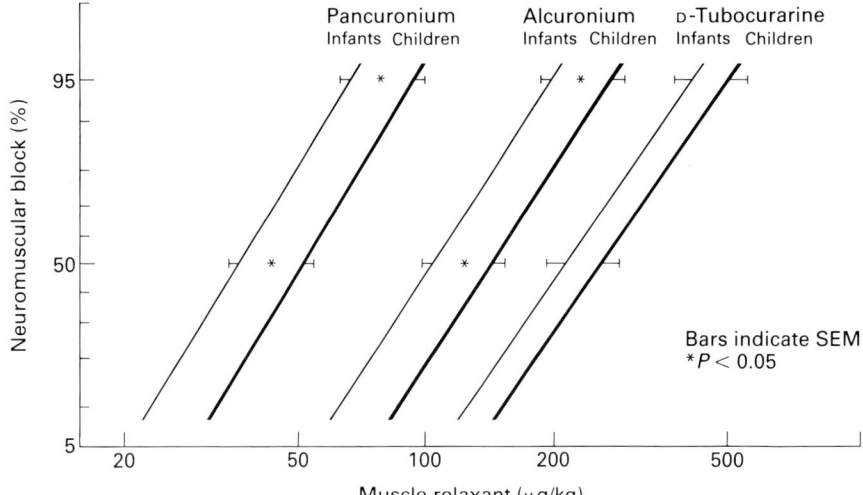

Fig. 2.6 Dose response for pancuronium, alcuronium, and D-tubocurarine in infants (under 12 months) and children (1–10 years), showing a significant difference between the age groups with pancuronium and alcuronium. (From Meretoja [93], with permission.)

muscular blocking drug is given on the basis of body weight (in mg/kg) the greatest dose may be required in children at the age when they have least fat and most muscle tissue compared to other age groups.

Figure 2.6 demonstrates the difference in dose–response between infants (1–12 months) and children (2–10 years), which was significant with pancuronium [107] and alcuronium [108] but not significant with D-tubocurarine [109]. Figure 2.7 shows that there was a significant difference in ED95 with atracurium and an even greater difference with vecuronium. The dose per kg in children is substantially larger than for infants under 1 year [111].

The onset time for non-depolarizing neuromuscular blocking drugs is more rapid the younger the patient (Table 2.2) and the larger the dose [93]. This is demon-strated for atracurium in Fig. 2.8 and applies to all non-depolarizing relaxants.

Recovery from non-depolarizing neuromuscular block is more rapid in children than in infants under 1 year (Table 2.3). This effect varies with the different drugs. It can be seen in Fig. 2.9 that the difference is small with atracurium and much greater with vecuronium, making it long-acting in neonates [93].

The search for a short-acting non-depolarizing muscle relaxant with a rapid onset continues. Mivacurium, a drug structurally similar to atracurium, has been on clinical trial [118]. Its ED95 in children during balanced and halothane anaesthesia is 110 and 90 μg/kg respectively [119]. These doses are 30–40% greater than the ED95 dose for adults [120]. It is probable that for a non-depolarizing relaxant to have as rapid an onset as

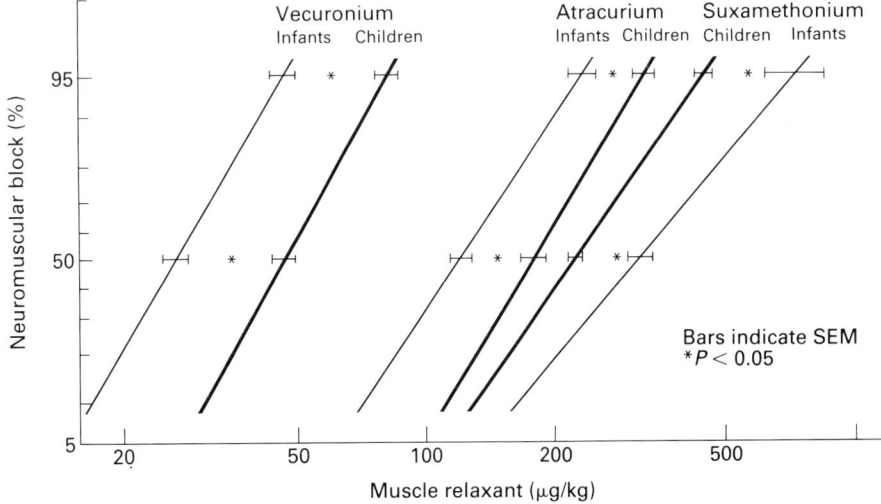

Fig. 2.7 Dose response for vecuronium, atracurium and suxamethonium, showing a significant difference between infants and children. (From Meretoja [93], with permission.)

Table 2.2 The onset time in minutes (time from intravenous administration to maximum response) of different neuromuscular blocking agents in paediatric patients. Data are collected from studies where at least two different age groups are compared

| | | Dose | Onset time in minutes | | | |
Ref.	Agent	µg/kg	Neonates	Infants	Children	Adolescents
[112]	D-tubocurarine	400	–	1.6	5.2	–
[113]	Pancuronium	70	–	1.3	2.7	3.4
[100]	Alcuronium	200	–	1.5	2.4	2.9
[114]	Vecuronium	70	–	1.5	2.4	2.9
[103]	Atracurium	300	1.4	1.7	2.3	2.8
[124]	Suxamethonium	500	–	–	0.6	0.7

The data for pancuronium and vecuronium for adolescents are from adults.
The data for atracurium are extrapolated from Ref. [103].

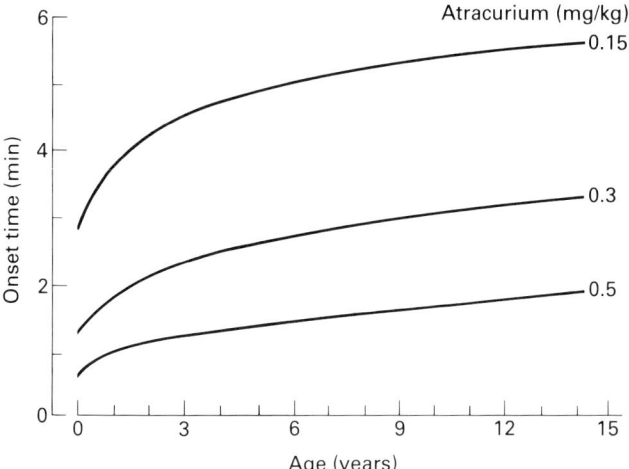

Fig. 2.8 Atracurium: rate of onset at different doses and ages. (From Meretoja [93], with permission.)

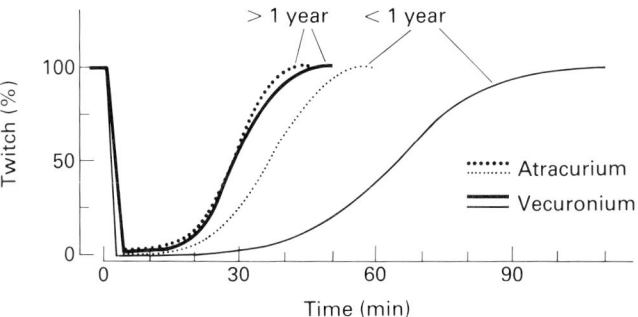

Fig. 2.9 Recovery from atracurium and vecuronium in patients over and less than 1 year of age, showing rapid recovery in the children and very slow recovery in infants who had vecuronium. (From Meretoja [93], with permission.)

suxamethonium, it will have to be given in a relative overdose, so that the receptor sites are rapidly flooded, but still be metabolized rapidly enough so that an unduly prolonged effect does not occur.

The maintenance dose requirement of non-depolariz-

ing muscle relaxants can be related to individual ED95 doses. The relationship is different for each relaxant. These amounts are summarized in Table 2.4 [93].

Suxamethonium

Suxamethonium is the only depolarizing relaxant commonly used in clinical practice [121]. For many years

Table 2.3 The recovery index (spontaneous recovery time from 25 to 75% twitch height) and the duration of effect (time from administration to 90–100% recovery of the twitch height) following vecuronium in paediatric patients. Times are in minutes

| | Recovery index | | | Duration of effect | | |
Ref.	Infants	Children	Adolescents	Infants	Children	Adolescents
[114]	20	9	13	73	35	53
[115]	18	10	–	–	–	–
[116]	29	11	–	78	33	–
[117]	21	7	9	98	35	45

Table 2.4 Maintenance dose requirement of muscle relaxants related to individual ED95 dose

Drug	ED95/h
Atracurium	2.0
Vecuronium	1.8
Vecuronium (infants)	1.3
Pancuronium	0.6
Alcuronium	0.4

it has been recognized that neonates and infants require a larger dose/kg than older patients. Walts and Dillon demonstrated that if dose was related to surface area, which is 2−2.5 times greater relative to weight in neonates, the requirement was constant [122]. Despite its wide usage it is only recently that dose−response studies have been undertaken. These show that the dose is significantly greater per kg in infants under 1 year than in older children [123, 124], that the ED95 is less in children over 11 years (270 μg/kg) than in children under 10 (450 μg/kg) and that the duration of action increases with age (Fig. 2.10) [124]. The fact that the usual recommended dose of 1 mg/kg is 2−4 times the ED95 indicates that a relative overdose is usually given. This hastens onset and provides a longer period of paralysis.

Suxamethonium has been used intramuscularly to facilitate intubation, especially in infants. The dose given is usually double the intravenous dose, so that in infants,

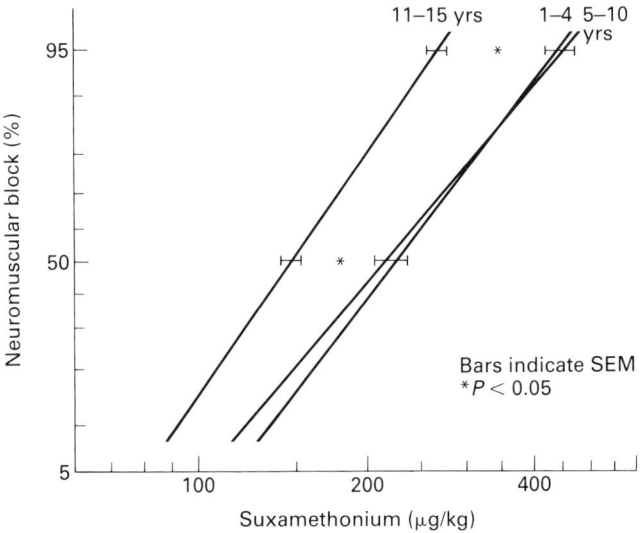

Fig. 2.10 Dose response for suxamethonium showing a significantly larger dose requirement in children from 1 to 10 years. (From Brown [124], with permission.)

3−4 mg/kg has often been recommended — probably more than is needed. Doses over 5 mg/kg tend to result in a change from depolarizing to dual block. This will also follow multiple doses or infusions.

Suxamethonium is structurally similar to two acetylcholine molecules and it therefore has an effect on the sinoatrial (SA) node, causing bradycardia. This response is exaggerated in children, especially after multiple doses. Atropine or glycopyrrolate should be given to prevent excessive bradycardia, especially in neonates with their rate-dependent cardiac output. Its action on the SA node is probably a factor in the interaction with digoxin, causing dysrhythmia.

Children can develop post-suxamethonium muscle pains.

Abnormal responses to muscle relaxants

1 Larger than usual doses of non-depolarizing muscle relaxants may be needed for patients with major burns (see Fig. 20.4), in children with malignant but not benign tumours [125], in some patients with severe cyanotic heart disease with a high haematocrit [126] and sometimes in patients with chronic infections.
2 Patients with myasthenia gravis usually require very small doses of non-depolarizing muscle relaxants; they should be given in small increments with monitoring of neuromuscular blockade, so that overdose is avoided [127] (see Chapter 25).
3 Some patients are sensitive to suxamethonium and will become paralysed with even small doses (0.1−0.2 mg/kg). These include patients with abnormal cholinesterase [128] (see p. 46), and patients during the second week after major burns, when they pass through a short phase of acute sensitivity to suxamethonium [129] (see Chapter 20).
4 Suxamethonium is a trigger agent for malignant hyperpyrexia in susceptible patients and may cause a rise in temperature, cardiovascular collapse or rhabdomyolysis in patients with Duchenne's muscular dystrophy (see Chapter 25).

Between the 2nd and 6th weeks following burns, suxamethonium will cause a significant rise in plasma potassium, the extent of which is related to the magnitude of the burn and the dose used (see Fig. 20.6). It should be avoided in very large burns, at least until grafting is complete. It can also cause hyperkalaemia following trauma and spinal injury.
5 Neonates and patients with myasthenia gravis are

resistant to suxamethonium and require larger than usual doses [127].

6 Suxamethonium's action is prolonged by interaction with some drugs such as anticholinesterases (e.g. ecothiopate) and cyclophosphamide.

LOCAL ANAESTHETICS

Pharmacokinetics

Volumes of distribution (V_D.ss) of amide local anaesthetics in neonates [134], infants [135] and older children [136] were all found to be about 2−3 times adult values. Clearance rates were 2−3 times faster in children than adults. In neonates, clearance of mepivacaine is slower due to decreased hydroxylation of the aromatic ring [137]. This prolongs elimination, making repeated doses hazardous. Clearance values of bupivacaine at birth are similar to adults, but increase during the neonatal period. The larger V_D.ss in neonates and children may be balanced by faster clearance, so that $T_{1/2}$ beta for local anaesthetics, apart from mepivacaine, is similar to adult values.

Adrenaline increases the duration of action of local anaesthetics by 50−100% in infants, declining to

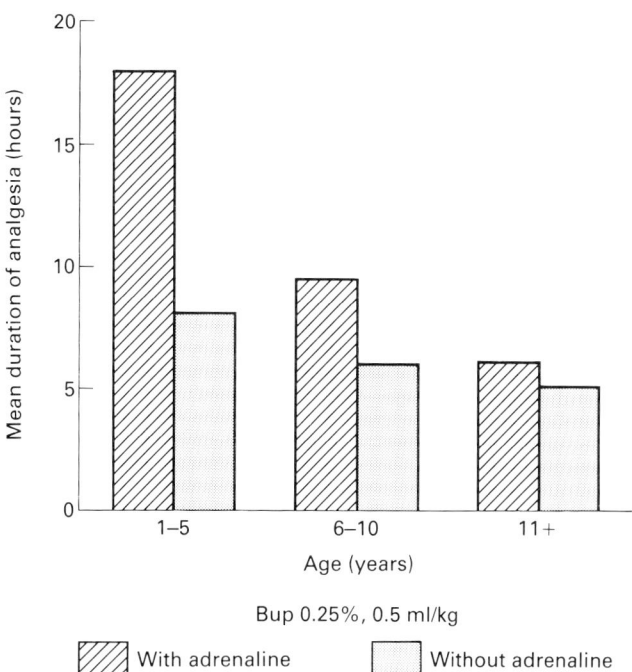

Fig. 2.11 The effects of adrenaline and age on duration of action of bupivacaine for caudal analgesia for inguinal surgery. (Derived from Warner [130].)

12−20% in adolescents [138, 130] (Fig. 2.11). It also decreases peak blood levels [138−140] (Fig. 2.12). Fresh adrenaline was added to the local anaesthetic in these studies; this mixture has a higher pH than the premixed commercial solutions. Higher pH increases the unionized portion, with resultant greater penetration of the local anaesthetic to the site of action inside the cell membrane [142].

Pharmacodynamics

Local anaesthetics act more rapidly, their effect lasts longer [130], and lower concentrations are needed to block nerve conduction in infants and young children than in adults [131]. Contributing factors may be incomplete myelination and the internodal distance. It has been suggested that a certain number of adjacent nodes of Ranvier must be bathed in local anaesthetic to block transmission [132, 133]. These are closer together in neonates and infants, making it easier to block nerves.

Toxicity

The manifestations of local anaesthetic toxicity are neurological irritability, culminating in convulsions and cardiac dysrhythmias, depression and arrest. Major toxic reactions may occur when usual doses of local anaesthetic are accidentally injected intravenously. In conscious patients apprehension, dizziness and circumoral tingling precede convulsions and dysrythmias following excessive absorption from other sites. Other dangerous complications can occur if large doses are injected into the wrong place, e.g. accidental total spinal anaesthesia following inadvertant dural puncture during epidural anaesthesia. Management of toxicity is discussed in Chapter 22.

Toxicity is related to the peak plasma level, which is dependent on the route of administration, age, addition of adrenaline and pH. It is lower following subcutaneous than epidural administration, and both are less than after topical spray of the trachea [143].

One of the important questions relating to local anaesthetics is to determine how much can be given safely. 'Toxic levels' have been determined in adult volunteers [144, 145] and relatively high doses have been used safely for blocks in both adults and children [147, 152]. Maximum safe doses have been stated for adults but have not been adequately defined for children, although many studies have been carried out in recent

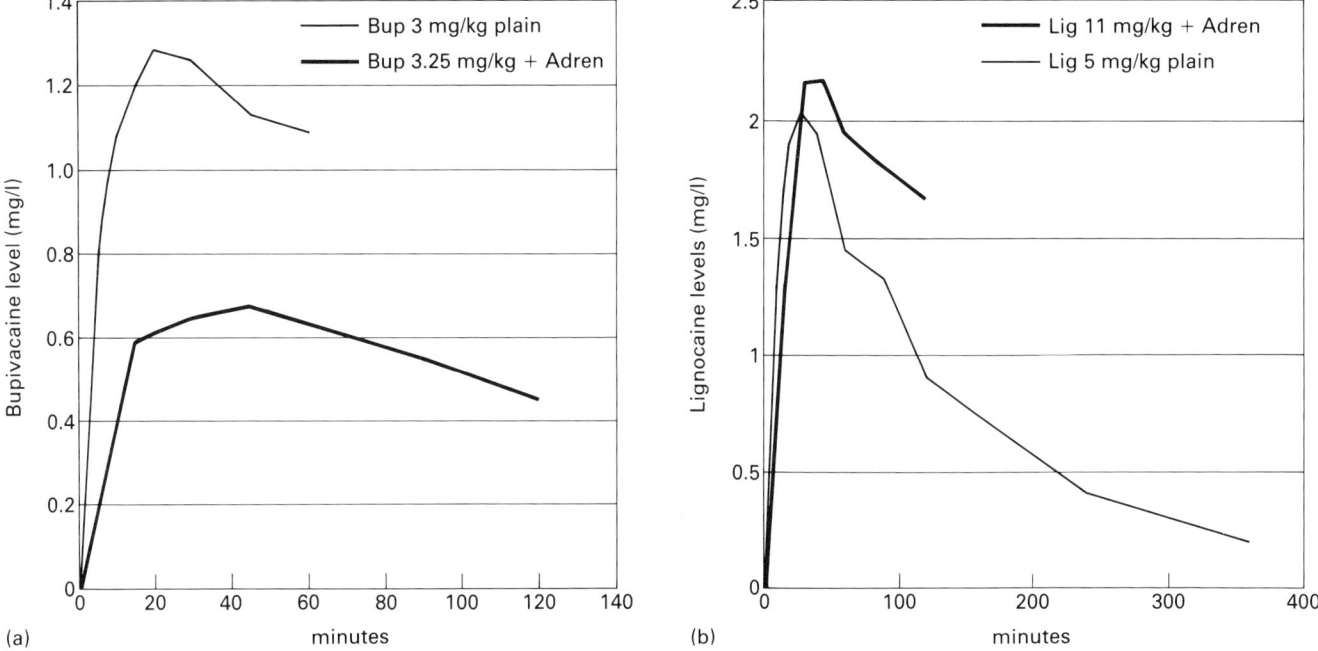

Fig. 2.12 The effect of adrenaline on absorption following caudal injection of (a) bupivacaine given in similar dosage — the plasma level was halved by adding adrenaline, and (b) lignocaine given in double the dose but achieving similar plasma levels. (Data derived from Eyres [141], Takasaki [139] and Ecoffey [140].)

years on blood levels after various blocks (Table 2.5). Sporadic high peak plasma levels reaching double the mean for the dose and age of the patient can occur (Table 2.6) [146]. That toxic manifestations (e.g. convulsions) have been rare suggests that the doses used are generally safe or that the signs have been suppressed by general anaesthesia.

In neonates, toxic levels of mepivacaine are about 8 μg/ml [148–150], similar to those found in adults. The situation is probably similar with lignocaine. Toxic levels of bupivacaine are not known, but may be influenced by changes in protein binding.

Neonates are sensitive to prilocaine. Significant methaemoglobinaemia has been reported after only

Table 2.5 Peak bupivacaine levels following blocks in children

Site	Dose mg/kg	Mean peak mg/l	Highest peak mg/l	+adr.	*n.*	Source
Intercostal	4	1.9	3.2	Yes	16	Rothstein [155]
Intercostal	3	1.4	1.7	Yes	5	Rothstein [155]
Axillary	3	1.8	2.7	No	20	Campbell [156]
Axillary	2	1.4	–	No	21	Campbell [156]
Ilio-inguinal	2	1.6	2.3	No	5	Epstein [157]
Ilio-inguinal	1.25	0.8	1.5	No	13	Stow [158]
Femoral nerve	2	0.9	1	No	14	Ronchi [159]
Caudal	3	1.3	2.0	No	45	Eyres [141]
Caudal	3.7	0.7	–	Yes	10	Takasaki [139]
Lumbar epidural	3.25	1.4	–	Yes	10	Ecoffey [136]
Penile nerve block	0.5 mg/kg/h	0.3	0.4	No	6	Sfez [160]
Lumbar epidural	0.2	0.6	0.8	Yes	6	Murat [161]
Intrapleural	1.25–2.5	3.4	7	Yes	14	McIlvain [162]

Venous plasma samples were used except by Rothstein, McIlvain, and Ecoffey who used arterial blood.

Table 2.6 Observations after tracheal lignocaine spray (4 mg/kg) in children [146]

Age (yrs)	No. of children	Mean peak plasma level	Highest peak plasma level	Mean time to peak in min
<1	13	5.2	10.1	6.1
1–3	21	5.7	7.2	6.5
3–5	23	5.8	10.1	7.9
5+	42	5.9	10.3	10.8

2 mg/kg [151]. Fetal haemoglobin is more easily oxidized to form methaemoglobin. If methaemoglobinaemia needs to be treated, ascorbic acid is safer than methylene blue because neonatal red cells are more easily haemolysed by reducing agents [153]. The absorption of prilocaine from EMLA cream (25 mg/g of both prilocaine and lignocaine) has been shown to be low in patients over 3 months of age [154].

ADDITIVES

Additives in drug preparations can cause toxicity or side effects. One example is the association of benzyl alcohol with intraventricular haemorrhage and kernicterus in premature infants. It is not certain how much has to be administered to produce these effects. Benzyl alcohol constitutes 9 mg/ml of the sterile water provided to dissolve vecuronium and it is present in atracurium, some brands of D-tubocurarine, midazolam and diazepam [163]. There are drugs which are formulated with benzyl alcohol by some companies and not by others [164].

PHARMACOGENETICS

There are many examples of genetically determined variation in the handling of drugs, mostly due to altered enzyme function. Some of these that are significant in anaesthesia will be outlined.

Cholinesterase variants

Suxamethonium (succinylcholine) is normally rapidly hydrolysed by plasma cholinesterase. Prolonged paralysis may be associated with low plasma cholinesterase levels (e.g. in liver disease) or be due to a genetic variant of plasma cholinesterase which metabolizes suxamethonium more slowly [165]. Four genes have been described — E_1u (usual gene), E_1a (atypical or dibucaine resistant), E_1f (fluoride resistant) [166–169] and E_1s (silent gene without cholinesterase activity) [170, 171]. A test was

developed in which the percentage inhibition of the plasma cholinesterase by an inhibitor, dibucaine (1×10^{-5} M), could be employed to distinguish between the usual and atypical enzymes [172]. Ninety-six per cent of the population is homozygous for the 'usual' enzyme, which is about 80% inhibited by dibucaine (DN80). The inhibition of homozygous atypical cholinesterase is about 16–25% (DN16–25) and the inhibition of the enzyme from heterozygous individuals is intermediate between these — about 50–65%. The reported frequency of people homozygous for the atypical gene has been 1:2000 [173] and 1:2400 [174]. Heterozygotes are relatively common. About 1 in 25 people are heterozygous for abnormal cholinesterase. Only 1 in 625 (1/25 × 1/25) couples will both be heterozygous and only 1 in 4 of their children will be homozygous for the abnormal genes (1/625 × 1/4 = 1/2500). The frequency of heterozygotes is about 2–4% but reports range from 7% in Czechoslovakia [175] to 1% in Australian aborigines [176].

Siblings who were heterozygous for the same genes have had widely divergent activity of the enzymes [177]. This suggested that there were other factors involved, or that the range of activity associated with a gene may vary, or that there are several atypical genes.

In dibucaine-resistant homozygotes, total paralysis lasts about an hour, and assisted ventilation may be required for up to 3 hours following 100 mg succinylcholine in adults [173]. Paralysis will occur with small doses (0.1 mg/kg) which can be used to differentiate heterozygotes from homozygotes by the different intensity and duration of block (Fig. 2.13) [178].

Genetic variants have also been described with increased pseudocholinesterase activity. The presence of an E_2+ gene at a separate locus controlling the C_5+ phenotype for cholinesterase is associated with a 30% increase in enzyme activity [174]. Another variant has been reported with about three times the cholinesterase activity normally present, which causes a marked resistance to suxamethonium [179].

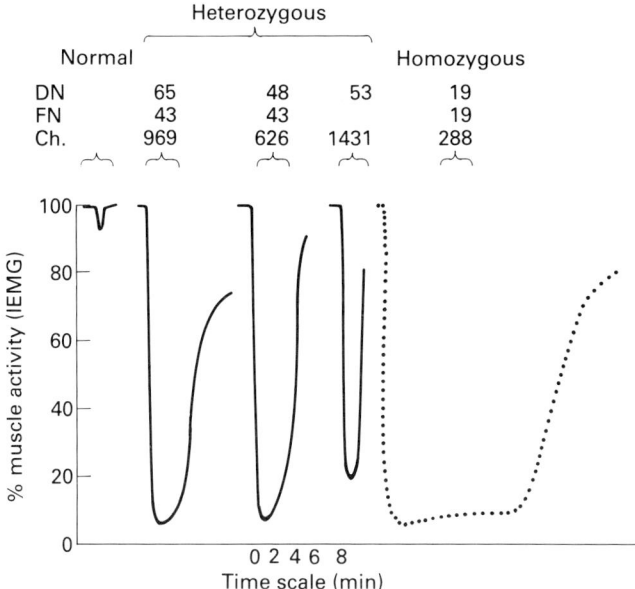

Fig. 2.13 Integrated electromyographic traces of percentage muscle activity in normal, heterozygous and homozygous patients with abnormal cholinesterase after 0.1 mg/kg suxamethonium i.v. The percent inhibition of dibucaine and fluoride and the cholinesterase activity are included so that they can be compared with the effect. The traces are on the same time scale. (From Brown [128], with permission.)

Procaine and several other esterase local anaesthetics are hydrolysed by plasma cholinesterase [180]. Prolonged action of these drugs has not been recognized in the presence of cholinesterase variants [181], probably because they are not often used nowadays and also because the rate of absorption into the circulation, which is relatively slow, determines the duration of local anaesthetic action.

Malignant hyperpyrexia

Malignant hyperpyrexia is a serious and dangerous complication which may develop during anaesthesia and requires urgent treatment (see Chapter 27). The condition presents in several forms, often with a family history. The first family was reported in 1960 by Denborough et al. [182, 183]. A mild or even subclinical myopathy may be a feature [184, 185].

Porphyria

There are several types of porphyria [186] but the genetically determined acute intermittent variety is the commonest of importance to anaesthetists, because it

may be exacerbated by barbiturates and sulphonamides [187]. These drugs increase the synthesis of the enzyme delta-amino-laevulinic acid synthetase which is the first and rate-controlling step in porphyrin biosynthesis. Increased activity of this enzyme leads to excessive production of porphyrins, which may precipitate the development of neurological signs including neuralgia and paralysis and may progress to respiratory failure [187]. Barbiturates should therefore be avoided in these patients, who sometimes present with abdominal pain and may have an unnecessary laparotomy carried out if the condition is not suspected.

G6PD deficiency

Glucose-6-phosphate dehydrogenase (G6PD) deficiency in red cells is commonly associated with drug-induced haemolysis. It is probably the most prevalent hereditary enzymatic defect of clinical significance. It is an X-linked trait of intermediate dominance. Exposure to certain drugs causes haemolysis, mainly of older cells, so that the process is self-limiting. The most common offending drugs are antimalarials, antipyretic analgesics, sulphones, synthetic vitamin K and nitrofurans as well as uncooked fava beans [188]. The common anaesthetic drugs do not seem to precipitate haemolysis.

Genetic influences on drug metabolism

Biotransformation of several drugs is influenced by genetic variation affecting their rate of metabolism. These include halothane [189] and several others not often encountered by anaesthetists, such as isoniazid and hydrallazine (slow acetylators) and phenytoin (Dilantin), which is hydroxylated [190].

REFERENCES

1 Walts I.E., Dillon J.B. The response of newborns to succinylcholine and D-tubocurarine. *Anesthesiology* 1969, **31**, 35.
2 Gallagher T.M., Black G.W. Uptake of volatile anaesthetics in children. *Anaesthesia* 1985, **40**, 1073.
3 Jantzen J.P.A.H., Tzanova I., Witton P.K., Klein A.M. Rectal pH in children. *Canad J Anaes* 1989, **36**, 665.
4 Kestin I.G., McIlvaine W.B., Lockhart C.E., Kestin K.J., Jones M.A. Rectal methohexitone for induction of anaesthesia in children with and without rectal aspiration after sleep: a pharmacokinetic and pharmacodynamic study. *Anesth Analg* 1988, **67**, 1102.
5 Cook D.R., Davis P.J. Pediatric anesthesia pharmacology. In: Lake C. (Ed.) *Pediatric cardiac anesthesia*, (1988) Appleton and Lange, East Norwalk, Connecticut, Chapter 8.

6 Kupferberg H.J., Way E.L. Pharmacological basis for increased sensitivity of the newborn rat to morphine. *J Pharmacol Exp Ther* 1963, **141**, 105.

7 Cheek D.B. Extracellular volume; its structure and measurement and the influence of age and disease. *J Pediatr* 1961, **58**, 103.

8 Friis Hansen B. Body composition during growth. *Pediatrics* 1971, **47**, 264.

9 Pasternak G.W., An Zhong Zhang, Teco H.L. Developmental differences between high and low affinity opiate binding sites: the relationship to analgesia and respiratory depression. *Life Sciences* 1980, **27**, 1185.

10 Cook D.R., Brandom B.W., Shiu G., Wolfson B.W. The inspired median effective dose, brain concentration at anesthesia, and cardiovascular index for halothane in young rats. *Anesth Analg* 1981, **60**, 182.

11 Lerman J., Robinson S., Willis M.M., Gregory G.A. Anaesthetic requirements for halothane in young children 0−1 month and 1−6 months of age. *Anesthesiology* 1983, **59**, 421.

12 Gregory G.A., Eger E.I., Munson E.S. The relationship between age and halothane requirements in man. *Anesthesiology* 1969, **30**, 488.

13 Cameron C.B., Robinson S., Gregory G.A. Minimum alveolar concentration of isoflurane in children. *Anesth Analg* 1984, **63**, 418.

14 LeDez K.M., Lerman J. The minimum alveolar concentration of isoflurane in preterm neonates. *Anesthesiology* 1987, **67**, 301.

15 Cole W.H.J. MSc Thesis, Melbourne University 1966.

16 Coleman S.A., McCrory J.W., Vallis C.J., Boys R.J. Inhalation induction of anaesthesia with isoflurane: effect of added CO_2. *Br J Anaes* 1991, **67**, 257.

17 Watcha M.F., Forestner J.E., Connor M.T., Duncan C.M. MAC of halothane for tracheal intubation in children. *Anesthesiology* 1988, **69**, 412.

18 Yakaitis R.W., Blitt C.D., Angiulo J.P. End tidal enflurane concentration for endotracheal intubation. *Anesthesiology* 1979, **50**, 59.

19 Morris P. Personal communication.

20 Murray D., Forbes R., Murphy K., Mahoney L. Nitrous oxide: cardiovascular effects in infants and young children during halothane and isoflurane anaesthesia. *Anesth Analg* 1989, **67**, 1059.

21 Murat I.M., Lapeyre G., Saint-Maurice C. Isoflurane attenuates baroreflex control of heart rate in human neonates. *Anesthesiology* 1989, **70** (Suppl 3), 395.

22 Warner L.O., Beach T.P., Garvin J.P., Warner E.J. Halothane and children: the first quarter century. *Anesth Analg* 1984, **63**, 838.

23 Johnston R.R., Eger E.I., Wilson C. A comparative interaction of epinephrine with enflurane, isoflurane and halothane in man. *Anesth Analg* 1976, **55**, 709.

24 Karl H.W., Swerdlow D.B., Lee K.W., Downes J.J. Epinephrine halothane interactions in children. *Anesthesiology* 1983, **58**, 142.

25 Badgwell J.M., Heavner J.E., Cooper M.W., Cockings E. The cardiovascular effects of anticholinergic agents administered during halothane anaesthesia in children. *Acta Anaes Scand* 1988, **32**, 383.

26 Murat I., Deleur M.M., MacGee K., Saint-Maurice C. Changes in ventilatory patterns during halothane anaesthesia in children. *Br J Anaes* 1985, **57**, 569.

27 Lindahl S.G., Olsson A.K. Respiratory drive and timing before and during carbon dioxide inhalation in infants anaesthetized with halothane. *Eur J Anaes* 1987, **3**, 427.

28 Tusiewicz K., Bryan A.C., Froese A.B. Contributions of changing rib cage: diaphragm interaction to the ventilatory depression of halothane anaesthesia. *Anesthesiology* 1977, **47**, 327.

29 Knill R.L., Gelb A.W. Ventilatory responses to hypoxia and hypercapnia during halothane sedation and anaesthesia in man. *Anesthesiology* 1978, **49**, 244.

30 Charlton A.J., Lindahl S.G. Ventilatory response during halothane and enflurane anaesthesia. *Anaesthesia* 1985, **40**, 18.

31 Larsson A., Andreasson S., Ekstom Jodal B., Nilsson K. Carbon dioxide tensions in infants during mask anaesthesia with spontaneous ventilation. *Acta Anaes Scand* 1987, **31**, 273.

32 Artru A.A. Effects of halothane, enflurane, isoflurane and fentanyl on resistance to reabsorption of CSF. *Anesth Analg* 1984, **63**, 175.

33 Wark H., Earl J., Chau D.D., Overton J. Halothane metabolism in children. *Br J Anaes* 1990, **64**, 476.

34 Wark H. Postoperative jaundice in children. *Anaesthesia* 1983, **38**, 237.

35 Warner L.O., Beach T.P., Garwin J.P., Warner E.J. Halothane and children. The first quarter century. *Anesth Analg* 1984, **63**, 838.

36 Kenna J.G., Neuberger J., Meili-Vergani G., Mowat A.P., Williams R. Halothane hepatitis in children. *Br Med J* 1987, **1**, 1209.

37 Wark H. Letter. *Br Med J* 1987, **2**, 117.

38 Wark H., O'Halloran M., Overton J. Prospective study of liver function in children following multiple halothane anaesthetics at short intervals. *Br J Anaes* 1986, **58**, 1224.

39 Egers E.I., Smuckler E.A., Ferrell L.D., Goldsmith C.H., Johnson B.H. Is enflurane hepatotoxic? *Anesth Analg* 1986, **65**, 21.

40 Joshi P.H., Conn H.O. The syndrome of methoxyflurane hepatitis. *Ann Intern Med* 1974, **80**, 395.

41 Cousins M.J., Mazze R.I. Anaesthesia, surgery and renal function. *Anaes Intens Care* 1973, **1**, 355.

42 Westhorpe R.N., Brown T.C.K. Unpublished data.

43 Stoelting R.K., Petersen C. Methoxyflurane anaesthesia in paediatric patients: evaluation of metabolism and renal function. *Anesthesiology* 1975, **42**, 26.

44 Mazze R.I., Cousins M.J. Biotransformation of methoxyflurane. *Int Anesth Clin* 1974, **12**, 93.

45 Hinkle A.J. Serum inorganic fluoride levels after enflurane in children. *Anesth Analg* 1989, **68**, 396.

46 Mazze R.I., Calverley R.K., Smith N.T. Inorganic fluoride nephrotoxicity: prolonged enflurane and halothane anesthesia in volunteers. *Anesthesiology* 1977, **46**, 265.

47 Westhorpe R.N. Anaesthetic agents and the ozone layer. *Anaes Intens Care* 1990, **18**, 102.

48 Sorbo S., Hudson R.J., Loomis J.C. Pharmacokinetics of thiopental in pediatric surgical patients. *Anesthesiology* 1984, **61**, 666.

49 Kingston H.G., Kendrick A., Sommer K.M., Olsen G.D., Downes H. Binding of thiopental in neonatal serum.

Anesthesiology 1990, **72**, 428.

50 Westrin P., Jonmarker C., Werner O. Thiopental requirements for induction of anaesthesia in neonates and in infants 1–6 months of age. *Anesthesiology* 1989, **71**, 344.

51 Jonmarker C., Westrin P., Larsson S., Werner O. Thiopentone requirements for induction of anaesthesia in children. *Anesthesiology* 1987, **67**, 104.

52 Brett C.M., Fisher D.M. Thiopental dose response relations in unpremedicated infants, children and adults. *Anesth Analg* 1987, **66**, 1024.

53 Duncan B.B., Zaimi F., Newman G.B., Jenkins J.G., Aveling W. Effect of premedication on induction dose of thiopentone in children. *Anaesthesia* 1984, **39**, 426.

54 Brown T.C.K. The principles of analgesic administration in hypovolaemic patients. *Med J Australia* 1972, **1**, 420.

55 Tibballs J., Malbezin S. Cardiovascular responses to induction of anaesthesia with thiopentone and suxamethonium in infants and children. *Anaes Intens Care* 1988, **16**, 278.

56 Bjorkman S., Gabrielsson J., Quaynor H., Corbey M. Pharmacokinetics of intravenous and rectal methohexitone in children. *Br J Anaes* 1987, **59**, 1541.

57 Valtonen M. Anaesthesia for CT of the brain in children: a comparison of propofol with thiopentone. *Acta Anaes Scand* 1989, **33**, 170.

58 Mirakhur R.K. Induction characteristics of propofol in children: comparison with thiopentone. *Anaesthesia* 1988, **43**, 593.

59 Purcell-Jones G., Yates A., Becker J.R., James I.G. Comparison of induction characteristics of thiopentone and propofol in children. *Br J Anaes* 1987, **59**, 1431.

60 Puttick N., Rosen M. Propofol induction and maintenance with nitrous oxide in paediatric outpatient dental anaesthesia. A comparison with thiopentone–nitrous oxide, halothane. *Anaesthesia* 1988, **43**, 646.

61 Patel D.K., Keeling P.A., Newman G.B., Radford P. Induction dose of propofol in children. *Anaesthesia* 1988, **43**, 949.

62 Hanallah R.S., Baker S., Casey W., McGill, Broadman L., Norden J.N. Propofol induction characteristics in unpremedicated children. *Anesthesiology* 1989, **71**, A1051.

63 Leslie K., Crankshaw D.P. Potency of propofol for loss of consciousness after a single dose. *Br J Anaesth* 1990, **64**, 734.

64 Westrin P. The induction dose of propofol in infants 1–6 months of age and in older children. *Anesthesiology* 1989, **71**, A1061.

65 Hickey P.R., Hansen D.D., *et al.* Pulmonary and systemic haemodynamic response to ketamine in infants with normal and elevated pulmonary vascular resistance. *Anesthesiology* 1985, **62**, 287.

66 Bourke D.L., Malit L.A., Smith T.C. Respiratory interactions of ketamine and morphine. *Anesthesiology* 1987, **66**, 153.

67 Shulman D., Beardsmore C.S., Aronson H.B., Godfrey S. The effect of ketamine on functional residual capacity in young children. *Anesthesiology* 1985, **62**, 551.

68 Cook D.R. Pharmacokinetics of ketamine in infants and small children. *Anesthesiology* 1982, **57**, A428.

69 Brown T.C.K., Cole W.H.J., Murray G.H. Ketamine, a new anaesthetic agent. *ANZ J Surg* 1970, **39**, 305.

70 Cole W.H.J. Midazolam in paediatric anaesthesia. *Anaes Intens Care* 1982, **10**, 36.

71 Payne K. The pharmacokinetics of midazolam in paediatric patients. *Eur J Clin Pharmacol* 1989, **37**, 267.

72 Ben-Shlomo I., Abd-El-Khalim H., Ezry J., Zohar S., Tuerskoy M. Midazolam acts synergistically with fentanyl for induction of anaesthesia. *Br J Anaes* 1990, **54**, 45.

73 Short T.G., Galletly D.C., Plummer J.L. Hypnotic and anaesthetic action of thiopentone and midazolam alone and in combination. *Br J Anaes* 1991, **66**, 13.

74 Kissin I., Mason J.O., Bradley E.L. Pentobarbital and thiopental interactions with midazolam. *Anesthesiology* 1987, **67**, 26.

75 Kay B. A clinical assessment of the use of etomidate in children. *Br J Anaes* 1976, **48**, 207.

76 Lynn A.M., Slattery J.T. Morphine pharmacokinetics in early infancy. *Anesthesiology* 1987, **66**, 136.

77 Gauntlett I.G., Fisher D.M., Hertzka R.E. Pharmacokinetics of fentanyl in neonatal humans: effect of age. *Anesthesiology* 1988, **69**, 683.

78 Davis P.J., Killian A., Stiller R.L., Cook D.R. Pharmacokinetics of alfentanil in newborn premature infants and older children. *Dev Pharmacol Ther* 1989, **13**, 21.

79 Greeley W.J., de Bruijin N.P. Changes in pharmacokinetics during the neonatal period. *Anesth Analg* 1988, **67**, 86.

80 Anand K.J., Sippell W.G., Aynsley-Green A. Random trial of fentanyl anaesthesia in preterm babies undergoing surgery: effects on the stress response. *Lancet* 1987, **1**, 62.

81 Collins C., Koren G., Crean P., Klein J., Roy W.L. Fentanyl pharmacokinetics and haemodynamic effects of preterm infants during ligation of patent ductus arteriosus. *Anesth Analg* 1985, **64**, 1078.

82 Robinson S., Gregory G.A. Fentanyl–air–oxygen anesthesia for ligation of patent ductus arteriosus in preterm infants. *Anesth Analg* 1981, **60**, 331.

83 Yaster M. The dose response of fentanyl in neonatal anaesthesia. *Anesthesiology* 1987, **66**, 433.

84 Koehntop D.E., Rodman J.H., Brundage G.M., Hegland M.G., Buckley J.J. Pharmacokinetics of fentanyl in neonates. *Anesth Analg* 1986, **65**, 227.

85 Hertzka R.E., Gauntlett I.S., Fisher D.M., Spellman M.J. Fentanyl-induced ventilatory depression: effect of age *Anesthesiology* 1989, **70**, 213.

86 Murat I., Levica T.C., Bey A., Saint-Maurice C. Effects of fentanyl on baroreceptor reflex control of heart rate in newborn infants. *Anesthesiology* 1988, **68**, 717.

87 Hickey P.R., Hansen D.D., Wessel D.L., Lang R., Jonas R.A. Pulmonary and systemic haemodynamic responses to fentanyl in infants. *Anesth Analg* 1985, **64**, 483.

88 Koren G., Butt W., Pape K., Chinyanga H. Morphine-induced seizures in newborn infants. *Vet Human Toxicol* 1985, **27**, 519.

89 Goudsouzian N.G. Maturation of neuromuscular transmission in the infant. *Br J Anaes* 1980, **52**, 205.

90 Goudsouzian N.G., Standaert F.G. The infant and the myoneural junction. *Anesth Analg* 1986, **65**, 1208.

91 Day N.S., Blake G.J., Standaert F.G., Dretchen K.L. Characterization of the train-of-four response in fast and slow muscles; effect of D-tubocurarine, pancuronium and vecuronium. *Anesthesiology* 1983, **58**, 414.

92 Keens T.G., Bryan A.C., Levison H., Ianuzzo C.D. Developmental pattern of muscle fibre types in human ventilatory muscles. *J Appl Physiol* 1978, **44**, 909.

93 Meretoja O.A. Neuromuscular blocking agents in paediatric

patients: influence of age on the response. *Anaes Intens Care* 1990, **18**, 440.

94 Fisher D.M., O'Keeffe C., Stanski D.R., Cronnelly R., Miller R.D., Gregory G.A. Pharmacokinetics and pharmaco-dynamics of D-tubocurarine in infants, children, and adults. *Anesthesiology* 1982, **57**, 203.

95 Matteo R.S., Lieberman I.G., Salanitre E., McDaniel D.D., Diaz J. Distribution, elimination and action of D-tubocurarine in neonates, infants, children and adults. *Anesth Analg* 1984, **63**, 799.

96 Brandom B.W., Stiller R.L., Cook D.R., Woelfel S.K., Chakravorti S., Lai A. Pharmacokinetics of atracurium in anaesthetized infants and children. *Br J Anaes* 1986, **58**, 1210.

97 Fisher D.M., Castagnoli K., Miller R.D. Vecuronium kinetics and dynamics in anaesthetized infants and children. *Clin Pharmacol Ther* 1985, **37**, 402.

98 Laycock J.R.D., Baxter M.K., Bevan J.C., Sangwan S., Donati F., Bevan D.R. The potency of pancuronium at the adductor pollicis and diaphragm in infants and children. *Anesthesiology* 1988, **69**, 908.

99 Goudsouzian N.G., Donlon J.V., Savarese J.J., Ryan J.F. Re-evaluation of dosage and duration of action of D-tubocurarine in the paediatric age group. *Anesthesiology* 1975, **43**, 416.

100 Meretoja O.A., Brown T.C.K., Clare D. Dose response of alcuronium and D-tubocurarine in infants, children and adolescents. *Anaes Intens Care* 1990, **18**, 449.

101 Goudsouzian N.G., Liu L.M.P., Gionfriddo M., Rudd G.D. Neuromuscular effects of atracurium in infants and children. *Anesthesiology* 1985, **62**, 75.

102 Goudsouzian N.G., Martyn J.J.A., Liu L.M.P., Gionfriddo M. Safety and efficacy of vecuronium in adolescents and children. *Anesth Analg* 1983, **62**, 1083.

103 Meakin G., Shaw E.A, Baker R.D., Morris P. Comparison of atracurium-induced neuromuscular blockade in neonates, infants and children. *Br J Anaes* 1988, **60**, 171.

104 Brandom B.W., Woelfel S.K., Cook D.R., Fehr B.L., Rudd G.D. Clinical pharmacology of atracurium in infants. *Anesth Analg* 1984, **63**, 309.

105 Smith C.E., Donati F., Bevan D.R. Dose−response curves for succinylcholine: single versus cumulative techniques. *Anesthesiology* 1988, **69**, 338.

106 Nightingale D.A. The use of atracurium in neonatal anaesthesia. *Br J Anaes* 1986, **58**, 32S.

107 Meretoja O.A., Luosto T. The dose−response characteristics of pancuronium in neonates, infants, and children. *Anaes Intens Care* 1990, **18**, 455−459.

108 Meretoja O.A., Brown T.C.K. Maintenance requirement of alcuronium in paediatric patients. *Anaes Intens Care* 1990, **18**, 452.

109 Shanks C.A. Pharmacokinetics of the non-depolarizing neuromuscular relaxants applied to calculation of bolus and infusion dosage regimens. *Anesthesiology* 1986, **64**, 72.

110 Meretoja O.A., Wirtavuori K. Influence of age on the dose−response relationship of atracurium in paediatric patients. *Acta Anaes Scand* 1988, **32**, 614.

111 Meretoja O.A., Wirtavuori K., Neuvonen P.J. Age dependence of the dose−response curve of vecuronium in pediatric patients during balanced anesthesia. *Anesth Analg* 1988, **67**, 21.

112 Smith C.E., Baxter M., Bevan J.C., Donati F., Bevan D.R. Accelerated onset and delayed recovery of D-tubocurarine blockade with pancuronium in infants and children. *Canad J Anaes* 1987, **34**, 555.

113 Bevan J.C., Donati F., Bevan D.R. Attempted acceleration of the onset of action of pancuronium. Effects of divided doses in infants and children. *Br J Anaes* 1985, **57**, 1204.

114 Fisher D.M., Miller R.D. Neuromuscular effects of vecuronium in infants and children during N_2O halothane anesthesia. *Anesthesiology* 1983, **58**, 519.

115 Motsch J., Hutschenreuter K., Ismaily A.J., von Blohn K. Vecuronium bei Sauglingen und Kleinkindern: klinische und neuromuskulare Effekte. *Anaesthetist* 1985, **34**, 382.

116 Schipers H.C., Bell B., Erdman W., Rees J.G. Pharmaco-dynamics of vecuronium bromide in anesthetized neonates, infants and children. *Anesthesiology* 1988, **69**, A760.

117 Kalli I., Meretoja O.M. Duration of action of vecuronium in infants and children anaesthetized without potent inhalational agents. *Acta Anaes Scand* 1989, **33**, 29.

118 Goudsouzian N.G., Alifimoff I.K., Eberly C., *et al.* Neuro-muscular and cardiovascular effects of mivacurium in children. *Anesthesiology* 1989, **70**, 237.

119 Sarner J.B., Brandom B.W., Woelfel S.K., *et al.* Clinical pharmacology of mivacurium chloride (BWB1090U) in chil-dren during nitrous oxide−halothane and nitrous oxide−narcotic anesthesia. *Anesth Analg* 1989, **68**, 116.

120 Savarese J.J., Ali H.H., Basta S.J., *et al.* The clinical neuromuscular pharmacology of mivacurium chloride (BW B1090U). A short-acting non-depolarizing ester neuro-muscular blocking drug. *Anesthesiology* 1988, **68**, 723.

121 Cook D.R., Fischer C.G. Neuromuscular blocking effects of succinylcholine in infants and children. *Anesthesiology* 1975, **42**, 662.

122 Walts L.F., Dillon J.B. The response of newborns to succinyl-choline and D-tubocurarine. *Anesthesiology* 1969, **31**, 35.

123 Meakin G., McKiernan E.P., Morris P., Baker R.D. Dose−response curves for suxamethonium in neonates, infants and children. *Br J Anaes* 1989, **62**, 655.

124 Brown T.C.K., Meretoja O.A., Bell B., Clare D. Suxamethonium−electromyographic studies in children. *Anaes Intens Care* 1990, **18**, 473.

125 Brown T.C.K., Gregory M., Bell B., Clare D. Response to non-depolarizing muscle relaxants in children with tumours. *Anaes Intens Care* 1990, **18**, 460.

126 Lucerno V.M., Lerman J., Burrows F.A. Onset of neuro-muscular blockade with pancuronium in children with cyanotic and acyanotic heart disease. *Anesth Analg* 1987, **66**, S108.

127 Brown T.C.K., Gebert R.G., Meretoja O.A., Shield L.K. Myasthenia gravis in children and its anaesthetic implications. *Anaes Intens Care* 1990, **18**, 466.

128 Brown T.C.K., Meretoja O.A., Bell B., Clare D. Responses to small doses of suxamethonium in four children with abnormal cholinesterase. *Anaes Intens Care* 1990, **18**, 477.

129 Brown T.C.K., Bell B. Electromyographic responses to small doses of suxamethonium in children after burns. *Br J Anaes* 1987, **59**, 1017.

130 Warner M.A., Kunkal S.E., Offord K.O., Atchison S.R., Dawson B. The effects of age, epinephrine and operation site on duration of caudal analgesia in pediatric patients. *Anesth Analg* 1987, **66**, 995.

131 Wolf A.R., Valley R.D., Fear D.W., Lawrence R.W., Lerman J. Bupivacaine for caudal analgesia in infants and children: optimum effective concentration. *Anesthesiology* 1988, **69**, 102.

132 Raymond S.A., Steffensen S.C., Gugino L.D., Strichartz G.R. The role of length of nerve exposed to local anaesthetic in impulse blocking action. *Anesth Analg* 1989, **68**, 563.

133 Fink B.R. The long and the short of conduction block. *Anesth Analg* 1989, **68**, 551.

134 Bricker S., Telford R., Booker P. Pharmacokinetics of bupivacaine following intraoperative intercostal nerve block in neonates and in infants less than 6 months. *Anesthesiology* 1989, **70**, 942.

135 Mazoit J., Denson D., Samii K. Pharmacokinetics of bupivacaine following caudal anaesthesia in infants. *Anesthesiology* 1988, **68**, 387.

136 Ecoffey C., Desparmets J., Maury M., Berdeaux A., Giudicelli J.F., Saint-Maurice C. Bupivacaine in children: pharmacokinetics following caudal anaesthesia. *Anesthesiology* 1985, **63**, 447.

137 Moore R.G., Thomas J., Triggs D.B., *et al.* Pharmacokinetics and metabolism of anilide anaesthetics in neonates. *Eur J Clin Pharmacol* 1978, **14**, 203.

138 Murat I., Delleur M.M., Saint-Maurice C. Effects of age and the addition of adrenaline to bupivacaine for continuous lumbar epidural anaesthesia in children. *Anesthesiology* 1986, **65**, A428.

139 Takasaki M. Blood concentrations of lidocaine, mepivacaine and bupivacaine during caudal analgesia in children. *Acta Anaes Scand* 1984, **28**, 211.

140 Ecoffey C., Desparmets J., Berdeaux A., Maury M., Giudicelli J.F., Saint-Maurice C. Pharmacokinetics of lignocaine in children following caudal anaesthesia. *Br J Anaes* 1984, **56**, 1399.

141 Eyres R.L., Hastings C.L., Brown T.C.K., Oppenheim R.C. Plasma bupivacaine concentrations following lumbar epidural anaesthesia. *Anaes Intens Care* 1986, **14**, 131.

142 Hilgier M. Alkalinization of bupivacaine for brachial plexus block. *Reg Anaes* 1985, **10**, 59.

143 Eyres R.L., Bishop W., Oppenheim R.C., Brown T.C.K. Plasma lignocaine concentrations following topical laryngeal application. *Anaes Intens Care* 1983, **11**, 23.

144 Foldes F.F., Molloy R., McNall P.G., Koukal L.R. Comparison of toxicity of intravenously given local anaesthetic agents in man. *JAMA* 1960, **172**, 1493.

145 Jorfeldt L., Lofstrom B., Pernow B., Persson B., Wahren J., Widman B. The effect of local anaesthetic on the central circulation and respiration in man and dog. *Acta Anaes Scand* 1968, **12**, 153.

146 Eyres R.L., Brown T.C.K. Observations after tracheal lignocaine spray in children. In: Cousins M.J., Bridenbaugh P.O. (Eds.) *Neural blockade.* (1988) JB Lippincott Co., Philadelphia, p. 673.

147 Moore D.C., Bridenbaugh L.D., Thompson G.E., Balfour R.I., Horton W.G. Bupivacaine: a review of 11080 cases. *Anesth Analg* 1978, **57**, 42.

148 Moore D.C., Bridenbaugh L.D., Bagdi P.A. Accumulation of mepivacaine HCl during caudal block. *Anesthesiology* 1968, **29**, 585.

149 Finster M., Peppers P.J., Sinclair J.C. Accidental intoxication of the fetus with local anaesthetic drug during caudal anaesthesia. *Am J Obst Gyn* 1965, **92**, 922.

150 Clark R.B., Jones G.L., Barclay D.L., Griffenstein F.E., McAninch P.E. Maternal and neonatal effects of 1% and 2% mepivacaine for lumbar extradural analgesia. *Br J Anaes* 1975, **47**, 1285.

151 Mandel S. Methemoglobinemia following neonatal circumcision. *JAMA* 1989, **261**, 702.

152 Melman E., Pennelas J., Maruffo J. Regional anaesthesia in children. *Anesth Analg* 1975, **54**, 387.

153 Menahem S. Neonatal cyanosis, methaemoglobinaemia and haemolytic anaemia. *Acta Anaes Scand* 1988, **77**, 755.

154 Engberg G., Damelsen K., Henneberg S., Nilsson A. Plasma concentration of prilocaine and lidocaine and methaemoglobin formation in infants after epicutaneous application of a 5% prilocaine/lidocaine cream, (EMLA). *Acta Anaes Scand* 1987, **31**, 624.

155 Rothstein P., Arthur G.R., Feldman H.S., Kopf G.S., Covino B.G. Bupivacaine for intercostal nerve blocks in children: blood concentrations and pharmacokinetics. *Anesth Analg* 1986, **65**, 625.

156 Campbell R., Ilett K.F., Dusci L. Plasma bupivacaine concentration after axillary block in children. *Anaes Intens Care* 1986, **14**, 343.

157 Epstein R.H., Larijani G.E., Wolfson P. Plasma bupivacaine concentration following ilioinguinal iliohypogastric nerve block in children. *Anesthesiology* 1986, **65**, A429.

158 Stow P.J., Scott A., Phillips A., White J.B. Plasma bupivacaine concentration during caudal analgesia and ilioinguinal/iliohypogastric nerve block in children. *Anaesthesia* 1988, **43**, 650.

159 Ronchi L., Rosenbaum D., Athouel A., Lemaitre J.L. Femoral nerve blockade in children using bupivacaine. *Anesthesiology* 1989, **70**, 622.

160 Sfez M., Le Mapihan Y., Mazoit X, Dreux-Boucard L.A. Local anaesthetic serum concentrations after penile nerve block in children. *Anesth Analg* 1990, **71**, 423.

161 Murat I., Martay G., Delleur M.M., Esteve C., Saint-Maurice C. Bupivacaine pharmacokinetics during epidural anaesthesia in children. *Eur J Anaes* 1988, **5**, 113.

162 McIlvaine W.B., Knox R.F., Fennessey P.V., Goldstein M. Continuous infusion of bupivacaine via intrapleural catheter for analgesia after thoracotomy in children. *Anesthesiology* 1988, **69**, 261.

163 Weissman D.B., Jackson S.H., Heicher D.A., Rockoff M.A. Benzyl alcohol administration in neonates. *Anesth Analg* 1990, **70**, 673.

164 Reynolds P., Wilton N. Inadvertant benzyl alcohol administration in neonates. Do we contribute? *Anesth Analg* 1989, **69**, 855.

165 Kalow W. Stanon N. On distribution and inheritance of atypical forms of human serum cholinesterase, as indicated by dibucaine numbers. *Canad J Biochem Physiol* 1957, **35**, 1305.

166 Harris H. Whittaker M. Differential inhibition of human serum cholinesterase with fluoride: recognition of 2 new phenotypes. *Nature* 1961, **191**, 496.

167 Simpson N.E. Genetics of esterases in man. *Ann NY Acad Sci* 1968, **151**, 699.

168 Lehmann H., Liddell J., Blackwell B., O'Connor D.C.J., Daws A.V. Two further serum pseudocholinesterase pheno-

types as causes of suxamethonium apnoea. *Br Med J* 1963, **1**, 1116.

169 Simpson N.E. C5 types of serum cholinesterase. *J Med Genet* 1967, **4**, 264.

170 Liddell J., Lehmann H., Silk E. A 'silent' pseudocholinesterase gene. *Nature* 1962, **193**, 561.

171 Kalow W. Pharmacogenetics and anaesthesia. *Anesthesiology* 1964, **25**, 377.

172 Kalow W., Genest K. A method for the detection of atypical human serum cholinesterase: determination of dibucaine numbers. *Canad J Biochem Physiol* 1957, **35**, 339.

173 Kalow W., Gunn D.R. The relation between the dose of succinyl choline and duration of apnoea in man. *J Pharmacol Exp Ther* 1957, **120**, 203.

174 Churchill Davidson C. The changing pattern of neuromuscular block. *Canad Anaes Soc J* 1961, **8**, 91.

175 Goedde H.G., Altland K. Pseudocholinesterase variants in Germany and Czechoslovakia. *Nature* 1963, **198**, 1203.

176 Horsfall W.R., Lehmann H., Davies D. Incidence of cholinesterase variants in Australian aborigines. *Nature* 1963, **199**, 1115.

177 Irwin H.L., Hein M.M. Substrate specificity of atypical cholinesterase in relation to phenotypes. *Biochem Pharmacol* 1966, **15**, 145.

178 Brown T.C.K., Meretoja O.A., Bell B., Clare D. Responses to small doses of suxamethonium in four children with abnormal cholinesterase. *Anaes Intens Care* 1990, **18**, 477.

179 Neitlich H.W. Increased plasma cholinesterase activity and succinylcholine resistance: a genetic variant. *J Clin Invest* 1966, **45**, 380.

180 Kalow W. Hydrolysis of local anaesthetics by human serum cholinesterase. *J Pharmacol Exp Ther* 1952, **104**, 122.

181 La Du B. Plasma esterase activity and the metabolism of drugs with their ester groups. *Ann NY Acad Sci* 1971, **179**, 684.

182 Denborough M.A., Lovell R.R.H. Anaesthetic deaths in a family. *Lancet* 1960, **2**, 45.

183 Denborough M.A., Forster J.F.A., Lovell R.R.H., Maplestone P.A., Villiers J.D. Anaesthetic deaths in a family. *Br J Anaes* 1962, **34**, 395.

184 Britt B.A., Locher W.G., Kalow W. Hereditary aspects of malignant hyperpyrexia. *Canad Anaes Soc J* 1969, **16**, 89.

185 King J.O., Denborough M.A., Zapf P.W. Inheritance of malignant hyperpyrexia. *Lancet* 1972, **1**, 365.

186 Lepinskie F.F. Porphyria as a problem in anaesthesia. *Canad Anaes Soc J* 1963, **10**, 286.

187 Peters J.H. Genetic factors in relation to drugs. *Ann Rev Pharmacol* 1968, **8**, 427.

188 Yoshida A. Haemolytic anaemia and G6PD deficiency. *Science* 1973, **179**, 532.

189 Cascorbi H.F., Vesell E.S., Blare D.A., Helrich M. Halothane biotransformation in man. *Ann NY Acad Sci* 1971, **179**, 244.

190 Kutt H. Biochemical and genetic factors regulating Dilantin metabolism in man. *Ann NY Acad Sci* 1971, **179**, 704.

3: Anaesthetic Apparatus

Safe anaesthesia requires reliable and appropriate equipment. In paediatric anaesthesia, a wide range of standard and specialized apparatus is needed because of the great diversity in sizes of children at various ages.

ANAESTHETIC MACHINES

Any standard anaesthetic machine, with the appropriate breathing system attached, may be used for paediatric anaesthesia. The machine should incorporate an oxygen failure warning device and be fitted with at least one reserve oxygen cylinder at least two-thirds full. A high-pressure relief valve should be fitted to protect the child's lungs from excess gas pressure should the expiratory limb of the breathing system become obstructed, or the oxygen flush device be used. The valve should be set to vent at $50\,cmH_2O$ pressure. The pressure-relief valve should be equipped with a manual override, so that higher pressures can be achieved on the rare occasions that they are needed. Use of the oxygen flush with a T-piece breathing system can result in much of the gas escaping via the pressure-relief valve. It can be useful to have the oxygen flush and manual override buttons near each other, by the fresh gas outlet.

The anaesthetic machine should be equipped with 'medical air' as well as oxygen and nitrous oxide. The nitrogen in air, being less soluble than nitrous oxide, splints the alveoli, thereby preventing their collapse. This is particularly useful when anaesthetizing premature infants (see Chapter 9) and in very prolonged anaesthesia.

Simple drawover apparatus may be used to anaesthetize children if the dead space and the resistance of valves and breathing systems are low.

BREATHING SYSTEMS

Many older children may be managed adequately with conventional adult breathing systems, but for smaller children, alternative or modified apparatus is needed. Factors that must be considered when adapting inhalation apparatus for small children are:
1 dead space;
2 resistance;
3 bulk of the equipment and its connecting tubing;

53

4 humidity of the inhaled gases;

5 disproportion between the patient's tidal volume and the capacity of the reservoir bag;

6 valves that may not respond to small tidal volumes.

The smaller the patient, the easier it is for these factors to have adverse effects. Increased dead space can be partly compensated for by intubation, controlling ventilation and increasing the tidal volume, but with spontaneous ventilation, the small tidal volume of the infant makes any apparatus dead space more significant. Apparatus resistance is of particular importance when small infants breathe spontaneously. Bulky equipment increases the chance of technical complications, in particular accidental extubation.

In high flow and non-rebreathing systems, dry gas may be inhaled directly into the trachea of an intubated patient unless artificial humidification is used.

The reservoir bag must be of a size that will not restrict tidal volumes, but if too large, its value as a monitor of ventilation is lost. In the same way, a valve system with a minor degree of incompetence may be adequate for large tidal volumes. This incompetence can result in some gas leaking past a closed valve, or in the escape of gas during the movement of the valve when ventilation is controlled. With small volumes the 'slip' (leak around the valve mechanism) may form a significant part of the tidal volume, and the system may not function as desired. Thus, when apparatus is used for inhalation anaesthesia for children, both the breathing systems and their application to the patient by face mask or endotracheal tube must be considered. Conventional gas machines with out-of-circuit vaporizers are satisfactory for use with these.

Breathing systems suitable for paediatric anaesthesia may be classified as:

Rebreathing absorption systems (using soda lime)

Rebreathing non-absorption systems (Mapleson systems)

Non-rebreathing systems

Drawover systems

Rebreathing absorption systems (circle systems)

Conventional adult circle systems are satisfactory for older children, especially with lightweight plastic breathing tubes, Y-connectors and adaptors. It is often recommended that these are suitable for children over the age of 4 years or about 20 kg weight. If ventilation is controlled, provided cardiopulmonary disease does not prevent increased tidal volume compensating for apparatus dead space, including that due to valve 'slip', these adult systems can be used for children who are more than about 10 kg weight or 1 year of age. For infants, or for children under 4 years or 20 kg who are breathing spontaneously, the system should be modified so that the effect of apparatus dead space is reduced or eliminated.

The effective dead space of an adult circle system can be reduced by inducing a continuous flow of gas around the circuit by means of a fan (e.g. Revell circulator) or a Venturi injector (Neff circulator). Alternatively, the dead space may be reduced by using small breathing tubes and connections attached to an adult absorber head. In the Columbia paediatric circle valve (Fig. 3.1), lightweight, one-way valves in a mount close to the patient are combined with a divided mask mount.

At the time when infant carbon dioxide absorption systems were being developed, cyclopropane was often used to anaesthetize infants. Economy and safety in the use of this expensive and explosive agent were obvious benefits. When cyclopropane became obsolete, the need for carbon dioxide absorption in anaesthesia for infants declined, but modern volatile agents are so expensive that there is renewed interest in these systems. Other advantages, including the conservation of moisture and reduction of atmospheric pollution, are offset by the fact that the humidification and venting of excess gases outside the operating area can now be achieved with high-flow systems. Carbon dioxide absorption systems are bulkier and less convenient to use than a T-piece system.

Rebreathing non-absorption systems

Mapleson [1] classified non-absorption breathing systems as outlined in Fig. 3.2.

MAPLESON A (MAGILL) SYSTEM

The Magill or 'Mapleson A' system was commonly used in the past. This is a continuous-flow system in which carbon dioxide accumulation is prevented if the fresh gas flow exceeds the alveolar ventilation during spontaneous breathing; during exhalation, 'alveolar' gas is vented through the exhale valve, while dead-space gas passes into the delivery tube to be inhaled in the next breath. During controlled ventilation however, a mixture of 'fresh', 'dead-space' and 'alveolar' gas is vented during the inspiratory phase, so that some rebreathing occurs, and prevention of carbon dioxide accumulation requires a fresh gas flow of 2−3 times the minute volume or up to

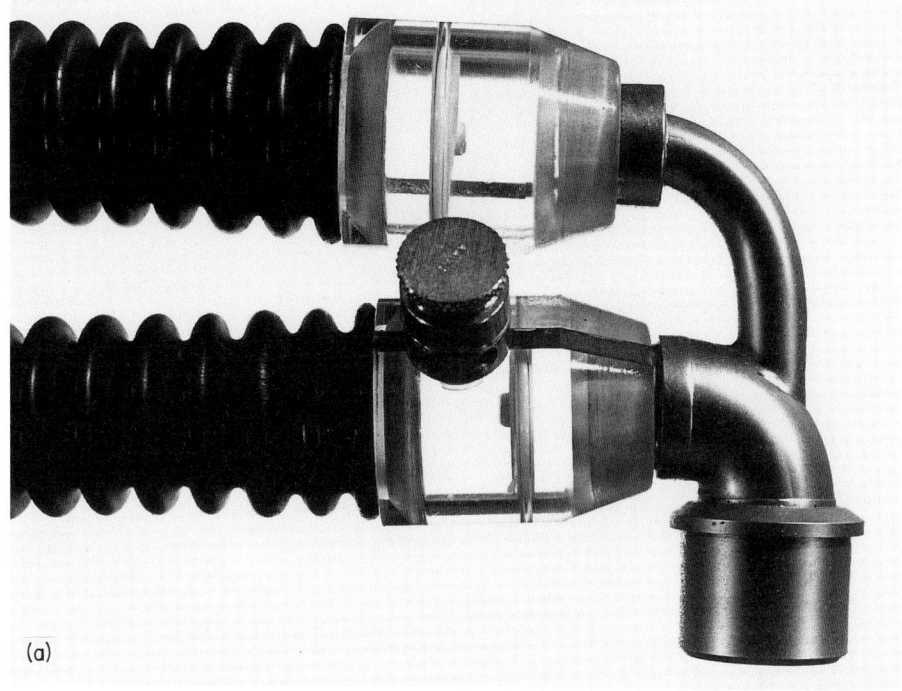

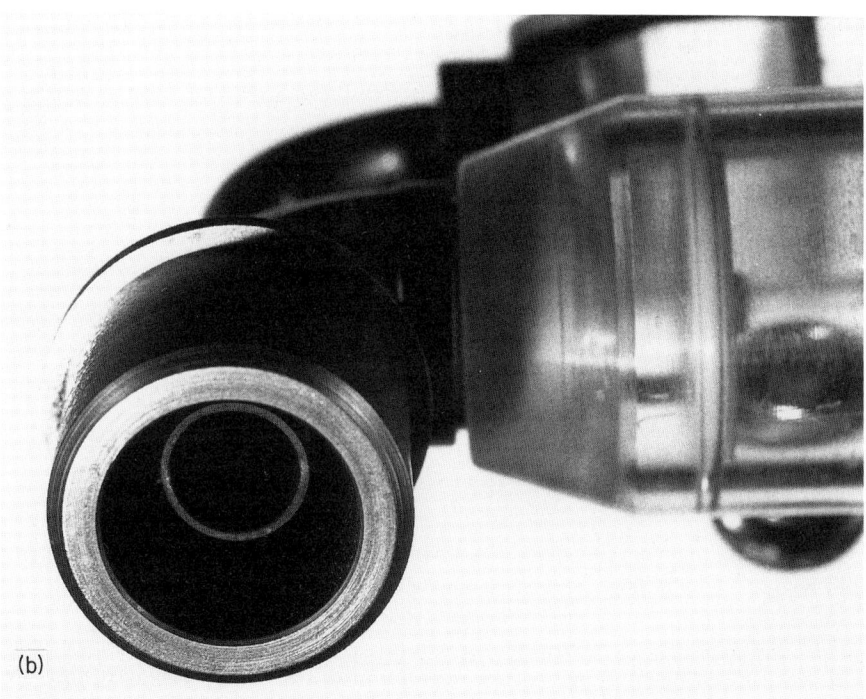

Fig. 3.1 (a) The Columbia paediatric circle valve; (b) inflow side of the circle delivering gas through central tube in the mask mount to reduce dead space.

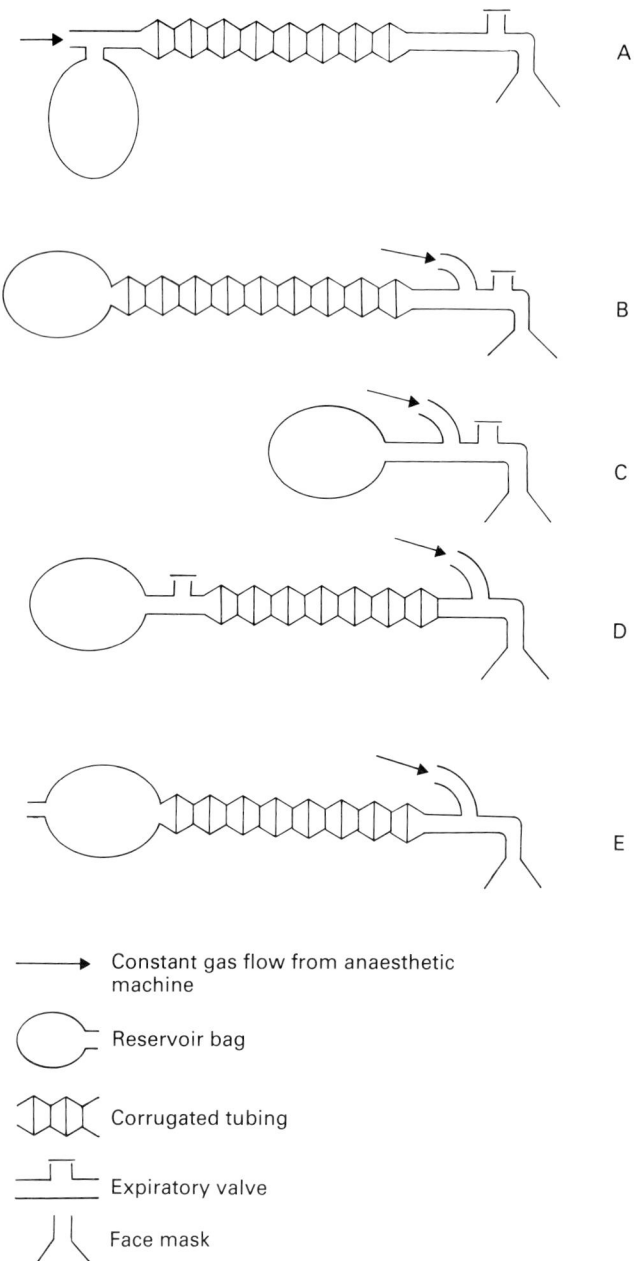

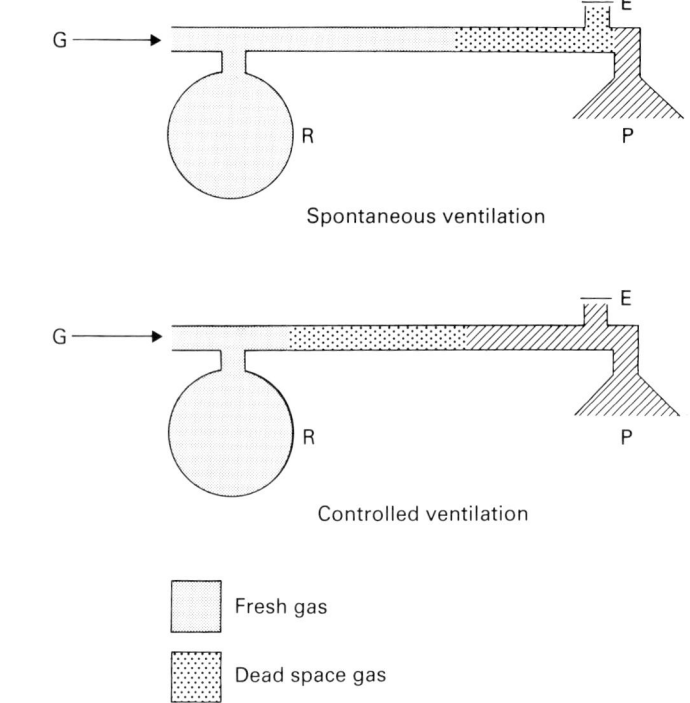

Spontaneous ventilation

Controlled ventilation

▪ Fresh gas

▪ Dead space gas

▪ Alveolar gas

Fig. 3.3 Mapleson A circuit, showing disposition of gases at end-expiration; G = fresh gas, R = reservoir bag, P = patient, E = expiratory valve.

⟶ Constant gas flow from anaesthetic machine

⟜ Reservoir bag

⟨⟩⟨⟩ Corrugated tubing

⊓ Expiratory valve

⋁ Face mask

Fig. 3.2 Classification of rebreathing non-absorption breathing systems [1].

600 ml/kg in an infant (Fig. 3.3). The popularity of this system has waned, probably because controlled ventilation is now used more frequently.

MAPLESON B AND C SYSTEMS

These systems are unsuitable for use during either spontaneous or controlled ventilation, since high fresh

gas flows are required to minimize carbon dioxide accumulation.

MAPLESON D AND E SYSTEMS

The Mapleson E system is commonly known as the 'T-piece' although the T-piece itself now forms only part of the system.

Ayre's T-piece and its modifications

The T-piece was introduced into anaesthesia in 1937 by Ayre (Fig. 3.4) [2], who used it for neurosurgical as well as hare-lip and cleft palate operations. The simple, open T-piece is similar to other open systems in which air dilution of anaesthetic gases can occur during spontaneous breathing, for example, a delivery tube with an open side hole. This system can be used to control ventilation by intermittent occlusion of the open limb of the T-piece. If an expiratory limb is added to the simple T-piece (Fig. 3.5), air dilution is prevented, provided the

A mechanical ventilator can replace the bag on the expiratory limb for controlling ventilation.

The Mapleson D system, popularized in recent years by Bain and Spoerel [5] (Fig. 3.6) is functionally identical to the T-piece system and may be used interchangeably with appropriate adjustment of the volume of the reservoir bag. The essential differences are the usual coaxial arrangement of the Bain system and the location of the expiratory valve. If the expiratory limb of the system, excluding the bag, has a volume in excess of the tidal volume, the position of the expiratory valve becomes largely irrelevant. In some versions of the Bain system, the fresh gas tube connection to the machine was concealed in the expiratory tube, so that if it became disconnected, rebreathing and hypoxia could occur before the disconnection was noticed.

Spontaneous breathing with T-piece or Mapleson D systems

A fresh gas flow of two and a half to three times the minute volume is needed to prevent the accumulation of carbon dioxide during spontaneous ventilation. The flows needed to maintain normocarbia in infants may be higher than expected because the metabolic rate (oxygen consumption and carbon dioxide production) is greater when related to body weight.

Although in practice, a flow of 3–4 l/min is commonly used in infants up to about 15 kg, increasing to 6 l/min for children of 20–25 kg, these flows are often higher than necessary (see below).

Controlled ventilation with T-piece or Mapleson D systems

There has been much confusion about the ideal or minimum fresh gas flows required to void hyper- and hypocarbia during controlled ventilation with these systems. With both systems, carbon dioxide elimination is almost entirely dependent on fresh gas flow, when administered minute volume is adequate.

It is best to consider the breathing system and the lungs as part of a single total system into which there is a flow of carbon dioxide generated by the metabolism of the body. Providing the minute volume of controlled ventilation is greater than the patient's normal minute volume (this is usually the case) then the efficiency of washing out of carbon dioxide from the system is dependent on the total flow of gas through the system,

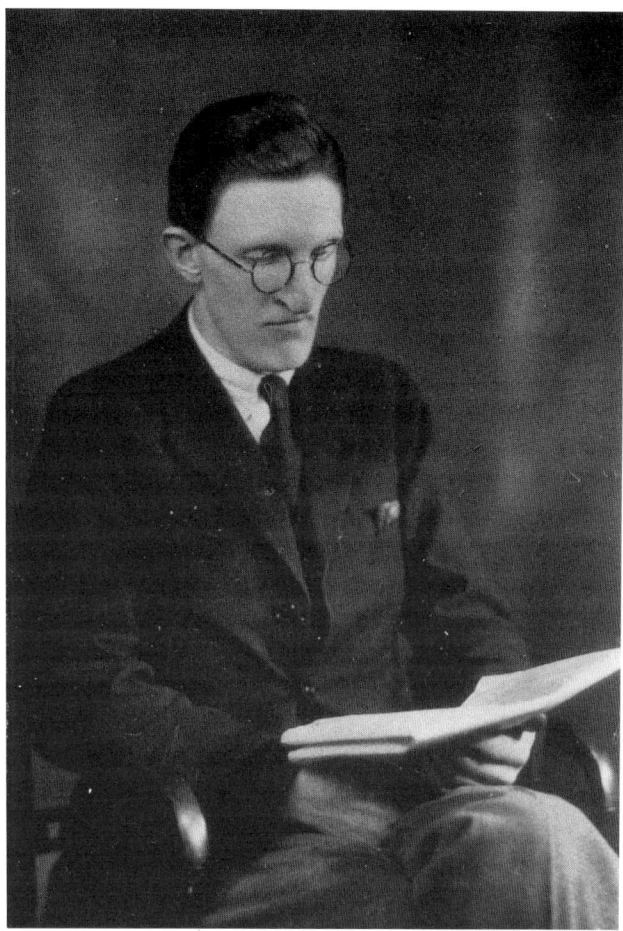

Fig. 3.4 Dr Philip Ayre.

volume of this limb approaches the patient's tidal volume. This allows accurate control of inspired concentration of gases and volatile agents.

The T-piece has the advantages of simplicity and low resistance because there are no valves. During spontaneous ventilation, there is the hazard that disconnection can go unnoticed. The addition, by Rees [3], of an open-tailed 500 ml reservoir bag (Fig. 3.5) allows visual monitoring of spontaneous breathing and ready control of ventilation if the open tail is partly or totally occluded by the thumb and index finger, or by the little finger compressing the tail in the palm. If the fresh gas flow is interrupted or disconnected, the bag will collapse. A valve, open during exhalation, may be used to occlude the tail of the bag during inflation. Alternatively, a hole in the bag may replace the open tail, as in the Montreal infant set. The hole is occluded by the thumb during inflation. A smaller bag may be used for newborn infants.

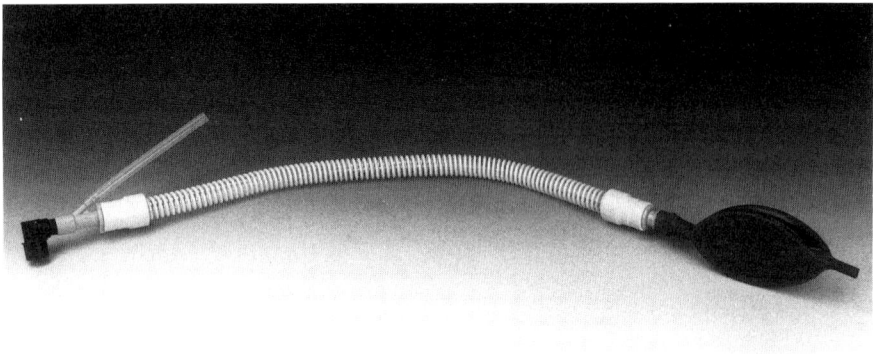

(a)

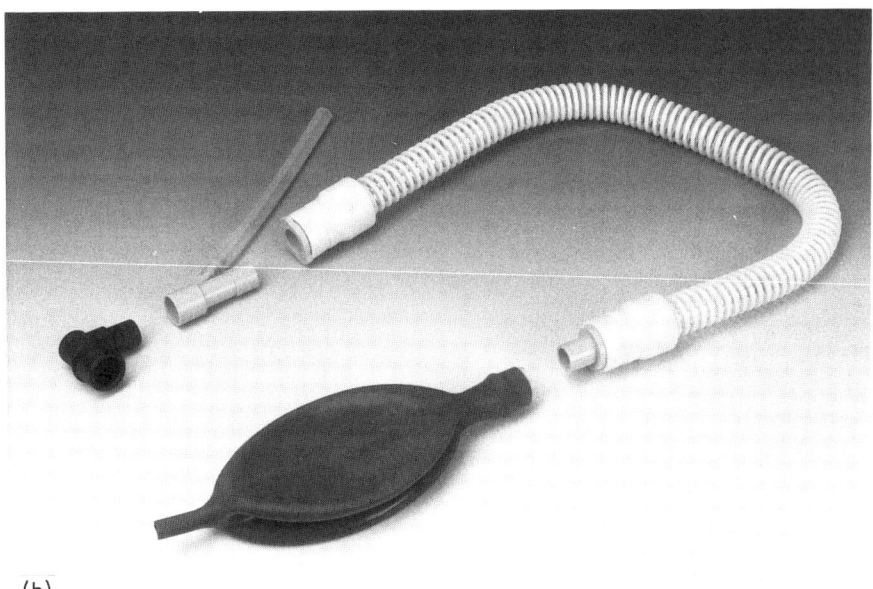

(b)

Fig. 3.5 T-piece breathing system: (a) complete; (b) showing component parts. Clockwise from left: right-angled mask or endotracheal tube connector; T-piece with portion of fresh gas hose; expiratory limb; open-tailed bag. All connections are standard 15/22 mm tapers.

i.e., the fresh gas flow. The mean level of carbon dioxide in the arterial blood is a result of two factors: CO_2 production minus CO_2 removal, and since CO_2 removal in a rebreathing non-absorption system is almost entirely dependent on fresh gas flow, arterial and end-tidal $Paco_2$ are determined by CO_2 production by the patient and fresh gas flow in the breathing system.

The rate or tidal volume of controlled ventilation is unimportant in relation to end-expired CO_2, providing the administered alveolar ventilation exceeds the patient's normal alveolar ventilation (see above). The inspired carbon dioxide level increases with increasing ventilatory rate because of the rebreathing nature of the system, and must be considered a consequence of the rate and fresh gas flow. It does not influence the end-expired or arterial carbon dioxide. The inspired CO_2

level may be reduced by simply reducing the ventilation rate.

The leak which occurs around an uncuffed endotracheal tube in a small child is of minimal importance in the determination of $Paco_2$, as is the small reduction in dead space achieved by cutting endotracheal tubes shorter.

Several formulae have been advanced to determine the fresh gas flow for individual patients, and these are outlined in Table 3.1. These formulae are represented graphically in Fig. 3.7 and demonstrate attempts to describe a predictable relationship between 'fresh gas flow' and body weight in achieving normocarbia with a T-piece circuit. They are based on the assumption that there is a constant and normal metabolic production of carbon dioxide. Normal metabolic rate in relation to

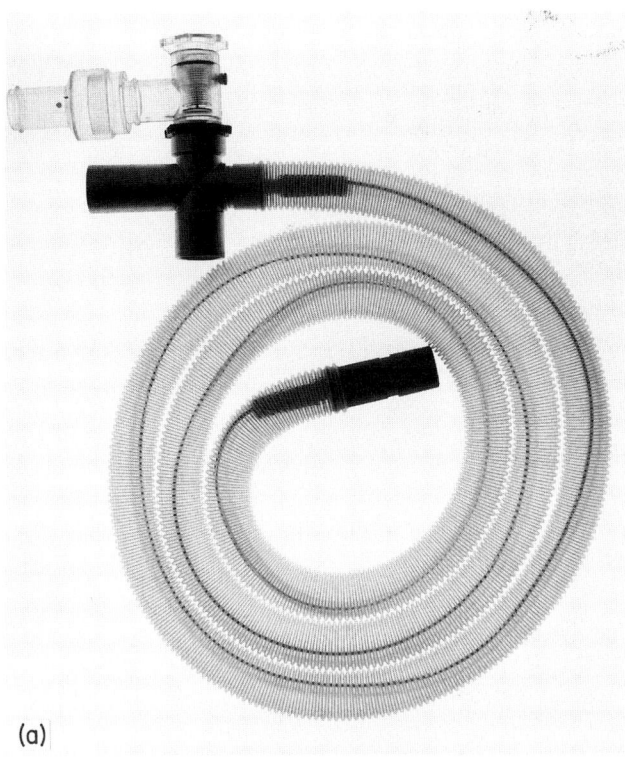

(a)

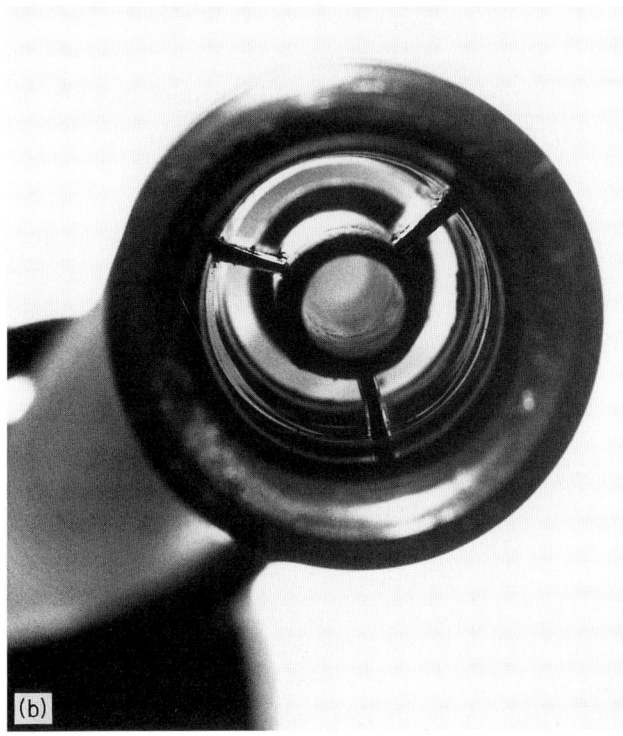

(b)

Fig. 3.6 The Bain system: (a) shows the system coiled up. The inner delivery tube can be seen as a darker line inside the outer expiratory tube. A bag mount is shown at the top left; (b) illustrates how the fresh gas delivery tube is fixed into the adaptor which connects to a mask mount or endotracheal tube.

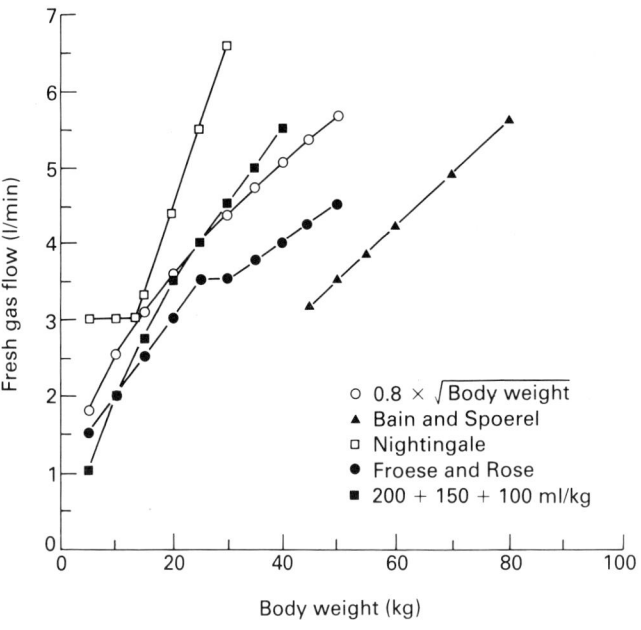

Fig. 3.7 Fresh gas flow requirements (l/min) with Mapleson D or E circuits to maintain normocarbia (or minimal hypocarbia), according to various formulae as outlined in Table 3.1.

body weight at different ages is shown in Fig. 3.8 and the similarity of some of the fresh gas flow plots in Fig. 3.7 to parts of that for metabolic rate in Fig. 3.8 should be noted. During anaesthesia, metabolic rate is usually

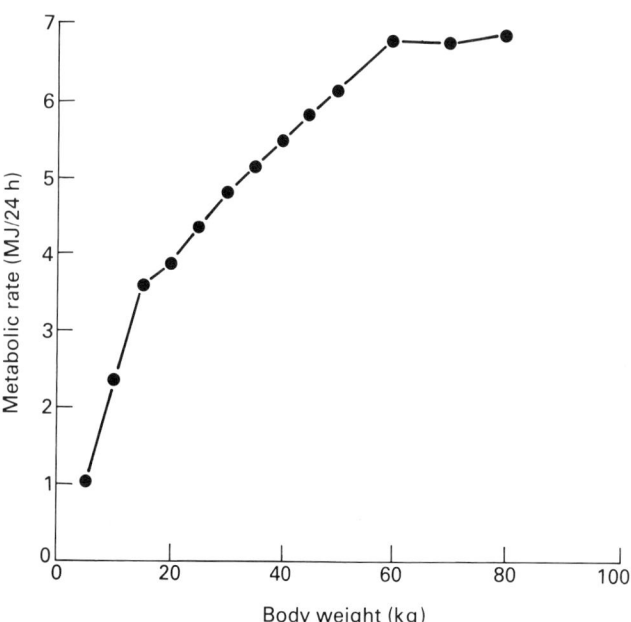

Fig. 3.8 Average metabolic rate at different body weights (Data derived from W.N. Schofield [18].)

Table 3.1 Fresh gas flow requirements for normo- or minimal hypocarbia with paediatric T-piece circuits

Gas flow	Patient group	Author	Reference
220 ml/kg/min (min. 3 l/min)	infant	Nightingale *et al.*	[4]
70 ml/kg/min (min. 3 l/min)	adult	Bain & Spoerel	[5]
200 ml/kg/min (min. 3 l/min)	<10 kg		
(2000) + 150 ml/kg/min (min. 3 l/min)	10–20 kg		
(3500) + 100 ml/kg/min (min. 3 l/min)	>20 kg		
(1000) + 100 ml/kg/min (min. 3 l/min)	<30 kg	Froese & Rose	[6]
(2000) + 50 ml/kg/min (min. 3 l/min)	>30 kg	Froese & Rose	[6]
$0.8 \times \sqrt{\text{Wt. in kg}}$ (l/min)	infant	Nightingale & Lambert	[7]
2.5–3 × minute vol.	infant	Harrison	[8]

basal, although influenced by the anaesthetic drugs commonly used, by changes in temperature and by the condition of the patient, who may be catabolic prior to surgery. Thus it remains that the only certain method of ensuring normocarbia during controlled ventilation with a rebreathing non-absorption system is to monitor the expired, arterial or transcutaneous CO_2 (see Chapter 4).

Advantages and disadvantages

The advantages of the T-piece and Mapleson D systems are:

1 The apparatus is simple and lightweight by comparison with many non-rebreathing and carbon dioxide absorption systems, and the only valves used are an exhale valve in the Bain system and those in an attached ventilator.

2 The dead space is small and can be further reduced by directing the fresh gas flow into the facemask.

3 Resistance is low. If the flow of fresh gases is directed slightly towards the patient, the resistance to breathing from this force is minimal and confined to exhalation. This slight increase in expiratory resistance acts like PEEP in slowing airway closure and may help to prevent a fall in functional residual capacity during prolonged anaesthesia.

4 The system may be readily used for spontaneous ventilation, or, if an open-tailed reservoir bag or a ventilator are attached to the expiratory limb, for controlled ventilation.

The disadvantages are:

1 A high flow rate of fresh gas is necessary.

2 Dry anaesthetic gases are inhaled, unless humidification is used.

3 Pollution of the operating theatres occurs unless special venting is arranged.

4 Nitrous oxide is not readily available in many parts of the world, and in these circumstances expense can be a deterrent to the use of high-flow systems.

5 The coaxial Mapleson D system makes inspection of the fresh gas line difficult. If the fresh gas line is obstructed or disconnected, this may not be apparent before rebreathing or hypoxia occur. There is, however, some warming of the inspired gases by the expired gas in the coaxial system.

Non-rebreathing systems

Non-rebreathing systems are those where the inspired and expired gases are completely separated, and include circuits which incorporate a one-way (non-rebreathing) valve, or ventilator circuits as part of a volume-controlled ventilator system.

The non-rebreathing valve may be used to replace the exhale valve and mask mount of a Mapleson A, B or C system, or used in conjunction with a self-inflating reservoir bag in a resuscitation or drawover circuit. Several such valves are available, including the Lewis Leigh (Fig. 3.9), Stephen Slater (Fig. 3.10), Ambu-E (Fig. 3.11), Ruben (Fig. 3.12) and Laerdal (Fig. 3.13).

Fresh gas flow should exceed the minute volume to keep the reservoir bag filled. Care should be taken to observe the bag in case of overdistension, which may occur if moisture in the exhaled gas causes the valve to stick. The inclusion of a low-pressure relief valve may be advisable when spontaneous ventilation techniques are used. The Stephen Slater valve is suitable only for spontaneous breathing, while the others are suitable for either mode. During controlled ventilation the fresh gas flow needs to be adjusted according to the minute volume and the amount of gas which may escape when the valve is operating (the valve 'slip').

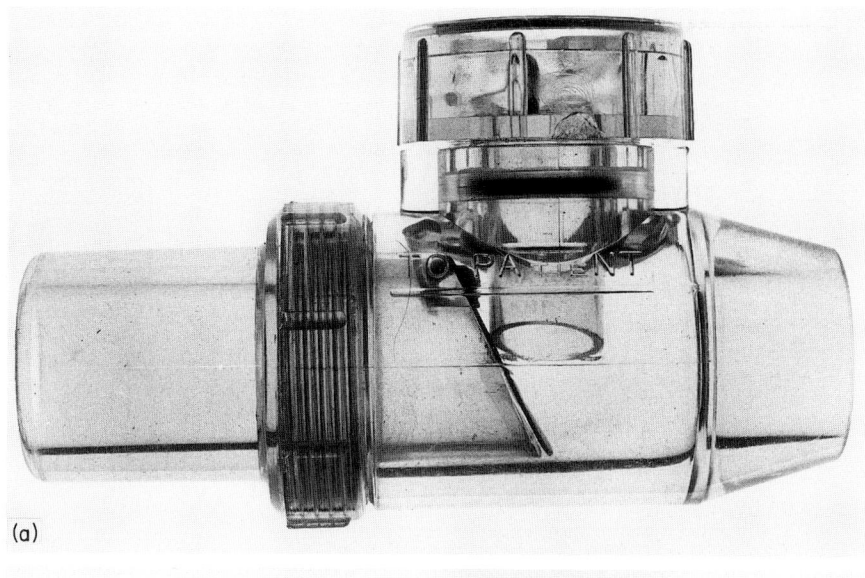

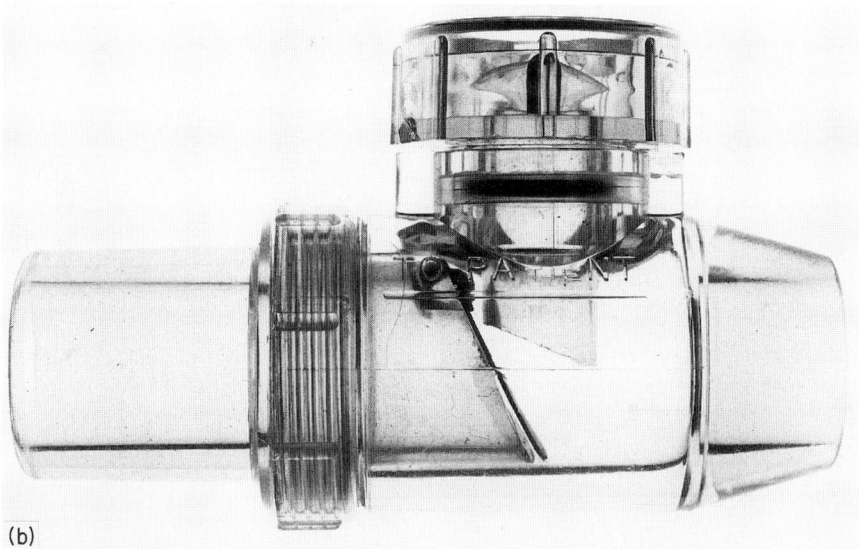

Fig. 3.9 Lewis Leigh non-rebreathing valve set for: (a) spontaneous ventilation; (b) controlled ventilation.

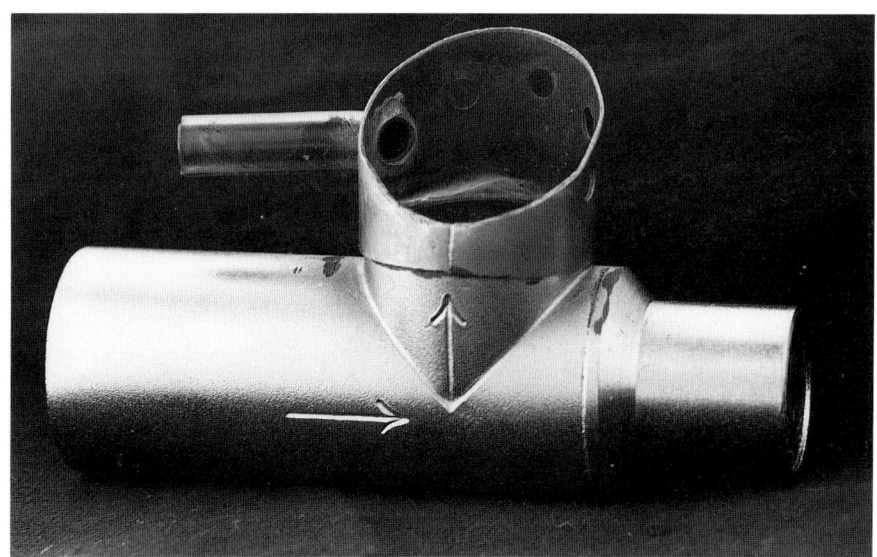

Fig. 3.10 Stephen Slater non-rebreathing valve.

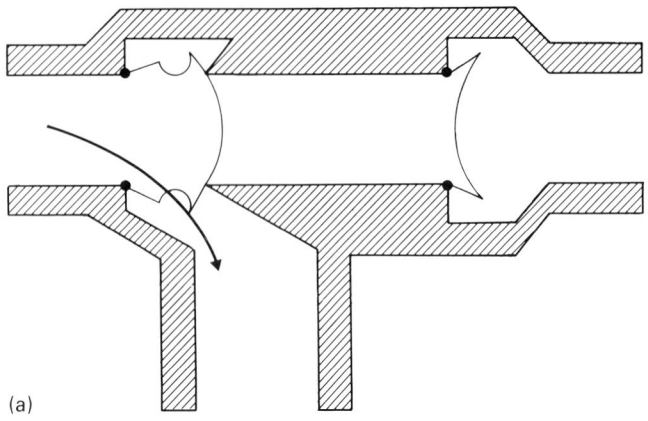

(a)

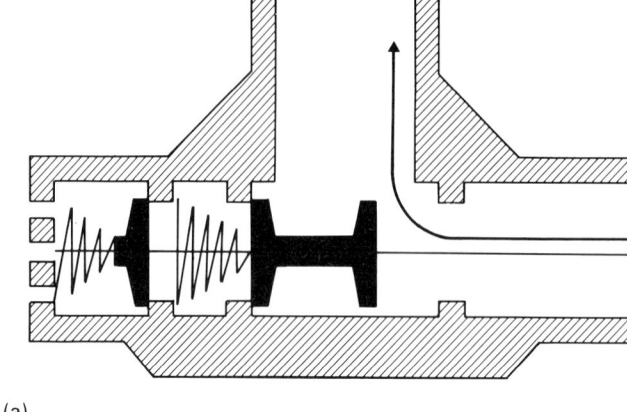

(a)

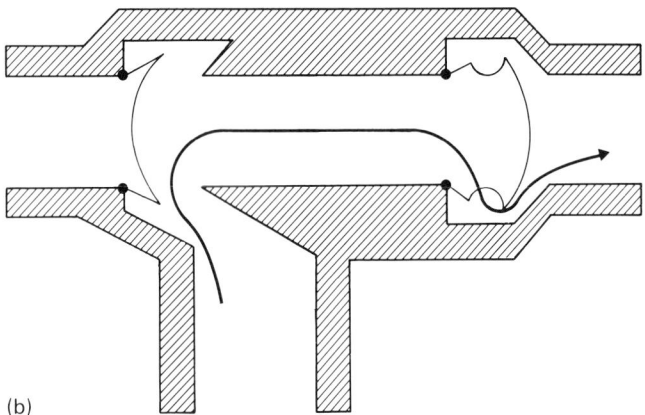

(b)

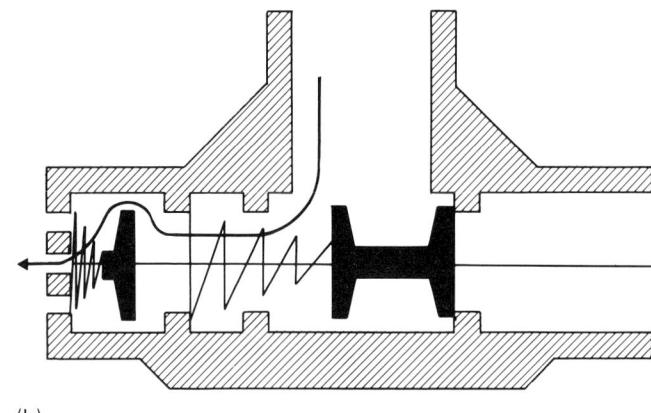

(b)

Fig. 3.11 Ambu-E non-rebreathing valve showing gas path during: (a) inspiration; (b) expiration. During the end-expiratory pause, fresh gas may pass through both valves, preventing excess pressure.

Fig. 3.12 Ruben valve showing gas path during: (a) inspiration; (b) expiration.

The advantage of these non-rebreathing systems is that carbon dioxide accumulation due to rebreathing is eliminated, but there are several disadvantages:

1 Valve slip may be significant if the valves are designed for the tidal volume of a larger patient.

2 The minute volume may vary, so that the fresh gas flow either needs frequent adjustment or must exceed the greatest minute volume, in which case a pressure-relief valve is needed, to prevent jamming of the valve.

3 Effective humidification is needed to prevent inhalation of dry gases, but condensation may interfere with proper valve function.

4 In some situations, especially with controlled ventilation, the system is not as convenient to handle as the T-piece or circle absorption systems. It is much easier to produce hypocarbia by hyperventilation in small children.

Emergency breathing systems

Lightweight sterilizable resuscitation or emergency breathing systems are available with non-return valves, standard 15 mm connectors and self-inflating reservoir bags (Ambu, Laerdal) (Fig. 3.14) with provision for adding oxygen. These should be available in every anaesthetizing location, recovery room, intensive care and emergency departments, and for patient transportation.

Drawover breathing systems

In situations where a ready supply of anaesthetic gases is not available, drawover apparatus using low-resistance vaporizers, e.g. Oxford Miniature Vaporizer (OMV), may be used. The use of a self-inflating reservoir bag and non-rebreathing valve is a convenient means of controlling ventilation. The inspired gas may be supplemented

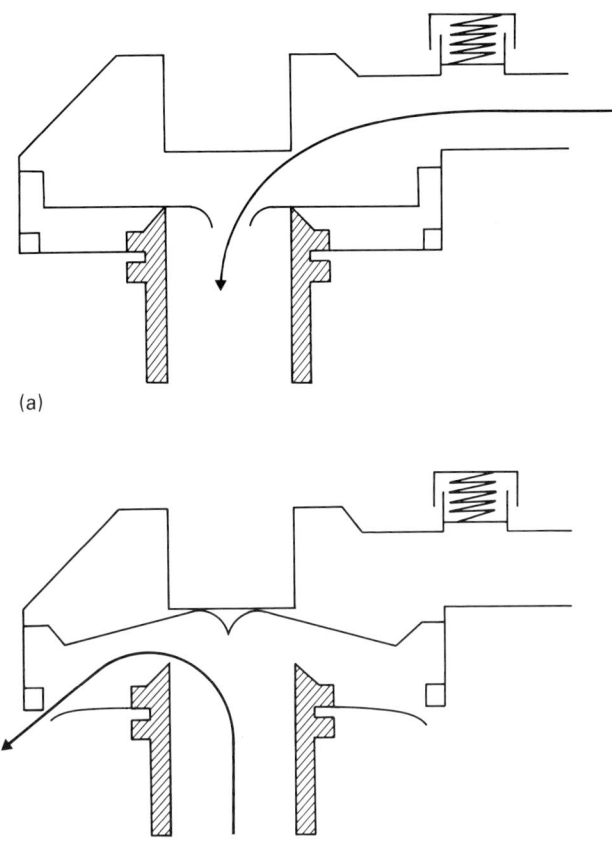

(a)

(b)

Fig. 3.13 Laerdal valve showing gas path during: (a) inspiration; (b) expiration. There is a pressure-relief valve, set at 45 cmH₂O with override.

with a low flow of oxygen via a T-piece on the air inlet, as in the Tri-Service apparatus [9].

Breathing system connections

Although there have been many connectors used over the years for paediatric anaesthetic breathing systems,

the International Standards Organization recommends the use of tapered 15 mm and 22 mm connectors. An alternative 8.5 mm ('Minilink') connector (Fig. 3.15) has been advocated for use in neonates and infants, to reduce bulk and turbulence at the end of the endotracheal tube. The system has proved to be useful in units dealing primarily with neonates. On the other hand, many anaesthetists find that the 15 mm connector is more universally suitable and avoids non-interchangeable connections.

There are obvious advantages in the tapers for paediatric use being interchangeable with those for adults. This is particularly important in adaptors for endotracheal tubes and mask mounts. Mask mounts for anaesthesia and resuscitation apparatus now have a male 22 mm taper on the outside and a female 15 mm taper on the inside; these can be used without additional adaptors.

Most connectors are now available in plastic, making them light, cheap and semi-disposable. They fit together with a more secure and suitable gas-tight seal, provided excessive force is not used such that the connector becomes cracked. The tapered fittings allow secure connections to be made if they are twisted when the male and female parts are joined.

HUMIDIFICATION IN ANAESTHETIC BREATHING SYSTEMS

There are two important considerations related to the humidity of inspired gas in paediatric anaesthesia. The dessicant effect of the inhalation of dry gases through an endotracheal tube, bypassing the heat and moisture exchange of the upper airways, and the influence of respiratory water loss on the heat exchange of the body.

Reduction of ciliary activity and mucus formation occurs in respiratory mucosa exposed to dry gases, and the use of added humidification to reduce complications during prolonged tracheal intubation is recommended

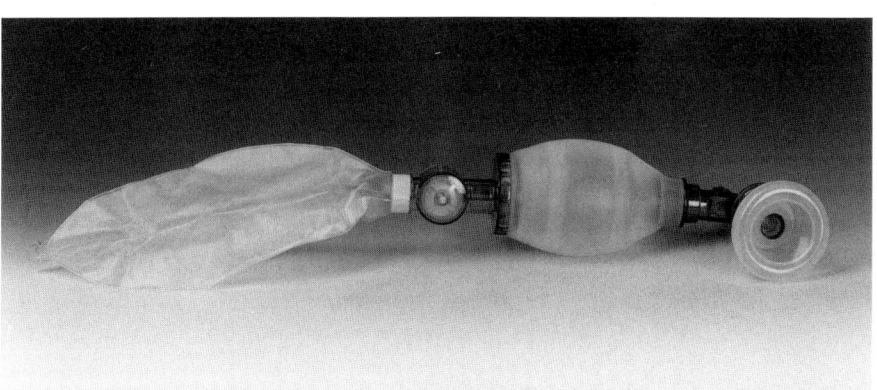

Fig. 3.14 Laerdal self-inflating resuscitation system, including optional reservoir bag which may be used to store supplemental oxygen.

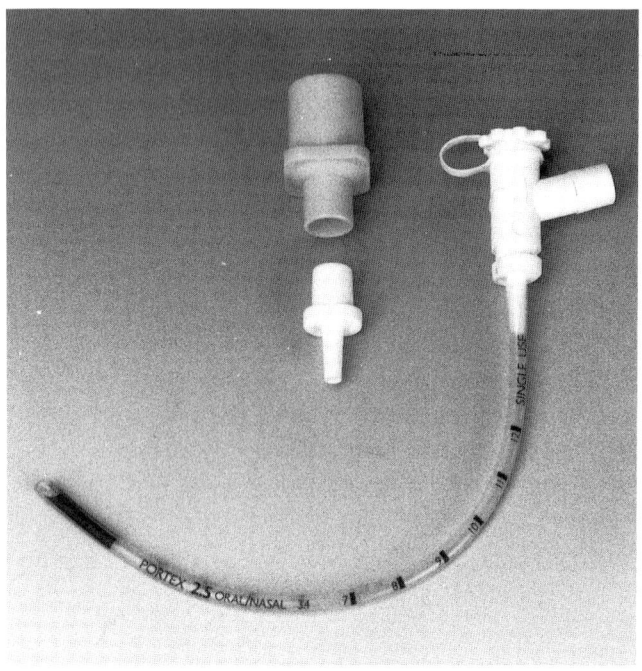

Fig. 3.15 A selection of 8.5 mm ('Minilink') endotracheal adaptors, including an adaptor for use with 15 mm connections.

[10]. In circle systems, the combination of the increased water content of the inspired gas with the heat and moisture exchange occurring in the endotracheal tube may prevent undue drying without added humidification, provided the fresh gas flow is not too high. A maximum of 3 l/min fresh gas flow is recommended in order to maintain humidity for adults, and smaller flows would be needed for children. Using high flow systems such as the T-piece, there is an appreciable reduction in the water content of the gases in the trachea unless the gas supply is humidified.

The maintenance of body temperature during anaesthesia and surgery can be significantly influenced by the use of warmed, humidified anaesthetic gases. The difference between respiratory heat loss when dry gases are inhaled through an endotracheal tube at room temperature and the loss when gas saturated with water vapour at 37°C is inhaled can amount to 20% of the basal heat production of an infant. Humidification is recommended during anaesthesia for all children, particularly infants of less than 10 kg or 12 months of age, and for all procedures likely to last in excess of 1 hour.

Various methods may be used to humidify gases. Nebulizers, both jet and ultrasonic, can be used to add water to the dry gases of the high-flow system,

but, because rain-out occurs in the delivery tube, jet nebulizers are relatively inefficient unless the tubing is heated.

In a heated tank humidifier, saturated gas is delivered to the T-piece by heating the humidification chamber to a temperature such that the gas delivered to the patient is between 32°C and 37°C and has fallen to dew point. The temperature to which the tank must be heated will depend on the gas flow and the length of the delivery hose. Condensation in the delivery tube results in 'rain-out', so that a water trap or periodic emptying is needed. The temperature of the gas in the patient's end of the T-piece must be measured to ensure that water vapour at high temperatures is not being administered. A sudden increase in flow through the system can cause a dangerous increase in the temperature at the point of delivery.

More recent and satisfactory versions of heated tank humidifiers provide a heated delivery hose, so that minimal temperature drop occurs over the length of the hose and rain-out is virtually eliminated. This allows the heated humidifying chamber to operate at a lower temperature and minimizes the effects of flow rate and tubing length on delivery temperature. The Nicholas and Fisher & Paykel (Fig. 3.16) models use a servo control with temperature probes at the delivery point and in the vaporizing chamber to ensure that the gas reaches dew point at the time of delivery.

With all heated tank humidifiers, extreme care must be taken to avoid the risk of introducing hot water into the inspiratory limb of the T-piece, and the unit should never be positioned higher than the level of the patient's head.

Heat and moisture exchangers (HME) have been available for many years but have been unsuitable for use in paediatric anaesthesia because of dead space. Recently, cheap, disposable HMEs with a low dead space (e.g. 6 ml and 2.7 ml) have been developed which are effective in providing humidification of inspired gases (Fig. 3.17) [11]: 80% relative humidity after 90 min with 6 ml HME and 85% relative humidity after 40 min with the 2.7 ml HME.

FACE MASKS (Fig. 3.18)

The Rendell Baker–Soucek (RBS) mask was designed for infants and young children. It moulds closely to the face, with a resulting dead space of approximately 4 ml when the smallest mask is used. These masks are available in five sizes (0, 1, 2, 3 and 4) and are widely used by

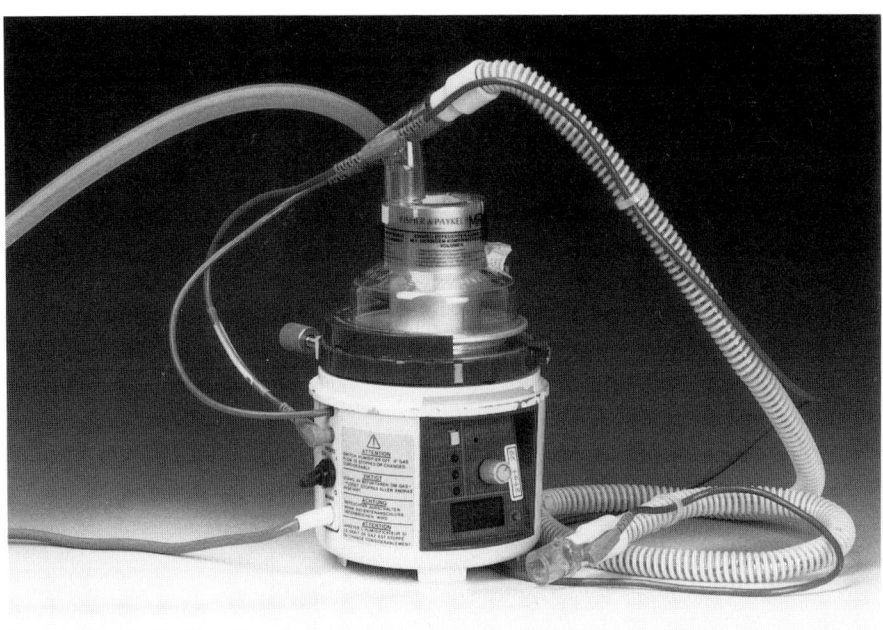

Fig. 3.16 Fisher & Paykel humidifier showing disposable humidification chamber and heated delivery hose with temperature probes at each end for servo control of temperature output.

paediatric anaesthetists. Although originally of antistatic black rubber, they are now available in clear malleable plastic. It is important to hold these masks near the mask mount as pressure on the rubber flanges causes leaks,

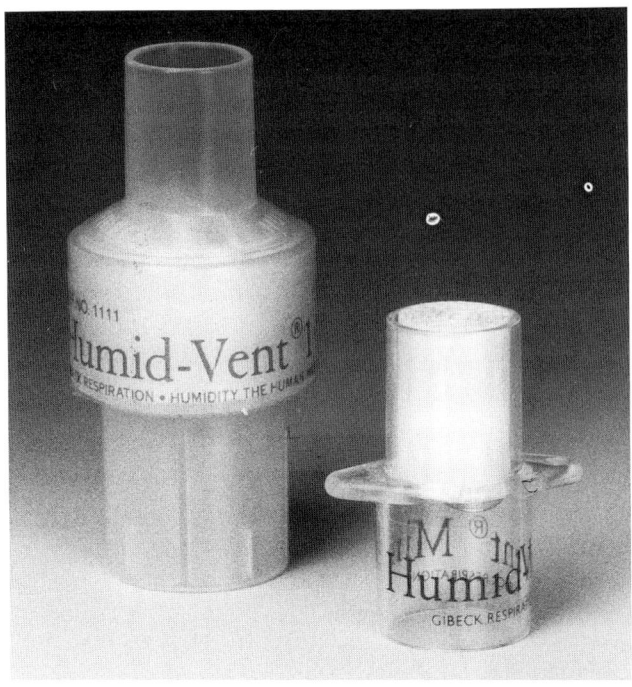

Fig. 3.17 Small disposable heat and moisture exchangers (HME) with standard 15 mm male and female tapers. Dead space is approximately 6 ml and 3 ml respectively.

and pressure on the nose can obstruct the infant's airway (see Figs 7.8, 7.9). Proper fitting, without leak, is difficult for occasional users. Placing the mask in the groove across the chin rather than below it makes it easier to obtain a good fit.

A divided mask mount reduces dead space above the mask. Further reduction in dead space will result if the fresh gas flow is directed through the mask mount into the mask as a jet. This principle is used in the Keats Elbow and the Hustead NRPR (non-rebreathing pressure relieving) elbow designed for infant resuscitation (Fig. 3.19). A standard hole in the latter allows the escape of fresh gas at such a rate that the maximum pressure in the system is limited by the fresh gas flow.

Cushioned facemasks of the BOC type have a large dead space and are generally undesirable for small children. For older children there is less need to reduce dead space under the mask and cushioned BOC masks in the smaller sizes are suitable. Disposable cushioned masks with reduced dead space are now available and can be used in infants (Fig. 3.18).

PHARYNGEAL AIRWAYS

Although various types of oropharyngeal and nasopharyngeal airways have been used, the Guedel oropharyngeal airway has replaced nearly all of these (Fig. 3.20). They are usually made from polyvinyl

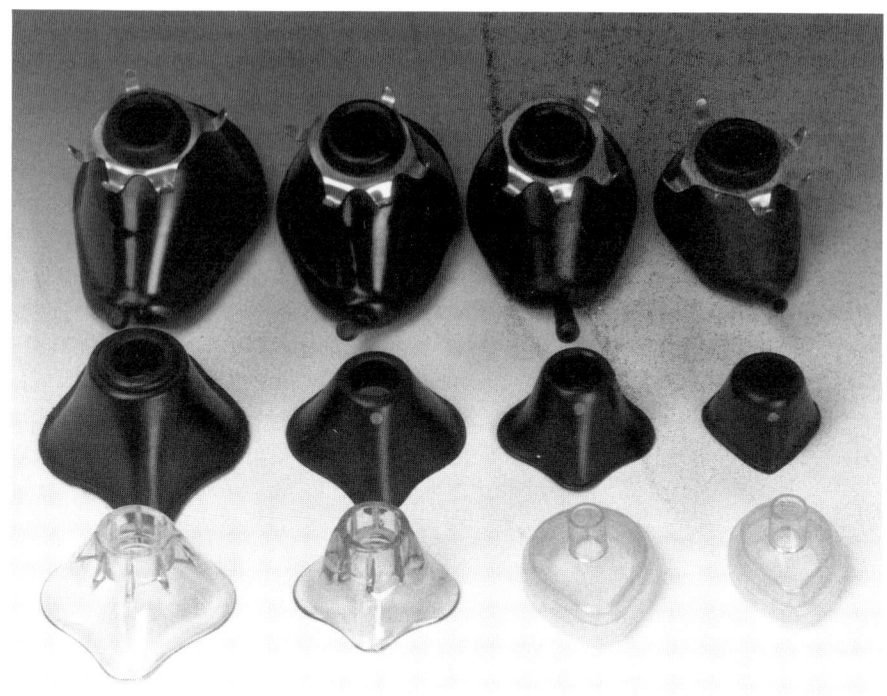

Fig. 3.18 A selection of paediatric face masks. From above down: British Oxygen pattern with air-filled cushion; Rendell Baker—Soucek masks; modern disposable clear plastic masks of both RBS pattern and low dead-space cushioned pattern.

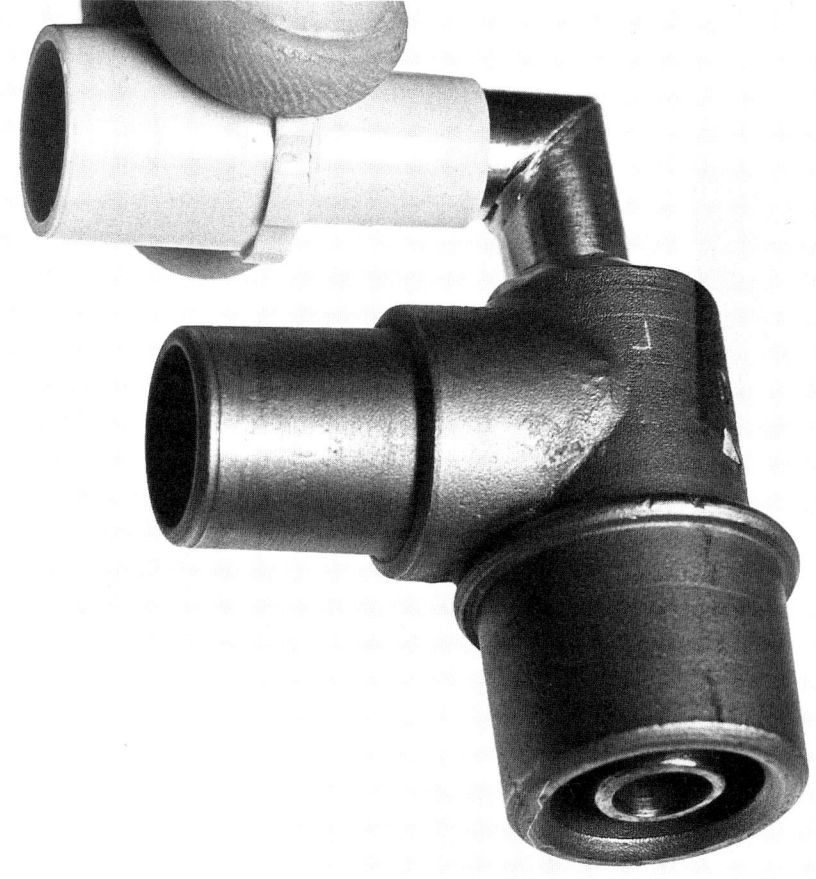

Fig. 3.19 The NPRR elbow in which the fresh gas enters as a jet.

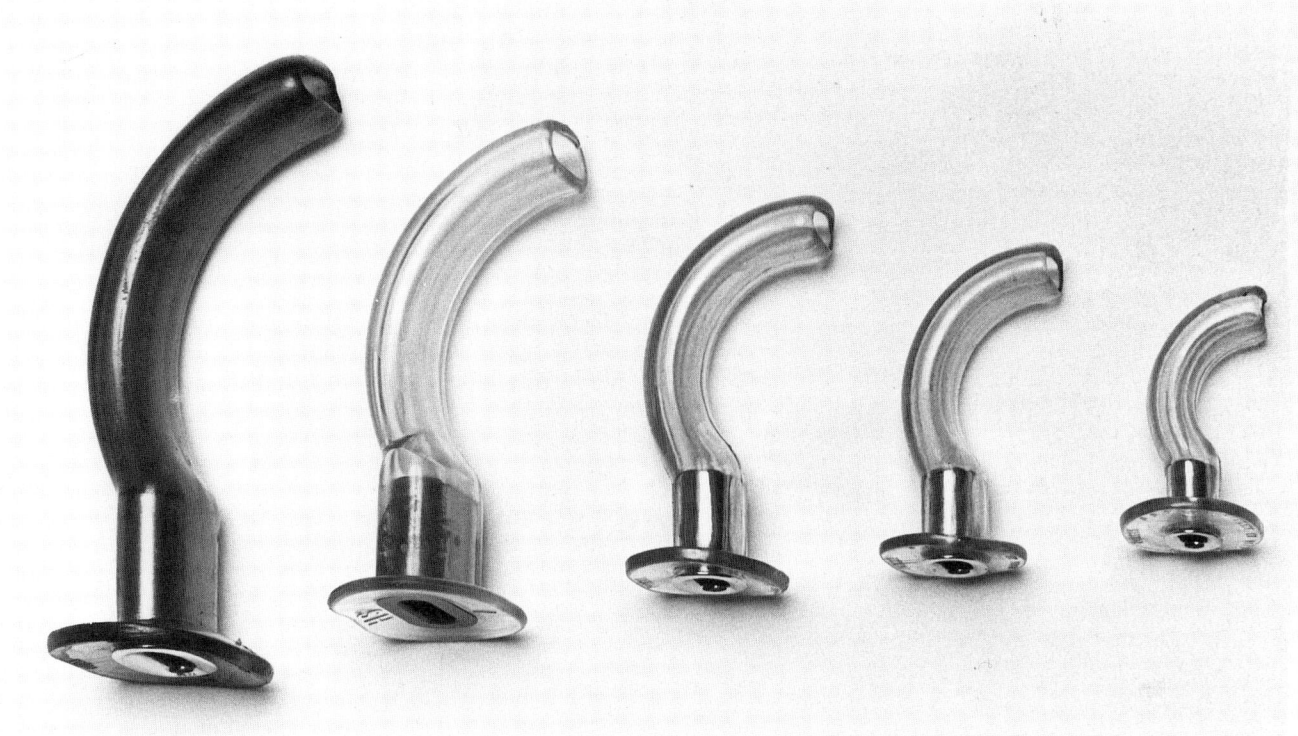

Fig. 3.20 Plastic Guedel airways, sizes from left to right: 2, 1, 0, 00, 000.

chloride (PVC) and need to have a metal or hard plastic insert which prevents occlusion by the teeth. The smallest sizes, 000 and 00, are made with an exaggerated curve to fit over the bulky tongue of small infants; unfortunately, the variability of the shape of the oropharynx makes it difficult to find an appropriate size and shape of Guedel airway in some infants. In most cases these airways are not necessary, especially if the mouth is held partly open under the mask by pulling the chin forwards and downwards (see Fig. 7.8). If a nasopharyngeal airway is needed, it can readily be fashioned from a Magill

endotracheal tube, although commercial versions in some paediatric sizes are now available (Fig. 3.21).

LARYNGOSCOPES

A wide range of paediatric laryngoscope blades is available (Fig. 3.22). For infants, a laryngoscope must be able to cope with the problems of size of mouth and airways, the anterior position of the larynx and the soft, mobile epiglottis. The blade should not be too bulky for the small mouth, but should prevent the relatively large

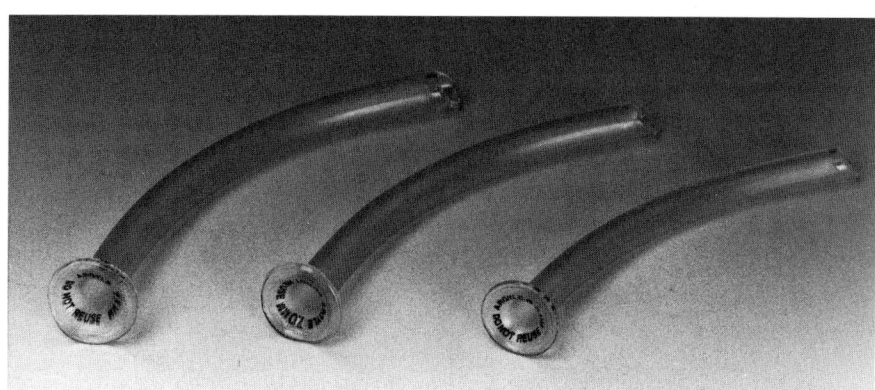

Fig. 3.21 Nasopharyngeal airways made of PVC.

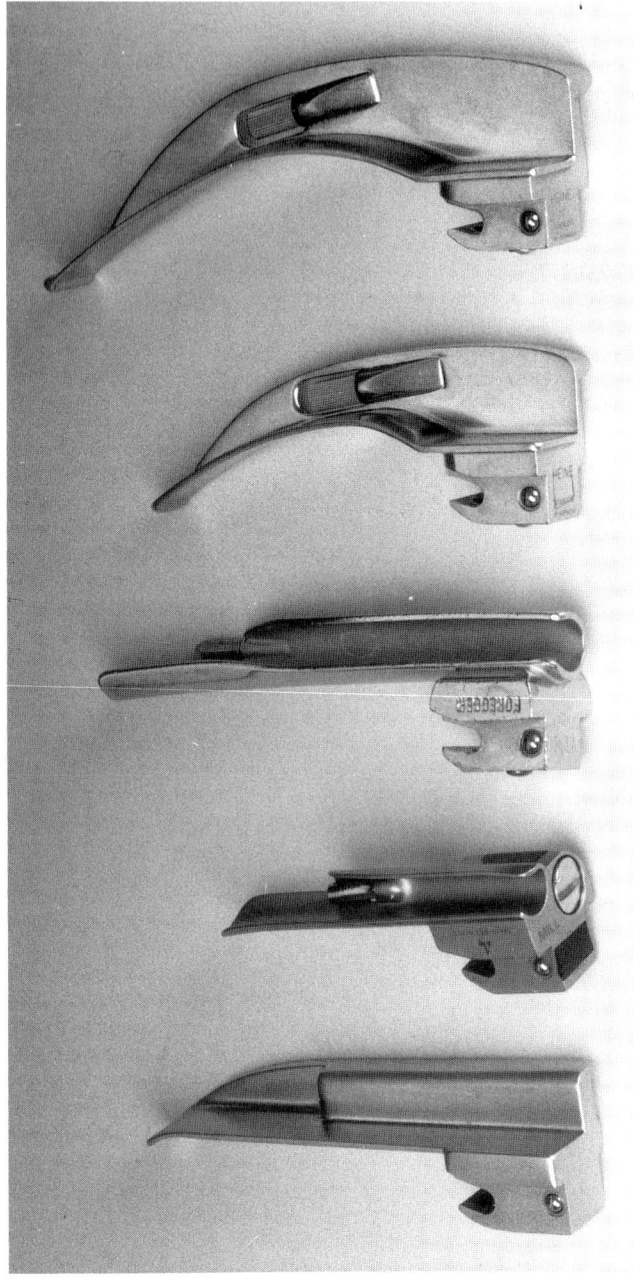

Fig. 3.22 Laryngoscopes suitable for paediatric anaesthesia. From above down: Mcintosh size 2; Mcintosh size 1; Wisconsin; Miller; Seward fibreoptic.

tongue from obscuring the view. The light should be near the tip of the blade so that it illuminates inside the mouth. Many prefer the adult Macintosh blade for all but infants while others prefer straight blades for all ages. Most anaesthetists use straight-bladed laryngoscopes for infants; some prefer to have a flange on the medial side to keep the tongue out of the way, as in the

Wisconsin blade, while others prefer a flat blade such as the Seward. A small version of the Macintosh type blade is available, but the design of this is illogical, because the thickest vertical part of the hub of the blade enters the mouth of an infant. If an adult blade is used, only the thin part enters, so that the small blade is less suited for infants than the adult one. Plastic laryngoscopes are available in two sizes and are suitable for resuscitation purposes at all ages, with the exception of very small premature infants. The choice of an appropriate blade depends largely on the personal preference and experience of the anaesthetist.

ENDOTRACHEAL TUBES

Most endotracheal tubes are now made of PVC. Favourable experience with PVC Magill tubes for prolonged intubation in intensive care units has led to their wider use in paediatric anaesthesia. If long, uncut tubes are used, then connections can lie beside or near the patient rather than being fixed to the face. Nasotracheal tubes made of PVC are particularly useful for neurosurgery and neuroradiology (see Chapter 14).

The stepped Cole endotracheal tube (Fig. 3.23) is used in some centres because the step is said to prevent insertion of the tube too far into the trachea, but in practice this carries the hazard of the shoulder being forced into the larynx and damaging it. Resistance to gas flow is not reduced by having a short narrow segment because of the turbulence caused by the step.

The preformed Oxford tube is now largely obsolete and replaced by the RAE tube. The major disadvantages of the Oxford tube lie in the thickness of the wall, the fact that unless a hole is cut opposite the bevel, the airway may become obstructed when the head is flexed, and (most important) the external diameter at the larynx is at least 1 mm greater than at the tip, so that a tube which passes the cricoid ring may easily be too large when fully inserted.

The RAE oral or nasal tube is made from PVC. It is shaped (Fig. 3.24) to fit into the mouth or nose without kinking, and has a bend located just as the tube emerges, so the connections to the breathing circuit are below the chin or on the forehead. The connections do not interfere with access for surgery in the head and neck. The tracheal portion has side holes. The tubes have a slightly thicker wall than the equivalent sized PVC Magill tube, but they are not tapered. The shaped bend is flexible enough to allow slight adjustment of tube position for an individual

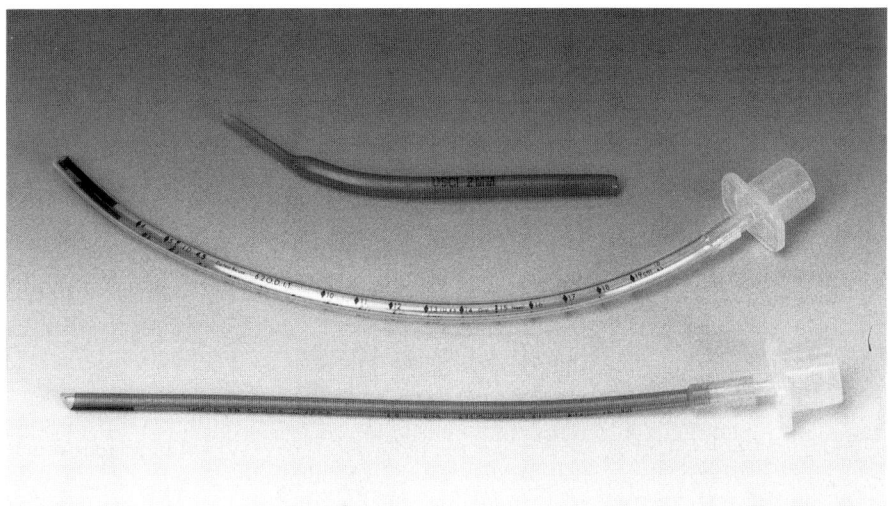

Fig. 3.23 Endotracheal tubes, from above down: Cole, Magill, wire-reinforced silastic tube to prevent kinking.

patient. Other preformed endotracheal tubes introduced in recent years are the child's anatomical tube (CAT) and the Polar tube (Fig. 3.24).

Care must be taken to ensure that bronchial intubation does not occur in growth-retarded children, where laryngeal diameter is commensurate with age but tracheal length is not.

Nylon- or metal-reinforced tubes of latex or silastic are relatively incompressible and unkinkable, except where they join the connection. Latex versions have a relatively thick wall and deteriorate rapidly when heat-sterilized. Modern silastic, reinforced tubes are more suitable. Accidental extubation is more likely to occur than with any other type of tube, while their floppiness makes them difficult to insert without a stylette. Nasotracheal intubation with a PVC Magill tube can usually avoid the need for a reinforced tube.

One of the problems which faces the newcomer to tracheal intubation of children is the selection of the appropriate tube. A number of axioms may be stated:

1 Tubes which are irritant (e.g. older forms of red rubber), or tubes which are still contaminated by chemical disinfectants (e.g. ethylene dioxide, glutaraldehyde, etc.) may cause subglottic oedema and are dangerous.

2 Formulae, such as (age/4 + 4) or general guides to tube size are useful (see Chapter 33), but variations in the size of airway in children are such that the final decision must depend on demonstrating a small leak around a non-irritant tube when a positive pressure of $15-20\,cmH_2O$ is applied. Thus a range of sizes of tube must always be available.

3 Cuffed endotracheal tubes are rarely needed for children and increase airway resistance when used in smaller sizes. After puberty, with growth of the trachea, the

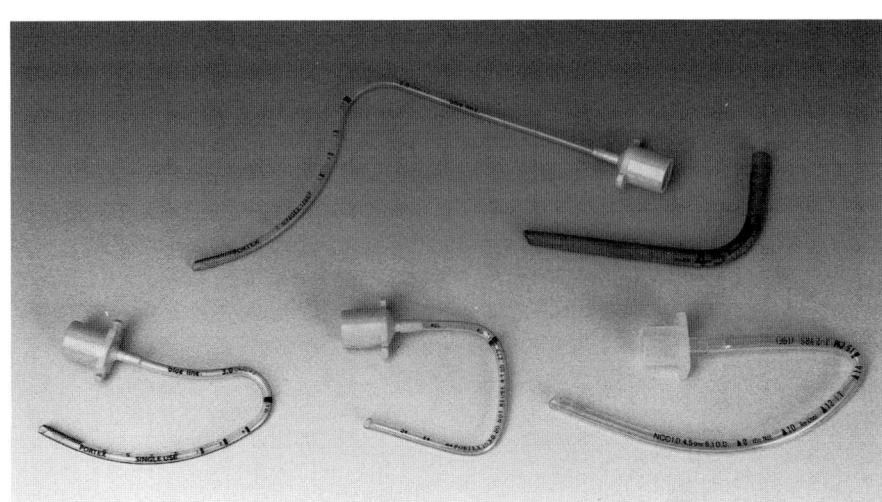

Fig. 3.24 Preformed orotracheal tubes. Clockwise from top left: North Polar tube, Oxford tube, RAE tube, CAT tube, South Polar tube.

cricoid ring ceases to be the narrowest part of the larynx. Cuffs are then needed to create an airtight seal for mechanical ventilation and to prevent aspiration. They should be inflated with the anaesthetic gas so that nitrous oxide does not diffuse into an air-filled cuff, thereby increasing volume and pressure.

In the past, attempts have been made to tailor the length of endotracheal tubes to the patients in the mistaken belief that the consequent reduction of dead space is important. With the exception of shaped tubes (RAE), modern tubes are longer than necessary but allow flexibility in fixation so that connectors are not placed next to the mouth, and the risk of accidental extubation by head movement is reduced. Markings on the tube to indicate how far it has been passed through the larynx during intubation as well as the distance at the lip or nostril are particularly useful. Accurate placement can be ensured in doubtful cases if a stethoscope is used to confirm intubation of one main bronchus and then the tube is gradually withdrawn until breath sounds are equal on both sides. If the tube is then withdrawn a little further (1 cm in infants, more in older children) the tip will be in the lower end of the trachea. In any case, it is always advisable to check that air enters both sides of the chest after intubation.

When it is necessary to clear an endotracheal tube by suction, disposable plastic catheters with multiple suction holes rather than an end hole, are readily available in sizes as small as 5 Fr gauge. They are less likely to cause suction biopsy of the mucosa. Negative pressures are generated within the tracheobronchial tree during endotracheal suction. These may be minimized by ensuring that the diameter of the suction catheter used should be no more than two-thirds of the internal diameter of the endotracheal tube. This effectively means that the cross-sectional area is reduced by a little less than half, and is conveniently remembered by using a suction catheter where French gauge is no more than twice the size of the endotracheal tube internal diameter in mm. (French Gauge Charrière is equivalent to three times the external diameter in millimetres.) During controlled ventilation, airway pressure may be maintained effectively by the use of a 'Stocks suction bullet' (Fig. 3.25), or an additional T-piece with a self-sealing rubber cap on the suction port (Fig. 3.26).

Laryngeal mask airway

This is a recent innovation and is available in three sizes suitable for children. Size 1 is suitable for infants up to 5 kg, size 2 for children 5–20 kg, and size 3 for larger children. The airway provides a convenient alternative to intubation in maintaining a secure airway. The device is also particularly useful in children who are difficult or impossible to intubate, and can be used effectively with positive pressure ventilation. It does not provide 100% security against aspiration.

SCAVENGING OF WASTE ANAESTHETIC GASES

Considerable attention has been paid in recent years to the possible hazards to operating theatre staff from volatile and gaseous anaesthetic agents discharged from breathing circuits. Many of the early studies incriminating these agents have been questioned and there remains little statistically valid evidence of any immediate or long-term sequelae.

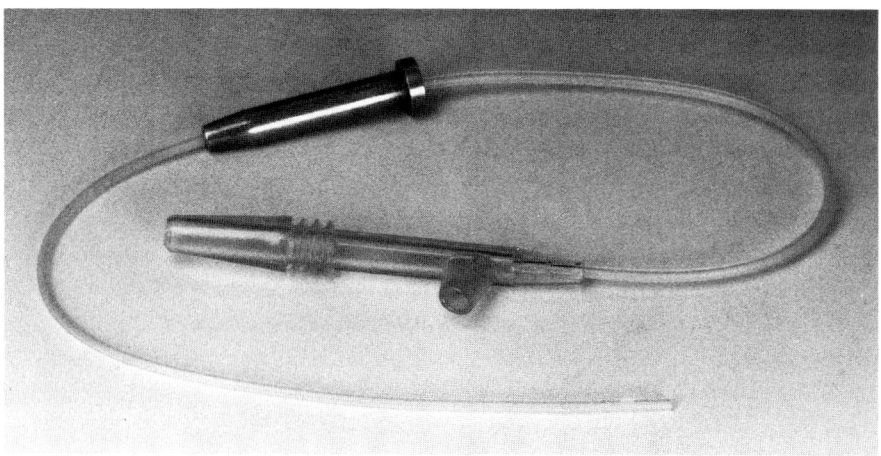

Fig. 3.25 'Stocks suction bullet' with suction catheter through lumen.

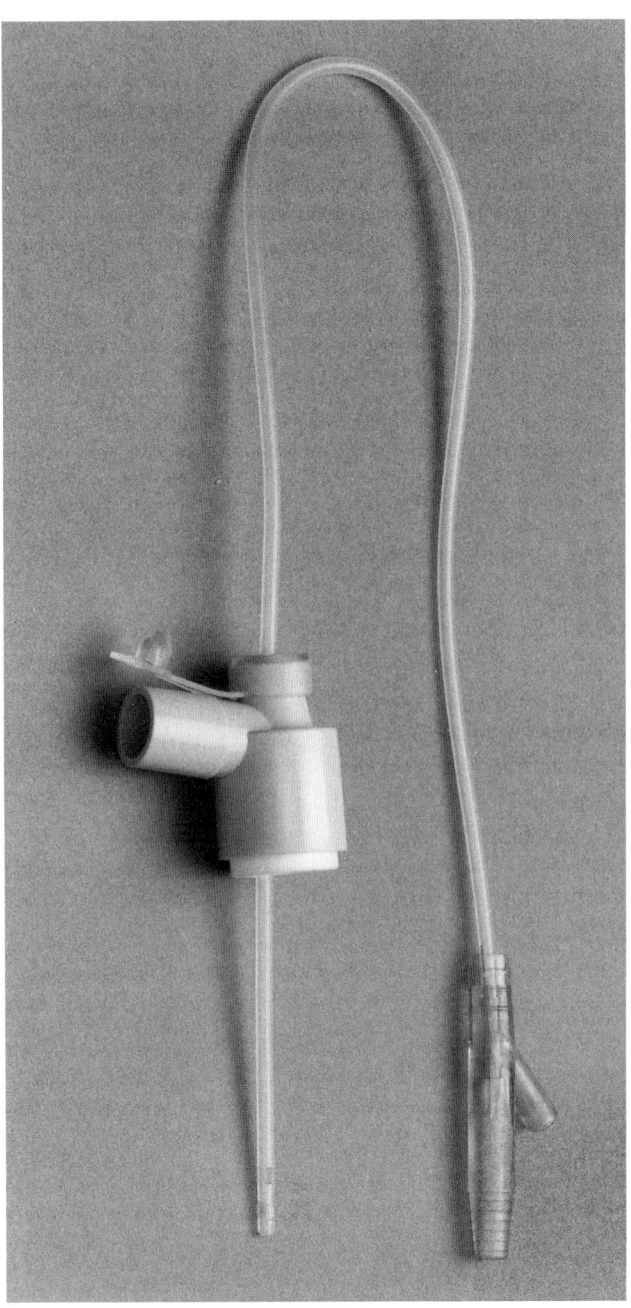

Fig. 3.26 15 mm endotracheal tube connector with sealing suction port.

Assuming that it is probably better to remove waste anaesthetic gases from the immediate environment, there are a number of methods and devices available. Normal operating room air-conditioning at 20 air changes per hour effectively removes gaseous contamination. The use of low-flow circle absorption systems reduces waste gas pollution.

Scavenging waste gas from a T-piece is more difficult, especially when using the open-tailed bag. The Steven scavenging valve, when connected to a low-pressure suction system with reservoir, is a simple and convenient method to use [12] (Fig. 3.27). Alternatives include the Berner valve with a closed bag, or high-volume suction systems placed near the open tail of the rebreathing bag. Scavenging from a mask may also be carried out using a high-volume suction system either adjacent to, or incorporated into, a shroud over the face mask.

Such scavenging systems are bulky and, especially with high-flow suction systems, cause cooling of the patient's head and/or the anaesthetist's hands when holding a mask. They have little to recommend them and add unnecessary complications.

VENTILATORS

Automatic ventilators can be used during anaesthesia for children as well as for adults. Almost any available operating theatre ventilator can be used with the T-piece system. Most ventilators designed for anaesthesia use a bellows or 'bag-in-bottle' to prevent the dilution of anaesthetic gases in the patient circuit with driving gas, and may be attached directly to the expiratory limb of a T-piece or Mapleson D in place of the reservoir bag. Such ventilators may be used without the bellows and connected directly to the expiratory limb of the circuit. The volume of the expiratory limb must be greater than the inspiratory tidal volume provided by the ventilator in order to avoid dilution of anaesthetic gases. The ventilator should have a means of disposing of excess anaesthetic gases during the expiratory phase.

A number of ventilators (e.g. Loosco, Sheffield) are specifically designed for use with a paediatric T-piece by intermittently occluding the expiratory limb. When these are used, the tidal volume varies directly with the fresh gas flow rate.

Jet ventilators for use in paediatrics have recently been developed by adapting the principle of jet ventilation to the T-piece circuit incorporating pressure control and means of humidification [13].

Ventilators must have a system pressure gauge or pressure-limit control. The ability to provide PEEP is a desirable feature. A ventilator disconnect alarm should always be used, as well as a high-pressure relief valve and/or high-pressure alarm.

INTENSIVE CARE VENTILATORS

Intensive care ventilators for infants younger than 1 year are usually T-piece occluders (see above), used with fresh gas flows 2–3 l/min in time-cycled, pressure preset mode. In older children, adult-type ventilators capable of time-cycled ventilation in volume preset or pressure preset modes are used. All intensive care ventilators used in children should ideally include:

low breathing system volume, compliance, resistance and weight;

minimal dead space;

accurate measurement of tidal volume;

independently adjustable inspiratory time;

respiratory rate up to 60/min;

fresh gas flows (in infant ventilators) of up to 20 l/min;

facilities to enable intermittent mandatory ventilation (IMV).

In either type of ventilator there should be a continuous flow of gas through the breathing system in expiration, to minimize respiratory work during spontaneous breathing.

WARMING DEVICES

In addition to humidification (see above), there are several other devices available to assist in preventing hypothermia during paediatric anaesthesia. These include heating blankets which use either circulating warm water or electrical heating. The latter are now available in a form resistant to fluids, and autoclavable. The temperature of the blanket should be monitored during use.

Warm-air mattresses covered with Gore-tex have recently been introduced. These are permeable to air but not to water. The warm air is pumped into the mattress from a floor-mounted heater, from where it passes through the cover to surround the patient and provide heat by both convection and conduction.

Overhead infrared heaters are useful during induction and extubation of small infants. Care should be taken not to subject the baby to excess heat from the device and the use of a skin temperature sensor is advisable [14].

APPARATUS FOR INTRAVENOUS USE

Needles

Intravenous induction of anaesthesia in children requires the accurate placement of a needle or cannula. Winged infusion sets are commonly employed and are available in sizes from 27 SWG (Table 3.2), although 25 SWG sets are usually used for neonates (Fig. 3.28). The wings enable secure fixation with a single piece of tape. The

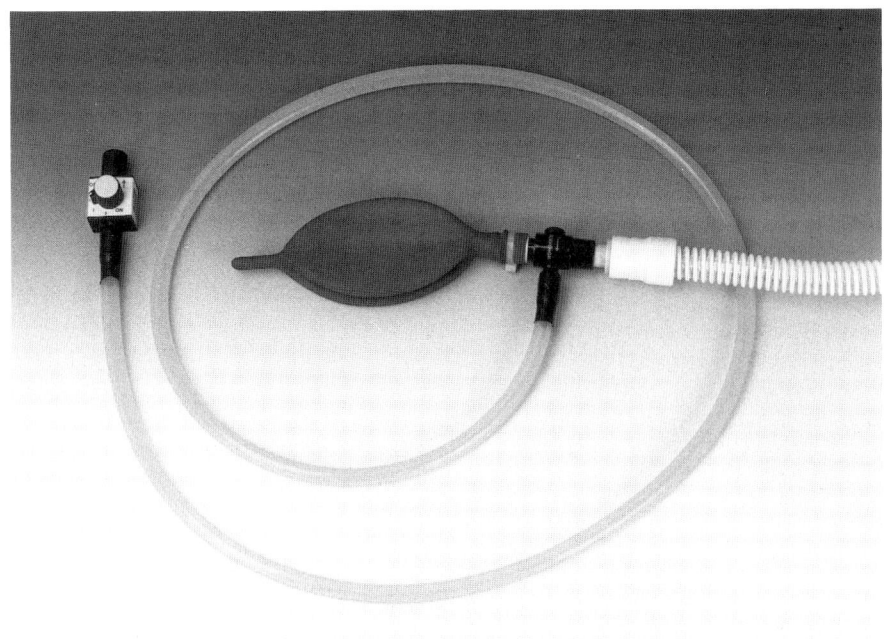

Fig. 3.27 Steven T-piece scavenging system showing connection placed between expiratory limb and closed-tail bag, and restricting valve for connection to low-pressure suction scavenging system.

Table 3.2 British Standard wire gauge (SWG)

Gauge no.	External diameter (mm)
12	2.642
13	2.337
14	2.032
15	1.829
16	1.626
17	1.422
18	1.219
19	1.016
20	0.914
21	0.813
22	0.711
23	0.610
24	0.559
25	0.508
26	0.457
27	0.417

flexible tubing should be short and have a small dead space to minimize the risk of injection of air. They can be used for prolonged infusion or rapid infusion of large volumes during surgery, but cannulae are more reliable since needles easily cut out of the vein when the patient is moved. The needle should be checked to ensure it is in the vein before drugs are injected.

For induction in infants and small children, a sharp fine hypodermic needle (27 or 25 SWG, 4–5 mm long) may be used. A clear plastic hub is advantageous so that the back-flow of blood can be detected early. Venepuncture with very fine needles requires some practice because the familiar 'pop' as the needle passes through the vessel wall may not be felt and the rate of 'flashback' or appearance of blood in the hub is slow.

Intravenous cannulae (Fig. 3.29)

Plastic intravenous cannulae of various designs are now available in sizes as small as 26 SWG. 24 SWG cannulae are usually suitable for neonates, with 22 SWG being used for infants and older children. They may also be used for arterial or central venous cannulation in appropriate lengths. Modern plastics are less likely to 'peel back' on insertion through the skin, and have low frictional resistance.

In some cannulae the needle protrudes much further past the tip than in others. When introducing these it is important that, once venepuncture has been achieved, the cannula is then advanced over the needle before the needle is withdrawn.

Secure fixation is essential, using tape in the longitudinal direction of the cannula, with care to leave the skin over the tip visible. Clear plastic adhesive dressings are now available, specifically designed for securing intravenous cannulae.

A minimum-volume extension set with a three-way stopcock can be attached to the cannula so that manipulation and administration of drugs will not dislodge the cannula. In addition, the use of extension sets enables the stopcock to be made more accessible during surgery when the cannula is covered by surgical drapes. The use of an injection site with a luer fitting, instead of a needle injection port, also helps to prevent accidental needlestick injuries.

Infusion systems

For accurate intravenous administration of small volumes of blood or fluid during surgery to neonates and small

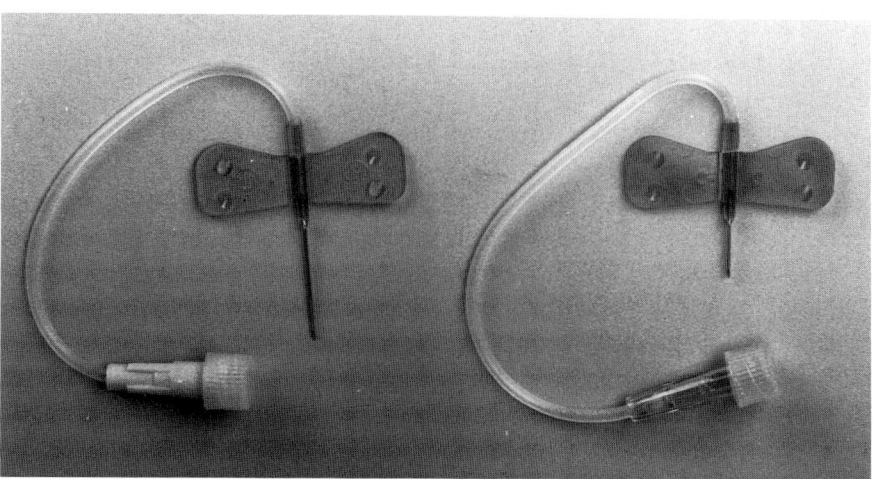

Fig. 3.28 Winged infusion sets, sizes 23SWG and 25SWG.

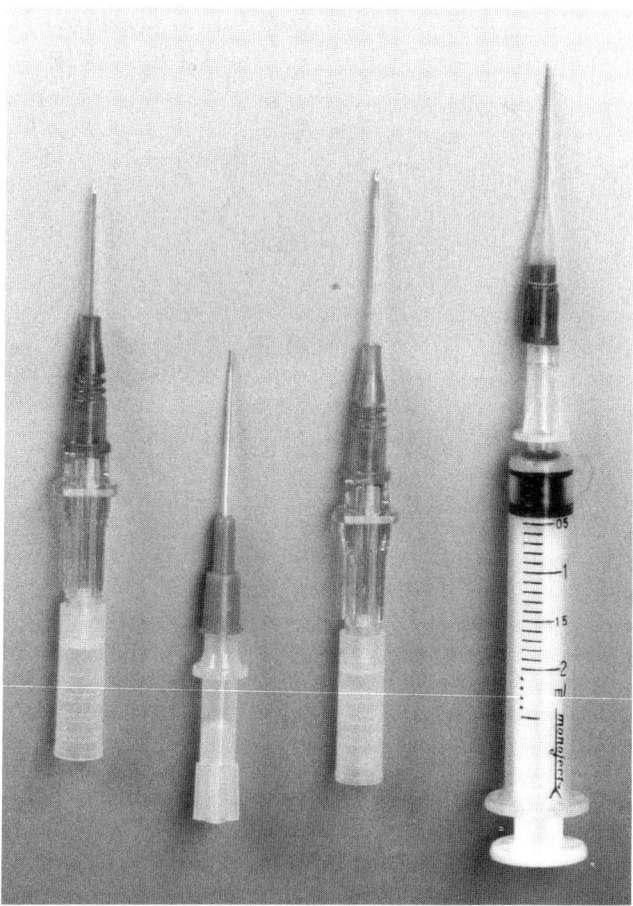

Fig. 3.29 Selection of intravenous cannulae of 22SWG and 24SWG (left).

infants, the use of 10 or 20 ml syringes in conjunction with the three-way stopcock is simplest and most accurate.

All intravenous infusion sets used in children should incorporate a burette of 100, 150 or 200 ml capacity marked in 1 or 2 ml divisions (Fig. 3.30). At the bottom of the burette there is often a valve to prevent air from running through the drip chamber and into the intravenous line when the burette empties. The burette should not contain more fluid than is needed for 2 hours, unless an infusion controller is used.

Drip chambers, often an integral part of the burette, may be either standard or micro-drip design. The micro-drip set allows 60 drops per ml compared with 15 drops per ml with the standard set, thus allowing finer control of the flow rate when used manually. An electronic controller or pump, incorporated into the infusion line, is now frequently used, especially postoperatively. Syringe pumps may also be used for small volumes or

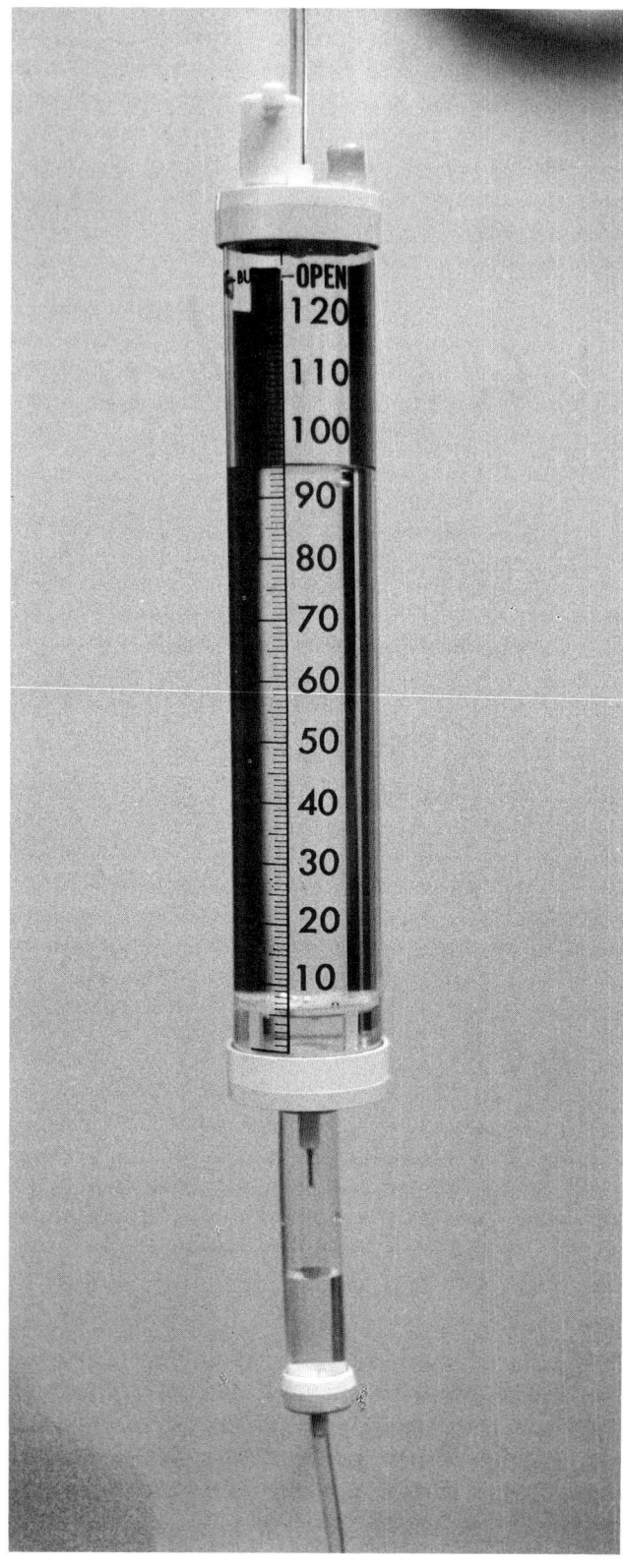

Fig. 3.30 A typical paediatric infusion set incorporating a burette (in this case 120 ml capacity) marked in 1 ml divisions, and a micro-drip which provides 60 drops per ml.

continuous drug infusions. All electronic infusion systems should be accurate and able to detect fault situations such as obstruction, runaway (loss of resistance indicating disconnection) and air bubbles, and should have a volume limit. It is important to ensure that the skin over the tip of the cannula is not covered by tape or bandages when an infusion pump is in use, so that extravasation may be detected early.

BLOOD-WARMING DEVICES

The infusion of cold blood or fluids is a significant factor in the cooling of patients and increasing myocardial irritability. The simplest method of warming solutions is to warm the container before administration using warm water or a special microwave heating unit. Otherwise, it is advisable to place a warming system in the intravenous line whenever blood, plasma or any other refrigerated solution is to be infused (other than slowly) and also when large volumes of crystalloid solution at room temperature are administered. A warming system is most conveniently inserted between the infusion set and the extension set and may be simply an extra extension under the warming blanket on which the patient is lying.

The usual method of warming infusions is by passing a coil of tubing through either a water bath or a dry-heat system, usually a heated grooved metal block (Fig. 3.31). These should aim to heat the blood to between 37°C and 41°C and incorporate a safety cutout with audible and visible alarms if the temperature rises to more than 2 or 3°C above the thermostat set point. The osmotic fragility of blood cells does not increase and significant haemolysis does not occur when blood is warmed for an hour at temperatures below 46°C [15].

Blood warmers for paediatric anaesthesia do not need to be as efficient as those for adults because flow rates are much lower, so that dry-heat systems may be suitable. Except when very rapid rates of infusion are used or the coil is next to the patient, blood or fluid warmed to 37°C by a warming device will cool to near room temperature by the time it reaches the patient. Thus it is advisable to use the shortest possible, preferably thick-walled, minimum volume extension set between the warmer and the patient. Long or additional tubing also increases resistance to fluid infusion.

DECONTAMINATION OF ANAESTHETIC EQUIPMENT

There should be a protocol for decontamination of all anaesthetic equipment, setting out the method and frequency. The first process for all equipment is cleaning, which is followed by either disinfection or sterilization [16].

Sterilization is defined as a process intended to kill or remove all living organisms, including bacterial spores.

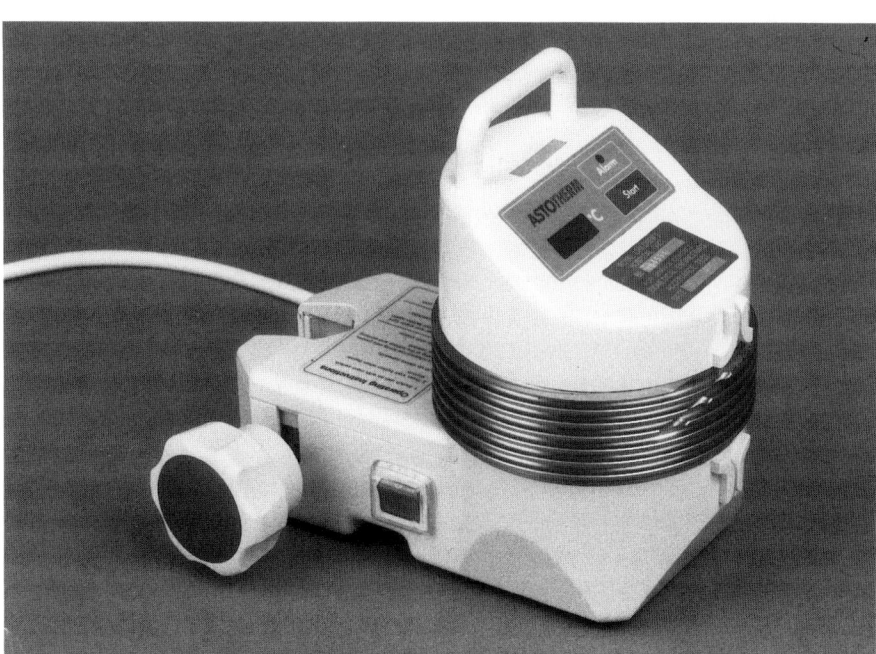

Fig. 3.31 Dry-heat blood warmer where ordinary drip tubing may be wound around core. A clamp is provided for attachment to the intravenous pole.

Disinfection is defined as a process intended to kill or remove disease-producing microorganisms, but not necessarily bacterial spores.

Items which are passed into the mouth and trachea should be sterilized after use, e.g. laryngoscopes and oropharyngeal airways which come into contact with saliva and/or blood. Endotracheal tubes, suction catheters, etc. should be sterile when used.

Respiratory equipment should be decontaminated. The question of the method and frequency provokes much debate. There is evidence that when no cleaning process is used, infection may result [17]. Pasteurization is a suitable method and will destroy most significant disease-producing organisms.

The method used for sterilization or disinfection will be dictated by the type of equipment, and information as to the correct method should be provided by the manufacturer. Disposable articles should be changed routinely.

Equipment standards

Many items of anaesthetic equipment are subject to internationally recognized standards. These stipulate design, manufacturing and performance criteria which should be met by the equipment. A list of some of these standards is included at the end of the book as Appendix 5.

REFERENCES

1 Mapleson W.W. The elimination of rebreathing in various semi-closed anaesthetic systems. *Br J Anaes* 1954, **26**, 323.

2 Ayre P. Endotracheal anaesthesia for babies; with special reference to hare-lip and cleft palate operations. *Curr Res Anesth* 1937, **16**, 330.

3 Rees G.J. Anaesthesia in the newborn. *Br Med J* 1950, **2**, 1419.

4 Nightingale D.A., Richards C.C., Glass A. An evaluation of rebreathing in a modified T-piece system during controlled ventilation of anaesthetised children. *Br J Anaesth* 1965, **37**, 762.

5 Bain J.A., Spoerel W.E. Flow requirements for a modified Mapleson D System during controlled ventilation. *Can Anaes Soc J* 1973, **20**, 629.

6 Rose D.K., Froese A.B. The regulation of $Paco_2$ during controlled ventilation of children with a T-piece. *Can Anaes Soc J* 1979, **26**, 104.

7 Nightingale D.A., Lambert T.F. Carbon dioxide output in anaesthetised children. *Anaesthesia* 1978, **33**, 594.

8 Harrison G.A. Ayre's T-piece: A review of its modifications. *Br J Anaesth* 1964, **36**, 115.

9 Houghton I.T. The Triservice anaesthetic apparatus. *Anaesthesia* 1981, **36**, 1094.

10 Berry F.A., Hughes-Davies D.I. Methods of increasing the humidity and temperature of the inspired gases in the infant circle system. *Anesthesiology* 1972, **37**, 456.

11 Bissonnette B., Sessler D.I., LaFlamme P. Is passive inspired gas warming as effective as active humidification in infants undergoing general anaesthesia? *Proceedings and Abstracts of the Second European Congress of Paediatric Anaesthesia.* May 1989, p. 99.

12 Steven I.M. A scavenging system for use in paediatric anaesthesia. *Anaes Intens Care* 1990, **18**, 238.

13 Chakrabarti M.K., Whitwam J.G. A new infant ventilator for normal or high-frequency ventilation: influence of tracheal tube on distal airway pressure during high-frequency ventilation. *Crit Care Med* 1988, **16**, 1142−1146.

14 Barnes J., Brown T.C.K. An overhead heater for use in infant anaesthesia. *Anaes Intens Care* 1985, **13**, 188.

15 Linko K., Hynynen K. Erythrocyte damage caused by the Haemotherm microwave blood warmer. *Acta Anaes Scand* 1979, **23**, 320.

16 Lumley J. Decontamination of anaesthetic and ventilatory equipment. In: *Bailliere's clinical anaesthesiology*, Vol. 2, No. 2, Bailliere Tindall, London, 1988, 391.

17 Nielsen H., Jacobson J.B., Stokke D.B., Brinklov M.M., Christensen K.N. Cross-infection from contaminated anaesthetic equipment: a real hazard. *Anaesthesia* 1980, **35**, 703.

18 Schofield W.N. Human nutrition. *Clinical Nutrition* 1985, **39C**, Suppl. 1, 5−41.

4: Monitoring

INTRODUCTION

Monitoring during anaesthesia is continuous observation of the condition of the patient, so that homeostasis and an appropriate depth of anaesthesia are maintained. It implies appropriate responses to any changes observed, so that adverse effects of anaesthesia and surgery are minimized. Observations made during anaesthesia and surgery must be carefully recorded, together with any changes of management in response to these. This record may be useful for management of the same patient in future surgical operations, for clinical audit or for medicolegal purposes. These observations and appropriate responses are the most important functions of the anaesthetist. They are only learnt by frequent practice during training, and must be maintained by meticulous application throughout the practising life of every anaesthetist.

The purpose of monitoring is to ensure that the patient is adequately but not too deeply anaesthetized and that there is an adequate supply of oxygen for metabolism. The latter implies a reliable source of oxygen, no disconnection in the breathing circuit, sufficient ventilation and an adequate cardiac output to transport oxygen and carbon dioxide to and from the tissues. The basis of effective monitoring is simple clinical observation, especially of colour, capillary refill, pulse rate, rhythm and volume, and ventilation.

Although the principles of monitoring in infants and children are the same as in adults, some methods need modification because of differences in size or physiology. The anaesthetist unused to working with children may find such monitoring difficult, but the difficulties can be overcome by a meticulous approach, willingness to learn, and determination to apply the principles safely.

A variety of apparatus is available to monitor many different functions in the anaesthetized child. The choice of these and the emphasis placed on their use depends on the preference and experience of the individual anaesthetist. The opinions of anaesthetists and the value placed by them on individual methods of monitoring vary widely. The essential task is to monitor important functions adequately, particularly pulmonary ventilation, oxygenation and the cardiovascular system. Complicated methods of monitoring must not be allowed to distract the attention from simple observation. There is a real danger that difficulty in setting up a monitor can distract the anaesthetist's attention from the patient.

CHECKING EQUIPMENT BEFORE USE

Before anaesthesia is induced, a thorough check of all apparatus upon which the patient's life may depend is essential. This includes the inspection and testing of gas supply and breathing circuits, to ensure that the required flow of gases can be delivered and that there are no leaks. Vaporizers should be in good order, filled with the appropriate agent, and turned off. There are protocols for checking the anaesthetic machine and these should be followed (see Appendix 6). Suction equipment must be tested, together with all ancillary apparatus such as ventilators and laryngoscopes.

In many countries the use of an oxygen analyser during anaesthesia is mandatory. The function of this device should be checked before use, verifying accuracy at both 21% and 100% oxygen concentrations.

MONITORING DURING ANAESTHESIA

During anaesthesia, a number of monitors will be in use, some monitoring primarily the anaesthetic delivery system, some the patient and others monitoring both or other equipment. Undoubtedly the single most important monitor of all is the anaesthetist using his or her senses continuously to care for the patient.

Observation

Although equipment, simple or complex, may be used to help the anaesthetist, direct observation of the patient without the use of such apparatus should continue throughout anaesthesia.

Cyanosis of skin or mucous membrane may be detected when the capillaries contain 4−5 g of reduced haemoglobin per 100 ml. Local causes (cold, venous obstruction) and general conditions (shock, reduced cardiac output or reflex vasoconstriction) can both result in cyanosis. Central cyanosis indicates low arterial oxygen tension, but peripheral cyanosis may result from stagnation in the capillary circulation, especially in the presence of polycythaemia. Vasoconstriction or reduction in cardiac output may also result in pallor.

By looking at the patient, the anaesthetist can detect changes associated with inadequate anaesthesia and insufficient muscle relaxation. Movement, lacrimation, sweating, or increased ventilation as well as tachycardia and a rising blood pressure with increased bleeding are signs of inadequate anaesthesia. The size and position of the pupils may also indicate depth of anaesthesia, moderately dilated central pupils signifying adequate depth for surgery. The respiratory movements are observed during both spontaneous and controlled ventilation. The detection of abnormalities in these movements in infants and small children requires practice and an appreciation

of differences in breathing patterns at different ages. On rare occasions seizures may be detected.

During the course of anaesthesia, the anaesthetist must continue to observe and check the apparatus frequently. Where cylinders are used, pressure gauges must be monitored to ensure that the gas supply remains adequate. Flowmeters must be seen to be working. It is important that vaporizers are adjusted to an appropriate concentration and are not empty. Excursion of the reservoir bag or of the reservoir of a mechanical ventilator must be watched.

Observation also involves the surgical field in order to determine blood or fluid loss; colour of tissues and blood; the progress of the operation; and to see if any steps can be taken which may improve the operating conditions. Examples of the latter include induced hypotension to reduce bleeding, changing the position of the lights, or of the patient, or the operating table to improve surgical access.

Listening

The anaesthetist is constantly monitoring the patient by listening. The use of a monaural stethoscope allows constant monitoring of the heart and respiration. The noise of the ventilator and audible pulse monitors often become part of the background and changes will alert the anaesthetist. Unusual noises may draw attention to obstructed breathing, leakage of gas supply lines, abnormal volumes of fluid passing through the surgeon's suction line and many other situations requiring prompt reaction. Even the surgeon's conversation should be monitored as comments relevant to the operation and anaesthetic may be made. Many monitors now incorporate audible alarms which must be listened for and attended to immediately.

Touch and smell

By touching the skin the anaesthetist can observe the temperature in different areas. A patient who feels hot should be monitored with a thermometer in case hyperthermia is developing. Cold extremities may be due to vasoconstriction or generalized cooling.

Touching the patient can give information about the circulation by observing capillary refill after pressure and by careful feeling of radial and other pulses. Anaesthetists unused to children may have difficulty in feeling the radial pulse of infants. A common mistake is to obliterate the pulse by pressing too hard. The superficial temporal or brachial pulse may be easier to detect if the radial is difficult. Frequent practice is again the key to successful monitoring; variations in pulse pressure and volume can alert the anaesthetist to changes in the circulation.

The anaesthetist may use his or her sense of smell to check the function of vaporizers or to detect leaks of excessive amounts of anaesthetic vapour.

MONITORS OF ANAESTHETIC DELIVERY SYSTEMS

Machine

In addition to regular observation of gas supply pressure gauges, flowmeters and the vaporizer dial and reservoir, there should be an oxygen failure warning device that is dependent purely on oxygen and shuts off the flow of nitrous oxide in the case of oxygen failure. This monitor should produce a characteristic audible alarm and may provide a small reserve supply of oxygen, as in the Howison alarm [1].

Anaesthetic breathing system

Breathing systems for paediatric anaesthesia should incorporate a pressure gauge and oxygen analyser. The oxygen analyser must be calibrated correctly and should have a fixed low concentration alarm at 17% or 18%, with audible and visible indicators. The types currently available include polarographic or galvanic cell electrodes and paramagnetic oxygen analysers, as well as mass spectrometry and acoustic spectroscopy. The three former examples are the most common and may be used either as mainstream sensors in the inspiratory limb of a high-flow paediatric system, or to sample a side-stream from anywhere in the system but preferably from the proximal end of the endotracheal tube. Paramagnetic oxygen analysers are now capable of a response time rapid enough to provide inspiratory and expiratory measurements from this site, but polarographic and galvanic sensors require simultaneous carbon dioxide measurement to distinguish inspiratory and expiratory samples. Polarographic and galvanic cells require replacement about every 12 months but may become non-linear prior to complete failure. Paramagnetic analysers have the advantage that there is no consumable component.

When using low-flow anaesthesia in a circle system, more information about oxygen uptake by the patient may be obtained by using the sensor in the expiratory limb. Condensation on the sensor may interfere with accuracy or may block the sample tube in a side-stream sampling system.

Ventilator disconnect monitor

The breathing system must incorporate a disconnection monitor because unrecognized disconnection of the breathing circuit when ventilation is being controlled is one of the common causes of tragic mishaps [2]. The ideal monitor should detect both disconnection and high circuit pressure. Alarm levels may be adjustable. For paediatric use, a peak pressure alarm should be available and set at $30-40\,cmH_2O$, or just above the peak cycling pressure if adjustable. On some disconnect monitors, cycling is detected by adjusting upper and lower pressure limits. If a single pressure is used to detect cycling, it should be between 8 and $12\,cmH_2O$ (this being lower than most peak inspiratory pressures and greater than the usual positive end-expiratory pressure). It should be noted that in the latter case, with high gas flows, disconnection or loose connection between the endotracheal tube and 15 mm adaptor may not be detected if the tube size is small. The apnoea delay should be about 10 seconds. The monitor may either be activated automatically or have an on−off switch, preferably as its only control. An automatically activated alarm should have a means of temporarily silencing the alarm.

MONITORS OF THE PATIENT

Stethoscope

The simplest and most reliable aid to monitoring for the paediatric anaesthetist is the precordial or oesophageal stethoscope, which may be used for continuous monitoring of heart and breath sounds. A stethoscope should always be used to check that both lungs can be inflated after intubation. An oesophageal or precordial stethoscope can be used continuously to monitor the rate, rhythm and intensity of heart sounds and respiration. A precordial stethoscope should be firmly strapped in position (Fig. 4.1). Provided the stethoscope does not move, a trained listener can detect changes in the intensity of heart sounds which indicate changes in cardiac output.

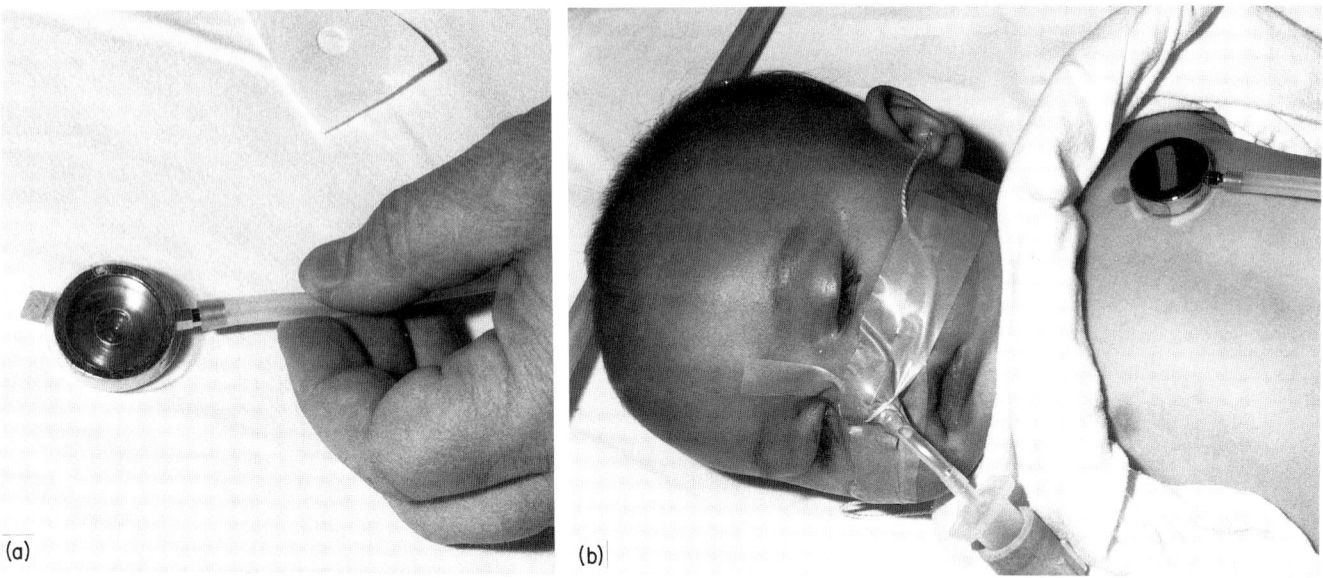

Fig. 4.1 (a) Precordial stethoscope showing application of double-sided adhesive disc; (b) precordial stethoscope in place.

An individual moulded single ear piece is more comfortable than an ordinary stethoscope and leaves one ear free.

Stethoscopes are available which incorporate a small microphone and FM transmitter, enabling the anaesthetist to use a receiver with headphones or monaural earpiece. These allow the anaesthetist much greater freedom of movement.

The use of a stethoscope should not inhibit an anaesthetist from using other methods of monitoring such as observation of the patient, feeling the pulse and taking the blood pressure.

Pulse oximetry

Pulse oximetry probably represents the most significant advance in patient monitoring since the Riva Rocci method of blood pressure monitoring. The ability to measure oxygen saturation continuously and pulse rate non-invasively has made paediatric anaesthesia considerably safer, because of earlier recognition and correction of falls in arterial oxygenation. Episodes of hypoxaemia and of hyperoxaemia in newborn infants that were not recognized in the past have been drawn to the attention of anaesthetists. These have influenced most, if not all, anaesthetists to modify their techniques.

Sensors are now available for use with the smallest of neonates and can be used in several sites (Fig. 4.2). Most

models are accurate down to 70% saturation, but below that level reliability varies. Accuracy below 70% may be unimportant except in cyanotic heart disease. Freedom from diathermy interference is important in the choice of a pulse oximeter and the sensor should be placed in a site where it will not be affected by surgery or the surgical

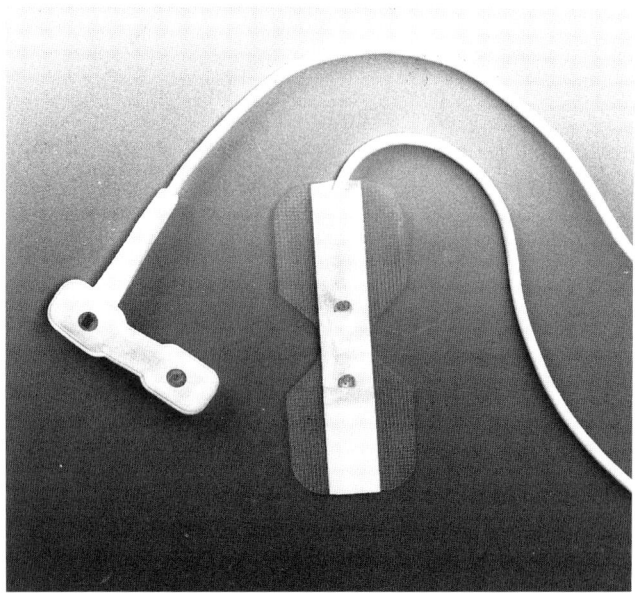

Fig. 4.2 Infant pulse oximetry sensors suitable for use on digits, palm of hand, or foot. Left: reusable sensor; right: disposable single-use sensor with adhesive fastening tape.

team. Desirable features include an indicator of adequacy of perfusion by pulse amplitude, and a modulated audible pulse tone which varies with saturation, enabling rapid recognition not only by the anaesthetist but by all members of the operating team. Artefacts may occur with low flow due to vasoconstriction or venous obstruction as well as from movement or extraneous light.

Pulse oximetry is especially useful in preventing hyperoxia and the consequent risk of retrolental fibroplasia in premature infants.

Arterial blood pressure

Arterial blood pressure should be measured at intervals during any anaesthetic procedure. A sphygmomanometer cuff may be used with either a mercury column or an aneroid gauge. The latter has the advantage that, when pulses are difficult to detect, pulsation conducted from the cuff to the needle of the gauge can be a rough guide to the level of systolic pressure. This principle is used more accurately with the Von Recklinghausen oscillotonometer. It is important that the sphygmomanometer cuff should be of an appropriate size for the child's arm. Cuffs are available in several sizes and should cover at least two-thirds of the upper arm. It is preferable that the inflatable bag should almost encircle the arm. If the cuff is too small, or if the material of which it is made is too stiff, a reading that is too high may

be obtained. The error with too large a cuff is less than with one too small.

Non-invasive blood pressure monitors using the oscillometric principle are now commonplace (Fig. 4.3). They are convenient and enable the anaesthetist to have his or her hands free for other tasks, but they must be recognized as being no more accurate than the manual method. Indeed at low pressures, when accuracy is needed most, they are poor indicators of true blood pressure. Non-invasive blood pressure monitors which use a standard cuff, and either a microphone to detect Korotkoff sounds or a Doppler sensor to detect flow, are still available.

An intra-arterial catheter or cannula and transducer are useful when continuous accurate monitoring of blood pressure is needed. This may be during open heart surgery, induced hypotension and other major surgery where blood loss may be sudden and massive. Percutaneous catheterization of the radial artery may be carried out using 20–22 gauge plastic cannulae in quite small infants. If pressure monitoring is not likely to be needed in the postoperative period, then winged needle devices with a short bevel may be used intraoperatively. Disposable pressure transducers are now available which are stable, accurate and relatively cheap (Fig. 4.4). A significant advantage is that they can easily be transferred with the patient from the operating room to the intensive care ward for continued postoperative monitoring.

Continuous flushing devices introduce some 3–4 ml of

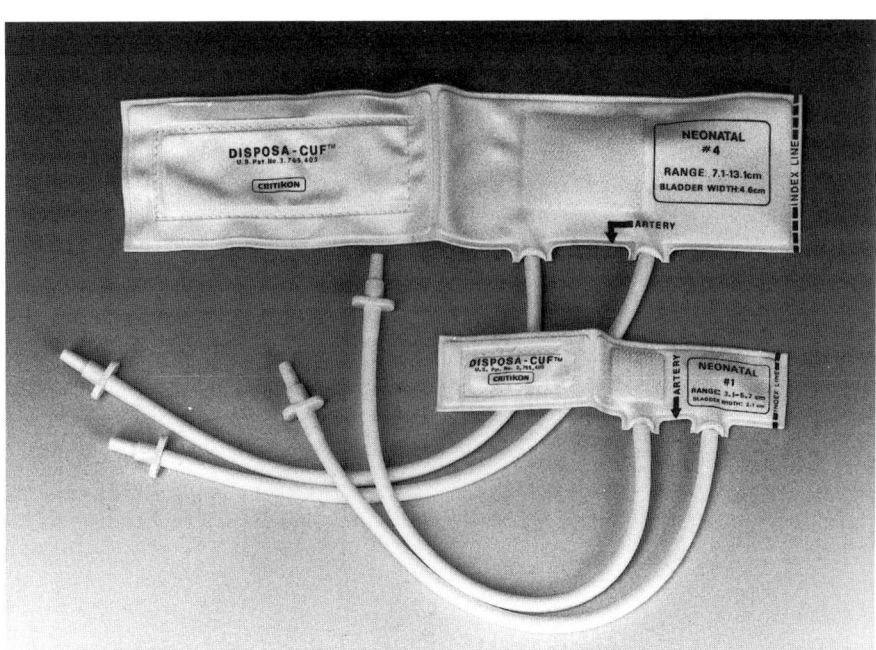

Fig. 4.3 Cuffs for use with non-invasive blood pressure monitors using the oscillometric principle. The smallest cuff is suitable for small premature neonates.

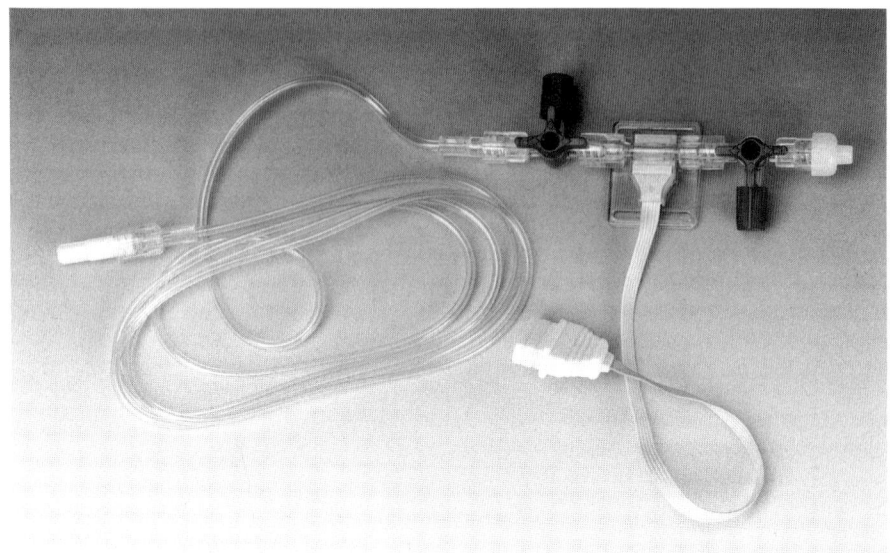

Fig. 4.4 Disposable pressure transducer.

fluid per hour into the patient. This must be added to the measured fluid intake. For small infants, the volume may be excessive and a constant infusion pump provides a means of continuous flushing while administering flows of as little as 0.5 ml/h.

When intermittent flushing is used, a 1 or 2 ml syringe used gently with a three-way stopcock is safer than an adult-type pressure-flush system. Not only may the latter infuse excessive amounts of fluid, but there may be retrograde flow of flushing solution into the aorta and cerebral vessels.

Electrocardiography

The electrocardiogram (ECG) is of less value in paediatric anaesthesia compared with older patients, except in children with pre-existing cardiac disease or those undergoing posterior fossa surgery. A normal ECG waveform gives no indication of cardiovascular integrity and changes in the waveform are late indicators of adverse circumstances.

Dysrhythmia occurring during anaesthesia which may be detected by ECG monitoring is easily detected by other means (stethoscope, pulse oximetry), and is almost always benign. The usual causes are hypercarbia, vagal reflexes resulting from surgical or anaesthetic manipulation (e.g. pulling on extraocular muscles), or inadequate or too deep levels of anaesthesia. Myocardial ischaemia due solely to coronary insufficiency is very rare in paediatric anaesthesia.

Pulse monitors

In places where pulse oximeters are not available, monitors that detect blood flow through the capillary bed by light reflection or pressure are useful. These monitors give information about the quality of the circulation and may be used in conjunction with a simple sphygmomanometer cuff to determine systolic blood pressure. If the capillary circulation is impaired, the light source may cause burns — the site of attachment of the sensor should be checked regularly in these circumstances.

Respiratory monitors

Simple means of monitoring respiration include observation of movement of the chest and the reservoir bag and the use of a stethoscope. A pressure gauge in the breathing system and ventilator disconnection alarm are needed during mechanical ventilation. Paediatric versions of the Wright respirometer, measuring smaller tidal volumes than the adult version, are now available, but care must be taken in high-flow circuits to place the device between the endotracheal tube and the breathing system to ensure accurate measurements. Water condensation may cause inaccurate readings, especially when humidification is added. Pneumotachographs for use in measuring small volumes are available, but are expensive and difficult to calibrate and maintain.

Capnography

The most effective and informative monitor of respiration is the capnograph. The end-tidal carbon dioxide level gives an indication (within $2-5$ mmHg) of arterial carbon dioxide and therefore adequacy of ventilation. Changes in end-tidal carbon dioxide are a useful early warning of problems related to gas supply, circuit integrity, ventilatory function and ventilation volume. Gas embolism or reduced cardiac output may be indicated by a fall in end-tidal CO_2 due to reduced pulmonary blood flow. A rise in end-tidal CO_2 may be the first indication of the onset of malignant hyperpyrexia. Early recovery from muscle relaxants may be indicated by small excursions on the capnograph in addition to the normal waveform.

Correlation between end-tidal and arterial CO_2 measurements is diminished with increasing V/Q mismatching, in particular with a large dead space. Children with congenital heart disease and large shunts show a poor correlation.

A large proportion of anaesthetic mishaps are the result of airway problems [2]. The combination of oximetry and capnography is the most effective means of detecting these and thereby reducing anaesthetic mortality and morbidity [3]. Capnographs are of two types, most using infrared absorption as the method of measurement. Mainstream capnographs use a cuvette in the breathing system with the infrared sensor placed over windows in the cuvette (Fig. 4.5). Cuvettes with low dead space (2 ml) are available and should be placed as near to the endotracheal tube as possible. Sidestream capnographs sample breathing system gas via a fine flexible catheter and perform the analysis within the monitor itself (Fig. 4.6). Monitors other than infrared also use this method of sampling, e.g. mass spectrometers, acoustic spectrometers. The sampling site should be as near to the tracheal end of the endotracheal tube as possible, particularly in neonates, but this is not always possible. Results from sampling at the breathing system end are usually satisfactory. Water condensation may occur with sidestream sampling but may be eliminated by a water trap on the monitor, or by the use of 'Aridus' tubing which is permeable to water but not to respiratory gas.

Although more bulky, the mainstream capnograph is more accurate when sampling at the breathing system end of the endotracheal tube. Accuracy of the sidestream capnograph may be increased by using a slow respiratory

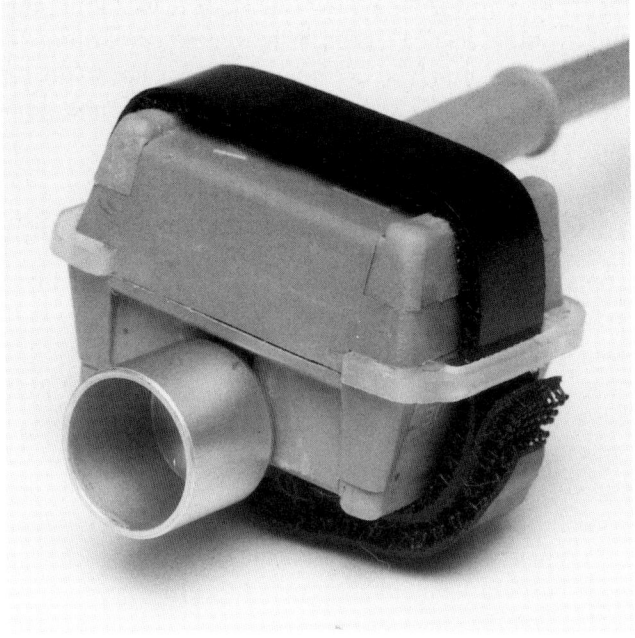

Fig. 4.5 Mainstream capnograph with low dead-space infant cuvette, which may attached directly to the endotracheal tube connector.

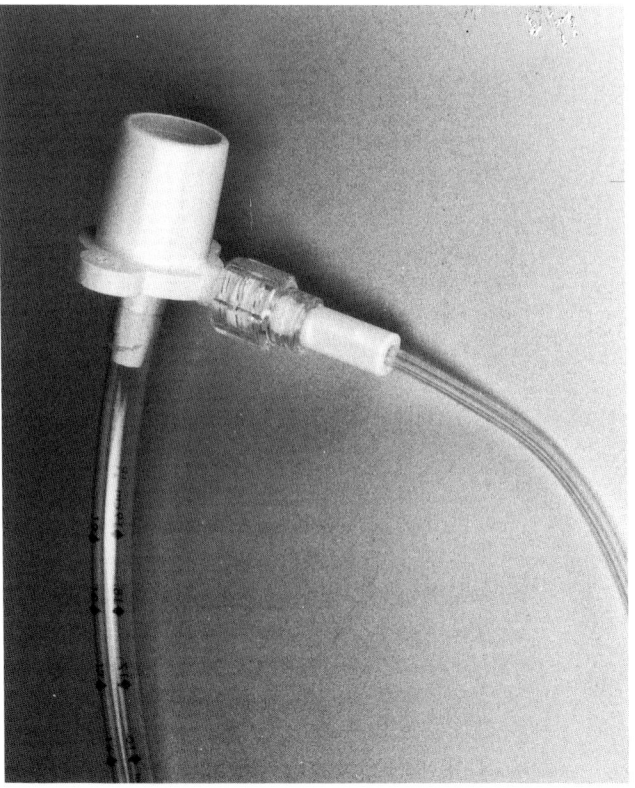

Fig. 4.6 Sidestream sampling system for capnography using a modified endotracheal tube connector.

rate, by using a sample flow rate of at least 100 ml/min and by introducing a sigh into the ventilatory pattern. It is useful to display the capnograph waveform, to be certain that the end-tidal measurement is a true indication of the plateau level.

Transcutaneous gas measurement

Transcutaneous oxygen ($TC.O_2$) monitoring is used less in anaesthesia since the advent of pulse oximetry. It is still valuable in the intensive care of neonates because it measures oxygen tension rather than saturation, but it is more difficult to use and has a slower response time than pulse oximetry. The sensors are heated and need to be moved frequently to avoid skin burns. Corrections are needed in the presence of halothane and nitrous oxide.

Transcutaneous carbon dioxide monitoring is also available, but many of the same difficulties apply to its use as to $TC.O_2$ monitoring.

Recent developments in the microtechnology of blood gas electrodes have produced an intravascular catheter to measure Pa_{O_2}, Pa_{CO_2} and pH directly and continuously. Further miniaturization will be required for use in paediatrics.

Inhaled anaesthetic agent monitors

Infrared detectors and mass spectrometers now enable accurate and continuous measurement of all the commonly used volatile anaesthetic agents. In addition, recent developments in photoacoustic spectroscopy enable the measurement of all anaesthetic gases. The place of these monitors in routine paediatric anaesthesia is yet to be established.

Temperature

Changes in body temperature during anaesthesia occur most frequently in infants, in patients who receive large infusions of cold fluid, and in those in whom hypothermia may be deliberately induced. Elevation in temperature is uncommon during anaesthesia but may occur in malignant hyperpyrexia, with infection, sometimes in patients with osteogenesis imperfecta and when infants are overheated with warming blankets, etc.

Some form of electrical thermometer is usual, most commonly a thermistor, although thermocouples and resistance thermometers are as effective. Usual sites for temperature probes to monitor central body temperature

are the oesophagus, the rectum, the nasopharynx and the tympanic membrane. Oesophageal probes must be placed in the lower third of the oesophagus if the readings are not to be unduly influenced by the temperature of the respiratory gases. It is essential to estimate the distance to which the probe must be passed by laying it against the nose and chest. The part of the probe which should be at the nose or mouth when properly inserted is then marked. Only in this way can the probe be correctly placed in infants and children of different sizes. In the same way a rectal probe should be passed so that its tip is well within the rectum. Axillary temperature probes may be used, provided the arm can be kept close to the side and that sudden induced changes of temperature are not expected.

Combination oesophageal stethoscope and temperature monitors are now available and some also include ECG electrodes.

If heating devices such as blankets and humidifiers are used, their temperature should also be monitored, as should the warmed humidified gas at the connection to the endotracheal tube. A skin sensor should be used if an infrared overhead heater is used with an infant.

The use of skin temperature sensors on the extremities may indicate the degree of vasoconstriction when the core−peripheral gradient is increased. During cardiac surgery, peripheral skin temperature gives a useful indication of the effectiveness of cooling and rewarming techniques.

BLOOD VOLUME AND FLUID BALANCE

It is essential that an exact record be kept of all intravenous fluid administered during anaesthesia. The rate of infusion and the amount of fluid or blood remaining in infusion burettes, flasks or bags must be checked regularly. During major surgery, such as open heart operations, or when cardiovascular status is unstable, measurement of hourly urinary output is useful to assess fluid balance as well as renal function, although this may be difficult in infants.

In many operations blood loss can only be estimated by clinical observation. Where blood can be collected in graduated jars in the suction line and the amount of added fluid estimated reliably, it is useful to measure blood loss. Small graduated suction traps are available to measure blood loss in children more accurately. Weighing of sponges and swabs (provided these are not soaked in large amounts of fluid) can be useful. The haemodilution method is still sometimes used when all swabs and suction material are mixed in a container of known volume (usually a modified washing machine), the haemoglobin content of the fluid then being used as a guide to blood loss. Whatever means are used to estimate blood loss, clinical observation of the patient with frequent assessment of cardiovascular status is the basis of management. The smaller the patient, the more difficulty may be experienced in measuring blood loss accurately. A rising pulse is often the first sign of hypovolaemia.

BIOCHEMISTRY AND HAEMATOLOGY

In some circumstances, estimation of blood constituents is valuable during operation. In premature infants and in the management of diabetics, estimation of blood glucose is useful. Glucose oxidase reagent strips are simple and can be useful provided the test strips are fresh. A drop of blood is placed on the strip, allowed to remain for 1 minute and then washed or wiped off. The resultant colour is then read in a reflectance colorimeter calibrated for the strips used. These measurements can be backed up where necessary by laboratory tests.

When bleeding has been excessive, haemoglobin or haematocrit estimations are useful as a guide to the appropriate replacement fluids. Abnormal bleeding may demand coagulation tests to enable appropriate management.

Blood gas measurements and estimation of acid−base status are indicated in the management of respiratory and resuscitation problems. Estimation of electrolytes, particularly of sodium and potassium, may be needed.

THE ANAESTHETIST

In practice, anaesthetists are often faced with incidents which could result in an adverse outcome for the patient. Although paediatric patients may be more resilient in recovery from potential incidents, the time delay in their progression tends to be shorter than in adults. Thus monitoring forms a vital component of good anaesthetic care.

Whatever apparatus is available to help monitor the patient's condition and make anaesthesia safer, the most important safeguard for the patient is diligent observation by the anaesthetist. The anaesthetist must continually evaluate all information from monitoring systems and use that information to make decisions regarding treatment. Careful selection and arrangement of monitors in the operating room is important so that all displays can be seen and the controls reached easily, without preventing access to the patient or other apparatus. All prime monitors should be concentrated in one area or on one screen, and the number of unnecessary visual and auditory monitoring signals reduced so that distraction is avoided and vigilance enhanced. The most important audible signal should be that from the pulse oximeter.

It is becoming increasingly clear that the combination of pulse oximetry, capnography and close clinical observation will detect most clinical incidents before any adverse outcome occurs. The introduction of, and adherence to, recognized standards or guidelines for patient monitoring (see Appendix 7) will help to ensure maximum patient safety during anaesthesia.

REFERENCES

1 Holmes C.McK. An oxygen failure warning and patient protection system. The Howison unit. *Anaes Intens Care* 1978, **6**, 71.
2 Cooper J.B., Newbower R.S., Kitz R.J. An analysis of major errors and equipment failures in anaesthesia management: considerations for prevention and detection. *Anesthesiology* 1984, **60**, 34.
3 Caplan R.A., Posner K., Ward R.W., Cheney F.W. Respiratory mishaps: principal areas of risk and implications for anaesthetic care. *Anesthesiology* 1987, **67**, A469.

5: The Child in Hospital

INTRODUCTION

Every child who enters hospital is an individual with his own personality based on inherent constitutional factors and on life experiences, but he is also a member of a family, a cultural group, a kindergarten or school and a society. He may then, often quite suddenly, have to become part of a hospital society with rules, people and procedures very different from those he has experienced before. All the things that happen to him will have an impact; kind supportive people can help him to understand, integrate and learn to accept these as being beneficial to him. Otherwise, he may learn that people do not care, they hurt without explanation and they leave him alone, frightened and lost in a confusing nightmare of nurses, trolleys, injections, smells, screens and suspicions. The paediatric anaesthetist has a most important role in relieving the child's fear of an operation and of being put to sleep. He can help the child feel that he is an important person to this doctor, who cares that

he understands what is happening to him, why a procedure is being done, and how he will feel before and after surgery.

The reaction of the child to hospitalization has been extensively studied by paediatricians, psychiatrists, anaesthetists, nurses and administrators, and some of this information is referred to in this chapter.

THE CHILD'S REACTION

Developmental age, family relationships, the child's inherent personality, the nature of the surgical condition, how well he has been prepared for hospitalization and the effect and timing of separation from parents all influence a child's response to hospital and surgery. The reaction to injections, fear of anaesthesia and operation and the effect of the hospital environment also need to be considered.

Developmental age

The young baby is too often regarded as a non-feeling individual who does not experience loss or separation, and on whom procedures may be carried out without preparation or consideration. Even babies a few weeks old are sensitive to their environment and it is important that they should be handled with gentleness and kindness.

The pre-school child is at the developmental stage of egocentrism and he relates everything that happens to himself. He often ascribes life to inanimate objects and he may believe that both his bad and good wishes come true. Children reason at this age according to their own preconceived ideas and show a different logic from that of adults. It is important to be aware of an individual child's beliefs, so that if a 4- or 5-year-old child is told that he is going to be put to sleep he should not deduce that you are going to treat him like his old family pet who was put to sleep — permanently. He should be told that he will be woken up after the operation. A child may stay awake all night because his mother has told him that the operation would be done when he is asleep.

Children attempt to rationalize their ill health as due to something bad they have done, such as disobeying a parent, stealing, or running instead of walking across the road, and that the operation is the deserved punishment.

The older school-age child is more aware of the events taking place around him, and tries to make sense from his observations about what has and what will happen to him. He may ask many questions and it is appropriate to answer these adequately and treat him as a sensible, co-operative person.

Family relationships

Every child brings into hospital the feelings of trust or mistrust acquired from his relationship with parents, and to a lesser extent with siblings. The child, secure in the affection of parents, can easily transfer this trust to the hospital staff, just as he can trust teachers when starting school. However, we live in a society where there are many emotionally impoverished families, where child maltreatment by neglect as well as physical injury is fairly common, and where broken marriages, frequent changes of home and lack of constancy of relationships occur with increasing frequency. Family attitudes differ according to racial, cultural and religious affiliations. Some children are brought up to fear the doctor and the hospital, just as some families believe that all unpleasant events must be hidden from children and they are protected from the news of family illness, hardship or distress. These children are often misled as to the reason for their visit to the hospital.

Personality differences

All parents are aware of the inherent differences in personality which distinguish their offspring. They comment not only on physical appearance but on different temperaments, and how some babies or children are nervy and highly strung, while others are placid and even-tempered. Children differ in their ability to respond to and receive affection. Some infants fail to make adequate emotional adjustments, even in the hands of a good mother [1]. Some children are more susceptible than others to family stresses.

Preparation for hospital

Part of the preparation of children for hospitalization should be to tell them why they are going to hospital and need an operation and anaesthetic. This can be explained by the surgeon and reinforced by parents.

Other methods of informing the child what to expect include extensive time-consuming programmes involving tours of the hospital, including the operating suite and recovery room, preparation protocols, like those described by Petrillo [2], the use of preparation booklets such as 'Humphrey's Visit to Hospital' [3], and videos showing what happens in hospital. It is useful if these are available preoperatively for hire.

Parents, particularly if they are familiar with hospitals and have been patients themselves, can often help their child considerably by explaining what happens in hospital and the series of events which the child might expect. Understanding parents can give an insight into hospital procedures without creating fear in their children. At the other extreme, parents may be frightened to tell their children anything, for fear of upsetting them. One father told his son, aged nearly 6, that they were going to the hospital to see the doctor, 'just a visit, because otherwise he would be scared'. He did not tell the boy that he was having an operation nor did he discuss it afterwards, because he did not want the child to cry. Preoperatively, this patient was withdrawn and the nursing staff regarded him as distressed. The anaesthetist thought he was timid. The anaesthetist then found that the premedication, although given at the appropriate time, was ineffective and that the child was very distressed at induction, and later developed bronchospasm. Postoperatively he was observed to be a quiet, withdrawn, frightened boy, and it is reasonably certain that, since he will not be given the opportunity to work through this experience, future hospitalization will be distressing to him.

The child's doctors, especially the surgeon, can help both the parents and the child by explaining adequately what procedures will be carried out, creating rapport and gaining the confidence of the child. The essential aspect of preparation is that the child trusts the person explaining events to him, and this trust is not destroyed by misleading information.

There are advantages in a 'pre-anaesthetic' class of 10–15 children scheduled for operation the following day. Twenty minutes can be spent in discussion with the children, encouraging questions and answering them truthfully [4]. Children gain from learning that others will experience similar procedures and that they are not alone in their fear; there is the added advantage of the opportunity to form friendships.

Since we live in an age of television and visual learning,

there is much to recommend a film as an introduction to the hospital environment and the events leading up to anaesthesia and recovery after surgery [5]. There are several films portraying a child's admission to hospital, the experiences he may encounter and parents' participation in his care.

Many other studies have been made of the effect of different forms of preparation for children entering hospital for surgery. The reports vary. Some found operative procedures were associated with a degree of 'psychic shock' in children who were inadequately prepared or misled about their hospitalization, or who came from disturbed family environments [6]. Others claim that over 90% of children were either scarcely affected or benefited from their hospital experience [7]. Behavioural disturbances that could reflect the attitudes and anxieties of the parents before and after discharge of their child from hospital, have been described [8].

Hospital environment

The awareness of the total hospital environment and the effect of each person coming into contact with the child is not fully recognized or acknowledged. Ward assistants, cleaners, clerks, theatre assistants, other parents and other children, all contribute to the hospital world and have an impact on the child. The advantage of a children's hospital or a children's ward in a general hospital, particularly if there is a children's operating theatre, is that the staff are generally attuned to the needs of infants and children.

Separation from parents

Anxiety about separation is understandably greater in the young child. To the young infant, toddler and pre-school child, their home and mother is to them the familiar and expected comforting world. Young children have little or no experience of big buildings, strange smells, big beds different from their own, and of people in uniforms with caps or white coats.

Mother and home are protective and offer security and no young child wants to be separated from them. Films and writings by the Robertsons (1956–1972) [9] have shown the emotional impact of hospitalization. Nurses and other hospital staff should be encouraged to include in their care the comforting normally undertaken by the child's parents. The majority of nursing and ward personnel are kind, responding people but sometimes

their technical training and the emphasis placed on scientific and procedural matters blunt their caring attitudes.

Whereas the common reaction of the young child is to protest, usually by crying when his mother leaves him, some children express their feelings by withdrawal. This reaction causes considerable distress to some mothers and is often misunderstood by inexperienced doctors and nurses [10]. It is important to correct this feeling of rejection, of 'he doesn't want to see me so I won't visit', or 'she can't be a good mum' and to recognize that this child needs, as much as the more openly expressive child, the presence and warmth of mother and the attention of nurses and doctors. It is important to recognize that the 'too good' child on the ward may be depressed, anxious or angry, but too frightened to display these feelings, and needs compassionate care. For some children separation is mainly experienced as loneliness, and in modern hospitals with their television sets it must be remembered that children need personal companionship and not just a picture.

The time of separation of the child from the parents has some bearing on the child's reaction, which is also related to the child's age, maturity and self-assurance. In younger children who are admitted the day before surgery, it is preferable if the parent can stay overnight with the child or at least be there preoperatively so that the child does not feel abandoned. The trend of bringing the child into hospital on the morning of the operation avoids the separation of the child from his parents before surgery.

The timing of separation varies and depends on many factors. In some hospitals a parent may accompany the child to the induction room and stay until anaesthesia has been induced. This can be advantageous, especially for pre-school children, if the parent is well adjusted and the anaesthetist is not stressed or hindered by their presence. In one study of children aged 2–6 years, those who were accompanied to the anaesthetic room and during induction by their mother were found to be better emotionally than a similar group who were unaccompanied. The behaviour of the mothers during the induction was assessed; all were enthusiastic about accompanying their child and behaved appropriately [11].

Some mothers are anxious and the anxiety may be conveyed to the child, who might not otherwise have been upset. Figure 5.1 shows that anxious parents are more anxious if they are with their child at induction, while with calm parents the opposite occurs. It is certainly undesirable having present a mother who cannot cope,

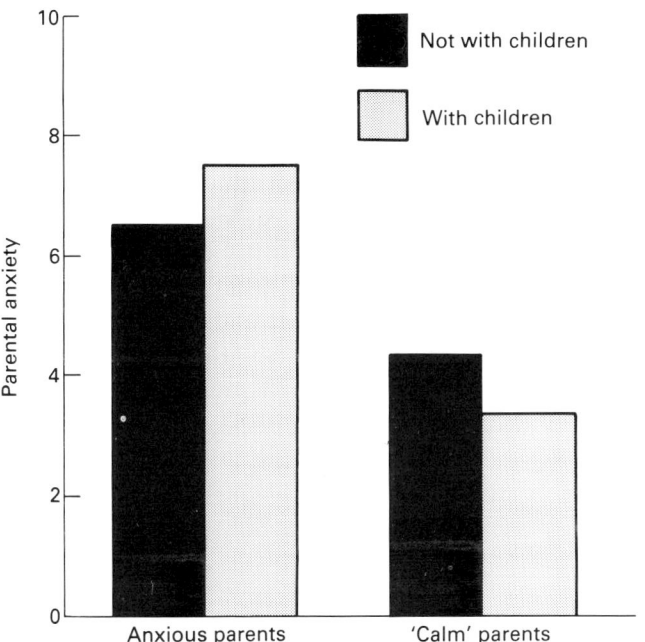

Fig. 5.1 The effect of parents accompanying children to induction on parental anxiety. It is increased in anxious parents and reduced in calm parents. (Data derived from Johnston [12].)

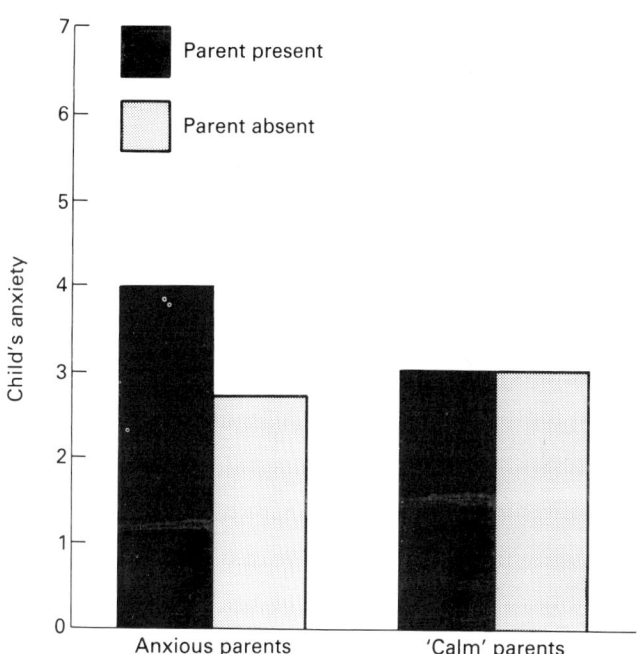

Fig. 5.2 The effect of parental presence on the child's anxiety at induction. Anxious parents have an adverse effect while with calm parents there is no difference. (Data derived from Johnston [12].)

or faints during induction of anaesthesia. As well as the distraction caused, someone then has to look after the mother. Some anaesthetists can perform their task comfortably in the presence of parents and happily accept them, while others, even some very experienced paediatric anaesthetists, feel more tense and uncomfortable and prefer not to have parents present. It has been demonstrated that child anxiety was increased when anxious parents were present compared to not being at induction, while children's anxiety was not influenced by parental presence when the parents were not anxious (Fig. 5.2) [12]. In some instances the child plays the anaesthetist off against the parent, which can interfere with a smooth induction. Experience in anaesthetizing children on several occasions, sometimes with and at other times without parents present, has shown that some children are more relaxed and more easily managed without their parents. This applies increasingly to school-age children as they grow older. This is illustrated in Fig. 5.3, which also shows that anxiety is significantly reduced with either sedation or parental presence [13, 14].

Not all parents wish to accompany their children to the induction room. Parental attitudes vary in different places. Where it is a socially accepted practice it is difficult for those who do not wish to accompany their

child. One way of resolving this difficulty is to say that they cannot accompany their child but to allow them to come if they say they really want to. In this way those who do not wish to go do not feel inadequate. One study found that half the parents wished to accompany their child to induction, either because of their child's anxiety or their own sense of duty. Thirty-two per cent of these changed their preference if the child was adequately sedated preoperatively; 18% did not want to accompany their children [15].

Having parents attending the induction of anaesthesia is easier where there are only one or two operating theatres, rather than a big theatre suite where there is a large turnover of cases − in the latter, the economic factors of having several extra people to supervise parents, and the cost of gowning them, become significant.

There are patients with communication difficulties due to deafness, blindness or other handicaps, where the parents' presence may be helpful both to the child and the anaesthetist. In hospitals where parents do not normally accompany their children to the induction room, there should always be an option to allow parents to come with such children.

When parents are not normally allowed to come into

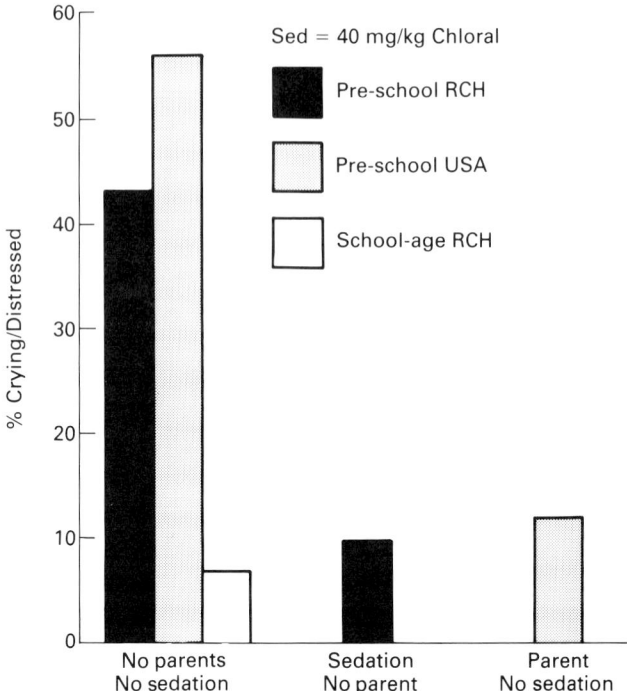

Fig. 5.3 This shows that unpremedicated pre-school children without parents present at induction are much more distressed than pre-school children who have been premedicated or have a parent present. Distress is uncommon in school-age children even without premedication or parental presence. (Data derived from Hannalah and Anderson [13, 14].)

the induction room, some hospitals allow them to come to the waiting area, but this will depend on there being a large enough area. The advantage of continuing parental support can be offset by the mothers becoming upset on separation [14]. It is easier to separate from a well-premedicated sleeping child.

When parents do not come into the waiting area or induction room, separation can occur after the premedication has taken effect, when the child leaves the ward or at the operating theatre suite entrance. If special staff are available to look after the children in the waiting area, separation in the ward is better than at the theatre entrance, where the problem of separation is compounded by entry into a strange area.

When all these points are considered, each hospital has to develop appropriate protocols. In general, pre-kindergarten children from the age of about 6−7 months, but especially 1−3-year-olds, benefit the most from parental presence. Before this infants are less discriminating while older children readily accept the support of others. Another important factor is to have caring staff who show an interest in the children at all times.

Transportation to the operating theatre

Some children are very anxious while they are being transported from the ward to the operating theatre. The fully awake child can talk to the nurse or attendant and be reassured as to where they are going and what is happening. An inadequately sedated child may be frightened, but too afraid to talk or indicate their feelings. Being shunted along corridors, into a crowded lift and sometimes left alone outside the operating suite without a kindly word may be very frightening. In one survey, a girl said that the worst part of her hospital experience was that nobody talked to her while she was waiting to go into the induction room. She felt very lonely and scared. It is very important for porters, nurses and other staff to talk to children when they are awake during transportation or while waiting.

Fear of venepuncture

School-age children, particularly those between 5 and 12 years, fear injections most. The application of EMLA (eutectic mixture of local anaesthetic) cream at the site of venepuncture has largely eliminated the discomfort. Although children of this age are better able to separate from their parents and to relate to other children in the ward, it is the fear of needles that worries them. Fear may be suspected in children who are inadequately premedicated when their veins are found to be very constricted, making venepuncture more difficult. Children should be told that venepuncture with a small needle causes little discomfort compared with other injections they may have had, especially intramuscular ones.

Fear of anaesthesia

The fear of anaesthesia may be the fear of not being fully asleep and thus feeling pain during surgery, or of not waking up after the operation [16]. A 13-year-old girl who had a splenectomy described her experiences: 'The effect of the needle [the premedication] made me panicky. Later I felt like going to sleep but I was still aware that soon I would have an operation and come back all scarred. I tried to keep awake to see everything was all right. If it was stronger that would have been better, because I was still conscious of being frightened. I had to sit in the hall, just left there, and everything was hazy. After a long time they moved the trolley into a room and everybody just seemed to talk pleasantly about the weather and their cases. That was awful because they didn't seem to have any concern for me. I was just another case, while really I was scared to death. I couldn't feel the next injection; it didn't bother me, but I thought they might start straight away, operating without really seeing that I was asleep. My eyes were closed because they were so heavy and I couldn't move my hand to show them that I was still awake, but I could hear. I was really afraid that I would wake up in the middle of it and feel the pain. They should have told me that everything would be all right.'

This illustrates how even an older child can be terrified because the staff do not appreciate her feelings. Anaesthetists should concentrate on their patients during induction, and reassure them that they will be looking after them during their operation.

Fear of surgery

It is not always realized that children fear the results of surgery. Even young children may have misconceptions about what the surgeon will be doing, and which part of their anatomy is to be removed. Earlier reports of children undergoing tonsillectomy showed that some expected an operation on their abdomen, particularly if they had pregnancy fantasies and their only knowledge of anyone going into hospital was to have a baby. A 10-year-old child admitted with a fractured arm said, 'Before going to theatre I thought I was a cripple, and you can't cure cripples, so I was very scared'.

Boys admitted for orchidopexy or circumcision may be especially worried that they might lose or suffer damage to their penis.

The adolescent is particularly concerned with his body integrity: it is the narcissistic age, the body beautiful time, when worries about pimples, greasy hair, height and figure — particularly breast development — assume enormous proportions. An understanding of this developmental stage explains why many teenage patients need more rather than less reassurance about the exact nature of the surgical procedure. They may be equally frightened by injections and many a healthy 6-foot youth has fainted during a venepuncture, despite the bravado of his conversation.

The outcome of heart and brain surgery may have more serious consequences, so these children need extra care and reassurance.

Parents' anxiety

Many parents are anxious about their child having surgery. It is often important to reassure them so that they do not transmit their anxiety to the child. Parents are often particularly anxious when their child is having a major operation where the result will determine the child's future. Parents usually expect the worst and their anxiety increases if operations take longer than expected, so they should be informed if it is progressing satisfactorily when the expected time has passed. This helps to reassure them and is much appreciated by the parents.

IDENTIFYING THE CHILD AT RISK OF EMOTIONAL DISTURBANCE

The concept of the child's vulnerability or resistance to stress such as hospitalization and surgery can be likened to the impact made on three dolls, one of glass, one of celluloid and a third of steel. If the dolls are hit with a hammer using equal strength, the first doll would break, the second scar and the third emit a pleasant musical sound [17]. Some individuals shatter easily, some are affected but recover, and some recover with additional strength shown in ways characteristic of the particular child. It should be possible to identify children who are at risk of adverse emotional effects from their hospitalization and operation. Several questions can be asked which will indicate increased vulnerability to stress and the need for extra support and care:

1 Has the child shown adverse reactions to previous separations?
2 Has the child had marked disturbances in feeding or sleeping behaviour?
3 Has the child revealed excessive fears — of the dark, of strangers, or of being left in new surroundings?
4 Does the child appear to be over-anxious in response to changes in routine or surroundings?
5 Did the child respond to the news of proposed hospitalization with excessive anxiety, asking many questions, or by withdrawal or refusal to talk about it?
6 Does the child mix well with other children?
7 Has the child been hospitalized before and how did he respond?
8 Have there been any recent crises or recent deaths in the family?

It is useful to try to assess how the parents relate to the child and how much they support and help in overcoming anxieties. One should also observe the parents' personalities and level of anxiety about their child and the hospitalization and surgery. The parent—child relationship is of unparalleled importance in the emotional development and the security of the child.

There are children undergoing major surgery or who have been severely injured or burnt, whose preparation may be inadequate. The postoperative course may be prolonged and involve extensive monitoring and other supportive treatment such as ventilation. These children will require additional care and extra efforts should be made, not only to provide good medical and nursing treatment, but also social and psychological services where these are indicated. It is regrettable that personnel involved in supportive care in many hospitals work only regular office hours, so that patient care at night and at weekends is often deficient, causing children additional stress. It is important that parents can be with such children, even in intensive care units, to give them support during the critical stages of their postoperative course.

THE ROLE OF THE ANAESTHETIST AND ASSISTANTS

The preoperative visit is an important part of the child's preparation for operation. As well as giving the anaesthetist the opportunity to check the patient's physical condition and other relevant details, it provides a chance to make himself known and to gain the confidence of the child, so that when the patient arrives in theatre there will be at least one familiar person there. The anaesthetist can use an identifying object, such as a toy, which the child can be shown at the preoperative visit and again in the induction room to aid recognition. The anaesthetist's approach will vary considerably, depending on the age of the child, but if he can talk about things with which the child is familiar and interested, some rapport can be developed. Little children, particularly if their parents are there for reassurance, can with encouragement be picked up or sat on the anaesthetist's knee, making them feel that he really wants to be their friend.

If the parents are present during the preoperative visit the anaesthetist can help allay their fears, which will benefit the child, as apprehensive parents can transmit their anxieties to the children. It reassures the parents if the anaesthetist can gain rapport with their child and it is often helpful to do this before turning attention to them to ask the necessary questions and answer their queries.

It is important that those involved in transporting children to the operating theatre, those who care for them while they are waiting to be anaesthetized and those helping with the induction, should all take an interest in the patient.

When the child arrives in theatre, the anaesthetist should speak to him while he is waiting. Before induction, the child should become the centre of attention and other small talk between the anaesthetist and assistants should cease. It should be remembered that the hearing is the last sense to be lost. In these ways the child will feel cared for, particularly if the anaesthetist continues reassurance.

Some babies and small children can be anaesthetized in the arms of their mother, nurse or the anaesthetist.

If the child is likely to remain intubated, have chest drains, catheters, intravenous cannulae, nose packed or the eyes covered postoperatively, the anaesthetist should explain this before the operation.

CHILDREN IN THE INTENSIVE CARE UNIT

There are many reasons for admission of children to an intensive care unit. They can be admitted with potentially short-term diseases, such as epiglottitis, where intubation is necessary for some hours, electively following major surgery where intensive monitoring and possibly ventilation are needed, following major trauma or with complicated life-threatening diseases. Patients with major trauma are a special category, because there is no opportunity to warn them that they may require intensive care, and other members of the family or friends may have been injured or killed. These patients may be unconscious or have been admitted because of cardiovascular or respiratory complications. Renal failure may occur if they have been in shock and they may need dialysis.

Medical patients may be critically ill, unconscious or require an artificial airway. Children may be unconscious following drug overdosage, requiring ventilation or monitoring for dysrhythmia. Monitoring may continue while the child recovers and he may suddenly become aware of abnormal and rather frightening surroundings.

Those requiring an artificial airway may be otherwise well and, if possible, should be placed in a part of the unit away from critically ill and dying patients.

Neonates may require respiratory support following surgery, e.g. infants with congenital diaphragmatic hernia or tracheo-oesophageal fistula. More and more premature infants are now being treated for the respiratory distress syndrome. In some hospitals, neonates are looked after in special neonatal units, while in others they are cared for in part of a general intensive care unit.

The psychological effects of being a patient in an intensive care unit vary depending on the patient's age. Neonates, attached to various pieces of apparatus and monitoring equipment, will suffer from lack of maternal contact and cuddling by nurses. It is important for parents to visit and spend time with their child and for staff to remember that their patients may become very lonely if not spoken to and treated with compassion and gentle handling. An anaesthetist who has been a patient himself in an intensive care unit has described the enormous difference made by people just being kind to him. The worst feeling he had was being 'out on his own', and he emphasized the importance of people giving him hope.

It is important for the staff to recognize that most of their patients are conscious and aware of their surroundings, and that they should talk to them and explain what is going on. Even if they do not appear responsive, they may appreciate more than is apparent. Children should be encouraged, and if they are getting better they should always be told. It is easy to talk about patients and their condition within their hearing and conscious effort should be made by staff to avoid this. Patients may hear things which increase their anxieties and feelings of isolation, as they know they are being discussed but not included.

Resuscitation is frequently required in an intensive care unit, and many patients have intravenous or intra-arterial cannulae, endotracheal tubes or urinary catheters. Although some may be unconscious or unable to appreciate or respond to these manoeuvres, others are aware that they are being performed and suffer discomfort, though unable to indicate this. Although these procedures may be life-saving, one should always remember that they are being carried out on people and not on physiological models, and that the sense of hearing is the last to be lost.

Intensive care units are frequently noisy places, with monitors, respirators, audible signals, alarms and repeated observations so that the infant or child is disturbed every 15 or 30 minutes. The lighting is never dimmed because of the importance of close observation, and hence sleep is difficult, although particularly necessary when recovering from the acute phase of an illness. Sedation is sometimes indicated in these situations and for children being ventilated, particularly if they also need to be paralysed. It is preferable to separate the conscious awake child, fearful but recovering, from the very ill or dying child and from those with intensive monitoring. Some of the excessive anxiety created by the atmosphere of the unit can be reduced by nursing the recovering child in a different area or separating by screens and by increased visiting.

The very ill child who may die, or survive as a sub-normal individual, presents serious moral, ethical and medical problems. The views of individual doctors as to how any patient should be handled vary considerably, and there are no fixed guidelines. The problem is that one cannot always tell which patient will make a good recovery and which will survive with a severe mental or physical handicap, placing an extra burden on the family and on the community, although intensivists have made significant advances in delineating positive and negative prognostic signs, which are sometimes helpful.

The medical staff of intensive care units, which frequently includes anaesthetists, have a responsibility not only to the patient and his family but also the nursing staff, who are expected to maintain a very high standard of efficiency and care, and to meet the incessant demands of the machines, the children and their parents.

When a child is cared for over a prolonged period, the staff inevitably form an attachment, which is broken when the child recovers and moves to another ward, or when he dies, and they are left with a deep feeling of loss. Thus the staff are subject to strain from their exacting work, frustration when their efforts do not produce the desired results, tension about the morality of sustaining life in apparently hopeless cases, and mourning when one of their patients dies. It is important for the Director of such a unit to be sensitive to these aspects and to ensure that his staff have access to support. In some units this may be a special individual or a group meeting with a psychiatric or paediatric colleague; in others it may be a general awareness of each other's level of stress and a sharing of this by communication.

THE DEATH OF A CHILD

Anaesthetists are rarely involved with death in the operating theatre, but are when this occurs in the intensive care unit. In the past, the dying child was often avoided, because of the doctors' interest in activities which prolong life and failure to understand the meaning of death to a child and to his family. Very simply, the child's fears of dying are that he will be left alone, abandoned, beyond hope or comfort. The parents do not want their child to suffer unnecessary pain and they are apprehensive of their anguish if the child dies. The child will always gain from contact with a concerned person; even when dying, the softly spoken word, the touch of a hand will convey comfort and care.

Families will respond to truthful explanations of how and why the child died, given as soon as possible after the event. Parents often seem to understand, better than the doctor, that no one is omnipotent or immortal. Even the angry parent who appears to blame the medical staff will be assisted by the opportunity to talk through this anger, which is often a defence for grief, and learn of the care the child received and the inevitability of death.

The anaesthetist has a role to play in supporting both the dying child and his family. It should not be presumed that this has been carried out effectively by other medical or nursing staff. Those doctors who are able to feel close to people and support them in times of crisis, will be appreciated by their patients and relatives to whom this compassion and concern is communicated. Sometimes this supportive understanding is provided by staff less directly concerned with the physical care of the child. A social worker, psychiatrist or hospital chaplain may be the most appropriate person to support a particular family. The family may include siblings who suffer unrecognized grief and have been neglected by their parents, whose energies were necessarily directed to the ill and dying child.

CONCLUSION

Despite the development of a more scientific approach to anaesthesia and the introduction of more equipment, the anaesthetist must remember that the patients are people and that, however young, they have feelings. Children will develop trust or distrust according to their experiences and how they are treated by all the staff who look after them.

REFERENCES

1 Lourie R.S. The first three years of life. *Am J Psychiatr* 1971, **127**, 11.

2 Petrillo M., Snager S. *Emotional care of hospitalized children.* (1972) Lippincott, Philadelphia.

3 Rule G. *Humphrey's visits to hospital.* (1972) Opal Books, Rigby, Adelaide.

4 Hodges R.J.H. Induction of anaesthesia in young children. *Lancet* 1960, **1**, 82.

5 Vernon D.T.A., Bailey W.C. The use of motion pictures in the psychologic preparation of children for induction of anaesthesia. *Anesthesiology* 1974, **40**, 1.

6 Pearson G.J.H. Effect of operative procedures on the emotional life of the child. *Am J Dis Child* 1941, **62**, 716.

7 Jackson K., Winkley A.B., *et al.* Behaviour changes indicating emotional trauma in tonsillectomized children. *Pediatrics* 1953, **12**, 23.

8 Prugh D.G., Staub R.M., *et al.* A study of the emotional reactions of children and families to hospitalization and illness. *Am J Orthopsych* 1953, **23**, 70.

9 Robertson J., Robertson J. Young children at risk: a problem of professional anxiety. In: British Psychoanalytic Society and the Institute of Psychoanalysis. *Scientific Bulletin*, 1972, **54**, 13.

10 Bowlby J., Ainsworth M., *et al.* The effects of mother–child separation: a follow-up study. *Br J Med Psychol* 1956, **29**, 211.

11 Schulman J.L., Foley J.H., *et al.* A study of the effect of the mother's presence during anaesthesia induction. *Pediatrics* 1967, **39**, 111.

12 Johnston C.C., Bevan J.C., Haig M.J., Kirnon V., Tousignant G. Parental presence during anaesthesia induction. *AORN Journal* 1988, **47**, 187.

13 Anderson B.J., Exarchos H., Lee K., Brown T.C.K. Oral premedication in children: a comparison of chloral hydrate, alprazolam, midazolam and placebo for day surgery. *Anaes Intens Care* 1990, **18**, 185.

14 Hannalah R.S., Rosales J.K. Experience with parents' presence during anaesthesia induction in children. *Canad Anaes Soc J*, 1983, **30**, 286.

15 Brande N., Ridley S.A., Sumner E. Parents and paediatric anaesthesia: a prospective survey of parental attitudes to their presence at induction. *Ann RCS (Eng)* 1990, **72**, 41.

16 Ramsay M.A.E. A survey of preoperative fear. *Anaesthesia* 1972, **27**, 396.

17 Anthony E.J. The concept of risk. In: Mussen R. (Ed) *Carmichael's manual of child psychology.* (1970) John Wiley and Sons, Inc. Vol 11.

6: Preoperative Preparation Including Premedication

INTRODUCTION

Children who are scheduled for an elective operation will have attended an outpatient clinic or surgeon's consulting room. At that time the surgeon should have informed the parents and, if appropriate, the patient, of the nature of the procedure to be undertaken and the reason for it. Many parents will have tried to prepare their child for the period in hospital and the operation. In some hospitals, orientation visits are held before admission to show the children what to expect, so that they are better prepared for hospitalization. When a child will need to stay in hospital for a few days postoperatively, admission the day before operation will give him time to become accustomed to the hospital environment. The staff should make every effort to make his stay as pleasant as possible.

Day surgery has become popular for children having minor procedures as it minimizes the period of separation from the parents. This is an important consideration in infants and small children. Parents are instructed about preoperative fasting, and in the interests of their child they will usually make certain that the instructions are followed. Day-care surgery requires adequate facilities for preoperative assessment by the anaesthetist, and for postoperative care. The preoperative assessment can be carried out in the outpatient clinic a day or two earlier. The timing of the operation must be such that the anaesthetist has the opportunity to assess the child preoperatively and there is sufficient time for full recovery before the day-care staff leave.

Emergency admission may impose a greater psychological stress upon patients, particularly if they have not been in hospital before. It may be easier for children to understand why they go to hospital in an emergency, but appropriate explanations are still important and efforts must be made to gain the patients' confidence.

Repeated procedures, such as dilatation of strictures, are particularly likely to disturb children unless great care is taken to establish rapport with them.

A bad experience, such as multiple attempts at venepuncture, may cause a fear of needles and a dread of further anaesthetics, making preoperative preparation more difficult the next time.

PREOPERATIVE VISIT AND ASSESSMENT

Whenever possible, the anaesthetist should see the child preoperatively to assess his condition and to become acquainted, so that at least one face is familiar to the child on arriving in the anaesthetic room. The anaesthetist should tell the child, where appropriate, and the parents, if present, what is involved — explain about preoperative fasting, the method of induction, postoperative discomfort, the recovery room where they will awaken and the intravenous drip or oxygen therapy if these are likely to be used. The parents can be asked to emphasize important points with the child and should know where to wait during the operation. It helps the parents if the anaesthetist reassures them and outlines what will happen to their child. Except where the child has recently been anaesthetized, he should not be expected to choose the type of induction (needle or mask), as he will not have the experience on which to base the choice. If it is necessary for another anaesthetist to make the preoperative visit it should be no less thorough, and full details of any unusual features must be passed on.

The visit is normally made on the evening prior to an elective operation, but where major procedures are planned the surgeon should inform the anaesthetist early, so that there is more time for assessment and consultation in preparing for the operation.

For emergency operations it may not always be possible for the anaesthetist to visit the patient beforehand. If this is the case, one of the surgical staff should inform the anaesthetist about the patient's condition. The anaesthetist should assess the child in theatre prior to induction and ensure that no essential preparation has been omitted.

The preoperative visit should include a review of the patient's clinical notes and an examination of the patient. The information sought by the anaesthetist and his assessment and preparations should include the following:

1 The patient's name for identification and establishing rapport, since children respond better to the use of their first name.

2 The patient's age, as this will give some indication of the anaesthetic equipment required for the operation.

3 The patient's weight will be used to calculate doses of most drugs. Errors in recording the weight do occur and can lead to under- or overdosage. The anaesthetist should assess the patient's size to judge whether the recorded weight is correct or compare it with the average weight for a child of that age. If a discrepancy is suspected, the child should be reweighed.

Consent for operation and anaesthesia should have been signed by a parent or guardian.

The nature of the proposed operation should be determined and its probable extent assessed. The anaesthetist should consider whether an intravenous infusion or blood transfusion will be needed, and ensure that blood is cross-matched or serum held for cross-matching if necessary. Previous anaesthetic charts should be reviewed, and a note made of difficulties or problems which may be relevant to this anaesthetic. Medication which the child may be taking should be noted. Will it affect the anaesthetic management of the patient, or is an important dose of a drug likely to be missed during preoperative fasting or the operation itself?

A history should be obtained of recent illness, incidental medical problems (discussed more fully in Chapter 25), previous anaesthetics with any problems encountered, drug therapy not recorded above and any family history of anaesthetic problems. The nature and time of the last oral intake is particularly important for emergency admissions and day cases. Stomach emptying may

be delayed after injury due to the autonomic nervous system response and/or to the administration of opioids, so that, although a fasting period of 5 or 6 hours is desirable before anaesthesia, there is still danger from a full stomach, particularly if the injury occurred soon after the last meal. The risk must be weighed against the disadvantages to the patient of delaying the procedure, and should be discussed with the surgeon.

Physical examination should be directed to the patient's general condition, colour, state of nutrition and hydration. If the child has an elevated temperature the source of infection should be sought, particularly in the respiratory tract. If the temperature is recorded several times during the day, a single spike may not be of clinical significance. If the last recording was high the temperature should be checked again.

The cardiovascular system should be checked for adequacy of the circulation, heart murmurs or evidence of heart failure. The anaesthetist may be the first person to recognize a heart murmur and should be able to decide whether it is innocent or whether the child should be referred to a cardiologist for an opinion (see Chapter 25).

Other abnormalities should be sought, particularly any which may affect the conduct of anaesthesia, especially maintenance of the airway or tracheal intubation. Micrognathia, a large tongue or abnormal facies associated with syndromes such as Hurler's, Hunter's (Chapter 25), Pierre Robin or Goldenhar (Chapter 17) may be associated with potential difficulties.

Veins should be inspected for possible sites for venepuncture or cannulation. One should be marked as the site where EMLA cream should be applied. It should be applied in a thick layer and covered with an occlusive plastic to maintain contact with the skin, as it requires at least an hour's application to produce adequate analgesia. It may at that time cause a blanching and vasoconstriction but if applied for longer (1.5 hours) the veins may dilate.

Haemoglobin estimation and urinalysis are common preoperative investigations and should be done whenever there is a clinical indication, and before major surgery. The need for the routine use of these investigations is not so great in otherwise healthy children undergoing less major surgery, where significant blood loss is unlikely. Other investigations may be relevant to the patient's condition, such as full blood count, electrolyte and acid–base examination, liver or kidney function tests, and chest X-rays should be reviewed and others ordered if needed.

Preoperative physiotherapy may be needed, especially before cardiac and thoracic surgery. If this has not been done and the patient would benefit from physiotherapy, it should be arranged.

Of other considerations, the most common dilemma for the anaesthetist is the presence of an upper respiratory infection. It may cause some airway obstruction, an increased tendency to laryngospasm [1], bleeding from the respiratory mucosa and bacteraemia. It may also increase the risk of postoperative pulmonary complications, especially if the child is intubated.

If there are purulent secretions and the child is febrile elective surgery should be cancelled. On the other hand, if the temperature is not elevated and the secretions are clear, it is probably reasonable to undertake short procedures where the child is not intubated. In the final analysis, a child who is developing a febrile illness may seem lethargic and not as active as one would expect. If the mother concurs with this assessment it usually means something is developing, and it is wiser to postpone the operation.

There is a whole range of situations which present and little information to guide the anaesthetist on whether or not to proceed with the anaesthetic. If the operation can be postponed without detriment to the child and undue inconvenience and expense to the family, it is preferable to play safe and wait until the child is well. The decision should be made jointly by the parents, the surgeon and the anaesthetist.

The operation may be part of the treatment of an infection, such as draining an abscess. Otherwise the presence of infection should lead to the postponement of elective operations until the infection is treated, unless there are compelling reasons to proceed, which are in the patient's interest.

Even after a full assessment of the patient, the anaesthetist may require further elucidation of some points before he can plan the details of his pre- and intra-operative management. Preoperative discussion with the surgeon may be invaluable for the anaesthetist to identify the nature and extent of the operation, and the presence of any unusual features or requirements. It is helpful if the surgeon warns the anaesthetist well in advance of major or probably complicated operations, so that there is time for proper assessment and a full work-up of the patient before surgery.

The timing of the insertion of an intravenous infusion may need discussion. If preoperative resuscitation and fluids are necessary, the infusion will be started in the ward beforehand. The type of fluid needed is discussed in Chapter 29.

If it appears to the anaesthetist that some further preparation for, or postponement of, the operation is necessary, he must discuss the matter with the surgeon. In emergency surgery the increased risks of inadequate preparation must be weighed against the urgency of performing the operation in deciding when to operate. The decision should always be based on what is best for the patient.

PREPARATION AND FASTING TIME

Studies of blood sugar levels immediately before induction of anaesthesia have shown that the mean values rise gradually with age (Fig. 6.1) and that despite quite long periods of fasting, hypoglycaemia is uncommon (Fig. 6.2). The lowest levels are most likely to occur in low-birth-weight infants [2] but can occur at any age. Those with low blood glucose levels cannot easily be predicted [3].

The question of how long children should be fasted before anaesthesia has received much attention in recent years. The results of studies have varied. Ideally the stomach should be empty when anaesthesia is induced. Some investigators have considered 0.4 ml/kg to be a significant volume in the stomach [4]. The problem is that any volume of fluid or solid material is significant if it is vomited or regurgitated and is aspirated into the trachea, causing respiratory complications, including

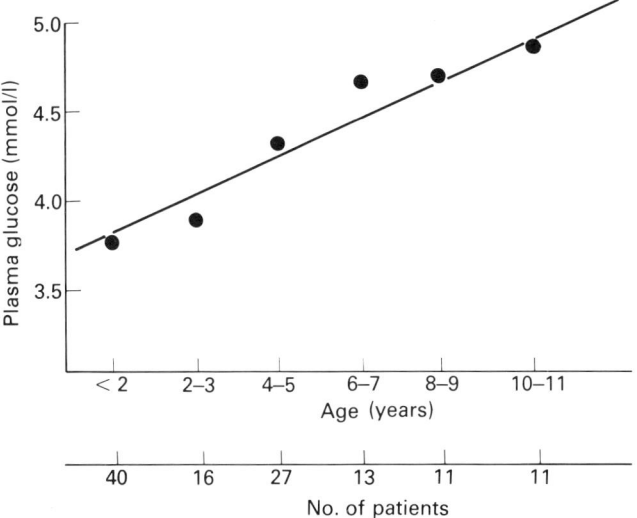

Fig. 6.1 Fasting plasma glucose measured at induction of anaesthesia, showing that the mean levels increase with age [3].

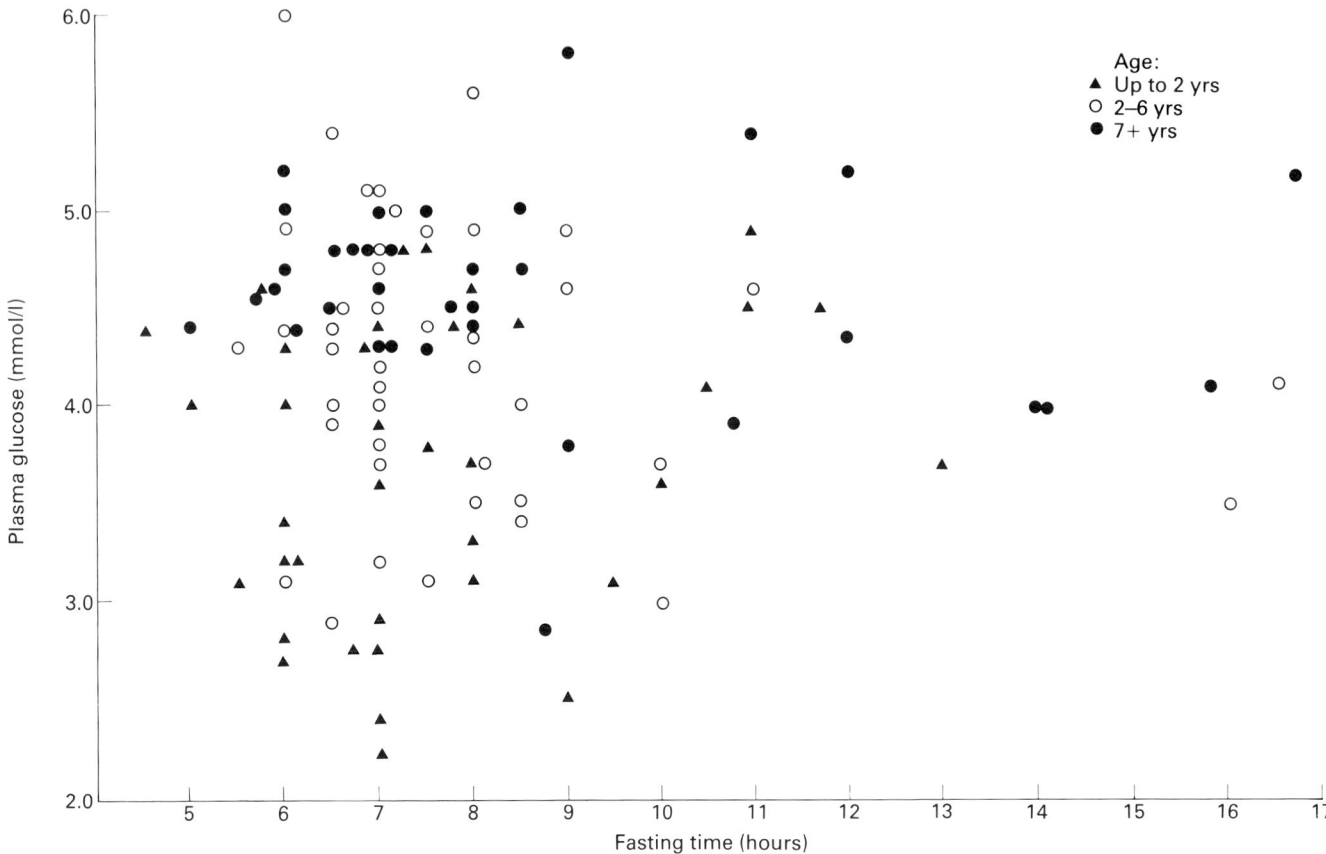

Fig. 6.2 Fasting plasma glucose levels with time of preoperative fasting. The age groups are differentiated and show that the lowest levels were in under-2-year-olds.

hypoxaemia. It is difficult to define beforehand which patients are liable to vomit or regurgitate during anaesthesia unless they have known gastro-oesophageal reflux. Patients who are anxious, in pain, have suffered trauma or have been given opioids may have increased gastric contents due to increased gastric secretions and/or delayed stomach emptying. Boys with torsion of the testis often have large volumes of fluid in the stomach, possibly due to pain. Recent studies have shown that children given a glucose drink, orange (5 ml/kg) or apple juice (5 ml/kg) had little left in their stomachs within 2 hours [5, 6]. The volume decreases exponentially with time — 80% is cleared in the first hour [5].

Although much attention has been given to the pH of stomach contents, clinical experience suggests that Mendelsohn's syndrome is rare in children, compared with obstetric patients. Respiratory complications from aspiration in children seem more likely to result from the volume of fluid or bulk of solids aspirated than to the pH of the fluid. pH can be raised by giving 0.3 ml/kg 0.3 M

sodium citrate immediately prior to induction [7]. H_2 blockers raise pH and may reduce gastric secretions [8–11]. Metoclopramide decreases gastric volume only [10], probably by hastening gastric emptying. Ultimately, the fasting time in patients having elective surgery should be a balance between the provision of oral fluids and calories to avoid hunger and thirst and waiting long enough for stomach emptying, so that the risk of aspiration is minimized. Despite all recommendations, the anaesthetist can never be completely sure that the patient's stomach is empty [12].

For elective procedures, babies under 6 months can be given clear fluids up to 2 hours before anaesthesia. Breast milk can be given up to 3 hours before, but cows' milk should not be given less than 4 hours before as it is less easily digested and absorbed. Using this regimen babies are more tranquil preoperatively, less prone to develop hypoglycaemia and, because they are usually fed every 3–4 hours, they will usually have emptied their stomachs by this time. Care must be taken not to give excessive volumes of fluid at these times, as overfed babies have occasionally vomited milk, although usually without serious consequences. A limit of 20 ml/kg is suggested.

Older children can tolerate longer periods of fasting and a rise in blood glucose is common in response to surgical stress. Solids are usually withheld after midnight for morning operations, and after a light breakfast for afternoon operations. Clear fluids can safely be given up to 3 hours before anaesthesia unless there is a reason such as trauma or opiate administration that will slow stomach emptying. Residual stomach fluid has been shown to be less in children given 10 ml/kg glucose-water drinks 3 hours preoperatively than in children fasted for more than 6 hours.

Before emergency surgery, an interval of at least 4 hours from the last meal is essential, unless the operation is so urgent that the risk of induction with a full stomach must be accepted. If the meal has been a large one, a longer period of fasting is indicated. After trauma, stomach emptying is likely to be delayed, so that even after 8–10 hours of starvation the stomach may still contain food, particularly if the trauma occurred less than 2 hours after the last meal [7]. The severity of trauma is an important determinant of gastric volume [13]. Recently, the use of metoclopramide (0.1 mg/kg) has been advocated to hasten the passage of food through the pylorus. Sitting up or lying on the right side may also facilitate stomach emptying.

PREMEDICATION

The doses and route of administration of the premedicant drugs should be written clearly on the patient's drug order sheet, dated and signed by the anaesthetist. If unusual orders are made, these should be pointed out to the nurse in charge. Sedative or narcotic drugs should *never* be ordered by telephone, as this greatly increases the possibility of error, particularly in young children, and it is illegal. The desired time of administration of drugs must be stated with the order, or the anaesthetist may indicate that he will inform the ward at an appropriate time during the list when the drugs should be given. The annotation 'on call' can be used to indicate this.

Premedication implies the use of drugs, but it should not be forgotten that psychological support is important and in some situations drugs may not be needed. The main purpose of premedication is to relieve the patient's anxiety and provide tranquillity before the operation. A child's attitude to an operation and anaesthetic will depend on age, previous experience, fear of being deformed or even of being put to sleep for ever like a family pet being 'put down' by a vet. Many of these fears will be allayed if the anaesthetist can explain what will happen, within the limits of the child's comprehension, and reassure the child that he will be well cared for. EMLA cream reduces the discomfort of venepuncture (provided, it is applied early enough — at least 1 hour beforehand) and reassurance on this point will allay one of the main fears of many children.

Small children cannot fully understand what is going to happen and it is in this group particularly that allowing a parent to accompany the child to the theatre may be helpful (see Chapter 5).

Premedication is adequate if it sedates the child so that he is sleepy, not caring what is happening and preferably amnesic as well. Oversedation can make a child become disorientated and more difficult to manage. It is easier to reassure an unpremedicated older child than one who is agitated because his inhibitions have been reduced by premedication.

The choice of premedication will also influence the conduct of anaesthesia. An inhalation induction will often be appropriate after oral premedication, while an intravenous induction is usually well accepted by children following morphine or papaveretum and hyoscine because they are euphoric, amnesic, analgesic and their veins are usually dilated, making venepuncture easy.

Many drugs have been used for premedication in children, by several routes of administration. Many factors need to be considered when comparative trials are assessed, but the fact that so many approaches to premedication are in use suggests that the perfect drug or combination is not yet available [14]. The sedation and tranquillity nearly always achieved by intramuscular morphine or papaveretum and hyoscine produces close to the ideal conditions for the anaesthetist at induction, but neither the nurses nor the children enjoy the premedication injections and the incidence of postoperative vomiting is tripled by the use of an opiate [15].

The various drugs used in premedication will be considered in groups according to the purpose for which they are given.

Psychic sedation

Formerly, barbiturates were used for sedation, but now

the most widely used groups of drugs are the benzodiazepines and phenothiazines, given 1–2 hours preoperatively as a suspension or tablet, depending on age. Diazepam (0.3 mg/kg) has been widely used but recently midazolam, temazepam, alpazolam, flunitrazepam and lorazepam have been tried. They may produce some amnesia, although lorazepam probably has the greatest effect. A trial in children over 4 years comparing the first four with paracetamol, all given orally, showed no significant difference between them and no difference between them and patients given placebo [16]. Midazolam is shorter acting than the others, particularly in children where the elimination half-life after i.v. bolus is 70 minutes [17]. It has been used for premedication intramuscularly (0.15 mg/kg) [17], orally (0.45–0.75 mg/kg) [17, 18], rectally and intranasally (0.2 mg/kg) [19, 20]. In the latter group, peak serum levels were reached in 11 ± 2 min [20].

Chlorpromazine (0.5–1 mg/kg) was introduced in 1960 by Laborit to suppress the stress responses to surgery. It was a landmark, as its introduction opened up the whole field of psychopharmacology. It is still a useful agent as a tranquillizer, antiemetic, sympathetic blocker (central and alpha-adrenergic receptors) and it is particularly useful when surface-cooling hypothermia is to be induced. Promethazine (0.5 mg/kg) is often used with pethidine, particularly for asthmatics. Trimeprazine (3–4 mg/kg) has been recommended [21] but the patients tend to be sleepy for too long postoperatively, especially for day surgery, and are often not suitably sedated for intravenous induction.

Chloral hydrate (40 mg/kg orally) and trichloral are good sedatives for infants and small children (under 4 years). They produce better sedation than benzodiazepines in this age group, but chloral hydrate has a bad taste and there is a significant incidence of restlessness before sedation occurs.

Rectal administration

Rectal administration of premedication is used in some centres, but is not universally popular. Rectal pH varies from 7 to 12, so that absorption will vary [26]. It has been shown that higher plasma levels of methohexitone are achieved with a 2% than with a 10% solution [27]. The doses normally used of thiopentone (30–45 mg/kg 10% solution) and methohexitone (15–20 mg/kg) are much higher than the intravenous dose. Continued uptake can lead to postoperative drowsiness unless the excess

drug is aspirated when the patient is asleep [28]. In many centres this route is not used, because children require closer preoperative observation due to the variability in response and degree of sedation achieved, and many children are upset by the rectal administration of drugs.

Analgesia

Analgesia can be obtained by the use of any of the commonly used opioid drugs. Morphine (0.2 mg/kg i.m.) and papaveretum (0.4 mg/kg i.m.) produce more psychic sedation than pethidine and have a longer action. They should be given 1–1.25 hours before operation for optimal effect before induction. Pethidine, with a more rapid onset and shorter duration of action, is often used when there is only an hour or less before emergency operations, and it is the preferred drug for asthmatics. These drugs all cause respiratory depression and should be given in reduced dosage if a prolonged inhalation anaesthetic with spontaneous respiration is contemplated. They should be avoided or used in smaller doses when the child has some airway obstruction (e.g. from very large tonsils and adenoids).

Orally administered analgesics such as buprenorphine and methadone have not yet been widely used in children. They are generally longer acting, but methadone has an irregular duration of action.

Pentazocine (0.5 mg/kg) is comparable to morphine for premedication, but care should be taken to ensure that, if it is used for premedication, it is also given for postoperative analgesia if required, because it antagonizes morphine-like drugs. The incidence of postoperative vomiting is comparable to the incidence after morphine [22]. Dysphoria can occur.

The opioids are not usually used in premedication under 6 months of age. If they are employed, the dose should be reduced so that respiratory depression and apnoea are avoided.

New approaches have been tried, such as fentanyl given in a lollipop so that the drug is absorbed transmucosally in the mouth. The optimal dose is 15–20 µg/kg. It causes dose-related respiratory depression, facial itching and vomiting [23, 24].

The transnasal route is currently under investigation for drugs such as sufentanil (2–3 µg/kg) [25].

Patients with raised intracranial pressure should not be given respiratory depressant drugs for premedication. A benzodiazepine provides satisfactory anxiolysis.

Drying of secretions

The commonly used antisialagogues are hyoscine (0.008 mg/kg), atropine (0.01 mg/kg) and glycopyrrolate (0.01 mg/kg). They are most effective for this action when given preoperatively, but it seems cruel to give atropine alone intramuscularly as it requires an injection, gives the patient a dry mouth and palpitations and offers no sedation. Hyoscine is more potent and also has amnesic, sedative and antiemetic properties, which make it a very useful drug to give with morphine or papaveretum. Hyoscine has also been given transdermally. Salivation was a problem with ether and is a nuisance during oral and pharyngeal operations. For other operations the new inhalation agents cause little of this effect and many anaesthetists feel that the routine use of a drying agent is unnecessary. In infants even small amounts of secretions can cause some obstruction in the narrow airways and there is therefore more justification for use of an antisialagogue.

Prevention of bradycardia

Atropine is the most useful premedicant drug to prevent bradycardia by vagal blockade, but is even more effective given intravenously. Hyoscine has some action on the heart rate but is less active than atropine.

Bradycardia can be caused by certain anaesthetic agents, such as halothane, at deeper levels of anaesthesia, and drugs such as suxamethonium, neostigmine and gamma-hydroxybutyrate. It may also occur during operations such as orchidopexy, cystoscopy and cleft palate repairs. Traction on the extra-ocular muscles in squint operations (see Chapter 16) and on the tonsil are other common causes. These reflex and drug responses are common in children and some parasympathetic blockade, such as atropine, is often used in the premedication or given intravenously at induction. Intramuscular atropine is most effective given about half an hour before induction of anaesthesia.

In conclusion, the choice of premedication is an individual one by the anaesthetist, taking into consideration the patient, the operation and the anaesthetic to be used. Often an anxiolytic or tranquillizer given by mouth will suffice. Sometimes heavier sedation or the inclusion of an opiate may be desirable, whereas in other situations, particularly in day surgery, premedication may be omitted. Greater emphasis on gaining rapport with the child and using parental support is needed when drugs are avoided.

OTHER MEDICATION

Patients who are receiving drugs for an associated condition such as asthma or epilepsy often present for surgery. It is important to know which drugs the patient is taking and to ensure that the last dose is given at an appropriate time before the operation. An asthmatic, for instance, may be given a salbutamol (Ventolin) inhalation at the same time as the premedication is given.

Prolonged treatment with corticosteroids may result in suppression of ACTH and hence adrenal cortical function. Patients who are being treated with these drugs should therefore be given hydrocortisone either preoperatively or intravenously at induction to counteract the stress of surgery. Adrenocortical function following steroid treatment usually returns towards normal within 2 months, so that it is unusual to need supplementary steroids after this time. When treatment has been stopped within this time, steroid cover may be needed, especially if large doses have been employed or treatment has only recently ceased. If steroids are withheld in these cases, hydrocortisone should be readily available during operation in case hypotension occurs owing to a poor stress response.

The response to insulin and consequent hypoglycaemia normally cause a cortisol induced opposite response. This can be tested by giving 0.15 μg/kg soluble insulin while fasting. A fall in plasma glucose exceeding 2 mmol/l suggests an inadequate response and that supplementary cortisol (hydrocortisone) may be needed [29].

REFERENCES

1 Olsson G.L., Hallen B. Laryngospasm during anaesthesia. A computer-aided incidence study in 136 929 patients. *Acta Anaes Scand* 1984, **28**, 567.

2 Lucas A., Morley R., Cole J.J. Adverse neurodynamic outcome of moderate neonatal hypoglycaemia. *Br Med J* 1988, **297**, 1304.

3 Brown T.C.K., Connelly, J.F., Dunlop M.E., McDougall P.M., Tibballs J. Fasting plasma glucose in children. *Aust Paed J* 1980, **16**, 28.

4 Meakin G., Dingwall A.E., Addison G.M. Effects of preoperative feeding on gastric pH and volume in children. *Br J Anaes* 1985, (ARS) 832 P.

5 Sandhar B.K., Goresky G.V., Maltby J.R., Shaffer E.A. The effect of oral liquids and ranitidine on gastric volume and pH in children undergoing outpatient surgery. *Anesthesiology* 1989, **71**, 327.

6 Splinter W.M., Stewart J.A., Muir J.G. The effect of preoperative apple juice on gastric contents, thirst and hunger in children. *Canad J Anaes* 1989, **36**, 55.

7 Henderson J.M., Spence D.G., Clarke W.N., Bonn G.G., Noel L.P. Sodium citrate in paediatric outpatients. *Canad J Anaes* 1987, **34**, 560.

8 Goudsouzian N., Cote C.J., Lin L.M.P., Dedrick D.F. Dose-response effects of oral cimetidine on gastric pH and volume in children. *Anesthesiology* 1981, **55**, 333.

9 Finlay G.A., Bissonnette B., Goresky G.V., Klassen K., Lerman J., McDairmid C., Pilato M., Schaffer E. The effect of oral ranitidine and preoperative oral fluids on gastric fluid pH and volume in children. *Canad J Anaes* 1989, **36**, S95.

10 Lerman J., Christensen S.K., Farrow Gillespie A.C. Effects of metoclopramide and ranitidine on gastric fluid pH and volume in children. *Canad J Anaes* 1988, **35**, S142.

11 Guay J., Santerre L., Gaudreault P., Goulet B., Dupurs C. Effects of oral cimetidine and ranitidine on gastric pH and residual volume in children. *Anesthesiology* 1989, **71**, 547.

12 Olsson G.L. Complications of paediatric anaesthesia. *Current Opinion in Anaesthesiology* 1990, **3**, 385.

13 Olsson G.L, Hallen B. Pharmacological evacuation of the stomach with metoclopramide. *Acta Anaes Scand* 1982, **26**, 417.

14 Van der Walt J. Premedication in children. *Current Opinion in Anaesthesiology* 1990, **3**, 346.

15 Rowley M.R., Brown T.C.K. Postoperative vomiting in children. *Anaes Intens Care* 1982, **10**, 309.

16 Anderson B.J., Exarchos H., Lee K., Brown T.C.K. Oral premedication in children: a comparison of chloral hydrate, diazepam, alprazolam, midazolam and placebo for day surgery. *Anaes Intens Care* 1990, **18**, 185–193.

17 Payne K., Mattheyse F.J., Liebenberg D., Dawes T. The pharmacokinetics of midazolam in paediatric patients. *Eur J Clin Pharmacol* 1989, **37**, 267.

18 Feld L.H., Negus J.B., White P.F. Oral midazolam: optimum dose for paediatric premedication. *Anesthesiology* 1989, **71**, A1053.

19 Wilton N.C.T., Leigh J., Rosen D.R., Pandit U.A. Preanaesthetic sedation of preschool children using nasal midazolam. *Anesthesiology* 1989, **69**, 972.

20 Walbergh E.J., Eckert J. Pharmacokinetics of intravenous and intranasal midazolam in children. *Anesthesiology* 1989, **71**, A1065.

21 Van der Walt J.H., Jacob R., Murrell D., Bentley M. The perioperative effects of oral premedication in children. *Anaes Intens Care* 1990, **18**, 5.

22 Sleeman K.W., Brown T.C.K. A comparison of pentazocine with morphine in premedication for adenotonsillectomy in children. *ANZ J Surg* 1971, **40**, 309.

23 Streisand J.B., Stanley T.H., Hague B., Van Vreeswijk H., Ho G.H., Pace N.L. Oral transmucosal fentanyl citrate premedication in children. *Anesth Analg* 1989, **69**, 894.

24 Feld L.H., Champeau M.W., Van Steenis C.A., Scott J.C. Preanaesthetic medication in children: a comparison of oral transmucosal fentanyl versus placebo. *Anesthesiology* 1989, **71**, 374.

25 Henderson J.M., Brodsky D.A., Fisher D.M., Brett C.M., Hertzka R.E. Preinduction of anaesthesia in paediatric patients with nasally administered sufentanil. *Anesthesiology* 1988, **68**, 671.

26 Jantzen J.P.A.H., Tzanova I., Witton P.K., Klein A.M. Rectal pH in children. *Canad J Anaes* 1989, **36**, 665.

27 Forbes R.B., Vanderwalker G.E. Comparison of 2% and 10% rectal methohexitone for induction of anaesthesia in children. *Canad J Anaes* 1988, **35**, 345.

28 Kestin I.G., McIlvaine W.B., Lockhart C.H., Kestin K.J., Jones M.A. Rectal methohexitone for induction of anaesthesia in children with and without rectal aspiration after sleep. *Anesth Analg* 1988, **67**, 1102.

29 Plumpton P.S., Besser G.M., Cole P.V. Corticosteroid treatment and surgery. *Anaesthesia* 1969, **24**, 3.

7: Anaesthetic Management

PREPARATION OF THE CHILD

After the preoperative visit by the anaesthetist (see Chapter 6), a child should be allowed to take part in normal ward activities until the premedication is given, or if not premedicated, until shortly before transfer to theatre. Care must be taken to ensure that nothing is taken by mouth after the time designated for preoperative starvation to begin, with the exception of oral medications ordered by the anaesthetist. This includes not only feeding by the staff but also by other sympathetic patients on the ward. A 'No nourishment' sign on the bed or 'Do not feed me' sign pinned to the small child's gown may be helpful. Once the premedication has been given the patient should stay in bed. Older children are often taken to theatre on a trolley, but the risk of falling out of bed is minimized if younger ones are brought to the operating theatre in their cots. It is reassuring to the children, especially the younger ones, if the parent can accompany them at least to the theatre waiting area.

Every precaution must be taken to ensure that the correct patient is anaesthetized. Each child should have name bands attached to a wrist and ankle on admission to hospital, and these should be checked prior to transfer to theatre. A system should operate for checking the patient's name and history before leaving the ward and again on arrival in theatre.

PREPARATION BY THE ANAESTHETIST

Before the patient is brought into the induction room, the anaesthetist should have checked the anaesthetic machine to ensure that:

1 the piped gases are attached to the machine or that the oxygen and nitrous oxide cylinders are turned on;

2 the vaporizer contains an adequate quantity of the inhalation agent to be used and that it is turned off;

3 the appropriate breathing system is gas-tight;

4 the necessary mask and endotracheal tubes are available;

5 the laryngoscope is functioning well. Preferably at least two should be available, with a variety of blades to cater for different sizes of patient;

6 the sucker should be checked to ensure that it is working and that, if it has a screw-on tip, it is not loose;

7 the drugs required during induction should be drawn up so that each syringe contains the expected dose required and is clearly labelled.

A child's dose requirement of drugs is reasonably predictable if calculated from body weight, but one must bear in mind special circumstances such as obesity, hypovolaemia and altered sensitivity to relaxants, as occurs in neonates, burns cases or cyanotic congenital heart disease. The practice of drawing up the appropriate dose will act as a safeguard against administration of an overdose, which is always possible when dealing with patients of widely varying ages and sizes. Particular precision is necessary in drawing up small doses for babies, especially of non-depolarizing relaxants. When the initial or incremental dose is small, greater accuracy may be achieved by diluting the drug in saline. An appropriate dilution of non-depolarizing muscle relaxant, for example, is 1 mg/ml. The syringe or ampoule containing the diluted drug must be carefully labelled. A 1 ml syringe is also useful.

When all has been prepared the patient is brought into the anaesthetic room, where he should be the centre of attention. People not involved with the induction of anaesthesia should be discouraged from attending, and unnecessary and irrelevant talk should not occur. The anaesthetist and his assistants should make the child feel the centre of attention and feel at ease and, where appropriate, they should explain what is happening.

The advantage of an anaesthetic induction room is that it can be kept quiet and there are not as many strangers around as there are when induction is performed in the operating theatre. Also, the presence of surgical instruments and equipment in addition to the anaesthetic equipment can frighten the child.

In view of the increasing hazard to anaesthetists of infection with HIV and hepatitis it is recommended that gloves be worn for procedures where there is a chance of contamination, such as venepuncture, intubation and pharyngeal suction.

INDUCTION OF ANAESTHESIA

The anaesthetist should always have an assistant during induction of anaesthesia. This person should preferably be a trained anaesthetic technician or nurse, but if untrained, the anaesthetist should ensure that the assistant knows what help will be expected of him or her.

The anaesthetist should talk to the child, as the distraction and reassurance which can be achieved in this way will make a smooth induction of anaesthesia easier. Some anaesthetists can almost hypnotize their patients by talking to them. This is particularly useful during an inhalation induction. Other people present tend to talk to the child at the same time. This should be discouraged, because it breaks their attention and causes arousal.

Anaesthesia can be induced (i) intravenously, (ii) by inhalation, (iii) occasionally with drugs such as ketamine which can be given intramuscularly, or (iv) rectally (not commonly used).

Intravenous induction

Intravenous induction is rapid and pleasant so long as the anaesthetist is adept at venepuncturing the small veins. This is almost painless with fine-gauge needles (27, 25 SWG). The introduction of EMLA (eutectic mixture of local anaesthetics) cream has reduced the fear of needles, as it anaesthetizes the skin if applied at least an hour beforehand. Occasionally children complain of discomfort as the needle enters the vein. Trainee anaesthetists, if working full-time in paediatric anaesthesia, can usually gain enough experience within a week or two successfully to puncture veins in most small children at the first attempt. It is a skill which does require continuing practice and therefore anaesthetists who only occasionally anaesthetize children often use inhalation induction for smaller children. The use of indirect angled light makes it easier to see veins because the distended vein casts a shadow (Fig. 7.1).

The common sites for venepuncture are the back of

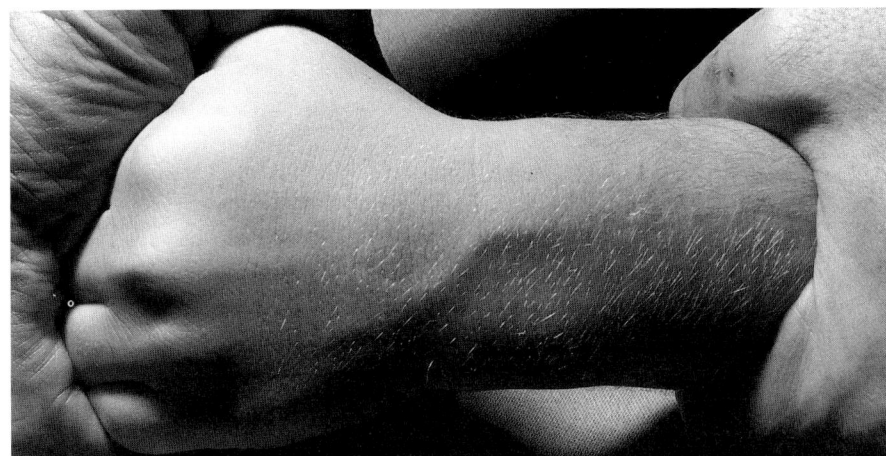

Fig. 7.1 The assistant constricts the wrist and puts proximal traction on the skin while the anaesthetist controls the hand. A light is shone at an angle so that the dilated vein casts a shadow, making it easy to locate.

the hand or the dorsum of the foot. Between about 6 months and 2 years of age, fat may partially obscure these veins from the inexperienced eye. In these patients it may be easier to puncture the very fine superficial veins which are present on the palmar aspect of the wrist. One must remember that the median nerve lies deep to these. Scalp veins can be used in babies and an elastic band around the scalp makes these stand out. Care should be taken to avoid needling scalp arteries, which are usually more tortuous, pulsate and can normally be traced back to the superficial temporal artery. One method of fixation is illustrated in Fig. 7.2. Another vein which often stands out in infants and small children lies on the dorsolateral aspect of the foot. The veins on the radial side of the wrist and in the cubital fossa may also be used. One should bear in mind the presence of the brachial artery and the possibility of an aberrant superficial ulnar artery in the cubital fossa. Blanching or severe pain suggests the possibility that the drug has been injected intra-arterially (see Chapter 27).

The availability of veins should be assessed and the one used for induction selected on the basis of whether this site will be used as the intravenous route for the whole procedure, or whether a cannula for infusion will be inserted later. It is important that the site to be used be convenient and accessible to the anaesthetist. If an intravenous cannula is to be inserted later, the anaesthetist may prefer to use a vein on another limb but the same vein may be punctured more proximally, particularly if the drugs given during induction cause the vein to dilate. A very small amount of nitroglycerine ointment applied to the interdigital spaces three-quarters of an hour beforehand, can make limb veins easier to see.

Having selected a site, the assistant should hold the limb one or two inches proximally, firmly enough to cause venous but not arterial obstruction, and with some proximal traction to help fix the vein. The anaesthetist should flex or extend the joint so that the skin is pulled taut and the vein does not move when the needle is inserted (Fig. 7.3). Excessive flexion or extension may empty the vein. The vein may stand out more if the wrist is flexed and extended a few times or if the skin over it is flicked or rubbed. For very small veins, an appropriate needle, such as 25 or 27 gauge, should be used. A winged needle ('butterfly') is often used to maintain venous access for the duration of the operation. In small infants it may be necessary to strap the needle and stabilize the joint on a miniature arm board, or over a sandbag. The assistant should immobilize the limb until the patient is anaesthetized so that sudden movements do not cause the needle to puncture the vein again or pull it out.

Cannulae are now more often used to maintain intravenous access and for infusions, particularly for longer and major operations. Since the advent of EMLA cream they have been used more for primary intravenous access, as they can be inserted through anaesthetized skin with minimal discomfort. In some small cannulae, the needle protrudes a significant distance beyond the plastic. When inserted into a baby, the needle may enter the vein and blood may run back but the cannula may still not be in the vein. For this reason once the needle is in the vein the cannula should first be advanced into the vein before the needle is withdrawn. If the needle is only partly withdrawn before fixation the cannula does not become kinked when the first piece of tape is applied. The needle is then withdrawn, the infusion attached and fixation completed (Fig. 7.4).

If the assistant is inexperienced, the use of a tourniquet

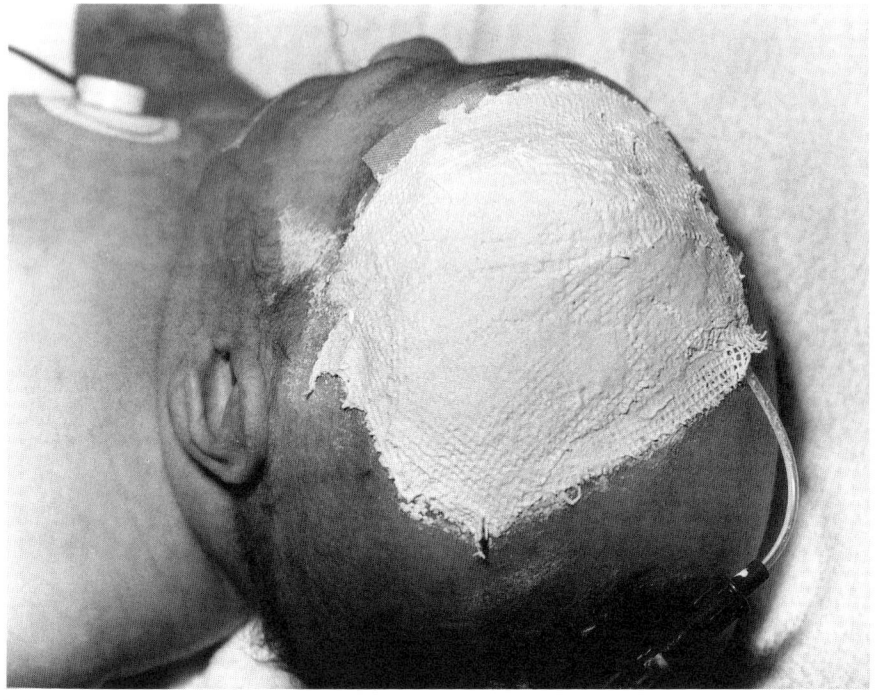

(a)

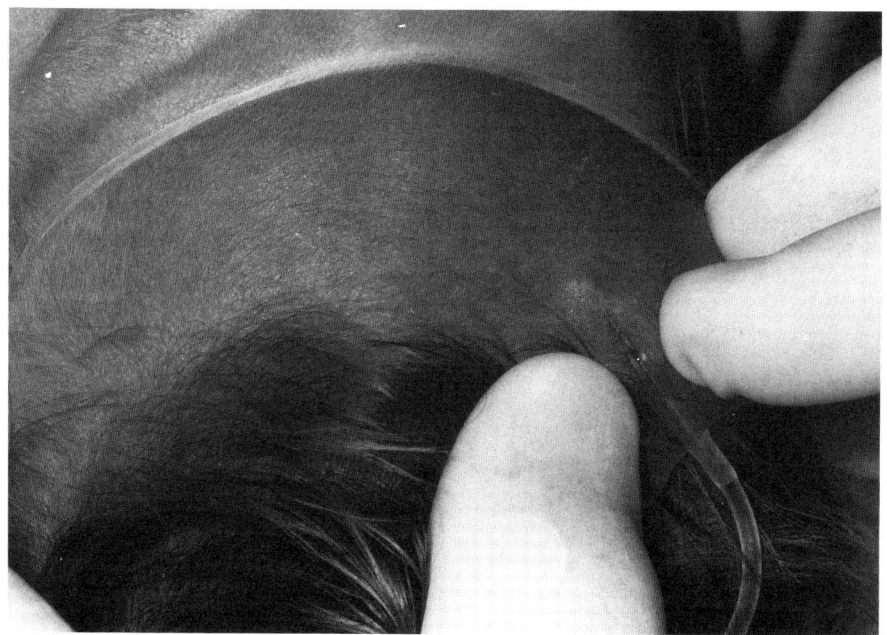

(b)

Fig. 7.2 Sometimes in infants a scalp vein provides useful intravenous access. Fixation is complicated and may be assisted by the use of plaster of Paris (a). The site of the needle tip should be exposed so that leakage into the tissues can be recognized (b). To make scalp veins dilate, an elastic band can be placed around the head making them easy to puncture.

or sphygmomanometer cuff may be a more reliable way of obtaining good venous distension.

Anaesthesia may be induced by a number of drugs, such as thiopentone, propofol, methohexitone and keta-mine. The dose will depend on age (see Chapter 2) and whether or not the patient has had premedication. If an opioid has not been given, some may be adminis-tered before intubation. Particular care should be taken with myocardial depressant drugs (e.g. barbiturates) in patients who are hypovolaemic because the plasma con-centration will be higher in the decreased blood volume and a greater proportion of cardiac output will reach the heart and brain, so that the usual dose will be a relative overdose. On the other hand, if a patient is apprehensive, the high level of circulating catecholamines will lead to a redistribution of cardiac output, with relatively more blood flow going to muscle and less to the brain, so that a larger dose of induction agent is needed. The dose per kg should be reduced in obese patients because the sleep dose is more closely related to lean tissue mass than body weight. In practice, intravenous induction agents are not usually used in the newborn, and doses per kg are reduced during the first 2 or 3 months of life (see Chapter 2). The decision to use an intravenous induction agent will depend on the size, maturity and health of the patient, and accessibility of veins.

Inhalation induction

An inhalation induction may be selected because the anaesthetist prefers to induce small children in this way. It may also be selected when the child is already asleep after premedication, when a suitable vein is unavailable or when attempted intravenous induction has failed. Sometimes a patient may volunteer a preference for an inhalation induction. The technique used will depend on whether the patient is co-operative, asleep from the premedication or apprehensive.

In the first situation the patient may accept the face mask and even hold it himself and can be allowed to breathe oxygen for a few breaths to denitrogenate the lung. A high concentration of nitrous oxide (80–85%) can then be introduced and after a few breaths this is reduced to 70–80% and the inhalation agent to be employed is introduced, gradually increasing the concentration.

When a patient is asleep or drowsy the gas may be blown on to the face from a mask held above, but not touching it. The anaesthetist's hands can be used as a mask until the patient can tolerate one without disturbance. Increased gas flow may be needed at first, to reduce air dilution. If the child comes to the induction room or operating theatre asleep, it may be frightening to awake during the induction.

The third approach is taken when the patient is apprehensive and may be crying, despite all efforts by the anaesthetist to calm him. In this situation the tidal volume and cardiac output are much increased and the rate of uptake of the anaesthetic agent is hastened. It is therefore desirable to use a high gas flow and fairly quickly increase the concentration of inhalation agent so that the patient

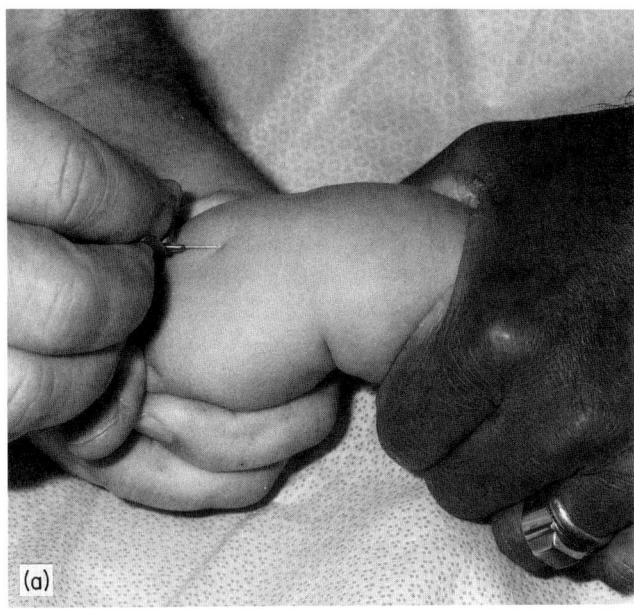

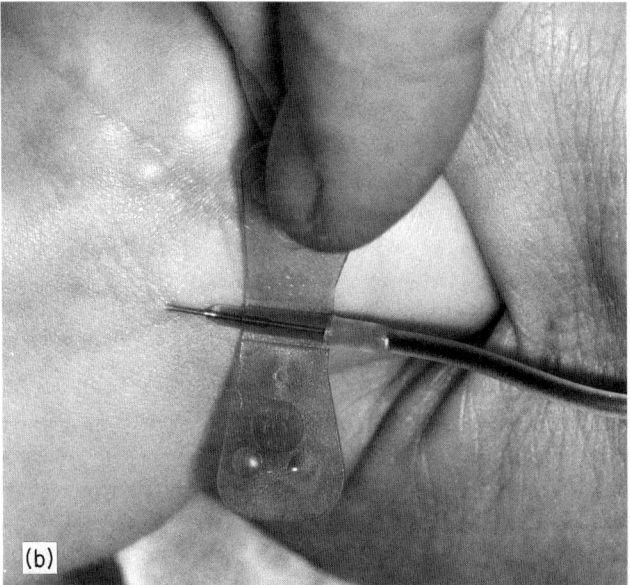

Fig. 7.3 (a) An infant's wrist is held by the assistant and the hand is flexed with the anaesthetist's left hand, which controls it. Infants between 6 months and 1 year often have subcutaneous fat that makes veins on the back of the hand more difficult to locate. Flexing the wrist a few times may make the vein stand out more. A winged needle is inserted at an angle through the skin. Fewer nerve endings are thus traumatized than if the needle is slid horizontally through the skin. Once the skin is penetrated, the needle can be inserted further on a plane more parallel to the skin until the vein is penetrated. (b) A winged needle inserted into a small vein on the palmar aspect of the wrist. These are sometimes more easily seen in older infants with chubby hands.

It is now recommended that gloves should be worn during venepuncture.

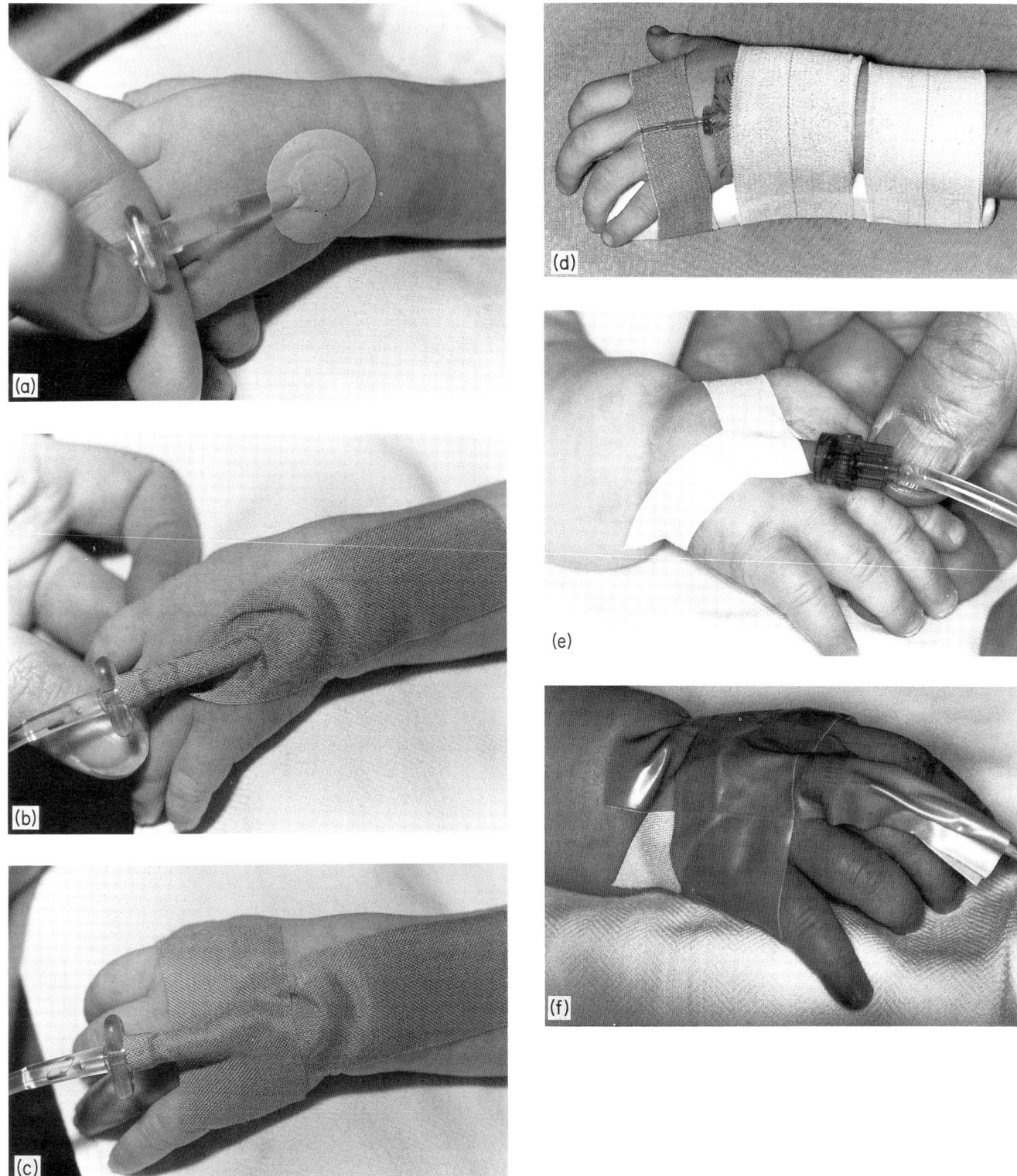

Fig. 7.4 (a), (b), (c) and (d) demonstrate one method of fixation of a cannula inserted into the back of the hand; (e) and (f) demonstrate an alternative approach to strapping the cannula. When a very fine cannula is used, kinking is avoided if the stilette is left in place until the first piece of strapping is applied. The stilette is then removed and the infusion set attached.

is anaesthetized rapidly. Using this technique with halothane the concentration can be increased as rapidly as tolerated to 4% until the patient becomes drowsy, when the anaesthetic concentration can be reduced.

During an inhalation induction there should be no noise in the induction room apart from the anaesthetist talking quietly and reassuringly to the child. Gentle stroking of the face also has a tranquillizing effect. If the child is upset, the anaesthetist can sit the child on his or her knee. A parent, if present, can hold the child during induction.

Of the currently available agents, halothane provides the smoothest induction as it is less irritant than isoflurane and enflurane. These agents induce anaesthesia rapidly because they have relatively low blood gas partition coefficients. Induction can be hastened by the use of nitrous oxide as the carrier gas.

Raising the concentration to 2, 3 or even 4 MAC during early induction enables maintenance levels of anaesthesia to be reached more rapidly. The concentration is then reduced as consciousness is lost. This technique is referred to as 'overpressure'.

Cyclopropane was widely used because of its very rapid induction due to its low blood gas solubility (0.46). It would be useful to have a non-flammable inhalation agent with similar physical characteristics and currently the search is for such an agent. Sevoflurane (blood: gas solubility coefficient 0.63) fulfils some of the desired characteristics but is not yet available world-wide. There is more detailed discussion of the inhalation agents in Chapter 2.

Intramuscular induction

Intramuscular ketamine can be useful when venepuncture is difficult or inhalation induction is contraindicated. The most common situation is in a severely burnt child, especially one with facial burns. Doses of 5−10 mg/kg are used but these larger intramuscular doses are associated with very slow recovery from anaesthesia. It is better to give 4−5 mg/kg and attempt venepuncture once the child is anaesthetized. Subsequent doses can then be given intravenously as boluses or by infusion.

Rectal induction

Rectal induction with thiopentone (40 mg/kg of a 10% solution) or methohexitone (15 mg/kg) is not often used.

Rate of uptake is variable. The time taken to lose consciousness is slower than intravenously so that a longer period of supervision during induction is necessary. Respiratory depression can occur and recovery is usually slow. The rate of uptake depends on the variable pH in the rectum and the faecal content. Better results are obtained if the patient is in the left lateral position, because the rectum is dependent, allowing better retention and spread of the drug. Recovery can be hastened if the excess drug is aspirated once the child is induced (see Chapter 2).

INTUBATION

The use of tracheal intubation in children has increased during the past 40 years and it is now widely used, although in some situations the laryngeal mask is an appropriate alternative.

Indications

The indications for intubation in infants and children are as follows:

1 Anaesthesia where muscle relaxants and controlled ventilation are used.

2 To secure the airway when awkward postures, such as the prone and sitting positions, are used.

3 During operations around the head and neck, so that the anaesthetic apparatus can be kept away from the surgical field.

4 To prevent the aspiration of vomitus during emergency anaesthesia.

5 To bypass an upper airway obstruction which would make the control of the airway otherwise difficult.

6 In operations on the mouth or pharynx to minimize interference with the surgical field and to prevent aspiration of blood, pus or debris.

Intubation is best avoided in the presence of upper respiratory infection or a history of croup and previous post-intubation problems, unless there are strong indications for it, and in day patients having operations that can be managed without.

Intubation reduces the cross-sectional area of the airway. In small infants the wall thickness of the tube is relatively greater, but the problem can be minimized by controlled ventilation.

Methods and drugs used

Intubation may be achieved under general anaesthesia with the aid of muscle relaxants, under deep general anaesthesia or with the aid of local anaesthesia to the larynx. In small neonates awake intubation is possible.

MUSCLE RELAXANTS

Suxamethonium

If muscle relaxation is needed for intubation, suxamethonium may be used, followed by spontaneous breathing with an inhalation agent or by a non-depolarizing relaxant. This allows intubation to be accomplished most rapidly. The onset of action is more rapid in infants than in older patients but it must be remembered that a slightly increased dose relative to body weight is necessary during the neonatal period (see Chapter 2). Suxamethonium may cause bradycardia, particularly following repeat doses; this may be prevented by intravenous atropine. It is usually used during induction in emergency anaesthesia when there is a possibility of a full stomach. In this situation, the patient is usually pre-oxygenated and cricoid pressure is used to compress the oesophagus during induction (Sellick's manoeuvre, Fig. 7.5), but

the pressure should not distort the trachea so much that the appropriate tube cannot be passed. This method of induction will minimize the chance of aspiration of foreign material before the tube is in place to protect the airway.

If venepuncture is a problem, suxamethonium can be given intramuscularly (2–3 mg/kg), with adequate conditions for intubation after about a minute. Suxamethonium should not be used between about 2 and 6 weeks after burns (see Chapter 20), when there has been major tissue damage such as after severe trauma, or in acute para- or quadriplegia, because hyperkalaemia may cause cardiac arrest.

Suxamethonium is preferred when there is doubt about the ability to intubate the patient, but only when the anaesthetist is certain that the patient's lungs can be adequately inflated. Its short action allows the anaesthetist to convert to a spontaneously breathing technique if intubation is unsuccessful.

The usual dose of suxamethonium in children is 1 mg/kg, although nearly all will be paralysed with 0.5 mg/kg (see Chapter 2). The larger dose gives a more rapid onset and longer period of paralysis.

Non-depolarizing relaxants

These provide suitable conditions for intubation in 1–2 minutes after injection, the onset of paralysis being more rapid in infants and when larger doses are given (see Fig. 2.8). The patient should be ventilated while the relaxant becomes fully effective. Initially it is best to assist the patient's ventilation and then gradually take over control.

DEEP INHALATION ANAESTHESIA

Most patients can be intubated during deep halothane anaesthesia. If the child is allowed spontaneously to breathe 4% halothane in oxygen for 5 minutes, intubation can be accomplished unless ventilation is reduced by respiratory obstruction. If attempts are made to intubate too soon (before the eyes have returned to a central position) there is a danger of laryngeal spasm. The above technique is useful when venepuncture is impossible, when relaxants are better avoided because of airway problems or when cost and availability of relaxants limit their use. During inhalation induction, monitoring with a pulse oximeter and/or precordial stethoscope is essential,

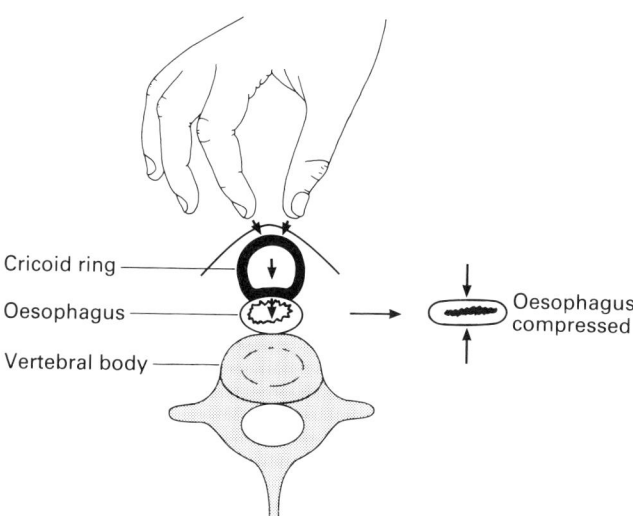

Cricoid ring

Oesophagus

Vertebral body

Oesophagus compressed

Fig. 7.5 Cricoid pressure being applied to the circular cricoid ring and pushing back to compress the oesophagus and prevent regurgitation.

so that bradycardia or diminution of the heart sounds can be recognized at once. Only when respiratory obstruction is present may the patient's ventilation be assisted gently to increase the tidal volume, but careful monitoring is mandatory. Deep halothane anaesthesia may cause significant bradycardia unless atropine or a similar drug has been given.

The same principles can be applied to the newer inhalation agents such as enflurane and isoflurane, that induce anaesthesia rapidly. In the past, cyclopropane produced rapid induction and intubation could be performed satisfactorily. This had to be done quickly, as awakening was rapid and laryngeal spasm was common during lighter levels of anaesthesia.

LOCAL ANAESTHESIA

The use of sedation and local anaesthesia for intubation has less application in paediatrics than in older patients.

AWAKE INTUBATION

Intubation without any pharmacological assistance may be employed in neonates, particularly when they are small or the anaesthetist is unsure of his ability to venti-late a paralysed baby, and in very ill or unconscious children. An experienced assistant is invaluable to hold the baby still. The shoulders can be held down with the arms by the side with the assistant's fingers stabilizing the head, or the arms can be held beside the head, using them to stabilize it (Fig. 7.6). There is some concern that a hypertensive response may occur, with the potential of causing intracranial haemorrhage in a very small baby.

CHOICE OF LARYNGOSCOPE

The adult **Macintosh blade** or a straight blade with a light near the tip can be used for children over 1 year of age, although pressure on the thyroid cartilage to bring the cords into view may be needed in younger children.

Under 1 year of age the larynx lies at a relatively higher level (opposite C3−4) and inclines more anteriorly than in older children (Fig. 7.7). The tongue is relatively large and the epiglottis is more U-shaped and narrower. Many laryngoscopes are available for infant intubation, but usually a straight blade or one with a slight curve at the tip is most suitable. As already mentioned, the light must be near the tip because if it is too far back the illumination within the mouth may be inadequate (see Chapter 3).

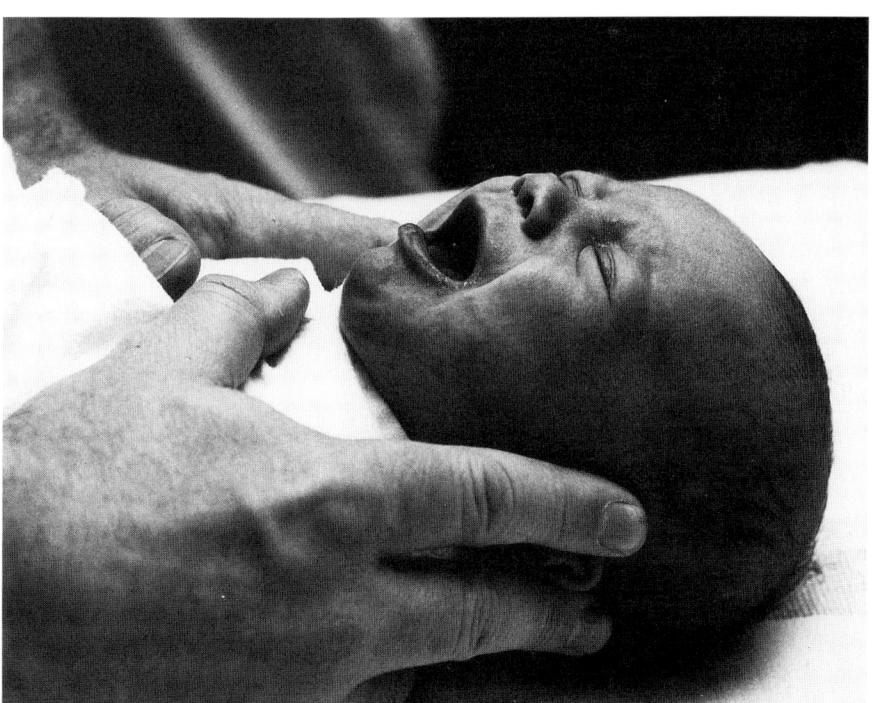

Fig. 7.6 If a small infant is to be intubated awake, an assistant must stabilize the head as shown and hold the shoulders down.

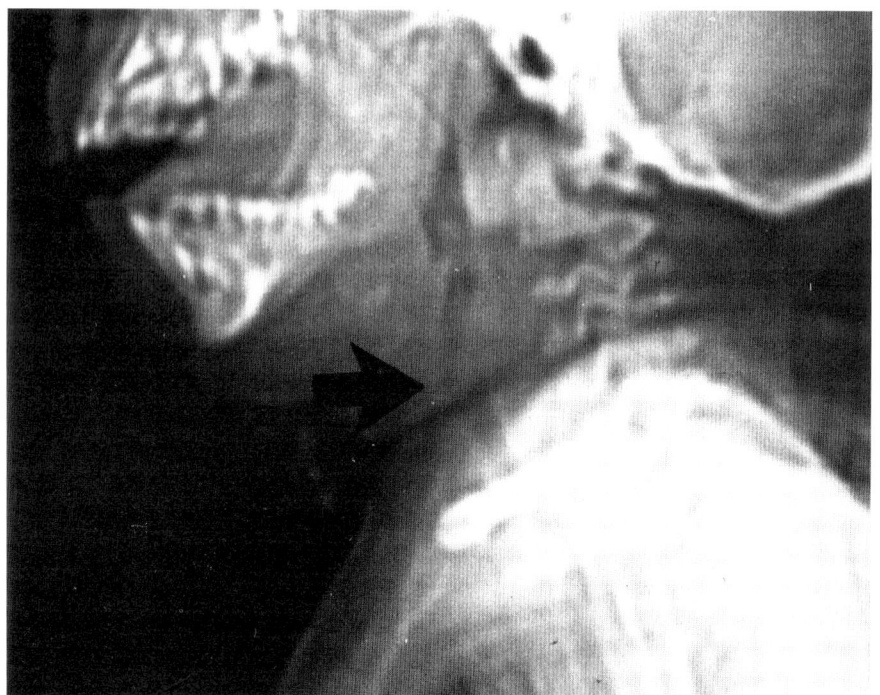

Fig. 7.7 This lateral CT scan demonstrates the anterior inclination of the trachea and explains why it is sometimes helpful to apply pressure as shown by the arrow, to bring the larynx into better alignment during intubation.

CHOICE OF TUBE

Endotracheal tubes are discussed in Chapter 3. Most anaesthetists develop personal preferences for specific circumstances. A disposable Magill tube is used for most procedures. The red rubber tube, despite its advantages of withstanding heat sterilization repeated many times and retaining its shape, is now rarely used. The PVC tubes soften at body temperature and mould to the airway. If they are being inserted nasotracheally, less trauma will result if they are warmed before use. Although they do not tend to kink when the head is flexed, they are compressible. PVC tubes do not retain their shape after use if heat sterilized, so if reuse is considered a stilette may be necessary for their insertion. Their shape is retained better if they are sterilized with ethylene oxide.

Oral RAE or 'south' Portex tubes are premoulded to lie over the chin while the nasal or 'north' Portex tubes curve up toward the forehead (see Fig. 3.24). These overcome some of the problems encountered with connections when one wishes the tube to run down towards the chest or up over the head.

Latex or silastic armoured tubes are resistant to kinking and compression if the connector is inserted into the armoured part of the tube. If this is not done, kinking can occur at the junction. A stilette is usually needed to insert them. It is usually a metal wire or teflon which holds its curve when inserted through the tube. It should not protrude beyond the tube as it is more likely than a tube to perforate the mucosa if pushed too hard.

Cole tubes (see Fig. 3.23) with a wide proximal and narrow distal part are of value in infants when a mouth gag has to be inserted, since they are resistant to compression, but turbulence increases the resistance to gas flow through them. They are not commonly used nowadays.

Cuffed tubes are not usually required before puberty because the narrowest part of the airway is the circular cricoid ring and it is only after puberty, when the subglottic area enlarges, that the triangular area of the vocal cords becomes the narrowest part. This means that the cuff is not needed to prevent aspiration or excessive gas leakage in prepubertal children and that postoperative laryngeal oedema, which might be caused by the cuff pressing on the mucosa, is avoided.

CHOICE OF SIZE OF TUBE

Tubes are now measured by their internal diameter (ID) in millimetres, and up to 6 mm they are also labelled with the external diameter. Some tubes are also measured in French gauge (external circumference in mm). A formula commonly employed to assess the expected size is age/

4 + 4 mm ID. Some anaesthetists using thin-walled tubes use the formula age/4 + 4.5 mm ID. There is a degree of variation around the average, so that a tube of the expected size and one size bigger and one size smaller are usually selected before induction. The size of tube which has a thicker wall (e.g. Latex Armoured) that will pass while still allowing a leak, may be one size (0.5 mm) smaller. It is most important to have a slight leak around the tube when positive pressure is applied to avoid mucosal compression and postoperative laryngeal complications.

Route of intubation

Endotracheal tubes are usually passed orally but there are indications for nasotracheal intubation. These include dental anaesthesia, neurosurgical and neuroradiological procedures, and in some instances when it is expected that postoperative ventilation will be necessary, especially in neonates and following complex open heart surgery.

Ventilation

If muscle relaxants are used, the patient must be ventilated by mask before intubation to ensure adequate oxygenation. Cessation of respiratory movements and increased compliance indicate that conditions are suitable for intubation. A cushion face mask is commonly used for older children as it is easier to obtain a gas-tight fit, although the dead space is greater than in the smaller Rendell Baker–Soucek masks.

A useful technique for small children is to apply the Rendell Baker–Soucek mask to the groove in the chin; the mouth is opened and the mandible pulled forward (Fig. 7.8a) and then the nasal part of the mask is placed over the bridge of the nose (Fig. 7.8b,c). When this technique is used, the open mouth allows ventilation with minimal pressure and tends to reduce the amount of air blown into the stomach; a pharyngeal airway is rarely needed. The airway through the mouth is obstructed if the tongue is pushed upwards by incorrectly placed fingers (Fig. 7.9). It is important in infants to use very gentle inflating pressures and not suddenly apply high pressure to the bag, so that the stomach is not distended with gas. This is important because gastric distension splints the diaphragm, preventing adequate ventilation.

There are several ways to control ventilation with an open-ended bag on the expiratory limb of the T-piece.

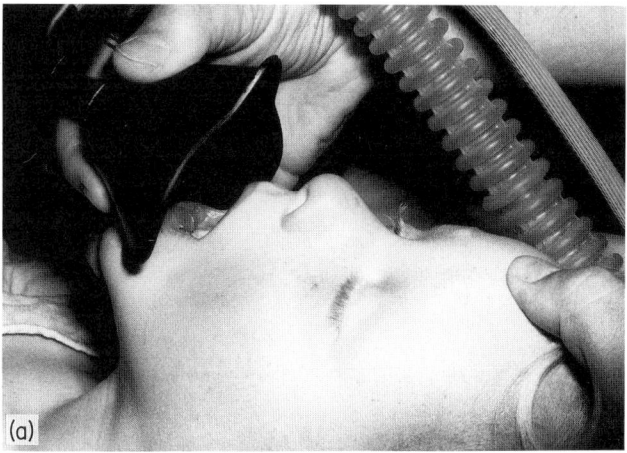

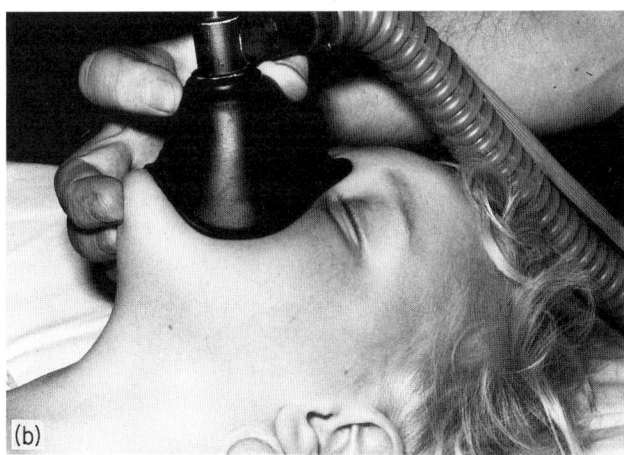

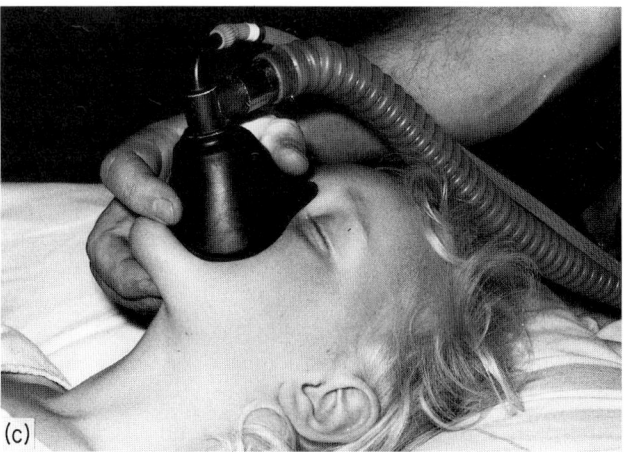

Fig. 7.8 (a) The Rendell Baker–Soucek mask is placed in a groove on the chin and the mandible pulled forward with the mouth open. (b) The mask is then placed back on to the face with the mouth still open. This shows the correct positioning of the thumb and index finger on the top of the mask pushing it back on to the face to obtain an airtight seal. (c) The incorrect positioning of the thumb and index finger causing splaying of the mask with an air leak at the side.

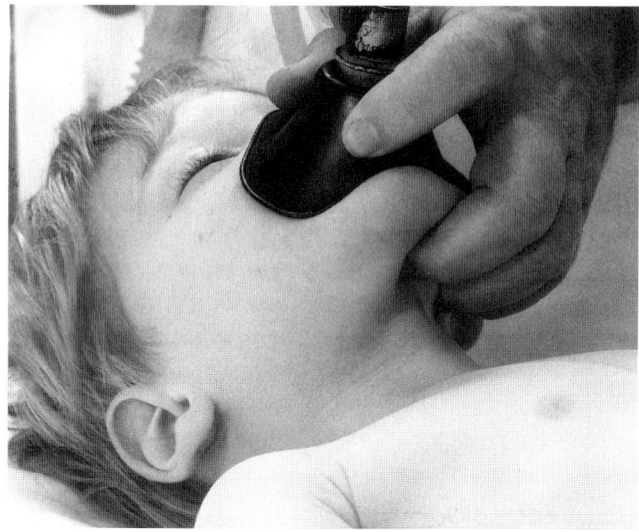

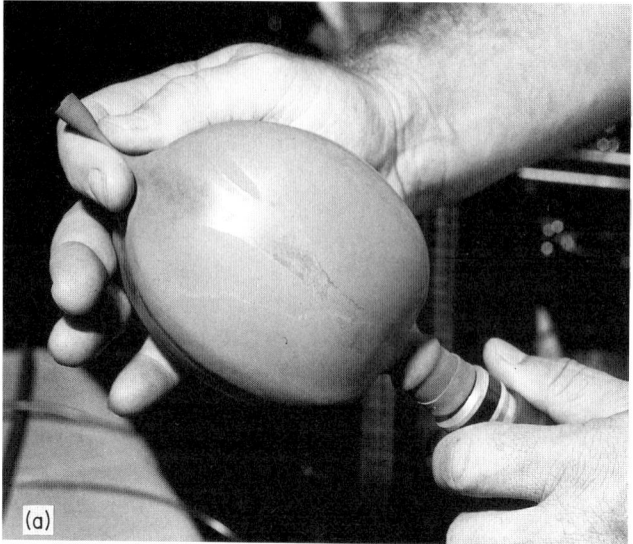

Fig. 7.9 Incorrect positioning of the fingers holding the jaw pushing the tongue upwards and thus blocking the oral airway. Ventilation is more difficult in children with enlarged adenoids or nasal obstruction when the mask is held in this way.

The one illustrated (Fig. 7.10) uses the pincer grip between the thumb and index finger to occlude the open face and the other three fingers to squeeze the bag during inspiration. This is an ergonomically efficient method that is less fatiguing than if the bag is held between the thumb and the proximal phalanx of the index finger.

Technique of intubation

When the patient is sufficiently relaxed for intubation, the following technique minimizes movement and cuts down intubation time. The heel of the right hand is used to steady the forehead of the slightly extended head and the index finger opens the mouth (Fig. 7.11). The laryngoscope is inserted with the left hand and passed down the right hand side of the mouth, ensuring that the tongue is displaced medially (Fig. 7.12). A straight blade can either be inserted between the tongue and epiglottis in the same way as a curved blade, or it can be passed

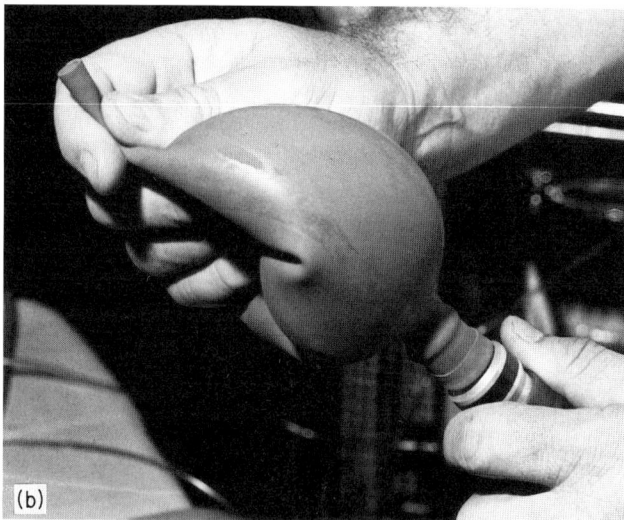

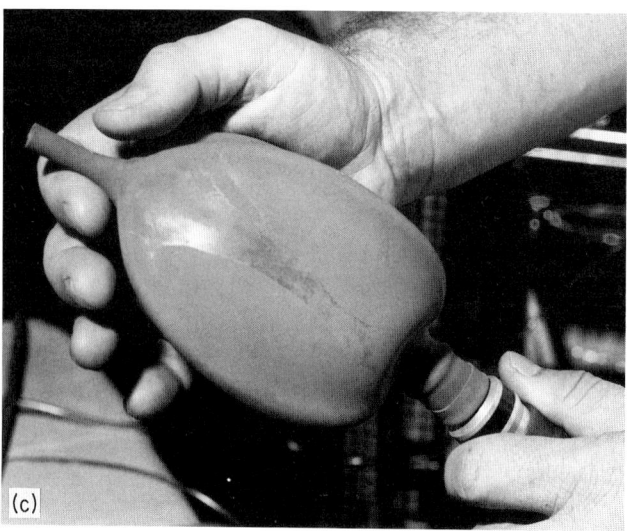

Fig. 7.10 (*right*) Manual ventilation using an open-ended bag on a T-piece. (a) The open end is compressed between the thumb and the distal phalanx of the index finger. This pincer grip is not easily fatigued. (b) The other three fingers compress the full bag to ventilate the lungs. (c) The pincer grip is released so that expiration can occur.

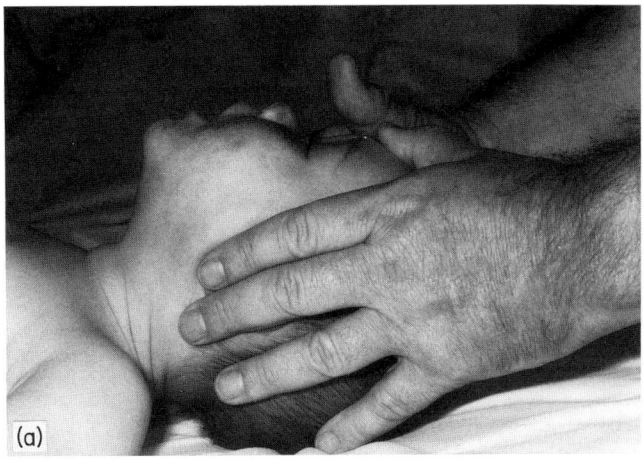

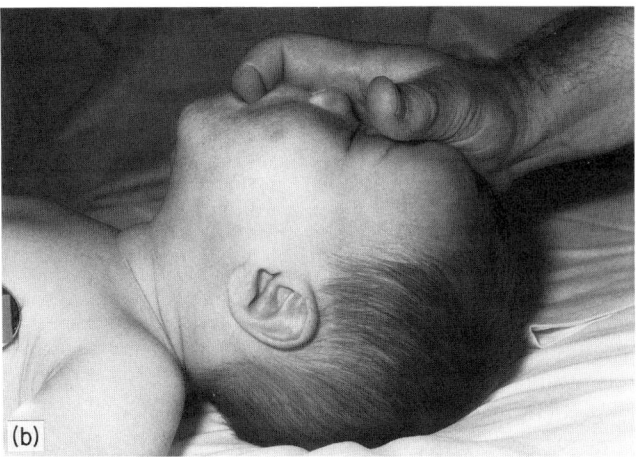

Fig. 7.11 (a) The head is slightly extended by the two hands placed on the side. (b) The right hand is rolled over so that the ball of the thumb stabilizes the forehead, while the index finger is used to open the mouth.

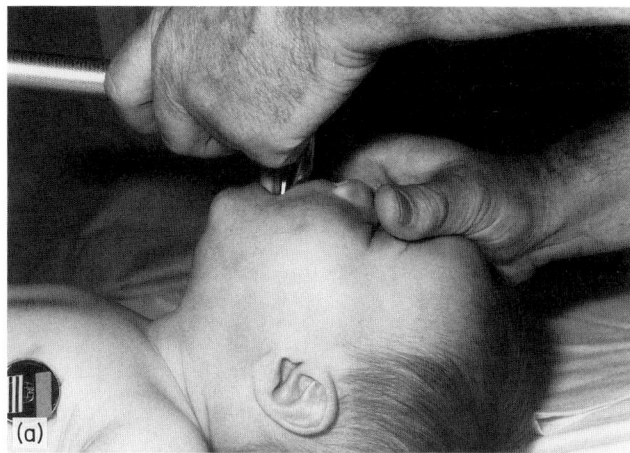

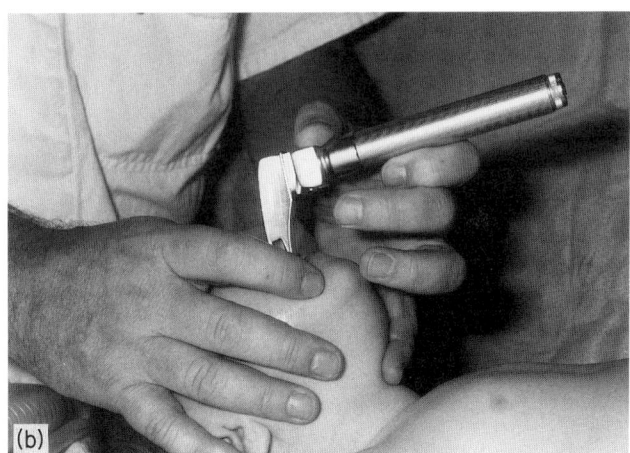

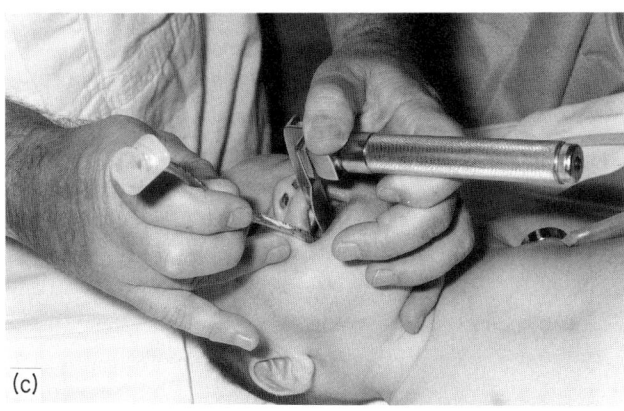

beyond the laryngeal inlet and then withdrawn until the arytenoids come into view and the epiglottis is held by the laryngoscope blade. The application of pressure on the larynx from the outside will bring the vocal cords clearly into view. An assistant can apply this pressure or it can be achieved in infants by the anaesthetist pressing the larynx back with the little finger of the left hand, if the laryngoscope is held between the thumb and index finger near the junction of the handle and blade, as shown in Fig. 7.12c.

ORAL INTUBATION

After the larynx is exposed by laryngoscopy the endotracheal tube should always be passed from the corner

Fig. 7.12 (a) The laryngoscope can easily be passed into the open mouth directly down to the epiglottis. (b) This demonstrates the method of holding the laryngoscope so that the fingers can be easily stretched to allow the little finger to press on the larynx. The laryngoscope blade is inserted down the right side of the mouth to keep the tongue out of the way when the tube is being passed. (c) The tube is now inserted from the right corner of the mouth so that the tip can be seen entering the larynx. It is important not to obscure the view of the larynx by passing the tube down the middle of the blade.

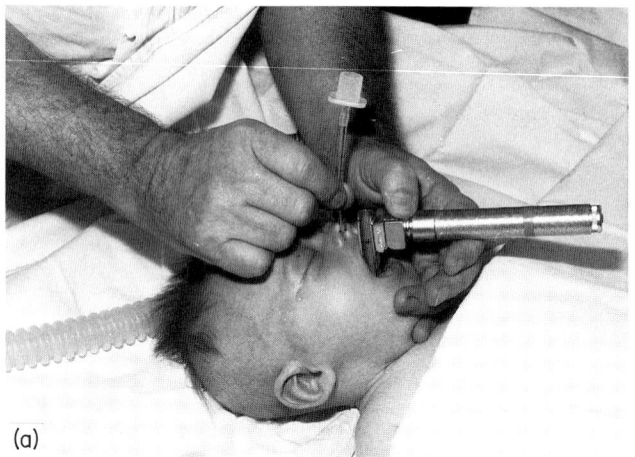

(a)

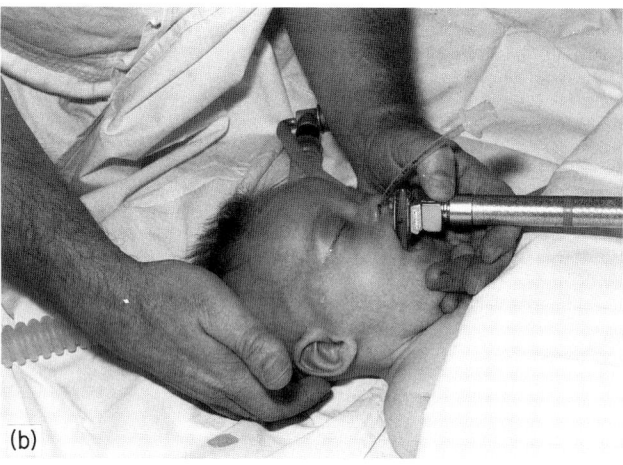

(b)

Fig. 7.13 Nasal intubation. (a) The tube is advanced through the nose towards the exposed larynx. The position of the larynx can be adjusted by pressure from the little finger of the left hand. (b) If the tube is passing posteriorly, flexion of the neck will often bring it into line with the larynx.

of the mouth so that it can be seen passing through the cords. If it is passed down the midline it will obstruct the anaesthetist's view and there will be uncertainty as to whether the trachea or the oesophagus has been intubated. This is a particularly important point to stress when teaching. In older children, leaving the head on a pillow and slightly flexing the neck will often bring the larynx into more direct line, so that less backwards pressure on the larynx will be needed. Air entry into both lungs should be checked before final fixation of the tube.

If the tube is too large (no leak with positive pressure ventilation) or too small (large leak), it should be changed, having first ascertained that turning the head to

the side will not provide an appropriate minimal leak. Before the tube is removed the laryngoscope should be inserted and the larynx visualized. The tube is then removed and another inserted with minimal delay. Alternatively if the tube is too small, a pharyngeal pack may reduce the leak sufficiently to avoid changing the tube.

If it is very difficult to visualize the larynx, the help of a second anaesthetist is invaluable. Although it is usual for the assistant to push on the larynx it is much more effective for the anaesthetist to manipulate the laryngoscope with one hand and to apply pressure on the larynx with the other. In this way optimum pressures can be applied to bring the larynx into view and the assistant can then insert the tube. This technique has enabled intubation of many patients previously regarded as difficult or impossible to intubate.

A variety of sizes and types of laryngoscopes should be available when difficult intubation is expected.

Fixation of the tube may be critical, particularly in neurosurgical procedures and operations around the head and neck, when the anaesthetist's apparatus is away from the patient. If a Magill tube is employed and kinking is to be avoided, the tube should be placed in the midline and strapped so that it runs straight back over the tongue. In this position it is unlikely to kink even when the neck is flexed, but if placed in the corner of the mouth it may kink over the angle of the mandible during flexion.

NASAL INTUBATION

When the tube is passed through the nose it should be warmed first to soften it. This can be done by placing the tube in hot water. It should be passed gently backwards, avoiding trauma to the posterior pharyngeal wall. If difficulty is encountered the tip of the tube can be guided through the nasopharynx over a fine catheter. The laryngoscope is inserted. When the tube is in the oropharynx, the anaesthetist must ascertain that it has not become blocked with adenoid tissue or secretions, before passing it into the trachea. Usually it can be guided into the larynx by flexing the neck slightly and pushing back on the larynx. If the tube is still tending to pass posteriorly, further flexion of the neck will often bring the vocal cords into line with the tube, which is then pushed through the cords (Fig. 7.13). If it catches on the edge, a 90° rotation bringing the bevel through the midline and then rotation back will usually take the bevel from the cords through the aditus into the trachea. If one is unable to pass the tube in this manner, forceps may be used to guide it into the laryngeal opening. Magill forceps which grasp the tube on the sides are most commonly used, although ones which grasp anteriorly and posteriorly are ergonomically more efficient (e.g. Lieberman).

The anaesthetist should check for marks on the endotracheal tube before insertion; it can be passed to a given point and then fixed appropriately. In a neonate who has a tracheal length of about 4 cm the tube can be inserted 2 cm beyond the cords without entering a bronchus. Having positioned the tube in this way, it is still necessary to watch for equal movement of both sides of the chest and to listen with the stethoscope to see that both lungs are ventilating. If in doubt, the tube should be passed into the bronchus and then withdrawn. It is advisable to listen laterally on the chest in infants, as transmission of breath sounds at the apices can be misleading.

Fixation of the tube is important, especially when it is to be left in postoperatively or where access will be impossible should it dislodge during the operation, as in neuro- or craniofacial surgery. One approach is to tie a thread firmly around the tube at the point of exit from the nose. Tincture benzoin compound protects the skin and increases adhesion of the tape. Figure 7.14 illustrates one technique for strapping a nasal tube securely.

Difficulties with ventilation and intubation

These include:
1 Structural abnormalities which make it difficult to position the head, such as encephalocoele, myelomeningocoele and gross hydrocephalus.
2 Anatomical abnormalities in the mouth and upper airway, such as micrognathia, macroglossia, grossly enlarged tonsils and adenoids, large teeth, cystic hygroma, tumours and large thyroglossal cysts.
3 External contractures such as burn scars on the neck or around the mouth.
4 Laryngeal obstruction such as papillomata, subglottic stenosis, web, haemangioma.
5 Patients with cervical spine injury or where there is potential for atlantoaxial or odontoid subluxation or dislocation, as in Down's syndrome, achondroplasia and Morquio's syndrome. Care must be taken with these to avoid excessive neck movement.
When difficulties with ventilation or intubation are anticipated, inhalation induction may be safer. After in-

duction, it is advisable to ensure that the patient can be ventilated adequately by mask before any relaxants are used. If the child can be ventilated easily, suxamethonium can be given and an attempt made to intubate the patient.

When intubation is difficult, it must be decided whether the patient has to be intubated for the operation, whether a laryngeal mask airway could be used instead (Fig. 7.15), or whether ventilation with a mask with, if necessary, an oral or nasopharyngeal airway would suffice.

If it is recognized beforehand that intubation will be difficult, a lateral X-ray of the neck is useful to assess the relation of the larynx to the vertebrae, because a superiorly placed larynx or abnormal vertebrae shortening the neck (e.g. Hurler's syndrome) makes intubation difficult.

If intubation is essential there is a number of methods which can be tried to visualize the cords or aid the passage of the tube if it is necessary:
1 The two-anaesthetist technique described above, where one manipulates the laryngoscope and larynx and the other inserts the tube, is often successful.
2 The epiglottis can sometimes be seen when a small straight blade is passed from the corner of the mouth. A stilette can sometimes then be directed into the larynx and the tube passed over it.
3 If an appropriately sized fibreoptic bronchoscope is available, it can be passed through an endotracheal tube. When the bronchoscope is passed into the trachea the tube can be passed over it through the larynx. The bronchoscope is then removed.
4 A laryngeal mask airway can be inserted and a stilette passed through it. Because of its shape this will usually pass into the larynx. The laryngeal mask is removed and the tube is placed over the stilette into the larynx.
5 Blind nasal intubation may be attempted when intubation under direct vision is impossible. It is usually attempted with the patient breathing spontaneously under inhalation anaesthesia. The neck is flexed, the tube is passed through the nose and advanced slowly while the larynx is pressed backwards and manoeuvred slightly from side to side until the intensity of the breath sounds is maximal and the expired gas can be seen condensing in the endotracheal tube. As the tube is advanced farther it may enter the trachea or it may require slight rotation to make it pass into the trachea. Additional flexion of the neck often facilitates tracheal intubation. If laryngeal reflexes are still active and the glottis closes, the tube may slip into the oesophagus. If

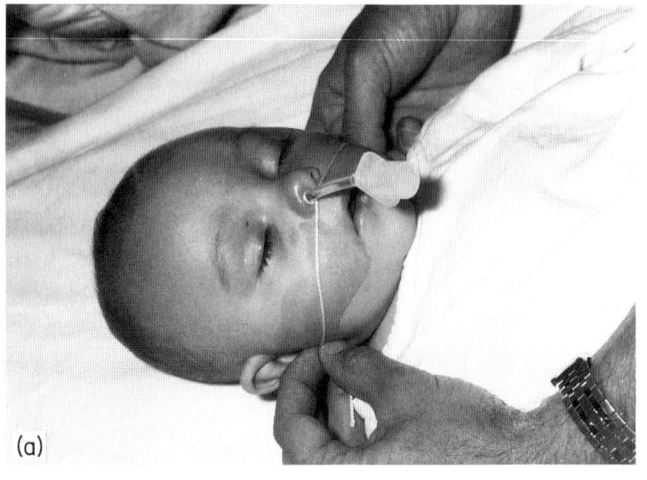

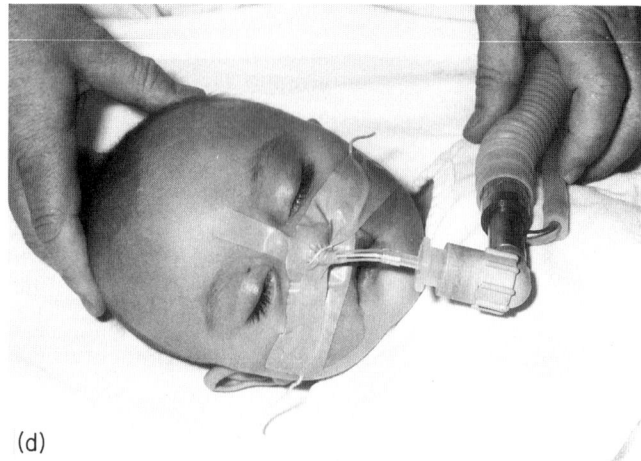

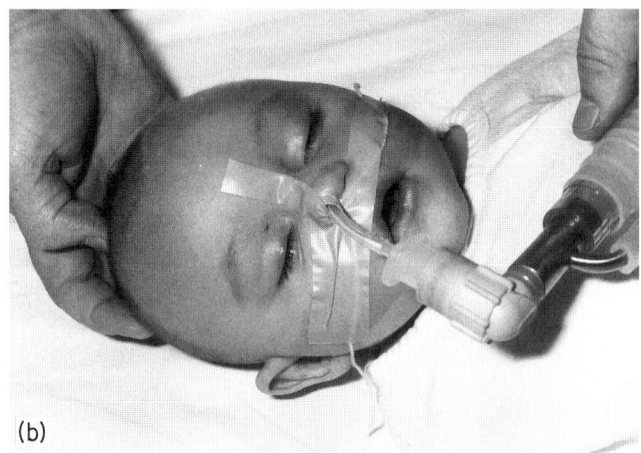

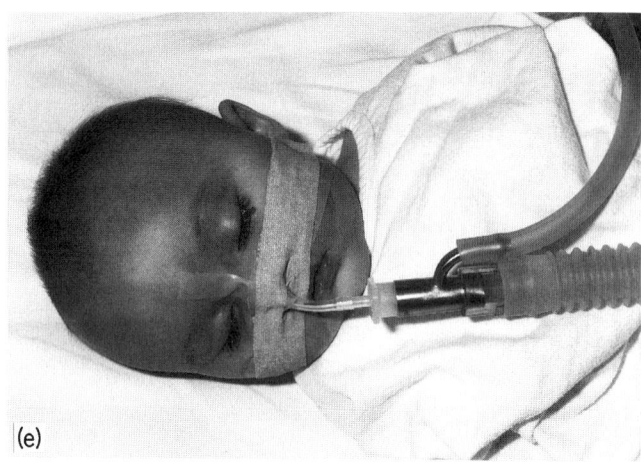

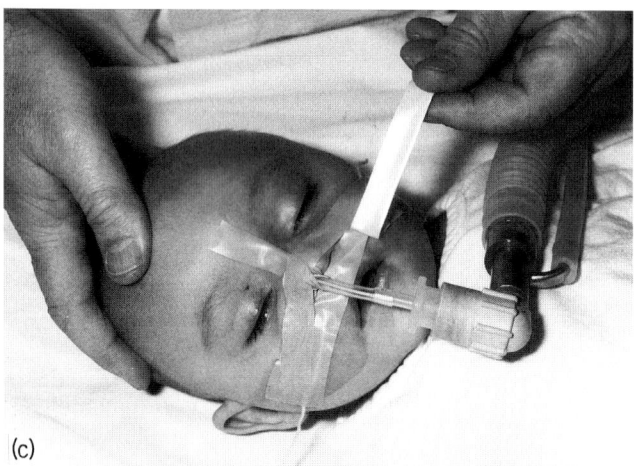

Fig. 7.14 Fixation of a nasal tube for prolonged intubation or where the airway must be guaranteed, as in neurosurgery. (a) A cotton thread is tied at the appropriate point in the tube and tincture of benzoin compound is applied to the face to increase adhesiveness and to protect the skin. (b) A split waterproof tape is placed first across the upper lip and the second leg is taped tightly around the tube and up the nose to provide counter-traction from a downward pull. (c) A second split tape is applied. The first leg, shown being held, is placed over the nose, thus fixing the previously placed upward tape and the second leg, shown being held, is then wound around the tube. (d) The two tapes in place showing a firm attachment to the tube. (e) A piece of elastoplast is placed over the waterproof tape and is attached to the side of the face. This should extend beyond the waterproof tape so that further adhesion to the face is achieved.

this occurs, anaesthesia can be deepened or a pool of local anaesthesia can be placed in the back of the pharynx. The larynx is then pressed back into it. This 'laryngeal dip' covers the larynx with local anaesthetic

obtunding the reflexes, and the remaining local anaesthetic can then be sucked out.

Anaesthetic techniques which can be used for blind intubation include deep inhalation anaesthesia, e.g.

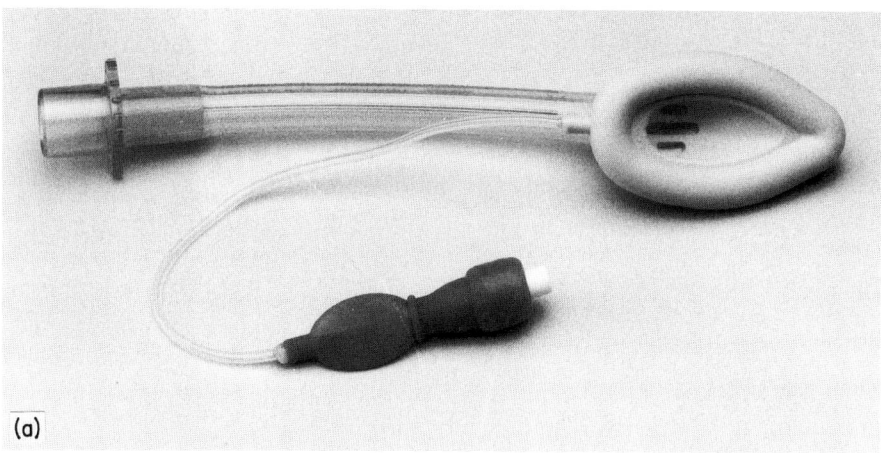

(a)

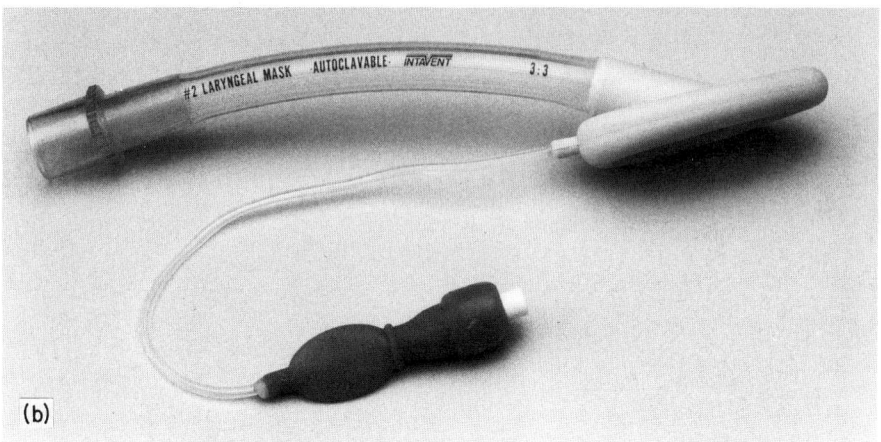

(b)

Fig. 7.15 The laryngeal mask which can be inserted through the mouth and over the larynx. When it is in position the cuff can be blown up, thereby providing a reasonably airtight airway.

halothane — 4% in oxygen for 5 minutes breathing spontaneously; gamma-hydroxybutyrate supplemented by inhalation anaesthesia or deep ether. The latter are of mainly historical interest because the drugs are not widely used but they were very useful methods.

Some anaesthetists who are very skilled at blind nasal intubation use muscle relaxants, but the advantage of hearing the breath sounds as the tube is advanced is lost. The anaesthetic can continue though the tube while it is being manipulated from the pharynx into the larynx.

6 A long intravenous catheter can be inserted through the cricothyroid membrane and passed up into the mouth, where it can be retrieved. The tube is then threaded over the catheter into the trachea. The catheter should be removed before the tube is passed too far down the trachea.

7 The use of image intensification or indirect laryngoscopy with a mirror to guide a stilette into the larynx are among other methods described. The latter is com-plicated because three hands are needed to manipulate the laryngoscope, the mirror and the stilette.

8 Another technique involves placing a fine stillette, with a curve near the end, through a tube which is then attached to a stethoscope. The tongue is pulled forward with one hand and the tube is inserted with the other, being guided blind by the breath sounds.

PHARYNGEAL PACKS

If it is likely that blood will accumulate in the pharynx during the operation, a moistened pharyngeal pack should be inserted gently. It should be placed so that some lies on either side of the tube and it occupies the area between the pharyngeal wall and the base of the tongue. Excess length can be cut off and, unless it is contraindicated by the nature of the surgery, a portion of it should remain outside the mouth, preferably tied to the tube or to clothing. If this is impossible, a note must be made that a pack is in the mouth to remind the anaesthetist to remove it before extubation. In some hospitals it is recorded with the surgical packs to be counted at the end of the operation.

A pharyngeal pack is sometimes used to reduce the leak around an endotracheal tube, but this is not usually necessary if the correct size of tube has been used.

DIFFICULT VENTILATION IN THE INTUBATED PATIENT

The differential diagnosis of this is extremely important in paediatric anaesthesia. The difficulty must be recognized and the cause corrected if more serious complications are to be avoided. It may be due to the following.

1 Kinking of the tube, usually in the pharynx where the kink may be felt, or at the junction of the tube with the connection.

2 Biting on the tube or compression by a mouth gag. The latter is usually associated with the use of a tongue blade which is too short, during tonsillectomy.

3 The bevel of the tube lying against the tracheal wall. This is most common with the now little-used Oxford tubes when the neck is flexed, and is overcome by using a tube which has a hole cut opposite the bevel.

4 The tip of the tube lying against the carina.

5 Intubation of a main bronchus. This is common in infants, as the trachea of a neonate is only about 4 cm long. A tube usually passes into the right main bronchus because it is slightly larger and in more direct line with the trachea, and also because the bevel tip is usually on the right side when the tube is inserted.

6 Blockage of the tube with secretions, blood, or adenoid tissue if passed nasotracheally.

7 Pulmonary causes such as pneumothorax or tension cyst. Pneumothorax is an occasional complication of anaesthesia most often occurring during controlled respiration, especially when high pressures are used. Accidental obstruction of the expiratory limb of the T-piece will generate high pressures, and can cause pneumothorax. This can be avoided by high-pressure limiting devices on the anaesthetic machine. Drainage by intercostal catheter may be necessary.

8 Chest-wall spasm sometimes occurs during light levels of halothane anaesthesia, especially if associated with stimulation of sensitive areas such as the larynx or carina. Deepening of anaesthesia will cause it to disappear. It may also occur with large doses of fentanyl if the patient is not paralysed.

9 Bronchospasm may occur, particularly in asthmatics who have been intubated while lightly anaesthetized. The use of D-tubocurarine has most often been associated with this problem. Before making this diagnosis one must be satisfied that the other causes of difficulty have been excluded. When it does occur, aminophylline (5 mg/kg) given slowly intravenously, will often relieve the attack. Salbutamol or other beta-2 stimulant intravenously or by inhalation may be helpful. Hydrocortisone may be beneficial, but its slower onset of action means the response will be delayed. If halothane is being given, deepening of anaesthesia may help. Ether and methoxyflurane are very effective bronchodilators which have been used in the treatment of resistant bronchospasm. Adrenaline may be effective but should only be used with extreme caution when halothane is being given. Bronchospasm may be a feature of an anaphylactic reaction (see Chapter 27).

10 Gastric distension with gas will splint the diaphragm. A particular problem occurs in oesophageal atresia with a large fistula, where the use of excessive inflating pressure or intubation of the fistula may lead to gastric distension and difficulty in ventilation. In the latter situation, withdrawing the tube into the trachea will often resolve the problem. Occasionally emergency gastrostomy will be needed if the fistula is very large.

OTHER COMPLICATIONS OF INTUBATION

These are:

1 Obstruction of the tube (as above).

2 Oesophageal intubation leading to gastric distension and hypoxia, owing to the lungs not being ventilated. It is important to listen for adequate air entry into the lungs. If in doubt, the tube's position should be checked by direct laryngoscopy or the tube removed and the patient ventilated with a mask. A fall in oxygen saturation and expired CO_2 also suggest that the lungs are not being ventilated.

3 Accidental extubation — the patient may become hypoxic and the lungs do not inflate when the bag is squeezed. The treatment is to remove the tube, ventilate with a mask and reintubate.

4 Extubation laryngeal spasm — oxygen should be administered with continuous positive pressure applied to the bag, so that when the cords open oxygen is forced into the lungs. If the positive pressure is applied intermittently the cords may open when the pressure is not

being applied. The spasm usually relaxes before the heart stops. If the spasm is severe, suxamethonium will relieve it but it should be given only when someone is available to draw it up and inject it before the patient becomes hypoxic. This will allow oxygenation before severe hypoxia occurs, which is desirable because bradycardia and arrhythmias are more likely when suxamethonium is given in the presence of hypoxia and hypercarbia.

5 Postoperative stridor and mucosal oedema are usually due to the use of too large a tube. If obstruction is severe, racemic adrenaline inhalation can be used, and if this fails intubation may be required.

6 Postoperative sore throat, especially if there has been much movement of the tube during the operation.

7 Traumatic laryngoscopy may injure the mucosa or lips. Teeth may be damaged or knocked out. A plastic mouth guard will prevent damage to teeth.

FURTHER PEROPERATIVE MANAGEMENT

Breathing systems

A T-piece or Bain system is used most often for children under about 25 kg. In larger patients the circle absorber conserves gases and reduces pollution. This subject is dealt with in full in Chapter 3.

Care of the eyes

When the eyes tend to open, or are not easily visible to the anaesthetist (e.g. in the prone position) or when drapes may cover the eyes, they should be taped closed to prevent corneal abrasions and drying. Before long operations, eye ointment should be used before taping to prevent corneal drying. The eyes can be completely covered and if the outside lower corner of the tape is folded back it makes it easier to remove at the end (Fig. 7.16). In neurosurgical patients, eye ointment, vaseline and a gauze cover may also be applied to give added protection.

Monitoring

This subject is dealt with in full in Chapter 4. All monitoring equipment should be in place and working prior to the patient being draped.

DIATHERMY

The diathermy plate should be attached. The principles of diathermy are given in Appendix 1.

INTRAVENOUS CANNULATION

If an intravenous cannula has not been inserted before induction and is deemed necessary, it should be inserted in the anaesthetic room. If the anaesthetist is going to insert the cannula after anaesthesia has been induced, he must ensure that a competent assistant is available to maintain the airway and ventilate the patient, and he must keep an eye on the patient's colour and ventilation while he is carrying out the venepuncture. A pulse oximeter is particularly useful at this time.

Peripheral vein cannulation is discussed in the intravenous induction section of this chapter. The internal jugular vein in the neck is most often used for central venous cannulation, but there are some circumstances such as neurosurgery where the infraclavicular subclavian approach may provide a more convenient site, away from the surgical field. The left subclavian approach is less likely than the right to be associated with the cannula entering the wrong vessel such as the jugular or opposite subclavian vein.

Central venous cannulation

Because of the comparative difficulty in cannulation of the central veins in children, the indications for the procedure should be examined thoroughly to see if a more peripheral access will suffice. The two basic indications for central venous cannulation are for measurement and for infusion.

Right atrial pressure can be monitored, as in adults, through a central venous cannula.

A central venous infusion may be used for resuscitation, during surgery or for administration of total parenteral nutrition (TPN).

The innominate, internal jugular, or much less commonly external jugular or subclavian vein approach is used where rapid access is required. The other alternative is the femoral vein just medial to the femoral artery in the groin. Percutaneous approaches to the internal jugular and innominate veins will be emphasized.

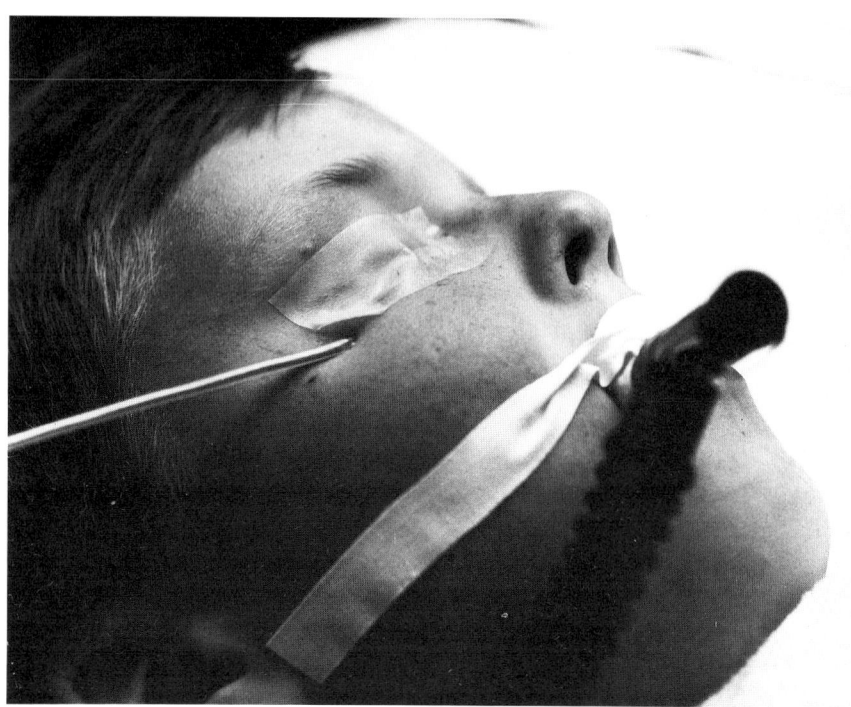

Fig. 7.16 A tape on the eyes closing the lids and preventing drying of the corneas. If the lower outer corner is folded in it makes removal easier at the end of the anaesthetic.

EQUIPMENT AND TECHNIQUE

Seldinger type and multi-lumen catheters suitable for smaller children and infants have become available only recently. Depending upon the purpose of cannulation, different cannulae are used. For neonates and low birth-weight infants, some form of Seldinger technique is probably the safest. The initial venepuncture is performed with a small-bore needle into which is fed a non-traumatic, soft, spring wire, and over this wire the definitive cannula is inserted. A dilator is passed over the guidewire first, so that the hole in the vein will accommodate the catheter. This avoids trauma from the initial use of a large-bore needle. If a large or multi-lumen catheter is advanced, it should be radio-opaque and made from a soft material (or material that will soften at 37°C) to avoid perforation of the great veins or cardiac chambers — complications that carry a high mortality.

BASIC PRINCIPLES OF TECHNIQUE

As most young children are not co-operative, central venous cannulation in the neck is best performed under general anaesthesia. This minimizes any potential for accidental air embolism and avoids the discomfort of maintaining a hyperextended position for a long time.

If the Seldinger technique is not used, the vein should first be identified using a fine needle. Fixation of the cannula is always difficult, and some form of suture is advisable. Subclavian cannulation provides the best and most comfortable fixation, but this approach is not popular for small infants. It is used in older children, particularly during neurosurgery. Subcutaneous tunnelling for long-term placement is possible but it is more difficult with percutaneous cannulation in very small patients. The popular method for fixation is the use of a clear plastic adhesive surgical drape such as Op-site over the cannula and adjacent tubing. A chest X-ray should always be used to determine the position of the catheter tip.

Sepsis is always a problem with central venous lines, the occurrence depending upon a number of factors, including:
maintaining sterility during placement;
meticulous care with placement and while in use;
the type of infusion;
the age of the patient.
Some catheters can be maintained sepsis-free for many months. Bacterial filters or antimicrobial ointments around the site of insertion have not been shown to prolong the sterility of the catheter.

Cannulation sites

INTERNAL JUGULAR—HIGH APPROACH (Fig. 7.17, point 3)

With the patient's head in the supine, head-down position, the neck hyperextended by a roll placed under the shoulders, and the head turned to the opposite side, a point on the skin is selected half-way between the tip of the mastoid process and the suprasternal notch. The initial direction of the needle is 10° lateral to the sagittal plane and at 30° to the skin until bony resistance is felt. This should transfix the vein and as the needle is withdrawn, slight negative pressure is exerted until blood appears in the syringe. Cannulation with a guidewire is then attempted. If the vein is not located at the first attempt, the next insertion of the needle should be 10° more medially. This can be repeated at 10° intervals until the jugular vein is located avoiding puncture of the carotid artery.

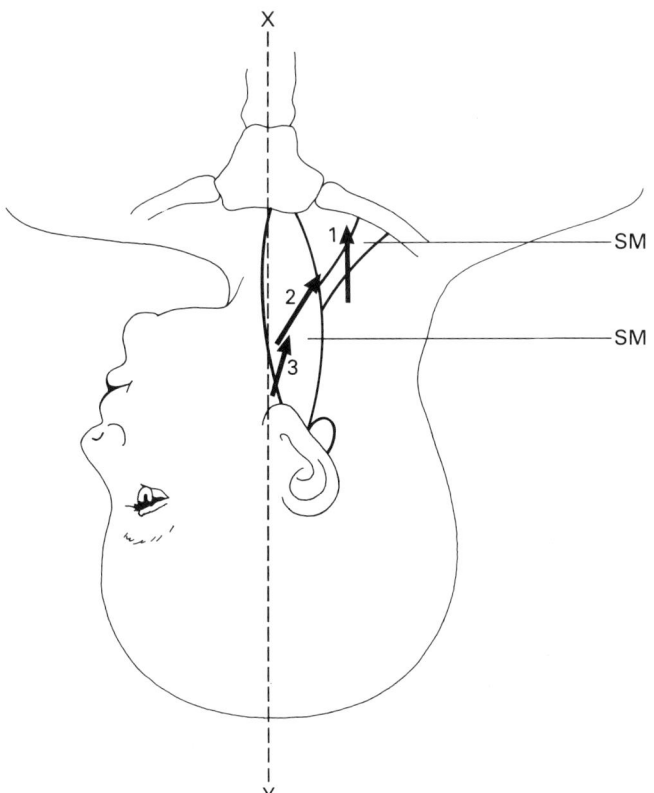

Fig. 7.17 Central venous cannulation. The head is turned to the side. The anaesthetist stands at the head and the three points marked demonstrate the angle at which the needle is inserted for the techniques described. SM = sternomastoid.

INTERNAL JUGULAR—LOW APPROACH (Fig. 7.17, point 2)

With the patient in the same position as before, using the apex of the triangle formed by the two heads of sternomastoid as the entry site, with the needle and syringe at 30° to the skin, they are directed towards the ipsilateral nipple. As the needle is inserted, the vein should be located superficially. The vein should not be intentionally transfixed with this technique. The anatomical reason for the direction towards the nipple is that at this point the internal jugular sweeps slightly laterally for its confluence with the subclavian vein to become the innominate.

INNOMINATE VEIN (Fig. 7.17, point 1)

This technique is useful for very small babies and premature infants, but carries a higher risk of pneumothorax. A notch is formed by the clavicular head of the sternomastoid on the medial end of the superior surface of the clavicle. Using the lateral margin of this notch or the attachment of the sternomastoid tendon to the clavicle as the entry site, the needle is inserted approximately 0.5–1 cm above the clavicle, down the sagittal plane of the body at 30–40° to the coronal plane. Direct cannulation may be attempted in the larger child, but transfixation is more common in the very small infant. Once mastered, this is one of the most reliable techniques in children and the most direct line to the right atrium.

FEMORAL VEIN

Femoral vein cannulation is less commonly used. Sepsis and thrombosis occasionally occur, but it is useful for short periods of 3–4 days. The femoral vein lies immediately medial to the artery in the groin. In small infants and babies a cannula over a needle or a Seldinger technique is used, as the needle is withdrawn into the vein after transfixation. If the patient is mobile the cannula must be flexible. If this approach is used during cardiac arrest it may be difficult to differentiate the femoral vein from the femoral artery, due to their close proximity, and resuscitation drugs (adrenaline, calcium, sodium bicarbonate) may be accidentally injected into the femoral artery.

SUBCLAVIAN VEIN

The infraclavicular approach to the subclavian vein can be useful when access to neck veins is awkward, as in neurosurgery. The vein is approached by inserting the needle medially and cephalad towards the sternal notch at an angle of 10−20° from the skin at the mid-point of the clavicle, so that it passes deep to the clavicle. The vein courses from the axilla and crosses under the clavicle at this point over the first rib and into the thoracic inlet. The needle should be attached to a syringe, with slight negative pressure being applied during insertion so that blood will be drawn back as soon as the vessel is entered (Fig. 7.18). It may help to turn the head away from the side of insertion. The catheter is more likely to enter the right atrium if inserted from the left side. There is a possibility of pleural puncture but this is minimized by inserting the needle at the angle upwards and medially between the clavicle and first rib. The other hazard is subclavian artery puncture, because bleeding cannot be stopped by manual compression.

A catheter can sometimes be threaded centrally from the cubital vein.

PERIPHERAL VEINS

The site will depend on its usage. TPN in small infants is often administered through a fine silastic catheter that has been fed centrally from a peripheral vein (scalp vein to internal jugular, saphenous to femoral vein). This is time-consuming, but long-lasting if maintained properly.

COMPLICATIONS

Complications of cannulation in the neck vary with the approach used, but the operator must be able to deal successfully with any complications. With internal jugular cannulation, perforation of either the carotid or the vertebral artery can occur, whereas with innominate vein cannulation pneumothorax, thoracic-duct perforation (on the left side) and pericardial puncture and tamponade are recognized complications. Phrenic nerve damage is a complication that often goes unrecognized after attempts at large-vein cannulation in the neck.

If the needle is inserted too far with the innominate vein approach pericardial puncture and tamponade can occur.

Infection is the main hazard of femoral venous cannulation, due to the difficulty in keeping the groin clean and dry.

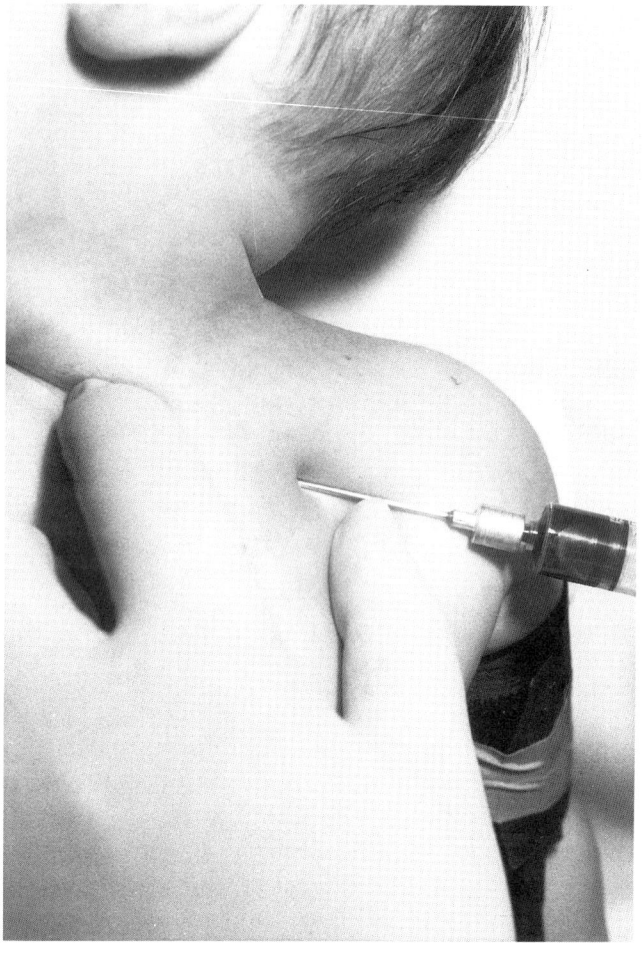

Fig. 7.18 Infraclavicular subclavian approach. The needle is inserted just medial to the mid-point of the clavicle, preferably on the left side, and angled up between the clavicle and the first rib in a medial direction.

POSTURING

The patient is now taken into theatre. Great care must be taken at this stage, and at any other time when he is being moved, to ensure that no traction is applied to the endotracheal tube or intravenous infusion or needle, which may cause them to come out. The head must always be stabilized when positioning, so that inadvertent neck movement does not occur. The patient should never be moved without the permission of the anaesthetist.

Once on the operating table, the patient is placed in the position appropriate for the operation. Whilst the limbs of children are usually freely mobile, it is nevertheless important that no excessive traction be exerted upon them, and that pressure areas are suitably padded, so that there is no danger of injury. Normally the head may be turned to one side, and the connections attached to the endotracheal tube immobilized over a sandbag (Fig. 7.19). The limb containing an intravenous infusion should, where possible, be brought out into a position where the anaesthetist can reach it, or an extension set should be inserted for injection of drugs. Any sandbags or folded towels are placed underneath, rather than on top of, a warming blanket. The posture, depending on the surgical needs, may be supine, lithotomy, lateral, prone or seated.

In the prone position, there is a danger that respiration may be embarrassed. Because of their large abdomen and small chest, infants are a little more difficult to posture than adults. However, an adequate respiratory excursion can usually be ensured by placing a relatively large sandbag under the pelvis, thus leaving the abdomen free, and some freedom of movement of the chest may be obtained by sandbag or rolled-towel supports under each shoulder. Another alternative for lower spinal surgery is the knee–chest position. In older children having spinal surgery, a special frame with hip and shoulder supports can be used (see Fig. 19.4).

The sitting position carries with it difficulties of access and an increased possibility of accidental extubation. Particular care must be taken that the endotracheal tube is firmly strapped in and that the breathing system is adequately supported so that it does not drag on the tube. The anaesthetist must have adequate access to the patient. All pressure areas need to be protected.

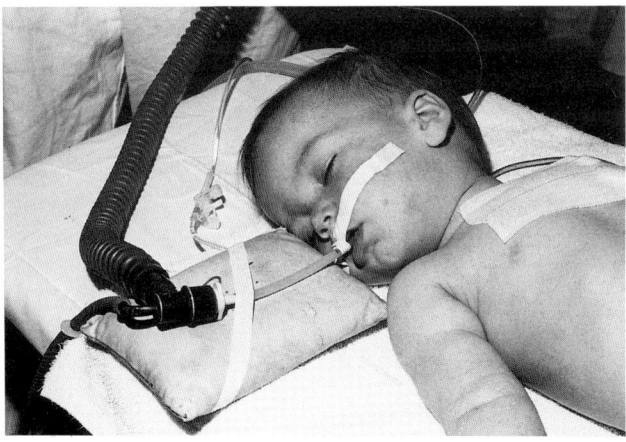

Fig. 7.19 The T-piece supported on a sandbag and fixed with a tape to stabilize the tube. Note the three-way tap for access to the intravenous infusion and the elastoplast holding the precordial stethoscope in place.

MAINTENANCE OF TEMPERATURE

Whenever cooling is likely to occur, the patient should be placed on a warming blanket, unless the nature of the surgical procedure makes this impossible. Exact guidelines are difficult to lay down, but a blanket should be used in every patient under 5 kg, in every patient between 5 and 10 kg having a long operative procedure, and in older patients if it is anticipated that large amounts of cold stored blood will be administered or large areas of the body will be exposed. Warming and humidifying the inspired gases is another important method of maintaining body temperature, especially in small infants (see Chapter 9). During induction and cleansing of the skin, an overhead heater is useful in infants. For neurosurgery, the exposure, shaving and application of cleansing solutions to the relatively large head are significant indications for such a heater.

MAINTENANCE OF ANAESTHESIA

Anaesthesia is usually maintained with a volatile inhalation agent, or by intravenous analgesic and hypnotic infusions. The aim should be to provide sufficient analgesia and to block adverse cardiovascular responses to surgery, which can increase bleeding. Nitrous oxide is frequently used with either of these, but is not essential. If muscle relaxants are used, additional doses, usually one-fifth to one-quarter of the original dose, are administered when required (see Chapter 2). Infusions, especially of the newer shorter-acting relaxants, can be used when neuromuscular blockade is monitored.

The anaesthetist is responsible for the provision of good operating conditions, the maintenance of the blood volume, circulation and ventilation, the administration of fluids and the overall care and monitoring of the patient. Particular aspects relating to the various specialties and techniques are dealt with in the relevant chapters.

CONCLUSION OF ANAESTHESIA

Anaesthesia is discontinued and residual paralysis from muscle relaxants, if they have been used, is reversed by neostigmine (0.03–0.05 mg/kg) or edrophonium (0.1 mg/kg) preceded or accompanied by atropine (half the dose used for neostigmine) or glycopyrrolate (10 µg/kg). These block the undesirable muscarinic (parasympathetic) effects of the acetylcholine, particularly

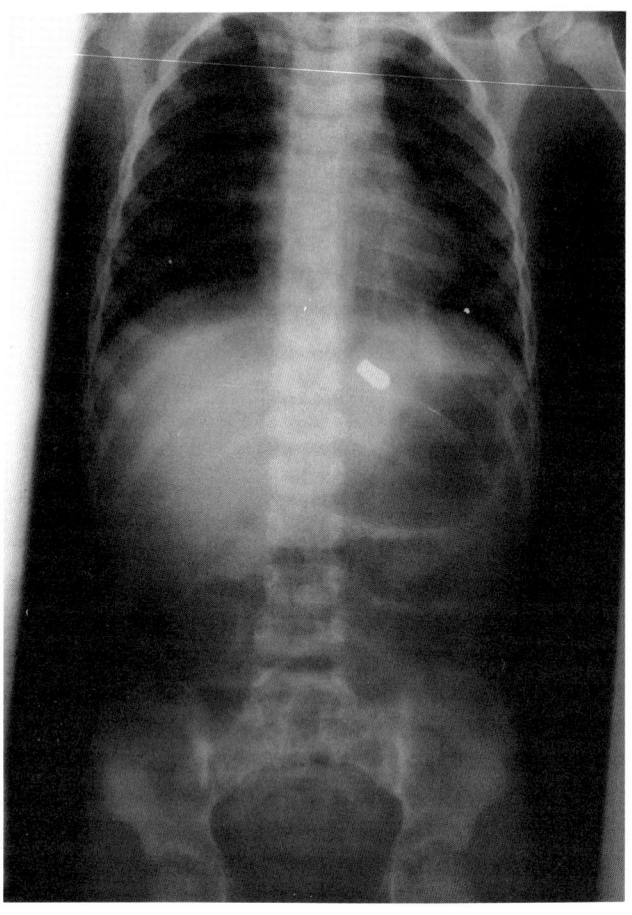

Fig. 7.20 A thoracoabdominal X-ray showing the tip of a sucker in the stomach. It is important to ensure that screw-on tips are firmly attached before suctioning.

bradycardia and production of secretions in the airway. Oxygen should be administered to prevent diffusion hypoxia caused by the elimination of nitrous oxide through the lungs. The patient's pharynx should be sucked out before extubation, ensuring that any loose sucker tip is securely attached (Fig. 7.20). The patient should then be turned on his side and the tube can be removed, when breathing is adequate. Extubation with positive pressure on the bag ensures that the patient exhales and clears the airway.

Extubation laryngeal spasm (see Chapter 27) may occur when the tube is removed at light levels of anaesthesia, especially with halothane, enflurane or isoflurane. It is more common in children than adults. This can be avoided by waiting until the child is almost awake before removing the tube or extubating while the patient is still deeply anaesthetized. The problem with the latter approach is that the patient may develop laryngeal spasm or stridor in the recovery room after the anaesthetist has handed the child over to the nurse.

The child should be on his side, unless there are reasons to the contrary, when going to the recovery room. The upper hand can be placed under the jaw to hold the head in extension so that the airway is maintained (see Fig. 10.3).

8: Pain Management

INTRODUCTION

In recent years anaesthetists have paid more attention to the management of pain and postoperative analgesia. This is particularly so in the youngest age groups, who were formerly considered not to require much analgesia. The ability to measure blood levels of analgesics and hence derive pharmacokinetic data for infants and children has led to improved control of pain. Analgesic infusions and the wider use of local and regional anaesthesia have provided more postoperative comfort for patients.

In this chapter the assessment of pain in children, its significance in newborn infants, and the means of controlling pain in infants and children will be discussed.

ASSESSMENT OF PAIN IN CHILDREN

The measurement and assessment of pain has proved difficult in the paediatric age group. Assessment and management are interrelated. If pain is assessed accurately, adequate and appropriate pain management should follow. Unfortunately no validated and totally accepted tools for measuring pain in children are available. Several methods which are available will be described (Table 8.1).

Physiological measures

Changes in pulse, blood pressure and respiration reflect autonomic arousal. Autonomic responses to pain occur in infants and children, and their measurement forms an important aspect of certain pain scales. As with neonates, it is difficult to correlate these changes with the perception of pain.

Metabolic changes, such as the release of catecholamines, growth hormone, glucagon, cortisol, aldosterone and increased concentration of β-endorphins, adrenocorticotrophin and vasopressin, have been documented in infants and children following noxious stimulation. These have decreased or been abolished by sedatives and analgesics. Such physiological changes may represent reaction to noxious stimulation without necessarily implying subjective distress and pain, but plasma cortisol has been shown to correlate with behavioural responses to noxious stimuli [1].

Self-reporting measures

Self-reporting measures are the best indicators of a child's subjective experience. Various methods have been used

Table 8.1 Methods used for paediatric pain assessment

	Self-report	Behavioural	Physiological
Infant/toddler		Cry characteristics Cry time Facial expression Visual tracking Body movement Response time to stimulus Behavioural state	Heart rate Blood pressure Respiratory rate Sweating

Pre-school	Faces drawings
	Oucher
	Poker-chip tool
	Ladder scale
	Colour scales
	Paediatric pain
	   questionnaire
		Children's Hospital of Eastern
		   Ontario Pain Scale
		Pain behaviour rating scale
		Pain behaviour check-list
		Observation scale of
		   behavioural distress
		Gauvain-Piquard *et al.*
		   scale	

School-age/
   adolescent
	Visual analogue scales
	Numerical rating scales
	Word scales
	Paediatric pain
	   questionnaire
		Objective pain scale
		Pain behaviour rating scale
		Pain behaviour check-list	

in children as young as 3 years. The basis of these methods is that the child identifies various levels of pain intensity using one of the numerous analogues available.

The 'Visual Analogue Scale' (VAS), the accepted method of measurement of pain in adults, is acceptable and provides reproducible results in children down to an age of 5 years. VAS uses a 10 cm length scale, marked 'no pain' at one end to 'excruciating pain' at the other end with 1 mm or 1 cm segments. Some investigators believe that a 100 mm segmented scale is better than 10 cm as fewer segments reduce the patient's choice to a limited number of grades. The child is asked to identify a point on the scale which corresponds to his pain. A score of less than 40 is no pain, less than 60 is tolerable pain and more than 60 needs medication. This scale requires patient comprehension and co-operation. Preoperative explanation of the method and its usefulness in alleviating patient's pain induces good co-operation.

This concept has been modified by different workers for ease of comprehension of children and usually gives fewer choices. These are the addition of smiling to crying faces along the scale (Fig. 8.1); a 10 cm pole or 10-step ladder with a monkey (toy) trying to climb it. The child is asked to locate the point up to which the monkey will be able to climb with the same degree of pain as the patient has.

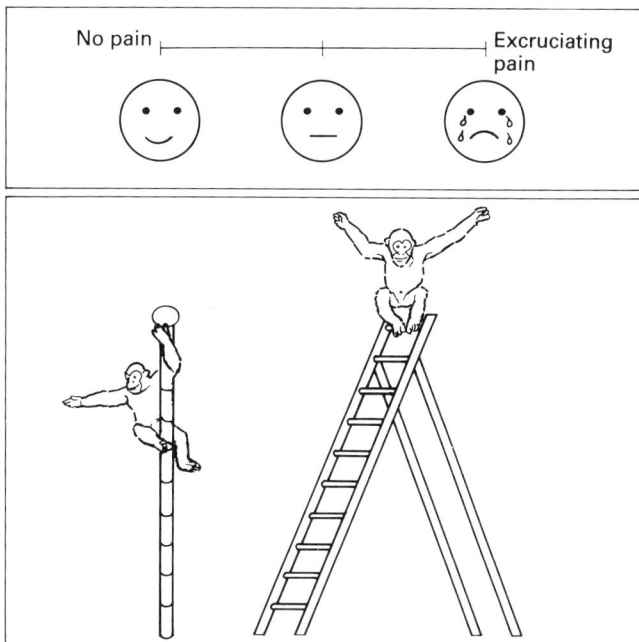

Fig. 8.1 (above) A simple visual analogue scale with three faces from smiling to crying. (below) Alternatively a 10 cm pole or 10-step ladder with a monkey climbing it can be used to locate the point.

The Oucher scale displays six photographs of a child's face showing increasing levels of discomfort. Children select the facial expression that best reflects their experience of pain (Fig. 8.2). Though the number of grades limits sensitivity, it is a useful scale for younger children as it does not require a high degree of cognitive development.

The Poker Chip Tool allows children to quantify pain when they select one to four poker chips to indicate the level of their discomfort.

For older children, a paediatric pain questionnaire has been developed as a modification of the McGill pain questionnaire used in adults.

Behavioural measures

This method of assessment relies on observation of behaviour and is more useful in the pre-school age group of children. A number of behaviour scales have been developed. They score the behaviours which represent the reaction to pain and scores are allotted according to the degree of alteration of a particular behaviour. The behaviours scored include vocal behaviours such as cry, scream, verbally expressed pain and anxiety, and non-verbal behaviours such as muscle rigidity, torso movement, leg movement, facial expression, the need to be restrained or carried.

The pain behaviour rating scale (PBRS) and Children's Hospital of Eastern Ontario Pain Scale (CHEOP) are two such scales. The observations in these scales can have an observer bias. The overlapping of scores for similar behaviours can give a falsely high score. Certain behaviours like cry, anxiety or muscle rigidity are taken for granted as being due to pain, which may not be true.

The objective pain scale (OPS) measures a physiological variable — blood pressure — along with behavioural changes. There is an overlapping of behaviours such as movement, agitation and body language, which gives a falsely high score.

Crying has often been attributed to pain only, whereas thirst and hunger can be important causes of cry. The All India Institute of Medical Science (AIIMS) pain—discomfort scale provides allowance for thirst and hunger, avoids duplication of behaviours and includes physiological changes such as heart rate and respiration, which can be measured without causing discomfort to the patient (Table 8.2). For these reasons it is a good, clinically relevant scoring system and has been validated against VAS in children up to 5 years.

Gauvain-Piquard described a behaviour rating scale for the assessment of cancer pain in pre-school children. In addition to pain and anxiety behaviours, behaviours indicative of depression, e.g. social withdrawal, were included [2].

Most of the pain scores described have been used in clinical research work. Their validity and role in clinical practice (except for VAS) is not well documented.

A simple, useful clinical method of assessment of pain in children is described as: severe — when the patient is too distressed to take a normal breath; moderate — when too distressed to take a deep breath; mild — when distressed while coughing; and no pain — when the

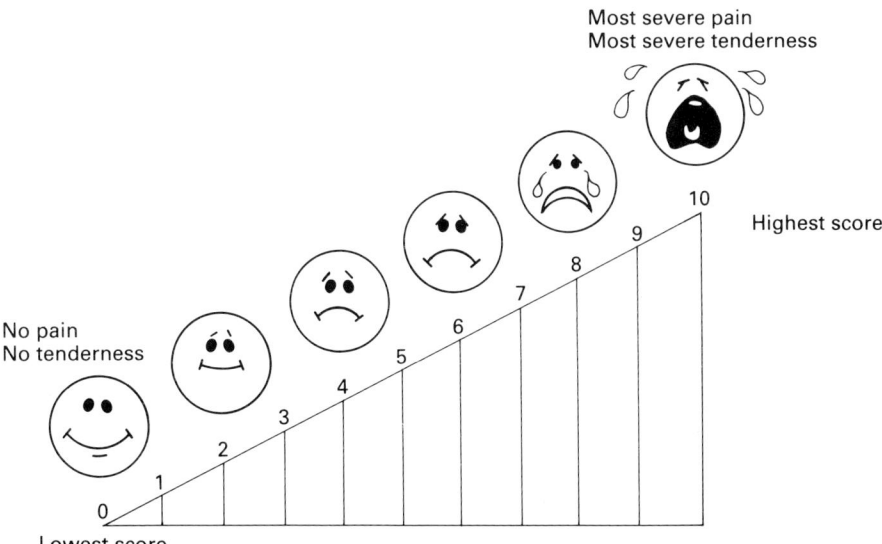

Fig. 8.2 An analogue scale with six faces indicating increasing discomfort.

Table 8.2 Pain discomfort scale (AIIMS)

Resp. rate	+ 20%	Pre-op	0
	+ 20–50%	Pre-op	1
	>+50%	Pre-op	2
Heart rate	+ 10%	Pre-op	0
	+ 20%	Pre-op	1
	+ 30%	Pre-op	2
Discomfort	Calm		0
	Restless		1
	Agitated		2
Cry	No cry		
	Cry respond to water, food, parental presence		0
	Cry respond to tender loving care		1
	Cry not responding to tender loving care		2
Pain at site of operation	No pain		0
	States pain vague		1
	Can localize pain		2

patient can cough without distress. For surgery of the limbs and lower abdomen, the latter two grades need no medication, whereas even mild pain is treated in postoperative patients following thoracic and upper abdominal surgery.

ASSESSMENT OF PAIN IN NEONATES

Development of pain pathways

The question of whether neonates feel pain has recently been looked at more closely. Maturation of the pain pathways in the human fetus and neonate would suggest that anatomical mechanisms are well enough developed for neonates to feel pain. Cutaneous sensory perception appears in the human fetus by the 7th week of gestation and is present in all cutaneous and mucous surfaces by 20 weeks [3].

A later development of the fetal nervous system is myelination, and as this occurs the conduction velocity of nerve impulses increases. The degree of myelination is used as an index of maturation [4]. Pain pathways in the spinal cord and brain stem up to the thalamus are developed by 30 weeks' gestation and the connection through the posterior limb of the internal capsule and corona radiata to the cortex are myelinated by 37 weeks' gestation. Thus the neural pathways conducting impulses from the periphery to the cortex are developed in fullterm infants [5]. In premature infants born before 37

weeks these pathways are not fully myelinated, so that conduction velocity will be slower.

By 20 weeks' gestation the cortex has a full complement of neurones. Evidence of functional maturity of the cerebral cortex in the fetus and neonate exists. Fetal and neonatal electroencephalographic patterns including cortical components of visual and auditory evoked potentials have been recorded in pre-term infants of less than 30 weeks' gestation [6, 7]. Measurements of cerebral glucose utilization have shown that the highest rates of metabolic activity occur in the sensory areas of the neonatal brain [8]. Thus human newborns do have the anatomical and functional components required for the appreciation of painful stimuli.

Assessment of pain in the neonatal age group has become one of the most challenging problems faced by paediatric anaesthetists. Assessment is by necessity indirect, as self-reporting measures are not applicable in this age group.

Parameters studied include physiological measures and behavioural changes.

Physiological measures

Physiological variables have been useful in examining the pain experiences associated with short-term medical procedures; however there are no physiological responses that directly reflect the neonate's perception of pain. In short procedures it is possible to detect physiological changes indicative of autonomic arousal, but adaptation may occur and autonomic responses return to normal.

HEART RATE

Increases in heart rate are seen in newborns when exposed to painful procedures such as heel-lance or circumcision. The heart rate returns to normal within 3–5 minutes following cessation of the painful stimulus.

RESPIRATORY RATE AND SYSTOLIC BLOOD PRESSURE

Both these parameters increase significantly in neonates subjected to painful procedures.

PALMAR WATER LOSS

Experimental studies have shown an increase in palmar water loss in neonates following heel-prick. Infants more than 36 or 37 weeks' gestational age had a 200–300% increase in palmar water loss, while in older infants the increase was nearly 500% [9].

Changes in transcutaneous oxygen tension occur in neonates during painful procedures. Both rises and falls in transcutaneous oxygen tensions have been seen in neonates. Most of the falls in oxygen tensions have occurred in the premature age group, and it is possible to conclude that healthy term infants and sick premature neonates may have differing responses to similar stimuli when measuring transcutaneous oxygen tension.

Behavioural changes

CRYING

Detailed characteristics of crying have also been used as indicators of pain/distress behaviour in response to noxious stimuli. Descriptive characteristics of cry patterns include changes in duration as well as pitch and intensity. Acoustic characteristics such as pitch were significantly higher for hunger than for pain cries. Researchers maintain that individuals can be trained to differentiate by ear different combinations of tenseness in neonatal cries, and perhaps in pitch and other important acoustic variables [10].

FACIAL EXPRESSION

Changes in facial expression associated with painful procedures in neonates are reliably recognizable, and a number of distinct facial behaviours have been noted. These include such things as brow bulge, eye squeeze, changes in nasolabial fold and changes in lip position. They may allow more accurate assessment of pain in this age group [11].

Further studies of behavioural changes in male infants undergoing circumcision have also proved interesting. Neonates who were assigned a category, either average, subdued or hyperactive, changed categories for at least 4 hours after circumcision and in a third of these children behavioural differences were maintained for up to 22 hours. The assumption that all subjects would become more active and irritable during and after circumcision was proved to be incorrect. Some infants react to the distress of circumcision by becoming less active. The diversity of responses to the stressful procedure of circumcision suggests that infants have unique coping styles from birth [12].

Neonates subjected to surgical stress show a substantial and prolonged postoperative catabolic reaction that is increased or more marked if no anaesthetic or analgesia is used. It has been argued that, although babies feel pain and mount a substantial stress response, this does not matter since the memory of the sensation is not retained and memory is necessary for the development of pain perception. This is really conjecture at the moment; long-term behavioural studies are needed to clarify the picture.

NEONATAL ANALGESIA

If we accept the accumulating data which suggest that neonates feel pain, what are the options for its management?

No analgesia

Some neonates having procedures that are not painful afterwards may require no postoperative analgesia, if they have been adequately anaesthetized. Avoiding unduly long preoperative fasting and resuming feeds as soon as practicable can reduce stress and hasten recovery.

Paracetamol

Paracetamol 15–20 mg/kg is the most useful drug for relief of postoperative pain in neonates and small infants. This may be given either orally or as a suppository. For short procedures, paracetamol may be added to oral premedication.

Local and regional analgesia

Local and regional techniques used in infants and older children can also be applied to the neonate for the relief of postoperative pain. Care must be taken in selecting the appropriate dosage of local anaesthetic in the neonatal period, as it has been suggested that the maximum safe levels of local anaesthetic, especially bupivacaine, may be slightly lower in the newborn than in older children. Intercostal block and local infiltration of wounds may be performed by the surgeon under direct vision to provide postoperative analgesia.

Opioids

Fentanyl causes less postoperative apnoea and shorter maximum periods between breaths in infants 3–12 months old compared to children and young adults. This is due to relatively lower plasma levels. It would seem that small doses of fentanyl can be used in neonates and may be the best choice for intraoperative analgesia (see Chapter 2).

Morphine up to 0.1 mg/kg intramuscularly, or as an infusion 10 μg/kg/h and perhaps codeine phosphate up to 1 mg/kg rectally or orally may be used in appropriate neonates for postoperative analgesia. These doses may cause respiratory depression in younger and less mature neonates, and should only be used in these patients if postoperative ventilation is planned. Neonates who require ventilation postoperatively may well require opioid infusions not only for the relief of postoperative pain but for continuing sedation to blunt the stress response that occurs in these neonates with handling and suction. This may be very important in the control of pulmonary hypertension in some neonates. In the first weeks of life, the distribution half-life of morphine is prolonged (6–8 hours). When patients have been mechanically ventilated, adequate time for opioid excretion must be allowed before weaning so that spontaneous breathing is not depressed. Adequate pain relief in the postoperative period in this group should not be traded for an increase in ventilator days, with possible associated morbidity.

Opioids used during the operation will continue to have an analgesic effect in the postoperative period and ablate stress responses in this age group. The danger of respiratory depression in the postoperative period must be emphasized. Careful nursing observation and appropriate monitoring are essential. In small and premature babies the sensitivity to opioids and slow elimination are determinants of opioid use. If the baby is to breathe spontaneously after operation, the margin of safety with these drugs decreases with the degree of prematurity.

If it is desirable to have the baby breathing spontaneously postoperatively, an inhalation supplement can be used, remembering that the MAC in neonates is lower than in older children, so that lower concentrations can be used to provide anaesthesia.

MANAGEMENT OF POSTOPERATIVE PAIN

Psychological

The management of postoperative pain begins preoperatively with appropriate teaching and guidance. Most children benefit from a simple and honest explanation of what they can expect following surgery. If the surgery planned is going to be painful postoperatively, these explanations should include a discussion of pain management and appropriate treatments.

Premedication

If analgesics are given with the premedication, their effect may last into the postoperative period. Successful premedication before surgery reduces anxiety and can help alleviate fear. Induction of anaesthesia is then easier. Rarely are intramuscular injections required if an effective oral premedication can be given safely.

Oral analgesics

These include:
Paracetamol 20 mg/kg;
Opioid, e.g. morphine, methadone, buprenorphine;
Combination;
Non-steroidal anti-inflammatory analgesics.

It is safe to use paracetamol in neonates because the immature neonatal liver forms less of the toxic metabolite than in adults. A single dose of 30 mg/kg will provide 8 hours' analgesia. Paracetamol is still the most useful drug for postoperative pain relief in children after minor procedures, and for day-stay patients. It is useful in combination with oral premedication in short procedures such as myringotomy and the insertion of grommets.

Oral opioids or drugs that combine opioids and paracetamol have had very little place in the management of postoperative pain in children. The opioids may cause gastrointestinal disturbance and adverse effects on the central nervous system. During long-term administration tolerance may develop.

The fourth category of oral analgesics constitutes the most important recent development in pain management with analgesic drugs. The newer peripherally acting, non-steroidal anti-inflammatory analgesics, some of which are clearly more efficacious than paracetamol compare favourably, not only with full doses of opioid combination products but even, in some cases, with strong injectable opioids. Some of these drugs have a much longer duration of analgesic effect than paracetamol. One example, diclofenac 2 mg/kg rectally, has been shown to be as useful as opioids in control of postoperative pain after tonsillectomy. Piroxicam is another example that can be used as a single daily dose, or at the most twice a day, for effective postoperative pain management.

The anti-inflammatory analgesics are particularly effective in dental pain, certain postoperative pain in adults and pain associated with acute musculoskeletal trauma. The potential use of these agents has not yet been completely explored by researchers or fully recognized and exploited in medical practice. Further studies need to compare non-steroidal anti-inflammatory drugs among themselves and determine their value in postoperative pain management in children.

Parenteral analgesics

These may be given either as intermittent intramuscular injections or by intravenous infusion. Intermittent injections have several disadvantages. Unless they are given frequently enough, and they rarely are, the plasma concentration reaches the therapeutic level only intermittently and a bigger dose which reaches the therapeutic level for longer periods may well increase the incidence of effects such as nausea and vomiting, or even respiratory depression (Fig. 8.3). The additional disadvantage in children is that their dislike and fear of needles and intramuscular injections may be so great that they may choose to suffer pain rather than ask for an injection.

Nurses may also be inhibited from giving injections because the child objects, or does not convey to the nurse that he has pain. Intermittent injections are probably appropriate where only one or two doses will be needed.

Opiate infusions provide more consistent analgesia with fewer side effects, because the plasma concentration can be maintained within the therapeutic range and below the toxic level (Fig. 8.4). Selection of the rate of infusion depends on factors such as age (neonates and infants should have lower rates) and the nature of the operation (major surgery, particularly orthopaedic, requires higher rates). If, after a loading dose, the infusion does not adequately control pain, the rate can be increased. A bolus can be given or the rate temporarily increased when a painful procedure, such as physiotherapy after a thoracotomy, is anticipated. If nausea, vomiting or drowsiness occurs and the patient is pain-free, the infusion rate should be reduced. Opiate infusions provide good postoperative analgesia even in infants, but the patient must be observed carefully for signs of respiratory depression.

Opiate infusions are usually run for up to 3 or 4 days postoperatively, but may be continued for longer periods in patients having multiple procedures such as burns grafting and dressing changes.

Suggested guidelines for opiate infusions are:

1 Morphine

0.5 mg/kg added to 500 ml of i.v. solution makes a solution containing 1 μg/kg/ml

Infusion rate: 10−40 ml/h

Initial bolus: 0.075−0.1 mg/kg i.v.

   or 0.1−0.2 mg/kg i.m.

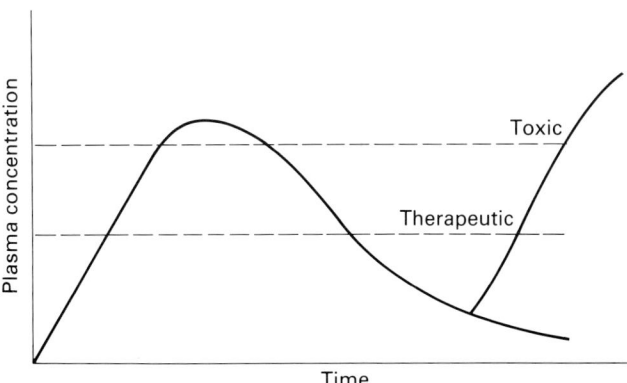

Fig. 8.3 A plasma concentration−time graph showing how there are periods when the levels are above the toxic level and below the therapeutic range following a single intramuscular injection.

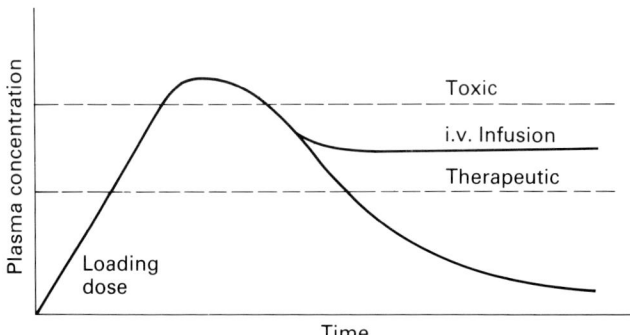

Fig. 8.4 A plasma concentration−time graph demonstrating how the use of a constant infusion after a loading dose can maintain the plasma level within the therapeutic range.

2 Pethidine

5 mg/kg added to 500 ml of i.v. solution makes a solution containing 10 μg/kg/ml

Infusion rate: 10–40 ml/h
Initial bolus: 0.5–0.75 mg/kg i.v.
or 0.75–1 mg/kg i.m.

Infusion rates are usually controlled by syringe pumps. If these are not available, infusion is still possible if an infusing burette and good patient monitoring is available. The hourly dose can be added to the burette — if, by accident, it runs through too quickly, serious complications are unlikely, provided the burette is not refilled until the hour is complete.

Patient-controlled analgesia (PCA) is a technique for managing postoperative pain which utilizes a programmable syringe pump to allow patients to self-administer their own intravenous narcotic medication. The syringe pump delivers morphine (or other opiate analgesic) in two ways. Firstly, by pressing a remote button the patient can deliver a programmed bolus dose as required. A lock-out period, usually 5–10 minutes, is set so that the machine will not respond for the set period of time. This allows each dose time to work before the patient can give himself another bolus, and it is this lock-out period which prevents overdosage occurring. In addition, a background infusion can be added to prevent peaks and troughs of pain relief and reduce the number of times the patient has to press the button. By putting the patient in control of his own intravenous pain relief, the analgesic therapy is tailored to individual requirements. Differences between patients is therefore well catered for. Patient-controlled analgesia, besides offering excellent analgesia for the majority of patients, has proved very safe, has high patient satisfaction and also reduces staff workload. Patients are instructed preoperatively about the PCA device and how it works. They are also instructed to use the PCA device in a prophylactic manner to avoid incident pain, which occurs during physiotherapy, dressing changes, ambulation and the like. It is difficult to set a lower age limit for the use of PCA devices in children but it has been used in 6–7-year-olds successfully. Any child who can understand the concept of pressing a button when they are in too much pain can well utilize this device.

Local and regional analgesia

Regional anaesthesia can be central or peripheral. The latter includes blocks for individual nerves. In children the blocks are performed either after the induction of anaesthesia or at the conclusion of the operation. In both circumstances they contribute to postoperative analgesia if a long-acting drug such as bupivacaine is used. There are no peripheral nerve blocks used in adults that cannot be used in children, although techniques must be adapted to the smaller patient (see Chapter 22).

Ilio-inguinal and iliohypogastric nerve blocks are useful for herniotomy and orchidopexy and are the most frequently used. The external oblique aponeurosis may be difficult to feel in small babies. In infants and for people not familiar with these blocks local infiltration of the wound may be as effective, provided recommended maximum doses of local anaesthetics are not exceeded. Blockade of the femoral, sciatic and lateral femoral cutaneous nerves can be used in lower limb surgery. Digital nerve blocks may be useful. Intercostal blocks can be useful even in small children. They can be performed under direct vision by the surgeon when the chest is open during thoracotomy, but if they are part of the anaesthetic they can be done following induction. Bupivacaine up to 3 mg/kg is an ideal agent for these blocks as it will give up to 5–6 hours' duration of analgesia, but care must be taken to avoid intravascular injection.

The relatively smaller size of the patient must be taken into consideration when assessing where to insert the needle. The correct plane for injection can be assessed by feeling relevant loss of resistance as the aponeurosis or fascia is penetrated, and using the fact that it is difficult to inject while passing through muscle. In small infants, fascia or aponeuroses are thin and less easy to feel even with a 45° bevel needle. An angled approach, for instance, when penetrating the external oblique aponeurosis during ilio-inguinal block, gives a greater thickness of fascia to feel.

Cervical plexus, brachial plexus, thoracic or lumbar epidural and caudal blocks are used to enhance operating conditions and provide postoperative pain relief.

Caudal extradural block is useful in lower abdominal, penile, scrotal and lower limb surgery in children. Bupivacaine 0.25% is useful in day-patient surgery as it provides good analgesia with minimal motor blockade, so that discharge from hospital is not delayed. The duration of analgesia can be extended by the addition of 0.05 mg/kg morphine [13].

Lumbar or thoracic epidurals can be used for more major surgery in children, either as a single injection or by continuous infusion. With newer equipment it is now possible to place indwelling epidural catheters, even in very small infants. Infusion of local anaesthetic can thereby be continued into the postoperative period. One such regimen uses 0.125% bupivacaine at a rate of 0.2 ml/kg/h with or without the addition of fentanyl (0.2 µg/kg/h). The solution can be made up in a 60 ml syringe for a syringe pump — 75 mg plain bupivacaine in 5% dextrose and fentanyl 60 µg. These infusions can be continued for up to 72 hours in the postoperative period. They offer good pain relief with few cardiovascular or respiratory complications. For success, the catheter should be inserted by an experienced anaesthetist, a dependable infusion pump is required and measures must be taken to prevent infection. If complications are to be avoided, the patient must be adequately monitored by nursing staff. Some potential complications of epidural infusions are: motor blockade, which can be reduced if a lower concentration of local anaesthetic is used; the signs of surgical complications may be masked especially in lower limb surgery when plaster casts are used; dural puncture and intravascular injection. These become less frequent as experience with the technique increases, but early detection is important so that total spinal anaesthesia or disastrous toxic overdose are avoided. The addition of opioids (most commonly fentanyl, pethidine or morphine) to local anaesthetic prolongs the duration of analgesia beyond that of the local anaesthetic alone. The commonest problems are nausea, vomiting and urinary retention, together with pruritis when morphine is used. So far there have been few reports of delayed respiratory depression after opioids combined with local anaesthetics in extradural blockade, but it is important that the maximum dose is not exceeded and that these patients are monitored very closely for respiratory depression for at least 24 hours postoperatively.

Opiate epidural infusions, for example with pethidine, are sometimes used, especially in spinal surgery where postoperative neurological assessment of leg function is necessary. The infusion rates used are similar to intravenous infusion rates, e.g. pethidine (0.1–0.4 mg/kg/h).

Newer techniques

New devices, concepts and techniques of drug delivery have been developed in recent years. Transdermal fentanyl patches have been used successfully in the management of postoperative pain. These patches achieve a steady plasma concentration of fentanyl, pro-

viding good postoperative analgesia with minimal side effects. Hyoscine patches have also been used for postoperative anti-emetic action.

Nasally administered sufentanil premedication has provided sedation, easier separation of children from parents, improved induction conditions and some postoperative analgesia. Although crying was common during administration and there was a high incidence of vomiting, there were few other side effects.

Fentanyl-impregnated lollipops are another possibility for use as a premedicant in children.

A morphine hydrogel suppository is being evaluated for control of pain in children. This suppository is a sustained-release rectal preparation which can be used to attain and maintain analgesic plasma concentrations of morphine.

Implanted drug delivery devices are also being developed, and these may be useful in the management of chronic pain in children.

These new delivery techniques should be convenient for the anaesthetist and the patient, providing a wide safety margin and improved bioavailability. Evaluation of the benefits of these systems should lead to more flexible and effective pain management and control of nausea and will almost certainly have an impact on anaesthesia in the future, as more agents and techniques are tested.

CHRONIC PAIN

Chronic pain in children relates mainly to malignant tumours and is usually managed by the oncologist, often with oral drugs. Patients with pain are sometimes referred to anaesthetists in the hope that a nerve block will relieve the pain or determine whether ablation of the nerve would be useful. Occasionally a single nerve block will break a pain cycle and cure a chronic localized pain, or at least provide relief for a prolonged period. On the other hand, a nerve block may relieve pain in one area but unmask pain somewhere else.

Coeliac plexus block may be useful in relieving severe malignancy-induced abdominal pain. It has proved very effective in patients with widespread malignant carcinoid tumour.

Debilitating limb pain is the most common type for referral to anaesthetists. In some patients this is due to reflex sympathetic dystrophy (see below).

Chronic pain is multifactorial and a variety of treatments may need to be tried. Appropriate texts should be consulted for a full discussion of chronic pain management.

Reflex sympathetic dystrophy

Patients with reflex sympathetic dystrophy are sometimes referred to anaesthetists for management of their pain, mainly by orthopaedic surgeons and neurologists. It is a condition which is uncommon before 10 years of age. It is characterized by a painful, tender foot or hand, which is cool and may be sweaty compared to the other side. The pulse on the affected side is usually weaker, and capillary refill slower. Long-standing cases may develop osteoporosis and oedema. Girls are more commonly affected than boys. There may be a history of trauma, which is often minor. Some of these patients, particularly young teenage girls, may have psychological problems. A slow intravenous injection of phentolamine (0.1–0.2 mg/kg) will temporarily relieve pain in reflex sympathetic dystrophy but will not if the problem is predominantly psychological. An intravenous infusion should be running when the injection is given, to prevent severe hypotension [14]. The diagnosis can be confirmed by demonstrating a delayed skin potential response on the affected foot and relief by sympathetic block [15]. If the diagnosis is made early, physiotherapy with a graduated exercise programme may be successful, but when it is delayed more aggressive treatment may be necessary. An intravenous regional guanethidine block with 10–30 mg of quanethidine in 20–30 ml saline injected into an exsanguinated leg with a tourniquet which is kept inflated for 15 minutes has been used with reasonable success [14]. Lumbar sympathetic block has produced good results when the foot is involved (Fig. 8.5). One or two local anaesthetic blocks may be curative and often have a beneficial effect lasting longer than the local anaesthetic action. On very rare occasions in children a phenol 6% block may be necessary. In one such child who was debilitated for several months, shortening of the tibia occurred [16]. Following successful sympathetic block, catch-up growth occurred over the next 6 months (Fig. 8.6). Early recognition and treatment is important if long-term disability is to be avoided.

Occasionally atypical cases present with a painful, tender foot for which no treatment has so far been successful. A phentolamine test may help to determine cases that might benefit from a sympathetic block, which is occasionally useful as a therapeutic test despite an unusual history.

CONCLUSION

The increased interest in pain in recent years has led to the development of new drugs and methods of adminis-

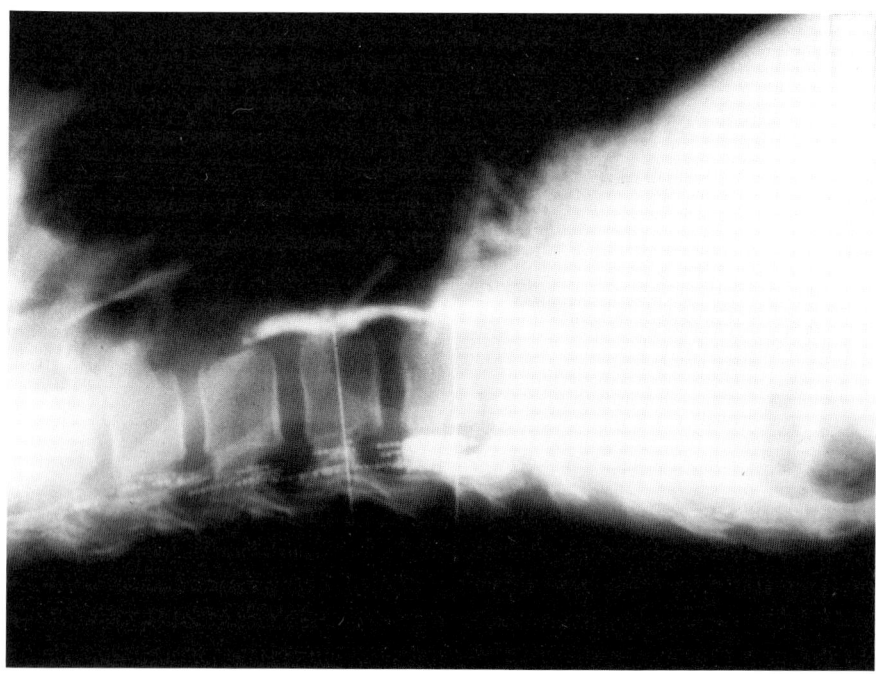

Fig. 8.5 A lateral view of the lumbar vertebrae showing the needles in place for a lumbar sympathetic block. The narrow line of dye indicates that the injection is in the correct layer. It should be noted that the space carrying the sympathetic chain is very narrow. The needle tip should be level with the anterior border of the vertebral body on the lateral view.

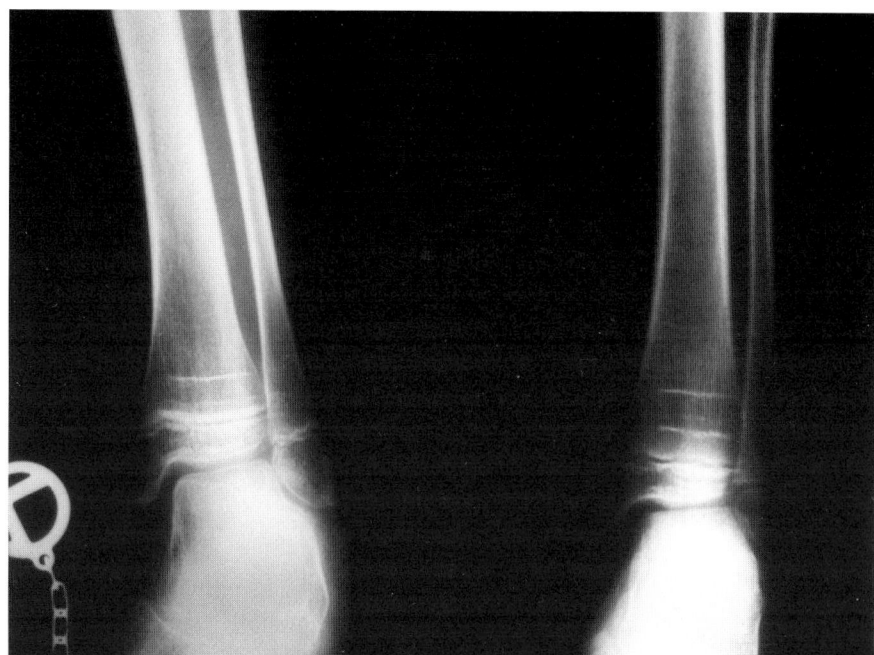

Fig. 8.6 X-rays of a 9-year-old girl with reflex sympathetic dystrophy. The left hand film was taken prior to lumbar sympathetic block and the right hand film 6 months later, indicating the segment of catch-up growth. (From Brown & Doolan, with permission, from *Anaesthesia and Intensive Care*).

tration and a greater emphasis on the recognition and assessment of pain in patients of all ages, including babies.

REFERENCES

1 Tennes K., Carter D. Plasma cortisol level and behavioural states in early infancy. *Psych Med* 1973, 121.

2 Gauvain-Piquard A., Rodary C., Rezvare A., Lemezle J. Pain in children aged 2–6 years: a non-observational rating scale elaborated in a pediatric oncology unit — preliminary report. *Pain* 1987, **31**, 177.

3 Humphrey T. Some correlation between the appearance of human fetal reflexes and the development of the nervous system. *Prog Brain Res* 1964, **4**, 93.

4 Tilnet F., Rosett J. The value of brain lipoids as an index of brain development. *Neurol Inst NY* 1931, **1**, 28.

5 Anand K.S., Hickey P.R. Pain and its effects in the human neonate and fetus. *New Engl J Med* 1987, **317**, 1321.

6 Henderson-Smart D.J., Pettigrew A.G., Campbell D.G. Clinical apnoea and brain-stem neural function in pre-term infants. *New Engl J Med* 1983, **308**, 353.

7 Torres F., Anderson C. The normal EEG of human newborn.

J Clin Neurophysiol 1985, **2**, 89.

8 Chugan H.T., Phelps M.E. Maturational changes in cerebral function in infants determined by ISFDG positron emission tomography. *Science* 1988, **231**, 840.

9 Harpin V.A., Rutter N. Development of emotional sweating in the newborn infant. *Arch Dis Child* 1982, **57**, 691.

10 Fuller B., Horjii Y. Differences in fundamental frequency, jitter and shimmer among four types of infant vocalization. *J Comm Dis* 1986, **19**, 111.

11 Grunau R.V.E., Craig K.D. Pain expression in neonates: facial action and cry. *Pain* 1987, **28**, 395.

12 Marshall R.E., Stratton W.C., Moore J.A. *et al.* Circumcision I. Effects upon newborn behaviour. *Infant Behav Dev* 1980, **3**, 1.

13 Wolf A.R., Hughes D., Hobbs A.J., Prys-Roberts C. Combined morphine–bupivacaine caudals for reconstructive penile surgery in children: systemic absorption of morphine and post-operation analgesia. *Anaes Intens Care* 1991, **19**, 17.

14 Olsson G.L., Arnar S., Hirsch G. Reflex sympathetic dystrophy in children. *Adv Pain Res Ther* 1990, **15**, 323.

15 Cronin K.D., Kirsner R.L.G. Diagnosis of reflex sympathetic dysfunction. Use of the skin potential response. *Anaesthesia* 1982, **37**, 848.

16 Doolan L.A., Brown T.C.K. Reflex sympathetic dystrophy in a child. *Anaes Intens Care* 1984, **12**, 70.

9: Anaesthesia for the Neonate

INTRODUCTION

Neonates differ from older patients in several ways which affect anaesthesia. Anatomical differences and the small size can make venepuncture, intubation and ventilation difficult. The response to, and requirements for, drugs vary with maturity within the neonatal period, and differ significantly from those of older children. Immature cardiorespiratory function, the relatively large surface-area-to-body-weight ratio that contributes to thermal instability, and the relatively large extracellular fluid compartment influence the management of anaesthesia. There is considerable difference in size and maturity between a premature infant and a baby 1 month old, so

that the anaesthetist must take into account the changes occurring during this dynamic period of growth (see Chapters 1 and 2).

PREOPERATIVE ASSESSMENT AND PREPARATION

Neonates requiring surgery usually have major anomalies. Often there are commonly associated malformations. They may be seriously ill due to the anomaly itself or other disease processes which may be associated with prematurity, delayed presentation or superimposed infection; infection may not be accompanied by pyrexia. In addition, the newborn infant is undergoing rapid changes in cardiorespiratory function associated with adaptation to extrauterine life. Before operation, it is important to assess cardiorespiratory stability, state of hydration, acid–base balance and electrolyte status. These should, if possible, be corrected before surgery.

Neonatal surgical patients are susceptible to intercurrent diseases and other problems that may influence the conduct of anaesthesia. These include the following:
1 Newborn respiratory distress syndrome (hyaline membrane disease) mainly affects premature infants. Lack of surfactant leads to alveolar collapse, hypoxaemia and increased work of breathing (see Chapter 1). The physiological disturbance can be mitigated by increased inspired oxygen, continuous positive airway pressure (CPAP) or continuous positive pressure ventilation (CPPV). Perforated necrotizing enterocolitis is the most common surgical condition associated with this disease. There are obvious implications for respiratory management during anaesthesia, such as the application of CPAP.
2 Unconjugated hyperbilirubinaemia is associated with maternal/fetal blood group incompatibility or prematurity. Affected infants may be sleepy and prone to apnoeic episodes. Caution must be exercised with drugs that are detoxified by the liver, such as barbiturates and narcotics, if liver function is depressed, and with drugs which can be displaced from their protein-binding sites by bilirubin.

3 Haemorrhagic disease of the newborn is now prevented by the routine administration of vitamin K_1 at birth. If there is doubt about the coagulation status of the infant, an additional dose should be given before surgery. Other coagulopathies, such as disseminated intravascular coagulation associated with septicaemia, may also occur.

4 Hypoglycaemia (below 2 mmol/l) occurs particularly in premature infants associated with reduced hepatic glycogen stores (Chapter 1) and starvation.

5 Hypocalcaemia (below 1.9 mmol/l, although symptoms rarely develop above 1.5 mmol/l) occurs in prematurity, sepsis, birth asphyxia and DiGeorge syndrome (hypoparathyroidism, thymic aplasia).

6 Birth trauma and asphyxia with central nervous system damage may be responsible for depression.

7 Infection may be present, especially septicaemia, pneumonia and meningitis.

Improvements in neonatal intensive care for newborns, especially the premature and very ill, have meant that the condition of many infants can be improved prior to surgery. The application of cardiorespiratory support has influenced the timing of major neonatal surgery. Specific groups of neonates that may be dramatically improved by intensive preoperative care include:

1 *Congenital heart disease.* Preoperative support with mechanical ventilation, prostaglandin E_1 (for babies with cyanotic heart disease and left-heart obstructive lesions, dependent for survival on a patent ductus arteriosus) and inotropic agents, combined with non-invasive cardiac investigation, allow such infants to arrive in the operating theatre in better condition. These developments have reduced the need for immediate surgery and thus the perioperative risk.

2 *Congenital diaphragmatic hernia.* It is now accepted that most infants with viable amounts of lung tissue can be stabilized with cardiorespiratory support, thereby separating the neuroendocrine effects of surgical stress from the stress associated with the birth process. Few infants undergo dramatic improvement as a result of surgical reduction of the hernia so that many are now operated upon semi-electively.

3 *Perforated necrotizing enterocolitis.* The condition of most infants can be improved with fluid resuscitation, inotropic agents, correction of acidosis, respiratory support and antibiotic therapy. Surgery can usually be delayed until the general condition of the infant is stabilized.

Improved neonatal resuscitation together with other technological advances have contributed to the reduced perioperative morbidity and mortality, particularly in patients needing neonatal open and closed cardiac surgery. Specific features of conditions requiring surgery in the neonatal period are covered in other chapters and are listed at the end of this chapter.

OTHER NEONATAL CONSIDERATIONS

Unlike in other branches of anaesthesia, the skill of the neonatal anaesthetist may have effects extending beyond the immediate perioperative period. Attention to preoperative assessment and management and high standards of intraoperative care can reduce perioperative morbidity and mortality.

A number of long-term sequelae may originate in the neonatal period and anaesthesia may contribute to their development. These may not be evident in the perioperative period, but their prevention requires carefully conducted anaesthesia and the avoidance of precipitating factors. Of particular importance are:

1 *Periventricular haemorrhage and ischaemic injury.* Fragile vessels in the germinal matrix are poorly supported and prone to periventricular haemorrhage, which may extend into the intraventricular space. The premature infant is especially at risk of intracerebral haemorrhage and this may be contributed to by hypoxia, hypercarbia, hypertension, rapid volume expansion and the administration of hyperosmolar solutions such as sodium bicarbonate. Cerebral blood flow is 'pressure passive' and the watershed areas of the germinal matrix and periventricular white matter are prone to underperfusion and cerebral ischaemia. It is important to avoid hypotension.

2 *Bronchopulmonary dysplasia.* This is a chronic lung disease likely to occur when immature lungs are exposed to high inspired oxygen tension and high airway pressure for prolonged periods. Infection may be an additional contributory factor. Barotrauma, evidenced by pulmonary interstitial emphysema, pneumomediastinum and pneumothorax may have its origins in the operating theatre and lead to bronchopulmonary dysplasia.

3 *Retinopathy of prematurity.* Arterial hyperoxia during surgical procedures has a potential role in the pathogenesis of the retinopathy of prematurity (retrolental fibroplasia). Intraoperative pulse oximetry and the use of air with the least amount of oxygen needed minimizes the risk of this complication developing as a result of anaesthesia.

4 *Hyperbilirubinaemia*. The threshold for kernicterus is reduced by superimposed acidosis and hypoxia.

ACCESS TO THE PATIENT DURING SURGERY

Access to these small patients is limited during the operation. Attention to detail is important: for instance, the anaesthetist should place the intravenous cannula so that he can ensure its patency, avoid extravasation and be able to inject drugs and volume expanders conveniently. It should be possible to pass a suction catheter through the endotracheal tube if necessary.

Even with oximetry, a light should be available so that skin colour and perfusion can be observed and an artery should be accessible to feel the pulse. A stethoscope is another valuable cardiorespiratory monitor.

VENEPUNCTURE

Venepuncture in neonates is a skill requiring regular practice. Those who anaesthetize infants only occasionally find it technically more difficult. When a cannula is inserted it should be firmly fixed so that it is not accidentally dislodged (see Fig. 7.4). If a three-way tap is used for injection of drugs it should be accessible during the operation. Drugs can be administered through injection sites in the infusion tubing, but these take longer to reach the patient unless flushed through with enough fluid to clear the dead space, and there is the danger of needle-prick injury from sharp needles.

VENTILATION

Ventilation with a face mask must be gentle to avoid inflation of the stomach, which splints the diaphragm if distended (Fig. 9.1). Neonates are dependent on diaphragmatic movement for respiration because the ribs are more horizontal and lack the bucket-handle movement of older patients. If the Rendell Baker–Soucek mask is placed on the face in the groove in the chin with the mouth open and jaw pulled forward, the lungs can be easily inflated with low pressure and distension of the stomach is avoided (see Figs 7.8, 7.9).

In the past, manual ventilation with a Jackson Rees modification of the Ayres T-piece was used so that changes in compliance could be monitored and positive end-expiratory pressure maintained by pressure on the bag. As ventilators for neonates have become more

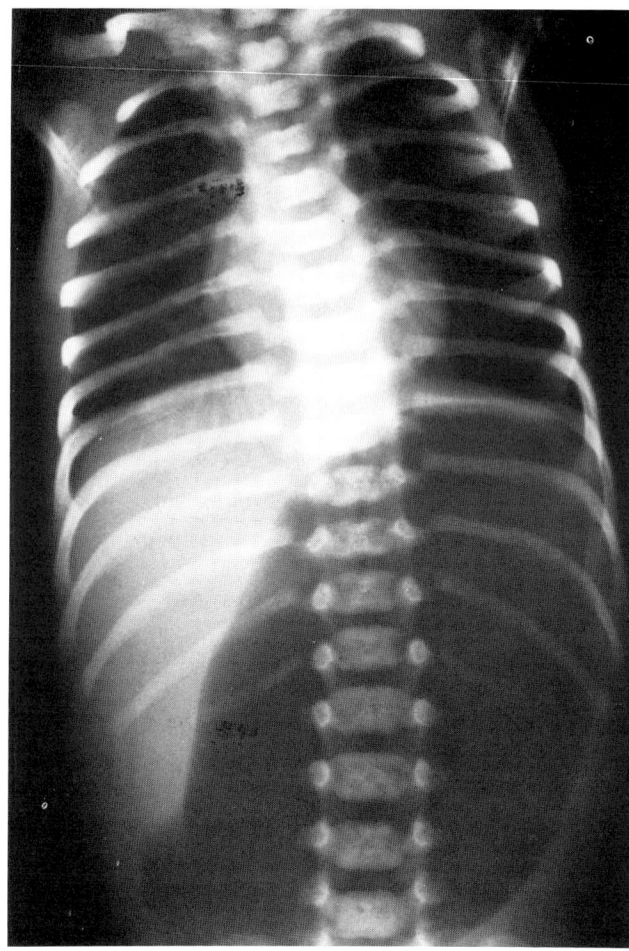

Fig. 9.1 Trunk X-ray of a neonate, showing gaseous distension in the abdomen pushing the diaphragm upwards. Note the higher flattened diaphragm.

versatile, they are being used more frequently in the operating theatre. Very sick neonates requiring critical ventilating pressures and flow patterns should have the same ventilator settings during operation. If possible the same ventilator can be used. Otherwise, skilful clinical assessment using either manual or mechanical ventilation will be needed. Great care is required when using either manual or mechanical ventilation when lung compliance changes during thoracotomy. If the breathing system has a large compressible volume in relation to tidal volume, hypoventilation can occur.

INTUBATION

Intubation may be difficult because of the anatomical peculiarities of the neonate. These include the small mouth, the U-shaped epiglottis and the larynx, which lies at a higher level (C3–4) than in adults (C5–6) (see Chapter 1) and has an anterior inclination (see Fig. 7.7). A laryngoscope with a short straight blade is usually preferred, and the light should be near the tip so that it illuminates inside the mouth. A 3 mm endotracheal tube is suitable for most neonates. It must be remembered that the cricoid ring is the narrowest part of the larynx. A small leak of gas is desirable around the tube when positive pressure is applied. A 2.5 mm tube is usually suitable for premature infants of about 1000 g or less.

Experienced anaesthetists usually use muscle relaxants to facilitate atraumatic intubation. The infant's head is extended and fixed with the heel of the right hand on the forehead and the index finger then opens the mouth, allowing the laryngoscope to be easily inserted by the left hand (see Figs 7.11, 7.12). The little finger of the left hand can be used to press on the larynx to bring it into view (see Fig. 7.12) or an assistant can help by pressing the larynx backwards. To enable the little finger to reach the larynx easily, the laryngoscope should be held between the thumb and index finger at the junction of the handle and the blade (see Fig. 7.12(b)).

Small neonates can be intubated awake without muscle relaxation after pre-oxygenation. This is less commonly done nowadays because of increasing awareness of the stress responses induced in the baby. In particular, hypertension may lead to increased anterior fontanelle pressure and the risk of periventricular haemorrhage. Increases in anterior fontanelle pressure are abolished by the use of general anaesthesia and muscle relaxation. In addition, if the patient is not relaxed, intubation may be traumatic and it is more difficult to visualize the larynx.

Awake intubation may be safer when the anaesthetist only occasionally anaesthetizes neonates and is not confident with neonatal ventilation and intubation. In such circumstances it is preferable to refer the infant to someone with more experience, but that is not always possible. An assistant should hold the shoulders on the table, stabilize the head and also press on the larynx if necessary (see Fig. 7.6).

A nasotracheal tube may be inserted during induction if it is expected or planned that the infant will require an artificial airway or respiratory support postoperatively. Such patients may include those with oesophageal atresia, diaphragmatic hernia, large exomphalos or gastroschisis. If the advancing tube tends to slide past the laryngeal opening posteriorly, flexion of the neck and pressure on the larynx often brings the tube into line

with the larynx. It is easier for the anaesthetist to control the pressure on the larynx with his little finger than for an assistant to do so. If these manoeuvres fail, Magill forceps can be used, although it is difficult to manipulate this instrument in the small mouth.

Failure to ventilate the baby adequately, or delay in intubation, will be quickly followed by hypoxia. Basal oxygen consumption increases from 4 to 7 ml/kg/min during the first 2 days, but it rises rapidly if the baby is crying, struggles during awake intubation or is exposed to a cool environment. Hypoxia and hypercarbia increase pulmonary vascular resistance. In neonates, especially the premature, this will result in a fall in left atrial pressure, opening of the foramen ovale and ductus arteriosus, with right-to-left shunting and reversion towards fetal circulation. The cyanosis that develops is due to shunting and does not respond rapidly to oxygen administration. This situation is sometimes referred to as 'transitional' circulation. A high concentration of oxygen should be given before attempts are made to intubate the baby and prolonged attempts without periodic ventilation should be avoided.

DRUGS

Drugs should be drawn up before anaesthesia is commenced, either in finely graduated 1 ml syringes or suitably diluted in 2 ml or 5 ml syringes, so that accurate doses can be administered. The pharmacological differences between neonates, who are generally more sensitive, and older children are considered in more detail in Chapter 2.

Premedication

Premedication is usually unnecessary in neonates. Although some anaesthetists give atropine (60–100 μg/kg) 30 minutes beforehand to reduce secretions, it can be given intravenously at induction or may not be needed. Although bradycardia does occur, it is not usually extreme unless the infant is hypoxic.

The immature central nervous system is more easily depressed by drugs than that of older patients (see Chapter 2). Depressant drugs are therefore not used for premedication.

Induction

Most neonates are induced with inhalation agents,

although thiopentone can be used, particularly in bigger babies, provided the dose is kept small (2–3 mg/kg; see Chapter 2).

Muscle relaxants

The response of infants to muscle relaxants differs from that of older children (see Chapter 2). They tend to be resistant to suxamethonium and require a dose of 1.5–2 mg/kg. If it cannot be given i.v., it will produce rapid onset of relaxation if given in a larger dose (3 mg/kg) intramuscularly.

Many studies have shown that neonates are more sensitive to depolarizing muscle relaxants, but these were usually done on peripheral muscles. The neonatal diaphragm is relatively less sensitive than peripheral muscle to non-depolarizing relaxants because the mix of muscle fibre types differs, so that the dose usual for an older infant may be needed to eliminate respiratory effort (see Chapter 2). Vecuronium, in contrast to atracurium, is a long-acting relaxant in neonates.

Analgesics

Narcotic analgesic drugs cause more central and respiratory depression in the neonate than in infants. If they are used in neonatal anaesthesia, it is better to use shorter acting drugs such as fentanyl and to decrease the dose, unless the baby is to be ventilated postoperatively.

Inhalation agents

Nitrous oxide has been used in neonatal anaesthesia, but the problems related to microatelectasis and decreased functional residual capacity that occur with anaesthesia are reduced if air is used instead as the carrier gas for the inhalation anaesthetic. Decreased oxygen saturation and increased work of breathing are thereby avoided. Normal oxygen saturation can usually be maintained when a neonate is ventilated with air (+ volatile agent) and a few cmH$_2$O PEEP. This is particularly important in premature infants. Nitrous oxide, because it is more diffusible than air, will also increase the gaseous distension of the gut or lung cysts.

The uptake of inhalation agents is more rapid and minimum alveolar concentrations (MACs) are lower in the neonate than in infants and older children.

TEMPERATURE CONTROL

With increasing age and maturity, temperature control improves. The neonate, especially when small and immature, has a narrow thermoneutral range. This is the range of environmental temperature where metabolic rate and oxygen consumption are minimal, usually 34–36°C. Below this range metabolism increases to increase heat production and maintain body temperature, also increasing oxygen consumption (see Chapter 1).

Several factors contribute to the tendency for neonates to drop their temperature. These may be aggravated by anaesthesia and surgery, and include:
1 immaturity of the thermoregulatory centre;
2 relatively large surface area (2–2.5 times greater relative to body weight when compared with an adult);
3 a thin layer of subcutaneous fat and thin skin (insulation);
4 lack of shivering, which is partly compensated by non-shivering or chemical thermogenesis (brown-fat metabolism);
5 exposure to a cold environment during induction of anaesthesia and preparation of the skin before draping the patient for surgery;
6 loss of the ability to respond to a cold stimulus when sick.
The baby should be placed on a warm-water circulating blanket and an overhead heater should be used during induction until the surgeon drapes the patient. During surgery, warming and humidifying the gases, using 'plastic' drapes, foil insulation and bonnets on the infant's relatively large head all help to maintain temperature. The operating theatre temperature can be raised, but not to a level where the operators are uncomfortable.

BLOOD AND FLUIDS

The extracellular fluid compartment is relatively larger in the neonate (40–45% of body weight; more in the premature infant). Fluid turnover is more rapid than in older patients. Intraoperative fluid requirements include:
1 maintenance fluids;
2 extra fluid to compensate for evaporative losses from an open body cavity — abdomen or thorax — and from the respiratory tract if the inspired gases are not adequately humidified;
3 replacement of third space and blood loss.
Neonates tolerate considerable variations in blood volume, as demonstrated by the substantial extra volume

that may be infused from the placenta at birth. They can safely be given 10–20 ml/kg of fluid of 4% dextrose in 0.22% saline in the first hour during surgery, plus replacement of blood loss. Initially, if the haemoglobin is high, a colloid, plasma protein or electrolyte solution is used. If large volumes of blood are lost, blood transfusion may become necessary. Smaller volumes of fluid are given in subsequent hours.

Estimation of blood loss in infants is difficult, even by weighing swabs or using dilution techniques. Experience helps in making a reasonable estimate. Careful observation of clinical signs such as rising pulse rate, falling blood pressure and decreased intensity of heart sounds should help in the recognition of hypovolaemia, if replacement is inadequate. Initially, the neonate compensates well for hypovolaemia by movement of the fluid from the large extravascular, extracellular fluid compartment.

The blood volume is about 80 ml/kg so that a 30 ml loss is over 10% of blood volume in a 3 kg neonate. Haemoglobin values are often 17–21 g/100 ml at birth, and the haematocrit about 60%, decreasing to between 35% and 45% at 2 weeks. Initial blood loss can be replaced with electrolyte (Hartmann's) or colloid solutions. Fetal haemoglobin delivers oxygen less readily to the tissues, but oxygen supply should still be adequate when the haematocrit exceeds 35–40%. Thus a newborn can tolerate more than 10% or even 20% loss readily if haematocrit is normal to start with, but the continuing decline in haematocrit during the first 3 months must also be considered when deciding at what stage to start replacing losses with blood. It is probably reasonable to begin giving blood if the infant (3 kg) loses more than 50–60 ml, provided haemoglobin and haematocrit were normal preoperatively. Polycythaemic infants are best treated with colloid solutions until the haematocrit falls to below 40%. If blood loss is not replaced with blood, iron therapy should be instituted to replace iron stores.

MONITORING

The newborn's clinical condition can change very rapidly. Colour and peripheral perfusion should be watched for evidence of hypoxia or hypovolaemia. The precordial or oesophageal stethoscope is invaluable to monitor heart rate, rhythm and intensity of heart sounds, which give an indication of cardiac output, and respiration. The pulse can be felt at the usual sites such as radial, brachial, axillary or superficial temporal arteries, or lower limb

arteries during neurosurgery. Blood pressure measurement has been made easier with the advent of neonatal non-invasive blood pressure monitors. The normal full-term neonatal systolic pressure is about 80 mmHg (10.6 kPa), but it is lower in premature infants. Pulse oximetry, when working reliably, has revolutionized monitoring, allowing closer observation of changes in heart rate and oxygen saturation and also allowing the inspired oxygen concentration to be controlled by lowering it to the point where the oxygen saturation just begins to decrease. This minimizes the risk of hyperoxic retinopathy in premature infants.

Capnography is useful as hypoventilation and marked hyperventilation, which can lower blood pressure, can be avoided.

Patient temperature should be measured in the oesophagus or rectum. The temperature of the warming blanket and inspired gases should also be monitored to prevent overheating or burning the baby.

Invasive arterial and central venous pressure monitoring is increasingly being used in babies having major procedures, particularly in those requiring pre- and postoperative intensive care (see Chapters 7 and 34).

CONCLUSION OF ANAESTHESIA

At the conclusion of anaesthesia, non-depolarizing relaxants should be reversed with atropine (25 μg/kg) and neostigmine (50 μg/kg). The endotracheal tube should not be removed until adequate ventilation has been re-established and the baby is awake and active. Delay in return of spontaneous ventilation may be a result of hyperventilation. The addition of CO_2 to the inspired gas usually causes a prompt return of respiration.

If there is evidence of respiratory insufficiency, postoperative respiratory support may be indicated, and a nasotracheal tube should be inserted, if not already in place, and strapped in carefully.

Postoperatively the baby should be kept warm, nursed in a warmed environment, such as a humidicrib, or under a radiant heater thermostatically controlled from an abdominal skin probe. A fall in body temperature should be avoided, otherwise energy requirements and oxygen consumption will be increased (see Chapter 1).

PREMATURITY

The premature infant poses many special problems which relate to physiological immaturity and the fact that fetal life was too short to lay down adequate stores of glycogen and iron. An anaemic patient is likely to need blood transfusion earlier, if blood loss occurs. Despite the stress response to surgery increasing blood glucose, some glucose should be given perioperatively because glycogen reserves are less than in more mature infants. Temperature-control measures are even more important, because they cool more rapidly.

Premature and ex-premature infants, up to a gestational age of at least 46 weeks, tend to have apnoeic spells, which can be aggravated by anaesthesia and surgical stress. The reduction in FRC following anaesthesia is a contributing factor that can be reduced by using air as the carrier gas for a volatile agent. If $3-5\,cmH_2O$ CPAP is also used, full oxygen saturation is sometimes achieved. Otherwise additional oxygen is added to provide adequate oxygenation. It is easy to over-ventilate very small babies when tidal volume is only 6 ml/kg. This reduces total body CO_2 so that the CO_2 drive may be lacking. Cardiac output is also depressed by hypocapnia. An increase in apparatus dead space will reduce CO_2 diminution. It is logical to add CO_2 to the inspired gas at the end of anaesthesia if hypocapnia is suspected.

Premature infants require smaller doses of drugs, and care should be taken to minimize their depressant effects. An inhalation agent is probably the best option if it is not planned to ventilate the baby afterwards.

Respiration should be monitored for at least 24 hours after anaesthesia in small prematurely born infants until they are 52 weeks post-gestational age. Intravenous theophylline (8 mg/kg) is often effective in stimulating respiration. Caffeine has also been used. Alternatively CPAP or CPPV may be necessary for a short period.

SPECIFIC CONDITIONS

Various neonatal conditions are considered in detail in the speciality chapters. These include:

Chapter 11
  Duodenal and ileal atresias
  Malrotation
  Imperforate anus
  Meconium ileus
  Cystic hygroma
  Exomphalos and gastroschisis
Chapter 12
  Oesophageal atresia
  Diaphragmatic hernia
  Congenital lobar emphysema
Chapter 13
  Congenital heart disease
Chapter 14
  Myelomeningocoele
  Encephalocoele
  Subdural haematoma
  Hydrocephalus

10: Recovery Room and Postoperative Care

INTRODUCTION

All operating theatres should have a recovery room, an area where patients are cared for as they recover from the immediate effects of anaesthesia and surgery. The recovery room is staffed by nurses with special skills in the care of the airway of unconscious patients and observation of cardiovascular changes after general and regional anaesthesia. A full range of resuscitation equipment, with oxygen and suction, is essential, as well as appropriate equipment for monitoring. After full recovery, the patient can be returned to the ward with less chance of a postoperative crisis.

The recovery room should have sufficient space to accommodate the number of patients being operated upon, so that each one can stay until the circulation is stable, breathing is adequate, airway reflexes have recovered and the patient is awake. It is recommended that there should be 1.5 to 3 bed spaces per operating theatre [1]. The length of stay will be influenced by the type of anaesthesia and the nature and duration of the operation. It will usually be at least half an hour and may exceed an hour. The use of long-acting sedatives and tranquillizers, especially if given in higher doses to ensure adequate preoperative sedation, may result in a sleepy patient who has to stay longer in the recovery room. Premedication is not used for many day-surgery patients, so that the period in the recovery room can be minimized.

The time taken for recovery depends on the nature and duration of action of the drugs used, as well as the dose and time of administration. The choice of induction agents and analgesic drugs can be important for short operations. Recovery from a 'balanced' anaesthetic is usually prompt, provided the muscle relaxant is adequately reversed. Volatile agents with high blood gas solubilities can slow recovery, but even with modern agents which have relatively low blood gas solubilities, awakening can be delayed if deep anaesthesia is used and the concentration is not decreased towards the end of the operation. Local anaesthesia combined with light general anaesthesia allows rapid recovery.

When ketamine is used in large doses (over 5 mg/kg) for operations lasting up to 2 hours, recovery usually takes as long again as the anaesthetic.

Children may be nursed on trolleys that can be tilted in the event of retching and vomiting, or in beds, cots or incubators. It is important that cots and trolleys have adequate sides to prevent the patients, particularly toddlers, from falling out.

RECOVERY ROOM REQUIREMENTS

There must be:

1 A sufficient number of nurses at all times to care adequately for all the patients in the recovery room. The children are transferred from the constant attention of an anaesthetist to the care of nursing staff, who may then be expected to look after more than one semi-conscious child at a time. Lack of sufficient staff to observe and care for the recovering patients unfortunately will sometimes result in episodes of hypoxia.

It is difficult to estimate the ideal number of staff for a recovery room because the numbers of patients fluctuate. The maximum number of nurses should be rostered during the peak times — ideally each unconscious patient should have a nurse, while one nurse can probably observe three patients who have recovered consciousness but are still too drowsy to return to the ward [1].

The recovery room staff should be able to communicate directly with theatre personnel, preferably by an intercom system. Medical staff should be available to deal with anaesthetic or surgical complications.

2 Suction and oxygen outlets and power points for each patient [2].

3 Suction handpieces and catheters.

4 Oxygen face masks and catheters.

5 A full range of face masks, pharyngeal airways, endotracheal tubes, and laryngoscopes.

6 A self-inflating resuscitation bag or an anaesthetic breathing system and bag for each patient.

7 A ventilator in case a child needs respiratory assistance for some time. Extra staff may be needed to monitor the child and perform suction.

8 Resuscitation drugs and drugs used to reverse neuromuscular block and respiratory depression (Table 10.1).

9 A selection of intravenous equipment, needles, cannulae, infusion sets, burettes and solutions (see Chapter 3).

10 ECG and defibrillator.

11 Monitoring equipment — pulse oximeter, blood pressure manometer or non-invasive blood pressure monitor, thermometer, nerve stimulator and stethoscopes.

12 X-ray and laboratory investigation, including blood gases, electrolytes and blood glucose available if needed.

13 Lighting conforming to the standards for recovery rooms [3].

14 An alarm system to summon aid in a crisis.

Table 10.1 Drugs which should be available in the recovery room

Emergency drugs	Reversal drugs	Others
Adrenaline	Neostigmine	Analgesics
Sodium bicarbonate	Naloxone	Parenteral suppositories
Calcium chloride	Flumazenil	Antiemetics
Atropine	Physostigmine	Anticonvulsants
Lignocaine		
Suxamethonium		
Glucose		
Hydrocortisone		

PATIENT HANDOVER

The anaesthetist must always personally hand the patient over to the recovery room nursing staff. It is essential that breathing is adequate and that the circulation is satisfactory. The nurse must understand the nature of the operation performed, the anaesthetic used, the need for intravenous fluids or blood transfusions, the state of the patient's consciousness and airway, any problems that have occurred and any complications which may be anticipated. The patient should be nursed on his side unless there is a reason for not doing so, in which case he must be observed with extra care in case airway obstruction or vomiting occur.

MONITORING

The recovery room staff should note:

1 the patient's colour;

2 respiration, by feeling the warm expired air on the hand and observing chest movements;

3 the circulation — pulse and blood pressure, as well as the peripheral perfusion reflected in the warmth of digits;

4 temperature;

5 drainage from operation sites;

6 the intravenous drip rate, if needed, to ensure that it corresponds with the postoperative orders;

7 pupil size and reaction to light in neurosurgical patients.

Advances in operating theatre monitoring are now being applied in the recovery room so that pulse oximetry, ECG and automatic non-invasive blood pressure devices are commonly available. A nerve stimulator is also useful to exclude residual paralysis in the differential diagnosis of respiratory insufficiency. Despite the use of monitoring devices, it is still essential that the staff personally observe the patients and that they understand and react appropriately to changes in heart rate and blood pressure. Observations should be recorded on a special recovery room chart. Significant trends such as increasing tachycardia associated with bleeding are then more easily noted and acted upon.

POSTOPERATIVE PROBLEMS

Pain and analgesia

Much attention has been paid recently to pain and its adverse effects. Paediatric anaesthetists are tending to use more intraoperative opioids, opioid infusions, regional anaesthesia and epidural infusions. Details of these methods are discussed in Chapter 8.

Postoperative pain may cause tachycardia and hypertension, with an increased tendency to bleeding. Restlessness may increase oxygen consumption and may cause disturbance of surgical dressings, particularly in plastic and burns surgery. The presence of pain may stimulate ventilation unless the surgical incision affects the muscles involved with respiration, when it may cause splinting of the chest wall. Crying will be associated with a sympathetic response which increases metabolic rate and hence oxygen consumption. It is easier to manage a patient who is relatively pain-free on recovery from anaesthesia than to gain control of established pain with opioids, which may also cause some respiratory depression and stimulate the chemoreceptor trigger zone, leading to vomiting. If opioids are given in the recovery room, the patient should remain long enough (at least half an hour) to ensure that respiration is not unduly depressed. If the patient is obviously in pain on arrival in the recovery room, the anaesthetist can give a dose of analgesic intravenously. If an infusion is not planned, part of the dose can be given intravenously and the remainder intramuscularly to prolong the effect.

The pain from some minor procedures such as myringotomy is less severe — oral paracetamol given with premedication will usually suppress the discomfort satisfactorily and more effectively than if it is given postoperatively (by suppository or orally).

Hypoxia

Some reduction in arterial oxygen tension is common in the recovery room. This may be due to hypoventilation from depression of the respiratory centre or obstruction of the airways, or to ventilation—perfusion mismatch associated with decreased functional residual capacity and variations in closing volumes (relatively higher in infants and small children, reaching a minimum relative to FRC at 8 years of age). The reduction in FRC due to denitrogenation of the lungs may be minimized if air is used in the anaesthetic mixture, so that some nitrogen remains in the alveoli, thereby preventing collapse. Decreased FRC may also occur with large abdominal and thoracic incisions.

The decrease in Pao_2 is often not dangerous, and attempts to administer oxygen often disturb the child, so that oxygen administration is impracticable and un-

necessary. There are situations where oxygen should be administered. These are:

1 after cardiac, thoracic, major abdominal and intracranial operations;
2 when the patient is unconscious for a prolonged period;
3 minor degrees of hypoventilation;
4 when oxygen consumption is increased, e.g. pyrexia, shivering, increased muscle tone and activity.

Care must be exercised in oxygen administration to the newborn, particularly premature infants, because of the danger of retrolental fibroplasia with the inhalation of high oxygen concentrations (see Chapter 32).

An oxygen mask (Fig. 10.1) can be used to raise inspired oxygen concentration to about 40%. Infants or small children requiring prolonged administration are more easily managed in an incubator or head box (Fig. 10.2).

It has been demonstrated that lower oxygen flows (1 l or less per min) are needed to raise Pao_2 when the catheter tip is placed in the nasopharynx than when it is placed in the nose. Care should be taken in infants to avoid inflating the stomach. If severe hypoxia develops, the cause must be sought. Direct laryngoscopy should be used to ensure that the airway is clear. The patient should be ventilated with oxygen and then, if necessary, intubated.

Respiratory obstruction may be due to the tongue obstructing the airway and can be corrected by pulling the jaw forward and tilting the head back; sometimes a

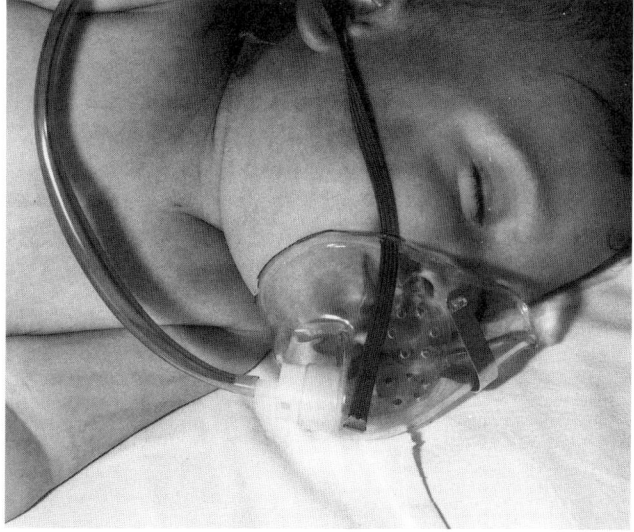

Fig. 10.1 Patient with a Hudson mask for the administration of oxygen. Some air dilution occurs through the side holes.

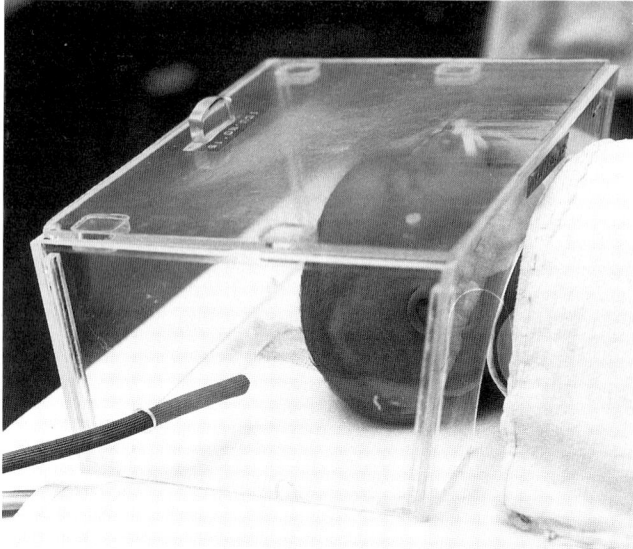

Fig. 10.2 A perspex head box into which additional oxygen can be administered to raise the expired oxygen for infants.

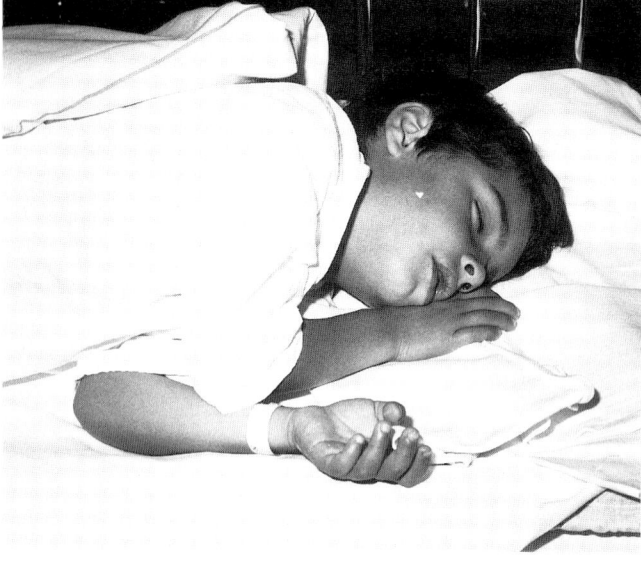

Fig. 10.3 A recovering patient placed on the side with the upper arm placed so that the hand supports the jaw and the head slightly extended. The head is not on a pillow so that there is free drainage out of the mouth.

pharyngeal airway is needed. Pharyngeal obstruction is less likely to occur if the child is nursed on his side with the head extended and held in that position by placing the hand of the uppermost arm under the jaw (Fig. 10.3).

Laryngeal stridor indicates some degree of laryngeal obstruction. Postoperatively it may result from irritability of the larynx, which occurs during lighter planes of anaesthesia with halothane, enflurane or isoflurane, and occurs most commonly following extubation under deep anaesthesia. Secretions or blood may act as irritants. Laryngeal spasm can occur in these circumstances (see Chapter 27). Stridor may also be a significant sign of incomplete reversal of neuromuscular block. Stridor due to laryngeal oedema develops following intubation, either traumatic or with too large a tube, or following repeated insertion of a bronchoscope. The onset is usually within half to 1 hour of extubation, and is unlikely after more than 2 hours. It can be treated with nebulized racemic adrenaline (0.05 ml/kg of 2.25% diluted to 2 ml. This is about 1 mg/kg so that 0.5 ml/kg 1:1000 adrenaline could be used instead) (Fig. 10.4). If the obstruction is not relieved, reintubation may be necessary, often with a smaller tube.

Stridor associated with laryngomalacia (infantile larynx) or other anatomical obstruction of the larynx is usually recognized beforehand.

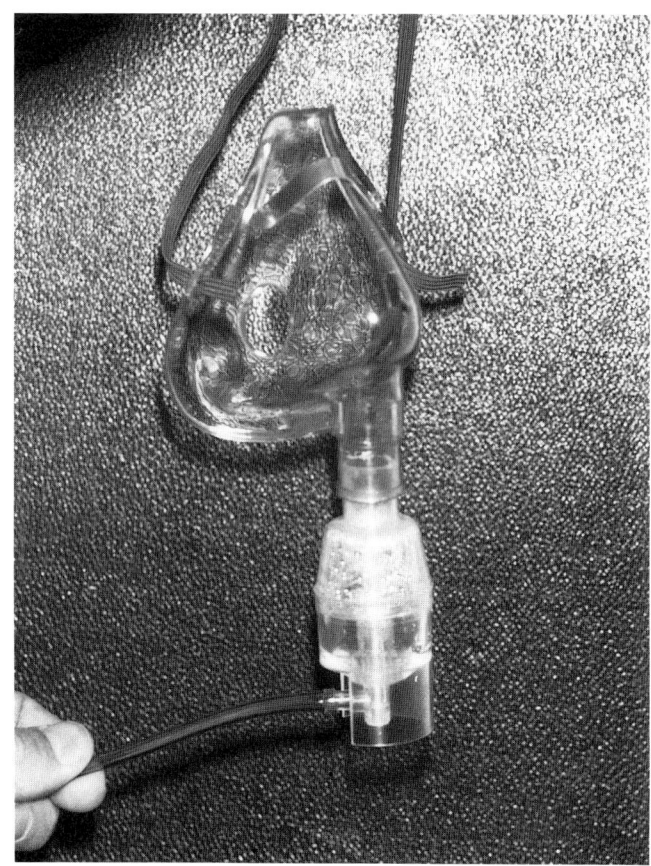

Fig. 10.4 Nebulizer for administration of adrenaline with attached mask.

Oxygen should be administered if the patient develops oxygen desaturation. The administration of oxygen by face mask with positive pressure may produce significant improvement in oxygen saturation.

Hypoventilation may be due to respiratory depression, residual effects of muscle relaxants, splinting of upper abdominal or intercostal muscles by pain, depletion of body stores of carbon dioxide by hyperventilation or mechanical factors such as tight dressings.

Respiratory depression due to anaesthetic agents will decrease as elimination occurs. If the depression is due to a narcotic analgesic, it can be reversed with antagonists such as naloxone. There have been a few reports of pulmonary oedema following naloxone. It is possible that this is associated with rapid reversal of analgesia. As the dose needed to achieve this may be very small in children, it should be titrated in small increments until the necessary arousal and improvement in ventilation occurs. Inadequate reversal of muscle relaxants is suspected when respiratory movements are uncoordinated and ventilation is shallow. Sometimes stridor is also present. A nerve stimulator can be used to test for fade and post-tetanic facilitation if residual non-depolarizing block is suspected. Neuro-muscular conduction can often be improved by additional atropine and neostigmine, but if there is any doubt the safest course is to assist or control ventilation until spontaneous recovery is complete. Respiratory acidosis from underventilation potentiates neuromuscular blockade.

Prolonged apnoea following suxamethonium may be due to a genetically determined abnormal cholinesterase, or to a drug interaction with a cholinesterase inhibitor such as isoflurophate (Dyflos, DFP), phospholine iodide (ecothiopate) eye drops or cyclophosphamide. These patients may require ventilation until the suxamethonium is hydrolysed and muscle power returns. Heterozygous cholinesterase abnormalities only cause paralysis for about 20–30 minutes, but in homozygous patients it may last 2–3 hours, depending on the dose.

Apnoeic episodes lasting 20 seconds or longer can occur in otherwise normal premature infants. They sometimes need to be stimulated to breathe. The frequency of attacks decreases with postnatal age and they are unusual after 46 weeks. Ex-premature infants may revert to their earlier tendency to have these episodes when exposed to anaesthesia (see Chapter 9). The incidence is reduced by using spinal anaesthesia, using air as the carrier gas for a volatile agent and reversing hypocarbia, if it occurs, with the addition of CO_2 at the end of the operation. Because of the hazard of postoperative apnoeic spells, these babies must be observed carefully and stimulated if they stop breathing. Apnoea alarms which respond to respiratory movement and alarm when it stops are useful for 24–36 hours after operation. Theophylline 8 mg/kg by slow intravenous injection or by infusion acts as a respiratory stimulant, and may prevent apnoea.

Nausea and vomiting

These are common and can occur after any anaesthetic. If patients are observed for 18–24 hours, the incidence of postoperative vomiting is often 20–30% or more, and most commonly occurs after return to the ward. Many factors influence the incidence, including:

1 Age — the incidence is lowest in infants and toddlers.
2 Sex — there is no difference before puberty, after which the incidence increases in females.
3 The duration of operation — the incidence increases with longer operations.
4 The anaesthetic agents used — this is probably dose-dependent with volatile agents, but the incidence was higher with some of the older agents such as ether, trichloroethylene and cyclopropane. Whether neostigmine used to reverse neuromuscular block significantly affects the incidence of vomiting is uncertain.
5 Narcotic analgesics — in a study of 1184 patients, 54% of those who had opioid premedication vomited, whereas the incidence was only 25% in patients who had other premedicants [5]. The concurrent use of hyoscine, which has antiemetic properties, with opioids may reduce the incidence [6]. The lowest incidence of postoperative vomiting that has been reported in children was in a group in which halothane induction was followed by caudal anaesthesia and sedation with diazepam [7].
6 Site of operation — ear, ophthalmic and upper abdominal surgery are associated with a higher incidence. Patients with burns have a lower incidence.
7 Movement — rough handling during movement of the patient after operation may cause vomiting.
8 Oral fluids given too soon after emergence from anaesthesia may precipitate vomiting.

A number of factors influence the incidence of nausea and vomiting and, although it is a frequent problem in the recovery room, many patients vomit for several hours after they return to the ward.

Vomiting is most hazardous during emergence from anaesthesia because of the danger of aspiration, particularly if the laryngeal reflexes have also been obtunded by local anaesthesia. As the duration of local anaesthesia is longer with higher concentrations [8], the 10% lignocaine spray packs should be avoided in operations lasting less than 1.5 hours. If vomiting occurs, the patient should be turned on his side. The patient can be tipped head-down and the pharynx should be cleared with suction. If it is suspected that the patient has aspirated, clinical examination of the chest and a chest X-ray should be carried out. The main danger is aspiration of very acid stomach contents, leading to Mendelson's syndrome (pulmonary oedema) or of solid material, which may cause obstruction of the airways. The incidence of the former is reduced by the administration of antacids or histamine blocking agents before operation (see Chapter 6). It seems to be a less common consequence of aspiration in children than in parturients.

While the patient may not be particularly upset by a single vomiting episode during emergence, prolonged vomiting can be very distressing. This can be reduced by employing drugs such as droperidol in low dosage or phenothiazines (e.g. prochlorperazine, 0.05 mg/kg 6−8-hourly) in the premedication or postoperatively. Metoclopramide (Maxalon) 0.12 mg/kg administered not more than 6-hourly is also useful.

The usual neurolept dose of droperidol is 0.15 mg/kg. Studies on low-dose droperidol have used doses of 5 μg/kg−75 μg/kg, the latter being shown to be associated with a significantly lower percentage of patients vomiting (16%) than 25 and 50 μg (40%) in strabismus surgery (controls 60%) [9]. 5 μg/kg reduced vomiting in children undergoing orthopaedic operations kept in hospital for more than 24 hours (25% − controls 34%) although the difference was significant only in the 11−15-year-old group [10].

Droperidol will not suppress vomiting in all patients, and the effective dose depends on the type of operation and whether the patient is a day case or not. Motion increases vomiting. Higher doses are more likely to cause unpleasant psychological effects. Care must be taken with phenothiazines (and other dopamine antagonists) as overdosage can cause extrapyramidal signs such as facial grimacing and athetoid movements. They can be treated with benztropine 0.2 mg/kg stat i.m. or i.v., repeated in 15 minutes if required.

In the large series mentioned above, 30 patients vomited more than 7 times (2.8%) [5]. It is important that repeated vomiting is reported to medical staff and treated with an antiemetic and, if necessary, an intravenous infusion.

Temperature

Temperature should be recorded on return to the recovery room. This will detect the delayed onset of hyperpyrexia following short procedures and significant lowering of temperature, which is particularly likely to occur in small infants. Patients who are hypothermic may be vasoconstricted, hypoventilate and recover slowly from anaesthesia. Oxygen consumption may be increased as the body attempts to increase temperature by increasing metabolic heat production. Patients should be rewarmed to normal or near-normal temperature before being returned to the ward. This may be achieved by warm blankets, mylar film, or occasionally, if very cold, by active warming with a heating blanket or overhead heater.

Shivering and muscle rigidity

Shivering or muscle rigidity is more common when the body temperature is lowered, but can also occur in normothermic patients after anaesthesia with agents such as halothane. The mechanism suggested is that there is a varying rate of recovery from anaesthesia of various parts of the brain, so that there is a period when muscle tone is increased. This will also tend to increase oxygen consumption.

Disorientation

Disorientation can occur following anaesthesia, and children may hallucinate. Physostigmine (0.025−0.05 mg/kg) is often helpful in stopping this confused behaviour and making the patient rational. It is possible that anticholinergics, especially hyoscine, may be a cause.

There is a significant incidence of dreaming and hallucinations after the use of ketamine in older children, particularly if other drugs such as benzodiazepines have not been used to suppress these effects. The problem is aggravated by rousing the patient too soon, and it is better to leave him to awaken slowly. Patients who normally dream frequently during sleep are much more likely to have dreams and hallucinations after ketamine. It is uncertain at what age ketamine hallucinations begin to disturb children, but probably they do so by 8 years of age or even younger.

Delayed recovery from anaesthesia

This may be due to:

1 *Drug effects*

overdosage with anaesthetic drugs;

failing to discontinue inhalation anaesthetics soon enough to allow adequate elimination for prompt recovery;

continuing action of long-acting premedicant drugs such as trimeprazine;

decreased body temperature, resulting in slowed drug metabolism and elimination;

unrecognized hypothyroidism, with associated increased sensitivity to central depressant drugs.

2 *Hypoglycaemia* — this may occur in neonates who have inadequate glycogen stores, neonates and infants receiving parenteral nutrition, but have received inadequate glucose intraoperatively, and insulin overdose in relation to glucose intake in diabetics.

Blood glucose can be checked with fresh reagent strips and if low, glucose 10% or 50% should be given.

3 *Tissue hypoxia* — an episode of hypoxia or inadequate cerebral perfusion during anaesthesia may result in delayed recovery. Such patients require intensive care management, so that the best possible outcome results (see Chapter 36).

4 *Cerebrovascular accidents* — very rarely, it is possible for an intraventricular haemorrhage to occur in a premature infant as a result of blood pressure or osmolality changes.

Cardiovascular complications

Hypotension may be associated with hypovolaemia associated with inadequate replacement of blood loss or inadequate fluid therapy. Other significant causes are hypoventilation and hypoxia, overdosage with anaesthetic drugs leading to myocardial depression, and transfusion reaction.

Hypertension may be due to CO_2 retention, pain or a distended bladder. It may be a warning sign of rising intracranial pressure in neurosurgical patients.

Dysrhythmia may be due to any of the factors causing these during anaesthesia, especially hypoventilation. Complications occurring in cardiac surgical patients are dealt with more fully in Chapter 11.

Cardiac arrest should not occur in the recovery room if the patient is observed adequately and complications are treated promptly. The management of cardiac arrest is described in Chapter 35. Following resuscitation, such patients are usually sent to an intensive care unit.

TRANSFER TO THE INTENSIVE CARE UNIT

Patients who go to the operating theatre from the intensive care unit will usually return there postoperatively. Some patients having major surgery, or who have borderline respiratory or cardiac reserve, will be sent electively to intensive care. Arrangements should be made preoperatively for these transfers. There remain a few patients who develop complications and who will be sent from the recovery room to the intensive care unit. These are most commonly children who develop upper respiratory obstruction following, for example, tonsillectomy, cleft palate repair or bronchoscopy.

PARENTS

Facilities for the parents to wait during the operation and to be interviewed after the operation by the surgeon, and sometimes by the anaesthetist, are desirable. Attitudes to parents visiting children in the recovery room vary in different units from allowing no visiting to fairly free access. Some flexibility is desirable.

Parents appreciate seeing their child after the operation. Some can be helpful in settling their child, especially preschoolers, in the recovery room, although occasionally the opposite occurs. In units where parents are allowed to visit, the nurses quickly become accustomed to their presence, but it is important that the handover from the anaesthetist and initial observations are completed before parents are admitted. Provided parents realize that they should not interfere with the nursing care of their child and that they may have to leave when requested — for instance if an emergency occurs — it is reasonable to allow them to visit.

REFERENCES

1 Faculty of Anaesthetists, RACS. (1989) *Guidelines for the care of patients recovering from anaesthesia in the recovery area.* p. 4.

2 Australian Standard 2120. (1977) *Suction systems for medical use in hospitals.*

3 Australian Standard 1765. (1981) *Code of practice for artificial lighting for clinical observation.*

4 Shann F., Gatchalian S., Hutchison R. Nasopharyngeal oxygen in children. *Lancet* 1988, **2**, 1238.

5 Rowley M., Brown T.C.K. Postoperative vomiting in children. *Anaes Intens Care* 1982, **10**, 309.

6 Riding J.E. Postoperative vomiting. *Proc Roy Soc Med* 1960, **53**, 671.

7 Busoni P., Audreucetti T. The spread of caudal anaesthesia in children: a mathematical model. *Anaes Intens Care* 1986, **14**, 140.

8 Robinson E.P., Rex M.A.E., Brown T.C.K. A comparison of different concentrations of lignocaine hydrocloride used for topical anaesthesia of the larynx of the cat. *Anaes Intens Care* 1985, **13**, 137.

9 Eustis S., Lerman J., Smith D.R. Effect of droperidol pretreatment on post-anaesthetic vomiting in children undergoing strabismus surgery: the minimum effective dose. *J Ped Ophth Strabismus* 1987, **24**, 165.

10 Lucide R., Mashallah G., Seleny F. Effect of low-dose droperidol on postoperative vomiting in children. *Canad Anaes Soc J* 1981, **28**, 259.

11: General Surgery, Urology and Liver Transplantation

PREOPERATIVE PREPARATION

Patients about to have an elective operation such as inguinal herniotomy will require only routine preoperative care unless there is obstruction or strangulation. Patients with more severe, acute conditions requiring emergency surgery may need to be resuscitated with fluids or blood before anaesthesia. The urgency of operation dictates to some extent how much time should be spent in preparing the patient, but, in the absence of severe haemorrhage or likelihood of tissues becoming gangrenous, the time taken to rehydrate the patient, to correct acid–base and electrolyte abnormalities and to allow antibiotics to take effect is well spent. The choice of intravenous fluid is dealt with in Chapter 29; the aim is to return the fluid, electrolyte and acid–base balance to normal.

The patient's clinical features, such as signs of dehydration, abdominal distension and the nature of vomited fluid, indicate the diagnosis and the resuscitation needed. For instance, pyloric obstruction results in projectile vomiting and the gastric contents are clear and acid in the unfed infant. Obstruction beyond the duodenum, causing bile-stained vomiting, is associated with less acid–base disturbance because the duodenal contents are alkaline and pancreatic secretions contain bicarbonate, which offsets the hydrogen ion loss from the stomach.

Diarrhoea may cause loss of fluid and electrolytes, and acidosis, which usually resolves with adequate rehydration. It should also be remembered that fluid may be lost into the lumen of the gut and that with peritonitis there may be substantial loss into the peritoneal cavity. These losses occur with trauma, perforation, acute inflammation, ulceration, or ischaemia, associated with malrotation, volvulus or intussusception. Major blood loss should be replaced with crystalloid or colloid solutions until cross-matched blood is available (see Chapter 29). When a significant volume of blood has been lost, or is likely to be lost during surgery, blood should be cross-matched before operation.

Abdominal distension can be due to bowel obstruction, gas in the stomach, pneumoperitoneum or ascites. It can cause respiratory embarrassment in infants due to splinting of the elevated diaphragm by the increased intra-abdominal pressure. A nasogastric tube is usually passed where there is upper gastrointestinal obstruction, vomiting or when stomach or duodenal surgery is to be performed. The volume of fluid aspirated should be taken into account when determining the amount of intravenous fluid required, and should be replaced with an equal volume of normal saline if nasogastric suction is continued. Before anaesthesia any fluid or blood loss should be replaced and acid–base and electrolyte disturbances should be corrected.

ANAESTHESIA

Intra-abdominal surgery requires muscle relaxation, tracheal intubation and ventilation. It is essential when a bowel obstruction is present. In emergency anaesthesia, pre-oxygenation followed by a rapid-sequence induction, usually with thiopentone, atropine, suxamethonium, cricoid pressure and intubation, is used.

General anaesthesia is often supplemented by local and regional anaesthesia, which also provides post-operative analgesia. Epidural anaesthesia, particularly in urological surgery, provides better operating conditions because the gut is contracted and bleeding is reduced. For cystoscopy, the sphincters are relaxed, making introduction of the cystoscope in small infants easier. Epidural and intercostal blocks have a place in upper abdominal surgery, while caudal anaesthesia is useful for rectal, perineal and penile procedures. For major intra-abdominal surgery the child should be intubated to protect the airway.

SPECIFIC CONDITIONS

An understanding of the common neonatal and paediatric surgical conditions is helpful to the anaesthetist.

Obstructions of the alimentary tract

NEONATAL

Neonatal intestinal obstruction may occur at any point in the intestinal tract due to a wide variety of congenital causes, such as intraluminal septum, bands, atretic segments of gut, and volvulus. If it is distal to the ampulla of Vater it presents with bile-stained vomitus, abdominal distension or delay in the passage of meconium.

Oesophageal atresia is discussed in Chapter 12.

Congenital hypertrophic pyloric stenosis

This is a common condition, typically presenting with projectile vomiting between 2 and 12 weeks of age. The infant, frequently a male, is often poorly nourished and dehydrated, the degree being dependent on the duration and frequency of vomiting. Significant hydrochloric acid loss from the stomach leads to hypochloraemic alkalosis. As well as some potassium and sodium being lost in the gastric juice, additional potassium is lost via the renal tubular compensatory mechanism, where hydrogen is retained in preference to potassium during non-respiratory alkalosis. In the assessment of replacement needs, particularly of chloride, the greater extracellular fluid compartment in infants of this age (40% of body weight) should be taken into consideration. The degree of dehydration is important in planning fluid replacement, but also in assessing the degree of haemoconcentration of the electrolytes when they are measured. If chloride is used as a guide to replacement, the amount needed will be:

$$\text{Cl deficit} \times \text{body weight} \times \left[\text{ECF (0.4)} + \text{dehydration factor} \left(\frac{10-20\%}{100} \right) \right]$$

In the presence of a significant deficit normal saline (154 mmol/l Cl) is used initially and then 0.5 N saline with dextrose (2.5%) is given. Potassium chloride must be given to correct the hypokalaemia and to allow the hydrogen ion to be retained to correct the non-respiratory alkalosis. Operation should be delayed, even for a day or two, until the dehydration and electrolyte disturbances have been corrected. A nasogastric tube is often inserted to drain the stomach contents preoperatively. These tubes are often long and narrow, two factors which increase resistance to flow. As a result, stomach emptying is often incomplete and it is better to change to a larger (12 Fr), shorter catheter before induction, to evacuate the remaining contents (often 20–50 ml). After the gastric tube has been removed (because it tends to make the cardio-oesophageal sphincter incompetent), a rapid-sequence induction is usual.

The operation is simple: the hypertrophic muscle is divided down to the mucosa. If it is suspected that the mucosa has been punctured accidentally, air can be injected via a catheter into the stomach, which is then compressed towards the pylorus to test for a leak.

Malrotation

Malrotation results from failure of the embryonic extra-coelomic gut to rotate fully on its return to the abdominal cavity, resulting in a narrow attachment of the small bowel which allows volvulus. This causes obstruction of the duodenum, with resultant bile-stained vomiting, and may lead to obstruction of the superior mesenteric blood vessels, causing gangrene of the entire midgut. Early recognition of the condition, with immediate surgery to untwist the volvulus, divide Ladd's bands and broaden the width of the small bowel mesentery, can save the gut. The small bowel is replaced in the abdomen on the right, and the colon on the left. Where volvulus and ischaemia are suspected, operative treatment is very urgent, otherwise most of the small intestine becomes gangrenous. Although some babies have been kept alive by long-term parenteral nutrition and special oral feeds, patients who have lost long segments of gut have a poor outlook unless an adequate length of viable small intestine remains.

Duodenal obstruction

This may be due to atresia, stenosis, an intraluminal septum or diaphragm, compression by Ladd's bands in malrotation or to an annular pancreas.

Jejuno-ileal obstruction

This is due to atresia, which may be single or multiple and are thought to be due to interference with the vascular supply during development.

Intestinal duplication cysts

These are uncommon but may cause obstruction from external compression of the main lumen by a large tense cyst attached to its mesenteric aspect.

Meconium ileus

Meconium ileus is an obstruction of the distal ileum by impacted inspissated meconium, and is often the presenting problem in an infant with cystic fibrosis (mucoviscidosis). These infants may present with abdominal distension and bile-stained vomiting. In selected cases a gastrografin enema may successfully relieve the obstruction by aiding the spontaneous expulsion of the meconium. Gastrografin is markedly hyperosmolar, so dehydration due to fluid shift into the intestine may occur if not prevented by rapid concurrent intravenous infusion. If the enema fails or meconium peritonitis (as shown by extraluminal calcification on plain X-ray) has developed, surgery is required, using the anaesthetic principles outlined. The respiratory secretions may be viscid and cause postoperative problems. It may be better to avoid atropine.

Hirschsprung's disease

Hirschsprung's disease is a functional obstruction of the colon due to the absence of ganglia in the distal colon and rectum. The usual treatment is a preliminary colostomy in the newborn, done proximal to the aganglionic segment, ideally determined by biopsy. At a later stage, when the child is a few months old, the aganglionic colon is excised and ganglionated bowel is brought down through the preserved sphincteric mechanisms. These operations may be time-consuming and require an abdominoperineal approach. Caudal anaesthesia may reduce blood loss, can be used to supplement general anaesthesia and provides postoperative analgesia.

Anorectal abnormalities

These result from embryological failure of differentiation of the cloaca and urogenital sinus. 'High' abnormalities lie above the levator sling, while intermediate ones lie on but not through the levator muscles. There is often a fistula into the vagina in the female, or into the bladder or the urethra in males. In either case, the usual treatment is a colostomy until the child is old enough for definitive surgery. Rectoplasty is usually performed at 10–15 months of age. An abdomino-perineal approach is used to bring the normal rectum down to the perineum.

In a 'low' abnormality the rectum passes through the levator muscles to end close to the perineum, almost always with a fistulous communication which can be identified by the escape of meconium. Low anorectal anomalies may be treated by a single perineal cutback along the fistula, or by incising the membrane when that is all that is present. This can be done in the neonatal period.

These lower gut operations are often performed in the lithotomy position, with upward compression of the diaphragm, or both supine and lithotomy for abdomino-perineal operations.

Intussusception

Intussusception is the telescoping of the bowel within itself, causing obstruction, and, if diagnosis is delayed, ischaemia and necrosis of the intussuscepted bowel may occur. In most cases intussusception may be reduced by a gas or barium enema, but, if attempted hydrostatic reduction fails or if it causes perforation, laparotomy is required. The presence of gangrenous gut will necessitate resection and may be complicated by excessive fluid loss and septicaemia.

Adhesions and bands

Following previous surgery or peritonitis these can lead to bowel obstruction. When the gut is distended, nitrous oxide should be avoided and volatile anaesthetic carried in an oxygen/air mixture should be used.

Perforation

Perforation of the gut can result from trauma, ulceration, infection or ischaemia. The site of perforation determines the nature of the material spilt; this, and the amount of soiling determine the degree and extent of the peritonitis which results. Preoperative resuscitation with intravenous fluids and treatment of peritonitis with antibiotics are required. The peritoneum can be lavaged with warm saline containing an antibiotic such as a cephalosporin, which does not prolong the action of non-depolarizing muscle relaxants.

Pneumoperitoneum may accompany perforation of the gut; gas under the diaphragm in an erect X-ray is diagnostic. A rare cause is gastric perforation occurring in infants who have been resuscitated with a face mask at birth. In such babies, abdominal distension may become severe enough to cause respiratory embarrassment. Needle aspiration of the peritoneal air may be necessary. During anaesthesia, nitrous oxide should be avoided until the abdomen has been opened.

The common type of peptic ulceration is rare in children, but may occur in neurosurgical patients or severe asthmatics treated with steroids, and in some cases of severe burns. Gastric mucosa may be present in a Meckel's diverticulum, and ulceration of adjacent ileum can lead to haemorrhage or perforation.

Necrotizing enterocolitis

Necrotizing enterocolitis is a condition most commonly associated with prematurity, hypoxia, respiratory distress, umbilical arterial catheters, or some other cause of perinatal stress. It is caused by intestinal ischaemia followed by bacterial invasion. The features include lethargy, vomiting, gastrointestinal distension, rectal bleeding and, if peritonitis supervenes, erythema of the abdominal wall with abdominal tenderness. The presence of air in the wall of the intestines (intramural gas) is diagnostic, but may not be present early in the disease. Ischaemic necrosis is followed by perforation with peritonitis, pneumoperitoneum and thrombocytopenia due to disseminated intravascular coagulopathy. Persistent acidosis resistant to correction with sodium bicarbonate is a bad prognostic sign. Surgery is indicated when there is pneumoperitoneum or evidence of dead bowel; it may be the only hope of survival in these babies, where deterioration can continue despite intensive resuscitation.

Appendicitis

Appendicitis is one of the commonest conditions requiring laparotomy in children. It is rare under 4 years of age, but perforation and peritonitis are more likely to have occurred at presentation in this age group than in older children. These children are sicker than older children with appendicitis and require preoperative intravenous fluids because they have usually lost fluid by vomiting, from intraperitoneal transudation and by insensible losses because they are febrile. They also need antibiotics, effective against both aerobic and anaerobic bacteria, to treat the septicaemia.

Uncomplicated appendicectomy and laparotomy to drain abscesses require a relaxed abdomen to allow easy surgical access. If the child has been vomiting or not drinking for some time and is dehydrated, intravenous fluids should be commenced preoperatively.

Inguinal hernia

Inguinal herniae in infants are five times commoner in babies born before 36 weeks' gestation. Prolonged compression of the testicular vessels by an incarcerated mass can lead to testicular atrophy. Attempts at manual reduction with pressure from outside is successful in 85% of cases. If unsuccessful, urgent operation is necessary. An infant who has had a hernia reduced should have a herniotomy within a few days to avoid recurrence. In infants less than 2 years of age, the contralateral side is usually explored because of the high incidence of bilateral inguinal herniae. A hydrocoele represents patency of the processus vaginalis, down which peritoneal fluid tracks to accumulate around the testis. Most resolve spontaneously in infancy, but if still present at 18 months may require herniotomy.

Herniotomy is usually performed after the hernia has been reduced. A number of anaesthetic methods are advocated. In the small ex-premature infant with a tendency to apnoea, spinal anaesthesia has been used (see Chapter 22) but general anaesthesia, preferably using air as the carrier gas to prevent a reduction in functional residual capacity, can be used, often supplemented by an ilioinguinal/iliohypogastric nerve block (see Chapter 22). If the patient is intubated and controlled ventilation is used, care must be taken not to overventilate excessively or very low $Paco_2$ levels may be reached, especially in small babies. The CO_2 stimulus to ventilation is thereby lost. Monitoring with a capnograph allows more accurate control of ventilation.

Genital surgery

This includes operations for undescended testis, torsion of the testis, circumcision and correction of hypospadias.

Orchidopexy for the correction of undescended testis is one of the commonest operations on boys. This operation is now often done earlier at about the age of 1–2 years. Failure of testicular descent leaves the testis in the groin, or occasionally within the abdomen. Traction on the testis when it is pulled down into the scrotum may cause reflex bradycardia, especially if the patient is inadequately anaesthetized and has not been given atropine. Local anaesthesia is sometimes used to supplement general anaesthesia — an ilioinguinal nerve block may cover the incision in the groin, and local injection into the scrotum may cover that area. If a caudal block is used it should reach $T12$ to cover the testicular nerve supply as well as the sacral nerves to cover the scrotum — this requires 0.7 ml/kg of local anaesthetic.

Torsion of the testis can be indistinguishable clinically from torsion of the appendix testis or, very occasionally, epididymo-orchitis. Operation is urgent if infarction of the testis is to be prevented. These patients should be intubated using cricoid pressure, because they tend to have an increased volume of acid fluid in the stomach, creating an increased risk of aspiration.

Penile surgery is often associated with some bleeding, with the problem of erection, and postoperative pain.

Circumcision performed during the first few days of life is now more often undertaken with some type of local anaesthetic penile block in the neonatal nursery. Anaesthetists are not commonly involved at this stage. When general anaesthesia is used, laryngeal spasm is likely to occur if the depth of anaesthesia with halothane, enflurane or isoflurane is inadequate. The boy may be very distressed on awakening from general anaesthesia if adequate analgesia has not been given. Caudal anaesthesia with bupivacaine given with a light general anaesthetic has become popular as it reduces bleeding, prevents erection, avoids laryngeal spasm, and provides postoperative analgesia for several hours. Bupivacaine 0.25% should be used to avoid postoperative leg weakness. An alternative is a penile block, where the dorsal nerve of the penis is blocked with local anaesthetic just below the symphysis pubis (see Chapter 22). When the analgesia wears off, the application of lignocaine ointment to the raw surface can provide continuing analgesia.

Hypospadias and chordee are conditions where the urethra does not reach the glans penis. The anaesthetic considerations for the repair, which may be done in one or two stages, are the same as for circumcision. Epispadias is an extremely rare anomaly in which the roof of the urethra is absent and the urethra is a groove lying on the dorsal aspect of the penis, between the corpora cavernosa. Corrective surgery, usually carried out at 2–3 years is aimed at providing a roof for the urethra and achieving continence.

Major intra-abdominal trauma

This subject is covered more extensively in Chapter 26. Usually, intravenous resuscitation has commenced before the abdomen is opened and blood should be cross-matched if there is time. On rare occasions, when continued bleeding is more rapid than replacement, prompt laparotomy is indicated to locate and control the source of bleeding. Another problem which occasionally occurs in a child who is apparently adequately resuscitated is a sudden and marked drop in blood pressure when the abdomen is opened. This results from the sudden reduction of the raised intra-abdominal pressure which has slowed the rate of haemorrhage by compression of the bleeding organ or vessel. Capacitance vessels which have also been compressed are suddenly relaxed, with a reduction in preload.

In the management of severe intra-abdominal bleeding, particularly when the liver is torn, there may be advantages in an approach which has theoretical and practical benefits in optimizing the operative conditions before beginning surgery. It is to infuse fluids through large-bore intravenous cannulae and compress the abdomen with binders or a MAST suit, provided ventilation is not embarrassed. Management may be easier if the patient is anaesthetized, intubated, ventilated and fully monitored. The patient can then be vasodilated to reduce the rate of haemorrhage and cooled to provide brain protection should circulatory inadequacy occur. When the patient is cooled and vasodilated, the abdomen can be opened and there is some hope that the catastrophic cardiovascular collapse sometimes seen will not occur. With massive intra-abdominal haemorrhage, it may be possible to use a cell saver and reinfuse the blood if it has not been contaminated.

Liver and biliary disease

Conditions which cause jaundice in infants and are amenable to surgery include:

1 *Biliary atresia.* This is a condition in which different segments of the intra- and extrahepatic bile ducts are missing, or present as solid fibrous cords. The proximal duct system is drained directly into a loop of small intestine, a procedure which should be performed well before the age of 3 months if a satisfactory result is to be obtained. Progression of bile-duct atresia and prolonged back pressure leads to failure of bile secretion, fibrosis, cirrhosis, portal hypertension, liver failure and death in untreated patients. Liver transplantation may now be an option for these patients in centres where it is available.

2 *Choledochal cyst*, an aneurysmal dilatation of the bile ducts, usually involves the common bile duct.

3 *Common duct stones or sludge*, rare in children before puberty except in the presence of a haemolytic anaemia.

ANAESTHETIC CONSIDERATIONS

Although halothane may cause hepatocellular disease and jaundice, this is very rare in children; it has been shown that halothane can be used in the presence of chronic liver disease in children without deterioration of liver function [1]. Alternatively, another agent such as isoflurane could be used.

When muscle relaxants are used, one which is excreted in the urine or is metabolized or breaks down outside the liver should be used, e.g. atracurium or vecuronium.

There may be a bleeding tendency in severe liver disease and in the presence of obstructive jaundice. This may be due to decreased absorption of vitamin K and reduced synthesis of coagulation factors II (prothrombin), VII, IX and X.

An adequate intravenous infusion should be in place.

These operations may be prolonged and therefore steps should be taken to minimize excessive heat loss.

PORTAL HYPERTENSION

Liver disease leading to cirrhosis may cause a rise in portal venous pressure with portal—systemic shunting and the development of oesophageal varices. Massive haemorrhage from oesophageal varices presents as haematemesis and shock, requiring blood transfusion. Initial treatment involves the injection of a sclerosant through an oesophagoscope, and occasionally insertion of a Sengstaken—Blakemore tube or administration of pitressin. Surgery to relieve the portal hypertension may be indicated if repeated haemorrhage occurs.

Preoperative investigation usually includes a splenoportogram and splenic pressure measurement, or mesenteric arteriogram (see Chapter 21). A portocaval or lienorenal shunt may be performed. As there may be significant blood loss, blood must be available. The anaesthetic considerations are similar to those for obstructive jaundice.

LIVER SURGERY

The surgery of the liver includes control of haemorrhage in trauma, the removal of tumours and hydatid cysts.

Liver trauma is often life-threatening from haemorrhage. A possible approach to its management is discussed above. Liver tumours are uncommon in children — their management is discussed in the section on abdominal tumours (p. 160). Hydatid cysts occur in communities where dogs eat infected offal (usually sheep) and thereby become intermediate hosts. The disease is rare when public health measures related to slaughtering animals have been effective. The cysts are often unsymptomatic until they rupture or cause other complications.

Splenectomy

Splenectomy is occasionally required when the spleen has been injured and rupture of the capsule has led to major and continued intraperitoneal haemorrhage. If haemorrhage is not severe following splenic trauma and intravenous resuscitation maintains cardiovascular stability, a conservative non-operative approach is followed. Raised intra-abdominal pressure may slow the haemorrhage if severe, but anaesthesia and opening the abdomen may cause the blood pressure to fall suddenly. Often the spleen can be repaired (splenorrhaphy), otherwise the splenic artery should be ligated and the spleen removed.

Splenectomy may be carried out electively in patients with haematological conditions, such as hereditary spherocytosis, idiopathic thrombocytopenia or thalassaemia. These patients may be anaemic preoperatively, but they compensate by increasing cardiac output and their increased 2.3 DPG levels play a role by increasing oxygen release in the tissues. When the spleen is massively enlarged, the splenic artery is ligated in the lesser sac prior to splenectomy. A significant autotransfusion is possible — usually raising the haemoglobin by 1−2 g/100 ml without transfusion.

Urology

The commonest developmental anomaly of the urinary tract requiring surgery is vesicoureteric reflux. Other developmental anomalies in the urinary tract may cause obstruction to the urine flow, which leads to dilatation of the ureter (mega-ureter) and the renal pelvis (hydronephrosis) if proximal to the bladder, and dilatation, hypertrophy and trabeculation of the bladder when a congenital obstruction affects the bladder neck or there are posterior urethral valves. Other abnormalities include ureters which drain ectopically into the bladder, urethra or vagina. A ureterocoele is an abnormal dilatation of the ureteric orifice. Where there is obstruction, the infant may be born with poorly functioning kidneys; continued obstruction and stasis leads to ascending infection into the pelvic calyces, and eventually parenchymatous damage and renal failure with azotemia, hyperkalaemia, acidosis and anaemia.

UROLOGICAL PROCEDURES IN CHILDREN

These are as follows:
1 Diagnostic, e.g. urethroscopy, cystocopy, ureteric catheterization.
2 Surgical correction of congenital abnormalities, e.g. vesicoureteric reflux, pelviureteric junction obstruction.
3 Removal of stones from the renal pelvis or ureter,

using techniques of percutaneous endourology or lithotripsy.
4 In patients with spina bifida or other types of urinary incontinence, urinary diversion, bladder augmentation (cystoplasty) and insertion of an artificial urinary sphincter are usually carried out. Construction of an ileal conduit is now rarely performed.
5 Partial or total nephrectomy following trauma.
6 Removal of tumour (see below).
The anaesthetic management should include consideration of the following points:
1 Preoperative assessment of renal function — patients with renal failure, hyperkalaemia and metabolic acidosis compensated by respiratory alkalosis, should be anaesthetized with care. Respiratory depression may lead to failure to compensate for the metabolic acidosis.

If anaemia is present, cardiac output will be increased and, of less importance, 2.3 DPG will be increased, facilitating oxygen release to the tissues. To ensure adequate oxygen transport, additional oxygen should be given and myocardial depression avoided.
2 For intra-abdominal operations, the same anaesthetic principles as outlined earlier in this chapter apply. Urological procedures such as pyeloplasty and ureteric reimplantation involve an extraperitoneal approach.

Epidural anaesthesia combined with general anaesthesia provides good operating conditions for these operations as it contracts the gut, tends to reduce bleeding and provides muscle relaxation with operative and postoperative analgesia. Continued postoperatively, it provides patient comfort, but also prevents bladder spasm in ureteric reimplantation.
3 Operations on the kidney may require a lateral approach with a raised kidney bar or a sandbag under the opposite side; this improves surgical exposure but may reduce ventilation in the dependent lung. The bar is lowered and the sandbag removed before closure of the wound so that the muscle planes can be closed without tension.
4 Blood loss during partial nephrectomy or pyelolithotomy may be considerable, and can be reduced by local cooling of the kidney and temporary cross-clamping of the renal vessels.
5 Cystoscopy in the lithotomy position can be done with an inhalation anaesthetic via face mask. Bradycardia may occur when the bladder is distended acutely with fluid.

Tumours

WILM'S TUMOUR

Wilm's tumour (nephroblastoma) is one of the most common solid malignant tumours of childhood. Over 70% present before 4 years of age. Modern treatment consists of a combination of chemotherapy (actinomycin D, vincristine and sometimes adriamycin) and surgery. Radiotherapy is limited to a few specific situations. There is about an 85% survival in patients under 5 years. The results are not as good in older patients and those with unfavourable histology.

The anaesthetist becomes involved with these patients during radiological investigations (e.g. CT scan), which are performed either under sedation or general anaesthesia, and during surgical excision of the tumour. An anterior transperitoneal approach is made, but sometimes requires a thoracoabdominal extension to provide better access when the tumour is massive. On rare occasions, when the tumour has spread via the renal veins into the inferior vena cava and right atrium, a femoroatrial or cardiac bypass may be required for removal.

Patients with Wilm's tumour who have not been treated with chemotherapy are usually resistant to non-depolarizing muscle relaxants [2].

NEUROBLASTOMA

Neuroblastoma arises from cells in the sympathetic nervous system derived from the embryonic neural crest. It is one of the most malignant diseases of childhood, but occasionally in infants it undergoes spontaneous remission. Most cases present during the first 5 years of life. The majority are abdominal, while a smaller number are thoracic or pelvic, and occasionally may involve the spine or extradural tissue, where they can cause spinal cord compression and paraplegia. A high proportion have disseminated by the time the child presents, and in the older child the prognosis is bad.

A neuroblastoma may secrete catecholamines, so that the patient may have hypertension, tachycardia, pallor and sweating. These symptoms should alert the anaesthetist to treat them in a same way as patients with phaeochromocytoma, with alpha- and possibly beta-adrenergic blockers and fluids to increase the blood volume. These drugs plus sodium nitroprusside should be available when a child with possible neuroblastoma is being anaesthetized. If catecholamine secretion is signifi-

cant, halothane should be avoided. Not all patients with neuroblastoma secrete adrenaline or noradrenaline, so hypertension may not be a problem. The possibility that such a tumour in a small child may be a catecholamine-secreting neuroblastoma should be borne in mind.

These patients often undergo CT scanning or angiography to locate and define the tumour. Total surgical excision is not always possible, but excision is usually attempted after it has been reduced in size by chemotherapy. Cyclophosphamide, which prolongs the action of suxamethonium, is one of the drugs sometimes used during chemotherapy.

LIVER TUMOURS

Liver tumours are usually benign in neonates, but thereafter hepatoblastoma is the commonest. A diagnostic feature of the latter is the presence of raised levels of alpha-fetoprotein in the plasma. Hepatoblastoma usually presents as a mass in the abdomen in children up to 3 years old. The size and site of the tumour can be demonstrated with ultrasound and CT scan. Occasionally, angiography is used to delineate the blood supply. A vena cavagram may show whether the inferior vena cava is compressed or invaded.

These patients exhibit a resistance to non-depolarizing relaxants, particularly to D-tubocurarine, if the tumours are malignant. Up to twice the normal dose may be needed to paralyse the child [3]. This resistance is absent with benign masses or when a malignant tumour has been successfully treated and shrunk with chemotherapy. Possible mechanisms are increased uptake by 'acceptor sites' present in the tumour, or the production by the tumour of some substance which modifies the neuromuscular junction.

Hepatic lobectomy to remove the tumour may be complicated by massive haemorrhage, which may be difficult to arrest if it comes from the inferior vena cava or hepatic veins. Slings placed around the vena cava prior to resection, which can be tightened to prevent bleeding, and inflow occlusion of the hepatic artery and portal vein during resection, can significantly reduce the blood loss [4]. If the inferior vena cava has been compressed by a large tumour, collateral veins develop so that vena caval occlusion is well tolerated. In such cases bypass, which is advocated by some groups, is unnecessary [5].

Hypothermia is a useful adjunct to liver tumour resection. Although surface-cooling hypothermia may take an hour to reach 32–30°C, the safety margin it provides against periods of low cardiac output or cardiac arrest from massive haemorrhage and vena caval clamping makes it worthwhile [5]. During partial liver resection one patient, who was hypothermic, recovered normally while another, who was normothermic, was brain-damaged following intraoperative cardiac arrest.

Vasodilators such as sodium nitroprusside may also help cooling, induce hypotension and reduce bleeding.

After major liver resection hypoglycaemia and hypo-albuminaemia are potential problems, unless infusion of 10% glucose and additional albumin is provided [6]. Other complications include transient jaundice and infection.

TERATOMATA

Teratomata may be posterior sacrococcygeal — usually evident at birth and benign — combined pre- and post-coccygeal (benign or malignant), pelvic (often malignant), retroperitoneal, ovarian (benign or malignant) or testicular (usually benign).

Sacrococcygeal tumours presenting in the neonatal period are almost always large and benign. Malignancy is more likely as age increases, when the tumour is rapidly growing, and when there is radiographic evidence of erosion of the coccyx or sacrum. Surgical treatment is excision, usually through a perineal incision with the patient prone. The coccyx is usually removed. In patients with a pelvic extension the perineal approach may be preceded by laparotomy and delineation and mobilization of the abdominal component of the tumour, which requires a change in position during the operation. Surgical excision is usually supplemented with chemotherapy.

During major tumour surgery, induced hypotension may be of value to reduce blood loss and to allow the surgeon a clearer view of the operating field. It may also make dissection of a major vessel surrounded by tumour safer by decreasing the tension on the vessel wall.

PHAEOCHROMOCYTOMA

Phaeochromocytoma is a tumour of adrenal medullary tissue which may secrete adrenaline and noradrenaline or, on rare occasions, dopamine. It causes intermittent hypertension, particularly when the tumour is handled during dissection. The principles of management are first, to increase the blood volume preoperatively to prevent dangerous hypotension following removal of the tumour, and second, to prevent dysrhythmias. Pre-operative preparation with an alpha-adrenergic blocker such as phenoxybenzamine, supplemented, if necessary, during operation by the vasodilator sodium nitroprusside, ensures that maximum vasodilatation is obtained. The increased capacity of the circulation should be filled by the administration of additional intravenous fluids, plasma protein solution or blood. If adequate blood volume expansion is achieved, intra- and postoperative hypotension, resulting from removal of the source of vasoconstricting catecholamines, is unlikely after the tumour has been removed. Tachycardia, due to the uninhibited beta-adrenergic effects of catecholamines on the heart, can be treated with a beta-adrenergic blocker such as atenolol. Hypertensive episodes occurring during operation can be rapidly controlled with an infusion of sodium nitroprusside; if dysrhythmias develop, these will usually disappear if the blood pressure is lowered. Labetalol, the combined alpha- and beta-adrenergic blocking drug, may also be useful.

The choice of anaesthetic technique becomes less critical once the patient has been adequately dilated, the vascular compartment filled, and beta-adrenergic blockers are available. Thiopentone followed by a relax-ant and nitrous oxide with an analgesic supplement is a satisfactory technique.

Abdominal wall defects

A variety of defects occur in childhood, some of which are large and present at birth. These include:

1 *Exomphalos* (or *omphalocele*), which is a protrusion of the abdominal contents within a thin-walled sac composed of amnion and peritoneum, as a central defect in the base of the umbilical cord (Fig. 11.1). Coexisting cardiac and renal anomalies are common. The Beckwith–Wiedemann syndrome (exomphalos, hemihypertrophy, macroglossia) may be associated with severe neonatal hypoglycaemia (from hyperinsulinaemia) and necessitate a 10% glucose infusion. The large tongue may make intubation difficult.

2 *Gastroschisis* is a protrusion of the abdominal contents through a defect at the side of the umbilicus. The bowel appears greatly thickened, matted together, oedematous and covered in exudate. Atresia and malrotation may coexist.

3 An *umbilical hernia* is due to a fascial defect beneath or just above the umbilicus, and becomes apparent after

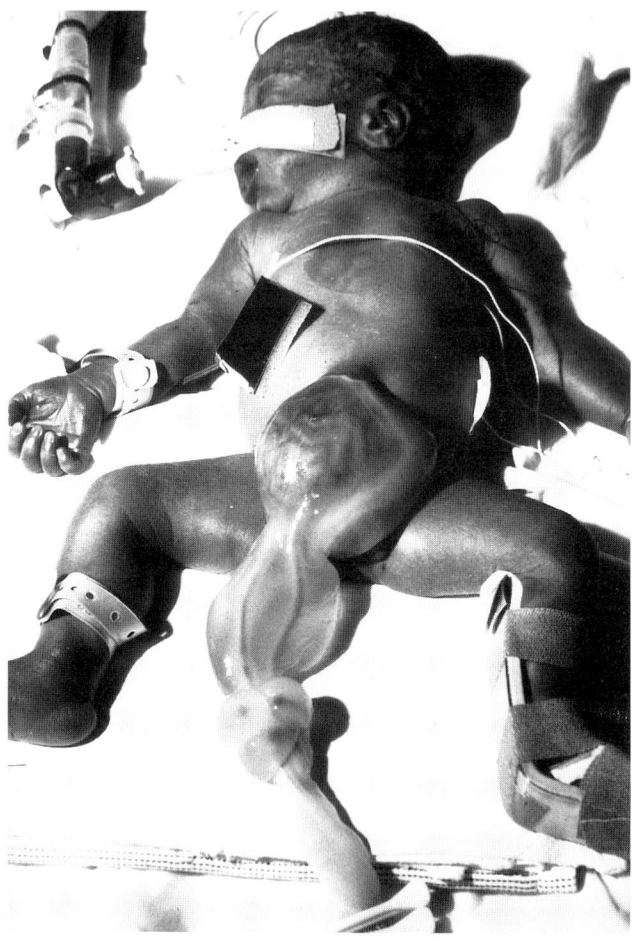

Fig. 11.1 A large exomphalos in a baby who has been monitored and ventilated preoperatively.

separation of the umbilical cord. Incarceration is very rare in children and repair is only indicated if the hernia persists beyond 2–3 years of age. An inhalation anaesthetic can be supplemented by infiltration of local anaesthetic or bilateral 10th-intercostal-nerve blocks to provide operative and postoperative analgesia.

4 *Prune belly syndrome* is a rare anomaly in which the abdominal muscles are deficient, associated with greatly enlarged ureters and bladder, bilateral undescended testes and wrinkling of the skin of the abdominal wall.

5 *Bladder extrophy* and *cloaca extrophy* are the result of disturbances in embryological development, with failure of midline closure causing anterior extrusion of the visceral structures involved. The pubic rami are widely separated.

The primary object of surgical management of abdomi-

nal defects and ectopia vesicae (bladder extrophy), is to correct the abnormality. Primary closure is preferred when the defect in exomphalos or gastroschisis is small enough, but when the amount of bowel and liver extruded is large or the sac is very large, returning the bowel (and liver) into the abdomen may be difficult; the increase in intra-abdominal pressure can lead to splinting of the diaphragm resulting in respiratory difficulties and the need for postoperative mechanical ventilation. In gastroschisis, if primary reduction is impossible, a prosthetic sheet of silastic or dacron can be sutured around the edge of the defect, enveloping the extruded abdominal contents. The prosthetic envelope is then reduced in size daily by tightening the dome of the sac over several days, until the contents have returned to the abdomen and the abdominal wall has accommodated sufficiently to allow secondary closure. A modification of this method may also be used in the large exomphalos.

Anaesthesia with intubation and muscle relaxation is desirable for these procedures. The stomach should be deflated with a nasogastric tube to reduce diaphragmatic splinting. Gaseous distension of the gut can be minimized by avoiding nitrous oxide. Blood loss can be considerable and may be aggravated by venous congestion when the abdominal contents are returned to the abdomen compressing the inferior vena cava. An intravenous cannula should be inserted into an upper limb or neck vein (rather than the leg) so that the flow is not obstructed by increased intra-abdominal pressure.

Head and neck surgery

ANAESTHETIC PROBLEMS

The anaesthetic problems in this area are mainly access to the patient for both the anaesthetist and the surgeon. The position of the anaesthetic equipment and the anaesthetist should allow the surgeon optimal access to the operative field without compromising patient safety. When the operation lasts only 5–10 minutes, an inhalational anaesthetic with a face mask may suffice as long as the anaesthetist's hands are out of the operative field. For longer procedures the airway should be secured with a laryngeal mask airway or by intubation. Precurved RAE, or Portex 'north' or 'south' tubes are often especially useful for these operations (see Chapter 3).

The anaesthetist's access to a vein requires either an extension set from the arm, which is either placed by the side or can be abducted, but in this position it may be in the assistant's way and in danger of hyperabduction with possible traction injury to the brachial plexus.

Monitoring may be more difficult, especially if the head is draped and the arms are at the side. A precordial stethoscope and pulse oximeter should be used. If the anaesthetist is at the head of the table, colour can be observed in the wound and a temporal pulse can sometimes be reached. Placed at the side of the table, the anaesthetist can easily monitor colour and pulse on an arm or leg. Blood pressure can be measured with a non-invasive blood pressure device or by direct pressure measurement.

For anterior neck operations the head is often extended to improve exposure and flexed at the end of the operation to assist in wound closure.

SPECIFIC CONDITIONS

Specific conditions to be considered which are not included in Chapter 15 (ear, nose and throat) and Chapter 17 (plastic surgery) are as follows:

Cervical abscess

Drainage is a short procedure which can be carried out using inhalation anaesthesia with a mask, but if there is any doubt about maintaining an airway, a laryngeal mask or tracheal intubation is preferable.

Ludwig's angina

This presents as a brawny induration which extends across the front of the neck, causing mandibular fixation with the mouth half open, inability to protrude the tongue and constriction of the airway between the tongue and posterior pharyngeal wall. This produces a high-pitched inspiratory and expiratory stridor. The basic lesion is either an abscess between the genioglossus and geniohyoid muscles which can be drained, or, less commonly, a median cellulitis. In the latter case response to antibiotics may be too slow and drainage ineffective — urgent tracheostomy may be necessary to prevent 'strangulation' by the swelling.

Anaesthesia is hazardous because of difficulty in opening the mouth adequately, and because the airway may already be constricted. An inhalation induction with a high concentration of oxygen is probably safest, but it will take longer if the airway is partially obstructed. The passage of a nasopharyngeal airway, if possible, will

improve the airway. It may be possible to insert a laryngeal mask. Tracheal intubation may be very difficult and even dangerous.

Local anaesthetic infiltration can be tried but may be less effective due to its reduced activity in the presence of infection and pus, which lowers pH.

Cervical lymph node biopsy

This is required when enlargement may be due to a tumour, tuberculosis or MAIS complex (mycobacterium avium−intracellulare−scrofulaceum). The latter may be clinically similar to tuberculosis lymphadenitis but has a more rapid course, is usually unilateral, does not have pulmonary lesions, is mantoux-negative and does not respond to antituberculous drugs. Treatment is therefore surgical excision. The anaesthetic considerations are the same as those mentioned above for neck surgery and depend on the expected duration of the procedure. Intubation is usual as they often take longer than expected.

Thyroglossal duct cysts

These may develop anywhere in the midline along the line of the thyroglossal tract between the foramen caecum of the tongue and the lower neck. They present as a swelling or as an anterior cervical abscess. Haemorrhage into the base of the tongue is an uncommon but troublesome complication, which can cause postoperative respiratory difficulties.

Branchial sinus, cyst or fistula

These are persisting embryological remnants of the branchial clefts. The fistula tracts upwards from a small orifice in the lower third of the neck, running between the internal and external carotid arteries to reach the lateral pharyngeal wall. Careful dissection should avoid damage to these vessels and haemorrhage.

Cystic hygroma

This is a congenital defect in the formation of the lymphatic channels that usually involves the neck. Some are small while others are very large (Fig. 11.2) and may extend across the midline, involve the floor of the mouth and descend into the mediastinum. Total excision is normally impossible because the lesion infiltrates into the

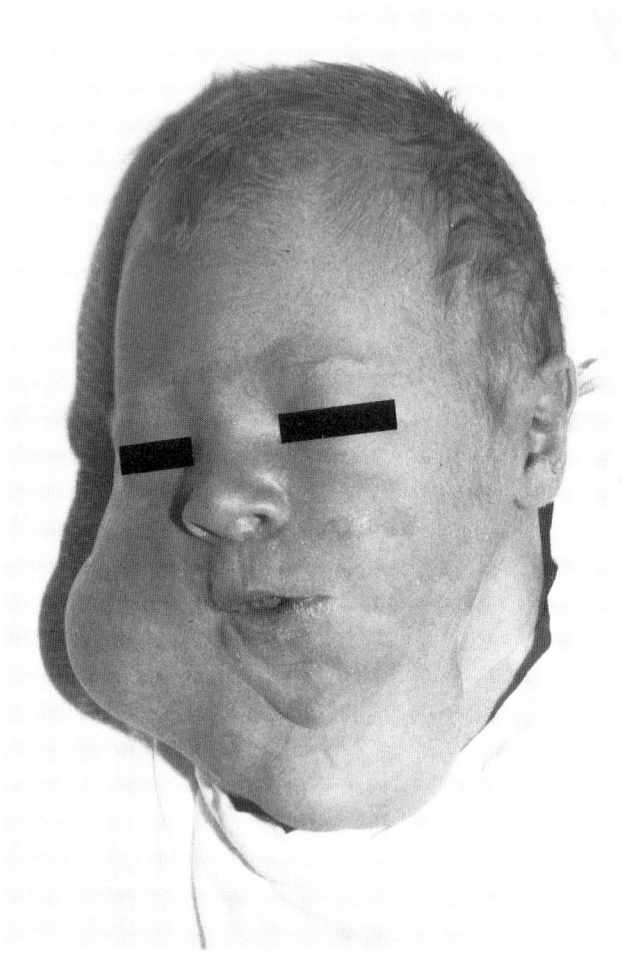

Fig. 11.2 A large cystic hygroma infiltrating the neck.

tissues at its periphery; vital structures in the vicinity may be endangered. An anterior midline or bilateral mass may be life-threatening if it is close to the airway, which it may distort or obstruct making intubation difficult. Removal of a large hygroma may take several hours and requires control of the airway and attention to fluid balance and temperature homeostasis.

Thyroid

Thyroid surgery is unusual in childhood, but thyroid abscess, and carcinoma following radiation earlier in life, do occur and may necessitate surgical removal. Thyroid function should be assessed preoperatively and, if abnormal, appropriate medical treatment begun. Untreated hypothyroid patients, for example, are very sensitive to anaesthetic drugs such as thiopentone and may become hypotensive or have delayed recovery. Possible problems

with the airway include compression of the trachea preoperatively by a tumour or abscess, or postoperatively by haemorrhage beneath the muscular layers of the incision. The latter can be relieved by cutting the sutures and opening the wound. Longstanding tracheal compression may result in tracheomalacia, which can cause airway problems postoperatively. Several small endotracheal tubes should be available in case the trachea is narrowed.

Liver transplantation

INTRODUCTION

Since the introduction in the early 1980s of cyclosporin as the primary immunosuppressive agent, survival after liver transplantation has improved dramatically. Currently the expectation is for approximately 80% 12-month survival. In addition, having reached 1 year post-transplantation, longer-term survival with near normal quality of life occurs in 90% of recipients.

Apart from improved immunosuppression, reduced morbidity and mortality are due to advances in surgical techniques, donor organ preservation, anaesthesia and perioperative care with vigilant postoperative management and follow-up.

INDICATIONS FOR LIVER TRANSPLANTATION
(Table 11.1)

The major indication for paediatric liver transplantation is biliary atresia, while in adults, post-necrotic cirrhosis is the most common. Children may present for transplantation either before 2 years of age or later in childhood or adolescence, when the effects of end-stage liver disease become apparent.

PREOPERATIVE CARE

Children considered suitable for liver transplantation undergo comprehensive assessment involving a multi-disciplinary approach. End-stage liver failure is a multi-system disease with many pathophysiological consequences (Table 11.2). As well as a detailed clinical assessment, a wide range of laboratory investigations is performed. Surgical work-up requires an assessment of liver size with ultrasound and CT scan, as well as liver blood supply with Doppler studies and occasionally digital subtraction angiography. Chest and abdominal

Table 11.1 Indications for liver transplantation

Children		Adults	
Indication	Frequency	Indication	Frequency
Biliary Atresia	50–55%	Cirrhosis	30–40%
Inborn errors	20–25%	Primary biliary cirrhosis	20–25%
alpha-1 antitrypsin deficiency		Sclerosing cholangitis	12–15%
Wilson's disease		Inborn errors	10%
Others, e.g. tyrosinosis		Fulminant hepatitis	5%
Cirrhosis	10%	Hepatoma	5%
Cholestasis (familial)	7%	Others e.g. Budd–	5%
Fulminant hepatitis	5%	Chiari syndrome,	
Others e.g. Budd–Chiari	5%	secondary biliary	
syndrome, sclerosing		cirrhosis	
cholangitis			

Table 11.2 Pathophysiological sequelae of chronic liver disease

Hyperdynamic circulation
Decreased effective plasma volume
Decreased renal perfusion and decreased free-water clearance
Ascites and peripheral oedema, low serum albumin
Gastrointestinal bleeding
Coagulopathy
Decreased functional residual capacity
Ventilation/perfusion mismatch
Decreased liver blood flow
Electrolyte disorders, e.g. hyponatraemia
Acid–base disorders
Hypoglycaemia
Encephalopathy
Increased risk of infection

measurements are also made, to help in selecting a suitable donor organ. Leucocyte compatibility (HLA) testing is not required for liver transplantation, where the major requirements are a suitable match for ABO blood group and size.

In the period leading up to a liver transplant, patients and their families are assessed psychosocially and given repeated counselling and education about liver transplantation. Most liver transplant programmes have a liver support group, which includes pre- and post-transplant patients and their families, social workers, pastoral care workers and play therapists.

SURGICAL TECHNIQUE

Donor organ management

The organ donor for liver transplantation will have been formally declared brain-dead. Apart from the usual criteria for organ donation, such as relatively stable cardiovascular function and negative screen for infection, liver function tests should be normal.

A separate surgical team is responsible for procurement of the donor liver. Before surgical removal, the donor liver is perfused with a preservative solution. After cross-clamping and removal, the organ is stored in ice for transport. The preservative solution contains high-dose potassium and other substances to minimize cellular metabolism during the ischaemic period. Current solutions (UW — Belzer's solution) allow up to 12 hours of ischaemia (see Table 11.3).

Recipient operation

A large bilateral subcostal incision with vertical midline extension to the xiphisternum is used to achieve the

Table 11.3 Components of University of Wisconsin solution for donor liver preservation

Substance	Amount per litre
K-lactobionate	100 mmol
K-H$_2$PO$_4$	25 mmol
MgSO$_4$	5 mmol
Raffinose	30 mmol
Adenosine	5 mmol
Glutathione	3 mmol
Insulin	100 units
Dexamethasone	8 mg
Allopurinol	1 mm
Hydroxyethyl starch	50 g
Penicillin	40 units

required exposure. Surgery is conveniently divided into three stages:

I *Pre-anhepatic*: Stage I involves mobilization and dissection of the native liver. This may involve considerable surgical bleeding, especially if there is portal hypertension with an extensive collateral circulation and/or adhesions due to previous surgery, such as portaenterostomy for biliary atresia.

II *Anhepatic*: The anhepatic stage commences when both portal vein and hepatic artery have been clamped. Removal of the liver is achieved after full mobilization, and a clamp is placed across the three main hepatic veins as they enter the inferior vena cava. Occasionally this will cause a degree of vena caval obstruction and resultant reduced cardiac output, but this is tolerated well by most patients. In adults the problem of vena caval clamping and splanchnic congestion is often overcome by veno-venous bypass (portal and femoral veins to axillary vein) but this is rarely used in paediatric liver transplantation.

After removal of the native liver, haemostasis is achieved and the donor liver is removed from ice, and the anastomoses between hepatic veins and inferior vena cava are performed. Next the liver is flushed with cold Ringer's solution to wash out ischaemic products and reduce the acid and potassium content.

The portal vein anastomosis is performed next, and then both portal and vena caval venous clamps are released and the liver is reperfused with portal venous blood, which is the start of Stage III.

III *Reperfusion*: Venous reperfusion of the liver invariably involves delivering a cold, potassium-rich, acid load to the heart.

After the liver has been reperfused from the portal vein, the hepatic artery is anastomosed. Occasionally this will require a graft (using donor vascular tissue) if direct anastomosis is technically impossible.

When all vascular work is completed and haemostasis secured, the bile-duct anastomosis is performed. If a direct choledochocholedochostomy is not possible, a choledochojejunostomy using a Roux loop is the alternative technique. A T-tube is placed in the bile duct, final haemostasis is achieved and the abdomen is closed.

INTRAOPERATIVE SEQUELAE (Table 11.4)

Liver transplantation imposes a major pathophysiological insult which involves five major categories:

Table 11.4 Biochemical sequelae during liver transplantation

Citrate intoxication
Metabolic acidosis
Hypocalcaemia
Osmolality changes
Plasma sodium increase
Hyperglycaemia
Rapid potassium flux

Cardiovascular changes

1 *Hyperdynamic circulation*. Patients with end-stage liver disease have a tendency towards high cardiac output, low sytemic vascular resistance and often a tachycardia. Sequelae are superimposed on this background.

2 *Blood loss*. The potential exists for massive bleeding during liver transplantation, so there is an ever-present threat of hypovolaemia.

3 *Effects of inferior vena caval obstruction*. Any degree of inferior vena caval obstruction, due to either partial or complete clamping or surgical manipulation of the liver, will decrease cardiac output.

4 *Reperfusion*. Initially there is usually a relative bradycardia and sometimes more serious dysrhythmias due to the potassium-rich, acidic cold blood reaching the heart. These effects are minimized by thorough flushing of the liver in Stage II, and correction of any metabolic acidosis and/or hypocalcaemia prior to reperfusion. This biochemical insult is transient and within $1-2$ minutes the rhythm is usually stable.

In some patients, a phenomenon called post-reperfusion syndrome occurs. This involves hypotension due to marked vasodilatation. Cardiac index usually remains high and systemic vascular resistance is very low. It is likely that various potent 'vasoactive' substances released from the ischaemic liver are responsible for this, but at present no specific cause is identifiable. These patients may require vasopressors (phenylephrine or metaraminol).

Biochemical disturbance

Many biochemical changes are likely during liver transplantation, and specific measures are taken to either prevent or treat them.

Patients who require large volumes of citrated blood, especially during the dissection and anhepatic phases, readily develop a metabolic acidosis. There is no hepatic function to metabolize citrate, so citrate intoxication with resultant hypocalcaemia occurs. Calcium chloride should be administered according to the measured changes in ionized calcium. Mild-to-moderate metabolic acidosis can be safely tolerated, but if base deficit exceeds 10, titration of alkali is recommended to reduce the risk of reperfusion arrhythmias.

It is important to minimize the dose of sodium bicarbonate because it has been shown that liver transplant patients are at risk from perioperative increases in plasma sodium. The resultant osmolality change imposes a risk of coma due to central pontine and extrapontine myelinolysis. An alternative buffer is THAM (0.3 molar solution of 2-amino, 3-hydroxy, 1,3-propanediol) which is useful for treating acidaemia without the risk of increasing plasma sodium concentration or producing extra CO_2, but it should be remembered that many of these patients are hyponatraemic preoperatively.

Blood glucose will tend to increase intraoperatively, associated with the dextrose load received from transfused blood. The major increase occurs after reperfusion and this is likely to be due to hepatic gluconeogenesis from the newly functioning graft. An insulin infusion is commonly required in Stage III. Plasma potassium may rise acutely with reperfusion, but subsequently it decreases and potassium commonly needs to be administered as well in Stage III.

Coagulopathy

There are multiple causes of abnormal coagulation during liver transplantation. Pre-existing coagulopathy is common in cirrhosis due to reduced synthesis of clotting factors, thrombocytopenia and sometimes disseminated intravascular coagulation. Massive transfusion dilutes coagulation factors and liver reperfusion is specifically associated with abnormal clotting. Fibrinolysis is almost universal during liver transplantation, and it may occur early in the operation. Debate exists as to whether this involves a primary fibrinolysis or whether it is secondary to consumption. Frequent monitoring of platelet count, clotting profile and indices of fibrinolysis such as fibrinogen level, euglobulin clot lysis time, fibrin degradation products and D-Dimer is required.

Thromboelastography has also been shown to be very useful in rapidly identifying a coagulation problem, and helps to rationalize the use of blood products such as platelets, fresh frozen plasma and cryoprecipitate.

Renal dysfunction

The kidneys are at risk during liver transplantation. Pre-renal factors involve large blood volume changes, as well as alterations in cardiac output due to caval manipulation. An additional important intraoperative stress is renal venous congestion secondary to portal cross-clamping. Some patients have abnormal renal function preoperatively, and all patients will be having nephrotoxic drugs such as cyclosporin. For these reasons, renal protection using low doses of dopamine (2.5 µg/kg/min) and mannitol (0.1 g/kg/h) are infused perioperatively. Aminoglycosides are avoided in favour of less nephrotoxic antibiotics.

Hypothermia

A long operation via a large incision involving massive fluid shifts and replacement requirements predisposes to hypothermia. In addition, at the time of reperfusion cold fluid from the previously cold-stored liver is released into the circulation and the cold liver continues to cool blood passing through it while it gradually warms up.

It is essential to minimize the fall in body temperature during liver transplantation, as hypothermia may further complicate the biochemical and coagulation disturbances. Cardiac dysrhythmia and arrest are more likely with co-existent biochemical disturbance, especially acidosis and hyperkalaemia. Many simple and practical methods are employed to reduce heat loss during liver transplantation, and these are especially relevant in children. They include increasing the ambient temperature (20–23.5°C), warming intravenous fluids, using a heated mattress, heating and humidifying the anaesthetic gases and covering all exposed skin.

Temperature is monitored via a nasopharyngeal probe and sometimes a pulmonary artery catheter thermistor. Environmental temperature should also be monitored, and there should be appropriate thermometers on the humidifier, water mattress and rapid infusion systems.

ANAESTHESIA MANAGEMENT

The major challenge facing anaesthetists involved with liver transplantation is prolonged physiological management of these patients, who are exposed to many problems already. It is important to use a technique with comprehensive monitoring that provides adequate anaesthesia for these often fragile children. In particular, the anaesthetist should take account of the fact that a newly grafted liver may take some time to function normally (from hours to days).

Premedication

Earlier visits by the anaesthetist during the assessment period will have achieved much in establishing rapport with the child. There is usually a high degree of antici-pation, anxiety and excitement associated with the 'news' of a donor liver. Heavy premedication is unnecessary and unpredictable and should be avoided. A small dose of short-acting benzodiazepine is often appropriate if a premedication drug is required.

Induction and maintenance

The risk of aspiration is increased, especially if ascites is present, therefore rapid-sequence induction is rec-ommended. After induction and intubation, anaesthesia is maintained with oxygen, air and isoflurane. A neuro-muscular blocking drug given as a continuous infusion (e.g. pancuronium $0.01-0.02$ mg/kg/h) is convenient. Fentanyl as a continuous infusion (approx 3.5 µg/kg/h) provides background analgesic supplementation. Iso-flurane at less than 2% inspired concentration has more favourable effects on liver blood flow and oxygenation than other volatile agents, and fentanyl pharmacokinetics are more predictable in liver disease compared with longer-acting narcotics.

Monitoring

After anaesthesia is established, multiple cannulae are inserted for infusion, transfusion and monitoring.
1 *Volume replacement.* At least two large-bore cannulae (up to $7-8$ Fr gauge) are inserted in the cubital fossa (cephalic or basilic veins) and/or the neck (internal jugular veins). These are linked to some device which allows for rapid infusion of warmed fluids.
2 *Arterial cannulae.* Bilateral radial arterial cannulae are used, one for direct blood pressure monitoring and the other for repeated blood sampling without interfering with monitoring.
3 *Central venous and/or pulmonary artery cannulae.* At least one multi-lumen central venous catheter is required for CVP monitoring and drug infusion. A pulmonary

artery catheter (e.g. 5 Fr gauge) may be useful. The right internal jugular vein is the preferred access.

Multi-system monitoring of the liver transplant patient is essential and is outlined in Table 11.5.

Laboratory investigations are performed hourly throughout the operation, and biochemical analysis of acid−base, potassium and calcium status as often as every 15-minutes during the anhepatic stage (Table 11.6).

POSTOPERATIVE CARE

After surgery is completed, the child is transferred to the intensive care unit for continued intensive monitoring management. Typically the post-liver transplant child emerges from anaesthesia relatively quickly and is usually awake within hours. Early extubation is important to reduce the risk of nosocomial chest infection.

Table 11.5 Patient monitoring during liver transplantation

Cardiovascular
ECG
Direct arterial BP
CVP ± PAP, PCWP, C. I
    ± calculated SVRI, PVRI
End-tidal CO_2

Respiratory
IPPV alarm
End-tidal CO_2
SaO_2 (pulse oximetry)

Renal
Urine burette

Temperature
Nasopharyngeal ± pulmonary artery
Airway temperature

Table 11.6 Laboratory monitoring during liver transplantation

Haematological
Haemoglobin concentration
Platelet count
Clotting profile; prothrombin, APTT
Fibrinogen level
ECLT (euglobulin clot lysis time)
FDP's D-Dimer

Biochemical
Arterial blood gases
Na, K, Ca^{++}, glucose

Analgesia can be achieved with low-dose opioids (incremental morphine or fentanyl), provided close monitoring of sedation is carried out.

Frequent assessment of liver-graft function is important and involves daily flow studies of the hepatic artery and portal vein, liver function tests such as bilirubin level, serum transaminases and prothrombin level. Clinical assessment is also important.

The early postoperative period may be complicated in three major ways:

1 Primary non-function of the graft. This will occur over hours to days as the graft failure is reflected by clinical and laboratory evidence of acute liver failure. Experimental support treatments such as prostaglandin E infusions are occasionally tried, but if the graft fails re-transplantation is the only option.

2 Technical problems.

(a) Bleeding. Meticulous haemostasis is important, but occasionally despite this, postoperative bleeding may occur and require re-exploration. Coagulation function usually recovers spontaneously in the early postoperative period.

(b) Hepatic artery thrombosis. The smaller arteries in children carry an increased risk of post-operative thrombosis. This will manifest as fever and progressive deterioration in liver function, and ultimately liver and multi-organ failure. Early detection is essential and is achieved by daily Doppler studies in the early postoperative period. If detected early, surgical intervention may be possible but if not, retransplantation is necessary.

(c) Bile leak may also occasionally occur and re-operation to correct the problem is usually required.

3 Infection and/or Rejection. Bacterial sepsis is an important risk, especially in the early postoperative period. Emphasis should be placed on prevention of infection by early extubation and the removal of invasive intravascular cannulae. Antibiotic prophylaxis (broad spectrum) is given for 48 hours perioperatively but should then be ceased, so that if sepsis occurs the offending organism can be cultured. Later in the postoperative period, the transplant recipient is at risk not only from bacterial sepsis but also from fungal and viral pathogens.

Various immunosuppressive regimens may be used, but these often involve a combination of therapy with cyclosporin, steroids and azothiaprin. From the time of transplantation onwards, great vigilance is required to differentiate infection from rejection, with the differing implications for treatment.

CONCLUSION

Anaesthesia for paediatric liver transplantation provides the personnel involved with a major challenge and requires commitment from not only the anaesthetists but a large number of other staff including nurses, technicians and laboratory staff. The reward of successful transplantation is to see the transition from a child with debilitating end-stage liver disease to one with new energy and anticipation of a normal life.

REFERENCES

1 Wark H., Earl J., Cooper M., Overton J. Halothane in children with chronic liver disease. *Anaes Intens Care* 1991, **19**, 9.

2 Brown T.C.K., Gregory M., Bell B., Clare D. Response to non-depolarizing relaxants in children with tumours. *Anaes Intens Care* 1990, **18**, 460.

3 Brown T.C.K., Gregory M., Bell, Campbell P.C. Liver tumours and muscle relaxants — electromyographic studies in children. *Anaesthesia* 1987, **42**, 1284.

4 Davidson P.D., Brown T.C.K., Auldist A.W. Elective hepatic resection in children. *Pediatr Surg* 1988, **4**.

5 Brown T.C.K., Davidson P.D., Auldist A.W. Anaesthetic considerations in liver tumour resection in children. *Pediatr Surg* 1988, **4**, 11.

6 Stone H.H. Major hepatic resections in children. *J Pediatr Surg* 1975, **10**, 127.

12: Anaesthesia for Thoracic Surgery

GENERAL PRINCIPLES

This chapter deals with thoracic procedures, excluding operations on the heart and major blood vessels.

Thoracic operations are commonly performed through a lateral approach between the ribs or sometimes through a midline incision with a sternal split.

Pneumothorax

The general principles of anaesthesia for thoracotomy mainly depend on the management of an open pneumothorax. When one side of the chest is open in a spontaneously breathing patient, the lung on that side will collapse, leading to hypoventilation. The mediastinum will shift towards the intact side on inspiration and in the reverse direction in expiration. Some of the expired gas from the intact side enters the collapsed lung and increases dead space as it is inhaled into the intact side again at the next inspiration. This phenomenon is called 'pendeluft' (Fig. 12.1). If the pleura are not opened during a midline approach, the lungs will not collapse as much and pendeluft does not occur. During thoracotomy, patients should be intubated and ventilated with positive pressure ventilation when the chest is open, to prevent the lungs collapsing.

Practical points

An intravenous infusion should be inserted in the uppermost arm to ensure that flow is not obstructed. It should be adequate to allow blood to be given rapidly if this is necessary.

A folded towel or sandbag is sometimes placed under the chest to aid separation of the ribs and improve exposure. When the chest is being closed it is removed to facilitate apposition of the ribs.

When the pleura is about to be opened, any pressure on the airways should be released so that the underlying lung will fall away and not be damaged. Likewise, during closure at the end of the operation the lung should be allowed to fall away while the pericostal stitches are being inserted. The lung should then be fully inflated after the final stitch is in, before it is pulled tight, particularly if a chest drain is not to be used.

Endotracheal suction should be carried out with a catheter at the end of the operation and during the procedure, if secretions accumulate. As suction may cause atelectasis, the lung should be well inflated afterwards.

Ventilation/perfusion disturbances are common when the lung is partially collapsed. Maldistribution occurs, so that there is a decrease in the V/Q ratio in some parts and an increase in others. The inspired oxygen concentration should be increased to compensate for the resulting fall in Pao_2. The common practice of maintaining a slight positive pressure on the bag when using the Jackson Rees modification of the Ayres T-piece, producing positive end-expiratory pressure (PEEP), improves ventilation. PEEP can also be applied when using a ventilator. Improved ventilation of the compressed areas of the lung reduces the V/Q differences and raises Pao_2 towards normal. The assessment of oxygenation has

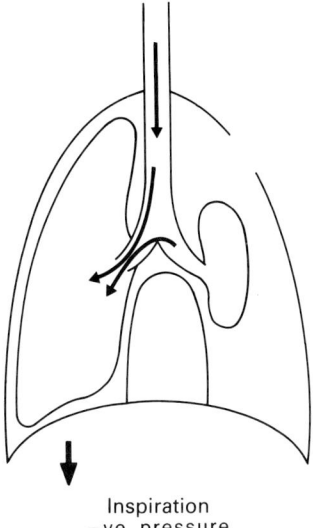
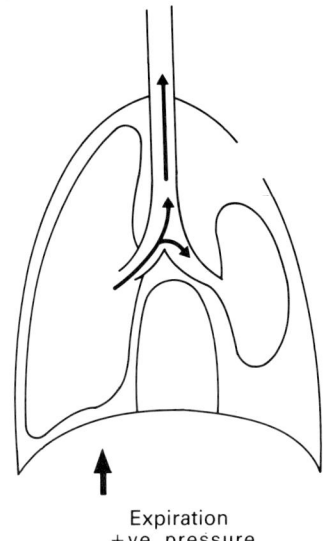

Inspiration
−ve pressure

Expiration
+ve pressure

Fig. 12.1 Diagram showing the effect of an open chest on the left side. On inspiration air is drawn from the trachea and from the contralateral lung to the intact side, while on expiration with positive pressure on the intact side air leaves via the trachea and into the collapsed side.

been simplified by the introduction of pulse oximeters.

It is useful to have a pressure gauge in the breathing system, particularly when operating on neonates. If the baby has been ventilated preoperatively, the pressures and FiO_2 which have provided appropriate ventilation and oxygenation preoperatively, can be maintained during anaesthesia but may need readjustment when the chest is open. Excessive pressures can also be avoided, especially in conditions such as diaphragmatic hernia where overdistension of the underdeveloped lung may cause pneumothorax.

One-lung anaesthesia

Bronchial intubation is not usually necessary or commonly employed in small children, with the result that paediatric surgeons are generally unaccustomed to the operating conditions provided.

One-lung anaesthesia is useful to prevent soiling from the lung which is unilaterally infected or bronchiectatic, particularly if it is by a resistant microorganism, or in the presence of a bronchopleural fistula. The methods of achieving this in small children are:
1 To block the bronchus on the operative side and place an endotracheal tube in the trachea. A Fogarty balloon catheter can be used as a blocker. A small Foley catheter placed in the bronchus would allow access for insufflation of gas or suction, as well as providing a balloon which can act as a bronchial blocker. The difficulty with these catheters is manipulating them into position, especially on the left side, unless a guidewire is used.

2 The insertion of a tracheal tube into the bronchus.
3 Double-lumen tubes are not available in small sizes, but a catheter with an angle tip, or alternatively a plastic catheter which has been curled up, can be manipulated into the bronchus on the operative side. The tracheal tube is then passed into the side which is to be ventilated. If both lungs need to be inflated at any stage of the operation, a second gas source can be attached to the catheter, taking care to avoid overdistension.

The right main bronchus can easily be intubated by passing an ordinary endotracheal tube more distally, because the right main bronchus is larger and is in more direct line with the trachea and because the tip of the bevel on the tube, being on the right side when inserted, is most likely to enter the right main bronchus. If this technique is employed, a hole should be made in the side of the tube so that the right upper lobe bronchus can be ventilated. Left bronchial intubation is more difficult but can be accomplished by moving the patient's head to the right and rotating the tube more than 90° anticlockwise, so that the curvature is towards the left side and the tip tends to slide to the left rather than the right side of the carina.

Chest drains

Chest drains are usually inserted at the end of thoracic operations for removal of any air, blood or lymph collecting in the pleural cavity. A few surgeons do not use chest drains routinely when air leak or fluid collections are unlikely. They rely on the lung being fully inflated between the insertion of the last periostial stitch and it being pulled tight and tied.

When an intercostal drain is used it is important to ensure that the tubing from the patient is connected to the tube placed underwater in the drainage bottle, otherwise incorrect connection may result in a tension pneumothorax (Fig. 12.2). The depth of the tube below the water determines the positive intrathoracic pressure necessary for air from the pleural cavity to escape. The tube is usually placed 2—3 cm into the water. Low-pressure suction is sometimes applied to the outlet tubing by attaching it to one inlet of a second bottle, with the other inlet open to air and submerged under a column of water (usually less than 10 cm) which determines the

level of negative pressure. The outlet tube is attached to suction. When the set level of suction is reached, air bubbles into the bottle and this negative pressure is applied to the chest-drainage bottle. This reduces the intrathoracic pressure required to allow drainage from the chest. In infants the drain tube should be narrow to reduce dead space, and may be partially occluded with a clamp to reduce the swing of fluid in the tubing from the bottle. Tidal volume will be reduced by the volume of swing in the tubing unless increased negative inspiratory pressure is generated to compensate. This will increase the work of breathing.

Postoperative analgesia

Thoracotomy can cause considerable postoperative pain. If not adequately managed this may result in inadequate ventilation and postoperative pulmonary complications.

An intercostal block with bupivacaine can provide analgesia for the first 6—8 hours. This may be performed by direct injection of the intercostal space under vision by the surgeon during the thoracotomy. It may also be performed before surgery, thereby providing some of the analgesia necessary for the operation. As a lateral thoracotomy often requires an incision reaching posteriorly, the block should be inserted medial to the usual site at the angle of the rib. The advantage of a more posterior injection is that when a larger volume of local anaesthetic is used, it can spread up and down for several spaces in the paravertebral gutter where the fascia is only loosely attached to the ribs. Alternatively, smaller volumes of local anaesthetic can be used by injecting two or three spaces at the level of the thoracotomy. Recently the use of intercostal catheters for intermittent injection or infusion of local anaesthetic has also been advocated to provide prolonged postoperative analgesia.

The most recent method for provision of postoperative analgesia is the insertion of an intrapleural catheter and injection of local anaesthetic through it. The potential danger of injecting large doses is that significant absorption and possible toxicity of local anaesthetic may occur.

Another option is the use of thoracic epidural analgesia, particularly in older patients. This should only be carried out by those skilled in the technique, but it is a useful method, particularly for the relief of pain following sternotomy. If an epidural catheter is left in place, analgesia can be maintained for prolonged periods.

The use of local anaesthetics for the relief of postoperative pain eliminates the problems of respiratory

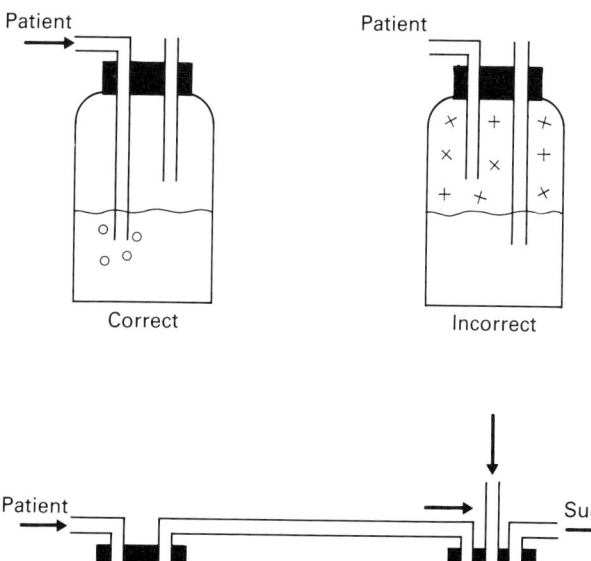

Fig. 12.2 Intercostal drainage. The correct position of the patient tube under water, so that air in the chest bubbles off when positive intrathoracic pressure exceeds the cmH$_2$O pressure at the end of the underwater tube. The right-hand diagram shows how air in the bottle cannot escape and creates a positive pressure, which is directly applied back to the patient if the tubes are connected incorrectly. The lower diagram illustrates how suction may be applied to a second bottle; the amount of suction pressure will be determined by the depth of the central tube under water.

depression associated with opioids. These can be added to the local anaesthetic for epidural use or an intravenous infusion can be used. Respiratory depression, nausea and vomiting are less with infusion than with intermittent intramuscular injections.

More details on postoperative analgesia are included in Chapter 8.

SPECIFIC CONDITIONS AND PROCEDURES

Congenital diaphragmatic hernia

Although this condition is usually repaired through an upper abdominal incision, it is basically a problem of underdevelopment of the lungs due to compression by abdominal contents. These usually enter the chest through a defect in the foramen of Bochdalek; 70–80% are on the left side. About one third of these babies are cyanosed at birth, due to having less than one third of a normal lung weight. This causes hypoxia, cyanosis and a generally poor prognosis. Patients who do not present with cyanosis or respiratory problems at birth usually have more lung and a better prognosis. They may develop respiratory problems due to increasing lung compression if the stomach and gut distend with air.

Occasionally a diaphragmatic hernia does not present for several months. These infants do not have obvious respiratory problems and may present with gastrointestinal symptoms, or be picked up on incidental chest X-ray. Some herniate through the foramen of Morgagni.

Clinically, neonates with diaphragmatic hernia have a scaphoid abdomen with a barrel chest due to the relocation of abdominal contents into the chest. Gastric distension may further expand the chest. A shift of the apex beat to the opposite side (usually the right), diminished or absent air entry and breath sounds or the presence of bowel sounds on the affected side are usual features. A chest, or preferably, a total trunk X-ray, will show abdominal contents in the thorax (Fig. 12.3).

Intrauterine diagnosis with ultrasound allows forward planning of delivery, so that the baby is born at a tertiary centre or can be transferred to one immediately after

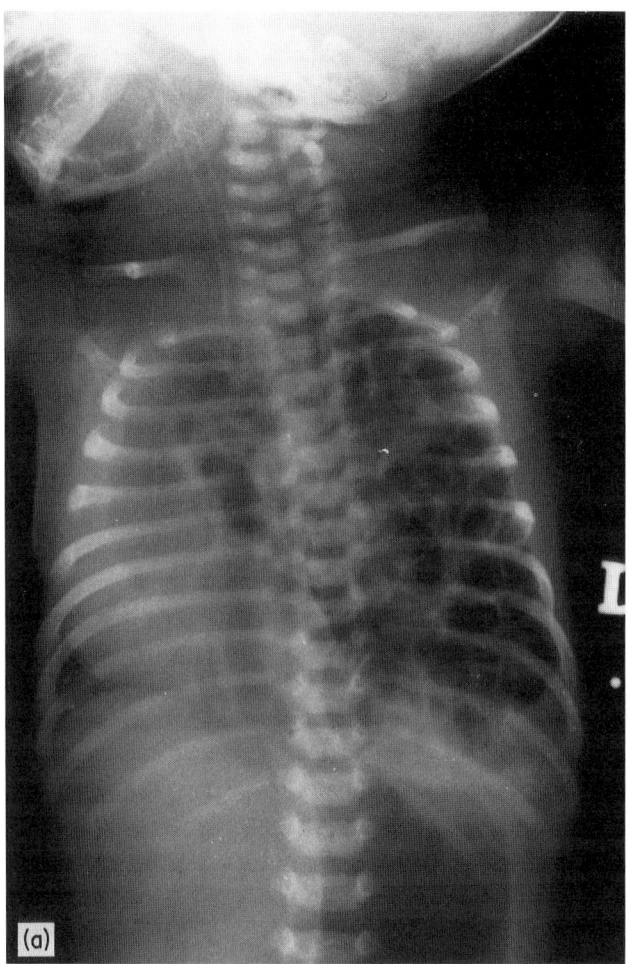

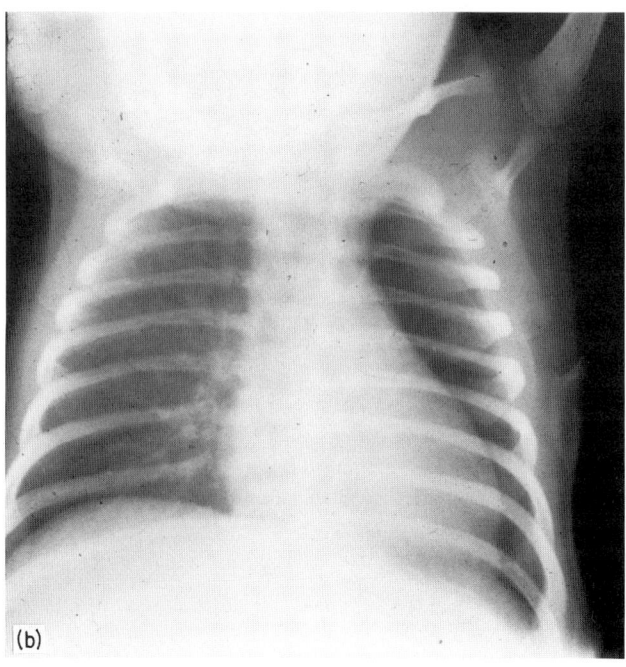

Fig. 12.3 (*right*) An infant with congenital diaphragmatic hernia. (a) Showing air in the gut in the chest and the heart and mediastinum shifted to the opposite side. Taken 24 hours after birth. (b) An X-ray of the same patient 12 days postoperatively.

delivery. Good perioperative care is essential if the cyanosed infants are to have any chance of survival. The current trend is to delay operation until the baby's condition is stable. The aim is to improve oxygenation, reduce acidosis and stabilize the circulation, which includes reducing pulmonary vascular resistance. Support with ECMO (extracorporeal membrane oxygenation) (Chapter 38) is used in some poor-risk babies. More detail on the perioperative care of sick neonates is given in Chapter 9.

During anaesthesia, the main points are adequate oxygenation and prevention of over-inflation of the underdeveloped lungs. Oxygenation can be easily monitored with pulse oximetry, so that the appropriate inspired concentrations can be selected.

An air–oxygen mixture plus an inhalational or opioid supplement is preferred because nitrogen, which diffuses slowly, stabilizes the alveoli. Nitrous oxide should be avoided because it will distend any gas-containing loops of gut, thereby increasing lung compression and making abdominal closure more difficult.

Ventilating pressures should be adequate to maintain oxygenation. Before the hernia is reduced, the gut will splint the underdeveloped lungs, preventing over-distension. The use of a ventilator similar to those used in the intensive care unit allows continuation of a ventilation pattern and airway pressures which have been

found to be optimal preoperatively. After the gut is removed from the chest, care must be taken not to over-inflate the lungs for fear of causing pneumothoraces. A pressure gauge in the breathing system is desirable.

If the lung on the affected side is very hypoplastic, the contralateral lung may also be hypoplastic. If the volume of the lung on the affected side is one third or more of normal, the prognosis is usually good. Although postoperative ventilation is not always necessary in these good-risk cases, there is a tendency to ventilate babies with diaphragmatic hernia in the early postoperative phase.

After reduction of the diaphragmatic hernia the lung will continue to grow.

Oesophageal atresia and tracheo-oesophageal fistula

This is the commonest non-cardiac neonatal condition requiring thoracic surgery. The types of anomaly and their incidence are illustrated in Fig. 12.4.

The general perioperative care of these neonates is discussed in Chapter 9. The present trend is to operate early on babies with oesophageal atresia, so that the respiratory complications due mainly to spillover from the upper pouch are minimized (Fig. 12.5). A metal bougie should be used if radiological assessment of the upper pouch is necessary (Fig. 12.6). Another occasional

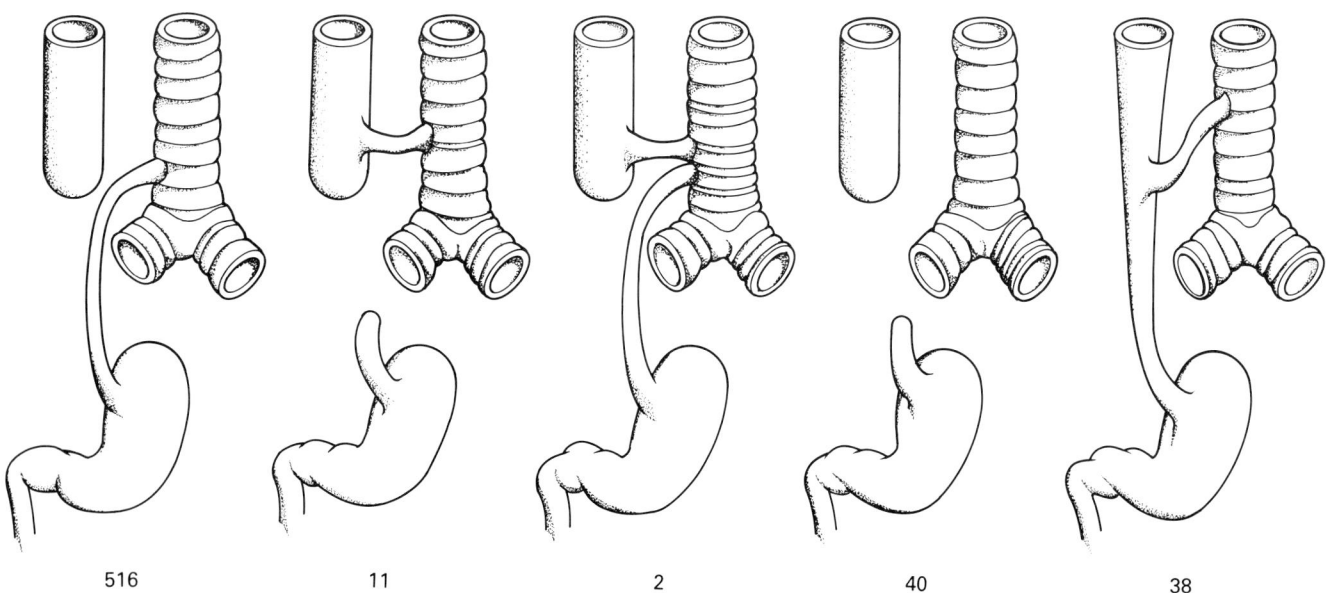

516   11   2   40   38

Fig. 12.4 Oesophageal atresia and tracheo-oesophageal fistula — types of anomaly and incidence (Royal Children's Hospital, Melbourne).

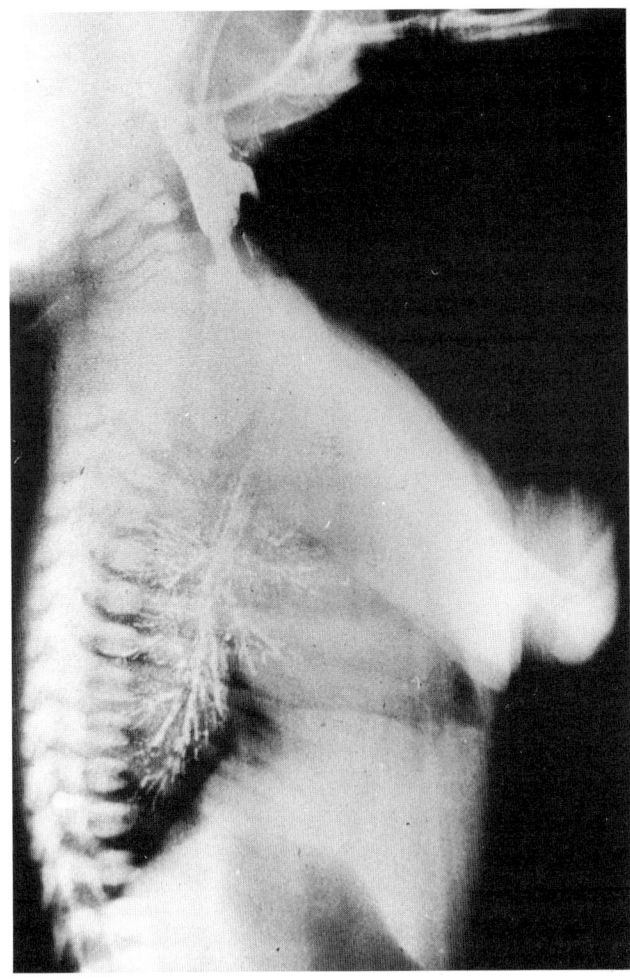

Fig. 12.5 An old X-ray showing how spillover from the upper pouch occurs — a barium installation.

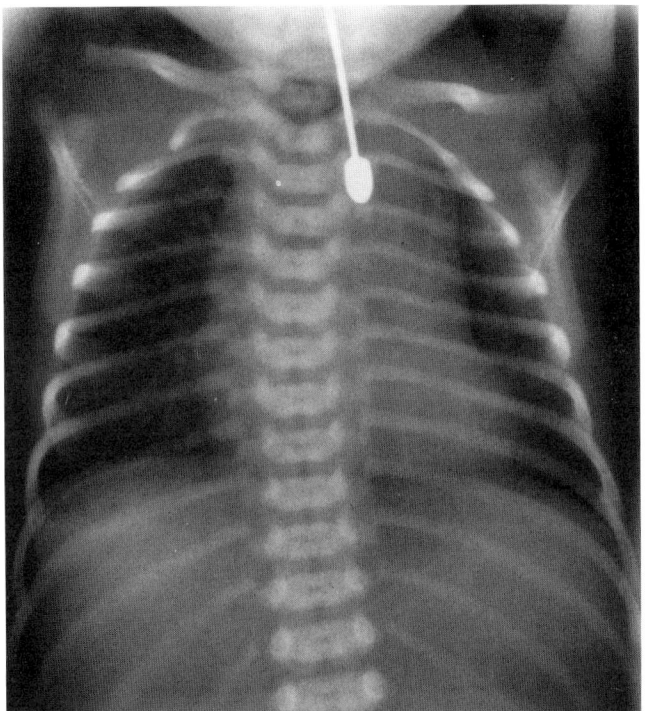

Fig. 12.6 A metal bougie demonstrating the depth of the upper pouch.

complication of delayed treatment is distension of the upper pouch with tracheal displacement (Fig. 12.7). Associated congenital anomalies occur in nearly half these infants. The most significant to the anaesthetist are congenital heart defects, but others include renal, vertebral and bony anomalies, and gastrointestinal obstructions including atresia.

Sometimes these babies need to be intubated preoperatively in the intensive care unit. If not, suction of the upper oesophageal pouch secretions should precede induction and intubation. Care must be taken not to pass the tube into the fistula. Sometimes, when the fistula is at or above the carina, the tube can be placed so that both lungs can be ventilated without inflating the fistula. Controlled ventilation can be used. The pressure employed must be sufficient to oxygenate the patient while avoiding significant inflation through the fistula and gastric distension. On rare occasions with a very large fistula, gastric distension may cause splinting of the diaphragm and difficulty with ventilation, necessitating urgent gastrostomy. This situation can be suspected if a lateral chest X-ray shows an air oesophagram greater than 2−3 mm diameter (Fig. 12.8). If the tube is in the fistula it should be aspirated and withdrawn. In some centres, bronchoscopy is performed before intubation so that the fistula can be located. If it is large, a blocker can be inserted to occlude it until it is closed at operation, at which time the blocker is withdrawn. A small Fogarty catheter may be used. It is wise to avoid nitrous oxide and use an oxygen/air mixture with an inhalation agent, so that distension of the stomach from diffusion of nitrous oxide does not occur.

A careful check must be made to ensure that the tube is in the trachea, that the fistula has not been intubated, and that ventilation of the left lung is adequate, since during the major part of the operation the right lung will be at least partially collapsed, because the trachea is usually approached through a right thoracotomy, often extrapleurally.

During the procedure, pressure from retractors or

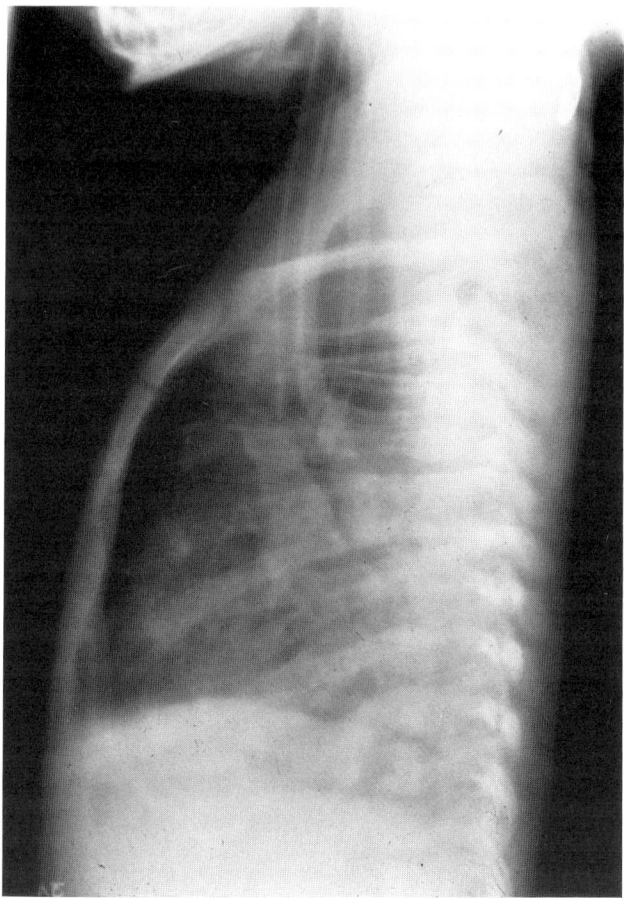

Fig. 12.7 A lateral X-ray showing the distended upper pouch displacing the trachea forwards. Nasotracheal intubation was necessary to overcome the tracheal compression.

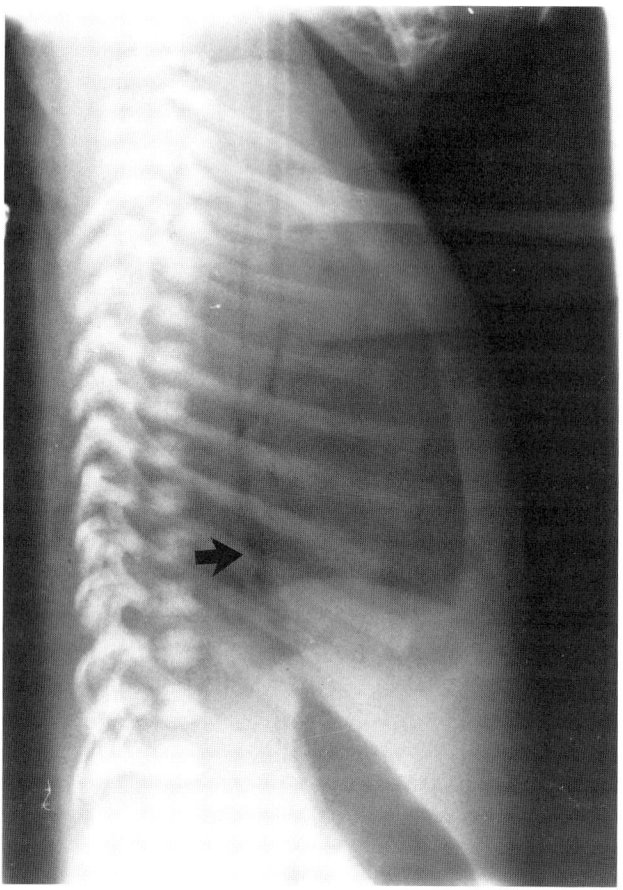

Fig. 12.8 A lateral chest X-ray demonstrating the air oesophagram (arrowed) in a tracheo-oesophageal fistula.

surgical dissection may compress the trachea and cause respiratory obstruction. This is detected by changing compliance when ventilating by hand, or by increased inspiratory pressures on the ventilator. It is important to inform the surgeon immediately if this occurs, so that the airway patency can be re-established. During the operation, when oesophageal anastomosis is being performed, the anaesthetist can assist the surgeon by pushing the upper pouch down with an oesophageal catheter (usually 10 or 12 Fr gauge).

In some patients where the two ends of the oesophagus cannot be approximated, a later major complex operation will be necessary to interpose a tube made from either stomach or colon. These operations need a long incision for exposure, and may be associated with significant blood loss. Attention to blood replacement and postoperative analgesia will therefore be important.

Fistula alone, between a continuous oesophagus and

trachea, occurs in 6% of cases (Fig. 12.9). Aspiration may occur and the diagnosis may be missed until a barium swallow or tracheoscopy are performed. The fistula is usually ligated by a cervical approach. An occasional complication is right recurrent laryngeal nerve damage causing vocal cord palsy and postoperative respiratory problems.

When there is a fistula from the upper oesophageal pouch into the trachea, soiling of the lungs is more likely. The operation is similar to the common type, when the fistula is closed before the anastomosis is performed.

Lung cysts

A lung cyst is usually a roughly spherical closed space containing air or liquid (Fig. 12.10). There may be one or several cysts and they may occupy the whole or part of a lobe, or only a segment. Cysts become symptomatic

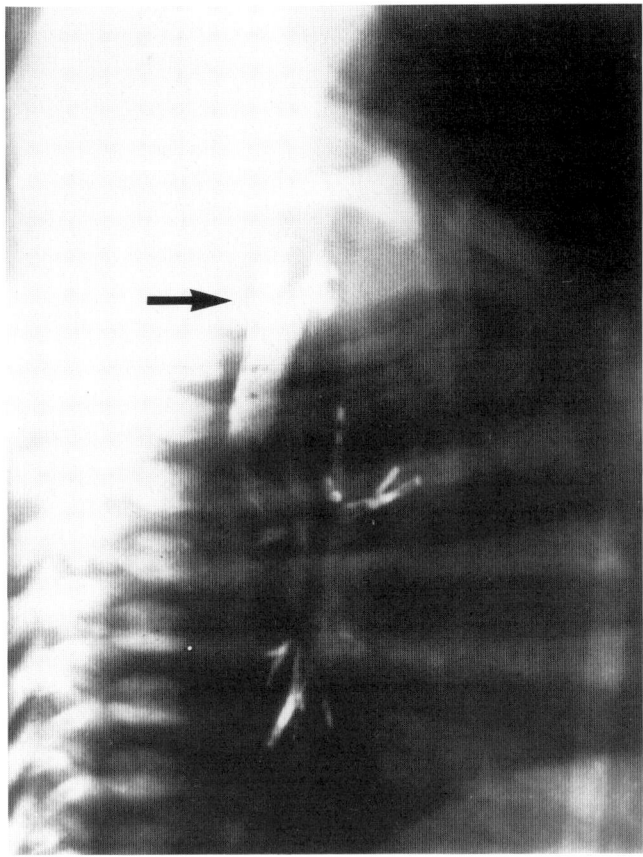

Fig. 12.9 A barium swallow demonstrating a fistula between the upper oesophagus and trachea (H type).

when they compress large airways, causing wheezing or a 'ball valve' distension of the lung distally, when large enough to be a space-occupying lesion, or if their contents discharge into the bronchial tree.

The anaesthetic problems include further distension of a gas-containing cyst if nitrous oxide is used, and possible difficulty in passing the expected size of tube if the trachea is compressed.

Lobar emphysema

Lobar emphysema is distension of part of the lung, most commonly the left upper or right middle lobe (Fig. 12.11), resulting from a variety of causes. These include overgrowth of the number of alveoli of one lobe or overinflation of abnormal segments by collateral ventilation when there is an atretic bronchus or a partial obstruction of a segmental bronchus, causing a ball valve with overinflation of the lobe or segment. Subacute cases not requiring surgical intervention may occur. The

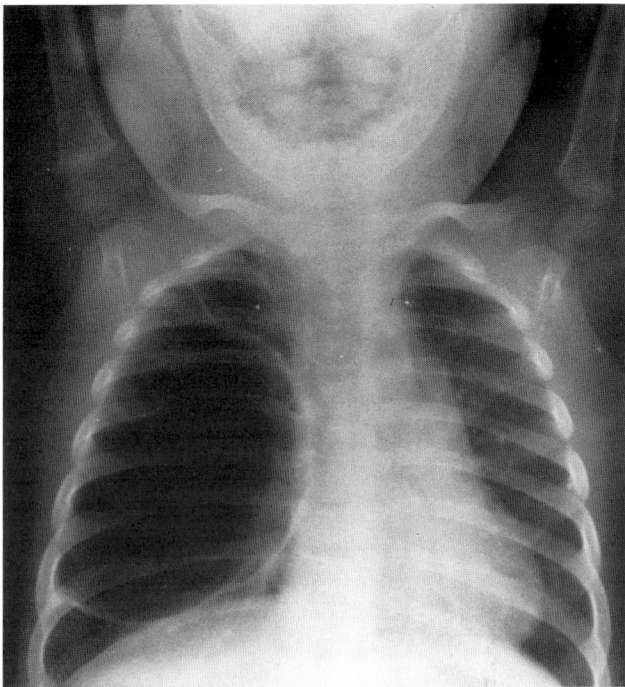

Fig. 12.10 Chest X-ray showing a large right-lung cyst.

clinical features include tachypnoea and dyspnoea, hyper-resonance, diminished breath sounds and prominence of the chest wall over the affected lobe, with relative immobility. There may be mediastinal shift.

If respiratory distress develops in lobar emphysema or

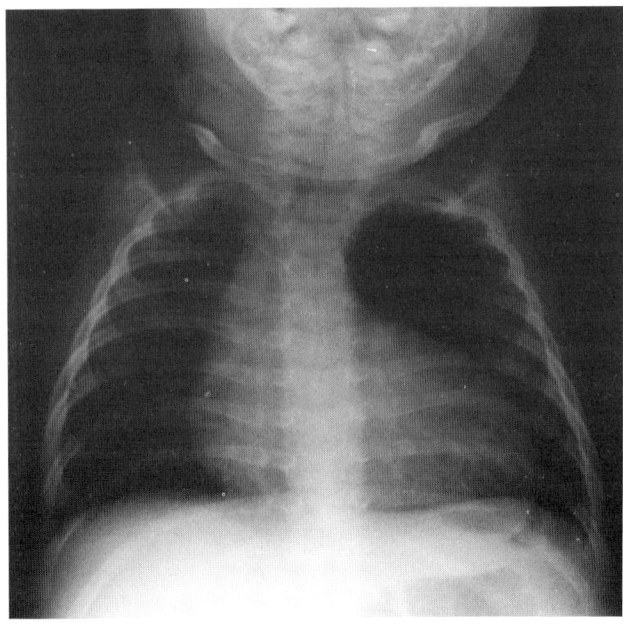

Fig. 12.11 Chest X-ray showing left upper lobar emphysema.

lung cyst, urgent treatment may be necessary. In very extreme situations, deflation of the emphysematous area by needle aspiration may be indicated. Ventilation of the contralateral lung via an endobronchial tube may help temporarily, but emergency thoracotomy under general anaesthesia with removal of the affected part is the definitive treatment. Further expansion of the lobe or cyst may be minimized during the early stages of the operation by avoiding nitrous oxide because it expands closed air cavities. If the distension is due to a ball-valve obstruction or bronchomalacia, the application of continuous positive airway pressure (CPAP) may occasionally allow the lung to deflate, but otherwise it could aggravate the problem.

Sequestrated lung segment

This is a condition where a normal segment of lung has an abnormal blood supply from a systemic artery, usually arising from the aorta either above or below the diaphragm. These segments may become infected. Pre-operative investigation usually includes angiography and sometimes bronchography (see Chapter 21). The general principles of anaesthesia for thoracotomy are followed if the lobe is to be resected.

Pulmonary interstitial emphysema

This is an iatrogenic disease of newborns with hyaline membrane disease who require ventilation with high inflation pressures. Air escapes into the lung tissues, producing blebs of air (Fig. 12.12). If these distend, they can compress lung and airways, aggravating the respiratory failure. If the disease is localized to one lobe and is causing a significant space-occupying problem, it may be excised. Alternatively, in some patients with widespread pulmonary interstitial emphysema, thoracotomy and 'scarification' of a lung, which involves rupture of these blebs, will release the trapped air and improve the patient's condition. Occasionally if the disease is localized to one side, intubating the other bronchus may decrease the pressure on the affected side, allowing the condition to resolve if severe hypoxia does not occur when only one lung is ventilating.

Bronchiectasis

Bronchiectasis was a common indication for thoracotomy and segmental resection, but with the more effective

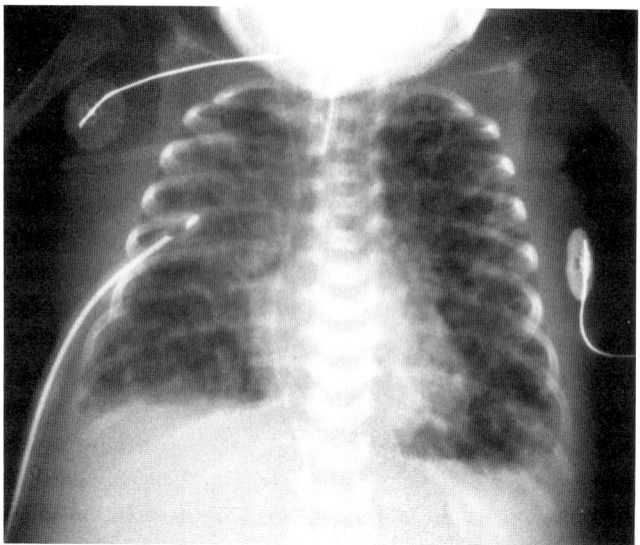

Fig. 12.12 Chest X-ray appearances of pulmonary interstitial emphysema.

treatment of infections with antibiotics this is now rare. It is usually preceded by bronchography. Resection is usually deferred until late childhood, to avoid or limit the risk of progressive disease in the remaining lobes. Before anaesthesia, physiotherapy, postural drainage and antibiotic treatment are intensified.

Empyema

Empyema is most common in children under 2 years of age when it follows staphylococcal pneumonia, usually resistant to penicillin. The clinical features are diminished movement of the chest, dullness to percussion and diminished breath sounds in a very ill child. The condition may suddenly worsen if a staphylococcal pneumatocoele bursts, causing a pyopneumothorax with a bronchopleural fistula. Immediate needle aspiration or insertion of an intercostal catheter may be necessary. Adequate drainage is required and this may necessitate thoracotomy and breaking down of loculi.

The patient is usually positioned with the affected side uppermost. If a bronchopleural fistula is present, the anaesthetist must be prepared to suck out the trachea as required. A large bronchopleural fistula can allow a considerable leak of gases, particularly when intermittent positive pressure ventilation (IPPV) is used. Fresh gas flow must be increased to maintain ventilation. Bronchial intubation may be helpful in this situation. Aggressive resection of necrotic lung and oversewing bronchopleural fistulae have resulted in the recovery of infants who formerly would have succumbed, due to their inability to ventilate stiff lungs with large bronchopleural fistulae. Drainage is best achieved with a large intercostal catheter, but this increases dead space and the swing should be controlled so that tidal volume is not reduced too much (see chest drains above).

Hydatid disease

This is now a rare disease in countries where effective elimination in the animal reservoirs has been achieved. The cystic stage of the tapeworm *Echinococcus granulosus* is hydatid disease, which occurs in sheep and occasionally in man. The host for this tapeworm is the dog. In children, the lung is the most common site of cysts, although they may occur in the liver and, rarely, in the brain. Cysts are usually single but they can be mul-

tiple. Investigations include radiography (Fig. 12.13a). Treatment is surgical. Lung hydatids are removed by incising the adventitial layer. The cyst, which consists of laminated membrane and attached germinal membrane, is then gently extruded from the lung by applying positive pressure to the anaesthetic bag (Fig. 12.13b,c). The open bronchus is closed and the cavity obliterated. Rupture of the cyst may result in soiling the trachea with daughter cysts. Prompt suction is necessary. This is a situation where a catheter can be placed in the affected side and the tube can be passed into the other bronchus. The catheter, 10–12 Fr guage if the child is big enough, can then be used for ventilation from a second gas source or as a sucker if required. Occasionally an anaphylactic reaction occurs when a cyst ruptures, and the anaesthetist must be prepared to treat this emergency with intravenous adrenaline (1:10 000) and colloid fluids, if hypotension occurs.

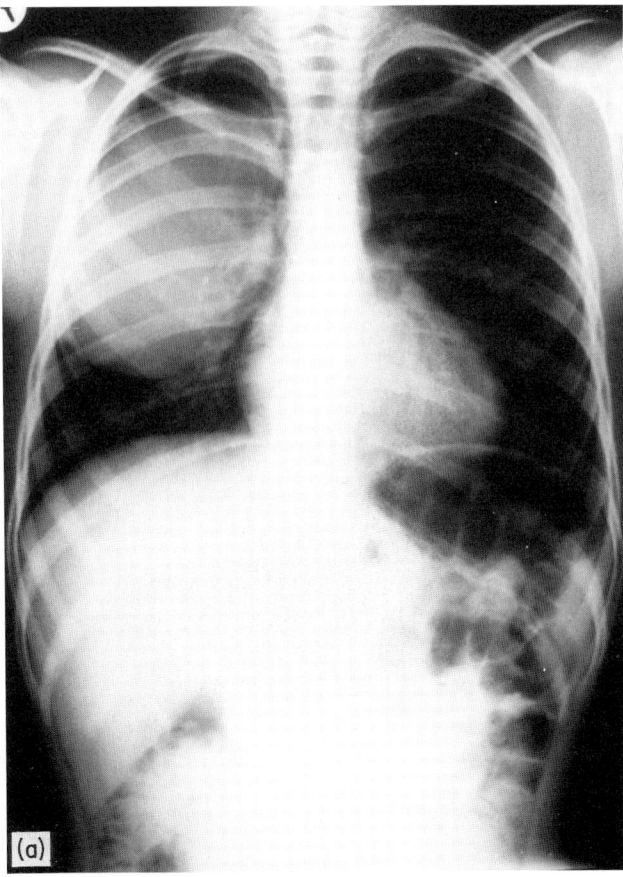

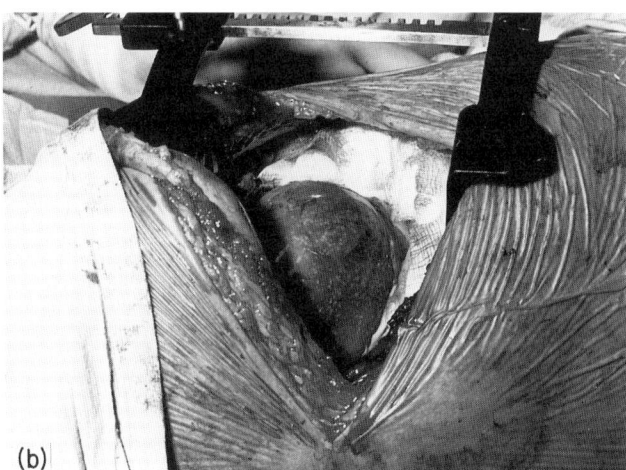

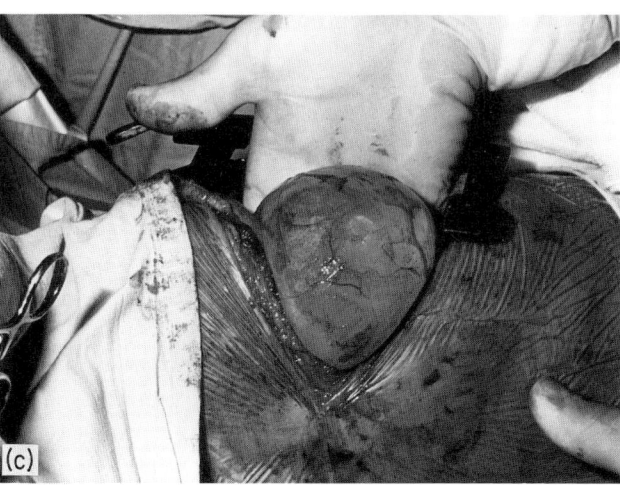

Fig. 12.13 (a) X-ray showing right-lung hydatid. (b) Lung hydatid through thoracotomy incision. (c) The delivery of the lung hydatid, which is achieved by the anaesthetist overinflating the lung once the outer layer is incised.

Lung biopsy

Occasionally lung biopsy is carried out. This may be done as a needle biopsy, when infection with *Pneumocystis carinii* is suspected, or as an open biopsy. The potential complication of pneumothorax following needle biopsy must be watched for, but is not common.

Mediastinal masses

These include tumours such as neuroblastoma, ganglioneuroma, thymoma or, rarely, anterior mediastinal teratoma. Cystic hygroma, which commonly involves the neck, may invade the mediastinum. Other masses may be bronchogenic cysts or duplication cysts of the alimentary tract.

Thoracotomy may be necessary for removal of any of these if they are malignant or are causing symptoms. The general principles of thoracic anaesthesia apply.

The presence of a large and rapidly expanding lymphoma in the mediastinum can present a major challenge to the anaesthetist. The problem centres around tracheal compression, which may become worse with the induction of anaesthesia, particularly if the patient is supine (Fig. 12.14). Respiratory depressants should be avoided in the premedication. It is preferable to induce the anaesthetic with an inhalation agent, ensuring that adequate ventilation can be maintained with a mask. If this is easily achieved and problems do not appear likely, a short-acting muscle relaxant can be used and the trachea intubated. If there are any doubts, the possibility of deepening anaesthesia, applying local anaesthesia by laryngeal spray or cricothyroid puncture, and intubating during spontaneous ventilation should be considered. If difficulties arise, the patient may be turned on to his side to relieve anterior compression of the trachea. One must always have a range of sizes of tubes, a stilette to facilitate the introduction of the tube, and possibly have available an armoured tube which will not be compressed. These patients usually present for a biopsy to determine the most appropriate chemotherapy. As this varies depending on the tumour, preliminary biopsy is essential. At the conclusion of the operation it is usually wise to leave the tube in if there has been any doubt about the patency of the trachea. Nursing the patient in the sitting position usually relieves some of the compression. The effect of chemotherapy is often dramatic and the shrinkage of the tumour is sufficiently rapid to allow intubated patients to be extubated within a day or two.

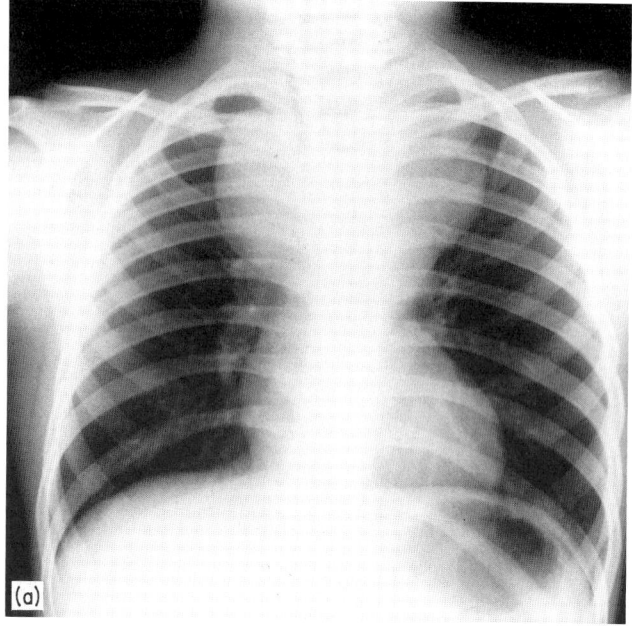

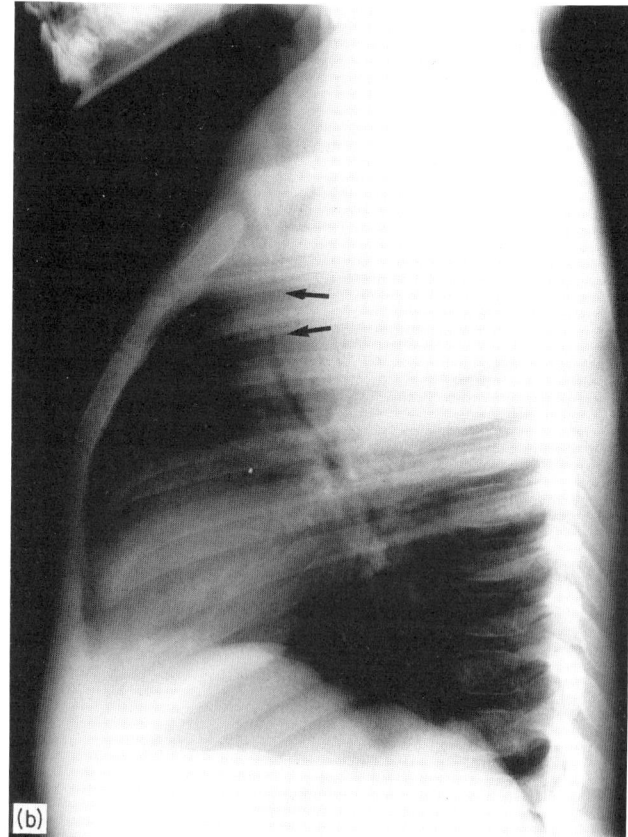

Fig. 12.14 X-ray of a mediastinal mass (lymphoma) causing tracheal compression. (a) AP, showing the trachea deviated to the right. (b) Lateral, showing compression of the trachea, which is aggravated if the patient lies supine.

Tracheal stenosis

Lower tracheal stenosis within the chest is approached by a midline sternotomy. The airway can be managed with a tube inserted to just above the stenosis (see Fig. 21.1). If a long-segment inlay graft is to be inserted, the tube can be advanced as soon as the trachea has been split. When posterior sutures have to be inserted, either in end-to-end anastomosis or during placement of a posterior cartilage graft, an alternative is to place a Portex Y-piece between the tube and breathing apparatus, and to pass a catheter through the side arm into the distal trachea. This can be attached to a high-pressure injector or gas source to ventilate the lungs until the sutures are in place. The endotracheal tube can then be advanced into the distal trachea, and the anterior suturing can be completed. A nasotracheal tube can be left in as a splint.

If the obstruction is intrathoracic, surgical access may be difficult, especially where the trachea lies behind major vessels. In some situations, cardiopulmonary bypass has been advocated, but another alternative that has been used successfully to provide additional safety is hypothermia. This will allow more time when a short segment has to be resected and the first posterior sutures are placed. If the muscle relaxant is allowed to wear off, the patient can breathe air for a few minutes through the tracheal opening, provided the stenosis has been approached through a sternal split. When the pleurae are intact the lungs do not collapse as much, and mediastinal swing does not occur as can happen in unilateral thoracotomy. Steps must be taken to ensure the patient remains anaesthetized and oxygenated while the trachea is open.

Anaesthesia for these operations is complex and requires careful planning with the surgeon, so that the best option is used for each particular operation.

Oesophagoscopy

This topic is discussed in Chapter 15.

Chest wall deformities

Sternochondroplasty is performed for pectus carinatum (pigeon chest) (Fig. 12.15), pectus excavatum (funnel

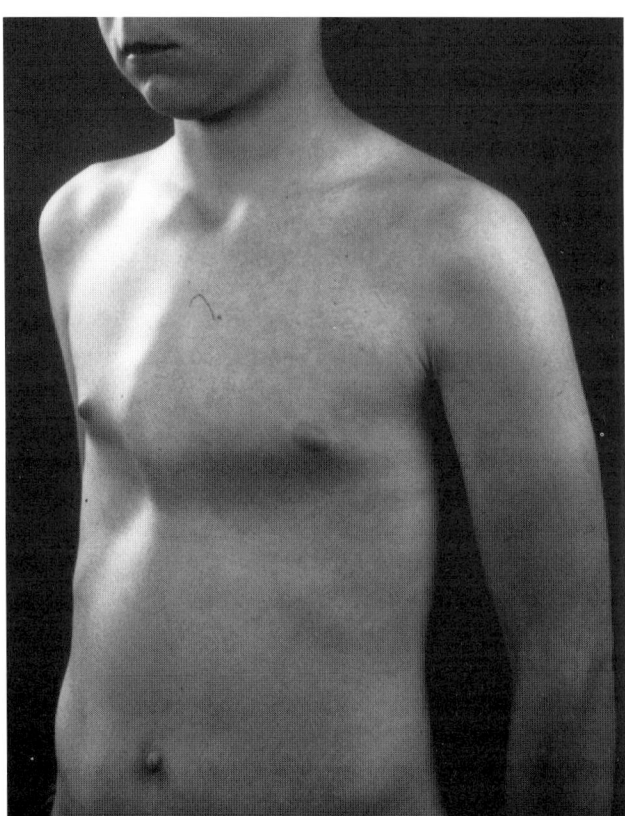

Fig. 12.15 A low protrusion deformity of the sternum situated just above the xiphisternal junction — pectus carinatum.

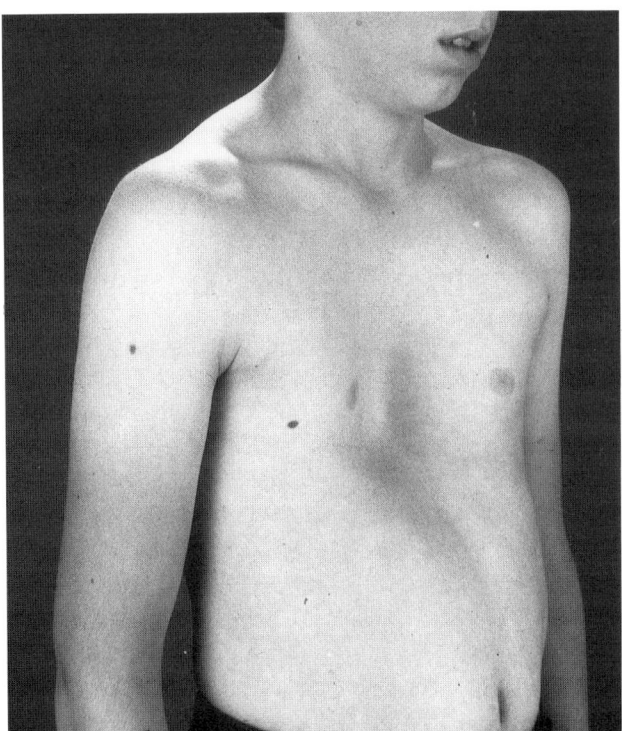

Fig. 12.16 A depression deformity of the chest wall — pectus excavatum.

chest) (Fig. 12.16) or local thoracic-wall deficiency. The operation consists of:

1 resection of costal cartilages to allow correction of the deformity with retention of the perichondrium to permit regrowth of the costal cartilages;

2 sternal osteotomy at the site of maximal deformity;

3 insertion of struts (of rib or of metal) behind the sternum, to hold it forward, in depression deformities. These operations are not usually done before 8 years of age and are often performed in the early teens.

The problems which may be encountered include:

1 Haemorrhage from the dissection or severed inter-costal vessels. A large-bore intravenous cannula should be inserted and blood must be available.

2 Pneumothorax — the main problem is recognition. It can usually be adequately treated by ensuring full inflation of the lung before the pleura is closed.

3 Paradoxical respiration is a rare complication due to an unstable sternal segment, which may require post-operative ventilation if it occurs.

4 Symmetry — the arms should both be placed at the side to prevent distortion. An intravenous extension set is needed for the injection of drugs.

5 Postoperative pain should be managed by an intra-venous opiate infusion or thoracic epidural analgesia.

13: Anaesthesia and Perioperative Care
for Cardiac Surgery

183

INTRODUCTION

Paediatric cardiovascular surgery is a rapidly changing field. Guidelines for management are presented in this chapter and problems that these patients may present to the anaesthetist are outlined. An understanding of congenital heart disease is essential for an anaesthetist, because the signs of a cardiovascular lesion may be discovered during a routine preoperative examination. This is further discussed in Chapter 25. Similarly a patient may present for incidental surgery with a known heart lesion, the specific haemodynamic problems and management of which are discussed in this chapter.

ANATOMY AND PHYSIOLOGY OF CONGENITAL HEART DISEASE

Congenital heart disease results from failure of the normal embryological development. Broadly, the problems result from (i) increased pulmonary blood flow causing pulmonary hypertension, (ii) right-to-left shunting which results in hypoxia and cyanosis if associated with reduced pulmonary blood flow, or (iii) flow obstruction, either within the heart (including valvular stenosis) or narrowing of a major artery, which causes proximal hypertension. Any obstruction causes hypertrophy of the cardiac chamber proximal to the obstruction, and may eventually lead to ventricular failure. In some complex conditions, more than one of these problems may exist. The anaesthetist is concerned more with the resulting physiological disturbances and the responses to drugs than with a purely anatomical classification.

TIMING OF OPERATION

The timing of the operation is important in congenital heart surgery. In the past, the size of the patient was an important factor in the decision of when to operate. With increasing surgical expertise and improved perioperative care, corrective operations are being performed at an earlier age to prevent progression of the detrimental effects of pulmonary hypertension, chronic hypoxia and flow obstruction which eventually lead to heart failure. Lesions with high flow and high pressures in the pulmonary artery will eventually result in a permanent increase in pulmonary vascular resistance, which may make the condition inoperable. The long-term pharmacological management of pulmonary hyper-

tension has been unsuccessful. The Switch operation for transposition of the great vessels with intact septum is usually performed during the neonatal period, before excessive involution of the left ventricle occurs as pulmonary vascular resistance falls. It was common to operate on Fallot's tetralogy in the third or fourth year of life, but more recently, the definitive operation has been performed in the first year of life thereby avoiding the need for palliative surgery.

ANAESTHESIA FOR CARDIAC INVESTIGATIONS AND INTERVENTIONAL PROCEDURES

Invasive catheterization with pressure measurements and the injection of contrast to demonstrate the cardiac anatomy is being increasingly replaced by non-invasive Doppler echocardiography. During echocardiography, sedation may suffice (e.g. oral chloral hydrate, diazepam or midazolam).

Anaesthetic requirements are altering. A large proportion of congenital heart disease is associated with high blood flow through the lungs. During cardiac catheterization, where pulmonary vascular resistance is to be measured accurately because the definitive operation may depend on the results, factors that most affect it, such as Pa_{CO_2}, Pa_{O_2} and pH, must be within normal limits for that patient. A satisfactory technique is intubation and ventilation to the patient's normal pH and P_{CO_2} under a very light general anaesthetic — thiopentone, fentanyl ($1-2 \mu g/kg$), muscle relaxant with a low concentration of a volatile agent which causes minimal cardiovascular effects, e.g. trichloroethylene $0.1-0.2\%$, satisfied these criteria but due to lack of availability isoflurane $0.5-0.75\%$ is being increasingly used. The patient is ventilated at a normal Pa_{CO_2} with an Fi_{O_2} of $0.28-0.3$. Alternatively, sedation with a combination of pethidine, promethazine and chlorpromazine (lytic cocktail) has been widely used, particularly when an anaesthetist was not available. The problem with heavy sedation in these patients is respiratory depression and/or airway obstruction with alterations in Pa_{CO_2} and Pa_{O_2}. Fluctuations in ventricular filling pressures may also result. In a small number of very sick infants it may not be possible to have the desired conditions, and the results are then interpreted in this light. Other problems which may occur during cardiac catheterization include blood loss, changing blood volume if hyperosmolar contrast medium is used, dysrhythmia due to catheter stimulation, myocardial damage during injection of contrast medium or even tamponade due to perforation, usually of the atrium. Because of these potential problems, there are advantages in an anaesthetist being present at these invasive investigations. For a more detailed account of the management of patients for radiological investigations see Chapter 21.

With the advent of new equipment, non-surgical percutaneous palliative or corrective procedures are more common, e.g. balloon septostomy or dilatation of stenotic valves and vessels. For these procedures an anaesthetist is needed to monitor and treat complications. Atrial balloon septostomy is a palliative procedure providing atrial shunting, which is performed on the newborn with transposition of the great vessels to promote increased mixing of saturated and desaturated blood in the atria. It is also used for pulmonary atresia and in patients with a single ventricle, or where the two ventricles function as one with a single outflow. Embolization of the collateral vessels and patent ductus arteriosus is being increasingly used. These procedures are performed in a catheter laboratory or a high-dependency area such as the intensive care unit. The babies should be managed as suggested above for cardiac catheterization, with paralysis and controlled ventilation. Analgesia, such as fentanyl, can be given. Higher doses (10–20 μg/kg) can be used when the patient is already being ventilated or will continue being ventilated after the procedure.

Complications of these procedures include blood loss, cardiac arrest and perforation of the myocardium with tamponade. Arterial pressure, ECG, Sp_{O_2} and ET_{CO_2} should be monitored and facilities for Pa_{O_2}, Pa_{CO_2} and pH measurement should be available. If acute cardiac tamponade occurs, it is difficult to evacuate the blood by needling, and surgical removal through a limited subxiphoid incision is advisable.

CARDIOVERSION

Life-threatening cardiac dysrhythmia is less common in children than adults, the most frequent being a supraventricular tachycardia. Drug treatment may consist of digoxin, drugs that affect calcium activity, such as calcium channel antagonists, amiodarone or even neostigmine. Cardioversion may be required and this is satisfactorily managed with careful administration of a sleep dose of a hypnotic (thiopentone, midazolam) followed by 2–5 μg/kg fentanyl by slow intravenous injection, with careful monitoring of respiration. This causes minimal cardiovascular disturbance and avoids intubation of the patient. The recommended energy levels for cardioversion are 1 J/kg body weight for atrial dysrhythmia and 5 J/kg body weight for ventricular dysrhythmia. Care must be taken with the use of calcium antagonists such as verapamil for dysrhythmia in very young infants, because of the possibility of cardiovascular collapse due to the difference in trans-sarcolemmal flux of calcium.

PHARMACOLOGY

Many drugs are potentially useful in cardiac anaesthesia. The anaesthetist should be thoroughly familiar with the pharmacology of the ones he uses, particularly their cardiovascular effects. The properties of commonly used drugs relevant to cardiac surgical anaesthesia are outlined below (Tables 13.1 and 13.2).

Table 13.1 Cardiovascular effects of anaesthetic agents

Agent	Myocardial contractility	Heart rate	Systematic vascular resistance	Pulmonary vascular resistance	Respiration
Thiopentone	⇊	↑	↑	↑ ?	⇊
Ketamine	⇈	↑	⇈	⇅	↓
Opioids	–	↕	↓ – ⇊	↓	⇊⇊
Benzodiazepines	↓	–	↓	–	↓
Volatile anaesthetics	↓ – ⇊	↓ – ⇊	↓ – ⇊	↓	↓ – ⇊

Table 13.2 The cardiovascular effects of anaesthetic agents

Thiopentone
is a myocardial depressant
may increase peripheral vascular resistance
decreases cerebral metabolism

Ketamine
is effective intramuscularly or intravenously
has analgesic properties
has a direct cardiac depressant action that is usually overridden by
   an indirect sympathetic response.
causes little change in pulmonary vascular resistance [1]
is associated with dreams and hallucinations during emergence that
   should be counteracted by other drugs such as diazepam

Benzodiazepines (diazepam and midazolam)
produce amnesia
do not cause much cardiovascular system instability
are often used with opioids

Opioids
direct cardiac depression is minimal
do not sensitize the heart to catecholamines
preserve autoregulation of blood flow in peripheral tissues
can be used with high oxygen concentration
respiratory depression is overcome by controlled ventilation

Morphine
1–3 mg/kg may be used for maintenance of anaesthesia/analgesia
   with some hypnotic effect
must be given very slowly to avoid hypotension due to histamine
   release

Fentanyl
is used as an induction agent because it disturbs cardiovascular
   stability less than morphine
the high doses (20–50 µg/kg) used for induction may increase
   muscle tone, which is prevented by the concomitant use of
   muscle relaxants
is a poor hypnotic and therefore supplements are needed to
   produce anaesthesia
when circulation is maintained by maximal sympathetic
   compensation, large doses may cause cardiovascular depression
   by suppressing this sympathetic compensation

Sufentanil
does not cause cardiovascular instability
has a longer duration of action than morphine but similar to large
   doses of fentanyl
can be used for induction

Pethidine and *alfentanil* are not popular in anaesthesia for cardiac
surgery because of cardiovascular instability.

Inhalation agents

The major effects on the cardiovascular system are shown
in Table 13.3.
   When anaesthesia is induced with an inhalation agent,

Table 13.3 Major effects of anaesthetic agents on the
cardiovascular system

Agent	MAC	Direct vasodilatation	Negative inotropic effect	Dysrhythmo-genicity
Halothane	0.7	+	+++	++
Isoflurane	1.4	+++	+	−
Enflurane	1.2	++	++	−+

the rate of induction may be modified by cardiac shunts.
Right-to-left shunts with reduced pulmonary blood flow
will slow uptake, especially of agents with low blood gas
solubility coefficients (Fig. 13.1) [2]. Anaesthetics with
high coefficients will be less affected.
   Nitrous oxide causes minimal cardiovascular depression and has minimal effects on systemic vascular
resistance. There is debate on whether it increases
pulmonary vascular resistance [3]. Because it is more
soluble than nitrogen it will increase the size of any air
bubbles entering the circulation. Prolonged exposure
may lead to depression of the immune system by in-
activation of methionine synthetase.

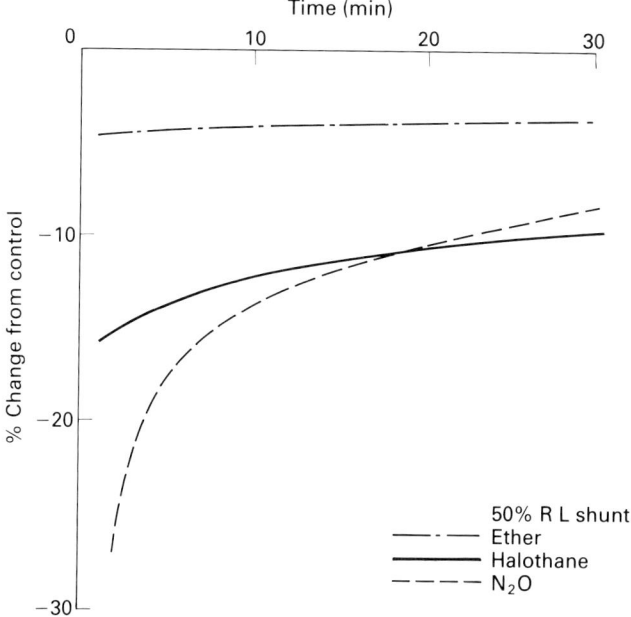

Fig. 13.1 Decrease in arterial-to-inspired concentration ratio for
three modelled anaesthetics (ether, halothane and nitrous oxide)
caused by a 50% right-to-left shunt, demonstrating delayed
uptake. The horizontal zero line represents the normal uptake
curve for anaesthetic agents. (Reproduced with permission from
Tanner *et al.* 1985 [2].)

Muscle relaxants

A non-depolarizing muscle relaxant is usually employed, often in larger than usual doses because of the length of the operation, the dilutional effect of the pump-priming fluid and because the onset of action of a large dose is more rapid. Pancuronium is the most popular non-depolarizing neuromuscular blocker for cardiac anaesthesia, unless tachydysrhythmia is a problem. Vecuronium also maintains cardiovascular stability and causes less tachycardia, but it is shorter acting, which is not an advantage for long operations when the patient is to be ventilated postoperatively. Drugs which release histamine such as D-tubocurarine and alcuronium may cause hypotension.

Vasodilators (see Chapter 23)

Vasodilators were introduced into paediatric cardiac surgery in 1972. Their main uses are to control blood pressure, to ensure even and rapid cooling and re-warming, to enable adequate filling of the circulation at the end of the bypass, to modify pulmonary vascular resistance and to improve left ventricular performance by reducing systemic vascular resistance.

SODIUM NITROPRUSSIDE

This is a potent vasodilator acting directly on vascular smooth muscle, affecting all vessels including cerebral and pulmonary. Its transient action makes it suitable as a trial, before using a longer-acting agent.

NITROGLYCERINE

This is a pulmonary vasodilator in infants as well as older patients.

PROSTAGLANDINS (PGE$_1$, PGI)

These have similar pharmacokinetics to sodium nitro-prusside and are useful as pulmonary vasodilators, because of the high first-pass elimination in the lung. PGE$_1$ will keep the newborn ductus open when a pre-operative life-preserving shunt is needed in obstructive right- and left-sided abnormalities. Prostaglandins may cause thrombaesthenia and apnoea. The dose range is 10–30 ng/kg/min.

PHENOXYBENZAMINE

This is a long-acting non-competitive alpha-adrenergic blocking agent which also inhibits autacoids such as histamine and serotonin. If the haemodynamic effect of vasodilatation is unpredictable, the effect of a short-acting agent (e.g. sodium nitroprusside) should be ascertained before phenoxybenzamine is used.

Inotropics

These are frequently employed following bypass. Dopamine and dobutamine are the drugs usually employed first; if a more potent agent is needed adrenaline or noradrenaline is used. Isoprenaline is used only for its chronotropic effect.

Recently, new phosphodiesterase inhibitor inodilators (amrinone, enoximone and milrinone) have become available.

PREOPERATIVE ASSESSMENT

Although these patients have usually had their cardiac defect thoroughly investigated preoperatively, the anaesthetist must still undertake a careful preoperative assessment of the patient to elucidate such problems as heart failure, dysrhythmias or infection.

Respiratory tract infection

Young children, particularly those with cardiac disease, are prone to respiratory tract infection. Intercurrent bacterial or viral infection may spread and can lead to bacteraemia. Although intercurrent infection often leads to postponement of the operation, there are some situations, such as a child with a resolving upper respiratory tract infection, where the disadvantages of postponing such an operation may justify proceeding with it.

Drugs

Cardiac surgical patients may be taking inotropic drugs, such as digoxin for cardiac failure, or a negative inotropic agent, such as a beta-adrenergic blocker for Fallot's tetralogy. The decision when and if to discontinue these agents is made in consultation by the anaesthetist, cardiologist and surgeon. Digoxin therapy predisposes the myocardium to dysrhythmia in the perioperative period. The serum level should be checked and should be below 2.5 nmol/ml. Beta-adrenergic blockade is usually continued and taken into account when inotropic drugs are used postoperatively.

Patient sensitivity to drugs

This must be ascertained, especially for antibiotics, as these patients will often have had multiple antibiotic therapy. Information about drug and other allergies must be sought.

Electrolytes

Patients treated with diuretics may be potassium- and magnesium-depleted in spite of normal plasma levels, unless supplements have been taken. Depletion of these tends to increase the incidence of dysrhythmia, especially at low temperatures and in the presence of digoxin.

Coagulation profile

Bleeding following bypass is treated empirically. Following routine heparin reversal with protamine, fresh frozen plasma (FFP) and then platelets may be indicated.

Patients with abnormal prothrombin time, activated partial thromboplastin time and/or platelet count should be investigated preoperatively and appropriate clotting factors should be available. Extra clotting factors are needed in very small patients (less than 10 kg) because of dilution by the extracorporeal prime, and in polycythaemic patients due to their increased fibrinolytic activity (Table 13.4). They may also be needed in patients undergoing repeated procedures, because there is often increased blood loss from division of adhesions.

Pulmonary hypertension

The cardiologist can assess the degree of hypertension and the risks implied. Precipitating factors such as hypercarbia and hypoxia should be avoided. The evidence that nitrous oxide and thiopentone increase pulmonary hypertension is contradictory.

Preoperative cardiac failure and shock (see Chapter 34)

Infants with severe heart failure not controlled by digoxin and diuretics should be transferred to the intensive care unit before operation and mechanically ventilated, using muscle relaxants to reduce the work of breathing. Monitoring is established and intravenous catheters inserted. Infusions of inotropic drugs, such as dopamine, and vasodilator drugs, such as sodium nitroprusside or phenoxybenzamine (see above), improve myocardial performance and organ perfusion and reduce systemic and pulmonary oedema. This approach allows the unstable child to recover from the handling associated with intubation and arterial and central venous cannulation before surgery.

In the first few days of life, shock due to obstructive left-heart lesions such as aortic stenosis, hypoplastic left-heart syndrome and aortic coarctation, requires urgent infusion of prostaglandin E_1 to open the ductus arteriosus

Table 13.4 The incidence of haemostatic abnormalities in patients with cyanotic congenital heart disease

Abnormality	No. of patients studied	Incidence	%
Thrombocytopenia	394	142	36
Defective clot retraction and platelet function abnormalities	152	88	58
Prolonged prothrombin time	357	71	19
Hypofibrinogenaemia	322	40	12
Prolonged partial thromboplastin time (or thromboplastin generation time)	123	23	18
Low factor VII	50	10	20
Low factor V	122	9	7
Low factor VIII	50	10	20
Accelerated fibrinolysis	142	14	10
Fibrin degradation products	112	4	3

and allow blood to flow from the pulmonary artery to the aorta. Metabolic acidosis should be corrected. Mechanical ventilation and dopamine infusion are needed to improve poor myocardial contractility.

There are other patients who benefit from intensive preoperative therapy, such as those with total anomalous pulmonary venous drainage, and neonates, particularly prematures, with large patent ductus arteriosus.

All patients managed in the intensive care unit before and after surgery should have blood glucose, electrolytes and acid−base state measured at least 4-hourly, and abnormalities corrected. Infants less than 5 kg weight should be nursed under an overhead heater, servo-controlled by skin temperature to maintain a neutral thermal environment, to reduce oxygen demand and myocardial work (see Chapter 1).

One of the difficulties encountered with these patients is maintaining the support and monitoring during transport from the intensive care unit to the operating theatre, when respiratory and circulatory instability may occur.

ANAESTHESIA

Premedication

Despite the trend towards oral premedication, these patients are often given an opiod/anticholinergic combination (papaveretum 0.4 mg/kg, hyoscine 0.08 mg/kg), an anticholinergic alone (e.g. hyoscine) or, in infants less than 6 months old, no premedication at all (see Chapter 6).

Induction

The general principles for both open (bypass) and closed (non-bypass) cases are the same. Closed cases where non-corrective procedures are attempted are often more difficult. Specific problems in certain conditions will be discussed below.

Intravenous induction is preferred, as venous access is essential for drug administration when complications occur. A safe combination of drugs includes fentanyl (20 µg/kg), and pancuronium with a volatile agent such as isoflurane. Care must be taken in all patients with right-to-left shunting to avoid introducing emboli (gas or particulate matter) into the vascular system because of the danger of paradoxical embolism to the brain and heart. The choice of ventilating gas (oxygen 100%, air/oxygen or nitrous oxide/oxygen) depends on the patient's

condition. For most of the routine cases nitrous oxide/oxygen has been found to be satisfactory in the pre-bypass period. Nasotracheal intubation is preferred because access may be difficult during the operation, and it is needed for postoperative ventilation, when stable fixation of the tube is very important.

Monitoring

Pulse oximetry, ECG and non-invasive blood pressure monitoring should be attached to the patient prior to induction.

Percutaneous arterial cannulation is better than open cutdown, which is more likely to cause permanent damage to the artery. Arteries that are likely to be occluded during operations for coarctation of the aorta or shunts must be avoided. Reliable access to major vessels is essential. As venous access is often difficult in children, it may be more expedient to cannulate a central vein or veins twice, one for central venous pressure monitoring and drug infusion, and the other for administration of drugs and fluids and venous sampling. It is convenient to cannulate an internal jugular or innominate vein, so that the anaesthetist has easy access for inspection during the operation and can minimize dead space when starting drug infusion. The techniques are described in Chapter 7.

Temperature is usually monitored at three sites to measure the gradients during active cooling and rewarming, and to ensure that the probes are appropriately placed. Commonly, the nasopharyngeal or tympanic membrane (representing brain temperature), oesophageal (indicative of heart temperature), and rectal or toe temperatures are measured (see Chapter 4).

A urinary catheter is inserted for bypass operations.

Equipment

The equipment that should be available for paediatric cardiac anaesthesia includes:

1 a gas delivery system that includes oxygen and air to allow fractional inspired oxygen without nitrous oxide down to 0.21; this allows nitrogen 'splinting' of the alveoli and avoidance of excessive oxygen exposure when there is a risk of retinopathy of prematurity;
2 a paediatric ventilator with PEEP mode;
3 a humidifier, preferably with heated delivery tube;
4 a heating and cooling blanket with a 10−40°C range. Direct contact between the patient and the irregular

surface of the blanket should be avoided by placing padding or a towel between them to reduce the chance of skin burns.

5 a DC defibrillator with both internal and external paddles and power output down to 5 J;

6 a pacemaker with sequential mode and rate facility preferably above 200 beats per minute to facilitate over-pacing of tachydysrhythmias;

7 syringe pumps for infusions (with batteries for transport);

8 a low-volume blood-warming device;

9 i.v. blood pumping facilities.

For additional information on equipment see Chapter 3.

OPERATIONS FOR CONGENITAL ANOMALIES

Surgery without bypass

Anaesthesia for non-bypass operations usually includes an intravenous induction agent, a non-depolarizing muscle relaxant, nitrous oxide and oxygen with fentanyl or isoflurane supplementation. Most patients who are to be ventilated postoperatively receive higher doses of opioid, usually fentanyl. When the neuromuscular block is to be reversed on the operating table, such as in patent ductus arteriosus, pacemaker insertion, pleurodesis or drainage of effusions, less opioid is given.

Blood should be cross-matched, and reliable intravenous access established for all cardiac operations.

LIGATION OF PATENT DUCTUS ARTERIOSUS

This procedure involves a left thoracotomy, exposure and ligation of the ductus arteriosus or less commonly, transection and suture of the ductus. Complications, which are rare, include haemorrhage due to a tear of the aorta or ductus arteriosus, damage to the thoracic duct leading to chylothorax and injury to the left recurrent laryngeal nerve. Examination of vocal cords at the end of the procedure is not recommended, as it is not always possible to assess function at this stage.

Intercostal nerve block for postoperative analgesia may be performed by the surgeon under direct vision, or by the anaesthetist preoperatively if it is to constitute part of the anaesthetic.

Recently, more premature infants of very low birth-weight have been presenting for ductus ligation. These patients are usually ventilator-dependent, in controlled cardiac failure, possibly with inotropic support, and needing total parenteral nutrition. Oxygen therapy is carefully controlled because of the risk of retinopathy of prematurity. These infants require particularly careful management. Specific points include:

1 continued inotropic support in the perioperative period;

2 continuous monitoring of FiO_2 and oxygen saturation, maintaining the latter between 88 and 92%;

3 replacement of parenteral nutrition during the operation with 10% dextrose solution and monitoring of blood sugar;

4 a muscle relaxant and an opioid or volatile agent anaesthetic. Their drug requirements and MAC are lower than older infants and children (see Chapter 2). Mechanical ventilation should be continued postoperatively.

Because these patients are so dependent on a stable environment, and because it is difficult to transfer them with all their monitoring equipment and infusions while being ventilated, it may be safer to perform ductus ligation in the intensive care unit.

AORTOPULMONARY SHUNTS

The modified Blalock–Taussig shunt is the most common method of improving blood flow through the pulmonary circulation, either to improve oxygenation or to enlarge hypoplastic pulmonary vessels for definitive repair. Instead of anastomosing the subclavian directly to the pulmonary artery, a Gore-tex graft is inserted between subclavian artery and pulmonary artery on the corresponding side. If the procedure is combined with transplanting coexisting major aortopulmonary collateral arteries (MAPCA), the operation is usually prolonged and may take over 5 hours. These patients are ventilated postoperatively. This allows assessment of oxygenation and pulmonary blood flow and enables acidosis to be controlled. This group of patients will vary in age between neonates with pulmonary atresia whose pulmonary circulation is sustained on PGE_1 infusion, and infants who are given a Blalock–Taussig shunt to increase the size of the hypoplastic pulmonary arteries. The general principles of anaesthesia with intubation and controlled ventilation have been outlined. As the patient is to be ventilated postoperatively, high-dose opioids (fentanyl) are appropriate. The position of the patient will either be lateral or supine, depending on the surgical approach. ECG, oxygen saturation, $ETco_2$ and intra-arterial and central venous pressure should be monitored. Care must be taken to insert the central venous pressure cannula at a site distant from where the shunt is planned to avoid damage to the subclavian artery. The arterial cannula should be on the opposite side to the shunt, as the subclavian artery will be clamped during anastomosis. Heparin 75−100 u/kg is given just before cross-clamping and continued into the postoperative period at a rate of 10 u/kg/h. Dopamine 5−10 μg/kg/min may be needed in the early postoperative period, because increased flow through the shunt and the low-resistance pulmonary circulation imposes a volume load on the left ventricle.

COARCTATION OF THE AORTA AND INTERRUPTED AORTIC ARCH

Coarctation of the aorta is often repaired in the neonatal period if the condition is diagnosed by an astute physician or presents as congestive heart failure. If the obstruction is complete, then the patient is dependent on the ductus arteriosus remaining open for blood flow to the lower part of the body. Infusion of prostaglandin (PG₁) at a rate of 10 ng/kg/min should be commenced preoperatively to keep the ductus open. Coarctation presenting in the neonatal period is best managed with intensive preoperative preparation with ventilation and inotropic support (see above).

Patients are positioned on the right side for a left thoracotomy. Monitoring is the same as for other closed cardiovascular cases. The arterial cannula should be in the right arm. A second intravenous cannula is inserted for the administration of vasodilators. If sustained extreme rises in blood pressure occur during cross-clamping, these are controlled with short-acting vasodilators such as sodium nitroprusside and a volatile agent. Induced hypotension is not warranted, and care must be taken to maintain blood pressure at a level necessary for perfusion of the organs distal to the aortic cross-clamp [4]. The surgeon should ensure that there is adequate pressure in the distal aorta and that the cross-clamp time is kept to a minimum (15−20 minutes). Moderate hypothermia (34°C) is sometimes used to protect organs in the lower body during aortic cross-clamping, especially in the older patient with only moderate coarctation and poorly developed collaterals. When the coarctation is narrow, collateral vessels enlarge so that marked hypertension does not occur when the aorta is cross-clamped. In neonates and infants the stricture is usually long and is enlarged with a subclavian flap, while in older children the stricture is short and an end-to-end anastomosis can be performed. When the cross-clamp is released, an adequate blood volume is necessary to prevent hypotension. The rate of vasodilator infusion and/or the concentration of inhalation anaesthetic is reduced a few minutes before the cross-clamps are removed. These are then taken off slowly, one at a time, to control bleeding and assess haemodynamic changes. In infants beyond the neonatal period, moderate postoperative hypertension is common. The real problem is stress on the surgical repair due to excessive swings in blood pressure. Antihypertensive treatment should be started intraoperatively.

PULMONARY ARTERY BANDING

The need for pulmonary artery banding to reduce pulmonary blood flow and pulmonary hypertension in the presence of VSD, complete A-V canal, etc. has been reduced as these lesions are corrected earlier in life. A new indication is emerging — that of 'conditioning' the left ventricle in preparation for an arterial switch for transposition. Pulmonary artery banding is a hazardous procedure with the possibility of sudden cardiac decompensation or ventricular fibrillation if the band is applied too tightly. Full monitoring is needed. A midline sternotomy is usual. Anaesthesia using a muscle relaxant and opioid is preferred, as most volatile anaesthetics have some negative inotropic effect that may add to ventricular decompensation or affect the intraoperative measurement of pressure gradient across the band. A dopamine infusion should be used postoperatively (5−10 μg/kg/min) for conditioning procedures. All patients are ventilated postoperatively.

VASCULAR RING

This is an anomaly in which two vessels (often a double aortic arch or aberrant subclavian, innominate or pulmonary artery) surround and compress the trachea, obstructing respiration. The treatment is to divide the vessel and, if necessary, reimplant it. Careful positioning of the endotracheal tube is necessary to prevent airway obstruction during the operation. There is also a danger of continuing postoperative obstruction due to tracheal softening. If the anterior arch is retained, this can be treated by surgical fixation of the vessels to the back of the sternum. An anomalous innominate artery compressing the trachea can be treated in the same way.

Anaesthesia for open heart surgery

Anaesthesia for open heart operations usually involves:
1 thiopentone, ketamine or midazolam. These may be used for induction and intermittent supplements;
2 high-dose opioids, such as fentanyl 20−50 μg/kg for induction, with further doses to a total of 50−80 μg/kg, or morphine 2 mg/kg infused slowly to avoid hypotension;
3 a volatile anaesthetic — halothane and isoflurane have different cardiovascular effects (see Chapter 2) so the choice depends on whether a negative inotropic effect (halothane) or vasodilatation (isoflurane) is needed;
4 a non-depolarizing muscle relaxant — pancuronium 0.2 mg/kg (unless there is tachydysrhythmia);
5 intubation and controlled ventilation.

All drugs should be given slowly and preferably diluted.

Anaesthesia for the more straightforward open heart operations (ASD, VSD) is similar to that previously described for closed cardiac operations.

AORTIC STENOSIS

Aortic stenosis may present at any age. In the older patient the left ventricle is hypertrophied. It requires adequate diastolic perfusion pressure and diastolic interval to allow adequate coronary blood flow to prevent ischaemia and myocardial irritability that may lead to ventricular fibrillation. Aortic stenosis in the newborn is often associated with heart failure and dilatation of the left ventricle without hypertrophy, but still with marked irritability.

The aim should be to avoid hypotension and tachycardia. The latter may be tolerated better than hypotension. Fentanyl (20−30 μg/kg given slowly), and pancuronium are used for induction and maintenance. Vasodilators are not started before cardiopulmonary bypass. Moderate hypothermia is used during bypass. Weaning from bypass may be complicated by recurrent or persistent ventricular fibrillation unless adequate perfusion pressure is maintained. Lignocaine is the antidysrhythmic of choice.

ATRIAL SEPTAL DEFECT (ASD)

Closure of an atrial septal defect is a short bypass procedure usually followed by only a short period of postoperative ventilation. For these reasons smaller doses of opioids are employed than for longer operations —

morphine 1 mg/kg or fentanyl 30−40 μg/kg total is used. This is supplemented by halothane or isoflurane. During final closure of the defect it is important to inflate the lungs to fill the left atrium with blood.

VENTRICULAR SEPTAL DEFECT (VSD)

A VSD that is significant in the first months of life will lead to pulmonary hypertension unless treated. The rate at which pulmonary hypertension develops varies, but the risk increases rapidly after 9−12 months of age. It was for this reason that deep hypothermia (18−20°C) with circulatory arrest was developed for safe repair of a VSD in infancy. Prior to this, the pulmonary artery was banded to protect the pulmonary circulation and the VSD was repaired at 2−3 years of age. Ventricular septal defects are now repaired in the first 6 months of life on cardio-pulmonary bypass with hypothermia. Vasodilator drugs are used before starting cardiopulmonary bypass. Some of these patients are being treated for congestive failure with digoxin and diuretics. If signs of congestive failure are present before operation, positive inotropic support using an infusion of dopamine or dobutamine is often helpful when bypass is discontinued.

TRUNCUS ARTERIOSUS

The right and left pulmonary arteries arise directly from the aorta, due to failed development of the aortopulmonary septum. The lungs are subjected to high flows and pressures which may result in heart failure in the neonatal period, or the early development of pulmonary hypertension. Surgery may be palliative with a pulmonary artery band, or corrective with a valved tubular graft extending from the right ventricle to the right and left pulmonary artery confluence. The usual sequence of anaesthesia for open heart surgery is followed, but when terminating bypass, hyperventilation and pharmacological pulmonary vasodilatation (see p. 200) are used. There is a high mortality associated with this condition, even with surgery.

COMPLETE ATRIOVENTRICULAR CANAL (CAVC)

This is an endocardial cushion defect resulting in an ostium primum ASD, VSD and a variety of deformities of the atrioventricular valves. Ninety per cent are associated with Down's syndrome. A pulmonary artery band or complete repair is performed in early infancy before pulmonary hypertension becomes established or heart failure develops. If pulmonary hypertension is present, hyperventilation and pulmonary vasodilatation are used when terminating the bypass.

TRANSPOSITION OF THE GREAT VESSELS

In this condition the aorta and pulmonary artery are transposed, so that they come off the right and left ventricles respectively.

The arterial switch procedure, which involves the translocation of the pulmonary artery and the aorta, is used more and more for correction of transposition. The major difficulty is kinking of the coronary arteries during translocation. The operation is performed before regression of the left ventricle occurs, usually in the first 3 weeks of life. The atrial switch procedure (Senning or Mustard) can be performed at a later age because it does not involve changing afterload on the ventricles, but if delayed too long, the problem of permanent pulmonary hypertension develops. Anaesthetic management involves a fentanyl and pancuronium induction, with opioid maintenance. These patients often need fluid loading after induction, to prevent hypotension. Deep hypothermia ($20-22°C$) is used for some or all of the correction. Vasodilation with sodium nitroprusside and/or phenoxybenzamine is usually started before bypass to facilitate cooling, and continued into the postoperative period to reduce afterload on the ventricles. At the end of bypass, dopamine $5\,\mu g/kg/min$ is routinely infused and $Paco_2$ is kept between 28 and 35 mmHg to control pulmonary vascular resistance. Attention must be paid following the switch operation to any ECG changes that indicate possible coronary artery occlusion due to kinking or air embolus.

FALLOT'S TETRALOGY

Fallot's tetralogy consists of a malaligned interventricular septum, so that a VSD lies below the aortic outflow, and increasing right ventricular outflow tract obstruction which develops in association with right ventricular hypertrophy. There is a variable right-to-left shunt through a non-restrictive VSD. The magnitude of the shunt will depend on the balance between the peripheral resistance and the degree of obstruction by the right ventricular outflow tract components — (a) valvular (fixed), and (b) infundibular (dynamic). The latter

increases as myocardial contractility increases and as right ventricular filling decreases.

Fallot's spells, attacks of increased cyanosis, may occur with a change in any one of these components but increased infundibular obstruction is the most important. Anxiety or any other cause of increased myocardial contractility will increase right ventricular outflow obstruction (infundibular), which will be relieved by beta-adrenergic blockade. If increased shunting occurs during the induction of anaesthesia, treatment, in sequence, consists of oxygen administration, volume loading, propranolol $0.05-0.1$ mg/kg slowly, and possibly a vasoconstrictor drug such as metaraminol. The myocardial depressant effect of halothane may also be used. The latter is useful if peripheral vasodilatation increases the shunting. The surgical procedure involves widening the right ventricular outflow tract, either with a patch or by surgical resection and closure of the VSD. This is usually done after the age of 6 months. Particular problems for the anaesthetist, apart from Fallot's spells, include a high haematocrit, the dangers of embolization through a right-to-left shunt, and the presence of beta-adrenergic blockade. Patients over 20 kg with a high haematocrit — over 45% — may be considered for autologous blood transfusion; the blood may be taken in the week preceding and/or during the period of stability following induction of anaesthesia. If the blood is taken in the weeks before, the reduced haematocrit leads to a reduction in the bleeding tendency, which is the physiological mechanism to prevent thrombosis in patients with very high haematocrits. The operation is performed with moderate hypothermia ($24°C$). The suggested anaesthetic management is induction with thiopentone (given slowly), fentanyl ($20-30\,\mu g/kg$) and pancuronium (0.2 mg/kg), followed by maintenance with fentanyl or morphine and pancuronium. Because of the likely increase in right-to-left shunt, vasodilators should only be used during bypass; sodium nitroprusside is the drug of choice.

DOUBLE-OUTLET RIGHT VENTRICLE (DORV)

This is a large ventricular septal defect with an overriding aorta so that part of the aortic valve is in the right ventricular outflow. Because of the increased pulmonary blood flow, pulmonary hypertension develops rapidly in a few months, unless total correction or a palliative pulmonary artery banding is undertaken. These patients may also need treatment for pulmonary hypertension in the immediate postoperative period.

TOTAL ANOMALOUS PULMONARY VENOUS DRAINAGE (TAPVD)

In this condition the pulmonary veins drain into any of the large venous systems above or below the diaphragm, instead of into the left atrium. Commonly they drain into a large vertical vein which runs into the left innominate vein. If an obstruction exists at this junction, pulmonary hypertension develops rapidly. Total correction should be undertaken as soon as the diagnosis is made. Deep hypothermic arrest is used while the confluence of veins is attached to the posterior aspect of the left atrium. Routine open heart anaesthesia is employed, and if pulmonary hypertension exists it should be treated with hyperventilation and pulmonary vasodilatation (see p. 200).

FONTAN PROCEDURE

The Fontan operation diverts systemic venous return passively through the pulmonary circulation without any intervening valves or pumping chamber. It was originally used for the treatment of tricuspid atresia, but is now used to convert any appropriate complex congenital heart disease to a univentricular situation, i.e. double-inlet left ventricle. Requirements for this operation are low pulmonary vascular resistance (or pulmonary artery pressure less than 16 mmHg), appropriately sized pulmonary arteries, and normally functioning A-V valves. It is usually performed after 1 year of age with moderate hypothermia (24°C). The usual anaesthetic for open heart surgery is appropriate.

If vasodilatation is needed, a short-acting vasodilator such as sodium nitroprusside is used. At the end of bypass, dopamine 5 μg/kg/min is routinely infused. A systemic venous pressure of 12−15 mmHg is needed to maintain cardiac output.

HYPOPLASTIC LEFT-HEART SYNDROME — NORWOOD OPERATION

The hypoplastic left-heart syndrome consists of a hypoplastic left ventricle, aortic and mitral valve atresia or severe stenosis, and hypoplasia of the aortic arch. Untreated, death usually occurs in the first week of life. The incidence is approximately 1% of all congenital heart disease. Methods for correction have recently been developed. The choice consists of a cardiac transplant or staged Norwood operations. The Norwood Stage I procedure incorporates the main pulmonary artery into the aortic arch, the right ventricle then becoming the systemic ventricle. The lungs are supplied by a separate shunt, such as a modified Blalock, performed at the same operation. The haemodynamics remain complex and death often occurs from heart failure following the procedure, because of pulmonary steal combined with poor coronary blood flow. If this shunt is too large and pulmonary vascular resistance is low, then pulmonary blood flow increases at the expense of systemic flow (pulmonary steal) and this can lead to cardiac failure and arrest. Part of the operation is performed with deep hypothermic arrest. A fentanyl−muscle-relaxant technique is suggested, with careful vasodilator therapy, e.g. nitroprusside. Immediately after bypass, hyperventilation with 100% oxygen is used until the patient is stable; thereafter the pulmonary-to-systemic flow ratio is balanced by avoiding reduction of pulmonary vascular resistance. This is achieved with a normal to slightly raised $Paco_2$, a low Fio_2 (0.21−0.3) and PEEP of 5 cmH$_2$O. When pulmonary and systemic blood flows are appropriately balanced, the oxygen saturation should be about 80%. The Norwood Stage II operation consists of conversion of the above correction into the anatomical configuration of the Fontan procedure. This is not performed until 3−4 years of age.

MITRAL STENOSIS

Mitral stenosis may be congenital, presenting in the very young, or acquired, from rheumatic heart disease, which is now uncommon in affluent countries and presents much later. In the very young, valvuloplasty is preferred, as this avoids the problems associated with valve replacement.

Open drainage of effusions

Pericardial and pleural effusions may need drainage or pleurodesis (obliteration of the pleural cavity). These effusions are more common after the Fontan operation. Patients with significant pericardial effusion and Fontan haemodynamics are unstable, and hence anaesthetic agents which cause myocardial depression or excessive vasodilation are to be avoided. Ketamine, fentanyl, pancuronium and judicious use of isoflurane are preferred for anaesthesia. Invasive monitoring is not essential, but pulse oximetry, ECG and non-invasive blood pressure monitoring are necessary.

ANAESTHETIC CONSIDERATIONS IN HEART TRANSPLANTATION

Heart transplantation in children may be undertaken in patients with end-stage cardiomyopathy, failure of previous corrective operations for congenital heart disease, and, combined with lung transplantation, in patients with significant pulmonary hypertension associated with serious heart disease. Transplantation is potentially useful for hypoplastic left heart syndrome and other complex abnormalities in neonates and infants. Its use in these conditions has so far been limited by lack of appropriate donors, mainly due to ethical considerations.

Patients requiring transplantation may have coexistent problems in other systems. They may have been given anticoagulants.

The timing of surgery is important, so that the delay between the arrival of the heart and the recipient being ready to receive it is minimal. As the heart may have to be brought considerable distances, communication between the team taking the donor heart and those anaesthetizing the recipient must be maintained to minimize this delay, and to avoid the recipient being on unnecessary long periods of bypass before transplantation. With the preservation techniques now available, ischaemic times of 3–4 hours have been followed by good myocardial function. Because the recipient is on standby and may not have much time for preoperative preparation, these patients may present with an inadequate period of fasting. An antacid should be administered preoperatively and a rapid-sequence induction using ketamine, suxamethonium, fentanyl, pre-oxygenation with cricoid pressure and intubation should be used. If the patient has fasted adequately, a fentanyl/pancuronium induction with monitoring similar to that for other major cardiac surgery is used. The patient is maintained on a high dose of opioid such as fentanyl. Inhalation agents are generally avoided as these patients are usually in cardiac failure. It is important to observe strict sterile precautions when placing invasive tubes, cannulae and catheters. These patients are immunosuppressed with cyclosporin A and azathioprine, and are therefore prone to infection.

Once the heart is transplanted it will usually function satisfactorily when coming off bypass, provided the donor heart ischaemic time has not been excessively prolonged. Postoperative support may include dopamine infusion and electrical pacing. The maintenance of an adequate blood volume is important as the denervated heart does not respond reflexly to hypovolaemia or hypotension. It is also unresponsive to anticholinergic and anticholinesterase drugs.

Postoperatively these patients must be nursed in isolation.

Anaesthesia for the patient with a heart transplant

The introduction of cyclosporin in 1982 to suppress rejection has increased the likelihood of successful heart and heart–lung transplantation.

PHYSIOLOGY OF THE DENERVATED HEART

These patients tolerate changing physiological demands well, but are usually on the low/normal range of exercise tolerance. They can increase cardiac output, but with a much slower response time. Because the heart is denervated, the resting pulse rate is often rapid due to the lack of vagal tone and continuing sensitivity to circulating catecholamines, both endogenous and exogenous. A change in cardiac output is usually due mainly to a change in stroke volume. The autonomically mediated tachycardia in response to hypovolaemia is obtunded. The myocardial adrenergic receptors appear to become more sensitive to catecholamines (up-regulation), but it is not known whether the receptors change. Another result of denervation is that the heart–lung recipient loses the normal cough reflex and needs frequent physiotherapy.

DRUGS USED TO PREVENT REJECTION

The basic triple therapy consists of steroids, azathioprine and cyclosporin.

Steroids (methylprednisolone, prednisone)

These drugs have been used to depress the rejection process since organ transplantation began. Relevant side-effects include predisposition to infection, poor tissue healing (especially heart–lung transplants), and growth arrest. It is because of these side effects that steroids are not used routinely in children, but only during phases of rejection.

Azathioprine (Imuran)

Azathioprine, one of the original immunosuppressants, is an imadazolyl derivative of mercaptopuran, and must be first metabolized in the liver to the active 6-mercaptopurine. It is also used in acute leukaemia, systemic lupus erythematosus and polyarteritis nodosa. Side-effects include serious white cell depression, particularly granulocytes, hepatotoxicity and the growth of lymphomas.

Cyclosporin

This was first isolated in 1970 from a fungus, *Tolypocladium inflatum*, and introduced for heart transplantation in 1982. Cyclosporin does not reduce the incidence of rejection episodes but decreases the severity. Side-effects of cyclosporin include nephrotoxicity and hypertension (which often requires treatment), hepatic toxicity, lymphoma and unattractive hirsutism. The ultimate metabolism of this drug is through the cytochrome P450 system, where it competes with other substrates such as steroids. It is available in both oral and intravenous formulations, the latter being dissolved in chremophore EL, which has been associated with anaphylactoid reactions of some intravenous anaesthetics, e.g. propanidid. The blood level of this drug must be closely monitored, but patients are often maintained in a wide therapeutic range, e.g. 300–1600 ng/ml.

Other drugs used during the rejection phase include ATG (antithymoside globulin) and OK23 (monoclonal antibody). The patient may also be given a number of ancillary drugs such as antibiotics and antihypertensives.

ANAESTHETIC CONSIDERATIONS

These patients present for anaesthesia for:
biopsy — heart and/or lung;
drainage of pericardial effusions;
pacemaker insertion;
other incidental procedures.
As these patients are immunosuppressed, sterility is very important; gloves should be worn, invasive monitoring limited, bacterial filters used on airways and further tracheal intubation employed only if really necessary. Depression of the immune system should be avoided if possible. Hypovolaemia should be corrected and a temporary transoesophageal pacemaker should be available.

RELEVANT PHARMACOLOGY

All anaesthetic agents directly suppress the cardiovascular and/or the respiratory system, and must be used with special care as these patients do not have the normal neurally mediated reflexes, such as increasing heart rate when cardiac output falls. Even ketamine, which normally maintains blood pressure and cardiac output, must be used carefully because these effects are normally achieved by sympathetic stimulation. All volatile agents cause direct myocardial depression in a dose-dependent manner, but no agent is specially contraindicated. Halothane is useful for lung biopsies of heart–lung transplants, but atropine will not antagonize the bradycardia it can cause at deeper levels of anaesthesia. Nitrous oxide is probably not contraindicated — its bone-marrow depressant effect occurs only after prolonged usage.

Pancuronium is the muscle relaxant of choice because of the direct myocardial stimulatory effect, while agents that release histamine such as D-tubocurarine, alcuronium and atracurium, should be avoided.

Fentanyl is preferred to morphine, because the latter releases histamine, causing some vasodilatation.

Neostigmine should still be combined with atropine to counteract the non-cardiac muscarinic effects. A direct depressant effect on the myocardium may be manifested.

Lignocaine is the preferred local anaesthetic, but there is no contraindication to the use of bupivacaine for nerve-block anaesthesia.

SUGGESTED METHODS OF ANAESTHESIA

Myocardial biopsy is preferably performed with the patient awake, using infiltration of the groin with local anaesthetic, if the patient is co-operative. Midazolam and fentanyl can be used for sedation. Non-invasive monitoring should be used. If the patient is unco-operative, then general anaesthesia with a slowly administered sleep dose of thiopentone or propofol, fentanyl and pancuronium, supplemented with isoflurane, which is the preferred agent because its cardiovascular effects are more peripheral than myocardial. It can be administered with air and oxygen.

Lung biopsy can be performed using a volatile agent such as halothane or isoflurane, and oxygen with topical lignocaine (up to 4 mg/kg) for intubation is an acceptable method. Alternatively, an anaesthetic using muscle relaxation and controlled or jet ventilation can be used.

Minor operations can often be carried out with a volatile agent such as isoflurane with nitrous oxide and oxygen, with the patient breathing spontaneously and adequately monitored.

Other operations which require intubation can be carried out with thiopentone, pancuronium, oxygen/nitrous oxide supplemented with fentanyl ± isoflurane. Epidural or spinal anaesthesia is not contraindicated, provided the patient is not hypovolaemic and the blood volume is maintained.

THE ANAESTHETIST'S ROLE IN CARDIOPULMONARY BYPASS

Apart from maintaining anaesthesia, the anaesthetist must prepare the patient for cardiopulmonary bypass. An anaesthetist may run the heart–lung machine or may be responsible for the supervision of a perfusion technician.

Cooling can be started early in the operation by reducing the temperature of a water blanket beneath the patient. The resulting decrease in patient temperature gives some protection if blood pressure or cardiac output decrease unexpectedly before bypass.

Vasodilator drugs can be started before bypass if indicated and if the blood pressure is stable. If the patient is hypotensive they should be withheld until bypass has commenced. The reason for vasodilating the patient during bypass is to promote even perfusion during rapid cooling, to control the mean perfusion pressure (about 35 mmHg in neonates; up to 60–65 mmHg in older children) and to reduce the afterload after bypass.

Anaesthesia during cardiopulmonary bypass can be maintained with a volatile agent (isoflurane) administered by the gas flow to the oxygenator, or with intravenous agents. Hypothermia reduces metabolism, cerebral activity and drug requirements. As the patient is rewarmed, requirements increase and further drugs, such as morphine or midazolam, are needed to prevent awareness.

Additional muscle relaxant should be given before bypass to ensure that the patient remains paralysed. The volume of the prime will effectively dilute the relaxant already present in the body, so a full paralysing dose should be used.

Heparin 3 mg/kg is given before bypass (1 mg, approximately 100 u. The pump prime is also heparinized. Hypothermia reduces heparin metabolism, so that further doses are rarely necessary but, if activated clotting time (performed hourly) decreases to three times control values, another 1 mg/kg should be given.

Ventilation is maintained until full flow (usually 2.2–2.4 l/min/m²) is achieved on cardiopulmonary bypass. The lungs should then be filled with air at a continuous positive pressure sufficient to keep them inflated (usually below 10 cmH₂O). The aorta is cross-clamped and cold cardioplegic solution is infused into the root of the aorta, and hence into the coronary circulation, to prevent myocardial activity. The aim of cardioplegia is to maintain the heart in asystole while preserving the myocardium (see Appendix 3). Cold lactated Ringer's solution is instilled into the pericardium to provide additional surface-cooling of the heart and mediastinum.

In children, unlike adults, because of the wide variation in heart size, cardioplegic solutions should be delivered in a separate controlled delivery system where flow, pressure and temperature can be monitored at the delivery site (see Appendix 3).

If the ventricles fibrillate and do not rapidly revert to a regular rhythm after the end of bypass, DC countershock of about 5–10 J may be given directly to the heart. If fibrillation persists, lignocaine 1 mg/kg is given before a further shock. If the rhythm is not regular after rewarming, temporary epicardial pacing may be needed.

Calcium chloride 10 mg/kg (0.1 ml/kg of 10% solution) may be used as a single-dose inotropic agent immediately after bypass. If it is anticipated that an inotropic infusion will be required, it is started before weaning from bypass, usually dopamine (about 5 µg/kg/min), or if pulmonary vascular resistance is high, dobutamine (in a similar dose).

After removal of the bypass cannulae, the heparin anticoagulation is reversed with protamine given in a dose 1–1.3 times the initial heparin dose. Hypotension may occur if protamine is given too quickly to a patient whose blood volume has not adequately been restored, or in a patient who has a sensitivity to the drug.

Postoperative bleeding is common. Predisposing factors include:

1 In small infants the blood volume is small relative to the volume prime of pump fluid, so that the clotting factors are diluted.

2 Prolonged periods on bypass lead to greater destruction of cells and platelets and denaturation of coagulation factors.

3 Patients having reoperation usually have adhesions which provide multiple bleeding points when divided.

Despite apparent surgical control of these, some continued oozing can occur from them.

4 Patients with cyanotic heart disease and a high haematocrit have increased fibrinolytic activity and thrombocytopaenia, which reduces the ability to clot (see Table 13.4).

5 Inadequate rewarming.

6 Bubble oxygenators cause more destruction of cells and platelets of blood than membrane oxygenators, due to the blood−gas interface. This becomes increasingly significant with prolonged bypass.

Bleeding can be reduced by:

1 adequate surgical haemostasis;

2 adequate heparin reversal;

3 administration of fresh frozen plasma (FFP) up to 10 ml/kg when bleeding persists or when predisposing factors are present;

4 administration of platelets when bleeding continues after fresh frozen plasma has been given.

POSTOPERATIVE CARE

After cardiac surgery, all children except for some straightforward closed cases such as ligation of ductus arteriosus, are managed in an intensive care unit where they can be monitored closely and staff are readily available to treat them when required.

Ventilation

Patients are usually ventilated after open heart surgery, often while still paralysed, until the cardiovascular system is stable. This reduces the work of breathing and allows adequate analgesia and sedation to be given to keep the patient comfortable during the early postoperative period.

Monitoring

The intensity of monitoring after cardiac surgery depends on the complexity of the operation. The ECG (usually lead II) and heart rate are monitored continuously after all operations.

Blood pressure is monitored by automated cuff after PDA ligation and pacemaker insertion, and by intra-arterial cannula after all other operations. Right atrial pressure is monitored by central venous catheter after all major cases (except repair of coarctation in older infants and children, PDA ligation and pacemaker insertion).

Left atrial pressure is monitored after all procedures on bypass, except the repair of ASD, small VSD and pulmonary valvotomy by a catheter inserted into the atrial appendage during operation. Pulmonary artery (PA) pressure is monitored by a catheter inserted directly into the pulmonary artery at operation when high PA pressure is anticipated, e.g. large VSD, A-V canal, truncus arteriosus, total anomalous pulmonary venous drainage, and transposition of the great arteries.

Cardiac output is often assessed clinically by observing blood pressure and indicators of organ perfusion such as urine output, conscious state, core−toe temperature gradient and acid−base balance. Cardiac output can be measured and the results compared with normal values for body size, but the measurements are of greatest value when repeated, so that they can give a trend of cardiac function. The methods include haemodilution, green dye dilution, Doppler or bioimpedance. As technology improves, oesophageal echocardiography will become more useful during and after surgery to monitor valve function and ventricular performance.

Fluid intake and output (losses from chest drains, urine and nasogastric tube) are monitored hourly. The state of hydration should be checked 3−4 times a day by clinical examination, and the fluid intake and diuretic administration adjusted accordingly.

Skin pulse oximetry gives a fairly accurate continuous indication of arterial blood oxygenation. Arterial blood gas tensions, together with sodium, potassium, haemoglobin and glucose concentrations, should be measured every 4 hours, and more often in unstable patients.

Total and differential white blood cell count and platelet count are measured daily. Clotting studies are performed once or twice daily as needed.

Plasma protein, magnesium and phosphate concentrations should be measured twice weekly, together with liver function testing.

POSTOPERATIVE COMPLICATIONS

The incidence and severity of complications tend to decrease with the time elapsed after cardiopulmonary bypass, but new problems can arise at any time. An explanation for any abnormalities must be sought. Hypotension, hypoventilation and dysrhythmia are particular risks during transfer from the operating theatre to the intensive care unit.

There are several problems that can occur after cardiac surgery which will now be discussed.

Low cardiac output

Decreasing cardiac output is common after open heart surgery. The signs are falling blood pressure and urine output, slow capillary refill, increasing core–toe temperature gradient and metabolic acidosis.

DECREASED PRELOAD

Ventricular filling and hence stretch of the ventricular wall in diastole are reduced by hypovolaemia, vasodilatation or cardiac tamponade. Hypovolaemia may result from bleeding with inadequate blood volume replacement or excessive urine losses in polyuric renal failure, or following the over-use of diuretics.

If the patient is hypovolaemic, the atrial pressures are low and fluid challenge with 10 ml/kg of blood or colloid will increase output, with minimal increase in atrial pressure.

Cardiac tamponade can develop rapidly in the first 24 hours after operation due to bleeding into the pericardium. The bleeding may be surgical, due to dilution of platelets and clotting factors by the bypass prime, or due to the residual effects of heparin. After 48 hours, serous pericardial effusion can cause the gradual onset of tamponade, especially when the right atrial pressure remains high, as in operations for Fallot's tetralogy or Fontan operations. Cardiac tamponade should be suspected and excluded whenever there is an unexplained decrease in cardiac output. Chest-drain losses may increase or suddenly cease. Milking the drains may improve the clinical state. An increase in atrial pressure after fluid challenge, with minimal improvement in blood pressure, suggests the presence of tamponade. In this case, immediate chest X-ray (to demonstrate a widening heart shadow), clotting studies and surgical consultation are needed. Urgent echocardiography will demonstrate pericardial blood. Immediate open drainage may be needed. Fairly high atrial pressures (12–15 mmHg) should be maintained and vasodilators avoided until the pericardium is drained.

DECREASED CONTRACTILITY

Decreased contractility at the end of bypass is due to pre-existing myocardial dysfunction, long aortic cross-clamp time, or ventricular oedema after ventriculotomy.

Later deterioration of ventricular contractility can cause blood pressure and cardiac output to fall and atrial pressure to rise. This may be due to myocardial oedema, especially after ventriculotomy, to reduced coronary blood flow (e.g. after switch operation for transposition), or to sepsis. Response to fluid challenge, chest X-ray, blood gases, blood culture and echocardiogram should be assessed before making this diagnosis. If cardiac output is low despite rising atrial pressures, tamponade, dysrhythmia, sepsis, ventilatory problems and electrolyte disturbance must be excluded. If these are not significant, inotropic drugs and, possibly, vasodilators are used.

Whenever haemodynamic deterioration cannot be explained, sepsis should be suspected and investigated early and thoroughly (see below).

INCREASED AFTERLOAD

Increased afterload due to systemic or pulmonary vasoconstriction may impair ventricular performance. Low cardiac output in the presence of normal or high atrial pressure may improve with the gradual introduction of a vasodilator drug such as sodium nitroprusside. The use of vasodilators is contraindicated when there is obstruction to the circulation. If this is within the heart (e.g. valvular stenosis or tamponade), vasodilators can cause a severe reduction in coronary perfusion pressure. Vasodilatation in the presence of aortic coarctation may critically reduce the perfusion of kidneys and spinal cord.

DYSRHYTHMIA

Sinus tachycardia up to 200/min and wandering atrial pacemaker can occur after any open heart operation, particularly in infants. They may be caused by factors such as pain, hypovolaemia, poor myocardial contractility, tamponade, hypoventilation, fever, hypoglycaemia, convulsions and pulmonary hypertensive crises. Some cases are due to drugs such as pancuronium and catecholamines. The precipitating cause should be sought and corrected, although in some cases no cause is found.

Supraventricular tachycardia after cardiac surgery is best treated by vagotonic manoeuvres, such as carotid massage or stimulating the pharynx with a catheter. If that fails, overdrive atrial pacing (increasing the rate with a pacemaker and then suddenly removing the pacing), DC shock or neostigmine (0.01 mg/kg i.v.) repeated if necessary at 2-minute intervals to a maximum of 0.05 mg/kg, should be tried. If the tachycardia persists, the patient should be digitalized. Verapamil should not be used. Amiodarone 5 mg/kg i.v. over 1 hour, then infusion of $5-15\,\mu g/kg/min$ may also be successful.

Premature ventricular contractions progressing to ventricular fibrillation are seen after repair of critical aortic stenosis, in patients with coronary artery abnormalities and in hypokalaemia and digoxin toxicity. Prophylactic lignocaine infusion is often used in these children, changing to oral quinidine or phenytoin after $3-4$ days. If ventricular fibrillation or tachycardia occurs, a DC shock should be given, followed by a bolus of lignocaine ($1\,mg/kg$) and then by an infusion.

Heart block and sinus bradycardia are most often seen:

1 in 'corrected' or L-transposition of the great arteries where the blood circulates RA>LV>PA and LA>RV> aorta because the Bundle of His may follow an irregular course and may be caught by a suture when the VSD is repaired;

2 after Fontan operations (see Appendix 4). In the latter cases the dysrhythmia is transient and may be treated with temporary A-V sequential pacing. In L-transposition, heart block is usually permanent, requiring permanent pacing.

PULMONARY HYPERTENSION

Congenital heart lesions that cause increased pulmonary blood flow (large VSD, atrioventricular canal, truncus arteriosus), obstruct pulmonary venous return (mitral stenosis) or both (obstructed total anomalous pulmonary venous drainage) impair the transition of the pulmonary circulation from its fetal to its adult form, and cause increased thickness and distal extension of the muscle coat in the small pulmonary arteries. These changes become more fixed with increasing age before correction. Postoperative acute right-heart failure may occur in any of these conditions if pulmonary vascular resistance remains high.

Hypoxaemia, hypercarbia, atelectasis, electrolyte disturbance, pain and sepsis can all increase pulmonary vascular resistance.

Pulmonary artery pressure should be monitored after operation in all children with lesions that increase pulmonary vascular resistance. Vasodilator drugs such as phenoxybenzamine should be continued from the time of operation into the postoperative period. In pulmonary hypertensive crises, pulmonary and systemic artery pressures and left and right atrial pressures rise acutely, and a marked tachycardia develops. Skin circulation deteriorates. In these circumstances, precipitating causes should be rapidly excluded and the patient gently hyperventilated with oxygen. If such crises are frequent, the child should be given a fentanyl infusion at $4-6\,\mu g/kg/h$. Dopamine infusion should be replaced by dobutamine, which has less tendency to increase pulmonary vascular resistance. A pulmonary vasodilator drug such as nitroglycerine ($1-10\,\mu g/kg/min$), sodium nitroprusside ($0.5-5\,\mu g/kg/min$) or prostacyclin ($5-30\,ng/kg/min$) should be infused.

Respiratory problems after cardiac surgery

Impaired gas exchange and increased work of breathing increase oxygen consumption, impair myocardial function and reduce oxygen delivery to all tissues. Hypoventilation will lead to carbon dioxide retention, with its adverse cardiovascular effects, and may also contribute to hypoxaemia. Some of the problems will be reduced by mechanical ventilation and adequate sedation, which will decrease oxygen consumption. Pulmonary oedema, lung compression and collapse will interfere with gas exchange and require treatment. Hypoxaemia may result from a right-to-left shunt in the lungs or heart. If $P\text{ao}_2$ remains below $140\,mmHg$ despite breathing pure oxygen, a significant shunt is present in the lungs or heart (Fig. 13.2). Contrast echocardiography is then indicated to exclude intracardiac shunt.

PULMONARY OEDEMA

If present before operation, pulmonary oedema often persists for $2-3$ days after correction of the lesion. The oedema may be cardiogenic (high left atrial pressure), the result of protein leak from pulmonary capillaries, or due to a combination of these.

The treatment of pulmonary oedema involves reducing left atrial pressure by fluid restriction, diuretics, venodilator drugs such as glyceryl trinitrate, inotropic drugs and possibly peritoneal dialysis. Capillary protein leak normally decreases $2-3$ days after bypass, in the absence of sepsis or prolonged shock.

PLEURAL EFFUSIONS

These occur in the presence of fluid overload, hypoproteinaemia or capillary leak, and after operations such as Fontan procedure and correction of Fallot's tetralogy, when the right atrial pressure is high, especially in older children. The effusion should be drained if it is interfering

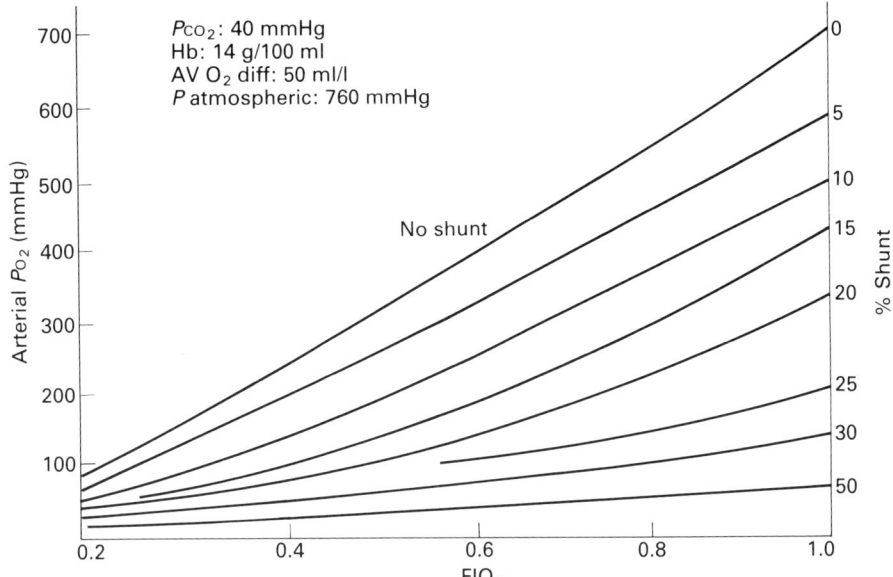

Fig. 13.2 Shunt diagram showing the percentage shunt for any given Pao_2 and Fio_2. For example, a child in 80% oxygen has a Po_2 of 300 mmHg; from this diagram this is a 15% shunt, and in 40% oxygen the child would be expected to have a Po_2 of 100 mmHg (in practice the Po_2 is usually less than the predicted value).

with ventilation. Otherwise, lowering the right atrial pressure by fluid restriction and diuretics may be sufficient.

ATELECTASIS

Atelectasis is common after cardiac surgery, particularly in the right upper and left lower lobes. It may involve a lung, one or more lobes, segments or sub-segmental areas. The usual causes are: poor clearing of tracheal mucus, which may be profuse with heart failure or respiratory infection; inadequate humidification of inspired gas so that secretions become inspissated; trauma to bronchial mucosa due to too vigorous suction; breathing at low FRC due to inadequate PEEP; and low tidal volume due to excess sedation or residual muscle relaxation.

Atelectasis may be managed with humidification, chest vibration and percussion to loosen secretions, posture (if tolerated), suction to remove secretions and over-inflation and deep breathing to expand the lung. Antibiotics are indicated if infection is present.

OTHER CAUSES OF RESPIRATORY PROBLEMS

These include blockage or displacement of the endotracheal tube and tension pneumothorax. After weaning from the ventilator and extubation, subglottic oedema, stridor, recurrent laryngeal and phrenic nerve palsies may occur. The problems are discussed in detail in Chapters 32 and 33.

Sepsis

After cardiac surgery, children have reduced defences against infection. Skin and mucosal barriers are invaded by vascular catheters, an endotracheal tube and the chest wound. Starvation and the hormonal effects of stress reduce immune responsiveness. Dilution and suppression of neutrophils and immunoglobulins occur [5]. Newborns are more susceptible to bacterial and viral infection than older children, and demonstrate few specific signs of sepsis. In all age groups, if there is unexplained deterioration, sepsis should be suspected and investigated with cultures of blood, urine and tracheal aspirate, and white-cell count with differential. Sites of infection include blood, wound, urinary tract, pleural and peritoneal cavities, middle ears, paranasal sinuses, lungs, bones, meninges and endocardium. The main organisms involved are *Staphylococcus aureus*, *Staphylococcus epidermidis*, Gram-negative bacilli and *Candida albicans*. If sepsis is suspected, antibiotics active against staphylococci and coliforms should be used until culture results are available.

Encephalopathy

Encephalopathy can occur after any cardiac operation. The signs are impaired conscious state, focal or generalized convulsions and localizing signs such as hemiplegia or cranial nerve palsies.

The causes of encephalopathy include focal or global brain ischaemia. Focal ischaemia is due to the entry of air or debris into the ascending aorta and cerebral vessels during operation, or to paradoxical air embolus (small air bubbles injected into a vein passed through a right-to-left shunt).

Global ischaemia may be due to cardiogenic shock before operation, prolonged hypotension during or after operation, or excessively prolonged deep hypothermic circulatory arrest. Both types of ischaemia are more likely to occur in newborn babies. Management involves ensuring the maintenance of adequate circulation and ventilation and the prevention of convulsions.

Convulsions are seen in 10% of newborns and in a smaller proportion of older infants in the first month after open heart surgery, especially after circulatory arrest with deep hypothermia. Unexplained tachycardia, hypertension and pupillary dilatation should suggest convulsions in ventilated patients. This can be confirmed by ceasing muscle-relaxant drugs and observing the child. Neurological consultation and investigation, including lumbar puncture, CT scan and EEG, may be necessary to diagnose intracerebral haemorrhage or brain infarction. Anticonvulsant drugs may be required. In a paralysed child, EEG may be monitored continuously using bitemporal electrodes.

Fluid and electrolyte disturbances

All children have oedema after open heart surgery because (a) the bypass circuit is primed with fluid with a low protein concentration, and (b) all children develop some capillary protein leak (see Chapter 34), which may follow long operations, deep hypothermia with circulatory arrest and any open heart surgery in the newborn. Sepsis is another predisposing factor. The protein leak may present as oedema of the lung, chest wall and extremities, as well as pleural and pericardial effusion and ascites. It results in hypovolaemia and haemoconcentration. Lung and chest-wall oedema impair ventilation. Venous return is reduced by ascites, which should therefore be drained. Capillary leak generally lasts 2−4 days: ventilation and circulation should be supported and drain losses replaced with fresh frozen plasma if clotting factors are deficient, or 5% albumin in saline. Peritoneal dialysis may reduce extracellular fluid without causing hypovolaemia.

To minimize the increase in interstitial fluid volume and deleterious effects on cardiorespiratory function, fluid intake should be restricted in the first 5 days after operation, paying attention to maintenance and cannula-flushing fluid. Blood and colloid should be given as required.

In children less than 6 kg body weight, fluid intake during the 24 hours after operation should be 2 ml/kg/h. In children between 6 and 40 kg weight, intake should be 1 ml/kg/h; in children heavier than 40 kg, intake should be 40 ml/h.

On the first postoperative day, fluid intake is increased to 60% of maintenance requirements (see Table 29.2). Thereafter, intake increases by 10% of maintenance per day until the child is taking normal fluid requirements.

Fluid intake should be restricted more severely and for longer periods for children with Fallot's tetralogy, or those who have ascites, pleural effusions, heart failure or clinical or radiological evidence of fluid overload. After Fontan operations, patients should be limited to 50% of maintenance requirements for several weeks.

In all infants, monitoring cannulae should be flushed continuously with heparinized fluid at no more than 1 ml/h (heparinized normal saline into peripheral artery cannulae, and heparinized 5% dextrose into all others — heparin 1 u/ml in prematures under 1500 g and 5 u/ml thereafter). If inotropic drugs are used, their concentration should be adjusted so that the lowest commonly used infusion rate (e.g. dopamine 5 μg/kg/min) is given in 1 ml/h, thereby minimizing fluid intake. This inotropic infusion can be heparinized and used as a cannula-flushing solution.

Hypokalaemia is common in the first 48 hours after bypass surgery and it should be corrected by the addition of potassium chloride to the intravenous fluids, to prevent dysrhythmias. Low plasma ionized calcium is also common, but does not usually require treatment.

Nutritional disturbances

Hypoglycaemia often occurs, particularly in small malnourished infants. An adequate glucose intake of 4−6 mg/kg/min is needed to maintain a blood glucose of 4−6 mmol/l. When fluids are restricted, this may mean using glucose concentrations of 10−20% in maintenance i.v. fluids, or even an infusion of 50% glucose through a central venous catheter.

Heart failure with failure to thrive is a frequent cause of malnutrition before cardiac surgery in children. Unless adequate nutrition is started within 2−3 days of operation in such children, the obligatory protein catabolism after major surgery will impair immunity, wound healing and respiratory and cardiac muscle performance. If enteral feeding cannot be started early, intravenous nutrition is often needed (see Chapter 37).

Acute renal failure

Renal failure after open heart surgery is more common in newborns, after long operations and when cardiac output and blood pressure have been low. Other predisposing factors are sepsis, haemoglobinuria and administration of nephrotoxic drugs, especially aminoglycosides. To prevent acute renal failure, blood pressure and cardiac output should be kept as near to normal as possible and aminoglyocoside levels should be monitored frequently. If the urine output falls below 0.5 ml/kg/h, prerenal failure should be suspected. The biochemical changes in the urine that differentiate established acute renal failure from prerenal failure are abolished by diuretics, so that the most reliable test of established acute renal failure in these children is a fluid challenge (10 ml/kg colloid i.v.) plus a bolus dose of diuretic (e.g. frusemide 1 mg/kg i.v.). A diuretic response indicates that acute renal failure is not established and that oliguria is probably due to hypovolaemia.

While metabolic acidosis can usually be controlled with sodium bicarbonate, and hyperkalaemia by restricting potassium intake and using ion-exchange resin enema, the decision to commence dialysis or haemofiltration is usually precipitated by a positive fluid balance. Nutrition, inotropic drug infusion and the maintenance of monitoring catheter patency require fluid intake: if this is not matched by urinary loss, fluid retention will cause pulmonary and systemic (including brain and myocardial) oedema. Azotemia alone is rarely the indication for dialysis after cardiac surgery.

If renal failure occurs, low volume (10 ml/kg) rapid cycle (30 minutes) peritoneal dialysis is preferred, because it allows more haemodynamic stability than haemodialysis or arteriovenous haemofiltration. After open heart surgery in children, peritoneal dialysis should be started as soon as it is clear that the oliguria or hyperkalaemia are not responsive to fluid challenge plus diuretic.

POSTOPERATIVE CARE AFTER SPECIFIC OPERATIONS

Ligation of patent ductus arteriosus

Postoperative problems are rare apart from haemothorax, pneumothorax or atelectasis. Very rarely, recur-

rent laryngeal nerve damage may occur. Newborn infants who were ventilator-dependent before operation often remain so for some days afterwards.

Repair of coarctation of the aorta

The major problem is postoperative hypertension, which stresses aortic suture lines and increases left-ventricular afterload. Possible causes of this hypertension include persistent renin production from kidneys which were underperfused before operation, and resetting upwards of baroreceptor reflexes. Treatment involves careful introduction of vasodilator and beta-adrenergic blocking drugs in the closely monitored child.

In the newborn, postoperative problems include pulmonary oedema, residual effects of preoperative cardiogenic shock, acute renal failure, liver impairment, disseminated intravascular coagulation, and paralytic ileus. Mechanical ventilation is usually needed for 1–2 days because of pulmonary oedema. The residual effects of shock are treated as required (see Chapter 34).

Palliative shunts

Blalock–Taussig (see Appendix 4), and other central shunts increase pulmonary blood flow in children with obstructive right-heart lesions. These children are often very cyanosed, with a high haematocrit, which may predispose to cerebral vascular thrombosis. In the newborn, oxygenation may be maintained before operation by keeping the ductus arteriosus open with infusion of prostaglandin E_1 (PGE_1) 5–20 ng/kg/min to allow blood flow from aorta to pulmonary artery. In any child with a right-to-left shunt, intravenous injection carries the risk of paradoxical embolus to the heart or brain. All air and clot must be removed from intravenous tubing before and after intravenous injections.

A palliative shunt must be large enough to allow for increased cardiac output with growth, and is likely to produce excessive lung blood-flow postoperatively, especially in infants. At least 2–3 days of left-ventricular failure and pulmonary oedema can be expected, with the need for inotropic drugs and mechanical ventilation to normocarbia, especially in the newborn.

Pulmonary artery banding

Pulmonary artery banding to reduce pulmonary blood flow and prevent secondary pulmonary vascular disease in lesions with a large left-to-right shunt may be complicated if the band is too tight. Signs of impending right-ventricular failure from this cause include cyanosis, bradycardia, premature ventricular contractions and soft heart sounds. Occurrence of any of these should lead to consideration of urgent surgery to loosen the band. Cardiac failure present before operation may persist for 2–3 days after operation, and may be exacerbated by too-early or too-rapid weaning from mechanical ventilation. Inotropic drug infusion is usually needed in the first 48 hours after surgery.

Total correction of Fallot's tetralogy

The main postoperative problems are those of biventricular failure, maximal 12 hours after operation, especially when there has been a long aortic cross-clamp time or a right ventriculotomy. Mechanical ventilation, inotropic drugs and infusion of sodium nitroprusside may be needed. Right-ventricular failure may occur if the pulmonary arteries are small, if there is residual pulmonary stenosis or a patch across the pulmonary valve annulus, the latter causing pulmonary regurgitation and right-ventricular dysfunction.

In a child who was very cyanosed, postoperative bleeding may be due to the physiological compensation which reduces the tendency for intravascular thrombosis in the presence of a high haematocrit. Platelet transfusion may be required for platelet dysfunction. Pleural effusion and ascites are frequent, due to high right-atrial pressure, and may interfere with gas exchange. Ascites also impairs venous return and cardiac output. Prophylactic drainage of the peritoneal cavity in Fallot's tetralogy reduces the incidence of postoperative haemodynamic instability. Pleural effusions are drained as necessary through a small-bore intercostal catheter.

Fontan procedure

After this operation, lung blood-flow and cardiac output (CO) are proportional to right-atrial pressure (RAP) minus left-atrial pressure (LAP) divided by pulmonary vascular resistance (PVR). If PVR increases, either CO decreases or RAP rises. If LAP increases, either CO decreases or RAP rises. Increased RAP causes congestion and dysfunction of the liver, pleural and pericardial effusions, ascites and oedema of the lung, chest wall and brain. After most Fontan operations, the RAP is 12–15 mmHg. To reduce pulmonary vascular resistance, the patient should be weaned from mechanical ventilation

as soon as stable (4–6 hours after operation), but hypoxaemia and hypercarbia should be avoided. The patient is nursed with head and feet raised. Effusions and ascites should be drained, and the losses replaced with 5% albumin in saline and fresh frozen plasma. Fluid intake is usually restricted to 50% of maintenance requirements for several weeks. In the first 3 days after operation, intake is restricted to 25 ml/kg/day. Paralyic ileus may last for several days and parenteral nutrition may be required after the second postoperative day for adequate nutrition. Bleeding may occur from long suture lines; clotting factors should be monitored. These patients usually require infusions of inotropic and vasodilator drugs for several days after the operation.

Switch operation for transposition of the great vessels

Coronary artery obstruction due to compression, twist or air may cause impaired contractility, premature ventricular contractions and raised ST segments. ECG and cardiac output are monitored closely. The coronary artery implantation occasionally needs urgent revision. Prolonged aortic clamping may also reduce myocardial contractility.

Pulmonary hypertension (see above) is an occasional problem in children with transposition and VSD. Most of these infants may be weaned from mechanical ventilation by 24–48 hours after operation, and most require inotropic drug infusion and vasodilator drugs such as phenoxybenzamine.

As a general rule, infants and children who have had cardiac surgery need careful monitoring, frequent assessment and prompt treatment of complications as and when they occur.

REFERENCES

1 Hickey P.R., Hansen D.D., Cramolini G.M., Vincent R.N., Lang P. Pulmonary and systemic hemodynamic responses to ketamine in infants with normal and elevated pulmonary vascular resistance. *Anesthesiology* 1985, **62**, 287–293.

2 Tanner G.E., Angers M.D., Barash P.G., Mulla A., Miller P.L., Rothstein P. Effect of left-to-right, mixed left-to-right, and right-to-left shunts on inhalational anesthetic induction in children: a computer model. *Anesth Analg* 1985, **64**, 101–107.

3 Hickey P.R., Hansen D.D., Strafford M., Thompson J.E., Jonas R.E., Mayer J.E. Pulmonary and systemic hemodynamic effects of nitrous oxide in infants with normal and elevated pulmonary vascular resistance. *Anesthesiology* 1986, **65**, 374–378.

4 Gelman S., Reves J.G., Fowler B.S., Samuelson P.N., Lell W.A., Smith L.R. Regional blood flow during cross-clamping of the thoracic aorta and infusion of sodium nitroprusside. *J Thorac Cardiovasc Surg* 1983, **85**, 287–291.

5 French MAC. Immunodeficiency. In: Oh T.E. (Ed), *Intensive care manual*, 3rd ed. (1990) Butterworths, London, pp. 392–400.

FURTHER READING

Burrows F.A., Klinck J.R., Rabinovich M., Bohn D.J. Pulmonary hypertension in children: perioperative management. *Canad Anaes Soc J* 1986, **33**, 606.

Ehyai A., Fenichel G.M., Bender H.W. Incidence and prognosis of seizures in infants after cardiac surgery with profound hypothermia and circulatory arrest. *JAMA* 1984, **252**, 3165.

Freeman R., Gould F.K. *Infection in cardiothoracic intensive care*. (1987) Edward Arnold, London.

Fyman P.N., Goodman K., Casthely P.A., Griepp R.B., Ergin A., Smith P. Anesthetic management of patients undergoing Fontan procedure. *Anesth Analg* 1986, **65**, 516.

Jones R.D.M., Duncan A.E., Mee R.B.B. Perioperative management of neonatal aortic isthmic coarctation. *Anaes Intens Care* 1985, **13**, 311.

Lowe E.E. Postoperative cardiac care. In: Lake C.L. *Pediatric cardiac anesthesia*. (1988) Appleton and Lange, East Norwalk, Connecticut, pp. 407–439.

Steward D.J. Afterload: non-surgical manipulation of the failing circulation. In: Swerdlow D.B., Raphaely R.C. *Cardiovascular problems in pediatric critical care*. (1986) Churchill Livingstone, Edinburgh, pp. 221–228.

14: Neurosurgical Anaesthesia

Physiology
  Intracranial pressure
  Cerebrospinal fluid
  Cerebral blood flow
  Cerebral venous pressure

Pathophysiology
  Intracranial pressure
  Cerebrospinal fluid
  Cerebral blood flow
  Regional cerebral blood flow
  Brain volume

Control of intracranial pressure
  Ventilation
  Cerebral dehydration
  Steroids
  Posture
  Drugs
  Hypothermia

Preoperative assessment

Anaesthetic management
  Premedication
  Anaesthesia and the choice of drugs
  The airway
  Ventilation
  Intravenous infusion and blood loss
  Prevention of injury to eyes and nerves

Posture
  Supine
  Prone
  Lateral
  Sitting

Monitoring
  Clinical signs
  The stethoscope
  Pulse oximeter
  Capnography
  Blood pressure
  Central venous pressure
  Temperature
  ECG
  Doppler flow detector

Air embolism

Neurosurgical conditions
  Hydrocephalus
  Subdural haematoma
  Extradural haematoma
  Skull fractures
  Intracranial space-occupying lesions
  Vascular malformations and aneurysms
  Moyamoya disease
    Treatment
    Anaesthesia
  Myelomeningocoele
  Encephalocoele
  Craniostenosis
  Spinal surgery

Postoperative care
  Monitoring
  Fluids
  Position
  Analgesia
  Treatment of convulsions
  Steroids

Special problems
  Inappropriate antidiuretic hormone secretion
  Diabetes insipidus

PHYSIOLOGY

Intracranial pressure

The cranium, lined with dura mater, contains the brain, cerebrospinal fluid (CSF) and the blood in the cerebral vessels. The interaction of the volumes of these determine the intracranial pressure in the closed skull. When the skull is open, the contents are exposed to atmospheric pressure and the intracranial pressure will fall. The factors influencing brain bulk and cerebral blood flow are still important in determining the operating conditions for intracranial surgery. It is difficult to retract a swollen or engorged brain to gain access to deeper pathology and to close the skull if the intracranial contents are not reduced in volume. CSF becomes less important because it drains away or can be aspirated.

206

Cerebrospinal fluid

The majority of CSF is formed by the choroid plexus in the ventricles. Some is derived from interstitial fluid which drains transependymally into the ventricles. The rate of production is constant and independent of intracranial pressure (ICP) up to 200 mmHg (26.6 kPa). It is reabsorbed through coiled microtubules in the arachnoid villi, and the rate of reabsorption is dependent on the pressure gradient between CSF and the pressure in the venous sinuses. The minimum pressure gradient required for reabsorption is 5.4 mmHg (0.7 kPa), and at greater pressure gradients the rate of reabsorption is linearly related to the gradient. CSF pressure varies with arterial and venous blood pressures and respiration, and is therefore influenced by the pattern of ventilation.

If intracranial volume increases, the pressure increase is limited by:

1 a reduction in intracranial blood volume by compression of veins;
2 a shift of CSF to the spinal subdural space which can increase its volume by compressing epidural veins,
3 an increased CSF reabsorption.

Cerebral blood flow

Cerebral (brain) blood flow is very sensitive to changes in Pa_{CO_2}, responding to hypercapnia with vasodilatation and an increase in cerebral (intracranial) blood volume and intracranial pressure. A reduction in Pa_{CO_2} causes cerebral vasoconstriction with a reduction in blood volume and intracranial pressure, which is the basis for the use of hyperventilation during neurosurgical anaesthesia.

Cerebral blood flow and intracranial pressure increase with hypoxia when the Pa_{O_2} falls below 50 mmHg (6.6 kPa). There is a slight decrease in cerebral blood flow when the Pa_{O_2} is raised.

Autoregulation is the mechanism whereby changes in arterial pressure between 50 mmHg (6.6 kPa) and 160 mmHg (21.3 kPa) are compensated by varying cerebral arteriolar tone, so that cerebral blood flow is maintained constant. Autoregulation may be abolished or disturbed by trauma, tumour, haemorrhage or following a phase of induced hypotension. It may also be modified by anaesthesia. In these circumstances, hypertension causes increased cerebral blood flow, intracranial pressure rises and cerebral oedema can develop.

Cerebral perfusion pressure is the difference between mean arterial blood pressure and intracranial pressure. In abnormal situations where intracranial pressure rises and/or blood pressure decreases, cerebral perfusion pressure may decline to a critical level where cerebral perfusion decreases and may finally cease. Vasodilating a patient thus lowering the blood pressure in the presence of cerebral oedema and raised intracranial pressure, may therefore be disastrous.

Cerebral venous pressure

An increase in intrathoracic pressure or central venous pressure can increase intracranial pressure directly by increasing cerebral venous pressure, and indirectly by distending the epidural veins which compress the dura and spinal CSF. Increases in intrathoracic pressure, for example due to coughing or crying, will thus cause a rise in CSF pressure.

When ventilation is controlled, the pattern of ventilation is important in determining the intracranial pressure, due to its influence on intrathoracic and hence venous pressure.

PATHOPHYSIOLOGY

Intracranial pressure

While intracranial pressure is low, slight changes in volume of one component of the cranial contents can be compensated by an opposite change in another. Cerebral swelling or mass, for example, can be compensated by decreasing intracranial CSF or blood volume. When further compensation is not possible, the critical volume is reached and intracranial pressure will rise (Fig. 14.1). Patients with intracranial pathology who are approaching this point are at great risk of developing cerebral ischaemia or coning through the tentorium or foramen magnum, resulting in compression of the vital centres. The aim in neurosurgical anaesthesia should be to avoid further rises and preferably induce a reduction in intracranial pressure.

The clinical features of raised intracranial pressure include headache, irritability, alteration in conscious state, vomiting, papilloedema, and when severe, bradycardia, hypertension, pupillary changes and respiratory depression. Infants and small children can expand their intracranial volume while the fontanelles and cranial sutures are open, and this affords them a greater margin of safety. Bulging of the fontanelle, which accommodates

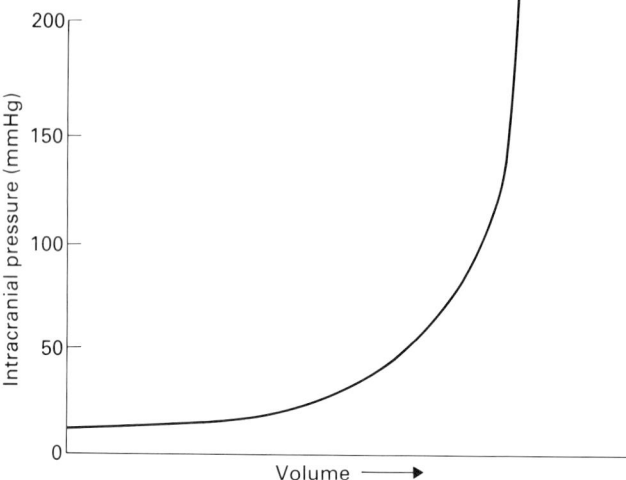

Fig. 14.1 Intracranial pressure–volume curve showing the relationship between intracranial pressure and volume of intracranial contents. This illustrates that a point is reached as volume increases where a small change results in a large rise in pressure.

some increase in intracranial volume, and proptosis, indicate that intracranial pressure is rising. Chronically raised intracranial pressure results in separation of the cranial sutures.

Cerebrospinal fluid

CSF volume can be increased by obstruction to flow in its normal pathways, by increased production or by impaired reabsorption through the arachnoidal villi into the venous sinuses. Raised venous pressure with arteriovenous malformations of the great vein of Galen results in decreased absorption of CSF. This leads to hydrocephalus. Increased production of CSF is rare, but may occur with choroid plexus papilloma.

Most infants with hydrocephalus have obstruction to CSF flow. There may be no communication between the subarachnoid space and the ventricles, which become distended, or the ventricles may communicate with the basal cisterns with obstruction between these and the subarachnoid villi in the region of the sagittal sinus. These obstructions may result from developmental abnormalities, or following infection or haemorrhage causing arachnoiditis, or be due to compression by tumour.

Cerebral blood flow

The cerebral blood flow can be increased by a raised Pa_{CO_2}. The increase which occurs in infants with, for example, bronchiolitis, can result in signs of raised intracranial pressure such as bulging of the fontanelle and, sometimes, proptosis.

Arteriovenous malformations in the brain cause a hyperdynamic circulation and increase cerebral blood flow.

Haemorrhage leading to hypovolaemia causes a reduction in arterial blood pressure and cardiac output, but cerebral and myocardial blood flow is preserved at the expense of other organs. Eventually compensation fails, cerebral perfusion pressure becomes inadequate for tissue perfusion and cerebral ischaemia results.

Regional cerebral blood flow

This is modified by local metabolism, CO_2 production and acidosis. In some pathological situations, the vessels in the affected area become unresponsive to the normal controlling factors such as CO_2. Blood flow may be adequate at rest, but if Pa_{CO_2} rises there is a relative increase in blood flow to the normal parts of the brain, while the unresponsive area does not increase its flow, which may reach a critically low level. This phenomenon of diversion of the blood away from an area with poor cerebrovascular control is known as cerebral 'steal'. Alternatively, when the patient is hyperventilated and Pa_{CO_2} is reduced, the abnormal part will receive a relatively greater proportion of the blood flow.

Brain volume

The volume of the brain can be increased by a tumour, cyst, abscess and by intracerebral bleeding. Also, trauma, cerebral ischaemia and water intoxication may cause cerebral oedema and brain swelling. In some patients following trauma, the swelling is due to hyperaemia and increased blood volume [1]. The resulting increase in volume may raise the intracranial pressure, causing symptoms.

CONTROL OF INTRACRANIAL PRESSURE

Several methods are available to reduce intracranial pressure. The volume of CSF can be reduced by aspiration; intracranial blood volume or brain bulk can be reduced by the methods outlined below. Some of these are commonly employed before, during, and after operation.

Ventilation

Hyperventilation is used to reduce Pa_{CO_2} and produce cerebral vasoconstriction. Nothing is gained by reducing Pa_{CO_2} below 25 mmHg (3.3 kPa) and it is probable that below 20 mmHg (2.7 kPa), cerebral oxygenation may be impaired.

Cerebral dehydration

Cerebral dehydration is achieved by raising plasma osmolality, thereby drawing interstitial and subsequently intracellular water out of the brain and into the circulation. The benefit of agents such as mannitol is derived from their osmotic diuretic effect, where they carry the extra water out in the urine. Urea also has an osmotic diuretic effect but its small molecule may diffuse into the brain, drawing water with it. This phenomenon of osmotically active particles drawing water back into the dehydrated brain is referred to as 'rebound' brain swelling. If a large piece of brain is resected this does not matter, but otherwise it will have detrimental effects on the patient.

Mannitol is now used in a dose of 0.5–1.5 g/kg intravenously. The first half of the dose is given quickly over 10–15 minutes and the remainder more slowly. When used during intracranial surgery, the infusion is begun while the skull is being opened. The effect lasts 4–5 hours and significant rebound does not occur. The dose can be repeated unless the patient has cardiovascular disease or is in renal failure. Cardiac failure may be precipitated if too much intracellular water is drawn into the circulation. The degree of initial brain 'shrinkage' with mannitol is not as great as with the previously popular urea, but it does not share with the latter the problems of rebound or local irritation and thrombosis at the site of infusion. Urea is now rarely used.

Glycerol has also been employed as an osmotic diuretic. It has the advantages of simplicity, no rebound or marked alteration of fluid and electrolyte balance even after prolonged use, and it provides calories because it is metabolized. It may cause haemolysis and haemoglobinuria when given intravenously. It can be given orally but it may cause nausea.

Other diuretics such as frusemide are becoming more popular because their effect does not require an intact blood–brain barrier, and they also decrease the rate of CSF production.

Steroids

Steroids have a beneficial effect on cerebral oedema, particularly that surrounding malignant tumours. They are no longer considered useful after trauma as they do not improve outcome unless given before the injury. They are usually begun preoperatively and continued into the postoperative period in cerebral tumour surgery. Dexamethasone is the most commonly used (0.1–0.2 mg/kg).

Posture

Head-up tilt or the sitting position can be used to improve cerebral venous drainage, but the possibility of air embolism is also increased. If venous pressure is high, this may minimize or prevent the resulting rise in intracranial pressure. Some elevation of the head is usual postoperatively, as well as after head injury. In the latter group, continuous positive airway pressure may improve ventilation in the patient who also has chest injuries, and some head-up tilt might be enough to compensate for the raised central venous pressure.

Drugs

Transient rises in intracranial pressure may be reduced by a bolus of thiopentone or lignocaine.

Hypothermia

Intracranial pressure may be lowered by hypothermia. This may be due to a decreased Pa_{CO_2} and hyperglycaemia, which often occurs to a level where glycosuria and an osmotic diuretic effect results (see Chapter 24).

PREOPERATIVE ASSESSMENT

The assessment of a child before a neurosurgical procedure should include an appraisal of his neurological status and general condition. The timing of surgery will be influenced by the patient's condition, the nature of the operation planned and its urgency.

Children for elective, non-urgent surgery require general preoperative assessment as for other operations. Before anaesthesia for investigations or operation, it is important to determine whether there is evidence of raised intracranial pressure, which should alert the anaesthetist to take special care to avoid raising the pressure further and to take steps to reduce it. Dexamethasone may benefit patients with cerebral tumours, while hyperventilation and diuretics may help to lower intracranial pressure when anaesthesia is induced.

Some neurosurgical procedures should be undertaken urgently to avoid irreversible brain damage or death. Distortion of the brain by an expanding mass or collection of blood herniates brain tissue through the tentorial hiatus or the foramen magnum. The most important sign of tentorial herniation is a progressive decline in the conscious state. This is the most reliable sign of damage to the reticular activating system, and it may be accompanied by changes in reactivity of the pupils and extra-ocular movements, as well as motor and sensory signs such as extensor plantar responses. Herniation at the foramen magnum is likely to result in depression of respiration and circulation, together with motor and sensory signs.

If any or all of the above develop, immediate investigation and treatment are needed. If these signs are ignored, the changes can cause permanent neurological damage or death.

The advent of CT scanning has made assessment of the pathology and site of the lesion more accurate. Repeat scans can be used to assess the response if necessary.

If unconsciousness following head injury is prolonged, brain damage is likely to be serious and may be complicated by intracranial haemorrhage. It is essential to assess the patient frequently, looking for changing levels of consciousness or signs of increasing intracranial pressure and possible herniation. After trauma, the steps outlined in Chapter 26 for assessment and management should be followed, paying attention to the airway, blood loss and other injuries as well as the neurological state. In infants, a significant amount of blood can collect under the intact scalp, and the extent of blood loss may not be immediately apparent. Blood loss must be treated promptly, as hypotension may lead to inadequate cerebral perfusion if intracranial pressure is raised. From the anaesthetist's point of view head injuries fall into three categories:

1 Closed head injury that does not require operation, but complicates other injuries for which general anaesthesia is necessary. The anaesthetist must remember that intracranial complications such as subdural haematoma and cerebral oedema can develop during surgery. Ideally these children should be assessed preoperatively by a neurosurgeon and, if possible, anaesthesia should be delayed 4–6 hours after the injury, until the patient's neurological state has stabilized, although this may not be possible when the operation for other conditions is urgent. It should be kept in mind that if epidural anaesthesia is used intracranial pressure may rise, possibly due to displacement of spinal CSF into the head.

2 Open or compound head injury or depressed fracture clearly need surgery. Unless there is uncontrolled bleeding, this is not an acute emergency and these patients usually benefit from preoperative resuscitation and stabilization until better anaesthetic and operating conditions are available.

3 Cerebral compression due to subdural, extradural or intracerebral haemorrhage. This is a real emergency and these children should be operated upon immediately. If there is easy access to a CT scanner, it may be helpful to have a scan on the way to the operating theatre unless there is danger of permanent damage or death as a result of the delay. If necessary, the anaesthetic can be started prior to the scan and the patient is intubated so that ventilation can be controlled during this critical period. Sometimes an unconscious patient may be intubated before or on arrival at the hospital.

Subdural haematomata in infants may be treated by aspiration. Resuscitation should continue while the haematoma is decompressed.

In the presence of intracranial bleeding, rapid reduction of intracranial pressure by osmotic diuretics may allow further bleeding to occur.

A rare complication of head injury is the development of severe vasoconstriction, leading to acute hypertension precipitating left-ventricular failure and pulmonary oedema. Central sympathetic hyperactivity following injury in or around the hypothalamus is the probable mechanism. The aim of treatment should be either to improve left-ventricular performance with a β_1-adrenergic agonist (isoprenaline infusion) and IPPV, or to reduce the afterload by vasodilatation [2]. The latter should be used only after careful assessment and consideration, because the reduction in blood pressure following vasodilatation will result in a decrease in cerebral perfusion in the presence of cerebral oedema, leading to cerebral ischaemia. Phenoxybenzamine, which is a long-acting alpha-adrenergic blocker, will cause some peripheral vasodilatation without causing cerebral vasodilatation. For this reason it is better than direct vasodilators such as sodium nitroprusside. It can be given in increments to normovolaemic patients, to produce some vasodilatation and a decrease in blood pressure which may not compromise cerebral perfusion. A dose of 0.5 mg/kg in children usually lowers the blood pressure by 15−25%.

ANAESTHETIC MANAGEMENT

Premedication

The preoperative visit is an opportunity to gain the confidence of the conscious child. Premedication should help to calm and sedate the patient.

Preoperative respiratory depressant analgesics are avoided in the presence of raised intracranial pressure. Most anaesthetists, if they are going to use premedication, prefer to use a tranquillizer or sedative which does not cause respiratory depression and an elevation in Pa_{CO_2}. These restrictions on premedication do not apply to extracranial and spinal operations.

Antisialagogues are often used in premedication or at induction because the presence of secretions in the respiratory tract, especially in the narrow airways of infants, can cause partial respiratory obstruction. Attempts to aspirate secretions may stimulate coughing, with a resulting rise in intracranial pressure.

Anaesthesia and the choice of drugs

A smooth induction is desirable because crying will raise intracranial pressure. An inhalation induction is acceptable in infants if the fontanelle and sutures are still open, otherwise an intravenous induction with thiopentone is preferred. The discomfort of the venepuncture can be minimized by the application of EMLA (eutectic mixture of local anaesthetics) cream at the venepuncture site at least an hour before operation.

Thiopentone has the advantage that it reduces cerebral metabolic rate and cerebral blood flow, and hence intracranial pressure. The vasoconstrictor effect appears to be associated with the thio (sulphur) component as it does not occur with the oxybarbiturate analogue, pentobarbitone.

Vecuronium has been recommended as the muscle relaxant with the least cardiovascular effect for use during induction, but the longer-acting relaxants have been used satisfactorily in children. If mild hypotension is considered desirable, alcuronium or D-tubocurarine can be used.

Attenuation of the hypertensive response to intubation may not be as critical in children as in older patients, but intravenous lignocaine, additional thiopentone or fentanyl may help to smooth intubation. With extracranial procedures or infants with open sutures, this is less critical.

The inhalation agent of choice is isoflurane. It reduces cerebral metabolism and causes less cerebral vasodilatation, and hence rise in intracranial pressure, than halothane or enflurane. It can reduce cerebral perfusion pressure by lowering peripheral vascular resistance. It is a useful agent if hypotension is desired because it can easily be achieved by increasing the inspired concentration. It also reduces the muscle relaxant requirement by about 40%.

The preferred anaesthetic for head-injured patients remains controversial. After periods of ischaemia, unsupplemented nitrous oxide may worsen the outcome while isoflurane in concentrations over 2% offers some protection. Barbiturates do not improve overall outcome, although they may lower raised intracranial pressure and reduce cerebral metabolism.

Halothane can increase intracranial pressure by cerebral vasodilatation and, although there is some evidence that this rise is temporary, it is undesirable for induction if the child's intracranial pressure is approaching the critical point where increased volume causes a marked rise in pressure (Fig. 14.1).

Anaesthesia may be maintained with an intravenous infusion of thiopentone or propofol, inhalation agents such as nitrous oxide and/or isoflurane, intravenous analgesics such as fentanyl, or a combination of these.

Total intravenous anaesthesia with thiopentone may result in delayed awakening, but after total doses of 10 mg/kg thiopentone given over 2−3 hours, children usually awaken promptly at the conclusion of anaesthesia. Propofol is more rapidly metabolized. It does not produce a prolonged effect due to active metabolites as occurs with thiopentone, but it has a very wide variation in dose requirement between individuals and is significantly more expensive.

Intravenous opioids can be used, but their administration and dosage should be adjusted so that they do not cause postoperative respiratory depression and do not affect pupillary reflexes and hence the neurological assessment of the patient. Morphine can be used if given at the beginning of the operation, but fentanyl is generally considered to be more satisfactory. The incidence of postoperative vomiting is increased after the use of opioids and sometimes occurs during emergence at the conclusion of anaesthesia.

Neurosurgeons often inject the site of the incision with local anaesthetic (logically a longer-acting drug such as bupivacaine) with adrenaline 1:200 000. This reduces bleeding and provides analgesia of the scalp, but temporarily increases blood pressure. Anaesthesia may need to be supplemented as the skull is opened and during closure at the end, but the intracranial part of the operation is not painful. Thiopentone can be given just before the brain is retracted, to provide additional cerebral protection, especially if the retractors are expected to be in place for some time.

At the conclusion of anaesthesia the pharynx should be aspirated and the relaxants reversed with neostigmine and atropine. Following intracranial surgery, the tube should be removed before the child's airway becomes reactive, as coughing will cause a rise in intracranial pressure. In the few cases where it is planned to ventilate the patient postoperatively, the tube is left in place. In these cases an intracranial pressure monitor is desirable because the clinical signs of raised intracranial pressure are masked.

The airway

In neurosurgical anaesthesia, it is of utmost importance that the airway is clear and unobstructed. This requires intubation, ensuring that the tube does not become kinked, and adequate fixation so that the tube does not become dislodged. An oral RAE or 'south' Portex tube which is moulded to pass down over the chin, a polyvinyl chloride (PVC) Magill or an armoured tube which is non-kinking can be used. If it is placed exactly in the midline and passed straight back over the middle of the tongue, which is soft, kinking is less likely, even when the neck is flexed (Fig. 14.2) than when the tube is placed in the corner of the mouth and passed over the side of the jaw. Nasotracheal intubation with a PVC tube allows easier fixation.

Most neurosurgical anaesthetists have their own technique for strapping tubes to ensure fixation. The use of benzoin tincture on the skin increases adhesion and protects the skin. Before applying tape, some people tie a piece of cotton around the tube to anchor it at the appropriate place (Fig. 14.3a). Many anaesthetists prefer a waterproof tape which is less likely to become unstuck (Fig. 14.3b,c). Excessive salivation in the prone position can reduce the adhesiveness of strapping and increase the likelihood of accidental extubation. A piece of elastoplast covering all the tape and attached to the

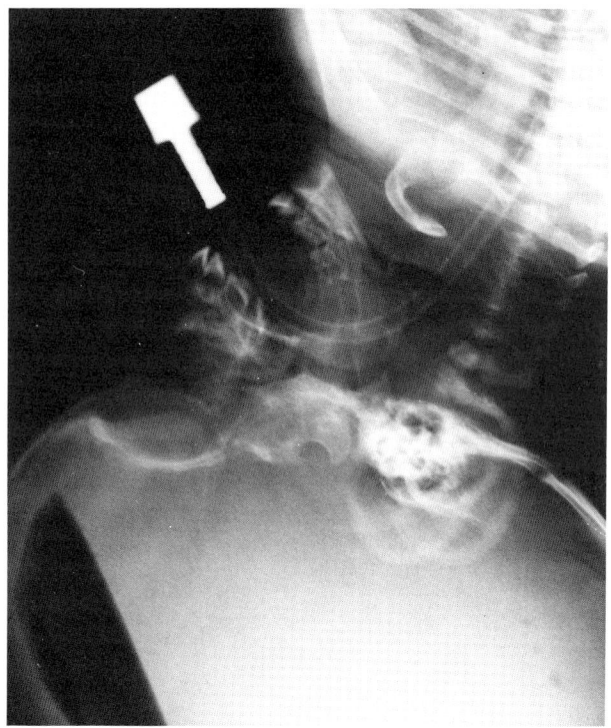

Fig. 14.2 A lateral X-ray to show that an orotracheal tube placed in the midline does not kink when the neck is flexed.

face almost to the ears will prevent this (Fig. 14.3d).

When the patient is prone, the head may be held by tongs or placed in a head rest. It is important when fixing the tube and attached breathing system to the head support or table, to ensure that the breathing system does not drag on the tube, thereby causing extubation. If the head sinks into the head rest, the tube may be pushed into a bronchus if it is fixed to a rigid structure. This will result in inadequate CO_2 elimination and distension of the cerebral vessels. It is wise to fix the breathing system where the expiratory limb is compressible, to avoid this problem (Fig. 14.4).

Ventilation

Most anaesthetists and neurosurgeons now prefer moderate hyperventilation during craniotomy, so that the resulting cerebral vasoconstriction helps to reduce 'brain bulk'. Occasionally a surgeon may prefer his patients to be breathing spontaneously during posterior fossa surgery, so that both respiration and ECG can be used to monitor the approach to the brain stem. The choice should be agreed upon beforehand.

Listening to the breath sounds with a stethoscope and

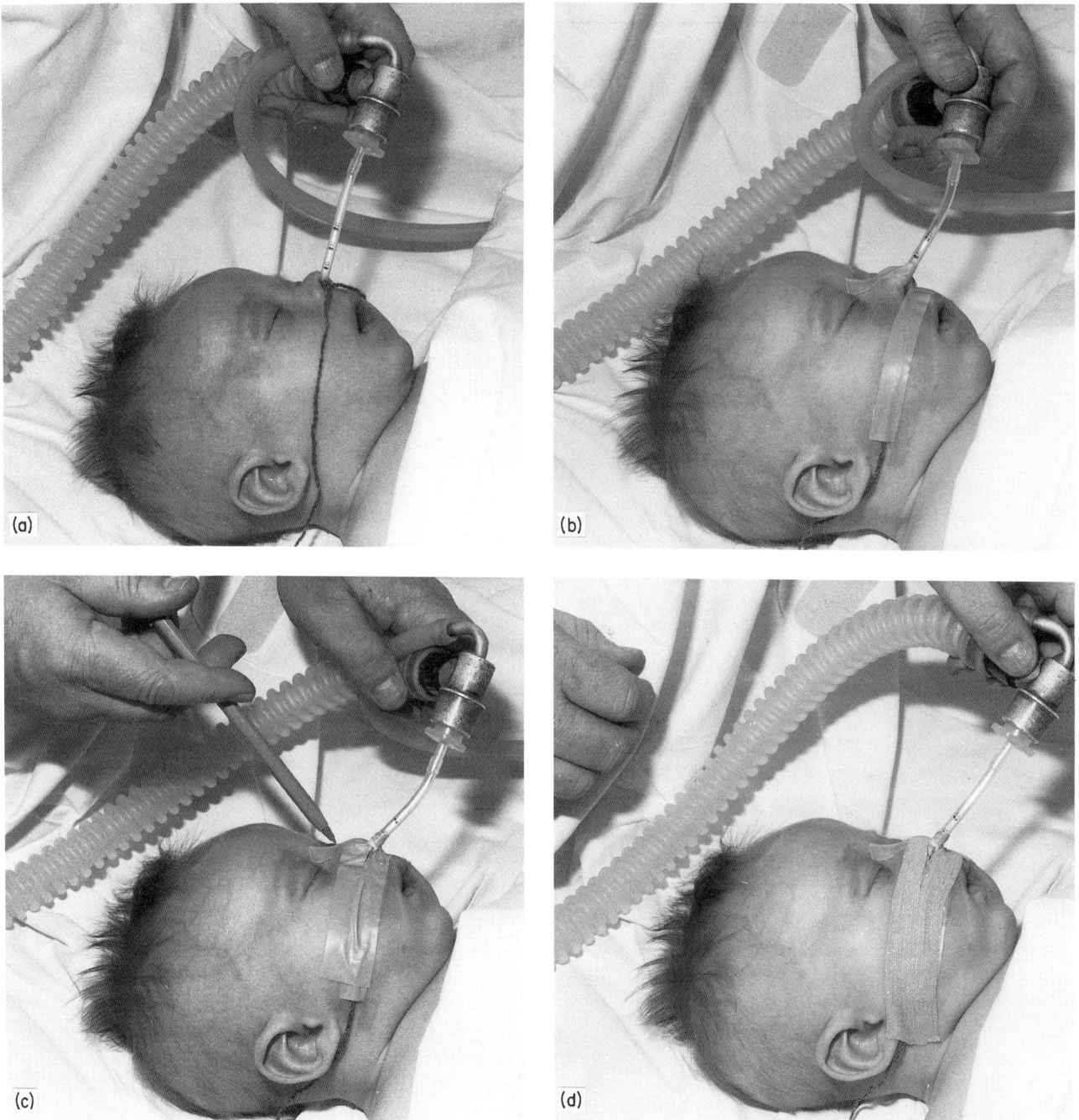

Fig. 14.3 Strapping a nasotracheal tube. (a) A thread is tied around the tube at an appropriate point to mark the correct position and to act as an anchor. (b) The first piece of waterproof strapping, which has been split down the middle, is laid so that one leg holds the thread in place and the other is wound round the tube and up the nose to provide counter-traction from a downward pull. (c) A second piece of split tape is laid over the nose and the other limb is wound round the tube and over on to the other side of the face. In this way the nasal strapping is secured to prevent dislodgement by a downward pull. (d) The tape is covered by a piece of elastoplast with a hole in the middle, attached so that it reaches the face beyond the edge of the waterproof tape, thereby giving extra adhesion.

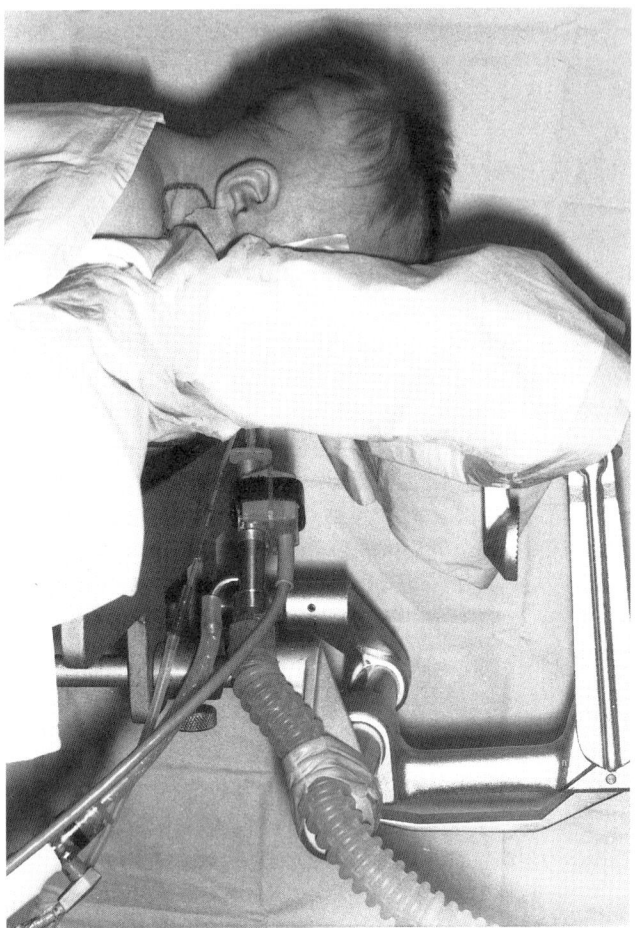

Fig. 14.4 The head placed in a head ring with padding to prevent pressure on the face. The endotracheal tube can be seen fixed into the capnograph sensor, which is then attached to the breathing system. Note that the breathing system is attached to the supports by a compressible part of the tubing. This prevents the tube being forced endobronchially if the head sinks into the head ring, which can occur if the breathing system is attached at a rigid point. An oesophageal stethoscope is also in place. It is important to ensure adequate padding so that pressure areas do not develop on the face, especially during long operations or when hypotension is used.

observing the chest movement allows the anaesthetist to assess the adequacy of ventilation. A capnograph is desirable to monitor ventilation and for air embolism. Capnograph readings can be checked by measuring Pa_{CO_2}. When the skull is opened, a bulging brain suggests that ventilation is inadequate, or occasionally that intrathoracic pressure is too high. This may occur with hand ventilation with a T-piece, when the pressure is not allowed to fall to zero in expiration.

The pattern of ventilation is especially important in intracranial and spinal surgery. Prolonged inspiration or high peak inspiratory pressure raises mean intrathoracic pressure, causing venous congestion. To avoid this, inspiration should be short relative to expiration and peak inspiratory pressure should not be excessive, but it must be sufficient to prevent hypercarbia. The once popular negative-pressure phase in expiration reduced venous congestion but is undesirable because it causes atelectasis and increases the chances of air embolism.

Intravenous infusion and blood loss

An intravenous infusion should be running during all intracranial operations and a large cannula should be inserted in any neurosurgical operation where the possibility of significant blood loss exists. It should be easily accessible to the anaesthetist. A right-atrial catheter positioned with X-ray control can be useful in the event of air embolus, because air can sometimes be aspirated from it. One should be considered for all major intracranial operations, especially when the patient is in the sitting position. It is also useful to measure central venous pressure as a guide to blood loss and replacement and to detect incipient circulatory overload.

Non-glucose containing electrolyte solutions should be used. Blood glucose tends to rise during surgery even when no glucose is given. Elevated glucose levels worsen the outcome following cerebral ischaemia or trauma.

Blood loss is difficult to estimate, because neurosurgeons frequently irrigate the wound. Although the methods commonly employed for assessing blood loss, including haemoglobin and haematocrit measurements, may be used, an intelligent estimate of losses based on observation and clinical signs, particularly a rising pulse rate, may be necessary as a guide to volume replacement.

Prevention of injury to eyes and nerves

Eye ointment may be used. The eyes should be closed and covered to prevent corneal abrasions. Vaseline may be used as an added protection to repel the solutions used for skin disinfection and prevent them from coming into contact with the eye (Fig. 14.5). Care should also be taken to avoid pressure on superficial cranial nerves and the eyes themselves. Adherent sponge is available to attach to the face to protect pressure areas. When a head rest is used, it should be well padded and the head positioned with care. The use of head tongs avoids these pressure problems. Positioning of the limbs so that peripheral nerves are not compressed is also important.

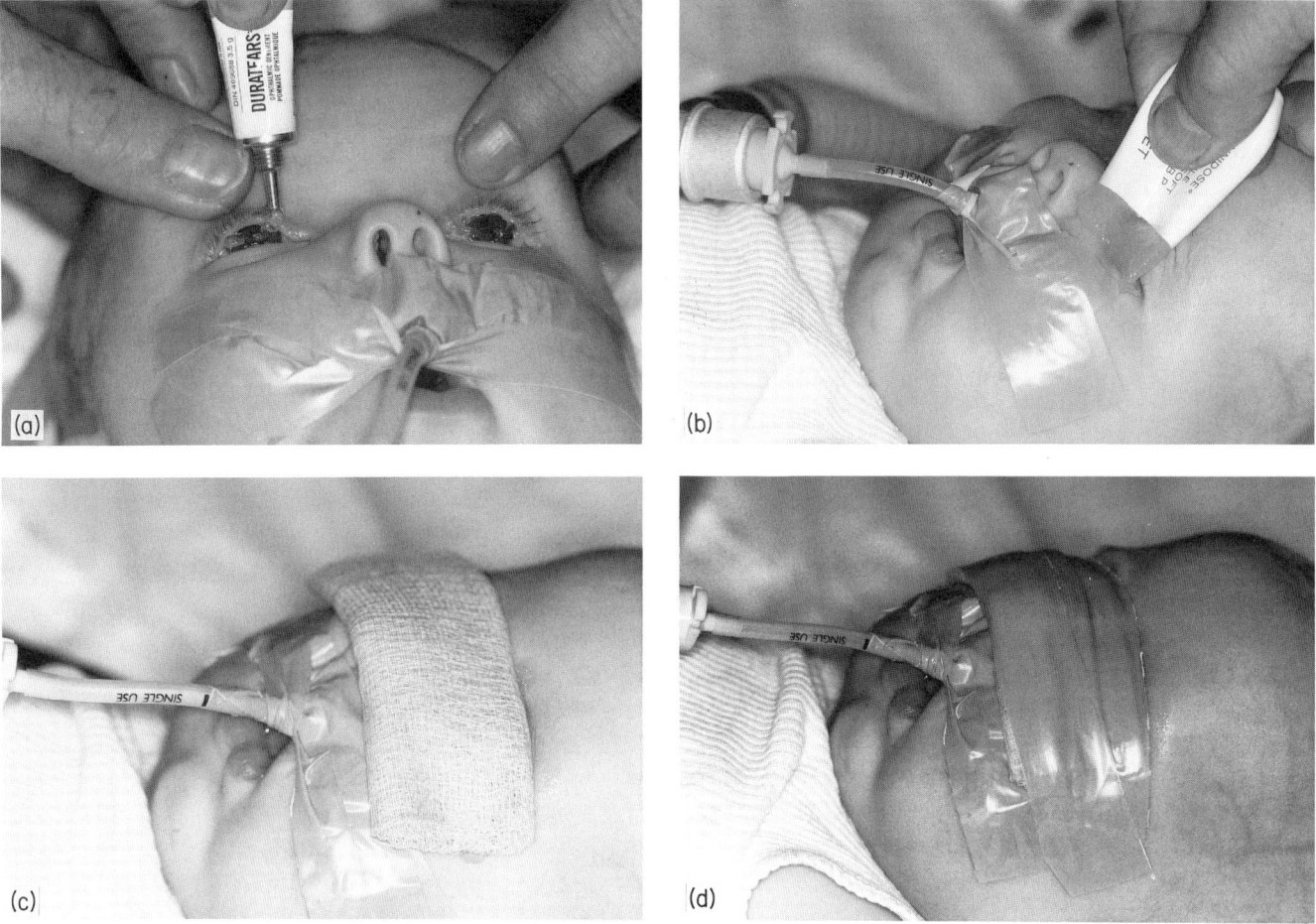

Fig. 14.5 Eye protection. (a) Ointment is placed in the eyes to prevent the cornea drying during a long procedure. (b) The eyelids are closed and vaseline placed over them to prevent antiseptic fluid gaining access to the cornea and conjunctiva. (c) A soft gauze pad is placed over this to prevent pressure being applied directly to the eyes. (d) This is covered with waterproof tape so that both pressure and access of irritant solutions is avoided. Note that the tube is placed centrally in the mouth so that it does not kink because it passes over the soft tongue in the midline.

POSTURE

The patient's position during a neurosurgical operation depends on the site of incision and the surgeon's preference. With some postures, head-up tilt may be used to facilitate cerebral venous drainage.

Supine

The anaesthetist is usually seated at the patient's side to allow free access to the head. The breathing system lies on the chest. The head may be turned to one side, so that the incision will be uppermost. Care must be taken to ensure that the neck veins are not obstructed. For ventriculoperitoneal shunts a sandbag is placed under

the shoulder to bring the neck forward, to allow easier passage of the trocar down over the chest wall to the abdomen.

Prone

Patients in the prone position are usually ventilated, but if the shoulders and iliac crests are supported to allow free respiratory movement, spontaneous respiration is acceptable in spinal surgery (see below). The support may be sandbags, rolled towels or a frame which has four supports to take the shoulders and iliac crests and can be adjusted to the size of the child. The latter has proved most satisfactory for bigger children (see Fig. 19.4). The knee−chest position is occasionally used for spinal surgery, where the flexion of the vertebral column separates the spines and laminae to provide good access and avoids compression of the abdominal wall.

Lateral

The anaesthetist and his equipment should be situated on the side of the table that the patient is facing for intracranial procedures. For spinal surgery in this position, the intravenous infusion should preferably be in the arm which is uppermost, because the venous return may be partially obstructed in the lower arm.

Sitting

The advantages of this position are good surgical access to the posterior fossa, gravity-aided cerebral venous drainage and a slight increase in the CSF accommodated in the spinal subarachnoid space. The problems are an increased danger of air embolism, pooling of blood with hypotension, and damage to the cervical spine. Bandaging the lower limbs helps to reduce peripheral pooling. Maintenance of body temperature is more difficult.

MONITORING

Clinical signs

Pulse, colour and peripheral perfusion should be observed. When hands and feet are not easily exposed, it may be necessary to use additional lighting so that a hand or foot can be adequately observed under drapes. Care must be taken to avoid contact between the light and the patient, especially if the table position is altered during the operation.

The stethoscope

The stethoscope is a simple, useful monitoring device which provides information on heart rate, rhythm and intensity of heart and breath sounds. The use of an oesophageal stethoscope is valuable in neurosurgical anaesthesia for the detection of air emboli, which cause an increase in the pulmonary second sound due to obstruction of the pulmonary arteries with air. A 'mill wheel' murmur may be heard when moderate volumes of air are aspirated. If a large volume of air is aspirated the murmur will disappear as cardiac output decreases.

Pulse oximeter

This should be a mandatory monitor, as it can give an audible warning of changes in oxygen saturation and pulse rate. It is particularly useful where the patient is covered with drapes.

Capnography

A capnograph is an important monitor in neurosurgery because of the importance of ensuring adequate ventilation, and because it is a sensitive monitor of air embolism. The expired CO_2 falls abruptly in proportion to the amount of air entrained.

Blood pressure

Blood pressure can be measured with a pressure transducer and arterial cannulation, a non-invasive blood pressure device or with a manually inflated cuff.

Postural changes influence blood pressure. This effect is maximal in the sitting position, when blood pools in the dependent parts of the body and cerebral arterial pressure may be lowered. This is not usually a clinical problem unless there is major blood loss, air embolism or hypotensive anaesthesia is being used. In the latter circumstance, intra-arterial pressure monitoring with the transducers set at head level will give an indication of cerebral arterial pressure.

Central venous pressure

Central venous catheters are more difficult to insert in infants and small children. A catheter in the right atrium may be useful for removing embolized air, measuring central venous pressure, as well as providing a line for infusion of fluids or blood.

Temperature

Maintenance of body temperature is a problem in neurosurgery because the operations are often prolonged and it is difficult to clothe the patient adequately. Wet drapes, which are sometimes used, tend to promote cooling by evaporation. It may be difficult to lie patients directly on warming blankets, particularly while prone with the shoulders and pelvis supported and in the sitting position.

Infants cool more readily than older patients. This

is particularly so in neurosurgery, where the head is exposed, because of its relatively greater surface area. Body temperature may fall several degrees unless some method is employed to maintain temperature. These include the use of a warm-water circulating blanket, warming and humidifying the inspired gases (see Chapter 3), wrapping the infant in cotton-wool, Mylar film (which is a plastic film impregnated with aluminium) (see Fig. 14.9b) or other plastic covering, and raising the operating theatre temperature. The use of an overhead heater during induction is worthwhile, especially in infants.

ECG

The ECG is an important monitor, particularly during posterior fossa surgery, when dysrhythmia may indicate that the surgeon is operating near vital brain-stem structures.

Doppler flow detector

A Doppler flow detector attached over the pulmonary artery is a very sensitive method of detecting air emboli, and will detect even small amounts which do not appear to cause significant clinical problems unless the child has a right-to-left shunt.

AIR EMBOLISM

Air embolism can occur when there is an open vein above atrial level and the venous pressure is low. This is most likely to occur with large veins or veins which are held open, as in bone, particularly in posterior fossa surgery in the sitting position. The head-up posture, whilst facilitating venous drainage so that the intracranial vessels do not distend, also facilitates air entry should a vein be opened. Any additional cause of decreased intrathoracic pressure will tend to suck air into an open vein.

A Doppler flow detector will sense even minute amounts of air in the veins. A capnograph is probably the most useful monitor for air embolism because the entrainment of significant amounts of air causes a fall in $FECO_2$ proportional to the amount of air entrained. A fall of 1% indicates an embolus of at least 1 ml/kg. A bolus of air tends to collect in the right side of the heart and produce an airlock, while with a slow infusion the air collects in the pulmonary arteries. The resulting diminution in pulmonary blood flow is associated with a

decrease in cardiac output and a fall in $FECO_2$. Central venous pressure rises, blood pressure falls and a compensatory tachycardia occurs — often an early sign of air embolus. A pulse oximeter will detect the tachycardia and decreasing oxygen saturation. Listening to a stethoscope, one may detect a loudening of the pulmonary second heart sound and sometimes a 'mill wheel' murmur, if sufficient air is aspirated and the cardiac output is not too low.

If a patent foramen ovale or right-to-left shunt is present, systemic air embolism can occur, with serious consequences if it goes to the coronary or cerebral circulation. The surgeon should be told as soon as an embolus is suspected, so that he can locate the open vein. He should flood the wound with saline. Pressure should be applied over the jugular veins if possible, and positive pressure should be applied to the airway to raise venous pressure until the offending vein is occluded. If nitrous oxide is in use it should be turned off, otherwise it will diffuse into the air bubbles and expand them. 100% oxygen should be used. If a central venous line is in place, immediate attempts should be made to aspirate the air. If successful, the abnormal signs will disappear, but quite often no air is obtained. The siting of the catheter tip is critical. If the cardiac output remains low, a positive inotrope infusion may help. Isoprenaline, being a β_1-adrenergic agonist and a pulmonary vasodilator, has advantages, at least theoretically, and it has been shown to be helpful in animal experiments. If these steps do not improve the patient's condition rapidly the patient should, if possible, be placed in the left lateral position, slightly head-down so that air can collect at the apex of the ventricle. This is usually impractical if the patient is in the sitting position.

NEUROSURGICAL CONDITIONS

Some of the conditions and their specific problems will be outlined in this section. The general principles of neurosurgical anaesthesia which are discussed above should be applied where appropriate.

Hydrocephalus

Hydrocephalus is usually due to obstruction to normal CSF flow resulting in increased volume and raised intracranial pressure. In infants this leads to enlargement of the head, bulging of the fontanelles and separation of the cranial sutures, but in older patients it may lead to an acute rise in intracranial pressure.

Hydrocephalus may be:

1 non-communicating, when there is obstruction to CSF flow within the pathways in the brain. This can be due to:

   (a) aqueduct stenosis between 3rd and 4th ventricles;

   (b) occlusion of the foramina of Luschka and Magendie;

   (c) tumours, cysts and vascular malformations compressing the CSF pathway, especially the aqueduct;

   (d) after certain inflammatory conditions.

2 Communicating hydrocephalus is the presence of ventricular enlargement due to obstruction of surface pathways outside the brain.

The common causes are congenital anomalies, inflammatory meningeal changes following haemorrhage or infection, and tumours.

The aim of surgical treatment is to provide a shunt through which the excess fluid can drain into a site from where it can be absorbed. The commonest shunt employed drains into the peritoneal cavity; other shunts drain into the right atrium (the lowest pressure part of the circulation), the pleural cavity and into the cisterna magna (Torkildsen shunt).

A ventriculoperitoneal shunt may drain the CSF from either lateral or fourth ventricle to the peritoneal cavity. The ventricular catheter is inserted through a burr hole, often on the right side. It is attached to a one-way valve,

which determines the pressure at which the CSF drains from the ventricle and can also be used as a pump. This is connected under the scalp to the peritoneal catheter, which may pass anteriorly or posteriorly over the chest wall before insertion into the peritoneal cavity through a small incision. A wedge or rolled towel under the shoulders makes it easier to pass the trocar subcutaneously from the head to the abdomen (Fig. 14.6). The advantage of this operation is that an additional length of tubing can be inserted, so that it does not need to be lengthened periodically during growth.

Ventriculoatrial shunts were popular but are now rarely used, because they needed repeated lengthening as the child grew and because embolization and pulmonary hypertension could develop. They are performed with the child supine and the head turned to the left side. A sponge-rubber wedge or rolled towel is placed under the neck to decrease the concavity and improve access to the common facial or internal jugular vein. The position of the tip of the catheter in the atrium is checked by X-ray or image intensifier.

The Torkildsen procedure (ventriculo-cisternostomy) is occasionally performed in older children to relieve non-communicating hydrocephalus. Spinoperitoneal shunt will relieve communicating hydrocephalus, but its popularity has waned due to a high incidence of complications and difficulty in assessing its function.

Further procedures may be required to relieve block-

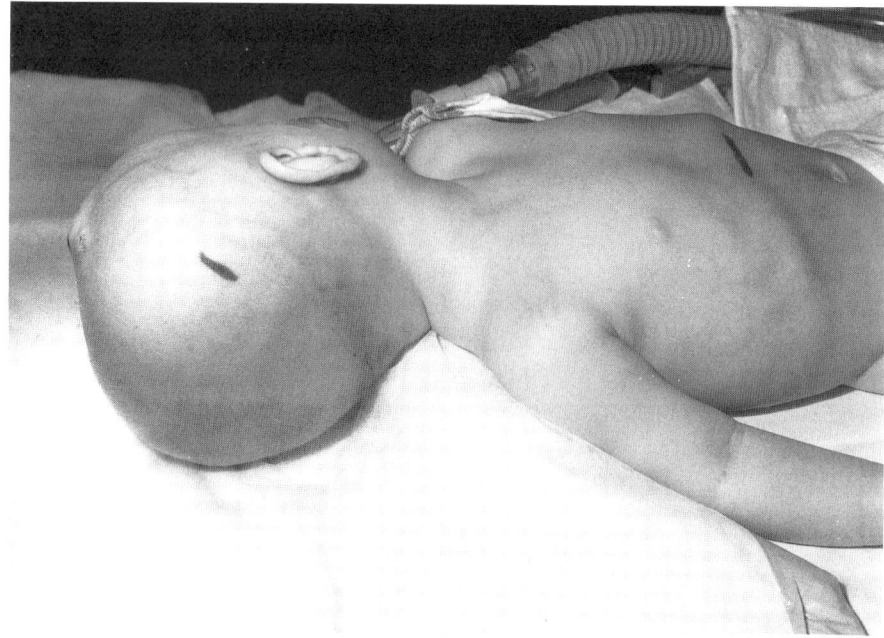

Fig. 14.6 Patient in position for a ventriculoperitoneal shunt with the head turned to one side. A rolled towel is placed under the shoulders to straighten the subcutaneous route for the passage of the trocar with the peritoneal tubing. The endotracheal tube is supported by a sandbag.

age, as part of the treatment ot shunt infection or for elective lengthening during growth, particularly of ventriculoatrial shunts. If a shunt blocks the child may become seriously ill, presenting with headache and vomiting due to the rising intracranial pressure. The obstruction must be relieved urgently.

Subdural haematoma

Subdural haemorrhage may occur at any age, but is commonest in children in the first year of life. Although trauma is the usual cause, thrombocyopenia is often an additional factor. Blood collects over the convexity of both cerebral hemispheres. The diagnosis is confirmed by ultrasound or CT scan. Subdural taps are the method of treatment to evacuate the fluid. This may be life-saving in acute traumatic subdural haemorrhage in infancy. In time, the blood changes to a yellow fluid which decreases in volume. In many infants repeated taps are the only treatment required, but in some patients surgical treatment such as burr-hole drainage or subdural—pleural or peritoneal shunt is necessary.

In the older child a chronic subdural haematoma may be evacuated through a burr hole, but for acute subdural haematoma a craniotomy is usually needed.

Extradural haematoma

Extradural haemorrhage in children can follow relatively mild trauma. The distortion of the thin skull at impact may tear meningeal vessels in the extradural space and lead to compression of the underlying brain. The features are a declining level of consciousness and the development of neurological signs, usually due to compression of brain structures herniating through the tentorium or the foramen magnum. A skull fracture is common but not invariable in children. If it crosses the course of the middle meningeal artery, the vessel may be traumatized and a haematoma may develop.

Progressive deterioration is an indication for urgent surgical decompression, because undue delay may result in irreversible neurological damage and death. An intravenous infusion should be running because haemorrhage may occur when the skull is opened. Blood should be cross-matched and available.

Skull fractures

A simple depressed fracture may require elevation if there is significant skull deformity. This is often a short procedure, especially in infants, where the skull is soft and can be easily elevated.

Skull fractures can be single or multiple and can be associated with trauma to the brain, meninges or blood vessels beneath the fracture. These injuries may be so severe as to be incompatible with survival. A CT scan is helpful in determining the degree of intracerebral damage. In some cases, particularly when CT scans are not available, burr holes may be made in the skull to exclude haemorrhage as the cause of unconsciousness, or to enable ventricular aspiration to relieve pressure.

Intracranial space-occupying lesions

These include tumours, cysts and abscesses. With the exception of leukaemia, the central nervous system is the commonest site of tumours in childhood. More than 40% present under the age of 5 years. More than 50% of these tumours are situated in the posterior cranial fossa and in the region of the third ventricle, causing obstruction to CSF flow and hydrocephalus. If intracranial pressure is increased, it may be relieved by shunting or drainage.

The principles of anaesthetic management have been outlined earlier. The control of intracranial pressure is of paramount importance. The posture required depends on the site of the lesion and, in posterior fossa surgery, is influenced by the surgeon's preference for either the sitting or prone position. The sitting position gives good access and facilitates cerebral venous drainage, but increases the possibility of air embolus. The prone position is now more widely used because the complications of air embolus and neck injury are less likely to occur.

When the sitting position is used, great care must be taken when posturing the patient. The head must be kept stable until it is fixed to the neurosurgical frame or head rest. The endotracheal tube must be strapped in carefully and the breathing system supported, so that accidental extubation does not occur. Fixation of the tube is easier with a nasotracheal tube. The blood pressure may drop when the patient sits up. This may be limited by bandaging the legs, administering intravenous fluids to fill the vascular volume and avoiding drugs with significant hypotensive action.

The intravenous infusion should be easily accessible to the anaesthetist. A central venous catheter should have a three-way tap attached so that it can be rapidly aspirated if an air embolus occurs. Intra-arterial pressure monitoring is desirable, so that changes in blood pressure can be observed instantaneously. The transducer should be set at head level so that the cerebral arterial pressure is monitored. This is particularly important should hypotension be used to reduce bleeding. Monitoring should include a pulse oximeter, stethoscope, capnograph and ECG, as well as arterial and central venous pressures.

The anaesthetist should warn the surgeon of the occurrence of dysrhythmia, marked changes in pulse or blood pressure, and alterations in respiration when the patient is breathing spontaneously, as these are indications that the surgery may be affecting the vital brain-stem centres.

Other intracranial operations are usually performed with the patient in the supine or lateral position (park bench) with the head positioned so that the operative site is uppermost. A sandbag under the shoulder may be helpful if the patient is supine and the head is turned to the side.

The anaesthetic should follow the principles outlined previously, but we have noted that some patients with cerebral tumours are resistant to some muscle relaxants, particularly D-tubocurarine. An additional dose may be required to hasten the onset of paralysis. In tumours at other sites, this phenomenon has been associated with malignancy, but with intracranial tumours the relationship has been less consistent.

Occasionally, bleeding becomes a problem and the surgeon may not be able to control its source because his view is obscured by blood. The anaesthetist then has the problem of keeping up with the blood loss. To avoid ending up with a massive transfusion and all parties stressed, a short period of induced hypotension will allow the surgeon to locate the bleeding point while the bleeding is diminished (see Chapter 23). The surgeon should pack the area and apply pressure, if feasible, to stop the bleeding, while the anaesthetist replaces the blood loss, if necessary, and then gives additional fluids before injecting a small dose of sodium nitroprusside in increments (50 mg is diluted in 500 ml and usually only a few ml of that is needed). As the pressure drops transiently the surgeon can locate and control the bleeding point. Bleeding can also be reduced by deepening isoflurane anaesthesia, but the transient action of sodium nitroprusside makes it ideal for overcoming this difficult problem.

Advances in intracranial surgery which influence the operation have seen the introduction and wider use of the operating microscope, the CUSA (Cavitron Ultrasonic Surgical Aspirator) which makes the dissection less traumatic, and stereotaxic location of tumours in association with CT scans. A special frame is attached to the skull for the latter. The lesion is located using CT scanning and the direction and depth for the insertion of a probe is accurately determined. The skull is then opened and the probe inserted — the surgeon can then follow it down to the lesion (Fig. 14.7).

Vascular malformations and aneurysms

The management of these conditions is changing with the advent of radiological embolization techniques, which provide either definitive treatment or make the lesions more amenable to surgery (see Chapter 21). There are sometimes particular surgical problems with cerebrovascular malformations, aneurysms and vascular tumours such as choroid plexus papilloma. These include difficult access, the potential for rupture, bleeding and increased pressure at the site when occluded or clipped. Ideally the anaesthetist should provide maximum safety for the patient with optimal operating conditions. This can be achieved with mild (33–34°C) or moderate (30–32°C) hypothermia, which provides safety by reducing cerebral metabolism, and the use of vasodilators to lower blood pressure and reduce bleeding. In the really difficult cases, phenoxybenzamine (0.3–0.5 mg/kg) will lower systolic arterial pressure by about 10–30 mmHg. Its advantages are that it is an alpha-adrenergic blocking drug and therefore does not raise intracranial pressure by dilating cerebral vessels. It is long acting, so that the arterial pressure rises slowly and rebound hypertension is avoided; and the vasodilatation helps the patient to cool and rewarm faster. Sodium nitroprusside normally causes some cerebral vasodilatation, but it can be used at the critical points of the operation because the skull is open and the doses required to lower the blood pressure further are smaller than usual if phenoxybenzamine has been used. Alternatively, isoflurane can be used for its hypotensive effect. The advantages of concurrent hypothermia are that it protects the brain if problems arise, it lowers intracranial pressure and it allows lower cerebral perfusion pressures to be used if bleeding is troublesome. This technique has been used successfully in some very difficult and potentially hazardous operations for vascular malformations and tumours. The extra time taken to induce surface-cooled hypothermia is well spent when the patient's safety and outcome are considered. The danger of dysrhythmia is negligible if the plasma potassium is kept normal. It usually decreases with hypothermia

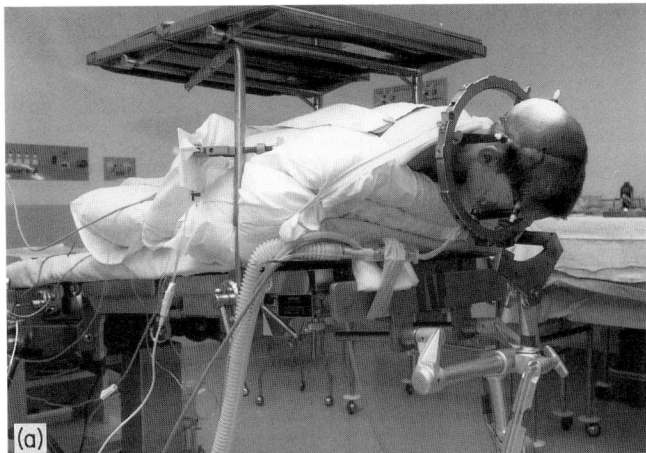

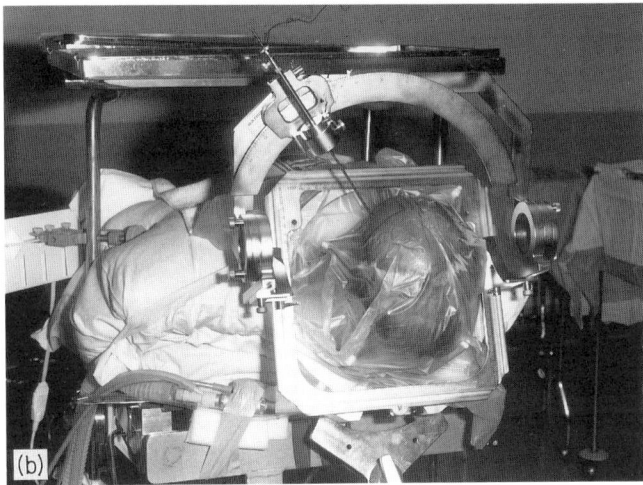

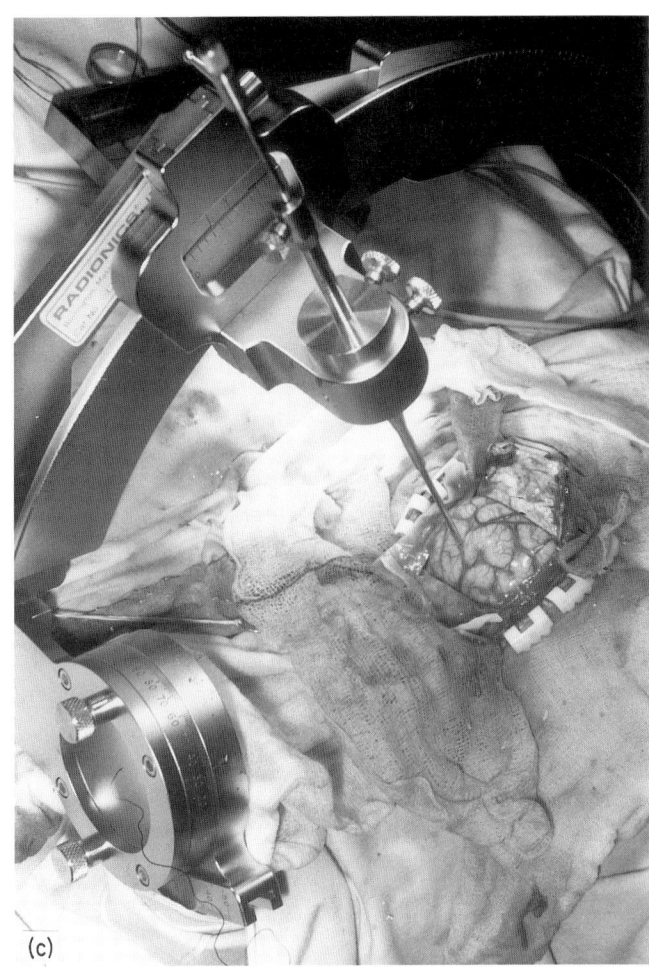

Fig. 14.7 The frame for stereotactic location of intercerebral lesions in place with the probe directed towards the lesion. (a) The attachment put on before CT scanning to locate the lesion. (b) The frame attached to provide accurate stereotactic location — the angles are determined by computer. (c) The probe directed towards the lesion.

(see Chapter 24). If dysrhythmia occurs, potassium chloride should be given slowly in small increments until normal rhythm is restored (see Chapter 24).

Moyamoya disease

Moyamoya disease is a rare cranial vascular disease which affects infants, children and young adults, and is characterized by the development of severe stenoses or the occlusion of major arterial vessels to the brain. Presentation is usually with ischaemic symptoms, such as speech disorder, hemiparesis, visual upset or epilepsy. Subarachnoid haemorrhage may occur, especially in adults. The disease runs a variable, fluctuating, unpredictable course, usually culminating in serious neurological deficits, but rarely a fatal outcome.

The aetiology is usually unknown, although some cases are associated with metabolic disorders such as homocystinuria. The disease is more common in girls and may be familial. Patients with Moyamoya disease have a predilection to cerebral aneurysms.

The Japanese term 'moyamoya', loosely translated, means 'puff of smoke' and refers to the characteristic appearance in the arterial phase of angiography of the 'puff' of contrast medium in the tiny collateral vessels in the region of the basal ganglia (Fig. 14.8).

Major narrowing or occlusion of internal carotid and vertebral vessels and their branches is seen, with marked collateral vessel formation in the basal ganglia, and often anastomoses from external carotid vessels such as the meningeal arteries to cerebral vessels.

ECG abnormalities such as ST-T wave changes, right

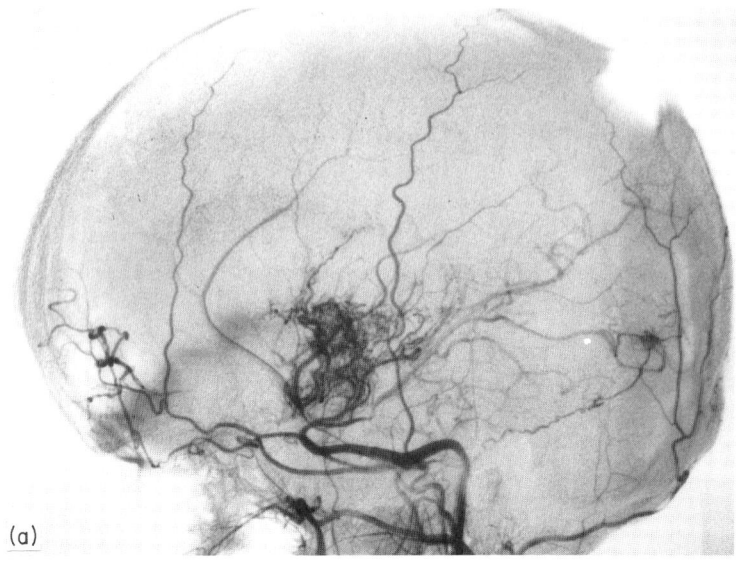
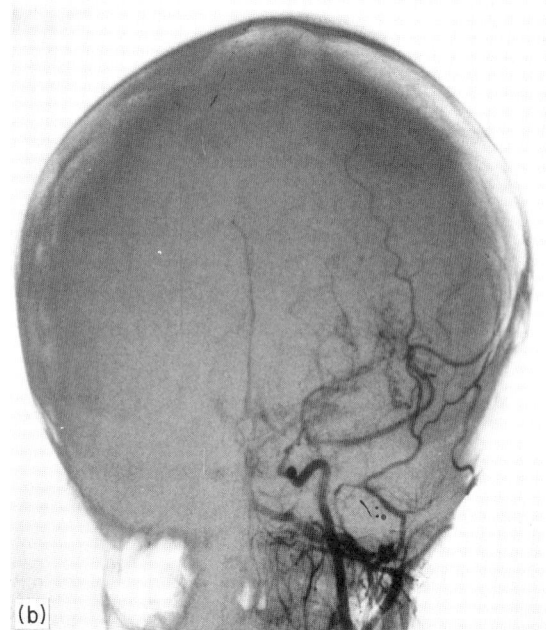

Fig. 14.8 X-ray appearances in Moyamoya disease, showing obstruction in major vessels and areas with multiple tiny collateral vesels. (a) Lateral view. (b) A-P view.

and left axis deviation, premature ventricular contraction, and evidence of ventricular hypertrophy are common.

TREATMENT

Treatment includes the use of antiplatelet drugs such as aspirin, avoidance of events which may precipitate cerebral ischaemia, such as hyperventilation (as in prolonged singing or shouting), exhaustion or hypotension. Surgical measures to increase cerebral blood flow include sympathectomy, external-to-internal carotid shunts such as superficial temporal or middle meningeal to middle cerebral anastomoses, temporal muscle or omental fat grafts, and more recently encephaloduralarteriosynangiosis. In this a mobilized but intact and flowing artery, usually the middle meningeal, is laid on the surface of the brain to allow development of a network of collaterals over ensuing months.

ANAESTHESIA [3, 4, 5, 6, 7]

Key points concerning anaesthesia of these delicately balanced patients are:
1 avoidance of hypocapnia which may produce cerebral

arterial spasm and, hence, ischaemic damage with delayed recovery;
2 avoidance of hypoxia and hypotension.

Myelomeningocoele

Myelomeningocoele presents as a swelling on the back and is external evidence of an anomaly of the central nervous system. It is a condition resulting from disturbance of neural tube closure between the third and fifth week of fetal life. The bony covering of the spinal canal is missing (spina bifida) and the neural elements are usually on the surface. There is usually sensory loss and paralysis which may involve the lower limbs and sphincters. Hydrocephalus, which may or may not be present at birth, is common and results from aqueduct stenosis or compression at the tentorium or foramen magnum.

In the past treatment was aggressive, including shunts for hydrocephalus, urinary diversion procedures and orthopaedic operations. Recently the trend has changed, so that treatment is not undertaken unless the lesion is relatively low, there is satisfactory movement in the lower limbs and the infant is assessed as having a chance of leading a reasonably normal existence.

The operation is performed in the prone position with the abdomen free so that ventilation is not inhibited, using supports under the pelvis and shoulders or the prone knee—chest position. It is preferable to intubate these babies lying on their side, but care must be taken to avoid rupture of the sac if the infant is placed supine. The skin edges may be injected with vasoconstrictors to reduce bleeding, which might otherwise be significant. The infant is usually nursed prone postoperatively.

Encephalocoele

This is similar to a myelomeningocoele at a higher level, involving the skull and brain. It is often situated in the occipital and suboccipital region, but occasionally presents in the midline just above the nose, causing lateral displacement of the orbits. Some are incompatible with life and are untreatable, but many can be excised. CT scanning helps to delineate the contents and the relationship to the ventricular system.

The main problem for the anaesthetist is positioning the infant during induction and intubation for the operation, especially when there is a large mass on the back of the head. During intubation the baby can be placed on the side, or the encephalocoele may rest in the ring of a head rest, or the head may be held by an assistant so that the mass is not compressed.

Hydrocephalus frequently complicates this condition and a ventricular shunt may need to be inserted some days after the repair of the encephalocoele.

Craniostenosis

This includes a spectrum of disorders due to premature closure of one or several cranial sutures. The shape of the head depends on which sutures are fused. The usual indication is cosmetic (to improve head shape). Occasionally, when more than one suture is involved, intracranial pressure may be raised as the skull cannot expand to accommodate the growing brain. The operation will vary according to which suture is involved. A strip of bone is removed parallel to the suture, and either the outer layer of dura is divided and turned back over the bone or a silastic strip is placed between the bone edges to prevent refusion. When the sagittal suture is fused, the patient may be placed as in Fig. 14.9, prone with the head extended and the table tilted head-up. Strips of bone are usually removed from each side of the midline because the sagittal sinus lies under the normal

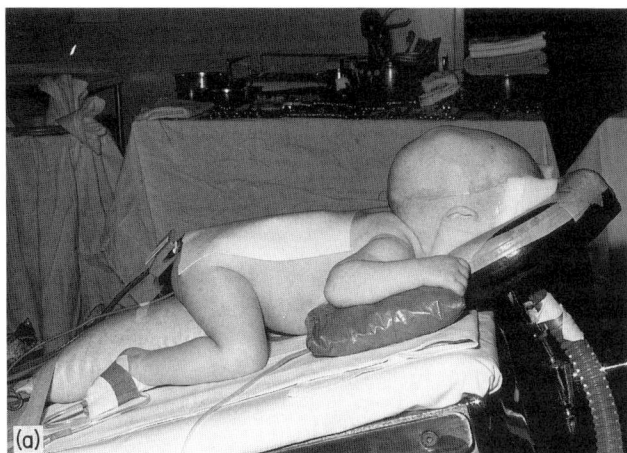

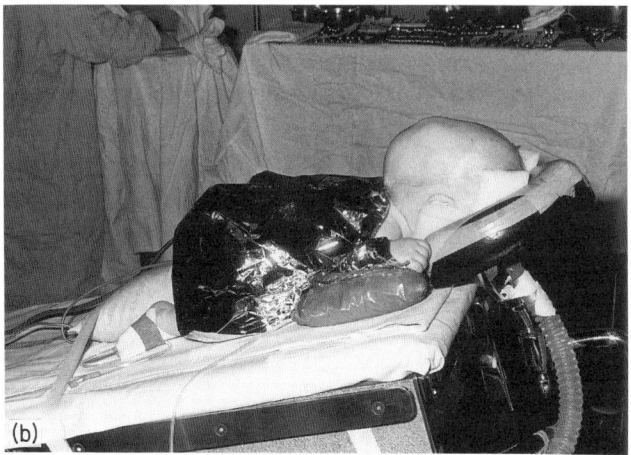

Fig. 14.9 (a) A position used for correction of sagittal suture synostosis. The head is extended and placed in a head ring, the table is tipped so that the top of the head is horizontal. A diathermy pad is placed on the back. The intravenous infusion is easily accessible from the foot. (b) The patient is covered with foil to prevent heat loss.

suture line, but there are several operative techniques. When the coronal suture is involved, the frontal bone may be flattened and a triangle of bone may be removed and refashioned to improve the cosmetic appearance of the forehead. The operation may involve frontal bone almost to the orbital margin. Care must then be taken with placement of the eye-protection tape, so as not to intrude on the surgical field. Operations on the lambdoid suture are done in the prone position. Elevation of the head helps to reduce blood loss, which is often sufficient to require blood transfusion. Blood should always be cross-matched. Parents often wish to donate blood for their child. Because the operation is cosmetic it can be staged if bleeding is excessive, but this is rarely necessary.

Spinal surgery

Laminectomy is usually performed to relieve compression of the spinal cord or nerve roots by tumour, blood clot or disc protrusion (uncommon in children). It is also necessary in the treatment of a number of congenital anomalies, including spinal-cord tethering by nerves at the lower end (spinal dysraphism), bony spur protruding through the cord (diastematomyelia), and dermal sinus or cyst. In diastematomyelia, profuse bleeding may occur from the artery supplying the bony spur. It is preferable to avoid suxamethonium if the patient is paraplegic.

The operations, which are done with the patient face down or on the side, require a clear operating field and thus efforts should be made to minimize bleeding. The patient should be positioned so that congestion of the epidural veins is avoided. Some surgeons use the lateral position so that blood drains out of the wound, but if the patient is prone, the use of the frame originally developed for scoliosis surgery (see Fig. 19.4) avoids abdominal compression and allows free diaphragmatic movement. Alternatively, abdominal compression is minimized by the use of supports under the pelvis and shoulders or by the knee−chest position.

Care must be taken to adjust the respiratory pattern so that venous congestion is avoided. It is usual to control ventilation in these patients in the prone position, although some surgeons believe that bleeding is less when the patient is breathing spontaneously. If bleeding becomes excessive, the use of induced hypotension is worth considering, to reduce blood loss and allow the surgeon a clearer view of the operating field.

POSTOPERATIVE CARE

Frequent observation and continuous monitoring are essential, especially after craniotomy and head injury. The anticipation and early recognition of adverse changes, with prompt treatment, will make the results of surgery better and improve the child's prognosis.

Monitoring

Routine nursing observations of pulse, blood pressure, respiration, conscious state and size and response of pupils to light are important.

Bradycardia and a rising blood pressure suggest increasing intracranial pressure. Hypotension, es-pecially if associated with reduced cardiac output, may result in impaired cerebral perfusion. The combination of hypotension and raised intracranial pressure can be disastrous. Dysrhythmia, which can be detected with continuous ECG monitoring, may result from brain-stem and other intracranial pathology.

Changes in respiration such as hypoventilation or Cheyne−Stokes respiration are significant. Hypo-ventilation leads to CO_2 retention, cerebral vasodila-tation and a rise in intracranial pressure. The airway should be checked to ensure that it is not obstructed, and if necessary ventilation should be controlled. After severe head injury, and sometimes following major intracranial surgery, it may be wise to leave the patient intubated and ventilated during the early postoperative period. In such cases intracranial pressure should be monitored.

Cheyne−Stokes breathing is often due to damage to the supramedullary nervous pathways, which normally inhibit either the respiratory centres or motor path-ways to respiratory muscles. It indicates a significant neurological problem.

Central cyanosis indicates hypoxia, although it may need to be distinguished from peripheral pooling. Hypoxia affects cerebral blood flow, initially causing it to increase. Because postoperative hypoxaemia is common, additional inspired oxygen should be given. Infants susceptible to retrolental fibroplasia should have the concentration carefully controlled. The conscious state is important. Deterioration of conscious state indicates serious complications, especially if associated with pupillary dilatation and loss of reactivity to light. The adequacy of ventilation should be checked and, if necessary, controlled ventilation and other steps to reduce intracranial pressure instituted. Surgical re-exploration may be urgently indicated. It is vital that the neurosurgeon is informed of these changes.

Temperature is usually monitored. When the patient inadvertently cools, peripheral vasoconstriction occurs, making the patient look pale and sometimes cyanosed. Drug metabolism can be slowed, so that recovery may be delayed. In the postoperative period the patient may shiver, thereby increasing heat production and oxygen consumption. In contrast, when a child has been cooled intentionally, and particularly when vasodilators have been used and the circulation has been well filled, the muscle relaxant can be reversed and the child can be extubated when the temperature is 34°C. As the patient's temperature is rising already, it will continue to do so provided he is covered with warm blankets or a reflective mylar film blanket. As the metabolic rate is rising, additional oxygen should be given. The adverse effects seen during inadvertent cooling do not seem to occur in patients who are rewarming from induced hypothermia. Slight overshoot may occur when the temperature reaches normal levels.

Postoperative temperature elevation occurs in some neurosurgical patients, and attempts should be made to promote cooling by exposure and the use of a net frame which allows free air circulation around the body.

Urine output should be measured following intracranial surgery and severe head injuries. Routine testing and, where indicated, measurement of urinary electrolytes and osmolality will help in the recognition and diagnosis of some potential postoperative problems (see below).

Intracranial pressure can be monitored directly with a ventricular catheter, a subdural bolt or an extradural pressure transducer screwed into a burr hole (see Chapter 36). The advantages of intracranial pressure monitoring are that early changes can be detected and treated before advanced signs such as dilated pupils develop, and the effect of treatment can be monitored. The aim should be to prevent the intracranial pressure reaching the steep slope of the pressure–volume curve (see Fig. 14.1).

The intraventricular method is useful when a craniotomy has been performed, but it is also used in head injuries with the catheter inserted through a burr hole. It can be used to monitor pressure and, if necessary, to permit therapeutic drainage of CSF. The catheter is linked by a closed system to a pressure transducer.

A significant problem is the risk of infection. Every precaution should be taken to avoid this and a closed system should be used. Daily aspiration of CSF for culture and sensitivity testing is a wise precaution and, should infection occur, immediate removal of the catheter is indicated.

When the mean pressure measured from the level of the catheter tip rises above 20 mmHg (2.7 kPa), CSF drainage, cerebral dehydration or hyperventilation can be used to reduce the pressure. This system can be modified so that when the pressure rises above this level, CSF will drain into a closed receptacle (Fig. 14.10).

There are many other pressure-detecting devices available, which can be situated extradurally or subdurally. These will be discussed in more detail in Chapter 36.

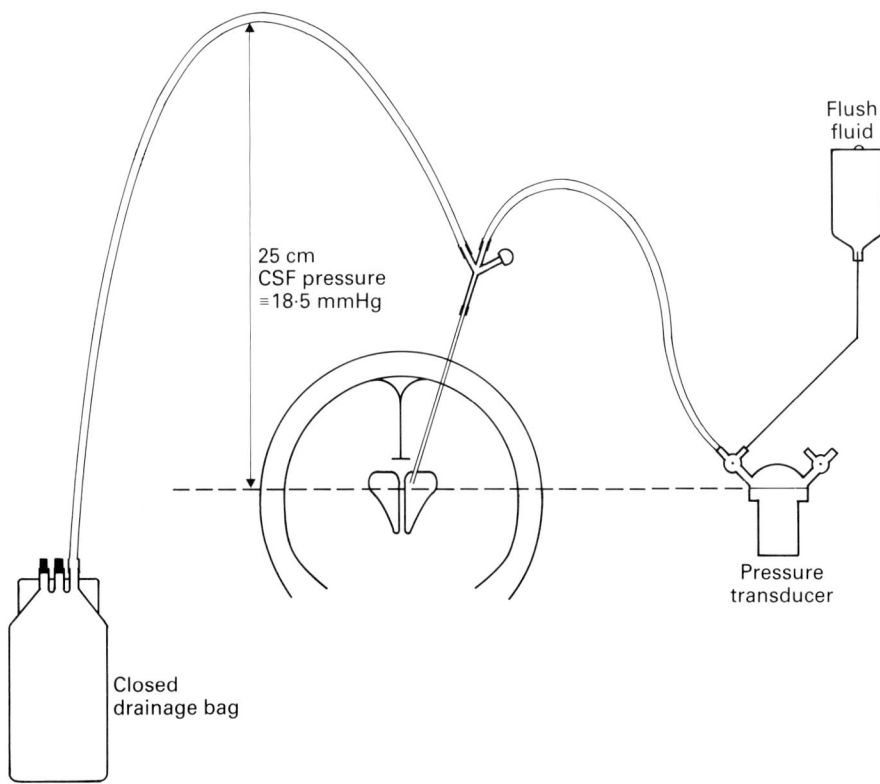

Fig. 14.10 The intraventricular method of monitoring CSF pressure, modified by a closed drainage bag which allows for CSF drainage when the pressure rises above 20 mmHg (2.7 kPa).

Flush fluid

25 cm
CSF pressure
≡18·5 mmHg

Pressure transducer

Closed drainage bag

Fluids

When the risk of cerebral oedema is present, intravenous fluids should be restricted to no more than half the normal maintenance levels and should not exceed 60 ml/kg/day, provided cardiac output and blood pressure are not reduced.

Position

The patient should be nursed on his side until consciousness is regained. Then some head-up tilt is desirable to facilitate jugular venous flow and to prevent cerebral venous congestion and a rise in intracranial blood volume. If the patient's clinical condition is satisfactory, the sitting position is ideal. If positive end-expiratory pressure (PEEP) is necessary, the back pressure on the jugular veins can be decreased by further elevation of the head.

Following meningomyelocoele repair, infants should be nursed prone. Special frames have been devised for them.

Following spinal surgery the patient is nursed flat, often for several days.

Analgesia

Analgesia is usually required in full doses following spinal operations. Pain following craniotomy is not severe and can usually be controlled with paracetamol or codeine. If severe pain or headache occurs, it suggests that either the bandages are too tight or an intracranial problem such as bleeding or cerebral oedema is developing which needs neurosurgical intervention. Occasionally sedation is required, and i.v. diazepam (up to 0.3 mg/kg) can be given.

Treatment of convulsions

These are usually treated with diazepam, midazolam or carbamazepine, and to prevent recurrence, phenytoin (Dilantin) or phenobarbitone may be used.

Steroids

Dexamethazone is usually continued in the early postoperative period if it has already been given to prevent cerebral oedema.

SPECIAL PROBLEMS

Inappropriate antidiuretic hormone secretion

More common than diabetes insipidus, this complication can occur following any craniotomy, particularly after trauma. The features include the passing of small quantities of concentrated urine, with subsequent water retention and dilutional hyponatraemia. The diagnosis is confirmed by plasma electrolytes showing an apparent decrease in sodium, potassium, chloride and often urea.

In the asymptomatic patient, the only therapy indicated is fluid restriction, often down to 20 ml/kg/day. In more serious cases there are signs of irritability, vomiting and then the level of consciousness deteriorates, followed by convulsions. This is due to the movement of water from the hypotonic extracellular space into the brain, causing cerebral oedema. The same occurs in acute water intoxication. Rapid intervention is necessary if the patient has symptomatic hyponatraemia. Plasma sodium should then be increased to above 120 mmol/l using hypertonic saline until symptoms resolve. (If a hypertonic sodium solution is needed and saline is not available, sodium bicarbonate can be used (8.4% = 6.7N)). After that, fluid restriction will usually allow gradual correction or a diuretic may be given. There is a danger of developing central pontine myelinolysis if correction is too rapid. Although the child's body sodium will be higher than normal in the presence of dilutional hyponatraemia, hypertonic saline is used to increase serum osmolality. If hypervolaemia with pulmonary congestion occurs, a diuretic such as frusemide should be given. It is more effective in the presence of an adequate or increased sodium load.

Diabetes insipidus

This is a life-threatening complication of surgery due to impairment of the hypothalamic−neurohypophyseal axis, so that there is a lack of antidiuretic hormone. Large quantities of dilute urine are passed. Hypovolaemia may rapidly follow unless appropriate replacement therapy is instituted.

Close monitoring of hourly urine output is essential and, should this rise, a sample should be analysed for electrolytes and osmolality. From these results, the constituents of the replacement fluid can be worked out. Low concentrations of sodium and potassium will be needed and, if glucose is used to maintain isotonicity, there is a danger of 'glucose loading' leading to hyperglycaemia because of the large volume of fluid involved.

REFERENCES

1 Bruce D.A., Abass A., Blaniuk L., Dolmskas C., Orbist W., Uzzell B. Diffuse cerebral swelling following head injuries in children: the syndrome of malignant brain oedema. *J Neurosurg* 1981, **54**, 170.

2 Loughnan P.M., Brown T.C.K., Edis B.D., Klug G.L. Neurogenic pulmonary oedema in man: aetiology and management with vasodilators based on haemodynamic studies. *Anaes Intens Care* 1980, **8**, 65.

3 Chadha R., Singh S., Padmanabhan V. Anaesthetic management in Moyamoya disease. *Anaes Intens Care* 1990, **18**, 120–123.

4 Yasukawa M., Yasukawa K., Akagawa S., Nakagawa Y., Miyasaka K. Convulsions and temporary hemiparesis following spinal anesthesia in a child with Moyamoya disease: letter. *Anesthesiology* 1988, **69**, 1023–1024.

5 Brown S.C., Lam A.M. Moyamoya disease — a review of clinical experience and anaesthetic management. *Canad J Anaes* 1987, **34**, 71–75.

6 Bingham R.M., Wilkinson D.J. Anaesthetic management in Moyamoya disease. *Anaesthesia* 1985, **40**, 1198–1202.

7 Sumikawa K., Nagai H. Moyamoya disease and anesthesia: letter. *Anesthesiology* 1983, **58**, 204–205.

15: Anaesthesia for Ear, Nose and Throat Operations

GENERAL PREOPERATIVE CONSIDERATIONS

The general considerations discussed in Chapter 6 apply. Some children needing operations to relieve upper airway obstruction may have a chronic upper respiratory tract infection. The anaesthetist should try to determine whether this infection is acute, and weigh up the disadvantages of the presence of infection, which include increased laryngeal and bronchial irritability, possible spread to the lower respiratory tract and increased bleeding at the operation site, against the chance that the operation may allow the infection to be cured.

There is another small group of children, usually young, who present for the removal of tonsils and adenoids, because these are grossly enlarged and causing airway obstruction. An allergic component may also be present. Some of these children have episodes of sleep apnoea, which are an indication for tonsillectomy and adenoidectomy. The degree of obstruction may be sufficient to cause chronic CO_2 retention and pulmonary hypertension. Preoperative oximetry has been useful for assessing the severity of this problem.

CARE DURING ANAESTHESIA AND THE OPERATION

Airway

In general, except for very brief operations not involving the mouth and for endoscopies, patients having ENT procedures should be intubated, so that the airway is secured and the anaesthetic breathing system is away from the operative field, leaving clear access for the surgeon.

Avoidance of pollution is difficult during endoscopy, when the anaesthetic gases are delivered via the side arm of the bronchoscope or insufflated. High-flow suction placed near the face, so that it draws gases exhaled from the open bronchoscope or the mouth, will reduce the degree of pollution considerably.

Some children with enlarged adenoids or allergic rhinitis, who normally breathe through the mouth, may be difficult to ventilate unless an oropharyngeal airway is used, or the mask is applied to the face with the mouth open (see Fig. 7.8).

Control of bleeding

Some sites, such as the nose, are very vascular. Vasoconstrictors, such as adrenaline 1:200000 or ornithine vasopressin (POR8), may be injected to reduce bleeding. Adrenaline has a direct action on the alpha-receptor and hence the onset of vasoconstriction is rapid. Topical cocaine (5%), as well as providing local anaesthesia produces adequate vasoconstriction on its own, but its onset of action is slower because it acts by blocking the reuptake of noradrenaline at the adrenergic receptor.

During microsurgery, particularly in the middle ear, even small drops of blood can interfere with the surgeon's

228

view of the operative field. Bleeding can be minimized by the use of vasoconstrictors, hypotensive anaesthesia (see Chapter 23), head-up tilt and ensuring that the patient is adequately anaesthetized and that hypercarbia does not develop.

POSTOPERATIVE

Postoperative vomiting is more common in patients after middle-ear surgery than after many other operations. An antiemetic may be given at the end of the operation (e.g. droperidol (0.03–0.05 mg/kg), prochlorperazine (0.02 mg/kg), or metoclopramide (0.12 mg/kg)).

Careful postoperative observation is necessary, as respiratory obstruction or aspiration may follow many ENT procedures. In particular, children who have had tonsillectomy and adenoidectomy for sleep apnoea must be watched carefully, as they may still have a tendency to obstruction due to mucosal swelling or laxity of the pharyngeal tissues. Children who have had chronic hypercarbia may be at added risk during the early post-operative period, during readjustment of the respiratory drive while $Pa\text{co}_2$ is declining to normal.

Pain should be controlled with analgesics, but care should be taken to avoid respiratory depression if there is any danger of airway obstruction postoperatively. Paracetamol (15–20 mg/kg) given with the premedi-cation is sufficient for less severe discomfort, such as that following myringotomy.

SPECIAL PROCEDURES

Tonsillectomy and adenoidectomy

Tonsillectomy with adenoidectomy was one of the most common operations in the past, but the occasional death and a more critical appraisal of the indications has reduced its incidence. The tonsils are now usually removed by dissection.

Tonsillectomy is an operation within the airway and the patient should therefore be intubated. The tube should be positioned in the midline (Fig. 15.1) so that it will lie comfortably under the split tongue blade of a Boyle–Davis gag (Figs 15.2, 15.3). Tubes such as the RAE oral and Portex 'south' tubes (see Chapter 3) have an angle which conveniently curves down over the chin for this purpose. Ventilation must be checked when the tongue blade is inserted because the tube may be kinked by the tip of a blade which is too short. Early awakening following tonsillectomy and adenoidectomy is desirable, so that the likelihood of aspirating blood or clots is lessened.

A technique with an intravenous induction, nitrous oxide, muscle relaxant and pre- or intraoperative opioid provides suitable operating conditions with rapid reversal

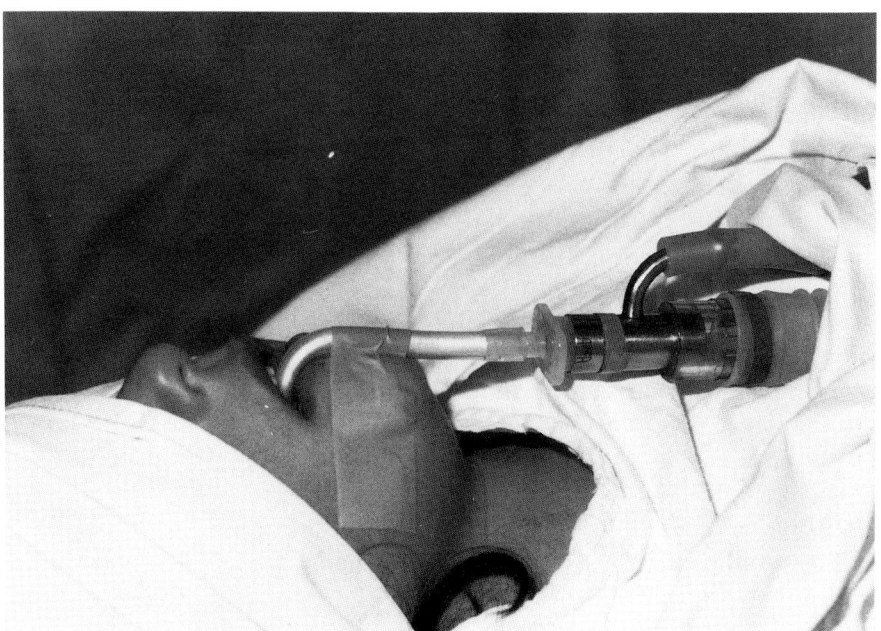

Fig. 15.1 A RAE endotracheal tube positioned in the midline before insertion of the mouth gag for tonsillectomy.

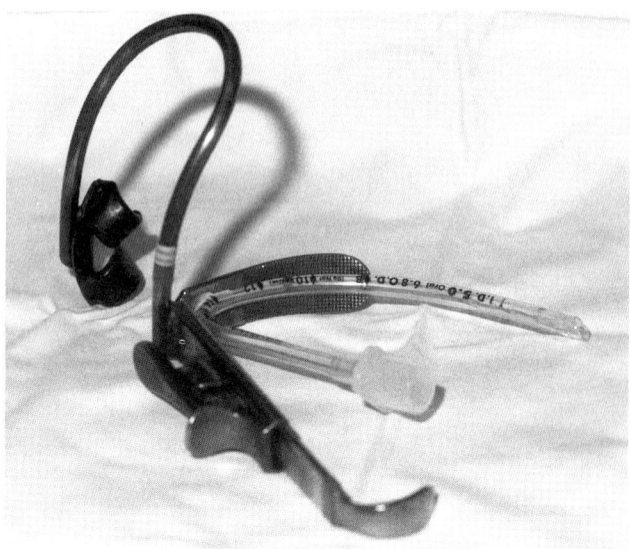

Fig. 15.2 Boyle–Davis gag showing how the RAE tube is accommodated under the tongue blade.

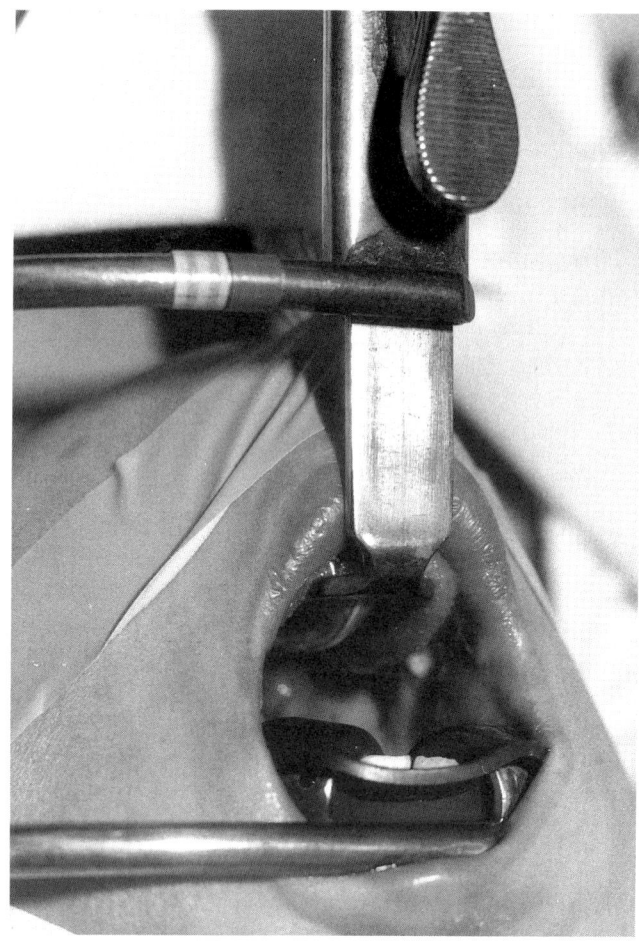

Fig. 15.3 Boyle–Davis gag in position for tonsillectomy, with the endotracheal tube showing in the split blade.

and recovery at the end. If there is any danger of preoperative sleep apnoea or obstruction, opiates should be given intravenously at induction rather than with the premedication. Halothane is used in many centres, but it is more likely to be associated with longer postoperative drowsiness, laryngeal spasm following extubation, particularly in inexperienced hands, and peripheral dilatation which may be associated with increased oozing, especially if hypercarbia develops.

Blood loss during tonsillectomy is usually increased by intercurrent infection, with very diseased and fibrotic tonsils and by rough surgical technique. Although an intravenous infusion is not essential during tonsillectomy, it is reasonable to administer fluids if blood loss exceeds the usual 2–5 ml/kg, if there has been a long preoperative fast or when the weather is hot and sweating is increased.

The discomfort following tonsillectomy can be reduced by spraying a few drops of bupivacaine 0.5% into the tonsillar fossae, ensuring that it does not spill over into the pharynx or on to the larynx. Bending the tip of a 21 G needle and using a 2 ml syringe provides a spray which will reach the upper and lower poles; 0.5–1 ml in each fossa is usually adequate (Fig. 15.4).

Alternatively, some surgeons inject bupivacaine with adrenaline prior to the operation. This helps to define the plane for dissection and provides analgesia and vaso-constriction.

The use of local analgesia in the tonsillar fossae enables the child to drink sooner because there is less pain on swallowing.

At the conclusion of the operation blood and secretions should be removed from the pharynx by suction under direct vision so that the tonsil fossae are not disturbed. Raising the head and flexing the neck should reveal any bleeding from the adenoid area before extubation. The patient should be turned on his side and positive pressure applied to the bag as the tube is removed to ensure that the patient immediately exhales so that any blood or clot in the trachea or larynx is expelled.

Management of post-tonsillectomy haemorrhage

It is important to watch for postoperative bleeding in the recovery room. If it becomes excessive or tachycardia, hypotension and pallor develop, treatment should be

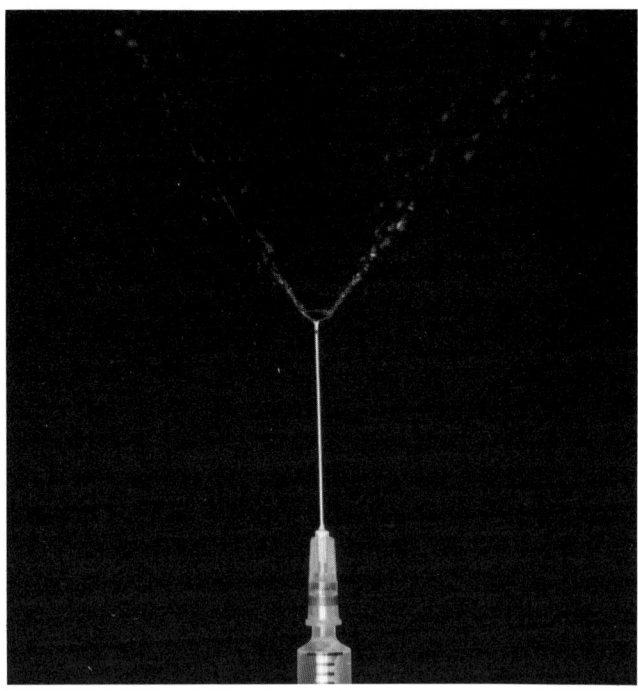

Fig. 15.4 Needle with bent tip, showing how the local anaesthetic sprays so that it can reach both poles of the tonsillar fossa.

started. Postoperative bleeding may occur as a continuation of operative bleeding or oozing, or a secondary bleed may occur some hours or days later, when clots break off and expose a bleeding point.

A less common cause of postoperative oozing is platelet dysfunction following the ingestion of salicylates during the preoperative period. If a history of aspirin ingestion is obtained and bleeding time (see Chapter 25) indicate platelet dysfunction, infusion of platelets will usually stop the continued bleeding.

If there is no history of salicylate ingestion and there is significant bleeding, it may occasionally be possible, if the child is co-operative, to pack the tonsillar fossa or post-nasal space. Otherwise the patient may have to be taken back to the operating theatre so that the bleeding can be controlled surgically. Any such patient will probably have lost a significant quantity of blood, and therefore an intravenous infusion should be running. Blood should be taken for cross-matching and, if available and transfusion is indicated, it may be started prior to the anaesthetic. It is difficult to assess the blood loss accurately after tonsillectomy because blood is commonly swallowed. If bleeding is rapid, the patient should be resuscitated with crystalloid solution or a plasma volume expander while blood is being cross-matched, and may be taken back to the operating theatre before the latter is ready. The potential problems to be faced by the anaesthetist are hypovolaemia, the presence of a substantial quantity of swallowed blood and clot in the stomach, and continuing bleeding in the pharynx.

Pre-oxygenation before the patient is paralysed is important, as positive pressure ventilation may result in the inhalation of blood. Cricoid pressure can be used to prevent regurgitation of already swallowed blood.

The main methods of induction for the child with post-tonsillectomy haemorrhage are:

1 Thiopentone, atropine and suxamethonium are given followed rapidly by intubation. If intubation is carried out with the patient supine, the anaesthetist must remember that blood may collect in the pharynx and be prepared to suck it out.

When an intravenous induction is used, the dose of induction agent may need to be reduced if the patient is still hypovolaemic, because there is a preferential blood flow to the brain and heart and therefore a smaller dose of drug is required to induce unconsciousness. Also, a given dose of thiopentone (or other i.v. agent) will produce a higher concentration if the blood volume is decreased. The administration of a normal dose of thiopentone could result in a serious fall in blood pressure if the patient is still hypovolaemic. There may still be some unmetabolized barbiturate in the body if it has been used for the first anaesthetic on the same day.

2 An alternative is to use an inhalation induction followed by suxamethonium and intubation. Because bleeding is continuing and there is a danger of aspiration, the patient is induced and intubated lying on his left side, so that blood will drain away and when the laryngoscope is inserted the tongue will tend to fall away from it.

Myringotomy

Myringotomies are usually performed to drain fluid or 'glue' from the middle ear in children with reduced hearing. Usually, tubes are inserted to allow aeration of the middle ear. This simple procedure can improve hearing significantly. Occasionally myringotomy may be needed in acute otitis media.

Elective myringotomy may be combined with tonsillectomy and adenoidectomy, or done as a single procedure. In the latter case, with a quick surgeon, a spontaneous-breathing inhalational technique with a mask can be used, but for multiple procedures the child should be intubated.

Antral washout

Chronically infected maxillary antra may be the source of suppurative nasal discharge. The operative procedure involves the passage of a trocar and cannula or a large needle into the anterior part of the antrum through the maxilla. The antra are washed out with saline. It is normally a simple procedure. There have been rare cases of collapse under anaesthesia during this procedure, which have not been adequately explained. It may be that air or septic embolism has occurred. Usually the patient is intubated, and a throat pack may be used to prevent aspiration of antral washings which may leak into the nose.

Cautery of turbinates

In this simple procedure the turbinates are cauterized to reduce mucosal swelling and obstruction. It is a brief procedure which if performed alone, can be done while the patient breathes halothane, the mask being removed while cautery is applied. The surgeon may occasionally use vasoconstrictors on the mucosa prior to the application of the cautery. Blood loss is usually insignificant. In patients with severe allergic rhinitis with nasal obstruction the turbinates may be trimmed.

Reduction of fractured nose

Prior to reduction of a fractured nose, the patient must be warned that the nose will be packed and that it will be necessary to breathe through his mouth postoperatively. The anaesthetic management includes the possibility of having to ventilate the child, until paralysed, with a mask with the nasal passages obstructed. If this happens an oropharyngeal airway may be inserted, or the mouth should be held open with the jaw forward to provide an adequate airway when the mask is placed on the face. When adequately paralysed, the patient should be intubated and a throat pack inserted to absorb blood. If blood loss has been considerable or is considerable during the procedure, appropriate replacement should be given. Early awakening is desirable and therefore a relaxant technique is preferable. Adequate supervision of the patient's airway is essential during emergence; if necessary an oropharyngeal airway can be inserted.

Septoplasty

The nasal septum is displaced to one side. Nasal obstruction on one or both sides occurs and normal airflow characteristics are lost. This operation involves an approach through the nasal mucosa and therefore a vasoconstrictor (e.g. adrenaline 1:200 000) is usually injected. Otherwise the principles of anaesthesia are similar to those described for reduction of a fractured nose. The blood loss does not tend to be as great as during rhinoplasty, which is a more major operation not commonly done in children.

Tympanoplasty

This operation involves laying a graft (often temporalis fascia) on to (overlay) or under (underlay) the eardrum. It may take about an hour, but can be longer. Intubation is necessary because access to the airway is limited. Several anaesthetic techniques are suitable for this procedure including thiopentone, nitrous oxide, relaxant with analgesic or inhalation supplement, or the use of inhalation anaesthesia with spontaneous ventilation.

Nitrous oxide is more soluble than nitrogen and expands the gas in air cavities. Its influence on the graft will depend on whether the graft is laid under the rim of the hole in the drum (underlay), in which case it will push it against the rim, or on the outside surface (overlay) in which case the nitrous oxide bubbles will tend to lift the graft while escaping. If the nitrous oxide is turned off as the graft is being put in place, the diffusion of nitrous oxide back into the bloodstream will lower the middle ear pressure and suck an overlay graft on to the rim. Anaesthesia should be continued with another inhalation agent.

Drainage of peritonsillar and retropharyngeal abscess

Fortunately these have become rare problems since the advent of antibiotics. The procedure requires drainage of the abscess into the pharynx with the possible danger of aspiration of pus. Intubation is desirable but may be difficult, particularly in quinsy (peritonsillar abscess), as trismus due to swelling around the temporomandibular joint cannot always be relieved by the use of relaxants. If drainage is attempted without intubation, the child must be on his side so that draining pus will not be inhaled. A mouth gag is inserted to gain maximum exposure. The anaesthetic can be continued by insufflation through a nasal catheter, which can be connected to a suction catheter, to remove any pus spilt into the pharynx when the abscess is opened.

Laryngoscopy

Laryngeal procedures include diagnostic laryngoscopy, removal of foreign bodies and the treatment of pathology such as papillomata, nodules, cysts, webs and other stenoses. Anaesthesia for diagnostic laryngoscopy will depend on the expected findings and the endoscopist. When it is suspected that pathology is minimal or that the larynx may be normal, all that may be required is a quick look at the larynx, which can be accomplished with thiopentone, atropine, suxamethonium and inflation with oxygen prior to laryngoscopy. If it is found that further treatment is necessary, then the anaesthesia can be continued using one of the other techniques to be described. This brief inspection of the larynx may also be sufficient for the removal of easily accessible laryngeal foreign bodies. These are often sharply angled, so that they become impacted. Eggshell, which shows up as a slightly curved opaque foreign body on X-ray (Fig. 15.5), is a special hazard as it may disintegrate when grasped with forceps. An anaesthetic which allows more time for gentle removal of the eggshell should be used.

Diagnostic laryngoscopy performed in infants with stridor may be a short procedure, and should preferably be carried out with spontaneous ventilation so that laryngeal movements can be observed. Laryngomalacia, or infantile larynx, is a common cause of stridor — the tip of the epiglottis is omega-shaped. This constricts and the arytenoids prolapse into the glottis on inspiration, narrowing the airway and causing stridor (Fig. 15.6). Stridor decreases under deep anaesthesia and when positive pressure is maintained on the airway (CPAP). This procedure can be performed under inhalation anaesthesia supplemented with lignocaine 2% spray (up to 4 mg/kg). If the depth of anaesthesia is initially too deep, it should be lightened to allow observation of the laryngeal movements under optimum conditions. Another alternative is to use suxamethonium, which allows easy inspection of the anatomy and the movements can be observed during recovery, which is rapid with a small dose (0.5 mg/kg). The patient must be oxygenated intermittently or continuously by insufflation. A pulse oximeter should be used.

The intravenous basal anaesthetic, gamma-hydroxybutyrate, is not widely available but it is a particularly useful induction agent in the presence of severe upper

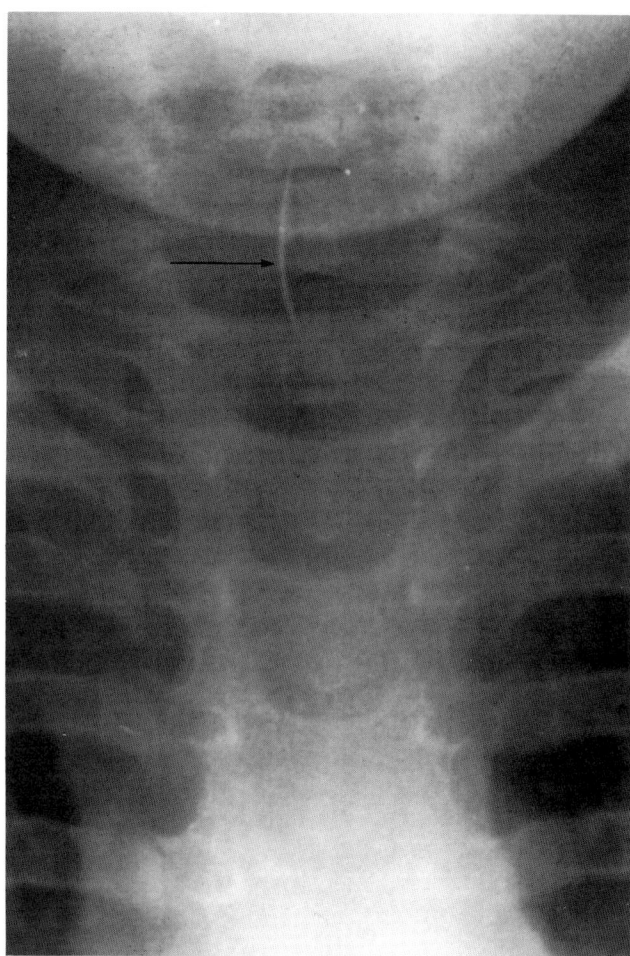

Fig. 15.5 An A-P view of the neck, showing eggshell impacted in the larynx.

airway obstruction, where an inhalation induction might be very prolonged. It provides jaw relaxation, slows the rate but increases the depth of respiration, and provides good visualization of the larynx. The usual dose is 40–

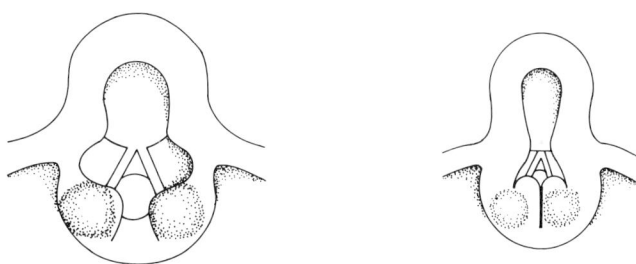

Fig. 15.6 Diagram showing the omega-shaped epiglottis and arytenoids during expiration (left) and inspiration (right), when the epiglottis constricts and the arytenoids flop into the glottic opening, causing partial obstruction.

50 mg/kg. Atropine should be given to counteract the bradycardia it causes.

Microlaryngeal surgery

The advent of the operating microscope has increased precision in laryngeal surgical techniques. Papilloma of the larynx, although a relatively rare condition, is a common indication for microlaryngeal surgery in children, as these patients require repeated anaesthetics. Others include the management of congenital or acquired glottic or subglottic stenosis.

The pathology in some of these patients may cause severe respiratory obstruction, which may be relieved by tracheal intubation but may require long-term tracheostomy.

The anaesthetic techniques for microlaryngeal surgery can be divided into two groups, depending on whether spontaneous or controlled ventilation is employed:

1 Spontaneous ventilation can be maintained after either intravenous or inhalation induction by the use of inhalation anaesthesia. Once the patient is adequately anaesthetized (pupils central) the larynx is sprayed with lignocaine. After insertion of the microlaryngoscope, inhalational agents may be delivered to the pharynx and larynx by insufflation, or a nasopharyngeal catheter may be used (Fig. 15.7). The concentration of anaesthetic or the gas flows may need to be increased to compensate for, or reduce, air dilution in the pharynx. Another method is insufflation via a catheter threaded down the light carrier of the microlaryngoscope, so that the gases are delivered at the laryngeal aperture. The advantage of the insufflation technique is that the view of the larynx is not obscured by an endotracheal tube. This is particularly important in the small airways of infants and children.

2 Controlled ventilation may be used with muscle relaxants and intermittent inflation by a high-pressure gas injection device, either through a needle attached to an operating laryngoscope or via a catheter passed into the trachea. The lowest pressure to provide adequate ventilation should be used, so that trauma from catheter movement is minimized. The other alternative, which is less appropriate for small children than for adults, is the insertion of a tube with a narrow lumen through the larynx, which allows the surgeon access to operate around the tube. In small children with narrow airways, such a tube may obscure the operative field.

When the patient has a tracheostomy, the breathing system can be attached and ventilation can be controlled

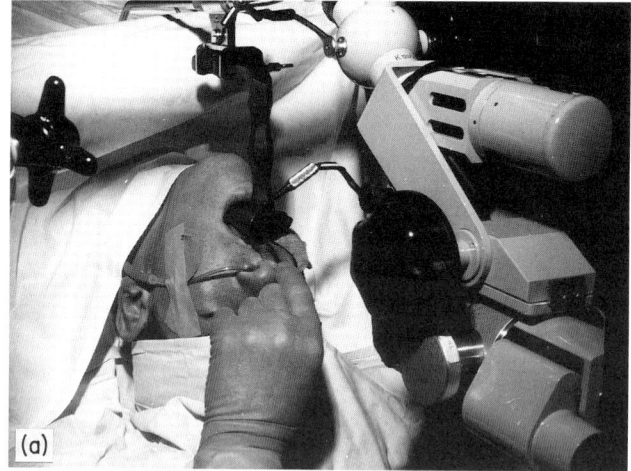

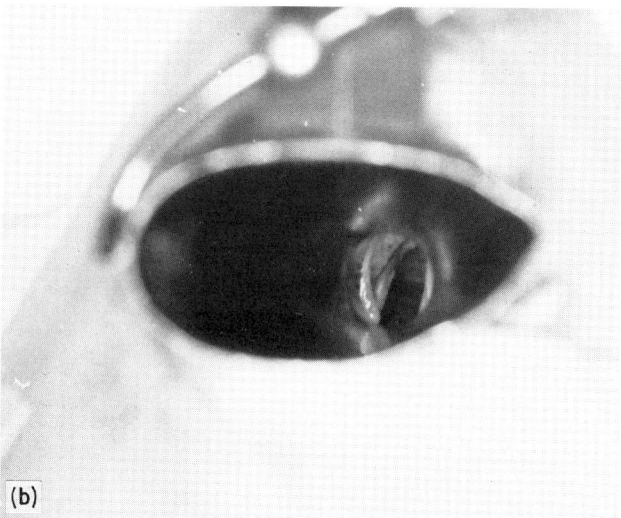

Fig. 15.7 (a) The microlaryngoscope in place with a nasopharyngeal catheter for insufflation of the anaesthetic. (b) A view of the vocal cords through the microlaryngoscope.

or spontaneous. In some older patients it is permissible to insert a small tube through the larynx and allow spontaneous respiration to continue through and around it, if there is no cuff. This would be possible for the removal of some anterior laryngeal lesions, where the presence of a small tube lying posteriorly would not interfere with surgical access. The details of some other techniques will be discussed at greater length in the section on bronchoscopy, as they are similar.

Lasers are frequently used for microlaryngeal surgery. They can destroy tissue with minimal pain or bleeding. The laser can ignite plastics, especially when there is an increased oxygen concentration in the enclosed environment (Fig. 15.8): it is therefore desirable to use the

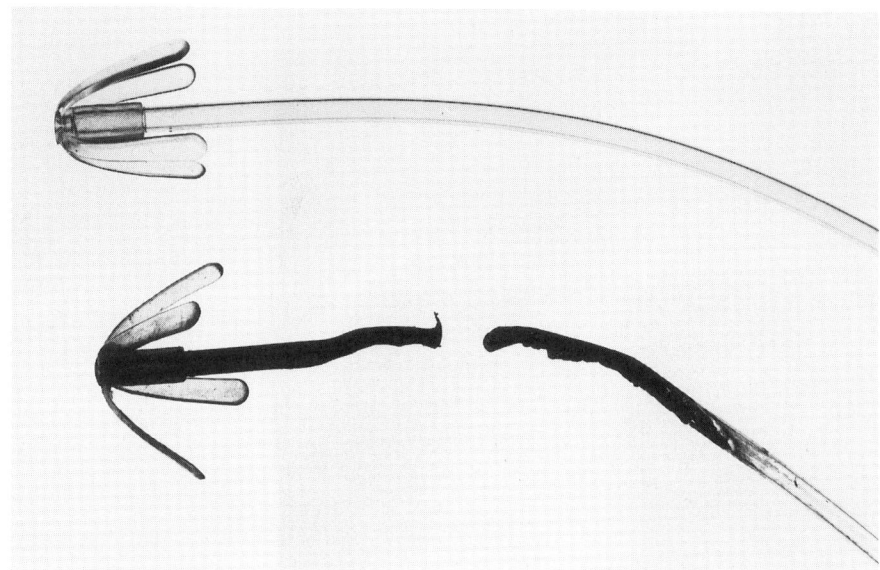

Fig. 15.8 A Benjet tube used in adult microlaryngeal surgery for delivery of gas into the trachea. The flanges prevent a whipping movement which would cause damage during inflation. Although claimed to be usable in the presence of laser, they will burn in the presence of a high oxygen concentration.

minimum concentration of oxygen that will maintain adequate oxygenation of the patient. This can now be easily monitored with a pulse oximeter. Whether breathing spontaneously or using an 'injector' to inflate the patient, air should be used as the anaesthetic carrier gas, with oxygen supplements if necessary. When a tube is used it should be metal or protected with aluminium tape. The laser must be applied accurately, as it can be reflected by metal.

Bronchoscopy

Bronchoscopy may be performed for diagnostic or therapeutic reasons. Diagnostic bronchoscopy may follow laryngoscopy in the investigation of stridor or airway obstruction, looking for such pathology as subglottic web, cartilaginous bar, haemangioma and compression of the trachea by a large vessel. It may also be part of the investigation of persistent segmental lung collapse or haemoptysis. Nowadays it is often performed with a fibreoptic bronchoscope.

Therapeutic bronchoscopy is usually performed to remove foreign bodies. These are most commonly inhaled in children between 1 and 3 years of age. A wide variety of foreign bodies are found, but in many countries peanuts are the most common — over 50%. The diagnosis may not be made for at least a week in as many as 15–30% of patients following inhalation. When vegetable material, particularly a nut, is inhaled the mucosal

reaction around the foreign body may cause swelling, leading to obstruction and infection.

Although the right main bronchus is slightly larger and more in line with the trachea than the left (see Chapter 1), foreign bodies are found on either side, but the majority are in the right. Larger foreign bodies in the trachea and multiple foreign bodies involving both bronchi cause the most serious obstruction that may be fatal if not rapidly relieved. In an emergency it would be possible to push a tracheal foreign body into one bronchus with a tube until the patient can be ventilated, and then it can be removed electively. A foreign body in one main bronchus is not usually an indication for such urgent intervention unless there is evidence of hypoxia.

A history of an episode of coughing and choking is usual when a foreign body has been inhaled. Subsequently the patient may develop a wheeze or evidence of decreased aeration of one lung. In some cases a ball-valve effect develops and hyperinflation of the obstructed lung may occur. This is caused by the normal dilatation of the bronchus during inspiration, allowing air to enter past the foreign body, and narrowing in expiration so that air cannot escape. The diagnosis of which side is involved usually depends on differential air entry to the lungs on auscultation, and on radiological examination in inspiration and expiration. This may be done by screening or by taking films in both phases of respiration. In these films the uninvolved side shows expansion in inspiration, whereas the involved side remains at about

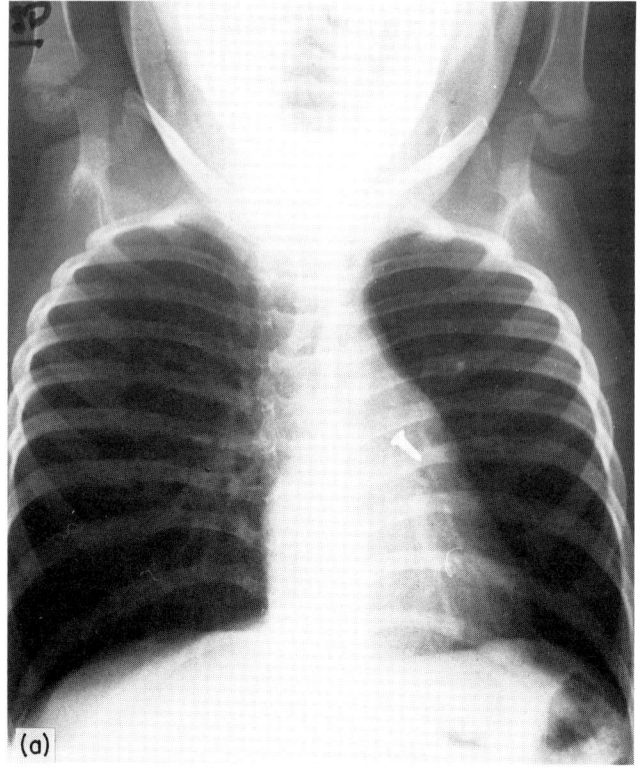

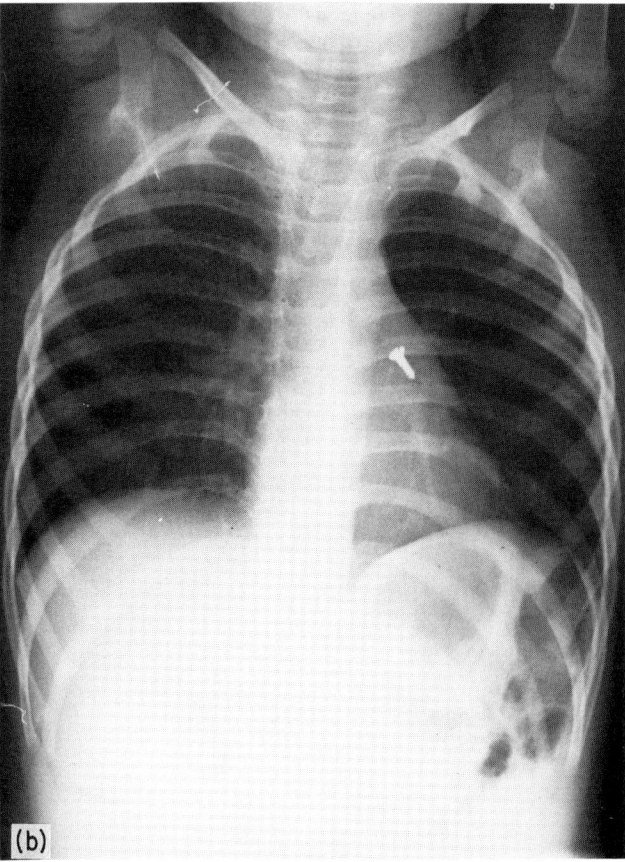

the same volume in both phases (Fig. 15.9). The lucency of the two sides will differ, increasing if the affected lung is hyperinflated.

If the foreign body has been present for some time and the child is febrile, intravenous fluids may be necessary preoperatively.

The anaesthetic techniques for bronchoscopy are summarized in Table 15.1. Premedication should be tailored to the technique chosen and the patient's condition. In the past, deep ether anaesthesia was used for this procedure. The tracheobronchial reflexes were suppressed and bronchodilatation occurred. Spasm of the larynx and airways was unusual, and the occasional cough during light anaesthesia could help to move the foreign body proximally. Its disadvantages are that it is an explosive agent with a pungent odour, and that induction is slow.

Halothane provides smooth induction and maintenance of anaesthesia in conjunction with a local anaesthetic spray (Fig. 15.10). Lignocaine (2% in smaller patients under 20 kg, 4% for older children) is the usual drug in a dose not exceeding 4 mg/kg. When the larynx is sprayed, a pool of local anaesthetic usually collects in the pharynx. Before this is sucked out the larynx can be pressed back into it, thereby giving it an additional coating of local anaesthetic. A dose of 4 mg/kg usually results in a peak plasma level of 5–6 µg/ml but occasionally levels over

Table 15.1 Anaesthetic techniques for bronchoscopy

Controlled ventilation: i.v. induction + muscle relaxant

Ventilating bronchoscope
Venturi attachment
Inflation via side arm
Inflation via a catheter in the trachea
Insertion of a tube into the end of the bronchoscope intermittently

Spontaneous ventilation: i.v. induction or inhalation induction

i.v. induction	+ inhalation agent	+ local anaesthetic
Thiopentone	Halothane–deep	(lignocaine)
Inhalation induction		+ local
Halothane		anaesthetic
		(lignocaine)

Fig. 15.9 (*left*) An inhaled screw in the left main bronchus.
(a) Inspiratory film showing inflation of the right lung.
(b) Expiratory film showing greater deflation on the right side than the left.

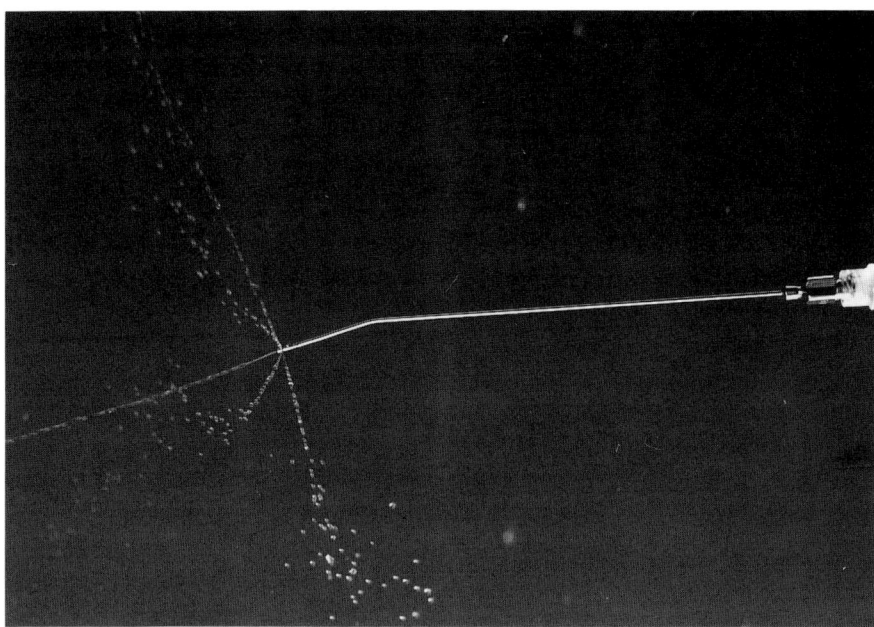

Fig. 15.10 The spray from a Cass–Waldie needle, which has an end opening and four terminal side openings, used for application of local anaesthetic.

10 µg/kg occur (see Chapter 2). Even at this level, convulsions do not occur when the patient is anaesthetized. This technique is suitable for fibreoptic or rigid bronchoscopy. Lignocaine 1–1.5 mg/kg intravenously will also suppress coughing and reduce airway reactivity.

Care must be taken to avoid inserting the laryngoscope and spraying too early, as laryngeal spasm can occur. On rare occasions when thiopentone has not been used, spasm of the thoracic and abdominal muscles can occur during light halothane anaesthesia. These are particular hazards when inhalation induction is slowed by partial airway obstruction and the pupils are not central, indicating inadequate depth of anaesthesia.

Any inhalation induction will be slowed by the presence of a foreign body obstructing one main bronchus, because one lung will be perfused but not ventilated. For this reason an intravenous induction may be helpful.

In another technique, muscle relaxants may be used following intravenous or inhalational induction. Ventilation can be achieved by one of several methods, of which the earliest was the intermittent insertion of an endotracheal tube into the end of the bronchoscope to inflate the lungs. This method is seldom used now because it interferes with the progress of the procedure.

Modern bronchoscopes allow attachment of a T-piece and delivery of gases down the side arm, and are suitable for endoscopy with spontaneous ventilation. This necessitates intermittent closure of the top of the bronchoscope. Ventilation must therefore alternate with surgical manoeuvres such as suction, biopsy and extraction of a foreign body. In spite of theoretical objections to such interruption of bronchoscopic manoeuvres, this system works well in practice, provided there is co-operation between surgeon and anaesthetist, each understanding the task of the other. Pulse oximetry indicates when the oxygen saturation falls to a level where the patient needs to be ventilated.

Another method is the use of a high-pressure gas source which entrains air to ventilate the patient. When it is used, care should be taken to reduce the inflation pressure for children, otherwise excessive intratracheal pressures may develop. With high inflation pressures hyperventilation also occurs and heat loss is increased. A pressure of 140 kPa (20 psi) through a 16 gauge needle, or a higher pressure through a 20 gauge needle attached to the bronchoscope inlet, will provide sufficient ventilation if an adequate frequency of inflation is maintained (over 20/min). Another high-pressure attachment which has a needle valve to control the pressure, a pressure gauge and an on/off button to control the frequency and duration of flow, can be adjusted to provide adequate ventilation with a reduced pressure (Fig. 15.11). These injector techniques allow controlled ventilation to continue regardless of surgical manoeuvres. This could be useful when there is difficulty removing a foreign body, because interruption of the surgeon's manoeuvres could

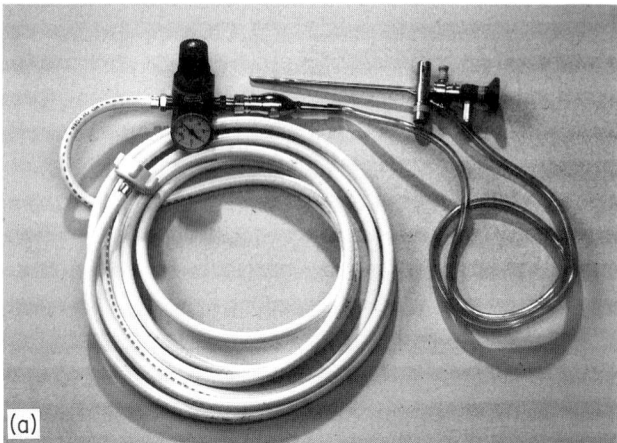

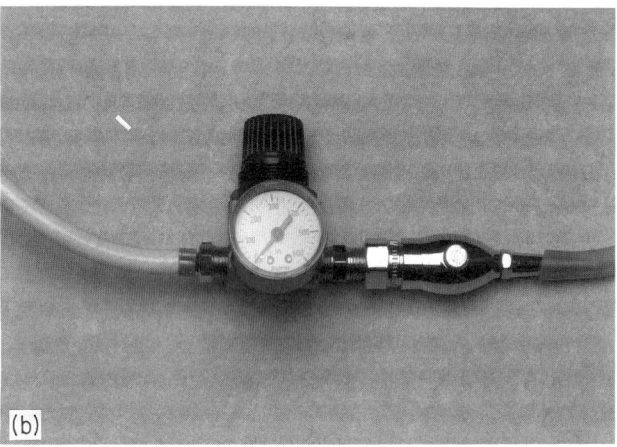

Fig. 15.11 (a) A bronchoflator with needle valve, pressure gauge and on/off button attached to the gas source at one end and bronchoscope at the other. (b) Close-up of the bronchoflator.

be inconvenient. The gas flow might blow the foreign body more peripherally and ventilation would be interrupted should the bronchoscope be removed from the trachea periodically.

It must be remembered that if prolonged suction is applied during these inflation techniques, it reduces the ventilation. The endoscopist should be told if this is happening.

If anaesthetic gases are being administered down the side arm of the bronchoscope, it is dangerous to inflate with a high-pressure gas source at the same time as the increased volume of gases reaching the lungs may raise the intrapulmonary pressures excessively, leading to pneumothorax or pneumomediastinum. This complication is rare but has occurred.

The factors influencing the choice of anaesthesia for bronchoscopy are:
1 the patient's age, general health and the reason for bronchoscopy;
2 the dexterity of the endoscopist and the likely duration of the procedure;
3 the anaesthetist should use a technique and drugs with which he is familiar.

The endoscopist and the anaesthetist must work together and they must understand their respective roles. If the anaesthetist or endoscopist are not experienced with children, or if a range of sizes of paediatric bronchoscopes is not available, it is wiser to refer the patient to a specialist centre.

Monitoring is important. Pulse oximetry provides immediately available information about oxygenation, and if this drops significantly the procedure should be interrupted until oxygenation is improved. A stethoscope is also useful in providing information about ventilation and the circulation.

Occasionally a non-vegetable foreign body which has been impacted for some time may have granulation tissue around it, making it impossible to remove. An open bronchotomy may then become necessary. It is sometimes performed in situations where adequate endoscopic equipment is not available and referral is not possible.

Laryngeal or subglottic oedema with stridor may develop after bronchoscopy in small children, especially if the bronchoscope is inserted several times, or too large a bronchoscope is used. This will usually develop within an hour of the endoscopy and can be treated with nebulized racemic adrenaline inhalations (0.05 ml/kg of 2.25% racemic adrenaline diluted to 2 ml in saline, or up to 0.5 ml/kg adrenaline 1:1000 — maximum 5 ml). Should the oedema not subside and significant airway obstruction develop, intubation may be necessary.

Operations for laryngeal and tracheal stenosis

CRICOID SPLIT OPERATION

Some children with laryngeal stenosis cannot be treated by microsurgery, particularly if the cricoid cartilage is small. In these patients, splitting the cricoid may be sufficient to relieve the obstruction, but a costal cartilage graft may be used to maintain the expanded circumference. The operation is carried out through the neck. If possible, a small endotracheal tube is passed through the stenosis and this is replaced by a bigger tube after the cricoid has been split, so that the airway is splinted. If the laryngeal opening is very narrow, a tracheostomy will probably have been done. An inhalational induction can be used via the tracheostomy. Once the patient is anaesthetized the tracheostomy tube can be replaced by a tube with an acute angled connector, or a non-kinking flexible tube which can be led down towards the chest and connected to the T-piece away from the operative site (Fig. 15.12). Following the operation, a naso-tracheal tube can be inserted to splint the larynx for at least 2 weeks.

If the opening is small but there is no tracheostomy, a fine non-occlusive catheter can be passed into the trachea, for insufflation of anaesthetic gas. There should be enough leak to allow the gases to escape. Later the nasotracheal tube can be inserted and advanced over the catheter and through the cricoid as soon as it has been split, thus providing an improved airway.

TRACHEAL RECONSTRUCTION

The site of the stenosis will determine whether the operation is intrathoracic or done through the neck. The length of the narrowing will determine whether the stenosis is resected with end-to-end anastomosis, or whether an inlay graft of costal cartilage is used to expand the stenotic segment. The anaesthesia for patients with subglottic stenosis and tracheostomy may be managed in a similar way to that described for cricoid split.

The tracheostomy tube is replaced by a special U-shaped tube, a short tube with an acutely angled connector, or a non-kinking flexible tube which is directed away from the neck to the side where the anaesthetist is situated, and attached to the breathing system (Fig. 15.12). The neck is opened and the trachea exposed. The stenotic segment is incised lengthwise anteriorly, and also posteriorly if the stenosis is very tight. A posterior costal cartilage graft, if needed, is then stitched in place. A stent is fitted so that it just protrudes to the level of the arytenoids above and to the end of the tracheostomy tube below. A hole is made at the appropriate point to insert the metal tracheostomy tube. The tracheal tube is then removed and the stent and tracheostomy tube are put in place (Figs 15.13, 15.14). The anterior graft of costal cartilage is then inserted to expand the circumference of the trachea and sutured in place over the stent. The latter is held in place by wire sutures passed through the skin and tied on the outside. After 6 weeks the tracheostomy tube is removed first, the wire suture is cut and the stent is removed from above through the larynx.

The management of tracheal stenosis within the chest is discussed in Chapter 12.

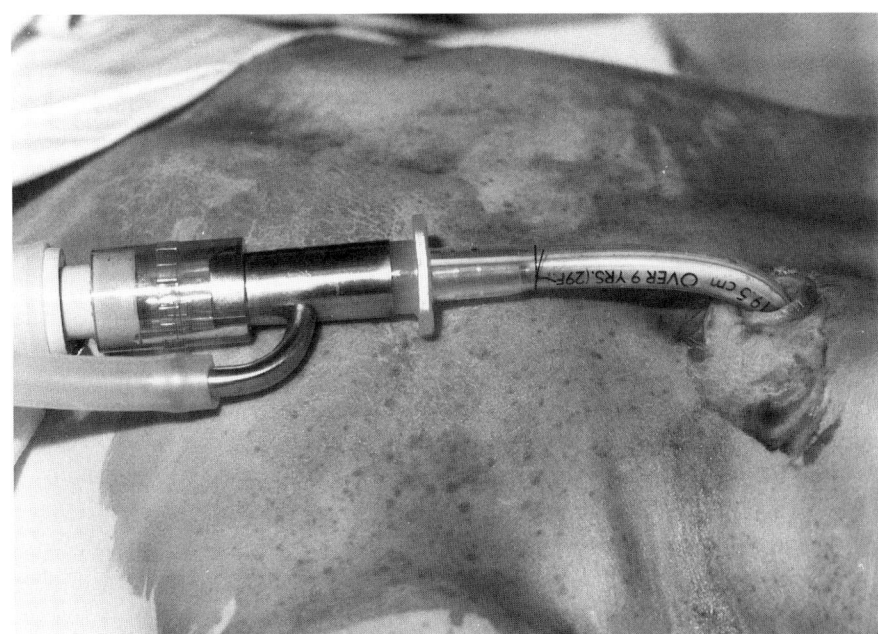

Fig. 15.12 A cutdown RAE tube in a tracheostomy in position for laryngotracheopexy, showing the attachment to the T-piece breathing system on the chest.

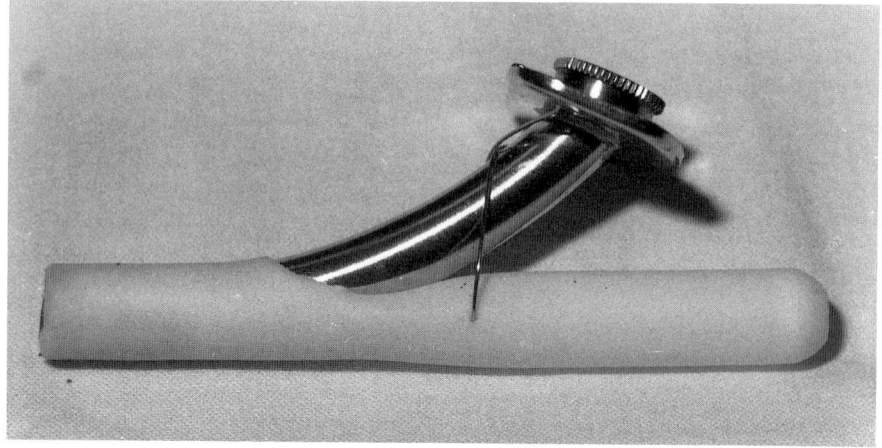

Fig. 15.13 Stent with tracheostomy tube sutured in place with wire as it would be positioned for laryngotracheopexy.

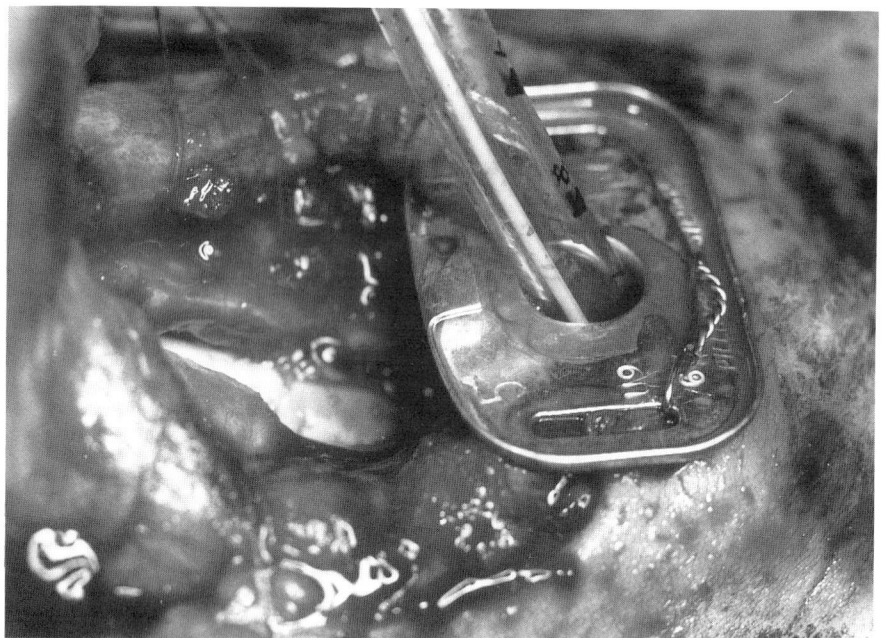

Fig. 15.14 The tracheostomy tube *in situ* with the stent showing through the anterior opening where costal cartilage graft will be sutured.

Oesophagoscopy

Oesophagoscopy may be performed to assess damage following corrosive ingestion, to remove foreign bodies or to dilate a stricture. In patients born with oesophageal atresia, strictures may develop at the site of anastomosis, but the use of less reactive suture material and the avoidance of sutures tied within the lumen has reduced the incidence of this complication.

Patients with a stricture are sometimes treated with steroids, and this should be ascertained preoperatively so that extra cover can be given if necessary. If the obstruction is complete, there may be food or fluid above it, which may be regurgitated during induction. If the obstruction has been present for some time, the patient may be dehydrated and should be appropriately rehydrated with intravenous fluids pre-operatively.

The anaesthetic requirements include aspiration of the oesophagus before induction if it is obstructed, adequate relaxation of the cricopharyngeal sphincter to allow easy passage of the oesophagoscope, and the prevention of coughing and straining, which may cause oesophageal rupture. The patient must be intubated and a suitable anaesthetic technique involves the use of thiopentone, nitrous oxide and a non-depolarizing relaxant with an analgesic or inhalation supplement. Suxamethonium may be used if rapid intubation is deemed necessary, or if the procedure is likely to be brief.

The hazards during the procedure include compression of the endotracheal tube by the oesophagoscope, and accidental extubation. The tube should be well fixed in the left-hand corner of the mouth. If the anaesthetist holds the tube or connection throughout the procedure, it is unlikely to be removed accidentally. Compression of the tube by the oesophagoscope is recognized by a rise in inflation pressure. The anaesthetist should tell the surgeon immediately if this happens so that the airway can be re-established.

Sharp foreign bodies such as pins may perforate the aorta or other major blood vessels. Reliable intravenous access for transfusion should be secured before inducing anaesthesia in these patients, in case haemorrhage occurs.

16: Anaesthesia for Ophthalmic Surgery

INTRODUCTION

Ophthalmic operations in children are usually performed under general anaesthesia, in contrast to adults where local anaesthesia is frequently used. They can be broadly divided into intra- and extra-ocular. Intra-ocular pressure and its control is important in intra-ocular operations, while the oculocardiac reflex may be significant in extra-ocular procedures, particularly strabismus surgery.

GENERAL CONSIDERATIONS

Intra-ocular pressure and the problems of the open eye

The normal intra-ocular pressure is $15-25$ mmHg ($2.0-3.3$ kPa) above atmospheric pressure. This pressure is maintained by a balance between the production and drainage of aqueous humour, which is secreted by the ciliary body. This maintains the globular shape of the eye and the optical properties of the cornea (the proper alignment and hydration of stromal fibres) and its even, constant curvature.

Factors which affect the intra-ocular pressure are summarized below. As these may be modified by anaesthesia, it is important to appreciate the steps which can be taken either to reduce the pressure or prevent it rising, especially when the eye is perforated or is to be opened. Rises in intra-ocular pressure with the eye open can have disastrous effects, including loss of vision.

AQUEOUS HUMOUR

The aqueous humour is formed by the ciliary body and its secretion is under parasympathetic control. It involves an active transport process for sodium, in which carbonic anhydrase plays a part. The carbonic anhydrase inhibitor, acetazolamide, may therefore reduce its production. Obstruction to the flow of aqueous can occur by:

1 Pupil block — apposition of the lens or vitreous (if aphakic) to the iris, preventing aqueous from entering the anterior chamber. This can be caused by displacement or swelling of the lens or vitreous following injury, or by adhesions which may develop in chronic inflammation.
2 Outflow obstruction at the irido-corneal angle or canal of Schlemm, secondary to injury, inflammation or tumour or, as in congenital glaucoma, due to a failure of development of the drainage pathways.

BLOOD PRESSURE

Intra-ocular pressure has been shown to some extent to follow changes in arterial pressure, but is markedly increased by venous obstruction or raised central venous pressure. The increase in venous pressure is transmitted directly to the eye as it distends the choriocapillaries and creates additional back-pressure on the 'aqueous veins' draining the canal of Schlemm. The increased pressure is cushioned only by the amount of aqueous which can be displaced and by the slight distension of the sclera. The highest intra-ocular pressures have been measured under conditions of venous obstruction. Even a mild cough, by raising intrathoracic pressure, produces enough venous obstruction to raise the intra-ocular tension by 30–40 mmHg (4.0–5.3 kPa) and heavy coughing can produce a large rise in both arterial and intra-ocular pressure. An induction complicated by coughing, bucking, hypoventilation or hypoxia will lead to a sustained rise in intra-ocular pressure, particularly in an abnormal eye, which may take more than an hour to return to normal. This is hazardous if the eye is to be opened, because of the danger of extrusion of intra-ocular contents, and may justify postponing the operation.

OCULAR MUSCLE TENSION

Contraction of the orbital muscles, including orbicularis oculi, increases eyeball tension.

ORBITAL SIZE AND CONTENTS

The infant's orbit is smaller and tension on the eye produced by the lids is greater than in older patients. An increase in orbital contents with haematoma or tumour will thus compress the eye, raise intra-ocular pressure and lead to more proptosis than occurs in older patients. This may be aggravated by hypercarbia.

THE VITREOUS

In infants this is a gel, which gradually liquifies with age. It is attached to the posterior capsule of the lens and its volume may increase with overhydration, or it may shrink with osmotic diuretics such as mannitol.

THE SCLERA

This is fairly rigid and limits volume expansion.

DIRECT PRESSURE

Direct pressure can be accidentally applied to the eye by a face mask, by a hand during intubation, or by adhesive tape used to close the eyes.

EFFECTS OF DRUGS

Suxamethonium raises intra-ocular pressure. The rise can be prevented or reduced by prior administration of acetazolamide (Diamox) or possibly by pretreatment with a very small dose of non-depolarizing relaxant. Drugs which reduce intra-ocular pressure produce a greater response if the pressure is already high. These include:

1 Miotics, e.g. pilocarpine, physostigmine (Eserine) or phospholine iodide, may be used in the preoperative management of congenital glaucoma. Beta-blockers in the form of eye drops, e.g. timolol maleate (Timoptol), are also used. They cause bradycardia.

2 Carbonic anhydrase inhibitors, e.g. acetazolamide (Diamox) 3–5 mg/kg intravenously. These are contra-indicated in the presence of liver or kidney dysfunction.

3 An osmotic diuretic such as 20% mannitol 0.4–1 g/kg infused intravenously 1 hour preoperatively.

4 Nerve blocks. Although these are not commonly used in paediatric ophthalmology, all blocks which reduce extra-ocular muscle tone lower intra-ocular pressure. Retrobulbar block interrupts the parasympathetic secretory innervation (ciliary ganglion). The facial nerve may also be blocked to prevent contraction of the orbicularis oculi.

5 Intravenous agents such as thiopentone and propofol and deeper levels of inhalation anaesthesia reduce intra-ocular pressure. Ketamine tends to raise intra-ocular pressure; it is not recommended for procedures with an open eye.

The oculocardiac reflex

The ophthalmic branch of the trigeminal nerve forms the afferent limb and the vagus nerve the efferent limb of this reflex arc. Reflex bradycardia or dysrhythmia can be caused by pressure over the eyeball, by traction on the medial or lateral rectus muscles and occasionally when the sclera is stretched or when a suture is placed through it. It occurs most often during strabismus surgery or enucleation. It is pronounced under general anaesthesia, particularly if there is hypoxia or hypercarbia.

The bradycardia may lead to cardiac arrest. As the efferent side of the reflex is parasympathetic, it can be blocked by atropine. Many anaesthetists give this (approximately 0.01 mg/kg) during induction for strabismus surgery. If it is not given, the degree of bradycardia can be reduced by gradually increasing the tension on the eye muscles to fatigue the reflex. If marked bradycardia does occur the anaesthetist must immediately request the surgeon to stop pulling on the muscle. The heart rate will usually increase and atropine can then be given if desired. The reflex bradycardia is reduced by neuromuscular blockers with anticholinergic effects (pancuronium or gallamine). It is particularly important to monitor heart rate and rhythm at times when the oculocardiac reflex may occur. If dysrhythmia occurs and does not resolve with removal of the stimulus, lignocaine may be indicated.

Occasionally the surgeon will seek the co-operation of the anaesthetist to monitor heart rate when he uses the oculocardiac reflex to identify a 'lost' extra-ocular muscle.

Preoperative preparation of the child

This is particularly important, and some time should be spent explaining the sequence of events to the child. Whenever the use of an eye pad is contemplated, it helps the child to adapt if the eye is covered preoperatively. Most eye operations, except for intra-ocular procedures, are not associated with any significant pain. Sympathetic handling of the child is the most effective measure, and judicious use of sedation may help. Narcotics are avoided because they aggravate the tendency to vomit postoperatively. A dose of paracetamol (20 mg/kg) an hour before the operation helps to control postoperative discomfort.

ANAESTHETIC MANAGEMENT

Anaesthesia for ophthalmic surgery has some special requirements. It is important, particularly in intra-ocular surgery, to avoid coughing, bucking, straining, vomiting or shivering during the perioperative period. Carefully administered anaesthesia which takes into account the points already discussed will be satisfactory for all operations on the eye.

When the eye is to be opened, or has already been perforated, there are advantages in using adequate premedication followed by thiopentone, nitrous oxide and a non-depolarizing relaxant. This can be supplemented by a volatile agent or an opioid to ensure an adequate depth of anaesthesia to obtund undesirable reflex tachycardia and hypertension. This approach reduces intra-ocular pressure and the tendency to coughing and bucking on the tube, particularly if the larynx has also been sprayed with local anaesthetic. If the induction is not smooth, intra-ocular pressure may rise, causing extrusion of the contents of the eye which may lead to permanent visual impairment.

Drug incompatibilities

These include incompatibility of halothane with adrenaline and with cocaine used in a nasal pack prior to dacrocystorhinostomy.

Drug interaction can occur between suxamethonium and cholinesterase inhibitors such as phospholine iodide (ecothiopate) which is used in eye drops as part of the medical treatment of glaucoma. Should the unwary anaesthetist give suxamethonium to a patient who has received these drugs during the past 4 weeks, prolonged apnoea may follow.

Bradycardia caused by timolol may be aggravated by suxamethonium unless atropine is given first.

Control of the airway

Control of the airway for most intra- and extra-ocular operations usually requires the patient to be intubated, taking care that the tube does not kink, has a firmly fitting connector and is well strapped in place.

During dacrocystorhinostomy, when blood or secretions can collect in the pharynx, it should be packed.

Some brief procedures such as examination under anaesthesia, the curettage of a Meibomian cyst, removal of sutures, or probing and syringing of lacrimal ducts can be performed using an inhalation anaesthetic administered by mask, insufflation through a catheter or via a laryngeal mask. It is important to have drugs and equipment available for intubation, as control of the airway may become difficult if secretions accumulate or laryngeal spasm occurs.

Monitoring the patient

The anaesthetist is usually positioned at the side of the operating table. A hand or foot is easily accessible for feeling the pulse and observing the patient's colour. Monitoring is important because of potential significant bradycardia due to the oculocardiac reflex. A pulse oximeter, stethoscope and ECG should be used and blood pressure measured periodically.

Protection of the eye not being operated upon

Whether or not the eye not being operated upon should be covered depends on the surgeon's preference. It is important that the cornea does not become dry or abraded. Some surgeons use a transparent drape with a hole over the eye being operated upon.

Stabilization of the head

Stabilization of the patient's head is important, particularly when the microscope is in use. This may be achieved by using a simple head ring or sandbags.

SPECIFIC OPERATIVE PROCEDURES

Examination under anaesthesia

This may include retinoscopy, tonometry, ultrasonography and other examinations. These patients can be managed using inhalation anaesthesia administered by a mask, or insufflation through a catheter. It is important to have the drugs and equipment available for intubation in case difficulties arise in controlling the airway, due to secretions or laryngeal spasm. It is desirable to have an adequate, even depth of anaesthesia with centrally fixed pupils, so that the conditions for tonometry are consistent.

Lacrimal drainage system

This may be infected when obstructed.

PROBING AND SYRINGING

This is often regarded as a simple procedure, but there are many ways of anaesthetizing infants for this operation and it is very important that the ophthalmologist and anaesthetist have a mutual understanding of what they are going to do. Probing can be done in infants with halothane anaesthetic. This may be administered by mask, but an alternative which gives the ophthalmologist more room to work is to use a Waters airway (Fig. 16.1), a pharyngeal airway with a catheter inserted through it, or a nasal catheter to maintain anaesthesia by insufflation. When using these methods halothane concentration may

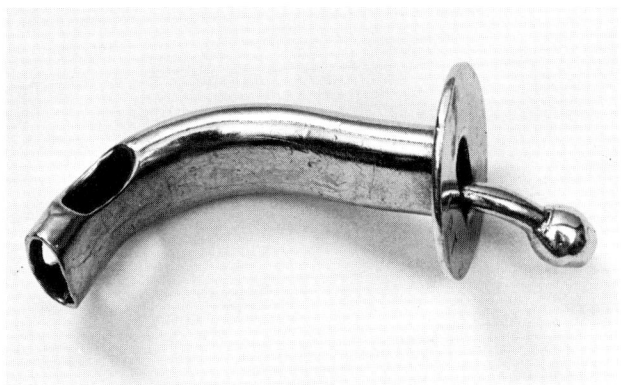

Fig. 16.1 Waters airway with an attachment for insufflation of gases.

need to be increased to compensate for air dilution. Although most ophthalmologists avoid syringing the ducts, if necessary a useful method to avoid spillage is to apply suction to a catheter passed into the nose on the side being syringed. The same catheter can be used for the anaesthetic until syringing begins. Gravity drainage with the child on his side and head-down can also be used. Alternatively, especially if the operation is likely to be prolonged, the patient may be intubated.

Most surgeons prefer to avoid syringing the duct after probing and confirm the success of the probing by passing another probe up the nose to meet the probe in the duct. Even with this method some bleeding may occur, and care must be taken to ensure that the airway is not compromised.

DACROCYSTORHINOSTOMY

In this procedure the obstructed lacrimal system is drained into the nose. It can be accompanied by substantial bleeding. A throat pack is used, and the nose is packed with gauze soaked with a vasoconstrictor, ensuring that the pack includes the middle meatus. Infiltration with adrenaline or ornithine vasopressin (POR8) added to bupivacaine produces effective vasoconstriction and prevents reflex tachycardia, which may increase bleeding.

CANALICULUS REPAIR

Following injury, this may be repaired using an operating microscope. A 0.6 mm silastic tube is threaded along the lumen and acts as a splint while the torn canaliculus is sutured.

Eyelid surgery

Ptosis may be due to muscle weakness or to damage to the innervation of the levator palpebrae superioris muscle. If the muscle contracts but is weak, it may be shortened. If the muscle is paralysed, a fascia lata sling is used to elevate the lid.

Tarsorrhaphy (suture of the lids together) is done to protect the cornea when the eyelids cannot be closed.

Strabismus

Strabismus surgery is common in children. It is important to have the patient adequately anaesthetized so that the muscles are relaxed before the operation begins. If a forced duction test is to be performed, to differentiate between paretic and adherent muscles, suxamethonium should be avoided, because the return of muscle tone to normal may be delayed.

The main problems in squint surgery are the oculo-cardiac reflex during traction on the extra-ocular muscles, and the high incidence of postoperative vomiting. This can be reduced by avoiding opioids and instead injecting 1–3 ml 0.5% bupivacaine subconjunctivally in the upper lateral fornix for analgesia, or giving 20 mg/kg paracetamol preoperatively. Antiemetics are commonly used to reduce postoperative vomiting.

Corneal surgery

Removal of imbedded foreign bodies, detailed diagnostic evaluation and the fitting of contact lenses are the commonest corneal problems requiring general anaesthesia.

Where corneal grafting is not indicated, a Gunderson conjunctival flap may be performed for chronic ulceration, an ulcer which is slow to heal, or for recurrent corneal ulceration interfering with the child's comfort and causing scarring. The operation involves removing the corneal epithelium and mobilizing a conjunctival flap and suturing it to the limbus on the side opposite to that from which the flap was mobilized.

Corneal grafting is usually avoided in very young children, but may be indicated if the cornea threatens to perforate and cannot be treated by the above procedures.

It is essential in corneal grafting to prevent a rise in intra-ocular pressure during surgery. The principles of anaesthetic management already outlined should be followed.

Perforating eye injury

A major problem confronting the anaesthetist is the child with a penetrating eye injury and a full stomach, who requires urgent operation. Fortunately most eye injuries are not acute surgical emergencies, and operation can be delayed a few hours. This applies especially if the ophthalmologist deems that the eye is unsalvageable. An adequate oral premedication with phenothiazine, which is also antiemetic, or diazepam given at least $1\frac{1}{2}$ hours preoperatively avoids an intramuscular injection and the crying that often accompanies it. EMLA cream allows painless venepuncture. Thiopentone induction is rapid, reduces intra-ocular pressure and prevents the struggling which may occur during an inhalation induction.

In other circumstances, when there is a full stomach, it is desirable to intubate patients rapidly with suxamethonium, applying cricoid pressure to prevent regurgitation and aspiration. Because suxamethonium causes a rise in intra-ocular pressure which may extrude the ocular contents, it should not be used unless preceded by a small dose of a non-depolarizing relaxant to prevent extra-ocular muscle contracture. Preoperative acetazolamide, 3–5 mg/kg intravenously, will reduce intra-ocular pressure and may offer some protection against a rise, but cannot by itself be guaranteed to prevent extrusion of orbital contents. As the rate of onset of non-depolarizing relaxants is related to dose, a reasonable alternative is to use a larger than usual dose of atracurium (0.6–0.7 mg/kg) and depend on cricoid pressure to prevent aspiration during inflation of the lungs until the child is sufficiently relaxed to intubate. Spraying the larynx with local anaesthetic before intubation may reduce any remaining tendency to cough and 'buck' on the tube, which might raise intra-ocular pressure.

Intra-ocular surgery

Incident-free anaesthesia is essential to prevent rises in intra-ocular pressure and extrusion of contents when the eye is opened. The microscope is commonly used, especially in anterior chamber surgery.

Intraocular operations are for:

1 Removal of foreign bodies which may enter through superficial or penetrating wounds. The anaesthetic problems have been outlined above.

2 Cataracts in children, which are either congenital or traumatic. The congenital types are either hereditary

or due to intrauterine infection, such as rubella or toxoplasmosis.

When the cataract affects the whole lens or is sufficient to cause severe visual impairment, early surgical intervention will produce the best long-term results. Thus, surgery may be undertaken within the first few days of life.

In young infants, the whole lens is removed, with part of the anterior vitreous, through a small incision in the cornea. The eye is not laid open and vitreous loss is controlled by the surgeon.

3 Glaucoma — high intraocular pressure resulting from obstruction to aqueous outflow. In congenital glaucoma an incision is made in the membrane that obstructs the drainage angle.

When glaucoma arises from pupillary block, iridectomy allows aqueous circulation and equalization of pressures between anterior and posterior chambers. This operation is also performed in association with cataract extraction.

In trabeculectomy part of the trabecular meshwork is excised through a scleral trapdoor, to allow drainage of aqueous.

4 In vitreous surgery or vitrectomy, the operator views the posterior chamber through the microscope and a contact lens on the cornea and manipulates the instruments which are passed into the eye behind the ciliary body. The main indication for vitreous surgery is haemorrhage. The vitreous is removed, providing a clear pathway for light to the retina. Vitrectomy may also be used in some cases of eye trauma and, if there is a cataract and vitreous damage, the cataract can be removed by the same route prior to removal of the vitreous. These developments offer some hope for patients with retrolental fibroplasia, as vitreous and retinal surgery may be combined through this approach.

Retinal detachment

Retinal detachment may be preceded by a breach in the retina, which may then become detached, due to abnormal fluid accumulating between the retina and the pigmented choroid. Surgery is monitored by ophthalmoscopy while the breach is sealed by cryopexy, applied through the sclera, or photocoagulation with a laser beam directed on to the tear. Then the retina is apposed to the pigment epithelium, frequently by evacuating the fluid. The sclera is buckled by attaching a piece of silicone sponge to reduce the volume of the posterior segment of the eye.

It is desirable to have a soft eye while this is done, so intra-ocular pressure is usually lowered by the administration of acetazolamide (Diamox) or mannitol.

When an air bubble is injected into the vitreous humour to facilitate mechanical re-attachment, nitrous oxide should be avoided or stopped at least 15 minutes before the injection of air, to prevent an increase in the size of the bubble, which can cause compression of the retinal vessels.

Tumours

Tumours of the eye and orbit are uncommon in childhood, malignant tumours being less common than benign tumours and swellings. The malignant tumours, rhabdomyosarcoma and retinoblastoma, usually present before 5 years of age. The sites of some tumours are illustrated in Fig. 16.2.

Rhabdomyosarcoma of the orbit tends to develop in unspecialized connective tissue, most often in the upper medial quadrant of the orbit, so that the eye is pushed down and outwards. Treatment has previously been by exenteration of the orbit, but recently good results have been obtained by radiotherapy, either alone or in combination with chemotherapy.

Retinoblastoma has a strong familial incidence and presents by the age of 3 years in two thirds of patients. There may be single or multiple tumours affecting one eye (70%) or both eyes (30%). Treatment may include enucleation followed by radiotherapy and chemotherapy.

Optic gliomas are usually benign tumours of the optic

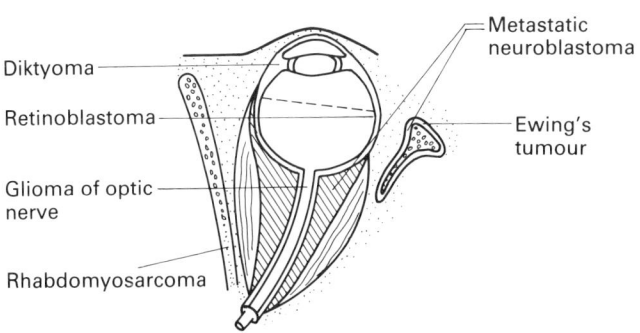

Fig. 16.2 Ophthalmic tumours.

nerve, which may develop in the orbit or intracranially. The most common age of presentation is 3 years. The tumour may be explored through a lateral orbitotomy. A biopsy can be taken and, if malignant or there is no useful vision and if there are gross cosmetic deformities, the tumour can be excised through the lateral orbitotomy or occasionally through a craniotomy. Unroofing the optic canal decompresses the nerve and appears to prevent further deterioration of vision.

In operations such as exenteration of the orbit, bleeding may obscure the operation site. The use of controlled hypotension will reduce bleeding and allow the surgeon a clearer view of the surgical field (see Chapter 23). For these operations the eye muscles should be relaxed, and care should be taken to avoid excessive traction on the optic nerve as bradycardia and cardiac arrest can occur.

Sympathetic ophthalmia

The management of a perforating injury causing prolapse of uveal tissue is always fraught with the risk of sympathetic ophthalmia. This is thought to be an autoimmune sensitivity to uveal pigment, with inflammatory change in the uninjured eye which can progress to total blindness.

Removal of the eye with prolapsed uveal tissue within 10 days of injury prevents the development of sympathetic ophthalmia, but this must be weighed against the possibility of useful vision following careful repair and retention of the injured eye.

POSTOPERATIVE COMPLICATIONS

Nausea and vomiting are common after ophthalmic operations, particularly following strabismus surgery. For this reason an antiemetic, e.g. low-dose droperidol, prochlorperazine (Stemetil) or metoclopramide, is often used with premedication or given during the operation. Vomiting is more frequent if opioids are used. As postoperative pain is not severe, paracetamol (10–20 mg/kg) or the use of local anaesthesia may be adequate.

Postoperative restlessness may be due to belladonna alkaloids, either injected or given as eye drops. This can be potentiated in infants receiving these alkaloids in 'colic' mixtures. Quiet emergence is the aim, particularly after intra-ocular surgery.

17: Anaesthesia for Plastic and Craniofacial Surgery

PLASTIC SURGERY

INTRODUCTION

It is desirable that the anaesthetist should understand the nature of the procedures and the surgical requirements to provide the optimum conditions for operation. The range in plastic surgery is wide, extending in age from the newborn to the teenager, and involving most regions of the body. In addition to elective procedures, much of the work follows trauma. This may be a localized injury or may involve multiple injuries and many surgical disciplines.

The principal considerations and requirements for satisfactory anaesthesia for plastic surgery will be discussed.

PREOPERATIVE ASSESSMENT

Elective surgery

Children scheduled for elective surgery should be assessed so that possible problems are recognized and the anaesthetist has a chance to plan an appropriate action in consultation with the surgeon.

Certain conditions may be accompanied by airway difficulties and intubation problems. Micrognathia, which may make ventilation and intubation difficult, is a feature of several syndromes requiring plastic surgery, such as Pierre Robin syndrome, Treacher–Collins syndrome (mandibulofacial dysostosis) (Fig. 17.1), and hemifacial microsomia (facio-auriculovertebral anomalad, Goldenhar syndrome).

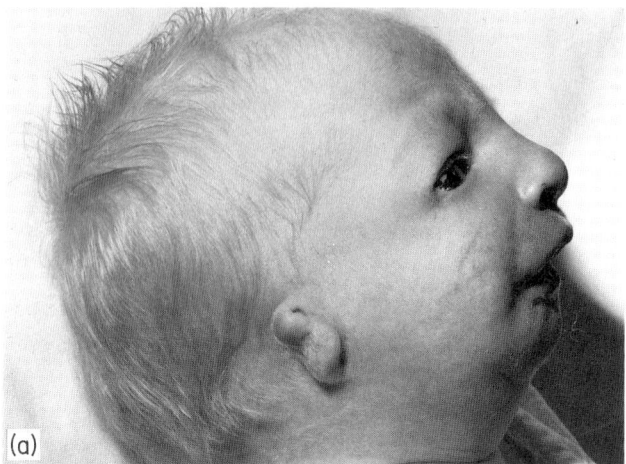

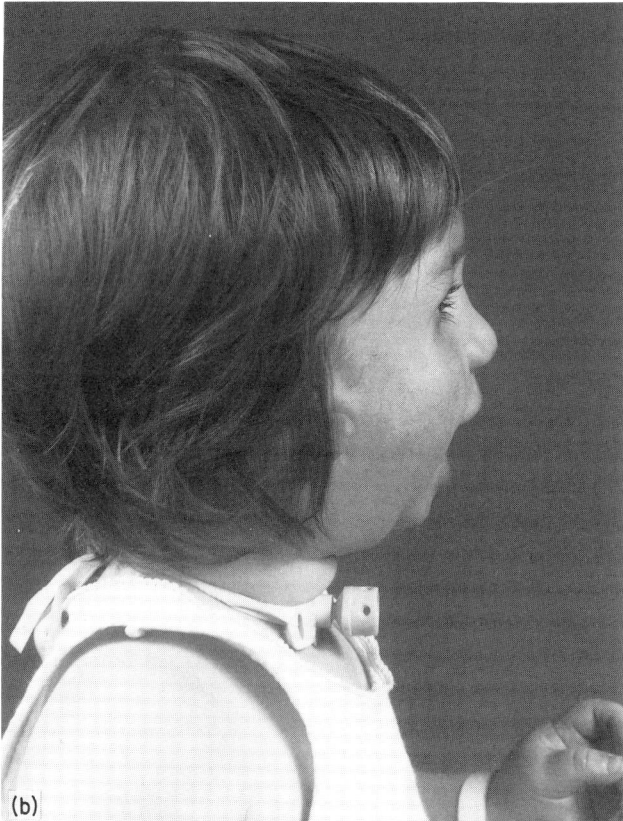

Fig. 17.1 Two patients with Treacher–Collins syndrome, showing the hypoplastic mandible and underdeveloped ears. (b) had a tracheostomy because of chronic airway obstruction, which can occur in patients with hypoplastic mandibles.

Some congenital abnormalities frequently have associated anomalies which require consideration by the anaesthetist, for example, congenital heart disease in association with cleft lip or palate.

Emergency surgery

For the patient with a minor localized injury, the preoperative examination involves an assessment of the general fitness of the patient for anaesthesia, the timing of the operation in relation to the intake of food and the urgency of the procedure (see Chapter 26). In severe injuries resuscitation will be necessary; early consultation between the anaesthetist and the various specialist surgeons involved should reduce the operating time and the number of operations.

CHOICE OF ANAESTHESIA

General anaesthesia is usually favoured in small children, except possibly for minor procedures. Nerve blocks used in association with general anaesthesia reduce the need for analgesic drugs, both during and following operation. Nerve blocks can be used in older, cooperative children, usually with sedation, which may be given intravenously. A variety of anaesthetic techniques is available, but one using thiopentone, nitrous oxide, an opioid supplement and muscle relaxant with controlled ventilation provides suitable conditions for most plastic surgical procedures. It is the preferred method when adrenaline is being injected for vasoconstriction. The problems of movement and postoperative shivering or rigidity are usually avoided, and the patient recovers rapidly after reversal of muscle relaxants at the conclusion of the procedure. Some anaesthetists use inhalation supplements; there is also a view that patients breathing spontaneously under inhalation anaesthesia bleed less.

Smooth, uncomplicated emergence from anaesthesia is desirable so that vomiting, shivering or muscle rigidity do not occur. Such complications could lead to excessive bleeding or haematoma formation, disruption of repaired tendons and nerves and interference with pedicles or attachments of flaps. These complications may be avoided by the use of local or regional anaesthesia for appropriate operations.

In most plastic surgical procedures, postoperative analgesic requirements are minimal if an analgesic has been given with the premedication or during anaesthesia, as postoperative pain is diminished by proper dressing and immobilization of the wound. Care should be taken to elucidate the cause of postoperative pain, particularly that due to excessively tight bandages or to haematoma formation, which will require intervention. Donor sites for split-skin grafts are painful. The use of long-acting local anaesthetic blocks of the nerve supplying the area or local infiltration provides several hours of analgesia. If these are not used it is desirable to provide postoperative analgesia, started intravenously before the end of the operation to avoid restlessness on waking. The use of occlusive dressings, e.g. 'Op-site' on the donor area may also reduce postoperative pain.

Regional anaesthesia is widely used in plastic surgery in adults but it is used less in children, mainly because children dislike needles and may be apprehensive in the theatre environment. Some regional blocks, such as axillary brachial plexus block, can be used without supplementary general anaesthesia in older children, when the anaesthetist can gain the child's confidence or the child is adequately sedated. Regional blocks may also be performed under light general anaesthesia. Axillary block is particularly useful when there is an isolated hand injury. If regional anaesthesia is employed and motor paralysis is achieved, the gradual return of power postoperatively prevents sudden tension being placed on repaired tendons. Similarly, caudal anaesthesia inserted during light general anaesthesia is useful for hypospadias repair as it prevents erection, reduces bleeding and provides postoperative analgesia (see Chapter 22). Nerve blocks are useful for head and neck operations as well, especially if they reduce complications such as coughing, laryngospasm and vomiting, which may cause bleeding, haematoma formation and impaired healing.

When the child is old enough to understand, it is helpful to warn him before surgery about such things as nasal packs, covered eyes and immobilized joints. This should be done by the surgeon but should be re-emphasized by the anaesthetist, particularly when the nasal airway will be obstructed.

A pharyngeal pack may be inserted to absorb blood and prevent tracheal soiling, provided it does not interfere with surgical access. If it does, the surgeon may pack the area with a surgical swab. If a pharyngeal pack is inserted, it must be recorded on the anaesthetic chart and a check made at the end of the procedure to ensure that it has been removed. Failure to remove the pack causes airway obstruction after extubation.

PATIENT IMMOBILITY

It is very important that patients do not move during the operative procedure and continue to remain still until the dressings are applied and immobilizing plasters are in place. Movement of a finger during suturing of a tendon or swallowing during repair of a cleft palate should be avoided. Furthermore, the operation is not complete until the dressings have been applied and the surgeon is satisfied with the state of the circulation, especially after a tourniquet has been removed.

SURGICAL ACCESS

The surgeon should have good surgical access; the positioning of the endotracheal tube and the anaesthetic equipment is important in providing this. When the operation involves the head and neck, the patient is usually intubated. A laryngeal mask airway is sometimes used. The tube and connection must be secured in place so that they do not come apart or become dislodged if the head is moved during the operation. Long PVC or RAE tubes allow the connection to be kept away from the site of operation.

The anaesthetist also requires adequate access to the patient, particularly to the airway if suctioning is required. The intravenous infusion may often be more accessible if sited in the lower limb.

CONTROL OF BLEEDING

Bleeding may prevent the surgeon from seeing clearly what he is doing. Methods employed to reduce bleeding include the application of a tourniquet for limb operations, the injection of vasoconstrictors such as adrenaline and ornithine vasopressin (POR8) and induced hypotension aided by posture (see Chapter 23). A tourniquet can be applied for an hour; unless the operation can confidently be expected to finish within a further half hour, the tourniquet should be released for 5 minutes at that time and then be reapplied for completion of the operation.

Moderate hypotension can be achieved with D-tubocurarine, volatile agents (particularly isoflurane) and posture, but sodium nitroprusside or other specific hypotensive agents can lower the blood pressure further and reduce bleeding more effectively (see Chapter 23). Maintenance of an adequate cerebral perfusion pressure is essential and requires careful monitoring.

Vasoconstrictors are used to reduce bleeding in procedures such as repair of cleft palate and nasal operations. When adrenaline is used it is preferable to avoid halothane, although the latter is used as a supplement by some anaesthetists with careful ECG monitoring and controlled ventilation. It is safer to use some of the newer agents with adrenaline (see Chapter 2). Cardiac dysrhythmia is more likely during nasal surgery, when the absorption of adrenaline is very rapid and may follow accidental intravenous injection. If halothane is to be used as the main agent, alternative vasoconstrictors such as ornithine vasopressin or phenylephrine should be substituted for adrenaline.

When significant blood loss is anticipated, an intravenous cannula should be inserted before surgery begins. It should be large enough to administer blood easily if required, although initially other fluids will be used.

SPECIFIC CONDITIONS AND OPERATIONS

Certain congenital abnormalities of the head and neck may be associated with major anaesthetic problems in plastic surgery. The commonest problem is difficulty with the airway during intubation and ventilation caused by particular anatomical features. Some of these congenital abnormalities will be described.

Choanal atresia

Choanal atresia is a soft-tissue or bony obstruction, usually at the level of the posterior border of the hard palate, which causes nasal obstruction and respiratory difficulty soon after birth, as neonates are essentially nose breathers. Temporary relief of the obstruction may be achieved with an oropharyngeal airway which can be strapped in place.

The object of the operation is to create a patent nasal airway by the passage of sounds through the soft tissue, or perforating the bony obstruction if present. Intubation is necessary, and the ability to ventilate the infant by mask should be established before using muscle relaxants for intubation. If the anaesthetist has difficulty ventilating the patient by mask, it may be safer to intubate the infant awake or under deep halothane anaesthesia with spontaneous ventilation (see Chapter 7). The tube is placed in the midline and the connections are led down over the chin. If a mouth gag is used, care must be taken to ensure that the tube is not kinked by the tongue blade. This will be detected by increased resistance to ventilation when the blade is put in place. Sounds are used to perforate the obstruction on one or both sides and nasopharyngeal tubes are passed from the nose through the newly created passages, and are usually left in place for some months until the danger of contracture has

passed. Cut-down endotracheal tubes are usually held in place by glueing a short segment of a larger tube over each end. Blood loss may be significant during this operation and an adequate intravenous infusion should be in place. The surgeon sometimes inserts a small pharyngeal pack to absorb blood.

These patients often return for further dilatation, and sometimes the insertion of larger tubes, until an adequate airway is established. It is sometimes difficult to achieve a good fit with a mask in the presence of the nasopharyngeal tube, and a variety of masks of different sizes should be available to overcome this.

Transpalatal repair of choanal atresia may be necessary when the passage of sounds is unsuccessful or recurrent obstruction occurs after the removal of the tubes. This can be associated with significant blood loss; adequate intravenous access must be obtained and cross-matched blood must be available.

Cleft lip (Fig. 17.2)

Congenital clefts of the upper lip occur because of failure of fusion of the maxillary and the medial and lateral nasal processes, which develop into the major components of the face between the 4th and 7th weeks of fetal life. They vary from a notch in the upper lip to a cleft through the lip and floor of the nose involving the alveolar ridge, or there may be a complete cleft of the lip and palate. The condition may be bilateral and is frequently asymmetric, being complete on one side and incomplete on the other.

Formal lip repair may be preceded by the preliminary procedures of lip adhesion and columellar lengthening. Lip adhesion is performed in patients with a wide unilateral cleft in order to reduce the gap and make formal lip repair easier. Columella lengthening is sometimes performed in patients with bilateral cleft lip. Both are usually performed at the age of 6 weeks; blood loss is generally not significant, but the principles of anaesthetic management are essentially those for cleft lip repair.

The timing of formal lip repair varies, but is commonly between 3 and 4 months of age, although some surgeons operate earlier than this. If there is an associated cleft of the anterior palate, it is often repaired at the same time.

These patients are often not premedicated. If opioids are used, reduced doses should be employed so that postoperative respiratory depression is avoided. The use of bupivacaine with adrenaline 1:200 000 – 1:400 000 will provide analgesia and reduce blood loss.

When a palate repair is included, care must be taken to ensure that the Kilner blade (Fig. 17.3) does not obstruct the tube. Intubation can be complicated by a prominent premaxilla or a deep cleft, if the laryngoscope blade becomes stuck in the cleft. Placing a rolled swab in the cleft helps to avoid this problem.

Bleeding may be significant; an intravenous infusion should be inserted, preferably in the foot because it will be nearer the anaesthetist. The use of a vasoconstrictor will reduce bleeding. A pack will be required and may be inserted by the anaesthetist, or alternatively the surgeon may place one or more swabs in the mouth.

At the end of the operation, a major problem is that of balancing adequate analgesia with a quiet but awake infant against respiratory depression and the possibility of airway obstruction. A tongue stitch is often useful to pull the tongue forward. The pharynx should be sucked

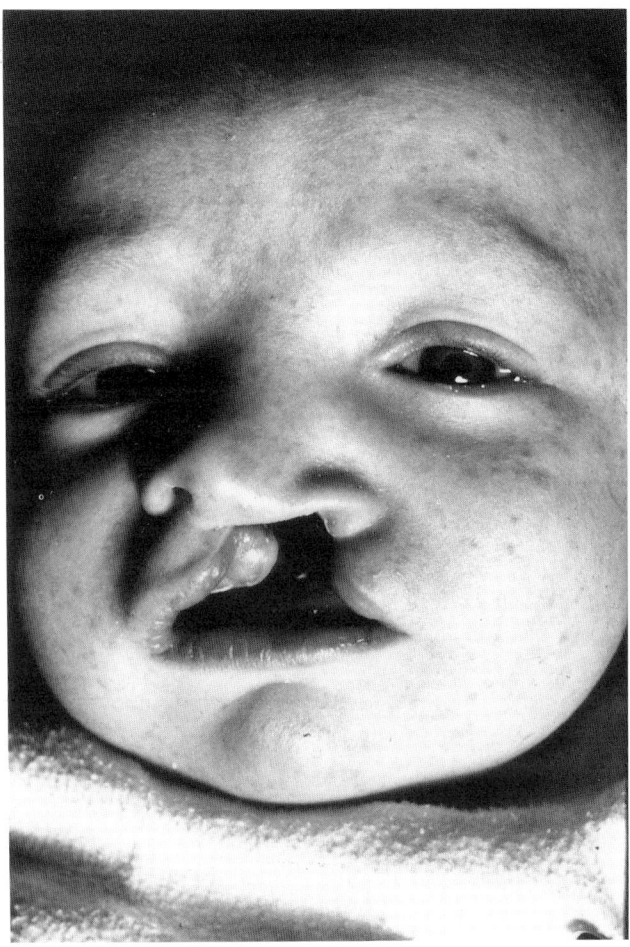

Fig. 17.2 Cleft lip.

In lip and alveolar margin surgery, special care should be taken to avoid trauma during intubation. Paralysing these patients provides better intubating conditions.

An intravenous induction followed by muscle relaxant and nitrous oxide with appropriate supplement provides satisfactory anaesthesia and rapid awakening at the conclusion of the operation. Alternatively, some people prefer to use spontaneous ventilation with the infant intubated, as they believe bleeding is less. It may be difficult to obtain a good seal with the face mask, particularly in babies with a hypoplastic nose and prominent premaxilla. This should be checked before paralysing the patient.

A RAE or Portex Polar 'south' tube, used with care to ensure it is not pushed into a bronchus, is brought down over the chin as the anaesthetist will be at the patient's side. If these tubes are not available, a tube cut to the correct length and an angle connector can be used.

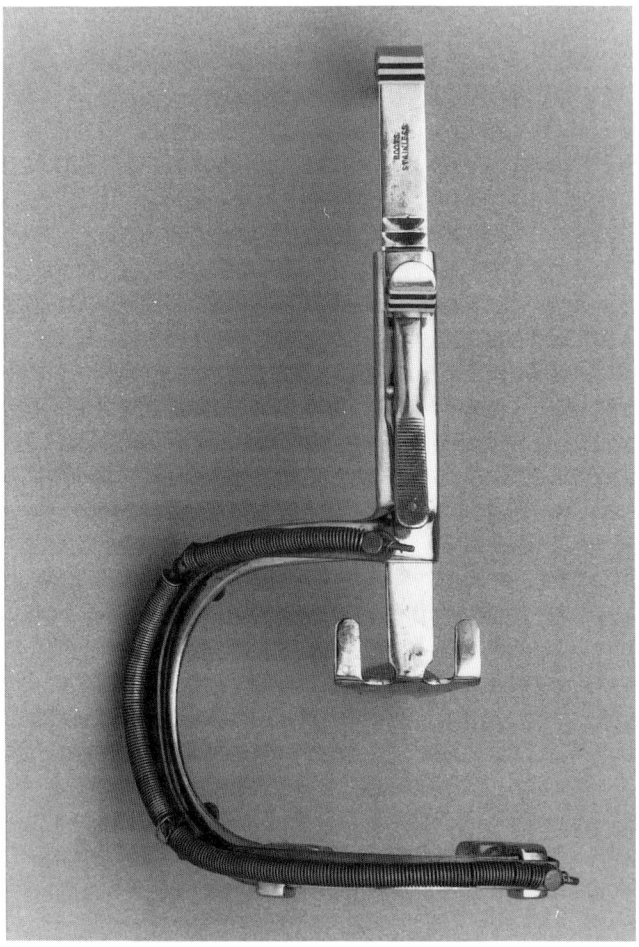

Fig. 17.3 A Kilner mouth gag and blade to hold the tube and tongue in place.

out under direct vision before extubation. A splint jacket is used to prevent the infant touching the operative site (Fig. 17.4).

Secondary procedures are often required at a later stage to improve the cosmetic result, especially of nasal deformities. In bilateral cleft, the upper lip may be short from side to side; this contrasts with a full and often pouting lower lip. In this situation, a segment of the lower lip, based on a pedicle containing the labial artery, is swung up and inserted into the midline of the upper lip to increase its width and simulate a philtrum. The pedicle of this Abbe flap is left for 2–3 weeks before division, so that a new blood supply can be established (Fig. 17.5). At the first operation the patient should be warned beforehand that he will not be able to open his mouth, as the lips are sutured together, and the endotracheal tube should not be removed until the patient's laryngeal reflexes have recovered and he is awake. The pharynx should be carefully sucked out with a catheter and the tube withdrawn into the pharynx. Suction should then be applied to the tube while it is removed from the pharynx, so that any irritating secretions or blood are removed. An antiemetic such as metoclopramide should be given to prevent postoperative vomiting. The patient should be well informed preoperatively and able to cooperate in the postoperative period. Adequate analgesia should be given; infiltration with local anaesthetic provides good operating conditions and postoperative analgesia.

These patients require an intravenous infusion postoperatively, as their oral intake is usually inadequate in the early postoperative period.

The pedicle can be divided at the next operation using ketamine or thiopentone anaesthesia, and then the patient can be paralysed and intubated before the surgeon completes the final setting of the flap. This procedure requires co-operation between the anaesthetist and the surgeon, and they should discuss beforehand how each will proceed. In the older and more co-operative patient, division of the Abbe flap is frequently performed under local anaesthesia supplemented with intravenous sedation.

Cleft palate

Isolated cleft palate is a different genetic entity from cleft lip and palate. The palatal structures develop during the seventh to 12th weeks of fetal life and failure of fusion may result in a central cleft in the posterior soft palate, varying from a bifid uvula and failure of muscle union only (submucous cleft) to a cleft involving the soft palate or extending forward through the hard palate as far as the foramen caecum. Children with cleft palates have a higher incidence of associated congenital anomalies than those with cleft lips.

The purpose of the operation is to produce a palate that will allow nasopharyngeal closure and, subsequently, good speech. It is done before speech develops.

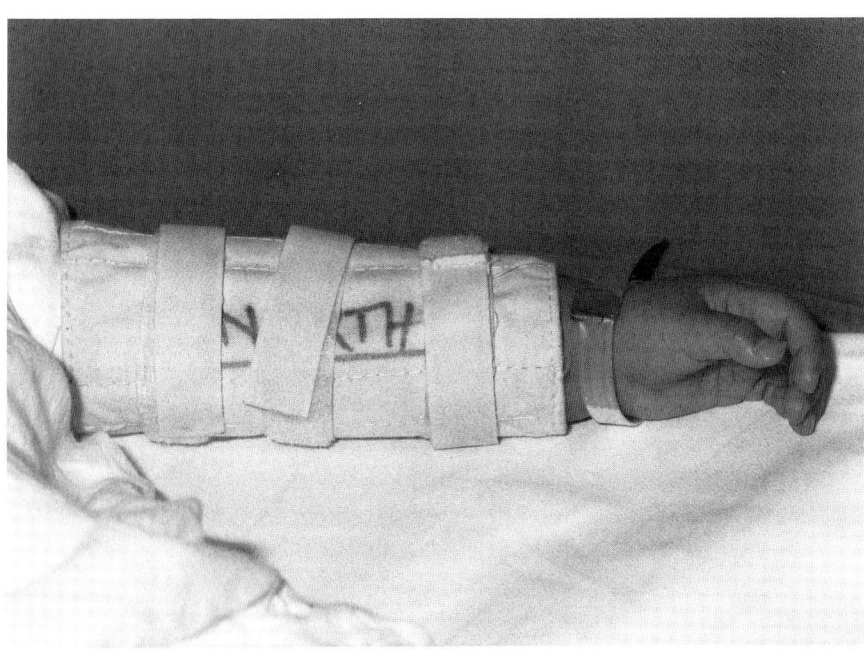

Fig. 17.4 Arm splints in a jacket to prevent the child touching the operative site following cleft lip repair.

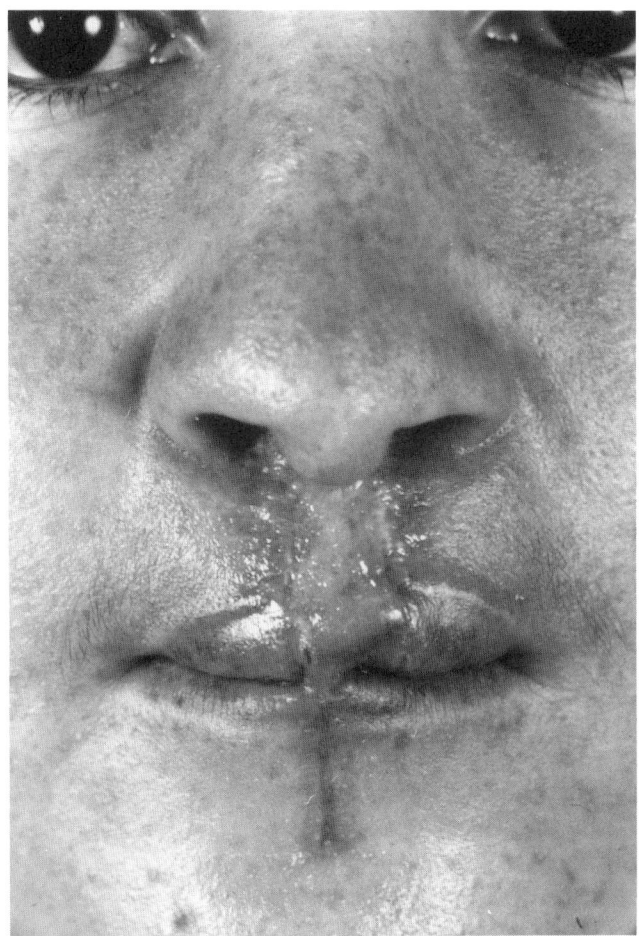

Fig. 17.5 An Abbe flap from the lower lip into the deficient upper lip. It is divided after the blood supply from the upper lip is established.

Repair is usually delayed until the age of 12 months, by which time the mouth has grown sufficiently to give reasonable surgical access and the palatal shelves have developed. There has been a recent trend towards earlier repair of the cleft palate, at 6–10 months of age.

Preoperative assessment is important because of the high incidence of associated anomalies and the frequency of otitis media and upper respiratory infection. A runny nose is fairly common and should not contraindicate surgery, unless it is purulent or has just developed as an accompaniment to a cold or fever.

The patient is usually premedicated. Papaveretum or morphine with hyoscine provides analgesia and dries secretions and is a useful combination, particularly when controlled ventilation is used during the anaesthetic.

Care must be taken to avoid depressed respiration at the end of the operation.

It is important that the endotracheal tube is fixed in the correct position so that it does not enter a bronchus or become kinked when the mouth gag is inserted. The tube should either have a preformed curve or an angled connection, so that it comes down over the lower lip where it is held in the midline by the mouth gag (Fig. 17.6). The surgeon will usually insert a surgical swab, rather than a throat pack, once the gag is inserted.

An intravenous infusion should be running. Blood loss is sometimes sufficient to warrant transfusion; blood should be cross-matched preoperatively. At the conclusion of the operation, the surgeon ensures that the pharynx and nasopharynx are cleared of secretions and the throat swab is removed. If there is any delay in removing the tube, the anaesthetist should check the

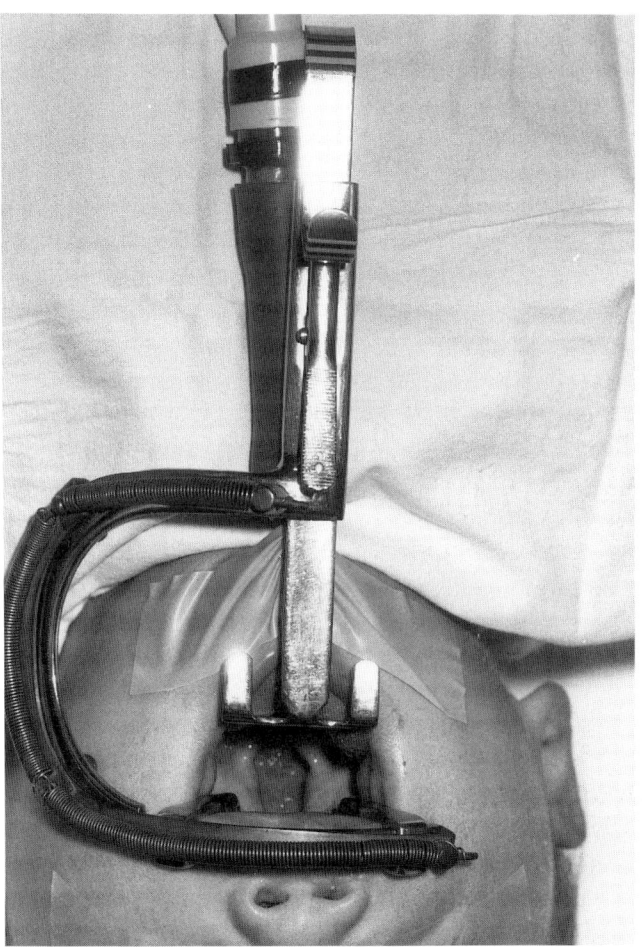

Fig. 17.6 A Kilner blade in place with the tube below the tongue blade, giving good access to the mouth and cleft palate.

pharynx again by laryngoscopy. Postoperative airway obstruction may occur and is more likely in the younger patient after a posterior palate repair. A tongue stitch and nasopharyngeal airway (inserted by the surgeon under vision) may be very useful in these patients.

Pharyngoplasty

A pharyngoplasty may be required either as a secondary procedure in children who have had a cleft palate repair or in children with primary velopharyngeal incompetence. The latter group are more likely to develop airway obstruction in the postoperative period. The creation of a pharyngeal flap in this operation is often associated with significant airway obstruction in the early postoperative phase. A tongue stitch is useful to pull the tongue forward and relieve obstruction.

Sleeping pulse-oximetry studies performed on patients having elective cleft palate repair and pharyngoplasty indicate that clinical airway obstruction and desaturation are quite common in the first 48–72 hours postoperatively (Fig. 17.7). Patients whose airway is compromised preoperatively, e.g. Pierre Robin syndrome, may have postoperative airway problems for a longer period, up to 7–10 days. Preoperative oximetry showing episodes of desaturation may be of value in predicting patients likely to develop significant airway obstruction postoperatively.

Insertion of a nasopharyngeal tube under direct vision by the surgeon at the completion of the operation is useful in maintaining a clear airway postoperatively. The patency of the tube must be maintained by regular suction and humidification.

Blood loss may be significant during this operation and transfusion may be necessary. The intravenous

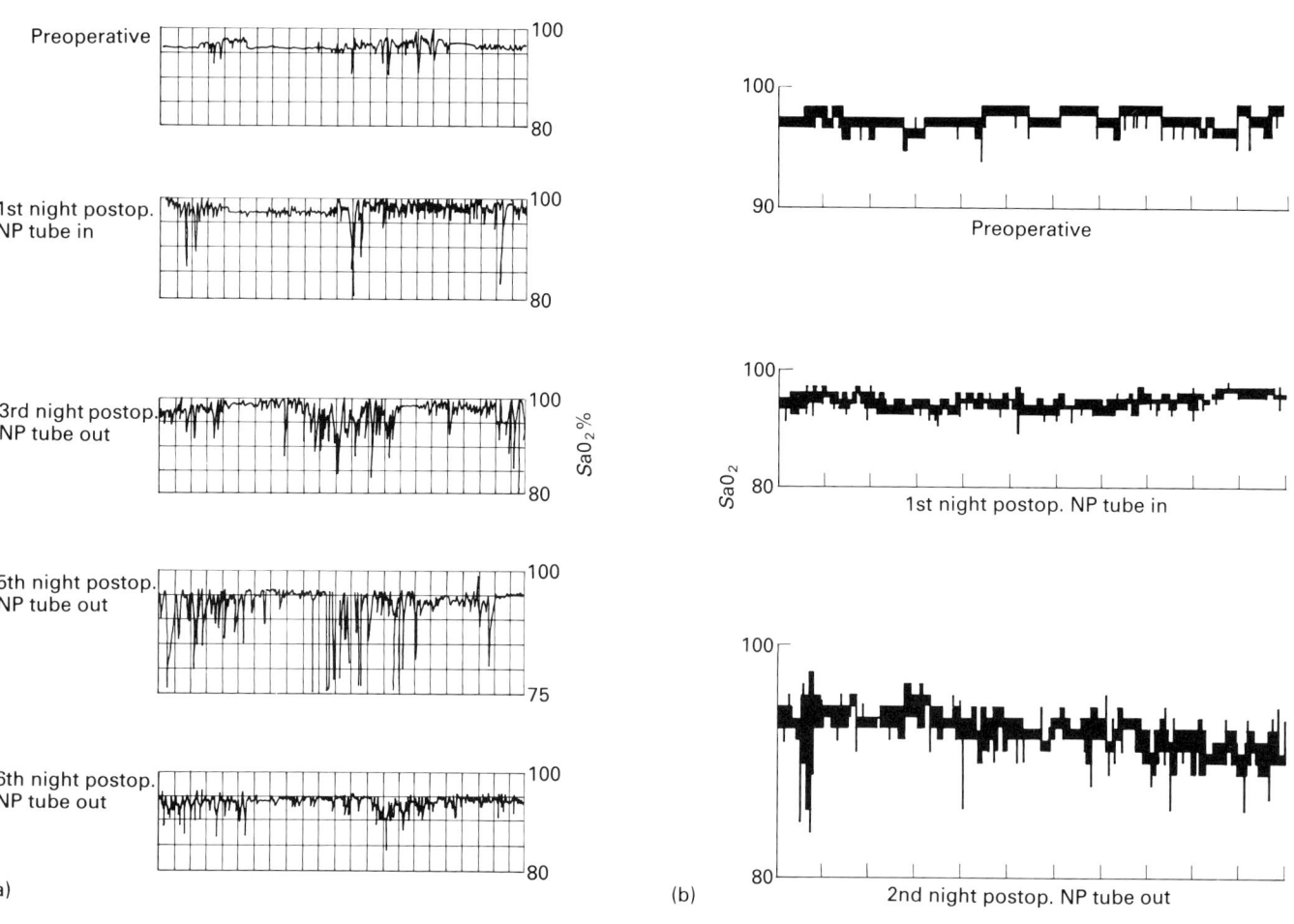

Fig. 17.7 Traces showing the value of pulse oximetry in the assessment and postoperative care of a child having (a) a cleft palate repair, and (b) a pharyngoplasty. It also demonstrates the value of a nasopharyngeal tube placed in position at the end of the operation and kept in for the critical early postoperative period — up to 2 or 3 days.

infusion should be continued for several days, as these patients find drinking difficult in the first days after their operation.

As this procedure involves suturing a flap from the posterior pharyngeal wall to the palate, the anaesthetist should be careful when nasal intubation is required in patients who have had a pharyngoplasty. Where possible, nasal intubation should be avoided.

Pierre Robin syndrome (Fig. 17.8)

This syndrome consists of micrognathia, glossoptosis and usually a cleft of the soft palate. The clinical features will vary with the severity of the micrognathia and may include airway obstruction, feeding difficulties with failure to thrive, chronic aspiration and pulmonary hypertension with subsequent right-heart failure, secondary to chronic hypoxia and hypercarbia.

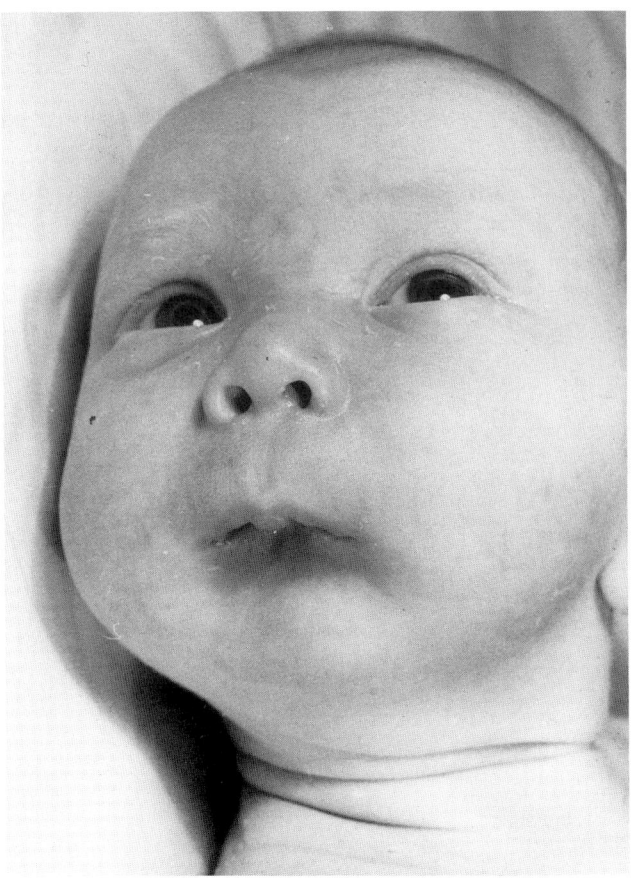

Fig. 17.8 A baby with Pierre Robin syndrome, showing the micrognathia which can make intubation difficult.

Airway obstruction, which is often not apparent until 4–6 weeks of age, is primarily due to the tongue impacting in the pharynx. It is further compounded by neuromuscular incoordination. The tip of the tongue may also wedge in the palatal cleft.

In less severely affected infants, the airway obstruction may be relieved by nursing prone, but severely affected infants will require a nasopharyngeal airway or even tracheostomy. The airway problem tends to resolve with age, but nasopharyngeal intubation may be required for up to 5 months, and the micrognathia may still cause difficulty with intubation when the cleft palate is repaired.

A variety of surgical techniques has been used in the past, including tongue–lip anastomosis. These have now been shown to be largely ineffective and have been discontinued.

The anaesthetist may be involved in the management of these patients in infancy, either to establish an airway or to provide anaesthesia for a tracheostomy or feeding gastrostomy.

These patients may be very difficult to intubate. In infancy, as one cannot always be sure of being able to ventilate them adequately if paralysed, it may be safest to undertake initial laryngoscopy awake. On the other hand, if ventilation by mask is easy, anaesthesia can be induced with an inhalation agent and, when deep enough, laryngoscopy attempted. If the larynx cannot be visualized easily, the use of a short straight blade from the corner of the mouth may enable intubation to be accomplished. Other techniques for difficult intubation are discussed in Chapter 7.

If the patient can be ventilated easily and the anaesthetist is competent at difficult intubation in neonates and infants, a short-acting muscle relaxant may be used.

Similar techniques for difficult intubation may still be necessary when the patient presents for cleft palate repair. There is a likelihood of airway obstruction after cleft palate repair in infants with Pierre Robin syndrome, which can be overcome by leaving a nasopharyngeal tube in for 2 or 3 days as described above.

Nasal operations

It is important to warn the patient that the nose may be packed postoperatively and that he must breathe through his mouth. Early recovery from anaesthesia is desirable. If the nose is obstructed, the anaesthetist will have to open the mouth or insert an airway when ventilating prior to intubation. After intubation a pharyngeal pack is inserted.

Vasoconstrictors are often used for elective nasal surgery. If adrenaline is used, there is a particular hazard of rapid absorption from the nasal mucosa, which will influence the choice of anaesthetic agent. Despite the use of vasoconstrictors, significant blood loss can occur and an intravenous infusion should be running.

Other head, neck and external ear operations

The patient should be intubated and the tube carefully strapped so that the airway is secured, enabling the anaesthetist to be out of the surgeon's way during the operation. Alternatively, a laryngeal mask airway may be suitable. If the head is turned from side to side, the anaesthetist must watch the tube or laryngeal mask airway to ensure that it is not dislodged accidentally.

Longer operations include ear reconstructions using costochondral graft. An intercostal block may be valuable for postoperative pain relief at the donor site. As these operations may take several hours, intravenous therapy is recommended.

Operations such as correction of 'bat ears' can be carried out under general anaesthesia or with sedation and local anaesthetic blocks (see Chapter 22).

Peripheral operations

Peripheral operations, such as nerve or tendon lacerations and correction of syndactyly and other hand and foot abnormalities, do not usually pose any problem with the airway and the anaesthetic can be given by mask or endotracheal tube. Brachial plexus or lower limb nerve blocks in combination with general anaesthesia provide analgesia and reduce the need for opioids. Blocks can be used, even in fairly young children, with adequate sedation.

Large haemangiomata

The problems which may be associated with large haemangiomata and their excision are:
1 hyperdynamic circulation and even heart failure, because they can functionally form an arteriovenous fistula;
2 thrombosis;
3 excessive blood loss during surgery.
Thrombosis in giant haemangiomata may consume platelets, and to a lesser extent other clotting factors, which in turn will lead to bleeding from mucous membranes or other areas unless the condition is recognized and treated. The anticoagulant heparin, aspirin (which prevents platelet aggregation), and cortisol may be required and have been successfully used for this condition.

Preoperative embolization of the vessels supplying the haemangioma, performed by an experienced radiologist under image intensification, helps to reduce the blood flow. The surgery may involve extensive blood loss and consideration should be given to the use of hypotensive anaesthesia. A large intravenous cannula should be inserted, blood should be cross-matched and fresh frozen plasma and platelets should be available. On very rare occasions these steps, including hypotensive anaesthesia, may be inadequate to control blood loss and cardiopulmonary bypass may need to be considered. It has been used occasionally.

Secondary surgery for burns

Patients with burns which have been previously grafted (see Chapter 20) may need release of scar contractures. This is a common operation. Multiple position changes may be required, to provide access for release of the contracture and harvesting of skin grafts. Blood loss during the operation may also be a complicating factor, particularly in operations on the scalp. A tourniquet can be used for peripheral limb operations.

The need to avoid postoperative restlessness requires adequate analgesia either using opioids, preferably by infusion, or local anaesthetic nerve blocks, particularly for donor skin areas. Occlusive dressings may also make the patient more comfortable.

In some burned children, particularly those who have not had the benefit of modern preventative prostheses and neck collars, neck contractures may be so severe that the head cannot be extended enough to allow intubation. It is then necessary to incise the contracture under local anaesthesia or ketamine, to allow neck extension and make intubation easier. An inhalation induction can be used, but it is often slower than usual, due to reduced uptake of anaesthetic caused by partial respiratory obstruction. Laryngeal spasm may occur if intubation is attempted too early. Return of the pupils to the central position indicates that an adequate depth has been reached. Intubation may also be achieved using a fibreoptic technique with either topical or general anaesthesia with spontaneous ventilation. In the former case, once the child is intubated, general anaesthesia can be administered and the operation completed.

Severe trauma

The plastic surgeon may be one of several specialist surgeons involved in the care of patients following trauma (Chapter 26). There must be interdisciplinary consultation so that the patient undergoes operative procedures at appropriate and optimal times, with a minimum number of anaesthetics.

MICROSURGICAL OPERATIONS

These operations are usually very prolonged and may involve the co-operation of the plastic surgeon with specialists in other fields, such as orthopaedics. The operations include the rejoining of severed limbs or digits, or they may involve transplantation of bone, soft tissue and skin flaps with their blood vessels which are anastamosed to vessels in the recipient area. It is important to maintain good perfusion of the tissues, which requires an adequate blood pressure and the use of dilators to prevent vasoconstriction and spasm.

The patient should be positioned so that pressure sores do not develop, although multiple position changes are sometimes necessary for the surgery. A warming blanket and humidified gases maintain body temperature. Intravenous therapy provides for the maintenance of fluid and energy requirements and the replacement of surgical blood loss if necessary.

Regional or local anaesthesia is useful, particularly if a catheter can be left in place to provide further top-up doses. The question whether the patient should be ventilated or allowed to breathe spontaneously is debatable, but some of the problems relating to prolonged anaesthesia may be avoided if air is included in the anaesthetic mixture, so that denitrogenation of the lungs, with alveolar collapse and reduction of functional residual capacity, is avoided.

Monitoring of these long cases may include a precordial stethoscope, intra-arterial pressure (which also gives access for arterial blood sampling), central venous pressure, urine output and temperature. The advent of pulse oximetry and capnography has been a major advance.

The vigilance of the anaesthetist is all-important, and the operation should not be undertaken unless there are two anaesthetists or unless there is adequate provision for periodic relief of the anaesthetist involved.

CRANIOFACIAL SURGERY

Craniofacial surgery may be defined as the correction of complex deformities of the cranium, orbit and face, which may be congenital, traumatic or neoplastic in origin. It may be undertaken for both cosmetic and functional reasons. The age at which surgery is performed and the scope of surgery varies widely — the latter ranging from a simple mandibular osteotomy to total reconstruction of the mid-face, orbits and cranium.

Both the concept of craniofacial surgery and the correction of these complex deformities are relatively new developments. Only palliative surgery was attempted until about 20 years ago. In 1967, Paul Tessier from Paris presented the results of his treatment of severe craniofacial anomalies over the preceding 10 years. He was able to demonstrate that radical new approaches would enable the correction of deformities hitherto thought impossible to treat. He developed the concept of the craniofacial team, by combining the techniques of plastic surgery, oral surgery and neurosurgery to expose the facial skeleton below and the cranial base and orbits above, thus allowing complete access to the orbits and mid-face, permitting multiple osteotomies, radical repositioning and reconstruction.

Before anaesthetizing these patients, it is essential to have an understanding of the underlying deformities and the surgical techniques used.

CLASSIFICATION OF DISORDERS

Hypertelorism

Hypertelorism may be defined as an increased distance between the orbits — usually the optic canal is in the correct position and the orbital canal is rotated outwards. Its occurrence may be secondary to:
1 craniostenosis of anterior cranial vault/base sutures;
2 midline frontal or basal encephalocoele;
3 facial clefts;
4 craniofacial dystostosis.
The eyeball attains 75% of its adult volume by the end of the second year and the optimal time for surgery is 2 years of age, when either an intracranial or extracranial

approach may be used, depending upon the underlying defect and the severity of the anomaly. The principle of surgery is to shift the orbits *en masse* and remove the enlarged central mass of nasal and ethmoid air cells.

Craniofacial dysostoses

This is a loose generic term applied to Crouzon's and Apert's syndromes (Figs 17.9, 17.10). They are different genetic entities, but there is little physical difference between Crouzon's and Apert's syndromes except for the presence of syndactyly in the latter. They are characterized by:

1 Craniosynostosis, which may affect all or some of the basal and vault sutures, coronal synostosis being the most common. The resulting intracranial hypertension may necessitate urgent shunting or bony decompression early in life.

2 Maxillary hypoplasia resulting in airway abnormalities and malocclusion.

3 Shallow orbits with exorbitism. There is a risk of corneal ulceration, keratitis and eye prolapse.

It is not clear to what extent the facial component is a primary facial bone dysplasia or secondary to the cranial component. Surgery which may be required includes:

1 Ventriculoperitoneal shunt — early in infancy.

2 Craniotomy with frontal and supraorbital rim advancement. The optimal time for surgery is 3—6 months of age because of the risk of intracranial hypertension developing and because early surgery may minimize the changes in facial growth.

3 Maxillary advancement (Le Fort III osteotomy) is usually performed at 8 or 9 years of age. Severe deformity resulting in airway obstruction or orbital prolapse may necessitate early surgery, and severe cosmetic deformity will require intervention before school age.

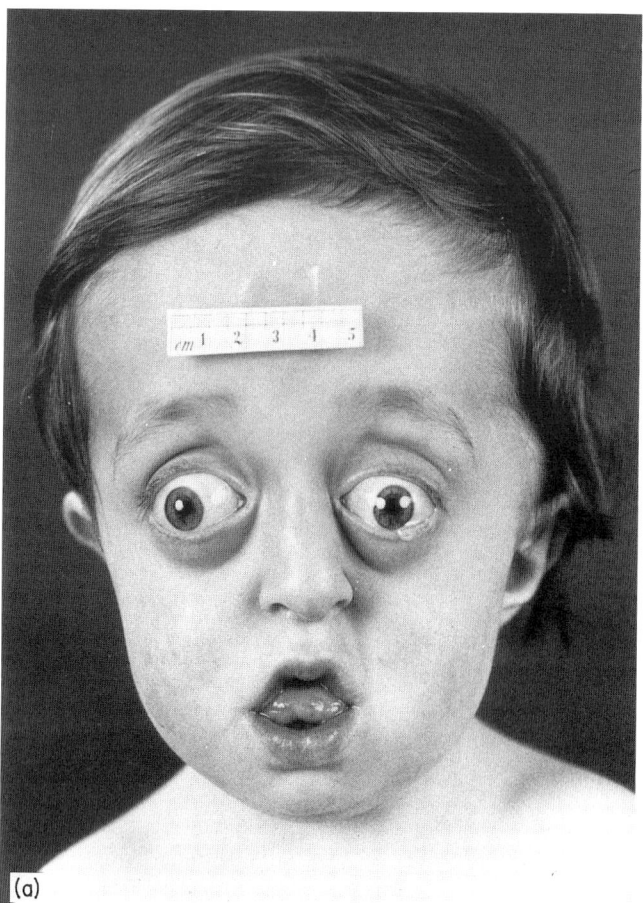

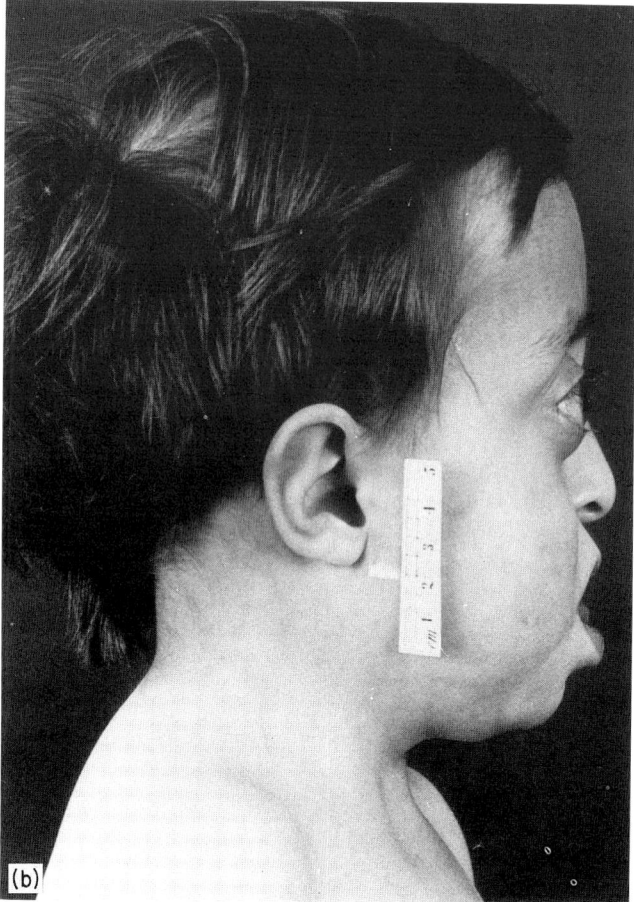

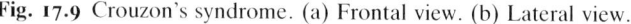

Fig. 17.9 Crouzon's syndrome. (a) Frontal view. (b) Lateral view.

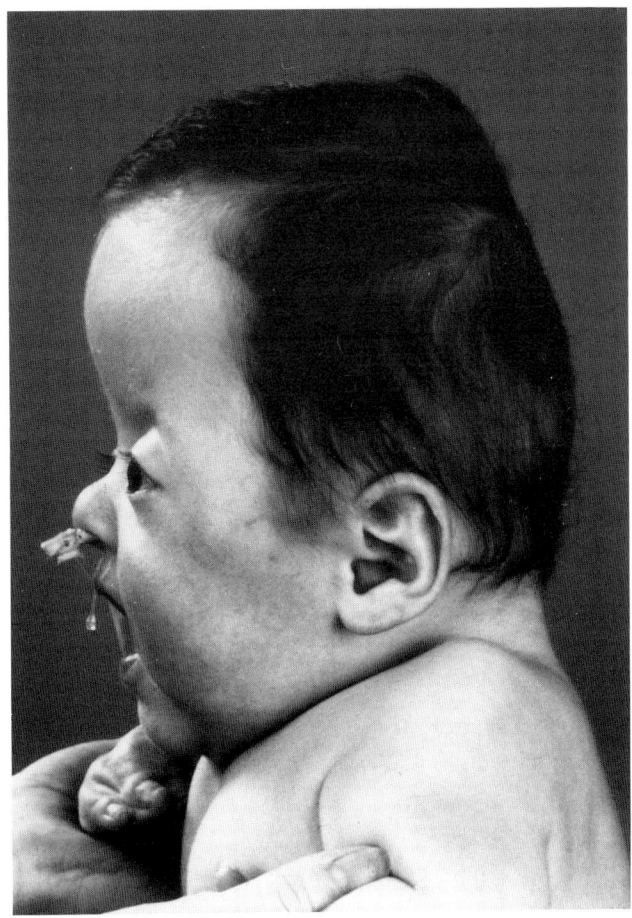

Fig. 17.10 Apert's syndrome.

Most children will require a Le Fort I maxillary osteotomy in adolescence for orthodontic management.

Maxillary hypoplasia

Maxillary hypoplasia may be idiopathic, occur as part of a variety of syndromes (e.g. Binder's) or, as in the majority of cases, be secondary to cleft lip and palate. Surgery in the form of Le Fort I and II maxillary osteotomies, and often associated mandibular osteotomies, is not undertaken until mid-face growth is complete in adolescence.

Rare facial clefts

A variety of defects may result from facial clefting, one of the better known being the Treacher—Collins syndrome (mandibulofacial dysostosis) which results from a lateral orbital cleft (see Fig. 17.1). Characteristic features include:

1 antimongoloid slant of the eyes, resulting from a zygomatic deficiency;
2 lower lid hypoplasia with a deficiency at the junction of the lateral and central third, and absent eyelashes;
3 deficient malar prominences;
4 small receding mandible with hypoplastic temporomandibular joints, which may make airway maintenance and intubation difficult;
5 ear deformities and often a cleft palate.
The timing of surgery is largely dependent on psychosocial factors, but the periorbital work is usually undertaken prior to school age, and the lower facial in adolescence.

Asymmetric disorders

UNICORONAL SYNOSTOSIS

Early suture resection and supraorbital advancement in the first 6 months of life is indicated to prevent progressive and severe facial deformity.

HEMIFACIAL MICROSOMIA (facio-auriculovertebral anomaly, Goldenhar syndrome; Fig. 17.11)

Features of this anomaly may include:
hypoplasia of maxilla, mandible and zygoma;
ear and temporomandibular joint anomalies;
lateral macrostomia;
cervical spine abnormalities (Fig. 17.12).
Initial correction is carried out before school age, but later surgery will be required in adolescence. These abnormalities, particularly the mandibular hypoplasia, may make intubation difficult.

SURGICAL OPERATIONS

Simpler procedures on the mandible and mid-face may be performed through upper and lower buccal incisions, but the more major procedures are usually approached through a bicoronal incision, which allows access to the cranium, orbits and face down as far as the level of the maxillary alveolus. The scalp is peeled forward and backwards in a single layer and extensive subperiosteal dissection is performed.

A frontal craniotomy allows extradural exposure of the floor of the anterior cranial fossa, thus giving access to the orbits from above.

The required osteotomies are performed — extensive

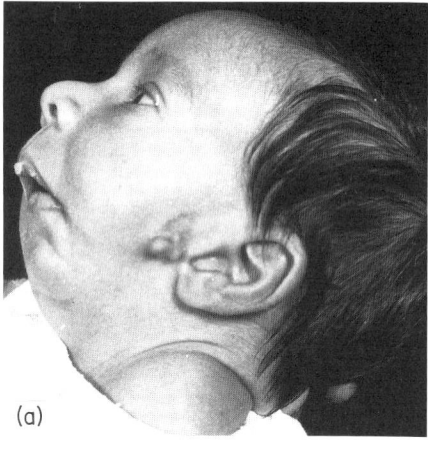
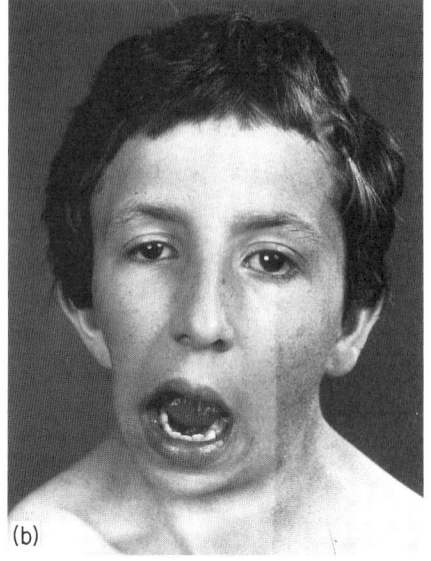
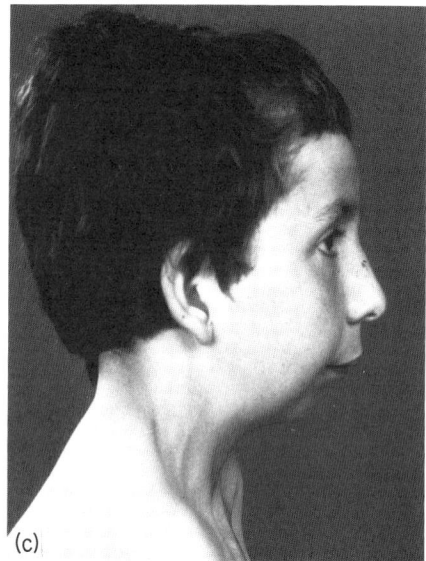

Fig. 17.11 (a) A baby with Goldenhar syndrome (hemifacial microsomia) showing severe micrognathia. (b) Frontal and (c) lateral views of an older boy with hemifacial microsomia, showing the micrognathia and unbalanced face.

areas of the craniofacial skeleton can be completely devascularized and repositioned, but still survive.

Bone grafts will usually be required to fill deficient areas. These may be taken from the cranium (particularly in infants), rib or ilium, the latter being associated with more pain and disability. Interpore, a synthetic bone substitute derived from coral, is frequently used in the mid-face and mandible.

Fixation of osteotomies must be rigid, and ideally osteotomies are performed so that they lock automatically when repositioned. When this is not feasible, fixation by direct wiring in the skull and orbits is usual. In the mid-face and mandible, direct fixation using miniplates and screws is usually possible, and the requirement for intermaxillary fixation is now rare. The latter is occasionally required and may be performed with orthodontic bands, cap splints or arch bars and acrylic bite wafers.

ANAESTHETIC CONSIDERATIONS

During these long and exacting procedures anaesthetic and perioperative care must be meticulous to avoid morbidity and mortality. Skills are required in neurosurgical and paediatric anaesthesia, management and intubation of difficult airways, and induced hypotension. Special consideration must be given to the following factors:

1 The variation in age of patients and the type and scope of surgery.

2 The association with a variety of congenital syndromes.

3 Difficulties with the airway and intubation, which may require fibreoptic laryngoscopy or the use of other special techniques for difficult intubation (see Chapter 7). Intraoperatively there is the possibility of kinking or severing of the endotracheal tube, or even extubation. Postoperatively, airway problems may arise due to bleeding, swelling or secretions.

4 The prolonged procedure poses problems for the patient, related to pressure areas, venous stasis, temperature control, fluid, caloric and electrolyte balance, and for the anaesthetist associated with fatigue, boredom and inattention.

5 Blood loss may be substantial and increases with the length of the procedure.

6 The oculocardiac reflex may be initiated by traction of the orbital contents and can be a warning to the surgeon that retraction may be excessive and the eye may be at risk. Atropine is not routinely used to prevent it.

7 Although the procedures involving frontal craniotomy are extradural, the principles of neurosurgical anaesthesia must be followed. Retraction of the frontal lobes is necessary to gain access to the floor of the anterior cranial fossa, and there is therefore a need for a relatively 'soft' brain. The principles of reduction of intracranial pressure, discussed in Chapter 14, must be followed.

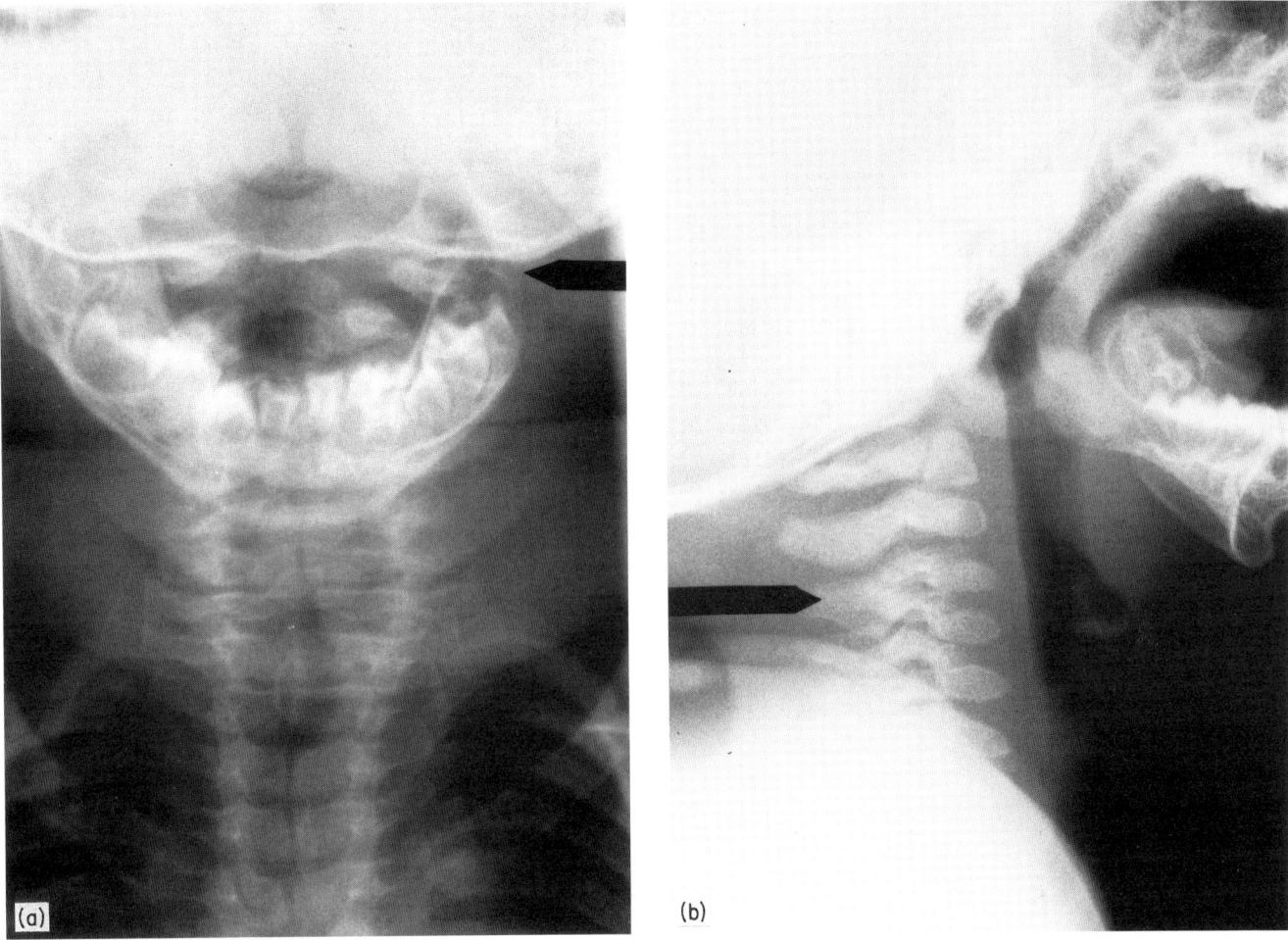

Fig. 17.12 Neck X-rays showing abnormal cervical vertebrae in Goldenhar syndrome.

8 Air embolism can occur through open veins or skull vessels when atrial pressure is low, as the patient is usually in a head-up position (see Chapter 14).

PREOPERATIVE ASSESSMENT

In the general assessment of the patient, associated anomalies should be noted. A careful assessment of the airway and the likelihood of a difficult intubation is required — past anaesthetic records and clinical examination are useful.

Preoperative investigations include full blood examination, clotting profile, urea and electrolytes, chest X-ray and lateral X-ray of the neck. The latter is particularly useful in assessing potential difficulty with the airway and intubation.

Sufficient blood to replace the patient's blood volume should be cross-matched for major procedures. Autologous blood may be collected in the month prior to the procedure, or may be collected immediately after induction with associated haemodilution. For more major procedures platelets and fresh frozen plasma may be required.

Many of these patients, particularly in the adolescent age group, are extremely anxious and require adequate premedication. A drying agent such as hyoscine is often advantageous when a difficult intubation is anticipated. Patients must be warned preoperatively if it is anticipated that intermaxillary fixation or a nasopharyngeal airway will be required. They should also be warned of postoperative facial swelling and the likelihood of pain from bony donor sites. Postoperative analgesia should also be discussed.

ANAESTHETIC MANAGEMENT

The anaesthetic technique of choice includes muscle relaxation following either an intravenous or inhalational induction. Nitrous oxide and oxygen are supplemented with isoflurane and fentanyl (up to 10 µg/kg). A low, antiemetic dose of droperidol should be given. The selection of D-tubocurarine for relaxation will aid the induction of hypotension.

When difficult intubation is anticipated, the patient may be induced with thiopentone or halothane and, after establishing that the patient can be ventilated with a face mask, suxamethonium is given. If intubation cannot be accomplished easily, different laryngoscope blades may provide better access, particularly if passed from the corner of the mouth, or one anaesthetist can manipulate both the laryngoscope and the larynx while the second anaesthetist can pass the tube once the glottis is exposed (see Chapter 7).

Alternatively, when conventional intubation is extremely difficult, fibreoptic laryngoscopy and intubation is the preferred technique. The patient is induced with intravenous or inhalation agents and deep anaesthesia established using oxygen and halothane with spontaneous ventilation. Initially the nose is packed with cocaine-soaked gauze. Local anaesthesia of the airway can be achieved using topical lignocaine via a pharyngeal catheter, cricothyroid puncture or internal laryngeal nerve block. Anaesthesia is maintained by insufflation via a small nasopharyngeal tube passed through the nostril not being used for intubation.

The choice of endotracheal tube will depend on the procedure. An oral RAE or Portex Polar 'south' tube will be satisfactory for procedures above the infraorbital margin, but for procedures involving the mid-face or mandible a nasal RAE or straight PVC tube with nasal Magill connector and flexible catheter mount will be required. All cuffed tubes should be of the high-volume low-pressure type and the cuff should be checked before insertion. Positioning and fixation of the endotracheal tube is important to avoid both bronchial intubation and, at the other extreme, extubation when the head position is changed or during surgical manipulation. Nasal tubes should be sutured in position at the external nares, as taping should be minimal to avoid intrusion into the surgical field. The face can be protected from the tubes and connections by adhesive foam; it is important that the anaesthetic breathing system be positioned and supported to prevent traction on the endotracheal tube.

The patient is ventilated to achieve normocarbia or mild hypocarbia. The gases should be humidified with a humidifier or an artificial nose humidifier–condenser.

A throat pack will be required in most patients to protect the airway and absorb secretions and blood. It will also help to fix the endotracheal tube in position. If intermaxillary fixation is used, the throat pack must always be removed by the surgeon prior to application of the fixation. A nasogastric tube will enable the stomach to be emptied at the end of the procedure.

A 15–20° head-up tilt is used in most instances. The eyes are protected with ointment and tape, or the lids are stitched when a bicoronal incision is performed. All bony prominences are padded and protected. A water-circulating blanket under the patient, an overhead heater at induction in infants, humidification and warming of inspired gases and warming of all intravenous fluids help to minimize the drop in body temperature. Antibiotics are administered routinely at induction. Dexamethasone is given to reduce soft-tissue swelling.

Maintenance fluid therapy is provided and third-space losses are usually replaced with Hartmann's solution, aiming to achieve a urine output of 1–2 ml/kg/h — usually approximately twice the maintenance rate is required. Estimation of blood loss is very difficult because of soiling of drapes and the use of large quantities of irrigation fluid. Blood loss replacement is usually based on changes in cardiovascular measurements, urine output and haematocrit.

The patient is positioned and the anaesthetic technique chosen to reduce blood pressure at the operation site and minimize bleeding; induced hypotension is often used as well. Sodium nitroprusside is infused to maintain mean blood pressure (at head level) at either 45–50 mmHg or two thirds of the original blood pressure. Isoflurane may also be used to lower blood pressure.

For major cases, monitoring should include all of the following: precordial or oesophageal stethoscope, intra-arterial blood pressure, central venous pressure, urine output, temperature, pulse oximetry, capnography, ECG and regular assessment of blood gas and acid–base status, electrolytes and haemoglobin.

If it is planned to extubate at the end of the operation it is sometimes wise, after aspirating the pharynx, to withdraw the tube into the pharynx and only extubate completely when the patient is fully conscious. This is a particularly valuable approach when the jaws are splinted together, such as following mandibular osteotomy, as it ensures the airway and allows easy pharyngeal suction.

POSTOPERATIVE MANAGEMENT

It is important that all patients be awake, orientated, co-operative and be able to sit up at the end of the procedure. They must be able to protect their airway but must also have adequate analgesia.

The majority of patients are extubated and go to the recovery room, where they are observed for several hours until they are stable with respect to their circulation, airway, analgesia and conscious state. Neurosurgical observations are made following intracranial surgery. Blood gas tensions, acid—base status and haemoglobin are repeated before the patient returns to the ward. After the removal of invasive monitoring, they return to a ward staffed by nurses familiar with the care of these patients.

All patients receive oxygen by face mask (intranasal cannulae are often contraindicated). In selected patients the airway may be aided by retention of the endotracheal tube as a nasopharyngeal airway, and the use of a tongue stitch, particularly in patients with intermaxillary fixation.

The decision to leave the patient intubated postoperatively must be made on an individual basis, but it should be considered in the following cases:
1 long, difficult procedures where excessive swelling of soft tissues and mucosa is likely;
2 when there has been excessive bleeding that is likely to continue postoperatively;
3 when impaired consciousness or cerebral swelling may necessitate ventilation;
4 when intubation has been particularly difficult and when swelling, bleeding or laryngeal oedema may necessitate reintubation.
Postoperative analgesia is provided with the use of a morphine infusion at a rate of 20—40 µg/kg/h, provided there is no neurosurgical contraindication. Intercostal blocks performed prior to extubation will also be useful in patients who have had ribs taken for bone grafting.

An antiemetic such as droperidol (low dose) or metoclopramide should be given as required. A large-bore nasogastric tube can be left in patients who have had intermaxillary fixation.

All patients are sat upright as soon as possible to minimize swelling and bleeding — cardiovascular stability is not usually a problem if intraoperative replacement of blood loss has been adequate. Early mobility and physiotherapy is important to prevent postoperative atelectasis. Facial, orbital and scalp swelling is usual, being maximal at about 24 hours.

Maintenance intravenous fluids will be required postoperatively, but patients are encouraged to drink as soon as they will tolerate fluids. Blood loss continues into the postoperative period, with ooze into the soft tissue and loss via mucosal breaches. Haemoglobin estimation should be repeated after 24 hours and the patient transfused as required.

COMPLICATIONS

The major complications of craniofacial surgery are death, brain damage and visual impairment; fortunately, these are rare. In a large multi-centre study, mortality was usually associated with uncontrollable intraoperative haemorrhage or airway problems. The more common complications are extensive blood loss, infection with consequent loss of bone grafts, pneumothorax following removal of rib grafts, and pulmonary problems. Other rare but potentially serious complications include cerebral oedema, inappropriate ADH secretion, diabetes insipidus, convulsions, CSF leak and extradural haematoma (see Chapter 14).

SUMMARY OF ANAESTHETIC REQUIREMENTS

1 Ensure an unobstructed airway and adequate ventilation, as an elevated Pa_{CO_2} may be accompanied by increased oozing.
2 The patient must remain still until the dressings are applied, including a plaster in limb operations, and the surgeon is satisfied with the state of the local circulation.
3 The anaesthetic equipment must be arranged so that the surgeon has good access to the operating field, and to allow for possible changes in position during the operation.
4 Steps should be taken, when required, to reduce blood loss and ensure adequate access to a vein if significant blood loss is expected.
5 When postoperative pain is expected, particularly after skin has been taken for grafting, analgesic drugs should be given before the end of the procedure, or local anaesthetic nerve blocks should be used.
A clear understanding of the patient's condition and the surgeon's requirements will help the anaesthetist to provide good operating conditions.

18: Anaesthesia for Dentistry

INTRODUCTION

Most dental treatment in children can be undertaken with local anaesthesia or no anaesthesia at all if the patient is managed well psychologically and is reassured adequately. A small proportion will benefit from pre-medication with a tranquillizer if they are very apprehensive, or from nitrous oxide sedation, but there will still be a few who require general anaesthesia.

VENUE FOR DENTAL SURGERY UNDER GENERAL ANAESTHESIA OR SEDATION

Dental treatment under anaesthesia may be performed in the dental surgery, in the outpatient department of a hospital, in a day-care unit or as an inpatient in hospital. Anaesthesia should be tailored to the situation, but rapid arousal is important in day-stay patients. In all places where patients are to be anaesthetized or sedated, including the dental surgery, full resuscitation equipment including suction, oxygen, bags, masks, laryngoscopes, endotracheal tubes and drugs must be available (see Chapter 35).

SEDATION

Some children can be managed satisfactorily with pre-medication. A method used by dentists is to give three doses of oral diazepam (i) the night before, (ii) at breakfast, and (iii) an hour before treatment, each dose either 0.1−0.15 mg/kg or 2 mg for young children and 5 mg for older children and adults.

A number of dental surgeons use intravenous or nitrous oxide sedation techniques. Skill is required to achieve this without obtunding airway reflexes. The single operator must be adequately trained in maintaining the airway and coping with a drowsy patient, and must have some means of monitoring the patient while working. An audible pulse oximeter is ideal. Sedation which makes the patient unconscious should not be used by a single operator.

PRE-ANAESTHETIC ASSESSMENT AND MANAGEMENT

Outpatients having dentistry under general anaesthesia, who are nervous and have not been given any pre-medication, need to be approached gently and reassured. Even though the dentist should have recorded a medical history, the anaesthetist should ask the mother about any known illnesses or allergies, or any undue tendency to bleed after injury or previous extractions. A careful preliminary examination must be carried out to discover associated medical conditions, in particular congenital heart disease, which may require antibiotic cover. Unrecognized heart murmurs should be evaluated. If they are innocent murmurs (see Chapter 25) one may proceed, otherwise a cardiologist's opinion should be sought. Any suspected respiratory illness should be assessed and a decision made whether or not to postpone the dental procedure until the illness has resolved (see Chapter 6).

Some children, who require extensive dental treatment, or who are unable to co-operate for management in the dental surgery, may have all their treatment carried out at one time under anaesthesia, often as a day patient. Inpatient treatment may be preferable for children with bleeding disorders, mental retardation or epilepsy, or when prolonged or complicated procedures are anticipated. Preoperative treatment with coagulation factors may require admission to hospital in advance (see Chapter 25).

Patients with congenital or acquired heart disease have an increased risk of acquiring infective endocarditis from the bacteraemia which follows any extraction or oral surgery. They should be given a prophylactic antibiotic (e.g. penicillin) to prevent the spread of streptococcal infection. When patients are on anticoagulant, therapy, it may need to be stopped or reduced preoperatively.

Some patients with medical problems (reviewed in Chapter 25) are also psychologically affected by their disease, so that they are unable to be treated without general anaesthesia. They may have had many hospital admissions and their parents' anxieties may have been transferred to them.

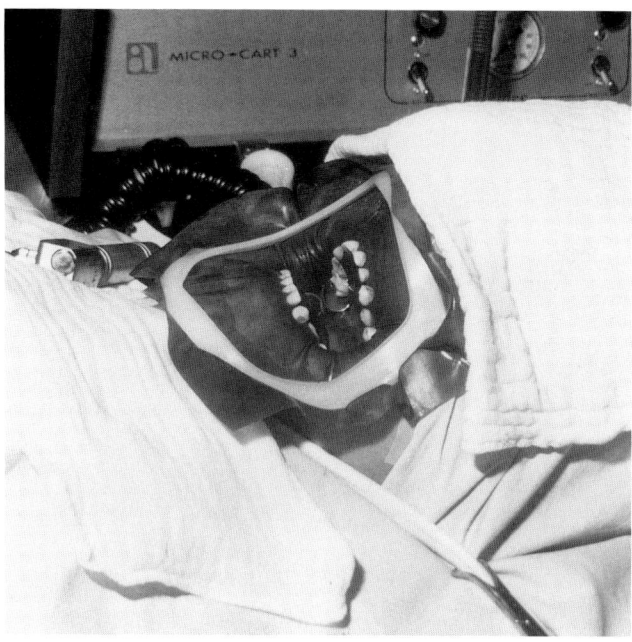

Fig. 18.1 Rubber dam in place with teeth protruding through it.

AIRWAY CONTROL

The most important aspect of general anaesthesia for dentistry is control of the airway. The patients should be intubated for all but very short procedures, such as simple tooth extraction. The latter may be performed under intravenous anaesthesia or inhalation anaesthesia using a nasal mask while the teeth are extracted.

Soiling of the airway with debris, blood and saliva should be avoided by:
1 tracheal intubation and a pharyngeal pack (this should be inserted so that it lies equally on both sides of the tube);
2 a rubber dam over all the teeth for restorative treatment (Fig. 18.1);
3 an absorbent plastic sponge in the back of the mouth, without blocking the nasopharyngeal airway, when anaesthesia is used without intubation (Fig. 18.2);
4 using an Erickson 'Vac-ejector' which has a plastic guard to provide clear access and to collect debris or fluid. It is attached to high-volume suction. It also has a bite block to keep the mouth open (Figs 18.3, 18.4).
Water, which is used as a coolant in high-speed drills and to irrigate cavities during conservative dentistry, should be sucked away with a high-volume, low-vacuum dental aspirator.

Another problem is the confined space of the small

mouth of a child, which makes access more difficult for the dentist, especially if an oral tube is used.

The sitting position, which was formerly widely used because it was claimed to make airway control easier when using a nasal mask, is not now recommended because of the problems of fainting in the chair and hypotension. The supine position is now usually used for most general dental procedures.

ANAESTHESIA WITHOUT INTUBATION

This is little used in modern dentistry and should be limited to very short procedures — usually a few simple extractions.

An intravenous induction can be used by those who can venepuncture children proficiently, or an inhalation induction with nitrous oxide (70%), oxygen and an agent such as halothane can be employed. A face mask can be used during induction, changing to a nasal mask or a small Rendell Baker—Soucek mask while the teeth are removed. The maintenance of the airway without an endotracheal tube requires some skill. The principle is to pull the jaw and tongue forward while the dentist places mouth packs to protect the pharynx from blood and debris, thus maintaining an airway through the nasopharynx. Anaesthesia is maintained with nitrous oxide, oxygen and halothane or another inhalation agent

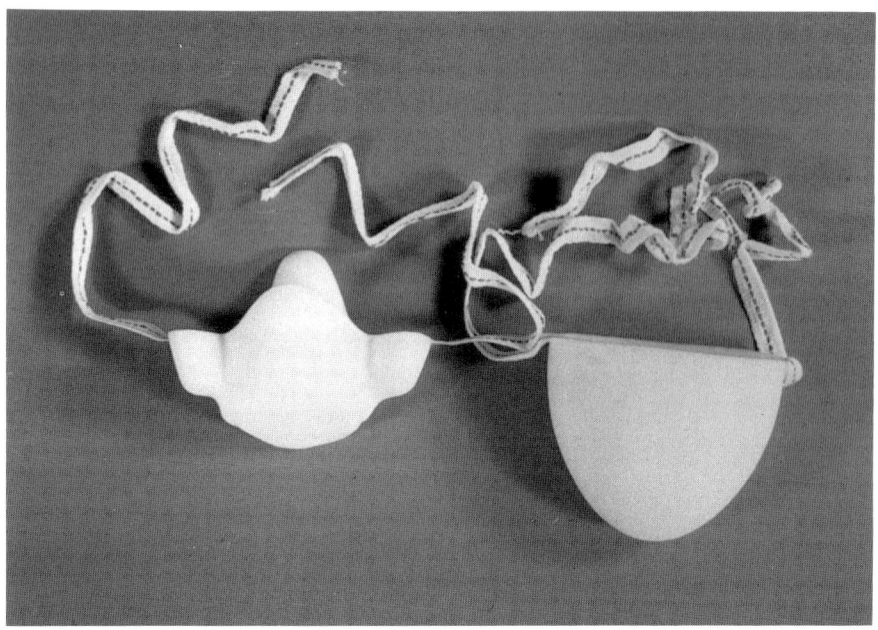

Fig. 18.2 Absorbent plastic sponges.

with a nasal mask. As the procedure nears conclusion, the halothane is turned off so that the child wakens rapidly. Alternatively intravenous anaesthesia with thiopentone or propofol can be used, with an analgesic supplement if needed, and inhalation of supplementary oxygen. Following extractions, packs are placed over the tooth sockets until bleeding stops. At the conclusion of the procedure the nitrous oxide is turned off and, after several breaths of oxygen, the packs are removed, any blood or debris is sucked out and the patient is turned on

his side to awaken quietly. If packs need to be left in place to control continued oozing, a folded and knotted pharyngeal pack with the ends taped to the face can be used; the anaesthetist must make certain that it is removed before leaving the patient.

If airway problems occur at any point during the procedure, the dentist should stop, preferably after quickly removing any partially extracted teeth or loose fragments, pack off any bleeding areas and allow the anaesthetist complete access to the patient to treat the

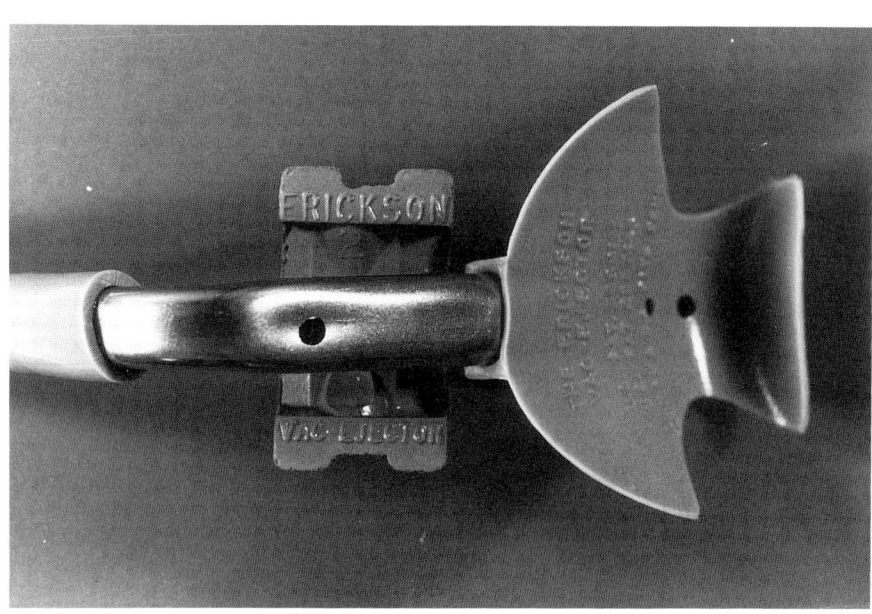

Fig. 18.3 Erickson Vac-ejector.

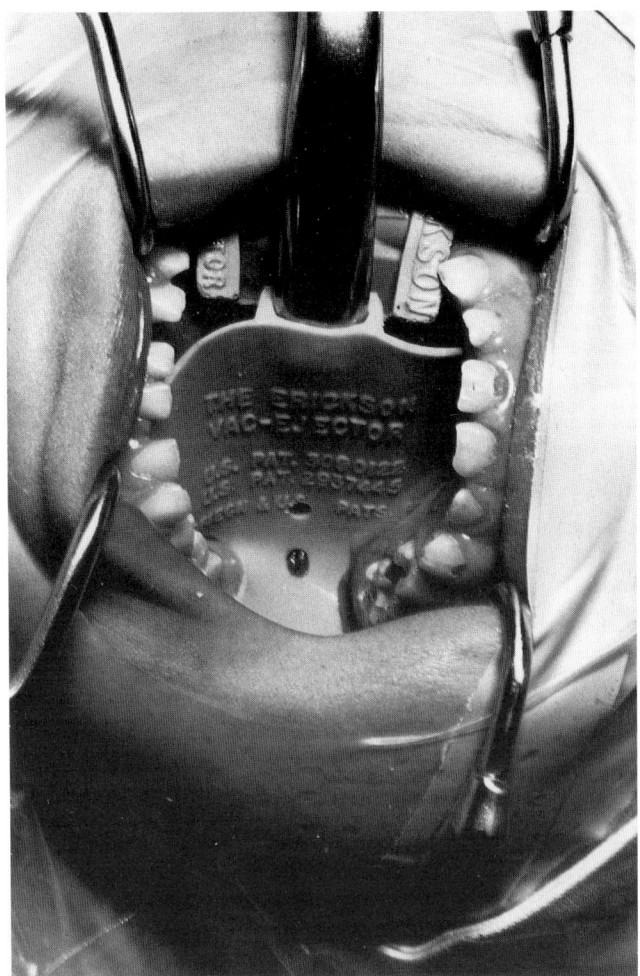

Fig. 18.4 Erickson Vac-ejector in place with plastic guard isolating operative area, the bite block keeping the mouth open and the suction connected.

problem. This may require ventilation, using an oral airway if necessary, clearing of debris or blood and, in some cases, intubation. Nasal and oral endotracheal tubes of appropriate sizes must always be available and the anaesthetist should not hesitate to insert one should respiratory difficulties persist. The decision to abandon the procedure if difficulties continue can be made more easily than other forms of surgery. It is most important to monitor ventilation and oxygenation.

ANAESTHESIA WITH INTUBATION

Endotracheal anaesthesia is the preferred method in children for all dental procedures which involve posterior teeth, or which last more than a minute or two. It is desirable to position the tube so that the dentist has the best access to the teeth. This is provided by nasotracheal intubation, but this is contraindicated in patients who have nasal obstruction, a tendency to severe epistaxis or a coagulation defect, including treatment with anticoagulants. Special precurved nasal tubes (e.g. Portex 'north' or RAE nasal) are available which attach to the breathing system over the forehead (Fig. 18.5). If care is taken to avoid kinking, a long nasal tube can be used if the others are not available. If an oral tube is used, a preshaped tube (RAE oral or Portex 'south') can sit in the upper right buccal sulcus behind the maxillary tuberosity, out of the dentist's way. The tube can be placed on the left side if it is more convenient. If the tube is to be moved from side to side so that the dentist has optimal access, the pharyngeal pack should be loose enough to allow the movement, or it can be changed when the tube is moved. Care must be taken to ensure that the tube is not dislodged. A less satisfactory alternative is to use a long PVC tube brought out of the corner of the mouth and turned in an appropriate direction, thus keeping the connection away from the mouth. The anaesthetist must watch out for potential problems such as compression or kinking of the tube during the operation. Plastic tubes become softer as they are warmed. Adhesive strapping may be loosened by secretions or the water coolant for the drill, with a resultant greater risk of accidental extubation.

The main problem associated with intubating young children as outpatients is the slight risk of postoperative laryngeal or subglottic oedema, usually due to the insertion of too big an endotracheal tube. This will usually become apparent with the development of stridor within 1–2 hours of extubation. A tube which allows anaesthetic gases to leak around it when positive pressure is applied to the airway should be used. Nasotracheal intubation may cause bleeding or removal of a piece of adenoid tissue when the adenoids are enlarged; the tip should be observed during larygoscopy to ensure that the tube is not blocked by such debris before it is passed into the larynx.

A slightly moist pharyngeal gauze pack should be inserted around both sides of the endotracheal tube to protect the trachea from debris. It should be an appropriate size for the mouth, so that the tongue is not pushed forward to protrude over the lower teeth. It should be packed in gently, as a firm gauze pack can cause a distressing pharyngitis. If the procedure is expected to be prolonged, ventilation may be controlled using a non-

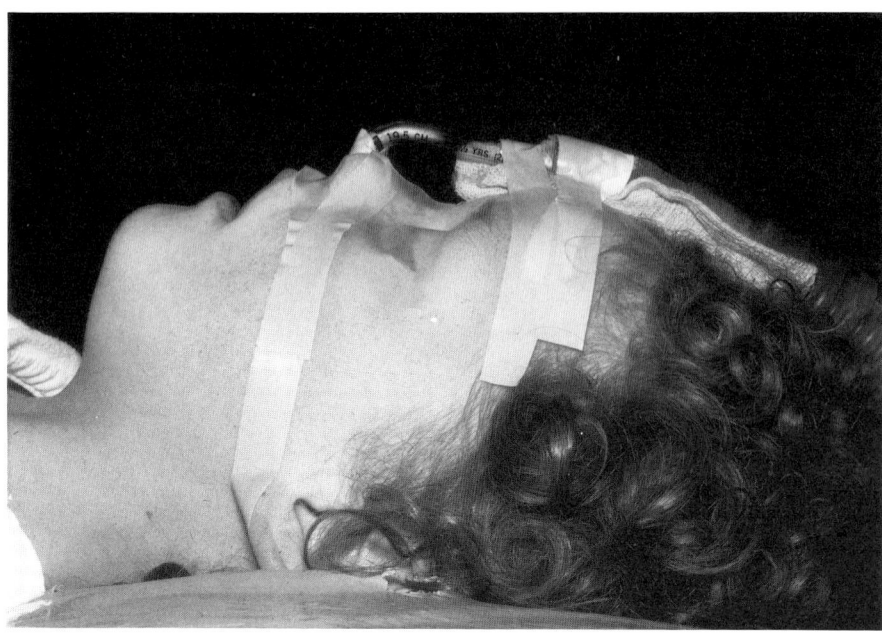

Fig. 18.5 Precurved nasal tube attached to the breathing apparatus over the forehead. A piece of gauze is placed to prevent the connection pressing on the forehead, and they are fixed with adhesive tape.

depolarizing muscle relaxant. For brief procedures, intubation using suxamethonium may be followed by spontaneous ventilation with an inhalation anaesthetic.

Intravenous fluids should be considered for longer procedures and are especially important if surgery or multiple extractions are to be carried out or in children with cerebral palsy, diabetes etc., to prevent dehydration.

At the conclusion of the procedure the patient should be turned on his side, the pharyngeal pack removed and blood or mucus aspirated before extubation. Following extractions, bleeding is usually controlled by placing small gauze packs over the sockets until it stops.

RECOVERY AND ADVICE TO PARENTS

When the children are awake after outpatient anaesthesia, they should be allowed to sit up with their parents for a further period until bleeding has stopped and they have recovered adequately from anaesthesia, before going home. When young patients have been intubated, their parents should be warned of the possibility of layngeal oedema developing. Although this is unlikely to develop more than 2 hours after extubation, they should be advised that if signs of respiratory obstruction such as stridor, rib retraction or tracheal tug occur, medical advice must be sought from the anaesthetist, their local doctor or the nearest casualty or emergency department if these are not available.

When suxamethonium has been used, particularly in older children, they should be advised to restrict activity for the remainder of the day in order to reduce the incidence of muscle pains. Alternatively a small dose of non-depolarizing relaxant can be given before the suxamethonium. This complication can be avoided by using a short-acting non-depolarizing relaxant such as atracurium.

After extensive dental procedures, oozing of blood may continue into the postoperative period. If it is swallowed, repeated vomiting may occur. The patient should be advised preoperatively and encouraged postoperatively to spit the blood out, as antiemetics are rarely helpful in this situation.

MANAGEMENT OF TRAUMA

Facial trauma may include fractures of the mandible, maxilla or teeth and their supporting bone, in addition to soft-tissue lacerations of the skin and oral mucosa. Its incidence increases with age during childhood. A brief description of the principles of management in these cases should help the anaesthetist to understand the requirements.

Fractures are frequently treated with cast silver (Fig. 18.6) or enamel-bond composite resin splints, or enamel-bonded titanium arch bars in infants and young children; anaesthesia is often not needed. Anaesthesia is necessary in the treatment of fractures where there is major displacement of the fragments, when

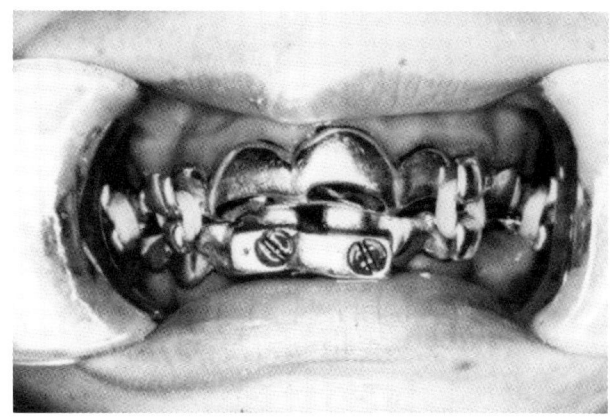

Fig. 18.6 Cast silver splints in place.

there are lacerations to be sutured or when the patient is unco-operative. Increasingly, low-profile titanium miniplate fixation is being used for certain types of fracture. In these cases the anaesthetist should discuss with the surgeon exactly what is planned. Surgeons appreciate maximum working space in the small mouths of children, and will prefer nasotracheal intubation if this is feasible.

If miniplate fixation is used, only one anaesthetic is needed. In difficult cases where cast splints, possibly in addition to wiring, are used, general anaesthesia may be required on two occasions. If custom-made casts of splints or arch bars are employed, impressions are taken and lacerations are sutured at the first procedure. The second stage is to cement the splints in place.

In displaced fractures, following reduction and fixation with splints or arch bars, immobilization of the mandible to the maxilla is achieved by intermaxillary elastic bands for 3–4 weeks. These high-strength elastic bands can usually be applied by the surgeon in the recovery room or in the ward after the child has recovered from anaesthesia. If the elastic bands must be applied before the end of anaesthesia, the throat pack must be removed and a check made to ensure that bleeding has stopped. The endotracheal tube can be left in place until the patient is awake, being withdrawn into the pharynx where it is left for a further period as a nasopharyngeal airway. A

suction catheter can be passed through it to remove secretions before final withdrawal. Short-bladed scissors are kept at the bedside or with the patient, when mobile, until the fixation is removed so that the rubber bands can be cut in the event of vomiting; this is very uncommon.

Comminuted or severely displaced maxillary fractures are usually treated with internal miniplate fixation and/or wiring, except in very small children where cast-splint fixation may still be used.

The problem for the anaesthetist is control of the airway while these are applied. Although nasal intubation may be more convenient for the operator, if the procedure involves intranasal or maxillary manipulation it is not always possible. The anaesthetist and the oral surgeon should always discuss which route is most appropriate for intubation in each patient.

The intermaxillary elastic bands can be removed in the ward or outpatient clinic about 1 week before the splints are removed. This allows return to normal mouth opening before general anaesthesia, should it be required, for splint removal. If fixation is maintained for too long the temporomandibular joint becomes stiff, but even then the jaw will open adequately if the patient is paralysed. This is rare where 3–4 weeks' immobilization is required for fracture union.

Elective operations such as maxillary and mandibular osteotomies, which are now quite commonly used to improve function or cosmetic appearance, are discussed in Chapter 17.

FURTHER READING

Bell J.M. Dental anaesthesia in children. *Anaes Intens Care* 1973, **1**, 540.

Bell J.M. *Dental anaesthesia.* (1975) Blackwell Scientific Publications, Oxford.

Hall R.K., Busowsky G. Ten-year survey of traumatic injuries to the face and jaws of children. 1970–1979: a computer analysis. In: Hjorting-Hansen S.E. (Ed) *Oral and maxillofacial surgery.* Proc. 8th Int. Conf. Oral and Maxillofacial Surgery. Chicago, (1985), pp. 143–150.

Rowe N.L., Williams J.W. (Eds). *Maxillofacial injuries.* (1985) Churchill Livingstone, Edinburgh, pp. 258–260, 538–558, 695–696.

19: Anaesthesia for Orthopaedic Surgery

INTRODUCTION

Patients requiring orthopaedic procedures range from normal healthy children with a fracture, to children with complex congenital abnormalities such as spina bifida, where the orthopaedic problem is only one of many. They can conveniently be classified as follows:

1 Trauma — simple, multiple or compound fractures which sometimes need an operation but often only need manipulation and immobilization, usually in plaster of Paris. Fractures are more likely where the bones have an abnormal structure, e.g. osteogenesis imperfecta.

2 Congenital or acquired deformity, as in patients with spina bifida, cerebral palsy, scoliosis, limb deformities, such as club feet and limb deficiencies, etc. Some of the acquired problems result from associated diseases such as muscular dystrophy (e.g. Duchenne) or arthrogryposis multiplex congenita.

3 Infection of joints or bones — septic arthritis or osteomyelitis, which are usually acute. Occasional chronic cases still occur.

4 Tumours, which may be benign, osteochondroma, bone cysts or granulomata, or malignant, Ewing's sarcoma, osteosarcoma, etc.

PREOPERATIVE ASSESSMENT

Children presenting for orthopaedic surgery should be visited and assessed by the anaesthetist in the usual way (see Chapter 6), but special consideration must be given to any causative or coincidental condition, such as those mentioned above.

Some of these children, particularly those with cerebral palsy or spina bifida, may be intellectually impaired. The presence of a parent or person who normally looks after the child is important at the preoperative visit and when the child comes to the operating theatre, as they are often the only people who can communicate with the patient.

Bone operations may cause severe postoperative pain. Patients may be very apprehensive, especially before major operations such as correction of scoliosis, or if they have had previous operations. They need effective premedication and may benefit from a sedative the night before.

ASSOCIATED CONDITIONS

Cerebral palsy

Cerebral palsy results from neurological damage occurring *in utero*, at birth, and sometimes later. It presents with spasticity, athetosis, ataxia or hypotonia. Most patients presenting for surgery are spastic (diplegic —

mainly affecting the legs — or quadriplegic — affecting the arms and legs). Spasticity of one muscle group leads to constant stretching of the opposing group, resulting in weakness. This leads to deformities. Surgery is performed to lengthen or weaken the spastic muscles to give the opposing muscles a chance to attain muscle balance. For instance, psoas lengthening and adductor release may reduce flexion and internal rotation of the hip and allow muscle balance, so that the femoral head stays in the hip joint. This improves the chance of walking or, in severe cases, facilitates nursing. Hypertonic hamstrings cause knee flexion, while spasticity of the calf prevents the child walking or causes a tendency to toe-walk. If physiotherapy and corrective splints cannot produce plantigrade feet, lengthening of the tendo Achilles may improve the position. The dorsiflexors can then function in a mechanically more advantageous range.

The aim of the operations is thus to help achieve functional position in less severe cases, or to make them easier to nurse and to seat in wheelchairs.

About half these children are intellectually impaired, some severely, but others may be of relatively normal intelligence.

Spina bifida

Spina bifida is a developmental abnormality of the neural tube. The size and location of the defect will determine the extent of the neurological deficit. There was a period when most patients were treated, but now there is a tendency not to treat severe cases because they lack bowel and bladder control, are completely paraplegic and possibly hydrocephalic, thus making their outlook dreadful. Patients with low lesions have more function and a better quality of life. Surgery is undertaken when unopposed innervated or spastic muscles, which work against flaccid muscles, cause deformity. The aims are to produce an extensor posture at the hip and knee, and plantigrade feet.

Spina bifida patients may have had several operations and may be less healthy than normal mobile patients. They may have urinary tract problems with infection. If they have significant neurological deficit, they may be more sensitive to some anaesthetic drugs such as thiopentone. Hypotension may occur if too high a dose is given. Their muscle relaxant requirements may also be reduced due to atrophy of their leg muscles.

Due to sensory loss, intravenous needles or infusions can usually be inserted painlessly in the legs.

Osteogenesis imperfecta (fragilitas ossium)

Osteogenesis imperfecta is a rare connective-tissue disorder mainly involving bones, making them more fragile. They can, for practical purposes, be broadly grouped into the milder tarda and the more severe congenita forms, although more complex classifications have been devised.

The mild tarda form is autosomal dominant with blue sclerae, but the bone and tooth abnormalities are relatively mild.

The severe form may have a small mandible and mid-face hypoplasia, dentinogenesis imperfecta, chest-wall and spinal abnormalities (prominent sternum and scoliosis) and severe fragility and deformity of the long bones (Fig. 19.1). Metabolic rate may be raised.

These patients most commonly present for treatment of fractures, or electively for the correction of deformities, particularly the Sofield osteotomy which consists of multiple osteotomies and insertion of rods into long bones, most commonly the femora (Fig. 19.2).

During anaesthesia, an intravenous infusion should always be running because even if blood loss is minimal, extra fluids are necessary to compensate for water lost by sweating.

Temperature should be monitored. It is either maintained or increases by a degree or two during the operation. The slight fall in temperature commonly associated with anaesthesia in normal patients does not usually occur. They are not predisposed to malignant hyperpyrexia [1]. Uncovering the patient will usually reverse the trend. These children have a normal response to the drugs commonly used in anaesthesia, including halothane and suxamethonium. In our large series the only drug commonly associated with a rise in temperature was hyoscine. It and atropine should only be used when really necessary.

The airway may be difficult to maintain with a mask in the more serious cases, because of the shape of the jaw and face.

Because of their weak chest wall, these children are less able to compensate for respiratory obstruction, so the airway must be watched with extra vigilance during recovery from anaesthesia. Care must be taken not to damage their fragile teeth.

There is a very rare complication where the base of the skull may collapse on to the cervical vertebrae, compressing the posterior fossa. Surgical decompression may be required. Care must be taken to avoid this serious

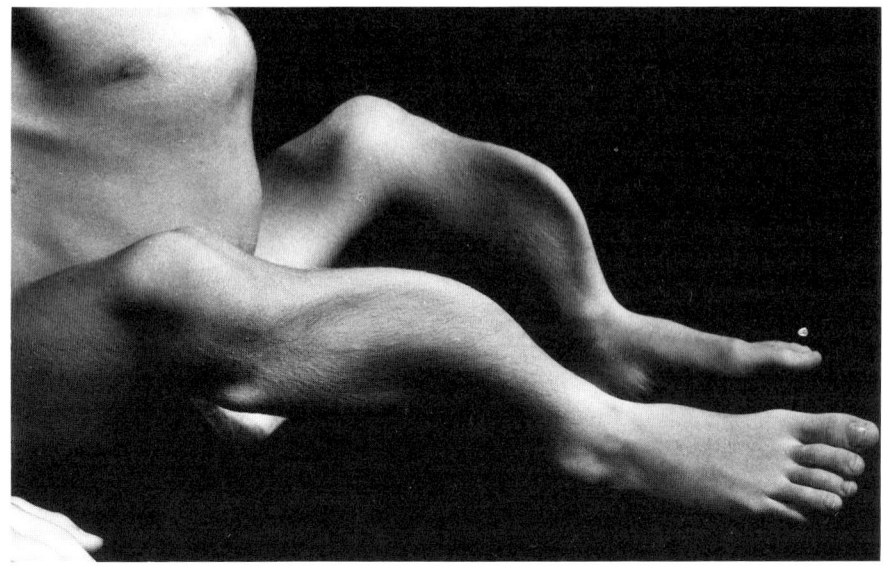

Fig. 19.1 Severe osteogenesis imperfecta, showing grossly abnormal legs (reproduced with permission from Hall *et al.* (1992) [1].)

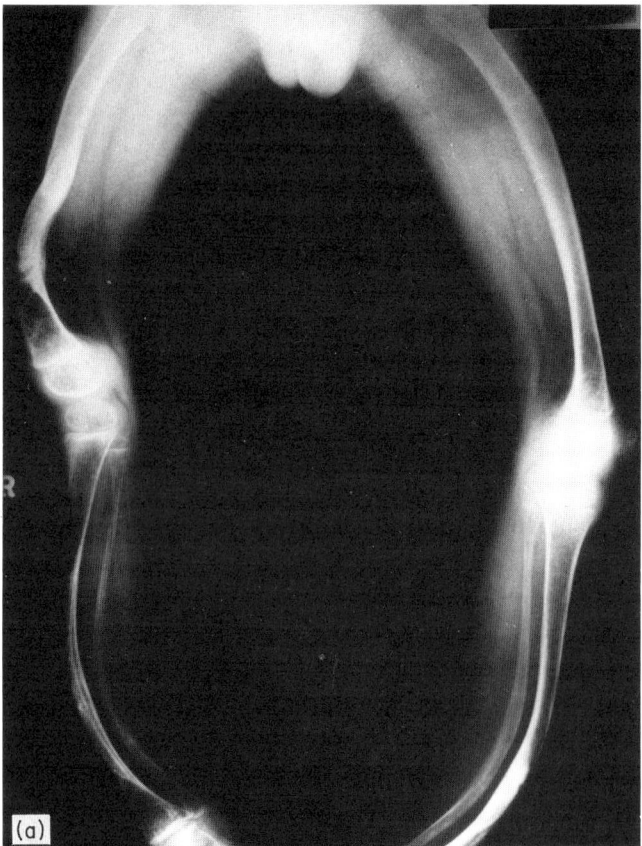

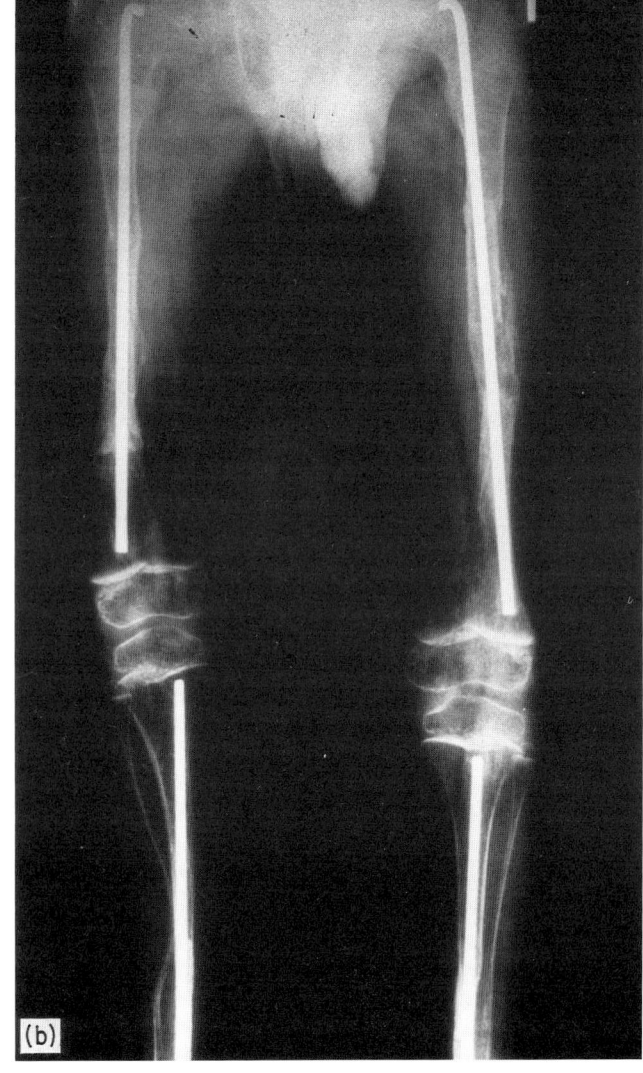

Fig. 19.2 (a) X-rays of legs showing the curved thin bones preoperatively. (b) X-rays following rodding to straighten the long bones. (Reproduced with permission from Hall *et al.* (1992) [1].)

complication during intubation and posturing the patient.

Great care must be taken in positioning these patients on the operating table so that pressure areas do not develop and other bone injuries are avoided.

Duchenne muscular dystrophy

Duchenne muscular dystrophy leads to progressive weakness and debility. The myocardium may be involved, and in the later stages respiratory reserve decreases. If vital capacity is less than 30% of normal, operation should not be contemplated. The patients also have a tendency to bleed more than usual during surgery, even if hypotension is induced. The mechanism is not known but an abnormality of the blood vessels is one possibility.

There have been several reports of cardiac arrest with and without pyrexia, particularly following suxamethonium. Some of these seem to be due to malignant hyperpyrexia and others probably to myocardial disease. These patients usually have high creatine phosphokinase levels, but do not necessarily develop malignant hyperpyrexia. It is safer to avoid suxamethonium.

Arthrogryposis multiplex congenita

This is an uncommon clinical condition in which there is contracture of the muscles. This may cause limitation of joint movement, wasting of some muscles, absence of some muscles, dislocation of joints (especially the hip) and absence of skin creases, producing a 'featureless' limb (Fig. 19.3). Limb involvement varies, and the spine and jaw may also be affected. These patients usually present for orthopaedic or plastic surgery.

The aetiology is probably due to immobility of the joints *in utero* as a result of a neurogenic abnormality or, less commonly, a myopathy.

The anaesthetist may encounter several problems with these patients. Their veins are often sparse, small and fragile and may be difficult to puncture, especially over the concavity of joints.

The commonly used anaesthetic agents, including halothane, suxamethonium and ketamine, have been used in these patients.

Intubation is sometimes more difficult than usual and occasionally impossible; the airway may only be maintained with some difficulty. It is advisable after induction of anaesthesia to ensure that the patient can be ventilated by mask before giving a relaxant. In the event of a long-acting relaxant being given and intubation failing, it is

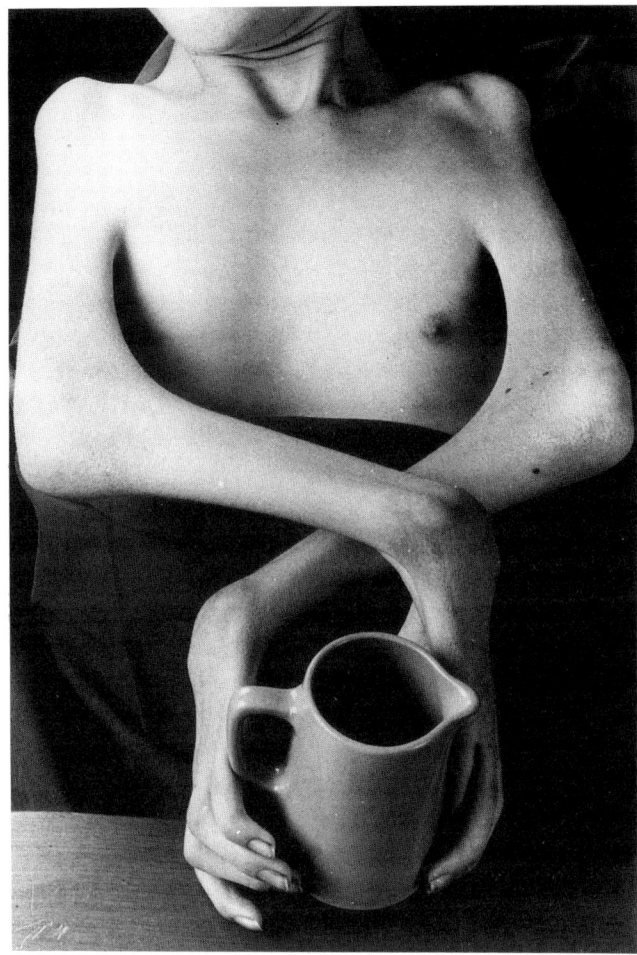

Fig. 19.3 Patient with severe arthrogryposis multiplex congenita, showing webbing of joints and muscle wasting.

better to ventilate by mask than to traumatize the mouth with repeated unsuccessful attempts at intubation. Alternatively a laryngeal mask may be tried.

The skin may sometimes feel hot during anaesthesia, but it is unusual for the temperature to be significantly elevated. It does not predispose to malignant hyperpyrexia [2, 3].

ANAESTHETIC MANAGEMENT

Anaesthetic management for most orthopaedic operations is not usually complicated. Problems may arise:
1 in the presence of other diseases such as those listed above, particularly if they affect respiratory or cardiovascular function or cause difficulty with ventilation or intubation (see Chapter 25);

2 when significant blood loss occurs;

3 in posturing the patient, as some operations are performed in the prone or partially rotated positions;

4 following trauma, where there may be multiple fractures (possibly compound) and the problem of a full stomach;

5 when a plaster is being applied. Movement may cause a crack in the plaster, making it useless. The anaesthetic should be continued until the plaster has set.

Choice of anaesthesia

General anaesthesia, either with inhalation agents and spontaneous ventilation, or 'with thiopentone, nitrous oxide, oxygen and relaxant supplemented with an analgesic or inhalation agent and controlled ventilation, is satisfactory for most procedures.

Regional anaesthesia can be used alone, but more commonly in children in conjunction with light general anaesthesia, to provide operative and postoperative analgesia, particularly for limb surgery. The surgeon must be aware that a block is being used and should be consulted beforehand because the ablation of pain, especially when a plaster is applied postoperatively, may prevent the recognition of pressure or ischaemia due to the plaster (see Chapter 22 for limb blocks). Intravenous regional anaesthesia (Bier's block) is useful for simple fractures and avoids the need for general anaesthesia.

Repeated anaesthetics may be necessary in children with multiple deformities requiring many operations, so that it is not uncommon for a child to have had ten or more anaesthetics before the age of 5 years. A kindly approach by the anaesthetist, giving consideration to the child's requests for a particular method of induction, will help to prevent emotional trauma. Although sensitization to halothane following repeated exposure may occasionally cause jaundice, it is extremely rare in children and it is unlikely if it has not occurred after two or three exposures to halothane. Many children have had multiple halothane anaesthetics (see Chapter 2).

Blood loss and its prevention

Blood loss may be considerable especially during spinal operations and pelvic osteotomy. When significant blood loss is expected, cross-matched blood should be available.

Autologous blood transfusion is being used increasingly to reduce the risk of infection (e.g. with human immune deficiency virus (HIV) or hepatitis) and because of the scarcity of blood. Blood may be taken preoperatively and stored, or it can be taken at induction with volume replacement using colloid or two to three times the volume of crystalloid solution. The blood can be returned later or at the end of the operation. A cell saver may also be used.

A large venous cannula should be inserted before the operation begins, so that blood can be given rapidly if necessary. A crystalloid solution such as compound sodium lactate solution (Hartmann's) is infused initially and may be all that is required unless gross blood loss occurs.

Difficulty may be experienced in finding a suitable vein in children who have had many operations, who are obese or who suffer from conditions where the skin or veins are abnormal, such as in arthrogryposis multiplex congenita, spina bifida or Ehlers–Danlos syndrome (see Chapter 25).

Tourniquets are frequently used for peripheral limb operations so that there is no bleeding in the wound during operation. This gives the surgeon a clear view of the operating field, reducing operating time and blood loss, although some bleeding may occur after the tourniquet is removed. The limb should be exsanguinated before a pneumatic tourniquet is applied with pressure exceeding arterial systolic pressure. When the tourniquet has been on for an hour, the surgeon should be informed. Most limb operations in children can be completed within 1–2 hours. The times of application and release of the tourniquet should be noted.

Blood loss and operating time can be reduced markedly in scoliosis surgery by the use of hypotensive anaesthesia with, for example, a sodium nitroprusside infusion (see Chapter 23). The control of blood loss has been most marked when the same surgeons and anaesthetist have worked together as a team.

After operation, a vacuum bottle (e.g. Redivac) communicating with the operative site via a catheter can apply continuous suction, pulling the tissue together so that a haematoma does not develop. In some instances, such as spinal surgery and operations where cancellous bone is exposed, continuous suction may lead to considerable blood loss. For this reason it is not so commonly used as formerly and, if it is, it may only be applied some hours later when clotting has occurred, or it may be used intermittently in conjunction with external pressure applied to the wound.

It is desirable to maintain the intravenous infusion until the following day, and to remove it only when it has been ascertained that excessive blood loss has been adequately replaced.

Posture

The choice of anaesthesia and whether or not to intubate the patient will be influenced by the position required for surgery. Optimum surgical access may require the lateral or prone positions.

A special adjustable Relton–Hall frame is available (Fig. 19.4) which supports the shoulders and iliac crests for spinal surgery in the prone position, so that compression of the abdomen causing venous congestion of the operative site is avoided.

Radiation

Image intensifiers or X-rays are used during some orthopaedic operations and corrections of fractures. It is easy to neglect precautions against radiation (see Chapter 21) but a lead apron should be worn when the anaesthetist is not able to move as far from the field as other theatre personnel.

FRACTURES

Simple

Simple fractures needing manipulation and plaster do not usually present anaesthetic problems, but if they are treated as an emergency there may be an increased risk of vomiting and aspiration, even though the patient has fasted for several hours, because stomach emptying may be delayed following injury (see Chapter 26). Where there is doubt, a gastric stimulant such as metoclopramide (Maxalon) can be given to hasten stomach emptying.

A regional technique or intravenous regional anaesthesia can be used in a co-operative child, or with the aid of intravenous sedation or Entonox. It has the advantage that the patient will not usually need to be admitted to hospital.

When intravenous regional anaesthesia (Bier's block) is used, care must be taken to follow the correct procedure. A double cuff on the arm is preferable, but is not always practical in children. It must be reliable enough to ensure that pressure will not drop inadvertently. A winged needle is inserted into the hand, and once the cuff is in place the arm is elevated. This will help exsanguination, particularly if the brachial pulse is occluded. The upper cuff, if two are used, is inflated above arterial pressure. Lignocaine or prilocaine (3 mg/kg as 0.6 ml/kg of 0.5%) is injected. Bupivacaine must *never* be used, as several fatalities have occurred with its use for i.v. regional anaesthesia. After 2 or 3 minutes the lower cuff is inflated and the upper one deflated. In this way the tourniquet pain is avoided because the area under the second cuff is anaesthetized. The cuff should not be let down for at least 20 minutes. This is usually sufficient time to manipulate the fracture and apply the

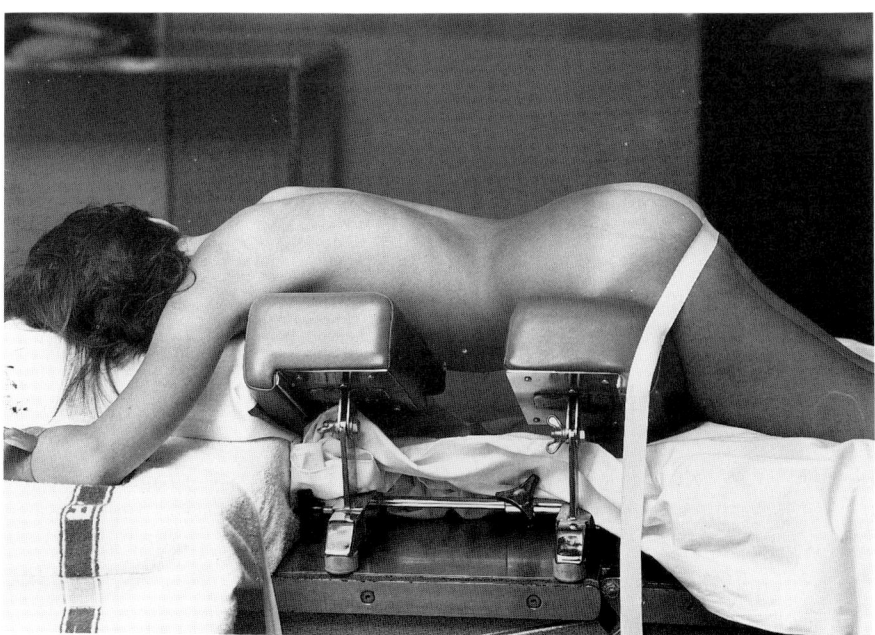

Fig. 19.4 Patient on the frame developed by Relton and Hall for scoliosis surgery, with the hips and shoulders supported.

plaster. Peak plasma levels of lignocaine, following de-flation of the cuff after 20 minutes, are only occasionally over 2 µg/ml. Oxygen, suction and resuscitation equipment must be available in case of cuff failure and the release of large amounts of local anaesthetic into the circulation. There should also be intravenous access in the opposite limb.

Fractures do not usually need to be treated urgently. Even supracondylar fractures of the humerus where the radial artery pulsation cannot be felt can be managed by elevation until the swelling goes down, provided the peripheral circulation and capillary refill following compression are satisfactory. Swelling is usually the cause of diminished pulsation on all but rare occasions when the artery may be traumatized. If prolonged ischaemia occurs, Volkmann's ischaemic contracture may develop.

Multiple

Major trauma may include multiple fractures and be associated with blood loss (see Chapter 26). Severe blood loss and shock are more likely to be due to internal haemorrhage than that associated with fractures, and other sources of blood loss should therefore be sought. The fractures can be splinted and then may be treated secondarily, after the patient has been resuscitated and more acute problems have been handled.

DEFORMITIES

Limbs

Many deformities can be treated without surgery. Correction may occur with growth (e.g. knock knees). Manipulation and stretching are often done without anaesthesia and the correction held in place with splints or plaster casts. About 50% of infants with talipes equinovarus (club feet) will require soft-tissue release operations to allow a good position to be achieved. These are usually carried out between 8 and 12 weeks of age.

Traction and wedged plaster may be used to correct deformity.

Soft-tissue operations to divide, lengthen or transfer tendons, or to divide or excise contracted fascial bands, may be undertaken as primary treatment or when more conservative measures have failed.

Osteotomy of the long bones is performed to correct malunion or malpositioned ankylosis. Arthrodesis can be performed to fix joints in a desirable position after the original deformity has been corrected.

When one limb grows much longer than the other, the epiphysis of one of the long bones can be removed (epiphysiodesis) to arrest growth.

Scoliosis

Scoliosis (lateral curvature of the spine) may be congenital, or may be associated with neuromuscular disorders or conditions such as Marfan's syndrome, neurofibromatosis or hemivertebrae, but the majority are idiopathic. Treatment may consist of a spinal brace or a plaster jacket, but more severe cases require spinal surgery. Older children with very marked deformity may have halofemoral traction for 2 weeks prior to surgery, to stretch and straighten the back. The metal halo is attached to the skull with four screws, under general anaesthesia. Local anaesthetic injected at the sites of insertion will provide early post-operative analgesia. At the later operation the halo may be removed after induction or after the patient is intubated, as it does not interfere with intubation.

Many patients are very apprehensive before scoliosis surgery and should have night sedation as well as adequate preoperative medication to calm them.

Anaesthesia is usually induced with thiopentone and muscle relaxant and maintained with nitrous oxide and an inhalation and/or intravenous analgesic supplement. In some centres, patients are awakened during the operation to ensure that the spinal cord is not damaged. This would require anaesthesia with short-acting drugs such as propofol, fentanyl and atracurium. Evoked potential recordings are now being used to avoid having to awaken the patient. Blood loss may be considerable unless hypotensive anaesthesia is used (see Chapter 23). This can be easily managed with sodium nitroprusside delivered through a second intravenous infusion, either with a flow control device or a syringe pump. D-tubocurarine or alcuronium tend to lower blood pressure, while isoflurane (or halothane) are useful supplements in hypotensive anaesthesia. Deep isoflurane anaesthesia can be used to induce hypotension as it has a significant vasodilator action, but older children often shiver when exposed to prolonged anaesthesia with these agents. Frequent or continuous monitoring of blood pressure and peripheral perfusion is essential. These operations are painful, and larger doses of opioids than usual are needed to provide analgesia, provided respiratory function is normal.

Epidural opioids such as pethidine or fentanyl have also been used with success as, unlike with local anaesthetics, neurological function can still be tested. This is essential at the end of, and sometimes during, surgery. Alternatively, intravenous opiate infusions can provide postoperative analgesia, but may need to be run at higher rates than after other surgery because the pain is more intense.

The corrective operations include:
1 The Harrington rod procedure, which was widely used but has been largely replaced by the Luque segmental instrumentation, and more recently by the Cotrel Dubousset procedure, which gives better correction.

The patient is placed prone on an adjustable frame with pelvic and shoulder supports (see Fig. 19.4). Hooks, threaded on to precurved rods, are attached posteriorly to various segments of the spine. The rods are then rotated to correct the deformity.

The postoperative course is short, requiring only 5–7 days in hospital. A brace or plaster jacket, which was formerly used for the Harrington procedure, is now not necessary.
2 The Zielke operation using a thoracoabdominal approach has largely replaced the Dwyer procedure. It is used to correct thoracolumbar curves. The discs and epiphyseal plates are removed and bone chips are inserted. The spine is placed in lordosis and the vertebral interspaces are packed to maintain lordosis. Derotation is also obtained by this process.
Patients with Duchenne muscular dystrophy form a special group. Spinal surgery is usually performed late in the disease, mainly to enable them to sit up in a wheelchair. They usually have a Luque segmental instrumentation, almost always reaching to the pelvis. They tend to bleed more than usual despite the use of hypotensive anaesthesia.

Congenital dislocation of the hip

This condition is more common in girls (80%) and in about 25% of patients both hips are affected. If the diagnosis is made in the first few days of life and treatment is begun, then the hip will usually develop normally. If the diagnosis is missed at birth, it may not be made until an abnormal gait is noted.

The basic principle of treatment is to achieve and maintain reduction. There are many ways of doing this with harness, splints or traction. If reduction is not achieved, the hip is examined, manipulated under anaesthesia and often an adductor tenotomy is performed through a skin stab. The position in 90° flexion and 60° abduction is maintained in a plaster spica. This can be done under inhalation anaesthesia with a mask. The infant may be rolled over for a brief period at the end so that the plaster can be tidied up.

If these methods fail, open reduction is necessary. The soft tissue between the acetabulum and the femoral head is removed and the hip is reduced. A plaster spica is then applied and, with periodic changes to accommodate growth, this treatment is continued for 3–4 months.

Occasionally innominate osteotomy is performed to increase the acetabular support for the femoral head, or a rotation osteotomy is necessary to correct persistent anteversion of the femoral neck. These operations may be accompanied by substantial blood loss. An intravenous infusion should be running and blood should be available for transfusion if necessary.

Perthes' disease

Perthes' disease is an avascular necrosis of the hip, in which the femoral head becomes softened and flattened if weight-bearing is permitted, or if the femoral head is partially out of the acetabulum. It mainly affects boys between 5 and 10 years of age. Treatment is usually conservative, but occasionally when the whole femoral head is affected, innominate osteotomy is performed.

Slipped femoral epiphysis

Slipped femoral epiphysis is most common in boys 10–15 years old. If it occurs acutely, the hip should be aspirated urgently so that the blood supply to the femoral head is not impaired by compression, and then placed in 90/90 traction (90° flexion of hip and knee). The femoral head should be pinned as soon as possible after 1–2 days of traction. This is usually done on a radiolucent table with a sandbag under the hip to aid positioning, and the pins inserted under image intensifier control. If these patients are not treated urgently, avascular necrosis of the femoral head will frequently occur.

ASPIRATION AND DRAINAGE PROCEDURES

Children may require aspiration of joints for blood or pus, and sometimes arthroscopy and even open arthrotomy will be necessary. Haemarthroses commonly occur in haemophilia (Factor VIII deficiency) and related diseases such as Christmas disease (Factor IX deficiency). They should be treated preoperatively as outlined in Chapter 25, to improve haemostasis.

As there is a high incidence of HIV infection in haemophiliacs, due to contamination of Factor VIII before the introduction of stringent blood testing, special precautions to prevent contamination of the operating theatre personnel and theatres must be taken.

When the child has suppurative arthritis or osteomyelitis he may be toxic and febrile. The X-ray changes of acute osteomyelitis may not be present for several days. A needle is inserted, usually under anaesthesia, to aspirate pus for diagnostic culture and sensitivity. An intravenous infusion is usually started so that fluids and antibiotics can be given. The limb is immobilized in plaster postoperatively.

BONE CYSTS AND TUMOURS

A number of bone conditions, including simple bone cyst and aneurysmal bone cyst, may present as swelling or pathological fractures. Benign lumps which may be painful are osteoid osteomata and osteochondromata. These should be excised.

Malignant bone tumours, including Ewing's and osteosarcoma, have had a much improved prognosis in recent years with chemotherapy before and after surgery. There is now about a 60% 5-year survival. When possible the tumour should be excised, preserving the limb. A prosthesis or a free vascular bone graft may be inserted into the deficit. The latter procedure will be a long operation taking several hours, because it involves dissection and transfer of the vessels to maintain the blood supply of the graft. When this course is contemplated, it is important that consent for operation should include amputation in case this turns out to be necessary. The anaesthetist should have an assistant or someone to provide relief. An epidural with catheter provides analgesia and sympathetic block, which may help blood flow in the vascular graft.

Chemotherapy may have an adverse effect on the patient's well-being and cause leucopenia. The blood count should be checked preoperatively. Psychological support will be needed, as the possibility of losing a limb is not easy to accept. It is important to ensure that the patient receives adequate sedation preoperatively when needed. Continued emotional support will be needed postoperatively.

Children with malignant bone tumours may be resistant to non-depolarizing muscle relaxants. It has been demonstrated electromyographically that the onset and degree of paralysis following D-tubocurarine and alcuronium are usually slowed and reduced when the tumour is malignant. When the tumour is removed or chemotherapy has been curative, the EMG response usually reverts to normal. The reliability of this finding as an assessment of the success of treatment is over 80% in bone tumours. Benign lesions have a normal response (see Chapter 2).

REFLEX SYMPATHETIC DYSTROPHY

This is a condition which often presents to orthopaedic surgeons with pain, tenderness and a cold hand or foot. It is associated with increased sympathetic nervous activity to that limb, causing a diminution of blood supply. If it is not treated or does not resolve spontaneously, additional features such as osteoporosis develop. Eventually long-term disability may become significant. It can be treated with physiotherapy and mobilization, transcutaneous electrical nerve stimulation, or sympathetic block. It is discussed further in Chapter 8.

REFERENCES

1 Hall R.M.O., Henning R.D., Brown T.C.K., Cole W.G. Anaesthesia for children with osteogenesis imperfecta. *Paed Anaes* 1992, **2**, 115.

2 Baines D.B., Douglas I.D., Overton J.H. Anaesthesia for patients with arthrogryposis multiplex congenita: what is the risk of malignant hyperthermia. *Anaesth Intens Care* 1986, **14**, 370.

3 Ode Y., Yukioka H., Fujimori M. Anaesthesia for arthrogryposis congenita multiplex — report of 12 cases. *J Anaes (Japan)* 1990, **4**, 275.

20: Burns

INTRODUCTION

The management of burns has changed in the last 20 years. Much earlier excision of the burn and grafting are now advocated, so that infection is reduced and earlier healing can occur. The development of deformities, contractures and prominent scarring have been minimized by the application of pressure suits. The problem of gastric ulceration has been reduced by early enteral feeding and the use of antacids and H_2 blockers. Despite these improvements, the tragedy of burn injury and the need for good care continues.

PSYCHOLOGICAL ASPECTS

The child who is badly burnt, especially if the face, hands or feet are involved, suddenly changes from a normal-looking person to one who has some disfigurement for life. It is a challenge to all those involved in treatment and rehabilitation to return the child to as near normal as possible. Apart from the discomfort involved, the realization of the consequences of the injury must be depressing, especially when a burnt face is first seen in a mirror. Psychological support from the staff is very important. In some instances the child feels that the burn is some sort of punishment; it may be a feature of the battered baby syndrome.

The treatment of burns by debridement, skin grafting, changes of dressings and baths is unpleasant for the child, and every effort should be made by the staff to provide compassionate support as well as adequate analgesia or anaesthesia as required.

Children with severe burns may be barrier nursed, and unless there are nurses, visiting parents or others around they can become lonely and have time to brood on their misfortunes.

The parents and family have problems too. Although some children are burnt in situations where no one can be blamed, the parents or adults caring for the child frequently develop guilt feelings, which can be disturbing, especially when others openly blame them for negligence.

Parents may spend much time visiting the child in hospital, and the other members of the family may feel neglected, leading to problems at home.

It is important to have psychiatric, psychological and social-work help for the children and their families as part of the team management of these patients. A caring and sympathetic anaesthetist also helps.

PATHOPHYSIOLOGY

The pathophysiology of severe burns involves many systems and will be briefly reviewed. Skin has an important protective function. The loss of large areas of skin will lead to loss of considerable amounts of fluid and heat, leaving the patient more prone to infection.

The burn injury causes an immediate local inflammatory reaction, with histamine and serotonin release, which leads to capillary dilatation and increased permeability. Fluid loss into the interstitial space causes burn oedema and there is increased evaporative loss. The fluid loss is proportional to the severity of the burn, and may be sufficient to cause hypovolaemia, leading ultimately to shock. This occurs during the first 48−72 hours. With the administration of fluids to maintain blood volume there is continued fluid loss into the tissues, aggravating the oedema. The fluid balance stabilizes and the oedema disappears after 3−4 days.

Haemolysis and the loss of red cells following heat damage in deep burns is related to the area and depth of the burn. In addition, spherocytosis with shorter red-cell survival and leucopenia may develop.

Upper airway damage may result from the inhalation of hot gases. The presence of charring around the nostrils, singeing of nasal hairs or facial burns should alert one to the possibility of airway obstruction developing which may require an artificial airway.

Lower respiratory tract damage may be associated with the inhalation of noxious fumes, steam or smoke. Steam may burn the respiratory mucosa, whereas noxious fumes may cause a chemical pneumonitis leading to pulmonary oedema. The latter may also result from fluid overload during resuscitation.

In major burns, pulmonary infections may follow sputum retention, particularly when there are circumferential burns of the trunk, or result from septicaemia.

Oliguria may result from hypovolaemia and hypotension and may be aggravated by the presence of haemoglobinuria. Unless the patient is promptly and adequately resuscitated, renal failure can become an additional problem.

Depression of liver function is proportional to the extent of the burn.

Burns cause a stress response, with increased corticosteroid secretion. The blood and urine corticosteroid levels are elevated for prolonged periods after major burns. Burn injury can cause a prolonged catabolic phase and it is not until later, when healing is occurring, that an anabolic phase develops. Gastroduodenal ulceration and erosion may occur. These ulcers show little inflammatory response and are predominantly in the fundus of the stomach.

Circumferential deep burns of the limbs or thorax may cause vascular and tissue compression beneath them as swelling occurs, with subsequent ischaemia of the limbs or limitation of ventilation when the chest is involved. Escharotomy needs to be performed urgently. This can be conveniently carried out under ketamine anaesthesia.

Albumin is lost during the initial period of increased capillary permeability. There is an associated decrease in the protein binding of drugs bound to albumin. Globulin tends to increase in response to infection. Basic drugs that are highly bound to acid glycoprotein may show a progressive increase in binding after burn injury.

Energy expenditure is increased. In patients with 30% or greater burns the evaporative insensible water loss can be as much as 200 ml/kg day. The latent heat vaporization of water is 580 J/g, so that any substantial evaporative water loss results in increased energy expenditure, which will require an additional caloric intake to compensate for it. It is estimated that in a 6−10-year-old child with 90% burns, 840 J/m^2/day (200 cal/m^2/day) will be required.

STAGES FOLLOWING BURN INJURY

1 The immediate post-burn or resuscitation stage:
(a) The initial phase of the first stage includes the first few hours following burn injury, when the patient is transported to hospital and resuscitation is begun.
(b) This is followed by a period of continued active resuscitation of 48−72 hours after the injury.
2 The second stage starts when resuscitation is complete, fluid and nutritional intake are stabilized and debridement is commenced. When it begins depends on whether the surgeons believe in immediate debridement or waiting for a few days (4−7) until the oedematous phase has subsided. The latter seems more logical, as it is better to anaesthetize and operate when the child is physiologically stable. Early grafting within the first week is now common practice, so that infection is minimized and early skin cover is achieved. The duration of this stage will depend on the extent of the burn and how long it takes to achieve skin cover. This may require only one operation for smaller burns, or up to 3 months of repeated operations for very extensive (80% or more) burns.
3 Following major burns there may be a further period in hospital for rehabilitation. The loss of fingers, stiffness of joints despite active physiotherapy, contractures, and psychological problems may need rehabilitation before

the patient can go home. Itching can also be a problem at this stage.

4 The reconstructive stage is when the child returns to hospital for operations to improve function and cosmetic appearance, and for injections of steroids to reduce prominent scar and keloid tissue.

Mortality from major burns has decreased where early effective resuscitation, earlier debridement and grafting and effective control of infection with cleansing silver sulphadiazine and antibiotics are achieved.

GENERAL MANAGEMENT

Initial post-burn phase (Stage 1)

On admission the extent and depth of the burn must be assessed and resuscitation commenced. First-degree burns affect only the epidermis. They are dry, do not blister and are erythematous and painful. Second-degree burns blister, are moist, mottled red and painful. These are now referred to as superficial burns and will heal in 10–14 days. Third-degree or deep burns reach the subcutaneous tissue. They are dry and the skin is pearly white or charred. They are not usually painful because the nerve endings have been damaged. There may be associated destruction to a greater depth involving fat, muscle and even bone. They will need to be grafted.

If deeper skin layers are not damaged and a viable blood supply remains, healing can occur by growth of epithelium from hair follicles and sweat glands and from the margin of the surrounding undamaged skin. This does not occur in full-thickness (third-degree) burns.

An estimate of the area involved should be made. The adult 'rule of nines' formula is not applicable to children because of the varying proportions contributed by the head and limbs at different ages. The alternative Lund and Browder chart is commonly employed for assessment of the burnt area in children (Fig. 20.1) [1].

Analgesics may be given if the patient is in pain, but sometimes they are not needed immediately following the burn. When narcotic analgesics are administered they should be given intravenously rather than intramuscularly, because muscle blood flow is reduced and absorption is slow during hypovolaemia. Small doses should be given because the blood volume is decreased, and a greater proportion of the cardiac output goes to the brain and the heart. Thus, normal doses would have an exaggerated depressant effect. If small doses are used

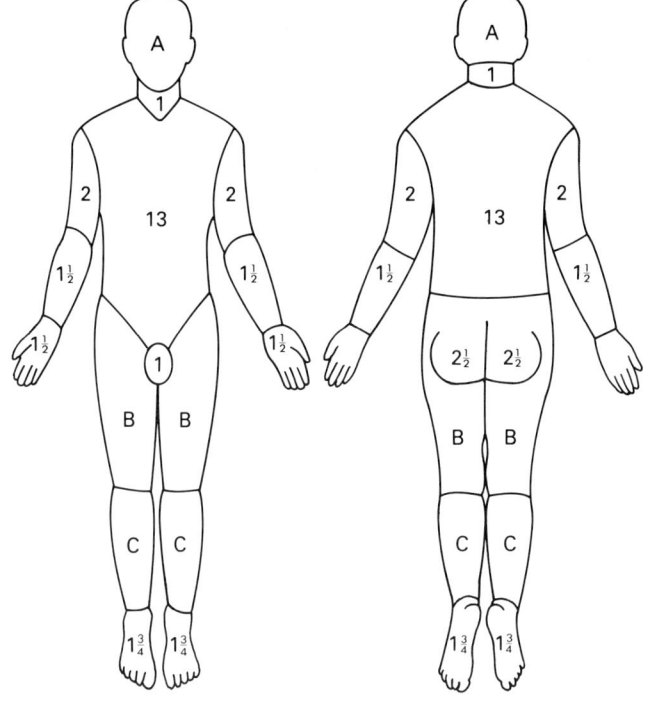

	Age (years)				
	0	1	5	10	15
A—½ of head	9½	8½	6½	5½	4½
B—½ of one thigh	2¾	3¼	4	4¼	4½
C—½ of one leg	2½	2½	2¾	3	3¼

Fig. 20.1 Modified Lund and Browder charts used to calculate area of burn.

and found to be inadequate, further small increments can be given. Once the patient has been resuscitated, an opioid infusion can be used beginning with a low infusion rate to avoid overdosage.

Resuscitation should include the insertion of a large intravenous cannula under sterile conditions, followed by adequate fluid replacement. Opinions vary regarding the proportions of colloid and electrolyte solutions used. Some units employ only electrolyte solutions initially, because they think that the colloid is lost into the damaged tissues and increases tissue oedema, whereas others argue that significant amounts of colloid must be given to maintain the intravascular colloid osmotic pressure. A reasonable compromise is to use colloid for a quarter to half the volume, depending on severity of the burn, with the remainder being given as a crystalloid solution such as Hartmann's solution in 5% dextrose. In severe burns, 3 ml/kg/per cent burn are given in the first 24 hours, half this volume being given in the first 8 hours. In addition, normal daily requirements and additional fluids to compensate for extra losses from diarrhoea, vomiting and pyrexia (10–15% per degree above 37°C) should be given. In less severe burns 2 ml/kg/per cent burn may be sufficient.

A catheter is inserted, and if fluid replacement is adequate and renal function is not impaired a urine output of 0.75–1 ml/kg/h should be expected.

A urine output below 0.75 ml/kg/h or a central venous pressure below 3–4 cmH$_2$O are indications for increasing the infusion rate, while a urine output over 1 ml/kg/h and a rising CVP over 7 cmH$_2$O call for a reduction.

Fluid requirements should be reassessed hourly for indications of under- or overinfusion.

After 24 hours, the type of fluid given will depend on urine output, haemoglobin, haematocrit and electrolytes. The volume of replacement fluid is reduced to about half that given during the first 24 hours. Oral fluids are begun with small quantities of milk any time after 4–6 hours following the burn injury. The patient may be given 30–60 ml per hour and this is gradually increased as tolerated. Unless the burns are very extensive or involve the face and mouth, most patients will be taking nearly all of their fluid requirements by mouth within 48 hours.

Blood transfusion is not usually needed during the initial resuscitation. Once the blood volume has been restored, anaemia can be corrected by blood transfusion.

The burn area is cleaned up and, depending on the practice in the particular unit, the burn is either dressed or managed by open exposure. Dressings are advantageous in small children unless the climate is hot, as they allow them to be nursed and to be mobile around their cot. Bacterial contamination of the burnt area can be reduced by the application of an antibiotic or antiseptic cream. Several of these have been used, but currently silver sulphadiazine cream containing 0.2% chlorhexidine gluconate has been found to be most effective for large burns. Tulle gras impregnated with chlorhexidine can be used for smaller superficial burns. The patient is bathed daily and the cream is applied. Tetanus toxoid is given on admission unless the child has recently been immunized, and nose and throat swabs are taken for culture and sensitivity.

When circumferential deep burns occur, early escharotomy may be necessary, to prevent vascular occlusion in the limbs or limitation of respiratory expansion of the chest.

Debridement and grafting (Stage 2)

Although in some patients superficial dead skin can be removed during bathing, anaesthesia will be necessary for preparation of deeper areas for grafting and for cutting of split skin. It is during these stages that the anaesthetist becomes most involved in the management of the burned patient. High nutritional intake, physiotherapy, occupational therapy and the general maintenance of morale are important. It is advantageous to have one anaesthetist involved throughout, to gain rapport with the child and appreciate the drug dose requirements, the patient's responses and accessibility to veins. Some children with major burns can have twenty or more anaesthetics.

Rehabilitation (Stage 3)

Once healing has occurred it is sometimes necessary to make moulds for pressure suits, which are worn to prevent contractures. When the face moulds are taken (Fig. 20.2) ketamine anaesthesia is often used.

Reconstruction (Stage 4)

Further anaesthetics may be necessary later to improve the mobility of joints by division of contractures, and to carry out cosmetic procedures.

ANAESTHETIC MANAGEMENT

Assessment

Children with burns of less than 10% of body surface area present no major anaesthetic problems unless the face or neck are involved.

Following extensive burns, the usual criteria of physical status for acceptance of a patient for elective anaesthesia are not relevant. Factors such as pyrexia, debility, infection, anaemia or respiratory tract involvement may have to be accepted as added risks, so that debridement and grafting may be undertaken at the earliest appropriate time. The preoperative assessment of patients with burns of the chest wall is further complicated if the chest is bandaged, because auscultation with a stethoscope and taking X-rays may be more difficult.

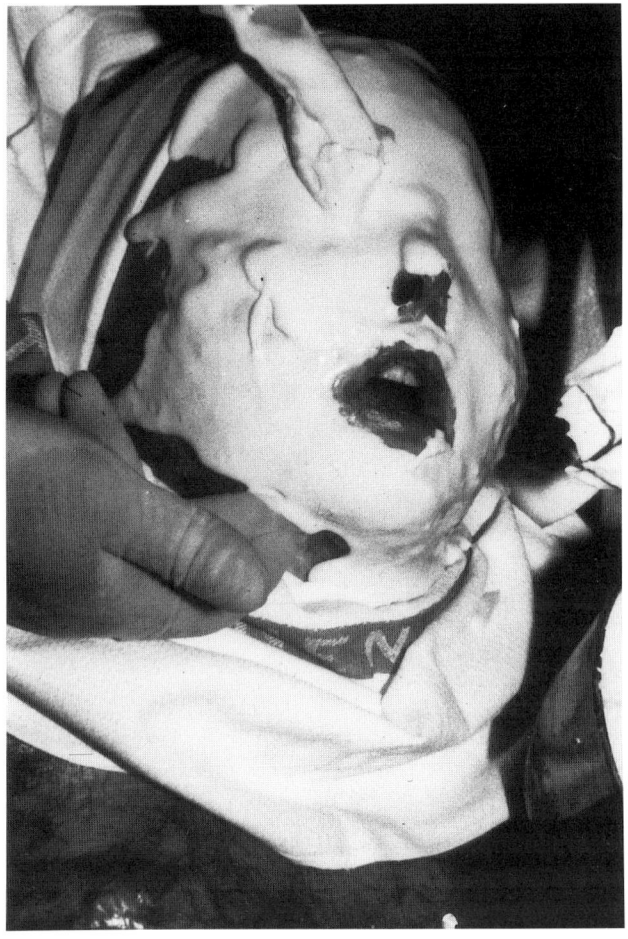

Fig. 20.2 The use of ketamine allows access to the face while a mould for a pressure garment is made.

The burn illness is a lengthy one, and rapport with the child is important, especially when many anaesthetics are required. This rapport is of particular value during induction. The method of induction is influenced by the availability of suitable veins and by the patient's choice, which is often expressed spontaneously after a child has had two or three anaesthetics.

It is better to limit the duration of the procedure to less than 2 hours and operate more often than to subject an already ill child to a prolonged operation, especially when there is significant blood loss.

Choice of technique

The choice of anaesthesia lies between an intravenous induction followed by a muscle relaxant, nitrous oxide, and opioid or inhalation supplement, an inhalation anaesthetic with agents such as halothane or isoflurane, and the use of ketamine. It will be influenced by the site of the burn, the area being operated upon, whether the patient's position will be changed during the procedure and whether the prone position will be necessary. Limited burns of a limb may be suitable for regional anaesthesia with sedation.

KETAMINE

Ketamine has been used in many centres for burn anaesthesia in children, despite the possibility of dreams and psychic problems. These seem to be less common or are not as well recognized in children and in patients with severe burns. The problem is reduced by the concurrent or premedicant use of diazepam or midazolam. Ketamine causes dissociation of the thalamo-neocortical and limbic systems. The brain-stem centres are not significantly depressed, so that laryngeal reflexes remain active, respiration is not depressed, and the cardiovascular system is stimulated [2]. Pulse and blood pressure tend to rise and cardiovascular decompensation in relation to blood loss is less with ketamine.

Postoperative vomiting is uncommon after ketamine anaesthesia, particularly in burnt patients. Ketamine causes salivation, which can be a nuisance, and many anaesthetists give an antisialagogue routinely, others only when required. Laryngospasm during ketamine anaesthesia is very rare but has occurred.

A particular advantage of ketamine is that postural changes are well tolerated, and it is easier to support the patient during posturing and while bandages are applied if some muscle tone is retained. The necessity for equipment around the face is eliminated. This is useful in the debridement and grafting of facial burns (Fig. 20.3).

Ketamine is also useful for the division and dissection of neck contractures prior to intubation.

Ketamine can be given intramuscularly if access to veins is difficult, but its action is prolonged when used by this route. An initial intramuscular dose of 3−5 mg/kg will usually allow time for an intravenous cannula to be inserted. Ketamine can be given intravenously as a bolus, followed by repeated increments or by an infusion. Further doses can always be given if necessary during infusion. Tolerance may follow the repeated use of ketamine.

Although ketamine is analgesic, even at subanaesthetic concentrations, it may not provide enough analgesia to prevent the patient moving during the intensely

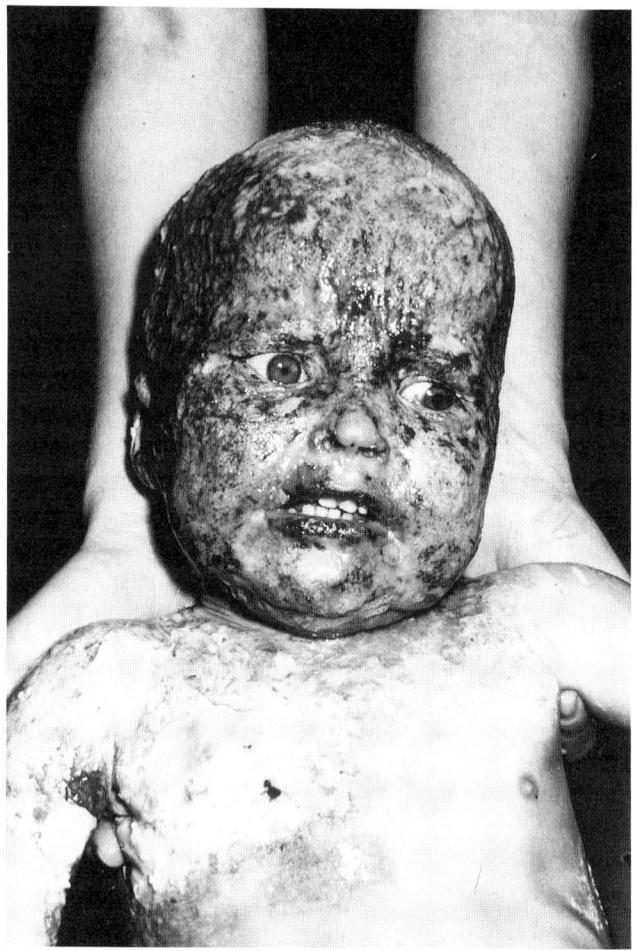

Fig. 20.3 A child with extensive facial burns. Ketamine anaesthesia allows the surgeon free access to the face.

painful procedure of taking donor skin grafts unless large doses have been used. These large doses prolong action and postoperative sleep time. Morphine can be used as an adjunct. When large doses of ketamine are used, a single dose of morphine given at the beginning of anaesthesia does not prolong sleep time but will prolong the effect of ketamine when the latter is given in small doses (less than 5 mg/kg total).

INHALATION

Inhalation anaesthesia, using a mask with an agent such as halothane, can be used for short procedures. The disadvantages of this technique include peripheral vasodilatation which enhances cooling and increases bleeding, prolongation of postoperative drowsiness, problems with ventilation if the patient is turned face-down during the

operation. Postoperative rigidity and shivering which may follow halothane is undesirable after skin grafting, as it may cause movement of the grafts. An inhalation induction may be requested by the patient and can help subsequent venepuncture by dilating the veins. If halothane is employed, any vasoconstrictors which the surgeon may wish to use must be compatible.

BALANCED ANAESTHESIA

The balanced anaesthesia sequence including muscle relaxants and tracheal intubation ensures adequate ventilation, which is particularly important if the patient is prone during the procedure. It allows access for tracheal suction. Venous access is essential for this technique, but a vein may not be readily available. It may not be the method of choice when skin grafting around the face is contemplated, because the anaesthetic equipment may interfere with the operating field.

Muscle relaxants

Severely burned patients respond abnormally to muscle relaxants. They have a decreased sensitivity to non-depolarizing relaxants [3]. The onset of this resistance may take 1−2 weeks to develop (Fig. 20.4). It has been reported that the effect lasts over a year [4], but studies in children show recovery occurring by 6 weeks (Fig. 20.5). The degree of relaxation produced by the usual dose of D-tubocurarine (0.67 mg/kg) is less, and full recovery occurs in a shorter time than usual. A dose of as much as 1 mg/kg D-tubocurarine, which is 1.5−2 times ED95, may be required to produce the usual degree of relaxation. It has been suggested that an increased binding to acid glycoprotein following burn injury may be a factor [5], but it is more likely that an increased number of acetylcholine receptors explains the altered response [6, 7].

The administration of normal doses of suxamethonium (1 mg/kg) to badly burned patients has been associated with cardiac arrest [8]. This is associated with a marked rise in plasma potassium following depolarization [9, 10]. The magnitude of this rise in plasma potassium is related to the extent of the burn injury, the dose of suxamethonium and the time elapsed since the burn injury. After 1 mg/kg it may be as much as 4−5 mmol/l when the burn area exceeds 25% and 1.5 mmol/l even in 10% burns following 1 mg/kg. The rise is much less when smaller doses are used (Fig. 20.6). It occurs between 10 days and

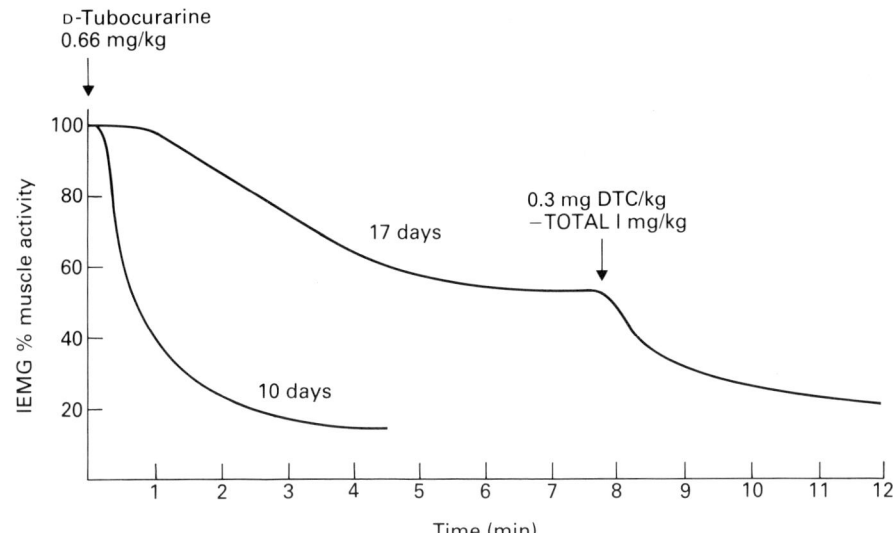

Fig. 20.4 Integrated EMG traces showing the changes in sensitivity to D-tubocurarine in a child with 27% burns between 10 and 17 days after burn injury.

8 weeks post burn, usually being maximal between 3 and 5 weeks [7, 12]. The duration may be related to the extent of the burn, starting earlier and going on longer in very severe burns. It is postulated that it is due to the

spreading of acetylcholine receptors throughout the muscle membrane [6, 7].

Patients with burns over 10% pass through a phase of acute sensitivity to suxamethonium some time between 4

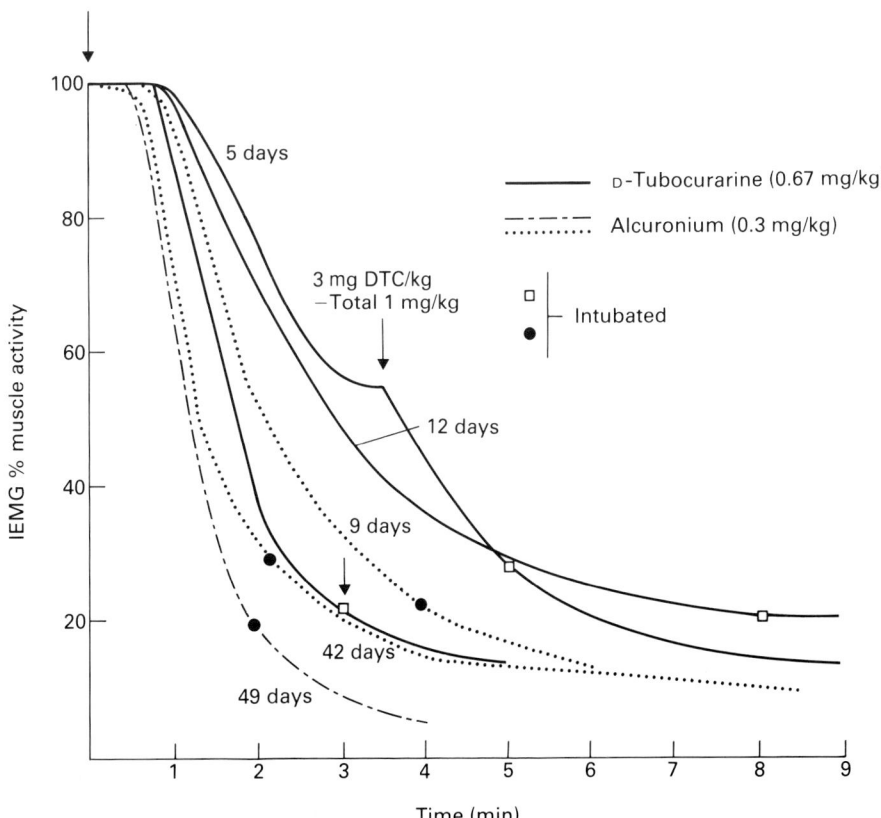

Fig. 20.5 Integrated EMG traces showing the changes in response to D-tubocurarine (solid line) and alcuronium (dotted line) during six anaesthetics on the same patient at different stages of the burn illness, returning towards normal after 6–7 weeks.

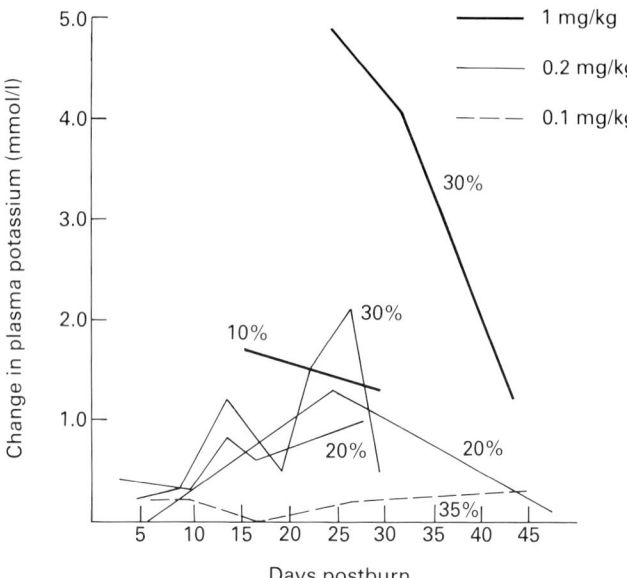

Fig. 20.6 Graph showing the relationship of the rise in plasma potassium after suxamethonium in six patients studied on several occasions, demonstrating the greatest changes with the biggest dose, with the larger burns and that the highest levels were reached between 2 and 5 weeks.

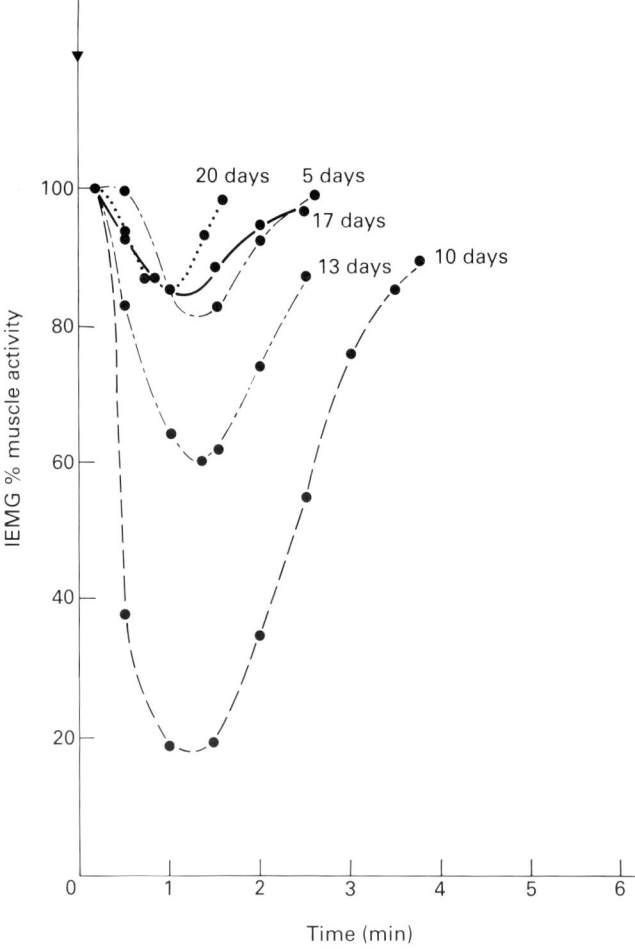

Fig. 20.7 Graph showing the variation in IEMG response to 0.1 mg/kg suxamethonium given on five occasions to a child with 30% burns. Note the acute sensitivity occurring at 10 days.

and 12 days post burn. This can be demonstrated using doses of 0.1–0.2 mg/kg. With these doses, patients may become paralysed at the time of maximum sensitivity (Fig. 20.7) [11]. It should be noted that this phase precedes the 'hyperkalaemic response' phase. Plasma cholinesterase is reduced at this time [12], but it tends to decrease earlier and last longer than the acute sensitivity phase to suxamethonium. In general, suxamethonium can be used in the immediate post-burn period, but it is safer to reduce the dose. After 10 days it is safer to avoid suxamethonium in large burns (over 10%).

Temperature control

Heat loss can be a problem, because dead skin or debrided areas allow excessive evaporation and because large areas of the patient can be exposed at any one time. Factors affecting heat loss include the area of the burn, the area of donor site if grafts are cut, wet packs, cold intravenous fluids or blood, a cool theatre and anaesthetics which cause peripheral vasodilatation.

Two important ways of reducing heat loss are to place the patient on a warming blanket and to cover the areas away from the site of the operation. An overhead heater

is useful, particularly in small children with extensive burns. Other methods include warming and humidifying inspired gases, warming blood, using warm wet packs, raising the operating theatre temperature and closing the doors to minimize draughts. If excessive cooling occurs, a mylar film or 'rescue' blanket which will reflect the patient's heat can be used intra- or postoperatively. Skin grafting early in the course of the illness and the application of dressings to donor areas immediately after the skin is cut also reduce heat loss.

Transfusion

The main reasons for blood transfusion in burns are to replace losses occurring during extensive debridement or the cutting of grafts and to correct the anaemia which follows severe burns.

The estimation of blood loss is difficult because of losses on to drapes and dressings, and because wet packs are commonly used. Reliance has often to be placed on clinical assessment, particularly heart rate, and an educated estimate of blood loss.

Blood loss can be reduced by the infiltration of vaso-constrictors prior to debridement. Ornithine-8-vasopressin (POR8) is an effective vasoconstrictor but needs at least 10 minutes to achieve full effect. It is usually diluted 1:50–1:70. It can cause a generalized pallor and hypertension, which may be confusing if one is relying on skin colour and perfusion as an indication of the patient's condition.

During debridement and grafting an intravenous infusion should be running in all children with burns exceeding 10%. Venepuncture can be technically chal-lenging because of the paucity of veins, particularly when the patient has already had many intravenous infusions or when all the limbs have been burned. In such situations veins on the trunk, shoulders or scalp may have to be employed, or central venous lines may have to be inserted at any available site. Venepuncture through a burnt area is undesirable because of the poten-tial infection and because underlying veins are often thrombosed.

Posture

During the changes in posture which may be necessary to expose burned areas or to gain access to healthy skin for grafting, particular care is needed to maintain the airway and ventilation, to prevent displacement of intravenous and monitoring lines and to prevent sudden hypotension.

Analgesia

Adequate postoperative analgesia is necessary, particu-larly when grafts have been applied, as restlessness may result in displacement of the grafts. Donor areas, where many nerve endings have been damaged, can be especially painful.

Ketamine provides some analgesia in the early post-operative period, as it has analgesic effects with sub-anaesthetic plasma concentrations.

Local anaesthetic nerve blocks of the areas where skin is cut provide better analgesia for 6–8 hours if bupi-vacaine is used. As skin is frequently taken from the thigh, the femoral, lateral and posterior cutaneous nerves of the thigh can be blocked separately, or, if both legs are involved, caudal anaesthesia can be used, although it will cause more bleeding due to vasodilatation (see Chapter 22 for details).

An opioid infusion provides constant analgesia for as long as required, and has advantages when major grafting has been undertaken (see Chapter 8). An extra bolus can be given prior to changes of dressing or baths to prevent discomfort.

Monitoring

It may be difficult to monitor some patients in the usual way, although a pulse can usually be felt and most patients have a finger, toe or ear to which a pulse oximeter can be attached. Greater reliance may have to be placed on clinical observation. If the chest is involved, an oesophageal rather than precordial stethoscope will have to be used but this is inconvenient with ketamine. If the limbs are burned it may not be possible to use a blood pressure cuff. An ECG can usually be attached, even if alternative sites have to be used for the electrodes to avoid the burnt areas, but it will not usually furnish any more useful information than the pulse oximeter or a stethoscope.

These patients may be febrile before operation. Temperature monitoring is useful to ensure that excessive cooling does not occur.

ANALGESIA FOR NON-OPERATIVE PROCEDURES

Children with burns may require some analgesia or sedation during Stages 2 and 3, for changes of dressings on the ward, baths, or physiotherapy which is aimed at maintaining joint mobility. Many drugs and combinations have been used. The importance of psychological support must not be forgotten. Kind, reassuring people can be very helpful. The combination of papaveretum and hyoscine has been satisfactory. The rate of an opioid infusion can be temporarily increased or an extra bolus can be given. Self-administration of Entonox (50% nitrous oxide) may be suitable for some, particularly older, children. Sometimes the discomfort is sufficient to warrant the use of ketamine. Oxygen and ventilating equipment should always be available in such circumstances.

STAGE 4 — PLASTIC SURGERY

Later operations to improve the function of joints or for cosmetic reasons can be undertaken even years afterwards. Generally the principles of anaesthesia for plastic surgery apply.

Severe contractures, particularly involving the neck, and deformities have been fewer since the advent of pressure garments, collars and splints.

Severe contractures of the neck (Fig. 20.8) may make intubation difficult. In these patients, inhalation induction may take longer than usual because there may be partial respiratory obstruction. The contracture may be divided rapidly following thiopentone or another intravenous agent; the relaxant is then injected and the patient

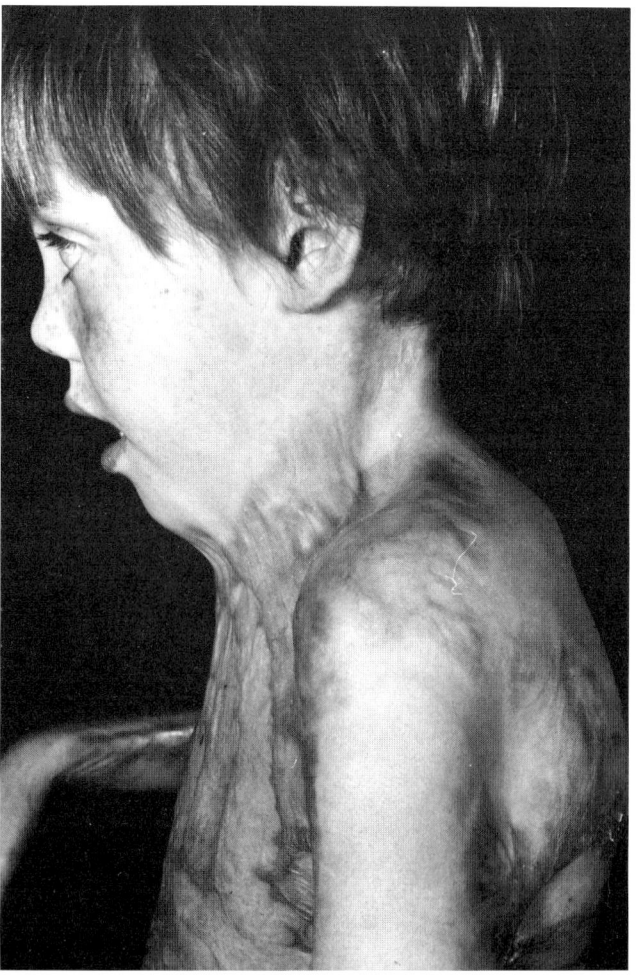

Fig. 20.8 A severe neck contracture following burns, which was divided under ketamine anaesthesia.

intubated. Ketamine has advantages in this situation because the airway is usually maintained, the patient is pain-free, and there is time to divide and dissect the scar before intubation is attempted. The surgeon should be standing by to divide the contractures when the patient is induced.

Although splints can reduce the degree of circumoral contractures which sometimes occur in facial burns, laryngoscopy and intubation may be difficult.

SUMMARY AND CONCLUSION

The anaesthetist who understands the burn illness and the associated anaesthetic problems can play an important part in the team caring for these unfortunate children. Continuity of care allows the development of rapport with the child, which enables the anaesthetist to advise on analgesic, anaesthetic and respiratory problems and to help in maintaining the child's morale.

REFERENCES

1 Lund C.C., Browder N.C. The estimation of areas of burns. *Surg Gyn Obs* 1944, **79**, 352.
2 White P.F., Way W.L., Trevor A.J. Ketamine — its pharmacology and therapeutic uses. *Anesthesiology* 1982, **56**, 119.
3 Martyn J. Clinical pharmacology and drug therapy in the burned patient. *Anesthesiology* 1986, **65**, 67.
4 Martyn J.A.J., Matteo R.S., Szyfelbein S.K., Kaplan R.F. Unprecedented resistance to neuromuscular blocking effects of metocurine with persistance after complete recovery in a burned patient. *Anesth Analg* 1982, **61**, 641.
5 Martyn J.A.J., Abernethy D.R., Greenblatt D.J. Plasma protein binding of drugs after severe burn injury. *Clin Pharmacol Ther* 1984, **35**, 534.
6 Grovert G.A., Theye R.A. Pathophysiology of succinylcholine hyperkalaemia. *Anesthesiology* 1975, **43**, 89.
7 Grovert G.A. A possible mechanism for succinylcholine hyperkalaemia. *Anesthesiology* 1980, **53**, 356.
8 Bush G.H. The use of muscle relaxants in burned children. *Anaesthesia* 1964, **19**, 231.
9 Tolmie J.D., Joyce T.H., Mitchell G.D. Succinylcholine danger in the burned patient. *Anesthesiology* 1967, **28**, 467.
10 Brown T.C.K., Bishop A.A. Anaesthesia for children with burns. *Proc. III AACA* 1970, p. 323.
11 Brown T.C.K., Bell B. Electromyographic responses to small doses of suxamethonium in children after burns. *Br J Anaes*, 1987, **59**, 1017.
12 Viby Mogensen J., Hanel H.K., Hansen E., Sorensen B. Serum cholinesterase activity in burned patients. I Biochemical findings. II Anaesthesia, suxamethonium and hyperkalaemia. *Acta Anaes Scand* 1975, **19**, 159, 169.

21: Anaesthesia for Radiological and Organ Imaging Procedures

GENERAL CONSIDERATIONS

In recent years many advances and changes have occurred — computed tomographic (CT) scanning, ultrasound, and magnetic resonance imaging (MRI) have been introduced, while pneumoencephalography, which required very demanding anaesthesia, has been superseded. Modern techniques have made some angiographic examinations unnecessary. Radiologists are undertaking more therapeutic procedures, such as embolization of vascular abnormalities, balloon dilatation of vascular stenoses and percutaneous organ biopsies.

Many anaesthetists feel uneasy in radiology or organ imaging departments unless they work there frequently, because they are remote from the familiar surroundings of the operating theatre.

Access to the patient during the procedure may be difficult due to the equipment used and the hazards of radiation. Visual access is diminished when the room is darkened for screening.

It is necessary to have an immobile patient while the examination is in progress. This requires a co-operative patient, usually aided by sedation, but co-operation may be lost if the procedure is painful. In some hospitals many procedures are undertaken under sedation, often intravenous pentobarbitone, administered by the radiologist. Although this may provide satisfactory conditions for the radiologist, the patient may be virtually anaesthetized and will require a prolonged period for recovery. Because many children, particularly small ones, cannot co-operate, general anaesthesia is often preferable.

The presence of an anaesthetist is advantageous for many procedures for the provision of appropriate anaesthesia or intravenous sedation if needed by the child, to monitor the patient and for resuscitation or treatment should serious complications occur.

THE PATIENT

The anaesthetist should aim to allay apprehension and prevent the child suffering unnecessary discomfort and, at the same time, provide optimum conditions for the performance of the investigation.

Small children cannot understand the procedures; it is therefore often preferable to anaesthetize them so that they will not recall the experience, which could otherwise be frightening to them. For some non-invasive investigations, a feed and sedation may allow a baby to sleep quietly throughout. When the investigation can be explained to a co-operative child, mild sedation may be sufficient for some procedures. Easy access to the patient enables intravenous sedation techniques to be employed, but where it is difficult, general anaesthesia with tracheal intubation may be preferable. In patients with raised intracranial pressure, sedation may lead to hypoventilation and a further rise in pressure, so that general anaesthesia with controlled ventilation is safer.

Patients requiring anaesthesia for radiological procedures must be assessed and treated just as if they are undergoing a major surgical procedure in the operating theatre.

THE ENVIRONMENT

The radiology or organ imaging department is frequently some distance from the operating theatre suite and anaesthetic department. As a result, adequate communication systems should exist between these three areas via telephone, intercom and emergency alarm to ensure prompt back-up in times of crisis.

Anaesthetic equipment in the radiology department should be comprehensive and well maintained. The space and layout of radiological investigation rooms may make the administration of anaesthesia difficult because of limitation of access.

Environmental temperature control should be an available option where paediatric anaesthesia is to be performed.

When the room is darkened for screening, a pulse oximeter is very useful to monitor oxygenation of the patient. A spotlight should be available to check flowmeters and monitors and for observation of the patient.

The large variety of electrical apparatus may cause interference with some monitors.

Air conditioning and scavenging systems should be as efficient as those in the operating theatre suite to ensure clean air for sterile procedures and adequate elimination of anaesthetic waste gases.

Radiation

This is a major hazard to both staff and patients. Maximum limits of exposure are recommended by the International Council for Radiation Protection. Limits for staff are 50 000 microSieverts (μSv) (unit of dose equivalent of absorbed radiation) per year and for patients 5000 μSv per year. X-rays have a wavelength of 10 cm − 100 m and travel in straight lines radiating from the source. The intensity of radiation diminishes by the square of the distance from the source.

Biological effects result from ionization as electrons travel through tissue, causing physicochemical changes in cell molecules. The effects may be somatic, affecting the exposed individual, or gonadal, affecting his or her progeny. The organs most at risk in the exposed individual are:

the red bone marrow, resulting in leukaemia;

the thyroid, with the risk of cancer — this is less in children than in adults;

the lens of the eye, producing cataracts — a cumulative effect.

Anaesthetists should wear lead aprons and thyroid collars and carry dosemeters while in the radiology department. The use of a ventilator, a long expiratory limb leading to the anaesthetic bag, or allowing spontaneous ventilation assists in reducing exposure to radiation.

Patient exposure can be minimized by reducing screening times, monitoring screening doses, and by the use of lead protection for sensitive organs.

Magnetic fields

The advent of magnetic resonance imaging (MRI) has presented a new hazard, that of high-strength magnetic fields. The magnet attracts ferromagnetic objects, the force of attraction increasing as the object moves closer to the centre of the field. Ferromagnetic components therefore need to be eliminated from the anaesthetic circuit and kept outside the '5 milliTesla (unit of magnetic flux) line'. This may be up to 5 metres from the core of the magnet with a 1.5 Tesla imager.

Oxygen, nitrous oxide and suction pipeline connections are desirable and should be mounted on the wall of the imaging room.

The magnetic field interferes with the function of some monitoring equipment and in addition, radiofrequency (RF) interference produced by many monitors causes deterioration in the imaging signal. A pulse oximeter compatible with MRI has recently become available.

ANAESTHETIC AGENTS AND TECHNIQUES

Anaesthetists must be particularly careful to check drugs and equipment before inducing anaesthesia in a radiology department which is separated from the operating theatres. For radiological procedures, the choice of methods lies between general anaesthesia and intravenous sedation with or without the addition of local anaesthesia.

General anaesthesia

Agents commonly used in radiological anaesthesia include thiopentone, nitrous oxide, halothane and isoflurane. Many anaesthetists use controlled ventilation with muscle relaxants, nitrous oxide and an inhalation supplement, but anaesthesia with spontaneous ventilation has advantages for some procedures. Patients with raised intracranial pressure must be carefully assessed, and in these patients controlled ventilation is preferable.

Flammable anaesthetics, although rarely used nowadays, should certainly not be used in radiology departments because of the presence of electrical equipment.

A period of apnoea may be necessary while the films are taken so that small vessels can be seen clearly, or during CT scanning of the thorax or abdomen. This can be achieved by paralysing the patient or by brief hyperventilation before holding the breath in inspiration, when ventilation is spontaneous. Sometimes, when the patient is breathing slowly and quietly, the films can be taken in the expiratory pause.

Sedation

The choice of drugs for sedation from the many available will depend upon the anaesthetist's preference and the patient's condition. Chloral hydrate in syrup form is a useful sedative in children under 4 years when given in a dose of 40–50 mg/kg 1 hour before the procedure. Papaveretum (0.4 mg/kg) and hyoscine (0.008 mg/kg) intramuscularly also sedates most children well and provides some amnesia, but tends to cause some respiratory depression and increases the incidence of postoperative vomiting.

Diazepam (0.3 mg/kg) is a tranquillizer which has been widely used in older children, but some of the newer benzodiazepines such as midazolam are being used more often for non-invasive procedures.

In younger children and infants, sedation may be used with or without the addition of inhalation anaesthesia.

Various forms of intravenous sedation are increasingly being used. These include intermittent thiopentone in small doses, propofol infusion, intravenous midazolam, and when pain is a problem, small doses of fentanyl (1–2 μg/kg) or similar drugs can be added. Low-dose

ketamine also provides some analgesia. These techniques are useful for investigations such as CT scanning, especially when contrast is injected, as it may cause discomfort.

The sedative effect of a feed may be sufficient to keep a baby still during non-invasive procedures, provided it is not intended to use other drugs and the part of the body being studied can be immobilized.

PROCEDURES

During radiological investigations, the patient must be still while needles are inserted, especially during spinal or cisternal puncture, during angiography while the contrast medium is injected, and when films or scans are being taken.

Non-invasive cardiological investigations

Echocardiography is now widely used in cardiological diagnoses and has reduced the number of patients requiring cardiac catheterization. Anaesthesia is not needed for this investigation. ECG-gated MRI is being used in some centres to outline cardiac anatomy.

Cardiac catheterization

Cardiac catheterization is invasive, involving the passage of catheters to record pressures, oxygen saturations and cardiac output, and to inject contrast medium for angiography. In infants with transposition of the great vessels, balloon septostomy may also be performed, while balloon dilatation is sometimes attempted to dilate stenotic vessels or valves.

The aim is to provide a physiological 'steady' state with sedation or anaesthesia.

The most widely used form of sedation has been the 'lytic cocktail', a combination of pethidine (25 mg), promethazine (6.25 mg) and chlorpromazine (6.25 mg in 1 ml) given in a dose of 0.05 ml/kg i.m. Others, such as intramuscular papaveretum (0.4 mg/kg) and hyoscine (0.008 mg/kg), have been used successfully, particularly in older children. Local anaesthesia, preferably bupivacaine, which is long-acting, is injected into the groin prior to the insertion of the catheters.

With all forms of sedation patient co-operation usually reflects rapport with the staff.

There is a risk with all forms of sedation that mild respiratory acidosis will occur, influencing the result of the study and possibly making accurate assessment of the patient's cardiac status difficult.

With the increasing tendency to early surgical correction in infants and the increasing complexity of anomalies being operated upon, more and often sicker infants are being investigated. Some of these who are in heart failure or generally poor condition benefit from some pre-catheter treatment in intensive care, which may include intubation and ventilation, correction of fluid, acid−base and electrolyte abnormalities and the infusion of inotropic drugs. They are usually sedated with an intravenous morphine infusion. They are then in better condition when subjected to the stress of catheterization.

When anaesthesia is employed, the infant or child should be paralysed, intubated and ventilated with air, enough supplementary oxygen to maintain reasonable oxygenation, and either an inhalation or intravenous supplement. The agent used should provide analgesia and anaesthesia with minimal physiological disturbance. Trichloroethylene ($0.1−0.2\%$), although now not widely used, provides stable cardiovascular conditions, although isoflurane, being the least myocardial depressant of the currently used agents, is an appropriate supplement in low concentrations despite reduced peripheral vascular resistance and blood pressure. Nitrous oxide is avoided because of the high concentration needed and the suggestion, still debated, but which many doubt, that it increases pulmonary vascular resistance. An analgesic such as fentanyl could be used, particularly if the patient is to be ventilated postoperatively.

Monitoring is important to ensure adequate oxygenation and a normal Pa_{CO_2} as hypoxia and hypercarbia increase pulmonary vascular resistance, while hypocarbia may be associated with a reduced cardiac output. Arterial pressure is usually monitored as part of the catheterization procedure. Monitoring methods should include pulse oximetry, capnography, ECG and temperature, although it must be recognized that PE_{CO_2} may not be an accurate indicator of Pa_{CO_2} in cases with large V/Q mismatch. The latter can be verified with an arterial sample.

COMPLICATIONS

1 Temperature maintenance, especially of infants, is a problem because the environmental temperature may not be well controlled. Cold solutions may be used to flush the catheters and, despite efforts to cover the child, large areas may still be exposed.

Steps which can be taken to overcome cooling are to raise the room temperature, warm the flushing solutions by passing them through a blood warmer, warm and humidify the inspired gases, and wrap the patient in insulating material. Radiolucent warming blankets using either circulating water or electrical heating are available for placing under the child.

2 Blood loss from repeated sampling and spillage may be more than is readily appreciated.

3 The injection of hypertonic contrast media may lead to fluid shifts from the intracellular to the extracellular space.

4 Access to the patient is often reduced by the radiological equipment; this can be a hazard if resuscitation is necessary.

Computed tomography (CT)

The exposure time required for CT scanning has been markedly reduced in recent years, so that the time during which the patient must keep still has decreased from $20−30$ minutes down to as little as 2 minutes.

Contrast enhancement is commonly used as part of the study. This requires an intravenous injection and may cause discomfort to the patient.

The anaesthetist's role is to keep the child still for the necessary period. In older children, co-operation or sedation is usually all that is needed. In very sick or unconscious patients no sedation may be needed but the airway and ventilation must be carefully observed. Intermittent injections or infusions of intravenous anaesthetics can provide satisfactory conditions in many patients. If airway or ventilatory problems are anticipated, intubation may be necessary.

If the patient is paralysed, a ventilator should be used so that the anaesthetist is not exposed to unnecessary radiation. He should wear a protective apron. The patient should preferably be monitored with a pulse oximeter or, if this is not available, a stethoscope with a long tube may be used.

Magnetic resonance imaging (MRI)

Problems arising due to the presence of the powerful magnetic field have already been mentioned.

Anaesthesia or sedation may be required for small and

uncooperative children. Patients, even adults, may feel claustrophobic in the imager. As each series of images takes about 8–12 minutes, with a brain study comprising 3–4 series, the total time needed may be 45–75 minutes.

Sedation with oral chloral hydrate (up to 60 mg/kg), diazepam or midazolam, supplemented by thiopentone or midazolam intravenous, has been used successfully.

For general anaesthesia, only plastic components must be used. A portable ventilator outside the 5 mT zone connected to the patient via a long non-distensible wide-bore tube and non-rebreathing (e.g. Laerdal) valve attached to the endotracheal tube, is a useful technique. An all-plastic ventilator has recently been developed, although standard ventilators have been used successfully [1].

Monitoring of children is difficult because they virtually disappear from view. Pulse oximetry is the most satisfactory monitor providing it is compatible with the imager, otherwise a non-ferrous precordial stethoscope may be used, together with close observation of an extremity. Some MR imagers are extremely noisy, making the use of a stethoscope virtually impossible.

Angiography

CEREBRAL

Cerebral angiography is usually performed under general anaesthesia because, if the patient is conscious, the injection of contrast may cause discomfort and consequent movement of the head at the critical time. Intravenous sedation with local anaesthesia at the catheter insertion site can be used in co-operative patients who have a normal intracranial pressure. The injection of contrast medium is frequently performed through a catheter passed percutaneously via a femoral artery. The advantage of an anaesthetic with controlled ventilation facilitated by muscle relaxation is that a $Paco_2$ of 30–35 mmHg (4.0–4.6 kPa) can be maintained. This prevents a rise in intracranial pressure, and the quality of the films is improved because of the slower flow of contrast through the brain. Halothane with spontaneous ventilation is unsatisfactory because $Paco_2$ may rise and it dilates the cerebral vessels, causing more rapid transit of the dye through the cerebral circulation. As this is important in timing the exposure of the films, the radiologist should know which anaesthetic technique is being used.

Spasm of the artery or dissection of the wall at the site of insertion of the catheter may make it difficult to manipulate the catheter, and will also reduce the blood flow. The injection of procaine, tolazoline (priscoline) or papaverine around the artery may reduce the spasm.

OTHER MAJOR VESSELS

Aortography with selective angiography of renal, hepatic or peripheral vessels may be needed to identify vascular abnormalities or to outline the vascular supply to tumours.

Vena caval studies may also be used to determine the relationship of tumours and possible venous extension, sometimes seen in nephroblastoma (Wilms' tumour). This can also give an indication of vena caval compression and the development of collateral circulation with large liver tumours. Less interference with cardiac output occurs if the vena cava has to be occluded during surgery and there is a good collateral circulation.

In the investigation of portal hypertension, the injection of 0.2–1 mg of sodium nitroprusside into the superior mesenteric artery, before the contrast is injected, improves the quality of the films in the venous phase.

When phaeochromocytoma is suspected, an acute hypertension may occur when the contrast medium is injected. The preoperative alpha-adrenergic blockade with phenoxybenzamine, accompanied by extra intravenous fluids to fill the expanded vascular space, should be considered and a vasodilator such as sodium nitroprusside should be readily available to treat severe hypertension. The catheter may also be used for intra-arterial pressure monitoring.

These investigations may be performed in older children using sedation, with local anaesthetic in the groin where the catheters are inserted. General anaesthesia is usual in small apprehensive children.

DIGITAL SUBTRACTION ANGIOGRAPHY

Digital angiography is a technique which requires the injection of smaller volumes of contrast into vessels and provides an immediate display of the image, so that the procedure is much shorter. Digital subtraction provides image enhancement. The technique provides more information than normal angiography, and can also be used in the study of cardiac function.

Embolization

This is a technique, performed preferably in association with angiography of vascular malformations and haemangiomata, where embolic materials are injected into the abnormal vessels. These include metal coils, polyvinyl alcohol sponge, gelfoam, concentrated alcohol, tissue glues and oils. The aim is to thrombose the vessels, or at least make the lesion less vascular as definitive treatment or preparation for surgical excision.

Peripheral investigations

Peripheral venography is performed with local anaesthesia, but peripheral arteriography is a painful procedure and should be done under general anaesthesia.

Lymphangiography usually takes half to one hour, and because children cannot keep still for that long a general anaesthetic is usually employed.

Splenoportography

This is part of the investigation of portal hypertension. It involves the insertion of a needle into the spleen and the measurement of splenic pressure, followed by the injection of contrast medium and removal of the needle. It is usually a short procedure which can be performed under general anaesthesia, with a period of apnoea induced by suxamethonium for the time during which the needle is inserted.

Myelography

Myelography is the study of the subarachnoid space in the spinal canal, using radio-opaque contrast media or air to outline abnormalities. Since the introduction of water-soluble contrast media such as metrizamide, the use of oil-based media (Myodil) has all but disappeared, and with it the risk of adhesive arachnoiditis. The contrast is normally injected through a lumbar puncture. When air is employed it is usually injected through a cisternal puncture with the patient tilted head-down. Postural changes include supine and prone positioning, head up and down, so that the contrast medium or air will move to the appropriate area within the subarachnoid space. These movements may involve steep inclines and the anaesthetist may have to help with posturing and holding the patient in position, as well as holding on to the endotracheal tube and connections.

When the contrast medium is injected via a lumbar puncture, the patient may only require sedation or an inhalation anaesthetic with a mask. If the patient is going to be tipped up and down, or cisternal injection is to be used, the endotracheal tube should be well-secured and the anaesthetist must continually ensure that it does not become disconnected from the breathing system. Care must be taken to protect the eyes, which should be taped closed, and to watch the arms so that nerve damage and other injuries do not occur while the patient is postured.

An oesophageal stethoscope should be used to monitor the patient, paying particular attention during the injection of air via a cisternal puncture, as accidental puncturing of the venous plexus may occasionally result in air embolism. After metrizamide, because of the risk of cerebral irritation, the child should be kept head-up in bed and given analgesics and intravenous fluids if necessary.

Bronchography

In earlier years, bronchograms were mainly used to delineate pathology such as bronchiectasis prior to surgery. Since the improved control of respiratory infections with antibiotics, the majority of investigations of the airways are now done to diagnose and delineate the extent of airway abnormalities (Fig. 21.1). These include abnormalities of the trachea or bronchi, and compression by major blood vessels. The severity of tracheomalacia or bronchomalacia can also be assessed by applying known amounts of positive airway pressure (CPAP) during the procedure to see how much is needed to keep the airways open (Fig. 21.2). The pressure can be recorded on the film by placing lead numbers on the patient.

Bronchography in children is best done under general anaesthesia with spontaneous ventilation. The child or infant can be intubated and a second Y-connector, as shown in Fig. 21.2, is attached, through the side arm of which can be passed an appropriately sized end-hole catheter (Fig. 21.3). With this arrangement the patient may either breathe spontaneously or be ventilated, and CPAP can be applied. The level of CPAP is measured on a pressure gauge. If local anaesthetic has not been applied before intubation, lignocaine 2% (up to 4 mg/kg) can be instilled down the catheter. It provides a non-reactive airway for about 20 minutes. It is important that the radiologist is available when the anaesthetic begins, otherwise the procedure may outlast the local anaesthetic and coughing occur, disrupting the procedure. The same

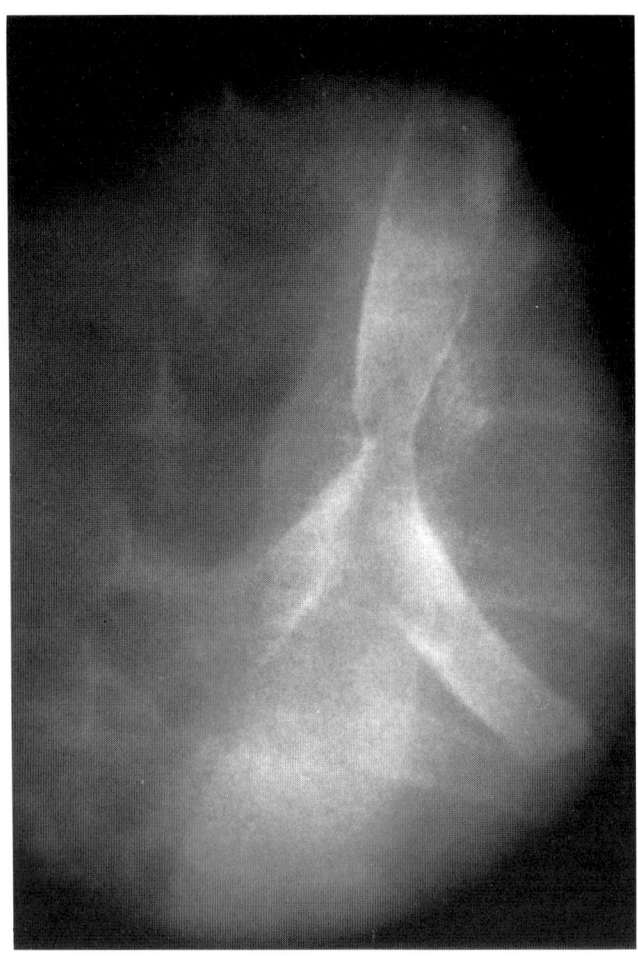

Fig. 21.1 Tracheobronchogram showing tracheal stenosis just above the carina.

catheter can be used to clear the airway of secretions or excess local anaesthetic before the X-ray contrast is injected. Gentle inflation will help to spread the contrast so that the airways are lined without using excessive volumes. Excessive inflation pressures will lead to alveolar filling with contrast medium, which cannot be sucked out easily at the end.

Ideally, the anaesthetist controls the airway and injection of dye, while the radiologist screens the patient during the injection of contrast and directs the positioning and taking of films, which may be single film or dynamic cineradiography or video. Co-ordination between anaesthetist and radiologist is essential. The films can be taken with spontaneous or controlled ventilation.

If bilateral bronchography is required, it is preferable to do one side at a time, sucking out as much contrast medium as possible from the first side before beginning the second side, so that oxygenation of the patient is not compromised. When the procedure is completed, as much contrast as possible should be removed by suction. Posturing the patient and physiotherapy (vibrations applied to the chest) will facilitate drainage.

Ultrasound

This is now a very widely used non-invasive, non X-ray modality which rarely requires anaesthesia. Most of these investigations can be performed with reassurance or some sedation such as chloral hydrate (50 mg/kg) or a benzodiazepine.

MONITORING

Patients must be monitored carefully and, when the room is darkened, a light should be available to check the child's colour. The methods of monitoring will vary. If the anaesthetist stays in close proximity to the patient or there are frequent changes in patient position, a precordial or oesophageal stethoscope is useful. The pulse oximeter is a reliable monitor which can be seen and heard from a distance during screening. An ECG monitor is used during cardiac and cerebral angiography.

A ventilator is desirable in a radiology department, so that the anaesthetist can move away from the area of high radiation intensity. A ventilator disconnect alarm is essential.

PROBLEMS WITH X-RAY CONTRAST MEDIA

Contrast media constitute a major hazard associated with radiological procedures, although the more recently developed agents are safer.

The injection of contrast media into a patient carries a risk of adverse reaction of approximately 1 in 20, and a mortality rate of 1 in 40 000 [2]. The reaction may be allergic or toxic.

Allergic reactions

These may vary from minor skin reactions, minor nasal irritation or nausea, through mild bronchospasm to anaphylaxis (usually anaphylactoid).

Anaphylactoid reactions to the injection of contrast are feared by radiologists because the effects can develop

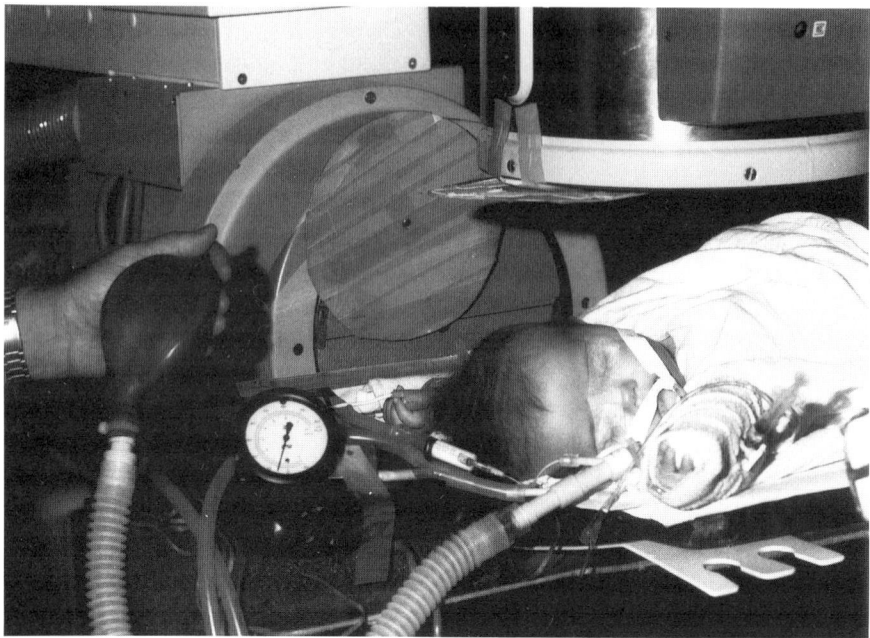

Fig. 21.2 Set-up for tracheobronchogram in an infant, showing two Portex Y-pieces in series — one with a catheter through which the radio-opaque dye is injected, and the other for the anaesthetic gases and the pressure gauge. The level of CPAP is controlled manually with the bag.

unexpectedly and progress rapidly to death if they are not treated immediately. The most dangerous features are bronchospasm and circulatory failure resulting from vasodilatation and increased capillary permeability. The latter results in loss of plasma causing oedema, which is dangerous if it involves the airway, and urticaria. At a cellular level, the defect is a reduction in cyclic 3,5-AMP.

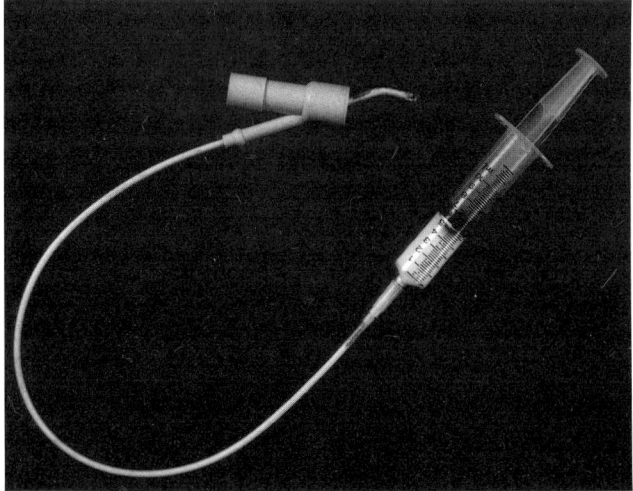

Fig. 21.3 A catheter passed through the side arm of the Y-piece. Note the angled tip on the catheter, which is useful for selective bronchography.

Treatment should consist of ventilating and oxygenating the patient, relieving bronchospasm, and improving the circulation, initially with adrenaline 0.015 ml/kg intramuscularly (1:1000) or slowly intravenously (1:10 000). Plasma loss should be corrected with intravenous fluids, which should include a plasma volume expander such as stable plasma protein solution (SPPS) modified starch solutions ('Haemaccel'), albumin or dextran to counteract the rapid loss into the tissues which results in hypotension.

If cardiac arrest occurs, the patient should be ventilated with oxygen, external cardiac compression should be performed, more adrenaline and intravenous fluids given and metabolic acidosis treated with sodium bicarbonate if severe (see Chapter 35).

Toxic reactions

The toxicity of contrast media depends on osmolality, cardiovascular effects, metabolic effects, neurotoxicity and renal toxicity. One of the major causes of problems with contrast media has been the high osmolality of the agents used, resulting in hypervolaemia, haemodilution, and rigidity and aggregation of erythrocytes.

In recent years there have been improvements in contrast media [3]. The conventional contrast medium is a monoacid, monomeric derivative of benzoic acid. The components are fully ionized in solution, the anion being either a sodium or meglumine ion together with the iodine-containing cation. The resultant solution such as angiografin has three iodine atoms per two ions, with a resultant high osmolality (Table 21.1).

The new generation contrast media are either non-ionic monomers such as metrizamide, iopamidol or iohexol, or monoacid dimers which have two of the iodine-containing rings joined together, and one of the carboxyl groups has been converted into a non-ionic radical. The latter solution, in contrast to the non-ionic monomers, is fully ionized but has six iodine atoms per two ions, and therefore for a similar iodine concentration will have a lower osmolality (Fig. 21.4). An example is sodium ioxaglate.

The cardiovascular effects of contrast media may be *electrophysiological*, resulting in bradycardia, A-V conduction delay and ventricular arhythmias. *Haemodynamic* effects are decreased ventricular contractility and alterations in coronary blood flow. All of these factors are more marked in patients suffering from coronary artery stenosis. The effects are considerably reduced with the new generation of contrast media.

Metabolic effects include binding of calcium ions, resulting in a decreased ionized calcium, and alteration in fatty-acid metabolism in the myocardium.

Neurotoxicity after intrathecal administration includes cerebral irritation and adhesive arachnoiditis, the latter being less likely with the newer contrast media.

Renal toxicity may occur in patients with pre-existing renal impairment, particularly with diabetes or myelomatosis.

Parasympathetic hyperactivity

This has been suggested as the mechanism for severe reactions to contrast media resulting in hypotension and

Table 21.1 Radio-opaque contrast media

	Iodine conc. (mg/ml)	Osmolality (mmol/kg)
Angiografin 65%	306	1530
Metrizamide	300	480
Ioxaglate	320	580
Iopamidol	300	680
Iohexol	300	690

bradycardia. It should be treated with intravenous atropine.

Finally, one must always remember the risk of inadvertent injection of air when contrast media are injected quickly under pressure from an automatic motor-driven syringe.

ISOTOPE STUDIES

Radioisotopes are employed for studies of the circulation of cerebrospinal fluid, liver scanning, locating bone lesions and confirming the diagnosis of a Meckel's diverticulum. These studies involve serial radioactivity counts over the organ being studied and may take several hours, although each count may only take a few minutes.

Older children may keep still for the necessary time, but small children may require some sedation (e.g. benzodiazepine) either given orally beforehand or intravenously in doses just enough to keep the child still.

These investigations are usually performed in the department of nuclear medicine, which is often separate from the radiology department. If heavy sedation is used, basic resuscitation equipment, oxygen and suction should be available.

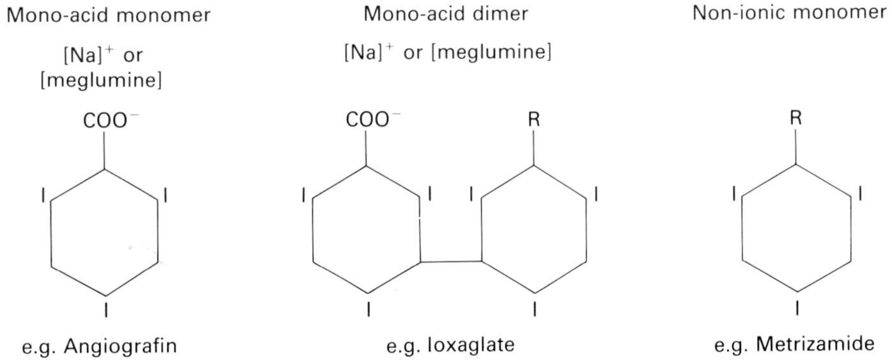

Fig. 21.4 The chemical structures of contrast media.

Mono-acid monomer

[Na]⁺ or [meglumine]

COO⁻

e.g. Angiografin

Mono-acid dimer

[Na]⁺ or [meglumine]

COO⁻   R

e.g. Ioxaglate

Non-ionic monomer

R

e.g. Metrizamide

REFERENCES

1 Mirvis S.E., Borg U., Belzberg H. MR imaging of ventilation-dependent patients: preliminary experience. *Am J Radiol* 1987, **149**, 845.

2 Ansell G. Adverse reactions to contrast agents: scope of problem. *Invest Radiol* 1970, **5**, 374

3 Dawson P., Grainger R.G., Pitfield J. The new low-osmolar contrast media: a simple guide. *Clin Radiol* 1983, **34**, 221.

22: Regional and Local Anaesthesia

INTRODUCTION

Local anaesthesia has been widely used for minor procedures such as suturing lacerations. Regional anaesthesia has been used less in children than in adults, although the earliest reports were by Gray 1909 (spinals) [1], Sievers 1936 (epidurals) [2], Campbell 1933 (caudals) [3] and Farr 1920 (brachial plexus block) [4]. Interest in regional anaesthesia has recently increased due to the development of longer-acting local anaesthetics such as bupivacaine, and a desire to improve the standards of postoperative analgesia. Also, these drugs do not pollute the operating theatre atmosphere, do not appear to be hepato- or nephrotoxic, and have been advocated on the basis that adequate neural blockade will abolish or reduce the stress response in major surgery.

Regional anaesthesia and nerve blocks can be used in children with sedation or light general anaesthesia, or as an adjunct to general anaesthesia.

The use of local anaesthesia alone in children is sometimes possible, when the patient is suffering from trauma such as a broken leg, or in a co-operative child who accepts an explanation of what will be done and does not mind needles. Adequate sedation will often facilitate its use. Self-administered 50% nitrous oxide (Entonox) is another option. Continued reassurance is essential while a block is being inserted.

When an anaesthetist contemplates using a local or regional technique in a small child, be should preferably have previous experience with the block and have studied the technique carefully, so that he is fully aware of the anatomy involved, the anatomical differences in children and the hazards and complications which may occur. In general, the smaller the child the narrower the spaces into which one attempts to place the needle and inject the local anaesthetic, and the shorter the distance to penetrate structures which may result in complications.

A good knowledge of the anatomy and the ability to locate the correct depth will allow the reliable performance of many nerve blocks without obtaining paraesthesia or using a nerve stimulator. The latter will be useful when one cannot easily locate the nerve accurately. For some therapeutic blocks, image intensification may be helpful.

The important aids to locating the depth of the nerve

are to use short-bevelled needles (45°) which help the anaesthetist to feel the resistance of fascia and aponeuroses and the loss of resistance as they are penetrated. They also reduce nerve injury. The other aid to determining depth is that it is difficult to inject as one pushes the needle through muscle, ligaments or thick fibrous tissue, and injection becomes easy when the needle enters the space deep to the structure. The nerves are often in such spaces.

The following sections highlight aspects of blocks which are useful in children. If further details are required, textbooks on regional anaesthesia should be consulted.

LOCAL AND REGIONAL ANAESTHESIA

The situations where local anaesthesia is useful for a child who is not anaesthetized are:

1 Suturing of minor lacerations.
2 Emergency procedures such as reduction of forearm fractures, or suturing lacerations, tendons or nerves when there is a danger of aspiration if general anaesthesia is used because the child has a full stomach.
3 When there is a family history of malignant hyperpyrexia or when the child is a respiratory cripple and it is desirable to avoid depressing the ventilation.
4 Spinal anaesthesia has been used in neonates and premature infants when there is a significant risk of postoperative apnoea, because general anaesthesia may increase this risk.
5 Cardiac catheterization or, in some cases, angiography in well-sedated co-operative children where the groin is infiltrated prior to femoral artery catheterization.

COMBINED REGIONAL AND GENERAL ANAESTHESIA

Except in some children having emergency surgery or with serious medical conditions, regional and local anaesthesia should be used in conjunction with general anaesthesia, especially in younger children and infants. When this is done the addition of local anaesthesia should offer some distinct advantages. The situations where local with general anaesthesia provides justifiable advantages are as follows.

1 To provide good operating conditions with reduced general anaesthetic requirement — this includes infiltration or nerve block for incision sites, caudal anaesthesia to decrease blood loss and prevention of erection in penile surgery and epidural anaesthesia to provide a contracted gut for urological surgery.

2 To block afferent stimuli so that general anaesthetic requirements are reduced and haemodynamic and hormonal responses to surgery are suppressed. The block provides postoperative analgesia and a smooth transition into the postoperative period.
3 To immobilize a limb for several hours after suturing tendons and nerves.
4 To reduce the requirements or eliminate the need for muscle relaxant drugs during anaesthesia.
5 Topical anaesthesia is often used to supplement general anaesthesia for bronchoscopy or laryngoscopy, reducing the incidence of operative and postoperative coughing.
6 Regional anaesthesia can block undesirable reflexes during anaesthesia, e.g. anal, testicular and penile reflexes causing bradycardia or laryngeal spasm.
7 In older children where sympathetic block causes some hypotension, blood loss may be reduced.

SPECIFIC BLOCKS

Central regional blocks

CAUDAL

This is often combined with a light general anaesthetic. It is particularly useful for penile surgery such as circumcision and hypospadias repair because it reduces bleeding, prevents erection and avoids laryngeal spasm sometimes seen in these operations under halothane anaesthesia; most importantly, it provides analgesia into the postoperative period when longer-acting local anaesthetics such as bupivacaine are used. This has transformed a sometimes stormy postoperative period into one of relative tranquillity and obvious patient comfort.

Caudal anaesthesia can be used for other procedures in the perineum, lower limbs and lower abdomen, such as hernia repair. Increasing the dose and volume will cause the local anaesthetic to spread higher for the latter operations.

Spread of local anaesthesia in the epidural space is more uniform in small children because the fat is less densely packed and the lobules are not separated by fibrous strands as they are in the adult. It has been shown that there is a reasonable correlation between volume/segment spread and age [5]. Lignocaine 1%, mepivacaine 1% and bupivacaine 0.25% requirements are about 0.1 ml/yr/segment (assessed by pin prick).

Another calculation is based on the findings of two studies using radiographic contrast which showed that

0.5 ml/kg spreads to at least L3 and often higher — up to T10–11 on occasions. A smaller volume will be adequate for circumcision, while a larger volume will be needed if reliable block is needed to T11 or higher (e.g. 0.7 ml/kg). Provided the total dose is kept to a maximum of 3 mg/kg, toxic blood levels are unlikely — measured peak plasma levels at this dose rarely exceed 2 µg/ml and averaged 1.4 µg/ml [6].

A third method of calculating dose, assessed by pinching, is to use the nomogram devised by Busoni (Fig. 22.1) [7].

Assessment of spread of local anaesthesia depends on the painful stimulus used. Pin prick is a less intense stimulus than pinching and thus will indicate a higher level of block, but pinching will correlate more closely with surgical stimulation.

The appropriate concentration will depend on whether or not motor paralysis is desirable. This will be achieved with 0.5% bupivacaine, but analgesia can be attained with lower concentrations. It has been shown that for operations below the umbilicus, 0.75 ml/kg of 0.25% and 0.125% bupivacaine will provide analgesia, but the ability to stand soon after recovery was inversely proportional to the concentration [8].

If combined general and regional anaesthesia is to be used, general anaesthesia is induced first; a trained assistant must be available to maintain the airway while the block is inserted. Access to a vein must be ensured so that fluids can be infused rapidly if necessary. The child is turned on his side with hips flexed. The skin over the area is cleansed and the sacral hiatus is located with the thumb by feeling the cornua and the sacral notch at the lower end of the vertebral column.

The skin is pulled up slightly so that the needle can be inserted at 60–90° to the skin at the apex of the hiatus through skin which has not been touched by the thumb (i.e. using a no-touch technique) (Fig. 22.2). At this point the sacrococcygeal membrane can be felt most easily as it is penetrated by the needle. It is also the deepest part of the sacral canal related to the hiatus, so the bevel of the needle is usually totally in the canal. The local anaesthetic can then be injected directly without leakage outside the epidural space. Some anaesthetists angle the needle after penetrating the membrane so that it is aligned with the sacral canal, and advance it into the canal (Fig. 22.2b). This should not be necessary if the bevel of the needle is wholly in the canal, and it is more likely to cause vascular and, rarely, dural puncture. In small infants and neonates it may be necessary to reduce the angle of needle insertion to 45° to facilitate entry into the shallower caudal space.

A large needle (21 SWG) is inserted so that blood or CSF will flow freely if a vessel or the dura are penetrated. The needle is inserted at an angle of 60–90° with the

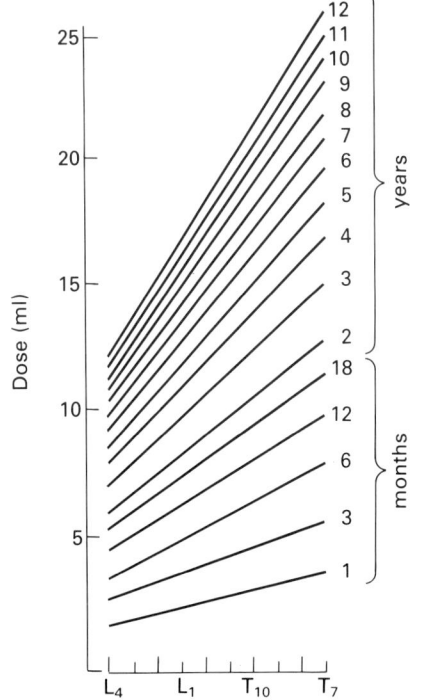
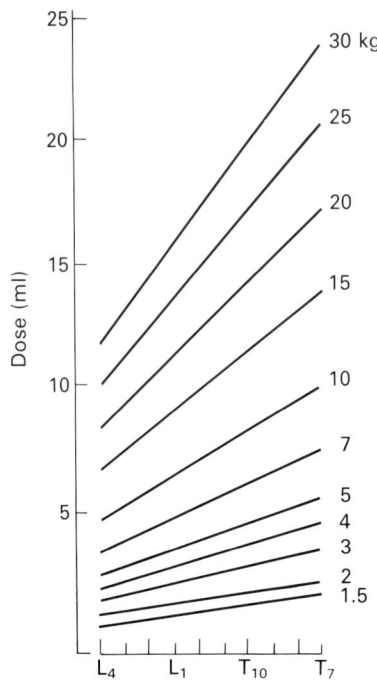

Fig. 22.1 Dose of 1% prilocaine (or lignocaine) for caudal anaesthesia. Nomograms based on age and weight for dose required to reach a predetermined height of block (after Busoni and Andreucetti [7]).

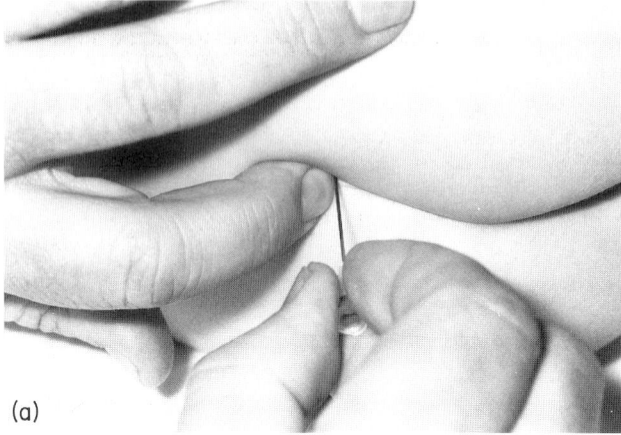

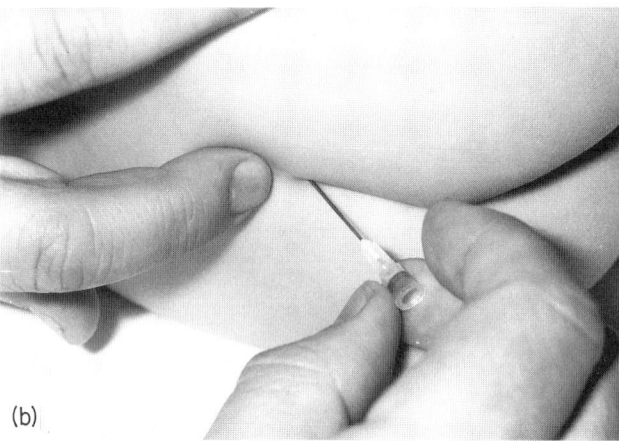

Fig. 22.2 Caudal anaesthesia — insertion of needle. (a) The sacral hiatus is located with the index finger of one hand. The needle is inserted perpendicularly through the apex where the depth of the canal is greatest. By pulling the skin cephalad, the needle can be inserted through a disinfected area of skin which has not been touched ('no-touch technique'). (b) Once in the canal some anaesthetists angle the needle (60°) into the bony canal to ensure it is correctly placed.

skin. The sacrococcygeal membrane is not easily felt with fine, sharp needles, which have the further disadvantage that they can more easily puncture bone without it being recognized. In neonates it may not be possible to feel the sacrococcygeal membrane. Aspiration before injecting the local anaesthetic is essential. It may show that the needle has entered a vein, the subarachnoid space or bone marrow. If the needle is in the correct space the drug should flow in easily. If bleeding occurs, the needle should be repositioned. If there is rapid uptake due to intravascular injection, a tachycardia will develop if the local anaesthetic contains adrenaline. An initial test dose can be injected to ensure that this is

not so. Repeated aspiration during injection is recommended. If the needle is not in the caudal canal, a subcutaneous swelling may be seen (Fig. 22.3).

The hazards of caudal anaesthesia include:
1 High plasma levels may result from accidental intravenous injection. Normally plasma levels are low following caudal anaesthesia in children.
2 The dura reaching lower than the usual level of termination at S2 (Fig. 22.4) or S3 in neonates, thereby increasing the possibility of dural puncture. This is more likely in infants. In our experience this occurs in 1:2000 to 1:3000 cases. If the total volume of local anaesthetic is injected into the subarachnoid space, a high spinal anaesthetic will result with vasodilatation, hypotension, inadequate ventilation and possibly unconsciousness. Intravenous infusion of fluids, to fill the dilated blood vessels, and ventilation must be established immediately to counteract these.
3 If the laminae of the lower sacral segments are incomplete, the needle may inadvertently be inserted at a higher level, with an increased chance of dural puncture. This abnormality also makes location of the caudal space more difficult. The anaesthetist must always look for this anomaly and it is advisable to avoid caudal anaesthesia in these patients.
4 Inadvertent intraosseous injection is easier with the soft bones of small children, especially when fine, sharp needles are used. The result can be similar to intravenous injection, producing high plasma levels.
5 If the needle is inserted too deeply, the local anaesthetic may spread around the pelvic fascia or into the pelvis (Fig. 22.5).
6 Additional hazards include the possibility of bleeding from punctured veins with haematoma formation.
7 Occasionally, a higher than usual block can occur.
All these problems are rare, but it is important that beginners should be shown the technique before attempting it themselves.

Contraindications to caudal anaesthesia are:
1 myelomeningocoele;
2 infected skin over or near the site of injection;
3 bleeding disorders;
4 uncorrected hypovolaemia;
5 local neurological disease.

Continuous caudal

Fine, narrow-gauge catheters inserted through the caudal canal, which can be advanced as far as the thoracic

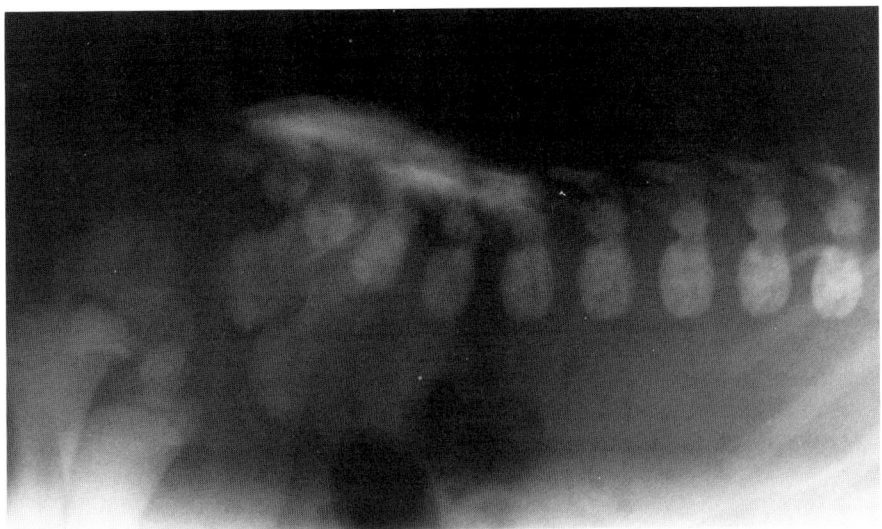

Fig. 22.3 Caudal: an incorrectly placed needle may result in subcutaneous injection of local anaesthetic.

region in infants and small children, can be used for continuous caudal analgesia by infusion or intermittent injection of local anaesthetic. The technique is probably more useful in small infants than in children, where the lumbar epidural route can be easily used. It has been used in neonates with oesophageal atresia where adequate postoperative care and ventilation were not reliably available [9]. The potential complications are haemorrhage, failure to place the catheter correctly and looping of the catheter.

EPIDURAL

Lumbar epidural block can be performed in children. Locating the appropriate intervertebral space depends on feeling the iliac crests and drawing a line between them. They are lower in infants (Fig. 22.6). The mean depth to the epidural space from the skin is approximately 1 mm/kg, although in infants it may be relatively greater (2 mm/kg at 10 kg, 1.5 mm/kg at 20 kg and 1 mm/kg at 40 kg with a range of ±20% [10]). The ligaments are soft and thin, but easy to feel as the needle is advanced. The epidural space is narrower in small patients, with a greater risk of dural puncture and possibility of inadvertent total spinal anaesthesia, particularly if the anaesthetist is inexperienced with this technique in children. If the anaesthetist is fully aware of the appropriate management of this complication by intubation, ventilation and the administration of intravenous fluids to fill the enlarged vascular compartment and hence prevent severe hypotension, the consequences should not be serious. Failure to recognize it or treat it adequately, usually due to inexperience, may result in a catastrophe. Experience with lumbar epidural anaesthesia in adults is desirable before using it in small children.

Epidural anaesthesia is a useful adjunct to general anaesthesia to reduce the stress response to surgery, to provide analgesia and, if an adequate concentration of local anaesthetic is used, muscle relaxation. Its additional advantages are that it improves blood flow for vascular flaps of the lower limb and it contracts the gut during urological procedures, such as ureteric reimplants and pyeloplasties, and other abdominal surgery. The hypotension which occurs in adults under epidural blockade is

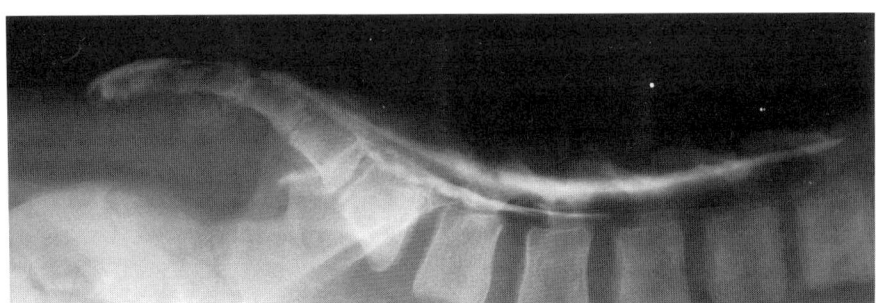

Fig. 22.4 Caudal: spread of radiopaque dye (0.5 ml/kg) injected caudally showing the dura reaching S2.

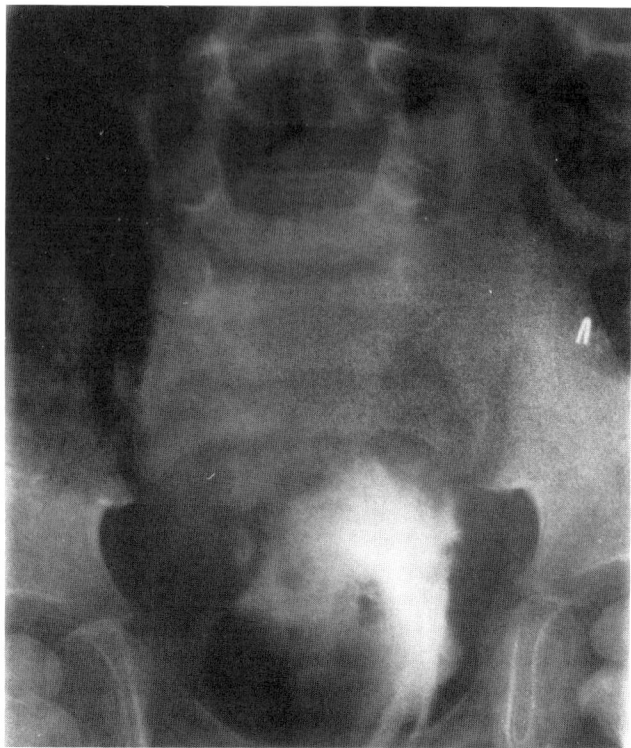

Fig. 22.5 Caudal: incorrect deep injection may spread around the pelvis.

uncommon in children below about the age of 8 years, but the block still seems to have a beneficial effect in reducing blood loss.

A variety of dose schedules have been suggested, including 0.1 ml/segment/year of age plus a little extra to

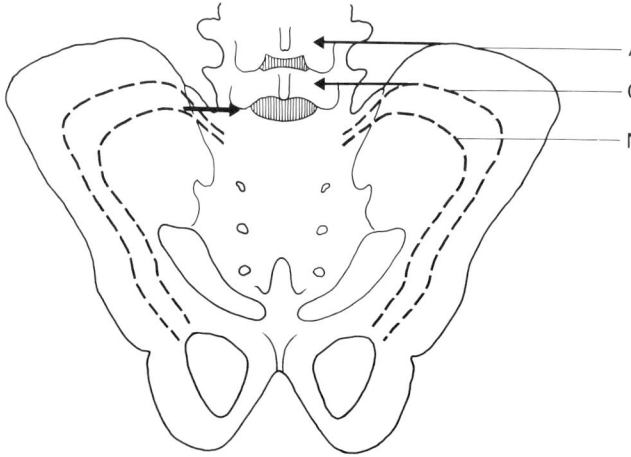

Fig. 22.6 Pelvis: the changing level of the iliac crest in relation to the vertebra. A: adult — L4, C: child — L4—5, N; neonate — L5—S1. (After Busoni).

cover individual variation and to ensure adequate spread. Another useful guide is that 2 mg/kg bupivacaine injected at L2—3 will reliably block to T6, and sometimes even higher.

The use of epidural catheters is increasing in children since the introduction of finer-gauge Tuohy needles and catheters (Fig. 22.7). Analgesia can be maintained for several days postoperatively by an infusion with a syringe pump, or with bolus injections if this is not available. A solution of plain bupivacaine 0.125% is infused at a rate of 0.2 ml/kg/h. If the addition of an opiate is desired, 1 μg/ml fentanyl is added to the infusion solution. At these infusion rates respiratory depression is not likely to occur, but particular care needs to be taken in infants and neonates. Usually the infusion can be discontinued by 72 hours postoperatively.

SUBARACHNOID

Spinal subarachnoid anaesthesia can be performed quite easily provided the anaesthetist can carry out lumbar puncture proficiently, but the technique has not been commonly used in children. The salient differences between small children and adults are that the intercristal line is relatively lower in infants because the iliac crest is less prominent (see Fig. 22.7), and the former have a relatively larger spinal fluid volume (4 ml/kg compared with 2 ml/kg in the adult); they thus require a relatively larger dose/kg to produce the same level of block. Five per cent lignocaine in 7.5% glucose is a hyperbaric solution providing about 45 minutes anaesthesia [11].

Tetracaine and bupivacaine have also been used for spinal anaesthesia in infants and children, providing 75—85 minutes anaesthesia [12, 13]. Various doses have been used. In infants, 0.15—0.2 ml 0.5% bupivacaine is used up to 5 kg, then 1 ml over 5 kg for procedures such as hernia repair. Doses of 0.3—0.8 mg/kg bupivacaine [12, 13, 14] and 0.4—0.9 mg/kg tetracaine have been reported.

The drop in blood pressure usually seen in adults with spinal anaesthesia is uncommon in children [12, 13], but has been reported to occur transiently [14].

Spinal anaesthesia has gained popularity in some centres for the management of premature infants with the aim of minimizing apnoeic episodes following general anaesthesia. Ketamine has been advocated for sedation with spinal anaesthesia, but cases of apnoea have occurred following its administration probably due to too-rapid injection or too large a dose [15].

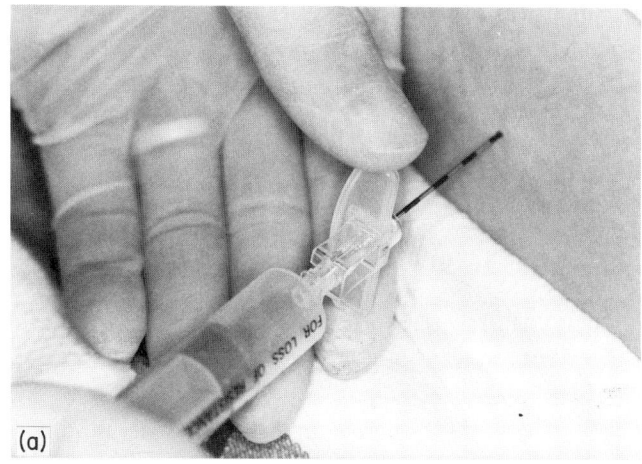

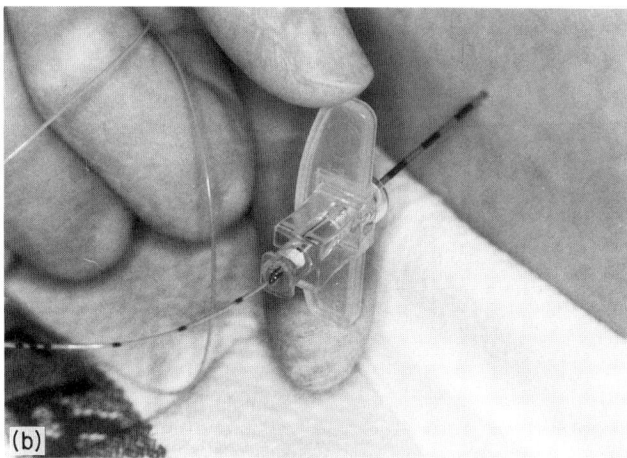

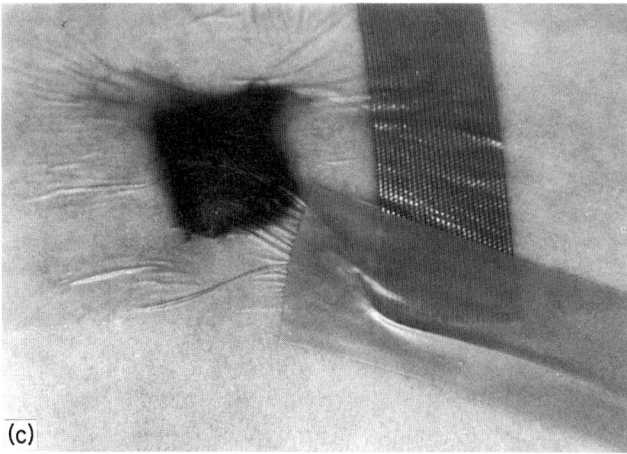

Fig. 22.7 Lumbar epidural. (a) Insertion of Tuohy needle with pressure on the syringe to detect loss of resistance as the ligamentum flavum is penetrated. (b) Insertion of an epidural catheter once the Tuohy needle is in the epidural space. (c) The catheter is passed over a small roll of gauze to prevent kinking on an acute angle while emerging from the skin. It is fixed by clear plastic adhesive and waterproof tape run up the back. This prevents accidental dislodgement.

Upper limb blocks

BRACHIAL PLEXUS

The axillary approach is the more commonly used method of blocking the brachial plexus in children [16] (Fig. 22.8). The medial, lateral and posterior cords of the brachial plexus surround the axillary artery, while the axillary vein lies on its medial side. These are all enclosed in a fascial sheath and the aim is to enter this sheath with the needle and deposit the total volume of local anaesthetic there (0.6−0.7 ml/kg with 1:200 000 adrenaline, lignocaine or prilocaine 1%, or bupivacaine 0.3−0.5%). The axillary or upper arm block is technically easy to perform, because the axillary artery can be easily palpated when the arm is abducted and externally rotated. The fingers of one hand should fix the artery while the needle is held and inserted by the other hand, which is rested on the skin for stability. An extension tubing from the needle to the syringe may help to prevent displacement of the needle once in place. A short bevelled needle (22 or 24 SWG) is inserted towards and slightly above the artery until the needle begins to pulsate, indicating proximity to the artery. If a short bevelled

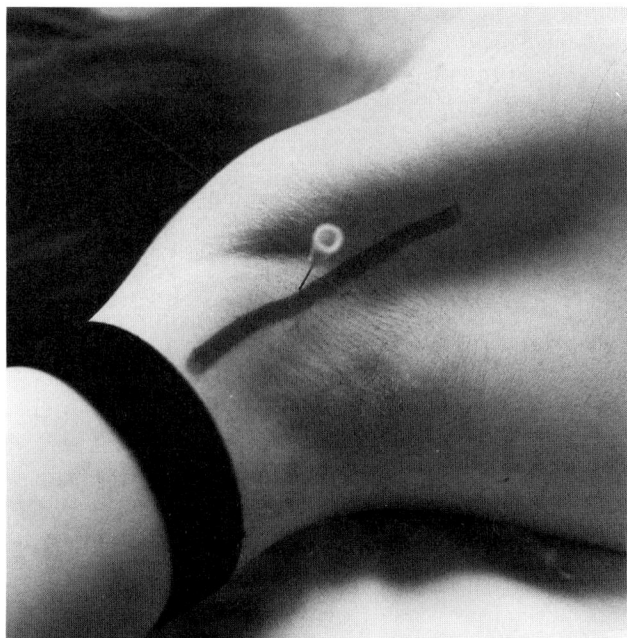

Fig. 22.8 Axillary plexus block. The needle is inserted beside the axillary artery, which may cause it to pulsate. A loss of resistance may be felt as the needle enters the sheath containing the nerves. The tourniquet or compression with fingers forces the local anaesthetic to flow proximally.

needle is used, a loss of resistance can be felt as the perivascular sheath is penetrated. As the plexus lies within this, the local anaesthetic can be injected easily. If there is resistance to injection, the needle is not correctly placed. One must always aspirate before injecting because the axillary artery and vein traverse the same space. The plexus lies fairly superficially. The commonest reason for failed block is injecting too deeply. Pressing distal to the injection site for a minute or two with the fingers used to locate the artery will prevent distal spread of the local anaesthetic. Because abduction and external rotation may cause obstruction of proximal flow by the head of the humerus, the arm should be internally rotated and adducted after the needle is removed, while still maintaining pressure so that proximal flow can be maximized. In this way the musculocutaneous nerve, which leaves the plexus proximally, will have the best chance of being blocked.

The supraclavicular approaches are less commonly used in children than the axillary approach, because the potential complication of pneumothorax is more easily produced, particularly when the first rib is used as a landmark to be located with the needle.

WRIST BLOCKS

These blocks are useful in the intra- and postoperative pain management of hand surgery. It is necessary to block the median, ulnar and radial nerves separately at the level of the proximal palmar crease. Depending on the site of surgery, only one or two nerves may need to be blocked.

Median nerve

To block the median nerve, the palmaris longus tendon is identified by flexing the wrist of the outstretched hand and moving a finger from the lateral to the medial side. The most superficially prominent tendon is the palmaris longus. Immediately lateral to the tendon (radial side) a short bevelled needle is inserted at right-angles. It is possible to feel the 'pop' of the flexor retinaculum. The nerve lies just deep to it — 2–3 ml of local anaesthetic is injected there.

Ulnar nerve

After identifying the pisiform bone on the medial (ulnar) side of the wrist, the flexor carpi ulnaris tendon is traced proximally as the wrist is flexed. The nerve emerges on the lateral side of the tendon at the proximal palmar crease on the wrist. The ulnar nerve is blocked by injecting 2–3 ml of local anaesthetic solution subcutaneously, as the nerve lies superficial to the flexor retinaculum.

Radial nerve

Though this nerve accompanies the radial artery in most of the forearm, it changes its course a few centimetres proximal to the wrist and becomes superficial. Fanwise subcutaneous infiltration of 2–3 ml of local anaesthetic solution at the 'anatomical snuff box' blocks the superficial branches supplying the medial side of the dorsum of the hand. Sometimes it is necessary to infiltrate up to the mid-point of the dorsal aspect of the wrist to block all branches.

Thoracic blocks

INTERCOSTAL

Intercostal blocks are useful for postoperative analgesia or after lateral and anterior rib fractures. During thoracic surgery the surgeon can inject the local anaesthetics under direct vision inside the chest, but if injected preoperatively they can constitute a useful part of the anaesthetic.

The intercostal space to be blocked should be located by palpation. A fine-bore needle is then inserted through the skin on to the rib above, ensuring that the hand holding the needle is resting on the back (Fig. 22.9). The needle is then moved progressively down the rib until the lower border is reached and the needle can be advanced further. There is often a grating sensation as the needle passes through the intercostal muscles into the intercostal space. This advance may only be 1–2 mm in infants, and increases in depth with growth. It is important to aspirate before injecting local anaesthetic, to ensure that a blood vessel has not been punctured. Although the vessels and nerve may be protected by lying in the groove on the under side of the rib, anatomical dissection and angiography (Fig. 22.10) show that the artery can follow a tortuous path along the intercostal space.

The traditional site for performing an intercostal block is at the angle of the rib, before the intercostal nerve gives off its lateral branch, where the innermost intercostal muscle provides some protection between the space and

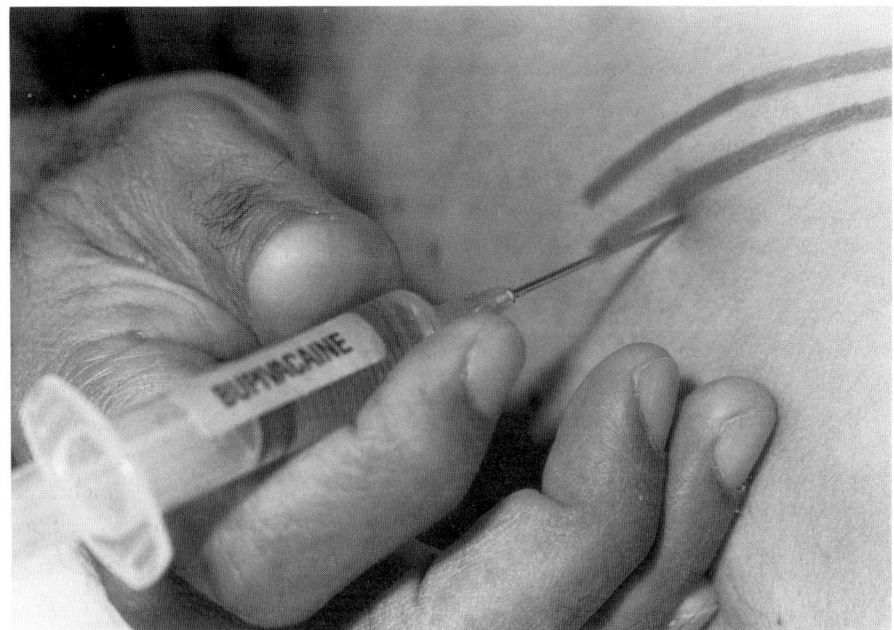

Fig. 22.9 Intercostal nerve block: this shows the hand placed on the back so that the position of the needle is kept fixed if the patient moves or coughs. The point of insertion shown is more medial than usual; injection at this point allows local anaesthetic to spread more readily to adjacent spaces, because the extrapleural fascia is less adherent to the ribs in this region. (It is advisable to wear gloves for protection.)

the pleura. In the posterior part of the space this muscle is absent, and the deep layer of pleura is only loosely attached to the ribs. It has been shown that a single large-volume injection can block several spaces, rather than using several injections of smaller volumes. The reason that this is successful is that the loosely attached posterior pleura allows spread along the paravertebral gutter to the neighbouring intercostal spaces. A lesser volume should achieve the same result if injected further posteriorly than the angle of the rib. It is possible that a

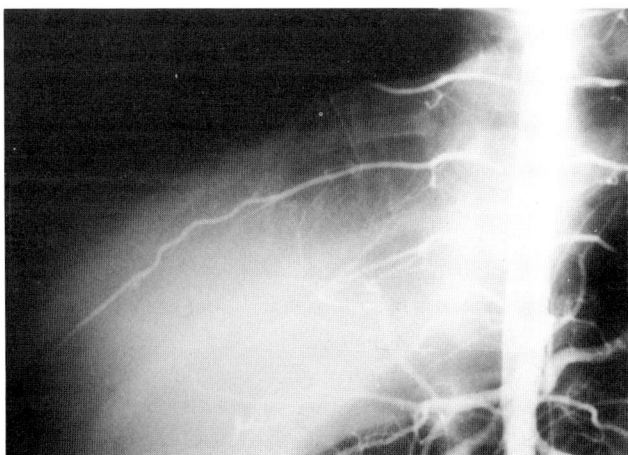

Fig. 22.10 An angiogram in an infant, showing an intercostal artery coursing through the middle of an intercostal space, and not as commonly stated in the groove on the lower border of the rib above.

large-volume injection could spread medially into the epidural space, resulting in an epidural block. Although intercostal blocks are commonly quoted as causing high plasma levels of local anaesthetics, a study in neonates (peak 0.8 μg/ml) and infants 1−6 months (peak 0.9 μg/ml) after 1.5 mg/kg bupivacaine does not bear this out [17]. Higher peak plasma levels may develop with the large-volume single injection method than with several small-volume injections into several spaces. In small infants 0.5 ml may be sufficient to block one space, while in adults 3−4 ml may be needed to ensure a good block.

Local anaesthetic toxicity can be minimized if intravascular injection is avoided and total doses are kept below the recommended maximum. The addition of adrenaline 1:200 000−1:400 000 will prolong the block and slow absorption.

Pleural puncture and pneumothorax are potential complications, and although more likely in small children with shallow intercostal spaces, pneumothorax should be avoidable by:
1 using fine-bore needles;
2 by inserting the needle through the skin directly on to the rib, moving it down the rib pulling the skin with it, so that when removed it will self-seal;
3 most importantly, by placing the hand on the back and stabilizing the needle in relation to the patient, so that even if the patient moves or coughs the needle maintains its position (see Fig. 22.9).
Intercostal blocks with long-acting agents such as

bupivacaine provide useful intra- and postoperative analgesia for thoracotomy, and upper abdominal and umbilical surgery. They are easy to insert and provide comfort without respiratory depression.

Intercostal catheters can be inserted so that further doses of local anaesthetics can be given to prolong blocks. The smaller the child the more difficult they are to place.

PARAVERTEBRAL

Paravertebral blocks are rarely used in children. In adults, thoracic epidural block achieves the desired effect, but in small children this is more difficult because the space is narrower, although catheters can be threaded up from below (see Caudal and Epidural).

The spinous process of the vertebra above the nerve to be blocked is located. The transverse process of the next vertebra below is level with this. The needle should be inserted lateral to the midline so that it hits the transverse process. It is then redirected slightly superiorly and medially and passed forwards to a deeper plane, missing the transverse process. The nerve passes from the epidural space posteriorly, which is deep, through the paravertebral space and crosses the costotransverse ligament into the intercostal space, which lies more superficially. The paravertebral space is therefore deeper than the intercostal space.

The distance from the midline and the depth that the needle must be inserted vary with the size of the child, which makes it a more difficult block to perform.

The danger with paravertebral blocks is the possible injection of local anaesthetic into the dural cuff, which occasionally extends further along the nerve into the paravertebral space. This may produce subarachnoid anaesthesia. A total spinal or significant epidural block from central spread is unlikely, but can occur if a large enough dose is injected.

A paravertebral block is most useful when a very posterior approach to the intercostal nerve is needed. This situation might occur postoperatively when a thoracotomy wound already reaches well round to the back and a normal intercostal approach is not accessible.

INTRAPLEURAL

Intrapleural block, in which an intercostal catheter is inserted into the pleural space, has been advocated for postoperative thoracic and upper abdominal analgesia.

The local anaesthetic is instilled into the pleural cavity and presumably achieves its effect by diffusing through the pleura to the intercostal nerves. It is claimed to be a simple, effective technique, but the possibility of pneumothorax must always be borne in mind.

Lower abdominal and penile blocks

DORSAL NERVE OF PENIS

The dorsal nerves of the penis emerge from under the symphysis pubis on the dorsal surface of the corpora cavernosa. They lie in a triangular compartment (lateral view) bounded by the symphysis pubis above, the corpora cavernosa below and the membranous layer of fascia in front (Fig. 22.11). When viewed in the anteroposterior view (Fig. 22.12) this space is divided by the suspensory ligament of the penis derived from the deep surface of fascia. The suspensory ligament then divides into two sheets which pass around the shaft of the penis. The nerves lie deep in the triangular space formed by the division of the suspensory ligament, and are accompanied by their arteries and vein.

There are potential pear-shaped spaces on each side of the suspensory ligament and it is into these that the local anaesthetic should be injected (Fig. 22.13).

The symphysis pubis should be palpated and the needle inserted at right-angles until it contacts it. The needle is then withdrawn and redirected below the symphysis, through the fascia into the space above the corpora cavernosa [18]. If the needle is inserted too deeply in the midline, it may enter the space deep to the suspensory ligament containing the nerves and vessels (Fig. 22.12). A good block should be obtained if the local anaesthetic is placed here, but there is danger of vessel puncture, haematoma and, if this is large enough to cause compression, ischaemia of parts of the penis. Radiological studies have shown that when the needle is placed in the midline it will usually enter the compartment on one side of the suspensory ligament (Fig. 22.13). Only occasionally is there communication between the two sides (Fig. 22.14). It is therefore best to inject on both sides, angling the needle about 15° and then redirecting to about the same angle on the other side for the second injection (Fig. 22.12). This approach avoids damage to the dorsal vessels of the penis and increases the chance of diffusion through to the nerves. An adequate volume of local anaesthetic is necessary to ensure a good block. It must *never* contain adrenaline. The ideal volume for

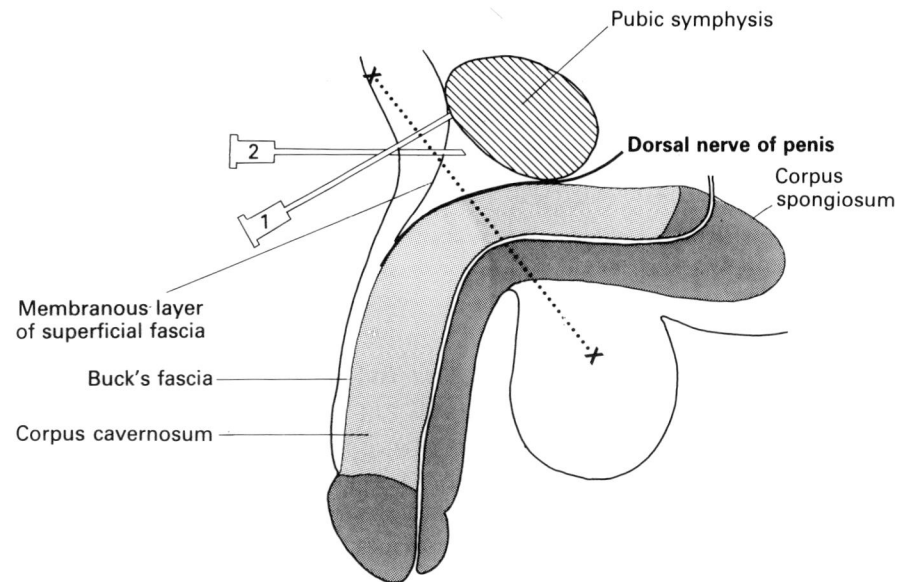

Fig. 22.11 Dorsal nerve of penis block — lateral view. The triangle bounded by the symphysis pubis, corpus cavernosum and membranous layer of superficial fascia through which the dorsal nerve of the penis passes and into which the local anaesthetic is injected. The needle is inserted to hit the symphysis [1] and then redirected through the fascia a few mm deeper [2].

use in children has not been defined, but 1.4−2 ml per side in a neonate, adding 1 ml/10 kg on each side for larger patients might be reasonable. The greater the volume the further posterior it will flow, making block of

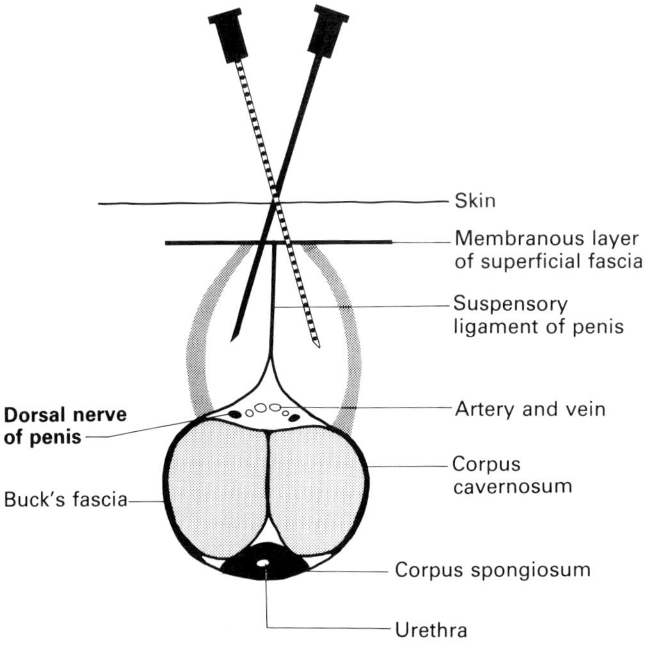

Fig. 22.12 Cross section through x−−−x in Fig. 22.11. It shows that the membranous layer of the superficial fascia divides to form the suspensory ligament of the penis. This divides to encircle the shaft of the penis. The nerves and vessels lie deep to the divided ligament. The needles show the bilateral approach for penile block which avoids vessel damage and potential haematoma.

the ventral branch, which supplies the frenulum, more likely.

The alternative to this approach is to perform a ring block of the shaft of the penis, ensuring that the dorsal vessels are not punctured. The ring must be complete to ensure that the ventral branch is blocked.

The advantage of the penile block over caudal anaesthesia for circumcision is that weakness of the legs and urinary retention do not occur.

ILIOINGUINAL AND ILIOHYPOGASTRIC NERVES

These nerves emerge through the internal oblique muscle to lie under the external oblique aponeurosis medial to the anterior superior iliac spine (Fig. 22.15). The nerves are blocked by inserting a short bevelled needle 1−2 cm medial to the anterior superior iliac spine, depending on the size of the patient. A 'pop' or loss of resistance is felt as the external oblique aponeurosis is penetrated. The local anaesthetic injected into this space will bathe the ilioinguinal and iliohypogastric nerves and anaesthetize them. If the needle enters internal oblique muscle it will be difficult to inject. As the needle is advanced further it will become easy to inject when the needle enters the space between internal oblique and transversus. Local anaesthetic injected in this space will track medially to surround the inguinal canal. Injection at both sites will provide surface and deep analgesia for inguinal hernia repair. In infants, when the aponeurosis is thin, loss of resistance may be difficult to feel. The apparent thickness

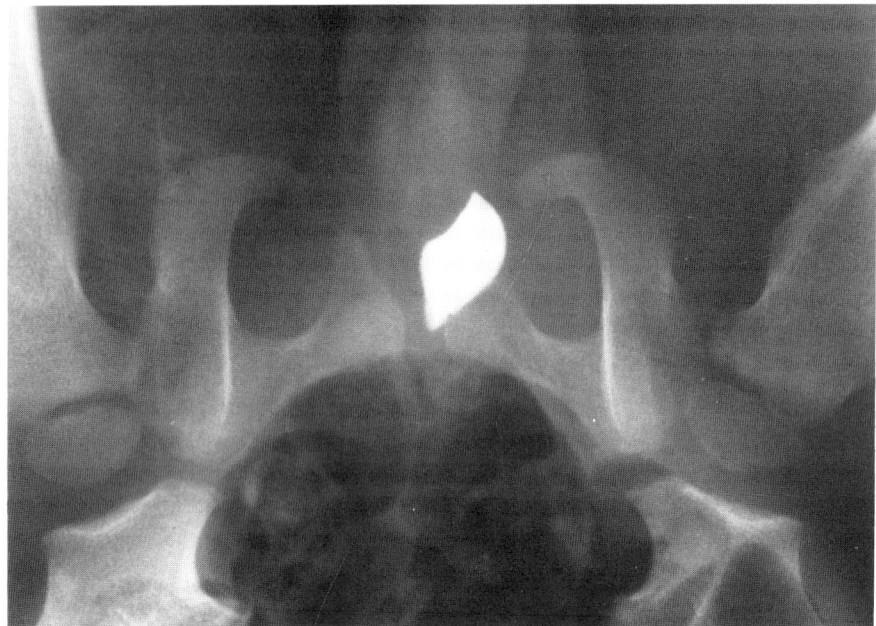

Fig. 22.13 Penile block: unilateral injection showing the potential space into which the local anaesthetic is injected. A midline approach usually fills only one side.

of the aponeurosis can be increased by passing the needle through it at an angle, thereby giving one a better chance of feeling the loss of resistance.

This block is useful for inguinal hernia repair, and because it lasts into the postoperative period further analgesia is not usually required.

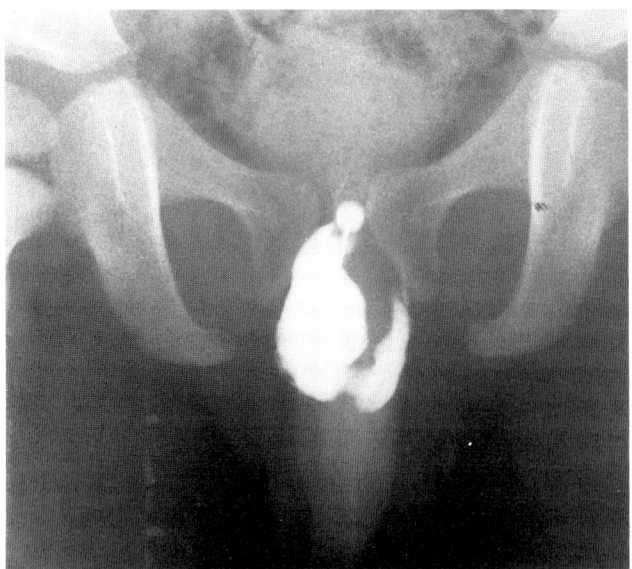

Fig. 22.14 Penile block: injection on one side spreading through a hole in the suspensory ligament to the other side — this is uncommon.

Lower-limb blocks

Although anaesthesia for lower-limb surgery can be provided by caudal anaesthesia, there are circumstances when one or several nerves can be blocked individually to provide analgesia. Examples include blocks around the ankle for foot surgery and blocks around the thigh for donor skin-graft areas in burns or plastic surgery.

FEMORAL NERVE

The femoral nerve lies lateral to the vein and artery in the groin. To locate it, the femoral artery is palpated immediately below the inguinal ligament. A short bevelled needle is inserted immediately lateral to the artery. As it is advanced, two distinct losses of resistance are felt as it passes through fascia lata and then the fascia iliaca to enter the canal containing the femoral nerve (Fig. 22.16). The artery and vein lie deep to the fascia lata but superficial to the fascia iliaca. Occasionally these two layers are fused, and then the needle may pass into the muscle lying deep to the nerve. As it is difficult to inject into muscle, the needle should be withdrawn with pressure on the syringe until easy injection occurs. If pressure is applied distally, the injected local anaesthetic should spread towards the lumbar plexus. If a large volume is used a three-in-one block can be achieved, anaesthetizing the lateral femoral cutaneous (lateral

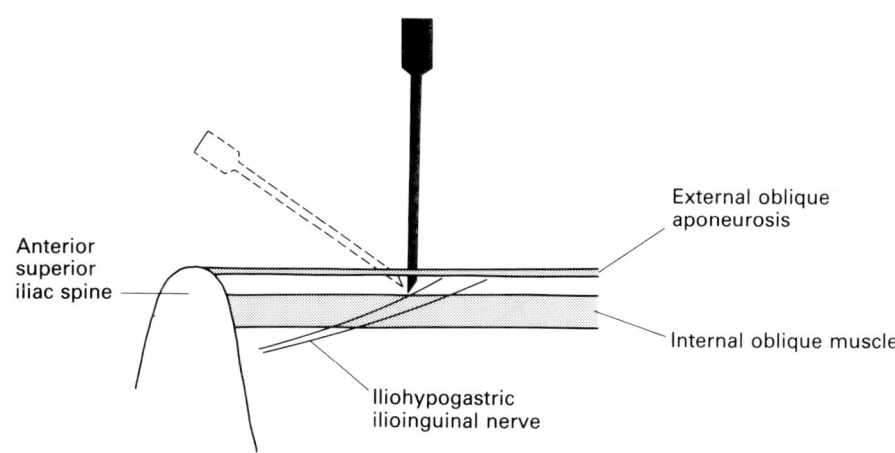

Fig. 22.15 Ilioinguinal block: a short bevelled needle is inserted 1–2 cm (depending on the size of the patient) medial to the anterior superior iliac spine. A loss of resistance is felt as the needle penetrates the external oblique aponeurosis. Local anaesthetic injected into this space spreads and blocks the ilioinguinal and iliohypogastric nerves as they pass through it. If a short bevelled needle is not available, or in neonates, the apparent thickness of the fascia can be increased so that resistance to penetration can be more easily felt if the needle is inserted at an angle (broken line).

cutaneous of the thigh) and obturator nerves as well. This two-'pop' or loss of resistance technique accurately locates the femoral nerve so that a nerve stimulator is not necessary [19]. The fanwise injection formerly recommended is not necessary if the anatomy is clearly understood.

Femoral nerve block can be used to provide analgesia and relieve muscle spasm in patients with fractured shaft of the femur. They can then be X-rayed and manipulated in comfort. The sensory distribution covers the anterior aspect of the thigh and leg, and blocks can be used to cover incisions or areas where split skin is being cut.

LATERAL CUTANEOUS NERVE OF THIGH

There are several ways of blocking this nerve, but the approach immediately adjacent to the anterior superior iliac spine (ASIS) is probably the best for accurate localization of the nerve [20]. A short bevelled needle is

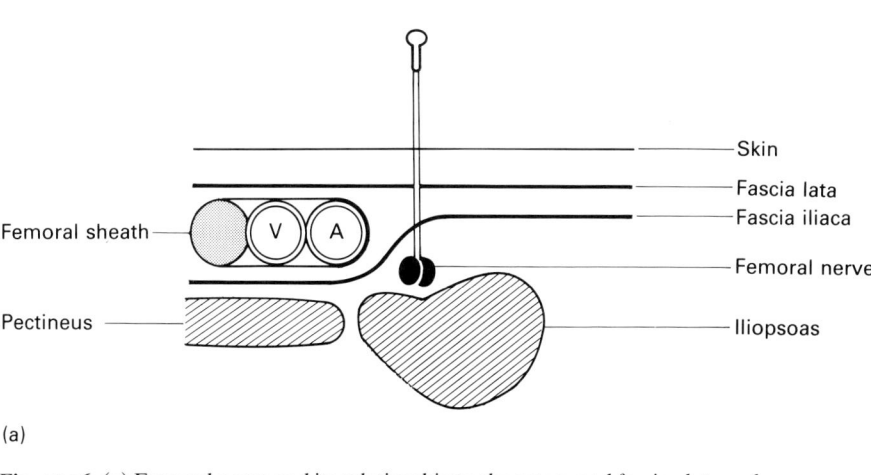

(a)

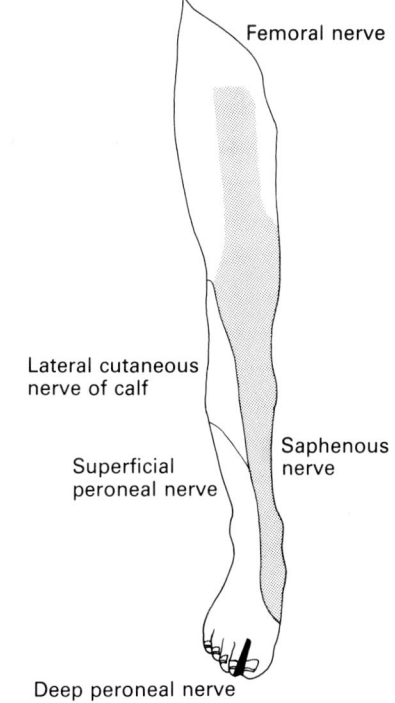

(b)

Fig. 22.16 (a) Femoral nerve and its relationship to the artery and fasciae lata and iliaca. (b) The cutaneous distribution of the femoral nerve.

inserted just medial to the ASIS. As it is advanced, a loss of resistance is felt as the external oblique aponeurosis is penetrated. The syringe should then be attached to the needle and it is advanced with pressure on the plunger. There is resistance to injection as the needle passes through the internal oblique muscle and then a second loss of resistance is felt and injection becomes easy as the

needle enters the canal carrying the nerve (Fig. 22.17). The local anaesthetic, when injected, will pass up and down the canal with the nerve on its course on the iliacus muscle and into the thigh respectively.

This block is useful for incisions on the side of the thigh and for taking donor skin grafts from the area of distribution.

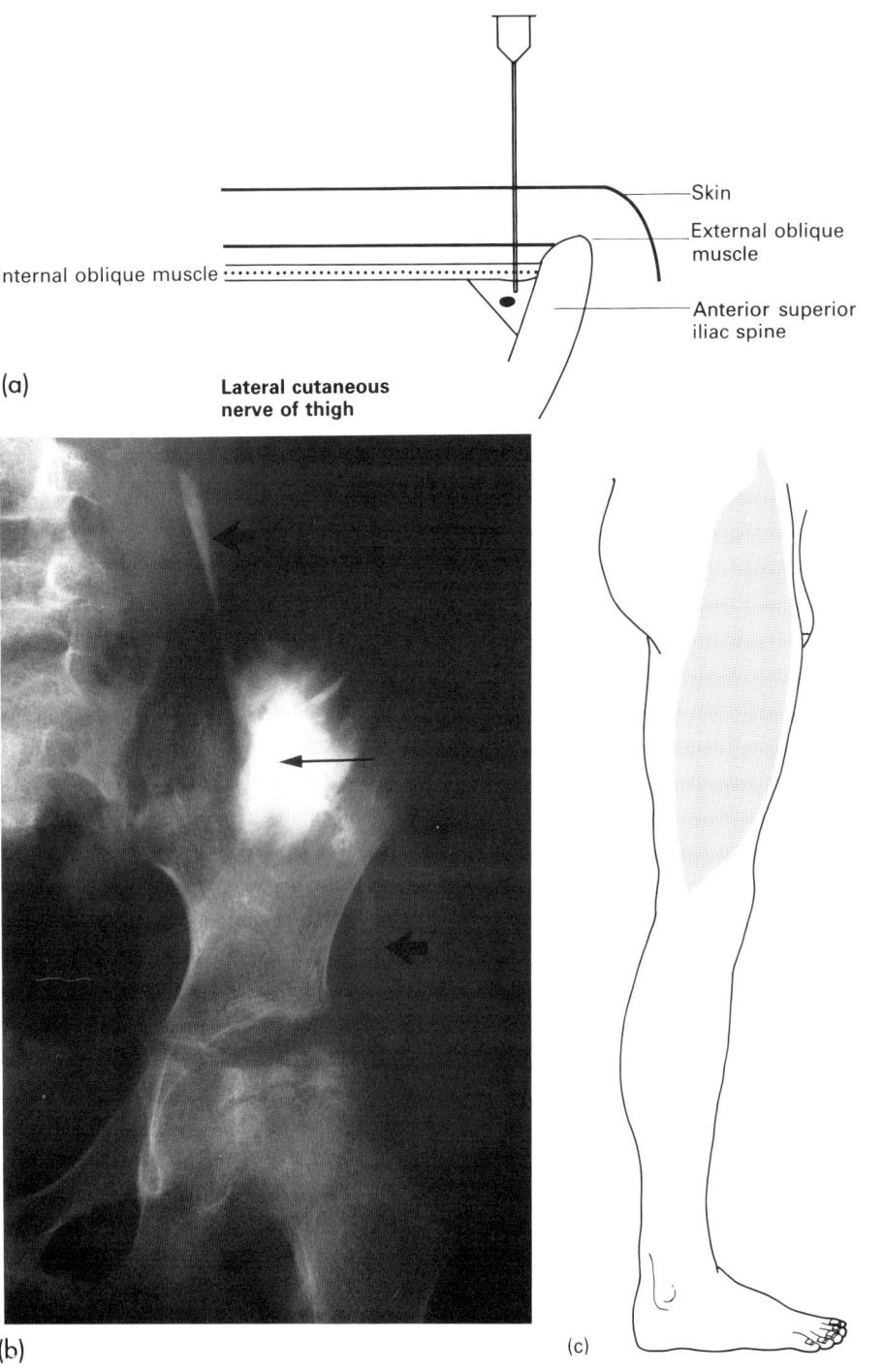

Fig. 22.17 (a) Lateral cutaneous nerve of the thigh in its canal medial to the anterior superior iliac spine and deep to the external oblique aponeurosis and internal oblique muscle. (b) X-ray showing the spread of dye along the course of the lateral cutaneous nerve of the thigh with injection as described in (a). (c) Cutaneous distribution of the lateral cutaneous nerve of the thigh.

POSTERIOR CUTANEOUS NERVE OF THIGH

This branches from the sciatic nerve near the sciatic foramen and diverges medially beneath the gluteus maximus. It breaks up into branches which emerge at the lower (medial) border of the gluteus maximus, some passing down to supply the back of the thigh to the knee, one passing medially to the perineum and some small branches turning up on to the buttock.

The hip is flexed to a right-angle. The block is performed by inserting the needle in the gluteal fold at a point vertically above a point one-quarter of the distance on a line from the ischial tuberosity to the greater trochanter (Fig. 22.18). As a short bevelled needle is advanced, a loss of resistance is felt as the superficial fascia is penetrated. The syringe is attached and the needle is advanced with pressure on the syringe. It is difficult to inject as the needle passes through a thick layer of fibrous fatty tissue. As it emerges on the deep surface, injection suddenly becomes easy and the local anaesthetic fills the potential space inferior to the gluteus maximus where the nerves emerge [21]. As this technique depends on bathing the nerves in a space, an adequate volume of local anaesthetic must be injected — about 4 ml in an infant of 1 year and about an extra 0.5 ml/year up to 12 ml for older children.

SCIATIC NERVE

The sciatic nerve can be blocked at various levels by several approaches.

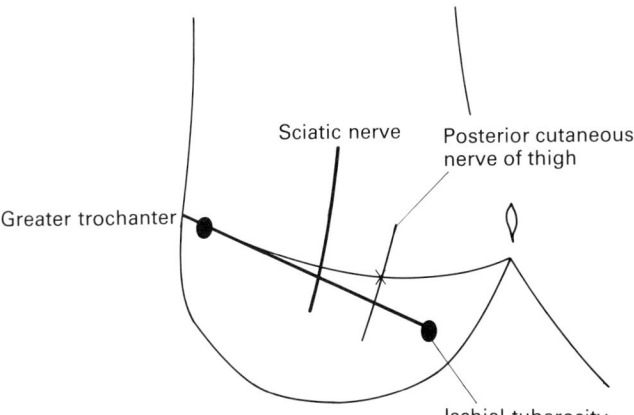

Fig. 22.18 Landmarks for the approach to the posterior cutaneous nerve of the thigh. With the patient either supine with the leg held vertically, or prone, the needle is inserted at point X in the gluteal fold one-quarter of the distance from the ischial tuberosity to the greater trochanter. The sciatic nerve can also be approached here through the mid-point of that line (lithotomy approach).

The posterior approach blocks the nerve as it emerges from the greater sciatic notch deep to the gluteal muscles and piriformis.

The lithotomy approach blocks it near the lower border of the. gluteus maximus. The needle is inserted at the mid-point between the ischial tuberosity and the greater trochanter. It is in a separate compartment from the posterior cutaneous nerve of the thigh at this point (Fig. 22.18).

The anterior approach, which is particularly useful in patients with fractured tibia when turning would cause discomfort, blocks the nerve in the upper thigh as it passes the lesser trochanter. A long needle is inserted at the point illustrated in Fig. 22.19a until it hits the femur. It is then withdrawn and redirected medially so that it just passes the bone at the level of the lesser tronchanter (Fig. 22.19b) (5 cm deeper in an adult — proportionately less in a child). If the syringe is attached it will be difficult to inject as the needle passes through muscle. A loss of resistance is felt as a large, or short bevelled needle penetrates the fascia deep to the adductor magnus. Injection then becomes easy and the local anaesthetic bathes the sciatic nerve which lies immediately posterior (or deep) to the fascia [22].

A fourth technique, blocking the nerve in mid-thigh, is useful for operations on the leg or foot. The sciatic nerve runs from the mid-point of the line between the ischial tuberosity and the greater trochanter, to the apex of the popliteal fossa. A line is drawn from the ischial tuberosity to the head of the fibula (the attachments of biceps femoris). The needle is inserted at the mid-point of that line where the sciatic nerve crosses deep to the muscle (Fig. 22.20). Pressure is applied to the syringe as it is advanced. It is difficult to inject as the needle passes through the muscle. The sciatic nerve lies deep to the muscle at this point, so that when the needle emerges from the muscle injection becomes easy and the nerve is bathed in local anaesthetic.

TIBIAL NERVE

The tibial nerve block was developed to relax the gastrocnemius in patients with extensor spasms following head injury. When the patient is recovering, manipulation of the feet and the application of plasters enable the standing position to be regained. When the patient is standing up, postural reflexes return. The application of plasters in the correct position is facilitated by reducing gastrocnemius tone. Tibial nerve block can be used in

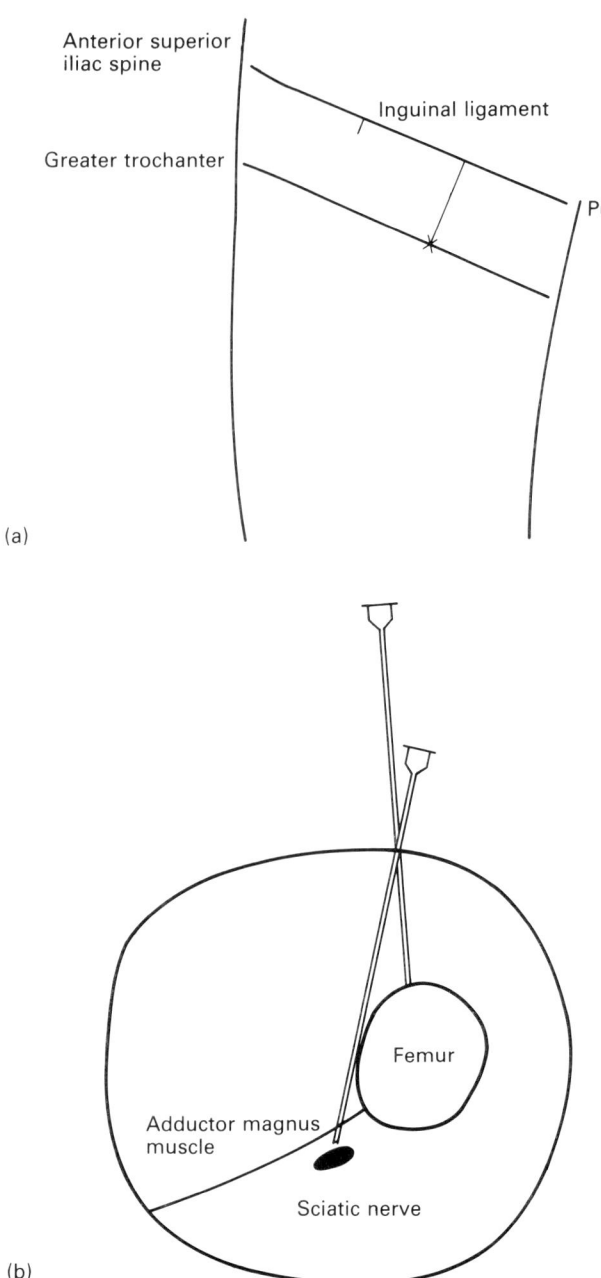

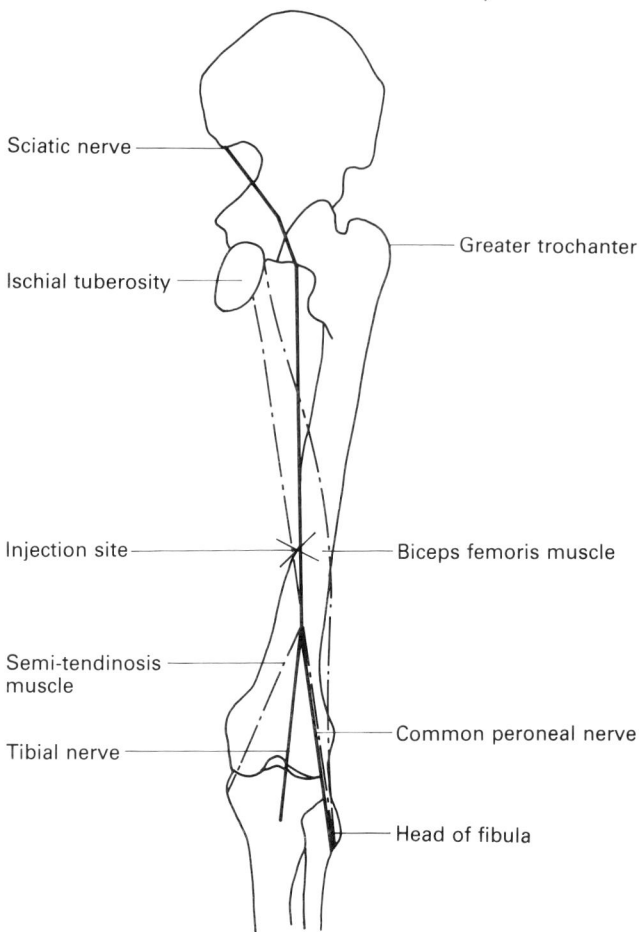

Fig. 22.20 Sciatic nerve — posterior mid-thigh approach (described by I. McKenzie). A line is drawn from the ischial tuberosity to the head of the fibula — attachments of the biceps femoris muscle. The mid-point crosses the sciatic nerve, running from the mid-point between the ischial tuberosity and the greater trochanter above and the apex of the popliteal fossa below, where it divides. The nerve lies immediately below the biceps muscle at this point.

Fig. 22.19 Sciatic nerve block — anterior approach. (a) Surface markings. A line is drawn from the pubis to the anterior superior iliac spine. A perpendicular is dropped from one-third of the distance between these points to a parallel line drawn from the greater trochanter. Where they intersect is the point to insert the needle. (b) Cross-section of the thigh showing how the needle is advanced to the femur, withdrawn and re-inserted past the medial side until it passes through the fascia posterior to the adductor magnus, where a loss of resistance can be felt.

conjunction with common peroneal nerve block (the two terminal branches of the sciatic nerve) for operations on the lower leg and foot as an alternative to sciatic nerve block [23].

The technique is to define the borders of the popliteal fossa with the patient lying prone or semi-prone. The needle is inserted at a point just lateral to the mid-point of a line drawn from the apex of the popliteal fossa to the mid-point of the intercondylar line (Fig. 22.21). It is advanced until the popliteal fascia is penetrated, which will be felt as a loss of resistance if a short bevelled needle is used. The nerve lies in a sheath about 3–6 mm deeper, depending on the size of the patient. It can be

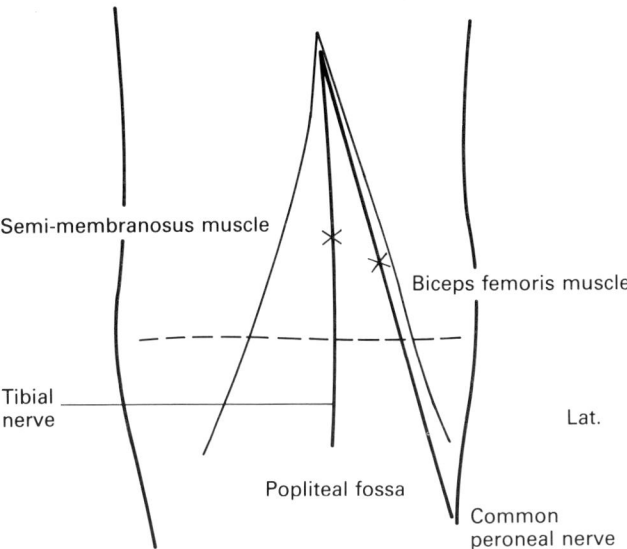

Fig. 22.21 The tibial and common peroneal nerves can be blocked in the popliteal fossa, which is bounded laterally by the biceps femoris and medially by the semimembranosus muscles. The needle is inserted at the points marked X.

accurately located by the use of a nerve stimulator. About 3–5 ml of local anaesthetic can then be injected. At this point the popliteal vessels lie medially and deeper and are therefore unlikely to be punctured.

COMMON PERONEAL NERVE

The common peroneal nerve can be blocked at a similar level to the tibial nerve where it lies immediately adjacent to biceps femoris on the lateral side of the popliteal triangle and at a similar depth below the popliteal fascia.

ANKLE BLOCKS

Nerve blocks around the ankle can be useful for minor operations on the foot, such as removal of ingrowing toenails or plantar warts, and suturing of lacerations. Three of these nerves are blocked by subcutaneous infiltration — the saphenous nerve immediately above and anteromedial to the medial malleolus (Figs 22.22, 22.23), the superficial peroneal nerve between the lateral malleolus and the mid-point between the malleoli (Fig. 22.23), and the sural nerve on the lateral side between the Achilles tendon and the lateral malleolus (Fig. 22.24). Because the nerves are subcutaneous, the needle is usually inserted across the area to be blocked and the local anaesthetic is injected during withdrawal. This ensures that all branches are blocked.

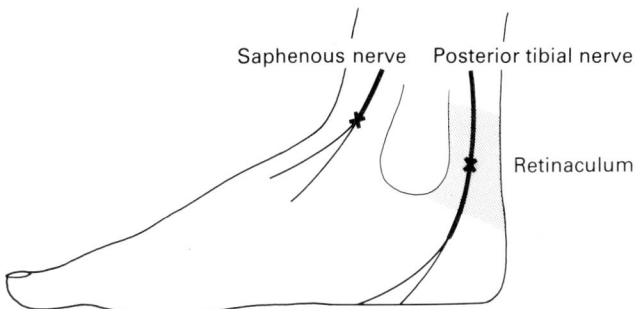

Fig. 22.22 The landmarks for blocking the saphenous and posterior tibial nerves at the ankle. Note that the posterior tibial nerve lies deep to the retinaculum (medial view of the ankle).

The posterior tibial nerve which supplies the anterior part of the sole of the foot lies deep to the retinaculum, between the medial malleolus and the Achilles tendon. It can be blocked by inserting the needle through the retinaculum. When the loss of resistance is felt as the needle penetrates the retinaculum, the local anaesthetic can be injected into the space (Fig. 22.22). It should be noted that the posterior tibial artery is also in this space and aspiration for blood should precede injection.

The deep peroneal nerve lies deep to the extensor retinaculum beside the anterior tibial artery, which can be palpated. The needle is inserted through the retinaculum just lateral to the artery (Fig. 22.23). This nerve

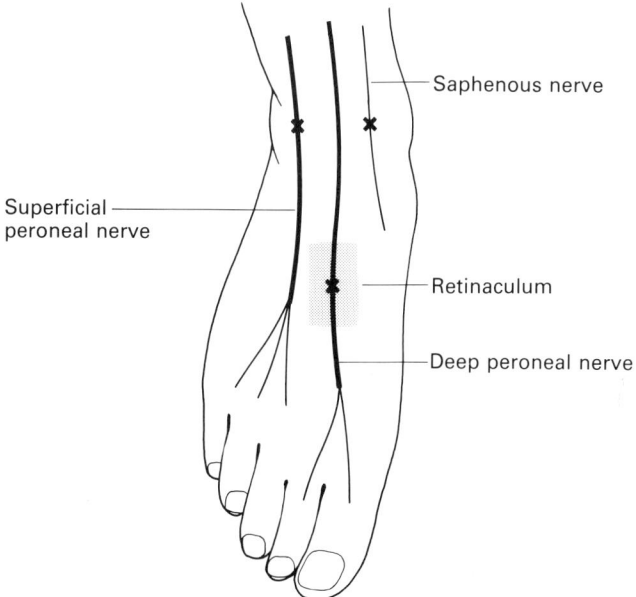

Fig. 22.23 The points for blocking the saphenous, deep and superficial peroneal nerves at the ankle are shown (anterior view).

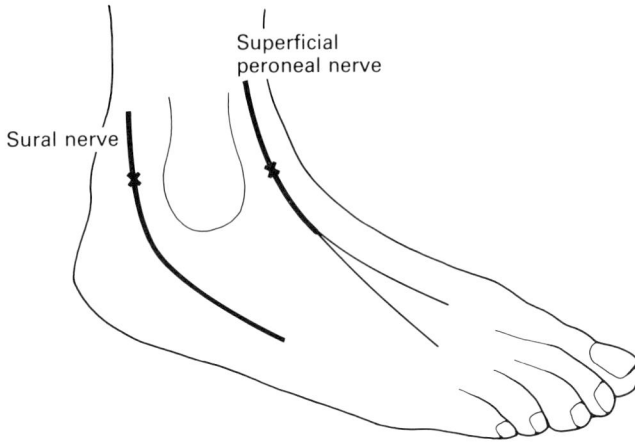

Fig. 22.24 The points for blocking the superficial peroneal and sural nerves at the ankle are shown (lateral view).

supplies the skin on the adjacent sides of the first and second toes.

Head and neck nerve blocks (Fig. 22.25a,b)

These can be used as adjuncts to general anaesthesia or with adequate sedation techniques, even in children. Their use provides postoperative analgesia and reduces the need for opioids, with their attendant disadvantages such as vomiting. The main indication is for plastic surgical procedures.

The sedation techniques usually employ combinations of a benzodiazepine, such as midazolam (30–50 μg/kg initially) with fentanyl (1 μg/kg initially) or alfentanil. The effect of the first doses of midazolam and fentanyl is assessed and further increments are given as necessary. An intravenous infusion of propofol or methohexitone can be added to provide moment-to-moment control over the degree of sedation.

Ketamine (1–2 mg/kg) may be useful to cover painful injections of local anaesthetic, followed by sedation as outlined above.

The methods of local infiltration and nerve blocks are similar to those used in adults, but allowance must be made for differences in the size of facial structures and the fact that bones may be softer in young children. The onset of blockade is more rapid than in adults. 24 SWG 45° bevel needles are recommended to avoid damage to nerve trunks.

Ring block may be used for operations on the scalp as all the nerves run up towards the top of the head.

Infiltration is superficial, except in the temporal region

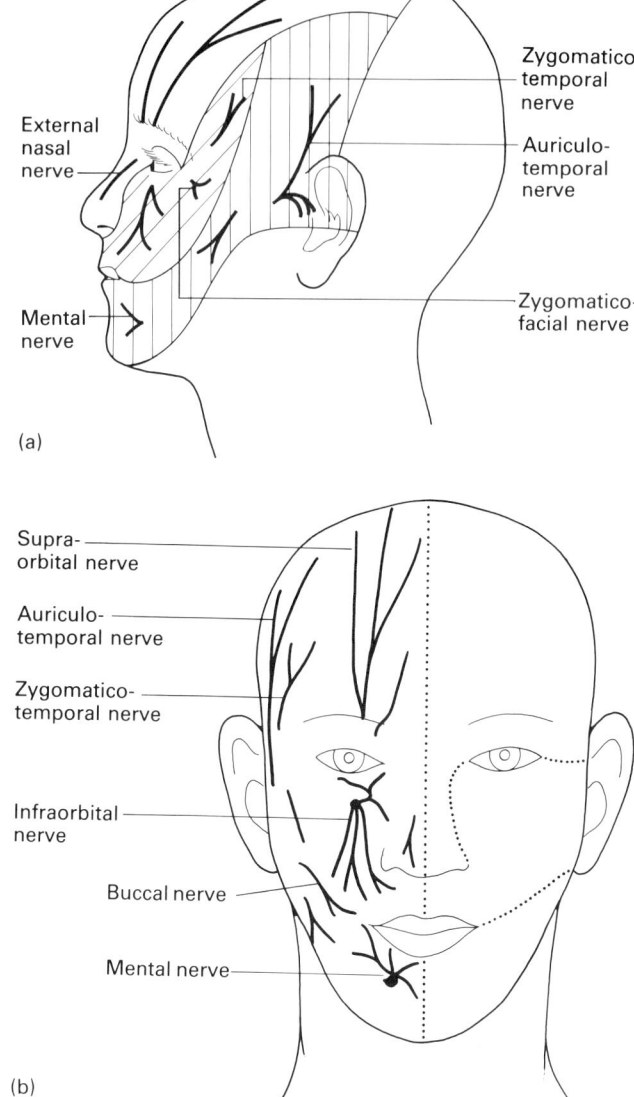

Fig. 22.25 (a) The nerves supplying the face (lateral view), showing the areas supplied by the branches of the ophthalmic (clear), maxillary (diagonal hatched) and mandibular (vertical hatched) divisions of the trigeminal nerve. (b) Frontal view, showing the nerves supplying the face.

where infiltration should also be deep to the deep fascia to reduce movement of the temporalis muscle during surgery.

The sensory nerve supply of the face is derived from the ophthalmic, maxillary and mandibular divisions of the trigeminal nerve (Fig. 22.25). It is common to block the branches of these nerves, and this can be done easily in children.

The forehead, upper eyelid and the upper part of the

nose can be blocked by inserting the needle into the orbit below the supra-orbital notch and directing it upwards away from the eyeball until the upper medial wall of the orbit is felt. Injection of 1–2 ml of local anaesthetic in this area will block the frontal, supratrochlear, infratrochlear and external nasal nerves (Fig. 22.26).

The infra-orbital nerve can be blocked as it emerges from the infra-orbital foramen. This lies below the orbit in a line directly below the supra-orbital notch, or in line with the pupil when looking straight ahead. It is often approached through the mouth behind the upper lip, the needle being passed upwards towards the thumb, which is placed on the skin over the foramen.

The zygomaticotemporal and zygomaticofacial branches of the maxillary division supply the side of the face anterior to the ear. They can be blocked by infiltration along the zygomatic arch.

The lower part of the face over the mandible is supplied by the buccal nerve and the mental nerve more anteriorly. The superficial branches of the buccal nerve will be blocked by infiltration along the lower part of the anterior border of the ramus of the mandible. The mental nerve and foramen lie on the lateral surface of the mandible in a line vertically below the supra-orbital notch and infra-orbital foramen.

The inferior dental (alveolar) nerve, which supplies the lower lip, and the lingual nerves can be blocked on the medial aspect of the ramus of the mandible, approached through the mouth.

The ear can be anaesthetized by blocking the auriculo-temporal nerve by infiltration along the anterior border of the ear (between the bony and cartilaginous parts of the anterior wall of the external auditory meatus). The lower and posterior parts of the ear supplied by the great auricular and lesser occipital nerves (branches of the cervical plexus), which emerge at the middle and upper posterior border of sternomastoid, can be blocked by infiltration over the mastoid process and injecting forwards along the lower border of the ear.

Although the maxillary and mandibular divisions of the trigeminal nerve can be blocked by the usual injections through the mandibular notch, blocks of the peripheral branches are simpler to perform and are effective. Depending on the size of the patient, the volume of solution needed for each of these peripheral blocks may be as little as 0.5 ml and rarely exceeds 2 ml.

The superficial part of the cervical plexus can be blocked by infiltration along the posterior border of the sternomastoid muscle. Some local anaesthetic must be injected under the deep fascia at the mid-point of the muscle to block the supraclavicular and transverse cervical branches.

More detailed descriptions of head and neck blocks should be obtained from special monographs [24] or reference books [25].

Nerve blocks for dental anaesthesia are not commonly performed by anaesthetists and reference should be made to appropriate texts for details [26].

Sympathetic blocks

Sympathetic blocks are occasionally useful in children to relieve vasospasm, and in the treatment of reflex sympathetic dystrophy. The lumbar blocks are usually done where the sympathetic trunk lies in front of the bodies of L2, 3 and 4. The needle is inserted from the lateral border of the paravertebral muscles and angled medially to hit the body of the vertebra. It is withdrawn slightly, and advanced just past the side of the vertebral body until the tip is level with the front of the vertebral body on the lateral view with the image intensifier. In the A-P view the needle tip should be anterior to the vertebral body. If it is in the correct plane, which is a very narrow space, X-ray contrast when injected will form a thin line on the anterior border of the vertebral bodies (lateral

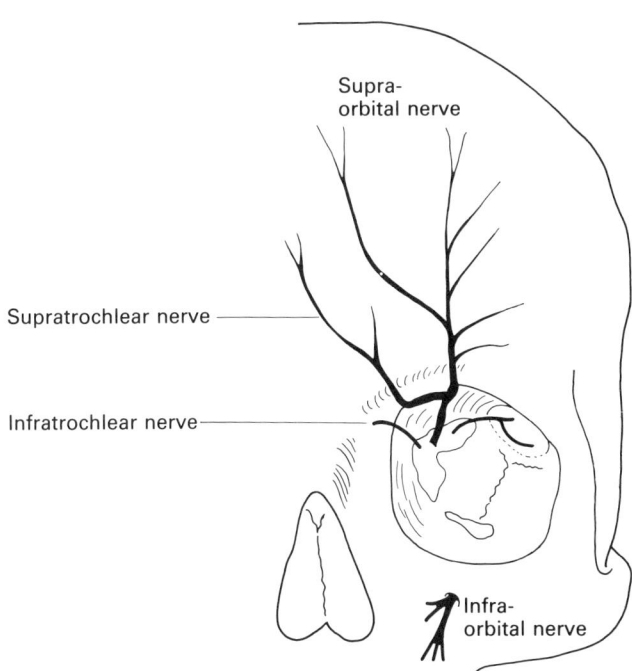

Fig. 22.26 Site of injection in the orbit to block the supra-orbital, supratrochlear and infratrochlear nerves.

view) (Fig. 22.27). The local anaesthetic can then be injected.

Miscellaneous

Other nerve blocks not described here can be used in children. The principles relating to patient size and dose have to be taken into account when they are used.

TOPICAL ANAESTHESIA

Local anaesthesia is sometimes used topically, especially for endoscopy and bronchoscopy. It is usually used as an adjunct to general anaesthesia and only occasionally with heavy sedation in children. Lower concentrations (2% lignocaine) are usually used in infants to avoid overdosage. Four per cent lignocaine is satisfactory for older children. These concentrations provide 20–30 minutes' anaesthesia. Higher concentrations last longer [27], which may be hazardous if the effect continues into the postoperative period. An upper dose limit of 4 mg/kg is recommended (see Chapter 2).

EMLA

Eutectic mixture of local anaesthetics is a mixture of equal amounts of prilocaine and lignocaine, which can produce surface anaesthesia when applied to the skin 1–1.5 hours before it is needed. It is widely used in

paediatric anaesthesia to make venepuncture pain-free, but in practice the needle is sometimes felt penetrating the vein.

INTRAVENOUS REGIONAL ANAESTHESIA

This procedure was originally described in 1908 by August Bier and reintroduced by Holmes of Dunedin, while working in Oxford in 1963 [28]. It can be used for peripheral limb surgery and reduction of simple limb fractures. It has been used successfully in children as young as 3 years [29]. Needles are inserted into a peripheral vein to inject the local anaesthetic and in the opposite hand, in case accidental overdose occurs. The limb is elevated for 30–60 seconds. Arterial occlusion by compression of the brachial artery will also aid exsanguination of the limb. A proximal pneumatic tourniquet which maintains the cuff pressure well above systolic pressure is applied to obliterate arterial blood flow. Prilocaine, chlorprocaine or lignocaine 0.5% (3 mg/kg) is then injected. The first two are safer because of more rapid metabolism, but all three drugs can be used safely. Although the child may become restless with the tourniquet, it should be kept on for 5–7 minutes if possible to obtain maximum effect. Another tourniquet is then applied distal to the first one, which is then removed. The fracture reduction or operation can then proceed. It has been shown that if the tourniquet is kept on for 20

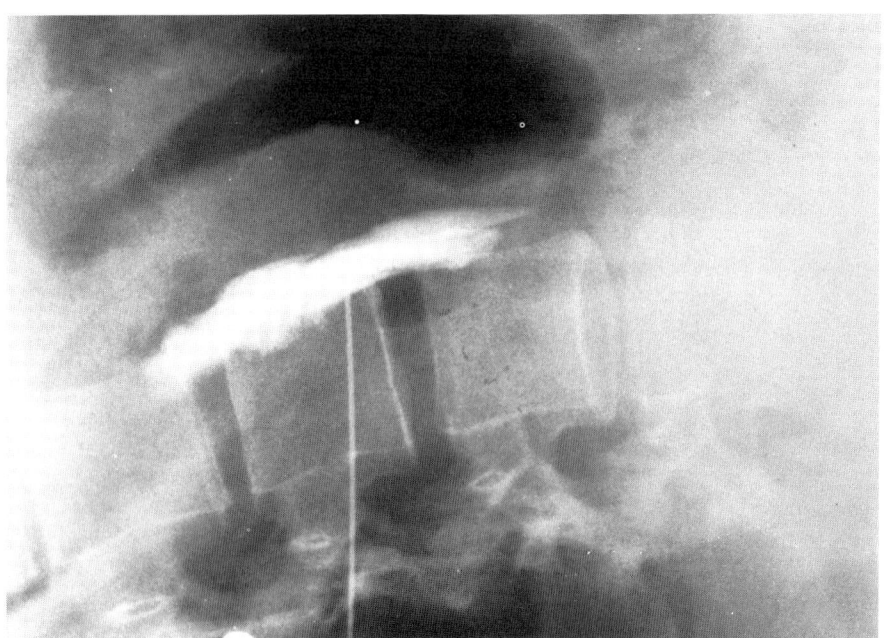

Fig. 22.27 Lateral X-ray showing spread of X-ray contrast and local anaesthetic when the needle is correctly placed, level with the front of the vertebrae for lumbar sympathetic block.

minutes the peak plasma levels of lignocaine rarely exceed 2 µg/kg, and are usually much lower following the use of 0.6 ml/kg of 0.5% lignocaine (3 mg/kg). Peak plasma levels of prilocaine are lower than lignocaine when the same dose is given [30]. Larger volumes have been shown to cause leakage, even when the cuff is adequately inflated [31].

The main hazard is the sudden release of large doses of local anaesthetic into the circulation if the tourniquet becomes incompetent, or is let down too soon after injection.

Bupivacaine must not be used for i.v. regional anaesthesia as a number of deaths have occurred when it has been used with this technique. The cardiovascular toxicity of bupivacaine has been difficult to treat, and there is no advantage in using a long-acting local anaesthetic which will rapidly diffuse away when the cuff is released.

DOSAGE OF LOCAL ANAESTHESIA

Recommended maximum doses

These are summarized in Table 22.1, but it must be recognized that larger doses have been used without apparent toxicity. The dose of bupivacaine and the blood levels associated with bupivacaine toxicity have not been accurately defined [32] (see Chapter 2). When deciding on the concentration and volume required for the proposed block, the total dose should always be calculated to ensure that it is below the maximum recommended dose.

BLOOD LEVELS

There are several studies on peak plasma levels and pharmacokinetics in children (see Table 2.5). In clinical practice, the peak plasma level is important in determining whether or not toxicity will occur. The levels at which various manifestations of toxicity occur have been delineated for lignocaine, e.g. convulsions about 10−12 µg/ml. Convulsions may be suppressed by concurrent general anaesthesia. The toxic levels are less defined for bupivacaine, although experimental data suggest it is four times as toxic as lignocaine. The problem is that convulsions are relatively rare and it is unusual for blood samples to be taken during the convulsion for assay of bupivacaine levels. Even if one is taken, one cannot be certain that it is the peak level or at what level the convulsion was triggered. A level of 7.5 µg/ml has been recorded during a convulsion following 'epidural' bupivacaine 2 mg/kg in a 12-year-old under general anaesthesia. Accidental intravascular injection had obviously occurred. As the convulsions were not suppressed by anaesthesia. It is concluded that 7.5 µg/ml is well above the convulsive level [33].

2 mg/kg is often quoted as the recommended safe dose of bupivacaine but there are studies showing that mean peak plasma levels did not exceed 2 µg/ml when 3 mg/kg were given by axillary [34], intercostal [35], caudal [36, 37] and epidural routes [38]. In the last group the mean just exceeded 2 µg/ml in children over 5 years.

Caudal lignocaine route (4 and 5 mg/kg) [39, 40] and subcutaneous lignocaine (4 mg/kg) produced peak plasma

Table 22.1 Maximum recommended doses of local anaesthetics

| Drug | Topical | | Injection | |
	Concentration	Dose	Plain	With adrenaline
Cocaine	3−10%	3 mg/kg	Not used for injection	
Procaine	Not used clinically		10−14 mg/kg	10−14 mg/kg
Amethocaine	0.5−2%	1 mg/kg	1.5 mg/kg	−
Lignocaine	2−10%	3 mg/kg	5 mg/kg	7 mg/kg
Mepivacaine	Not used clinically		5 mg/kg	5 mg/kg
Bupivacaine*	0.5%		2 mg/kg	2 mg/kg
Etidocaine	1%		4 mg/kg	4 mg/kg
Prilocaine	Not very effective		5 mg/kg	9 mg/kg
	4%	5 mg/kg		
Cinchocaine	0.2−0.5%	1 mg/kg	2 mg/kg (subarachnoid use)	−

* Clinical experience suggests that the maximum safe dose may be higher.

levels up to 2.2 μg/ml, while topical lignocaine 2−4% (4 mg/kg) in the trachea produced mean plasma levels of 5−6 μg/ml with occasional (4%) patients exceeding 10 μg/ml [41]. 3 mg/kg 10% lignocaine spray in the trachea produced maximum venous blood levels of 3.2 μg/ml [42].

It would seem that 4 mg/kg topical spray is safe, but higher doses have been used without apparent complications [43].

Factors which affect plasma levels include:

1 Route of administration — topical lignocaine in the airway reaches higher levels than other routes.

2 Vasoconstrictors slow uptake by reducing the blood flow through the area. The resultant prolongation of action is greatest in the youngest age group (see Chapter 2). The benefit of this is that larger doses of local anaesthetic can be given safely.

3 Neonatal factors — lignocaine has been shown to be 50−60% and bupivacaine 30% less bound to plasma proteins than in adults, making more available for tissue uptake [11, 44]. Hydrolysis of procaine is reduced in infants [45]. The enzymes which degrade amide local anaesthetics are present but less active in the newborn; they increase during the neonatal period [46]. These factors plus the more rapid uptake of local anaesthetics from some sites suggest that the toxic doses may be lower in infants.

Manifestations of toxicity

These are related to the plasma levels and their occurrence will depend on the rate of absorption. Plasma levels will be higher following inadvertent intravenous injection.

Toxic effects of local anaesthetics include central stimulation with anxiety, confusion and excitement, going on to twitching and convulsions. Central depression with loss of consciousness and respiratory and vasomotor depression may follow.

Other effects include direct myocardial depression, and with drugs such as lignocaine which slow conduction, bradycardia may develop.

Some patients may exhibit abnormal sensitivity, idiosyncrasy or allergic reactions to these drugs but these are uncommon.

It has been shown in mice that the toxicity of lignocaine related to the convulsion threshold varies widely with circadian rhythm, which adds further complexity to the study of toxic doses [47].

Management of toxic effects

Convulsions: oxygen should be administered so that neuronal damage does not result from the sudden increase in metabolic activity. It is likely that they will cease as soon as the peak concentration falls, but if not thiopentone or diazepam may be given, realizing that they will add to the central depression caused by high levels of local anaesthetic.

Coma requires support of ventilation and oxygenation.

Cardiac manifestations are associated with the membrane-stabilizing action of local anaesthetics, causing slowed conduction and a negative inotropic effect. A drug such as adrenaline, which has positive inotropic and chronotropic effects, may be necessary to support the circulation.

Ventricular dysrhythmia is less likely to occur in infants and children than hypotension.

CONCLUSION

For the safe practice of regional anaesthesia in children, it is important to keep below the recommended maximum doses, to have a clear idea of the anatomy involved and to take the additional precautions outlined, which relate mainly to smaller size and spaces in children.

The anaesthetist's first consideration in deciding whether to add a regional block technique to the anaesthetic management should always be what is best for the patient.

REFERENCES

1 Gray H.T. A study of spinal anaesthesia in infants and children, from a series of 200 cases. *Lancet* 1909, **II**, 913.

2 Sievers R. Peridural anaesthesia zur cystoscopic beim. *Kind Arch Klin Chir* 1936, **185**, 359.

3 Campbell M.F. Caudal anaesthesia in children. *Am J Urol* 1933, **30**, 245.

4 Farr R.E. Local anaesthesia in infancy and childhood. *Arch Paediat* 1920, **37**, 381.

5 Schulte-Steinberg O., Rahlaphs V.W. Caudal anaesthesia in children and spread of 1% lignocaine: a statistical study. *Br J Anaes* 1970, **42**, 1093.

6 Eyres R.L., Bishop W., Oppenheim R.C., Brown T.C.K. Plasma bupivacaine concentrations in children during caudal epidural analgesia. *Anaes Intens Care* 1983, **11**, 30.

7 Busoni P., Andreucetti T. The spread of caudal anaesthesia in children: a mathematical model. *Anaes Intens Care* 1986, **14**, 140.

8 Wolf A., Valey R., Fear D., Roy W., Lerman J. Bupivacaine for caudal anaesthesia for infants and children: the optimal

effective concentration. *Anesthesiology* 1988, **69**, 102.

9 Bosenberg A.T., Bland B.A.R., Schulte-Steinberg O., Downing J.W. Thoracic epidural anaesthesia via caudal route in infants. *Anesthesiology* 1988, **69**, 265.

10 Dalens B. Regional anaesthesia in children. *Anesth Analg* 1989, **68**, 654.

11 Gouveia M.A. Raquianesthesia para pacientes paediatricos. *Rev Bras Anest* 1970, **4**, 503.

12 Parkinson S.K., Little W.L., Mueller J.B., Pecsok J.L., Malley R.A. Duration of spinal anesthesia using hyperbaric bupivacaine with epinephrine in infants. *Anesthesiology* 1989, **71**, A1020.

13 Gallagher T.M., Crean P.M. Spinal anaesthesia in infants born prematurely. *Anaesthesia* 1989, **44**, 434.

14 Mahe V., Ecoffey C. Spinal anaesthesia with isobaric bupivacaine in infants. *Anesthesiology* 1989, **68**, 601.

15 Welborn L.G., Rice L.J., Broadman L.M., Hannallah R.S., Fink R. Postoperative apnea in former preterm infants: prospective comparison of spinal and general anesthesia. *Anesthesiology* 1989, **71**, A1025.

16 Eriksson E. *Illustrated handbook in local anaesthesia*. Astra, (1969) p. 78.

17 Bricker S., Telford R., Booker P. Pharmacokinetics of bupivacaine following intraoperative intercostal nerve block in neonates and in infants aged less than 6 months. *Anesthesiology* 1989, **70**, 942.

18 Bacon A. An alternative block for post-circumcision analgesia. *Anaes Intens Care* 1977, **5**, 63.

19 Khoo S.T., Brown T.C.K. Femoral nerve block — the anatomical basis for a single-injection technique. *Anaes Intens Care* 1983, **11**, 40.

20 Brown T.C.K., Dickens D.R.V. Another approach to the lateral cutaneous nerve to thigh. *Anaes Intens Care* 1986, **14**, 126.

21 Hughes P.J., Brown T.C.K. Posterior cutaneous nerve of thigh block. *Anaes Intens Care* 1986, **14**, 350.

22 McNicol L.R. Sciatic nerve block by the anterior approach for postoperative pain relief in paediatric practice. *Anaesthesia* 1985, **40**, 410.

23 Kempthorne P.M., Brown T.C.K. Nerve blocks around the knee in children. *Anaes Intens Care* 1984, **12**, 14.

24 McIntosh R.R., Ostlere M. *Local analgesia: head and neck*. E & S Livingstone, Edinburgh, (1955).

25 Murphy T.E. Somatic blockade of head and neck. In: Cousins M.J., Bridenbaugh P.O. (Eds) *Neural blockade*, 2nd edn. Lippincott, (1988) pp. 533–558.

26 Bennett C.R. Neural blockade of oral and circumoral structures: intra-oral approaches. In: Cousins M.J., Bridenbaugh, P.O. (Eds) *Neural blockade*, 2nd edn. Lippincott, (1988) pp. 561–576.

27 Robinson E.P., Rex M.A.E., Brown T.C.K. A comparison of different concentrations of lignocaine hydrochloride used for topical anaesthesia of the larynx in the cat. *Anaes Intens Care* 1984, **73**, 137.

28 Holmes C.Mc.K. Intravenous regional anaesthesia. *Lancet* 1963, **1**, 245.

29 Turner P.L., Batten J.B., Hjorth D., Ross E.R.S., Eyres R.L., Cole W.G. Intravenous regional anaesthesia for the treatment of upper limb injuries in childhood. *ANZ J Surg* 1986, **56**, 153.

30 Eriksson E. The effects of intravenous local anaesthetic agents on the central nervous system. *Acta Anaes Scand* 1969, **36** (Supp), 79.

31 Rosenberg P.H., Kalso E.A., Tuominen K.K., Linden H.B. Acute bupivacaine toxicity as a result of venous leakage under the tourniquet during a Bier block. *Anesthesiology* 1983, **58**, 95.

32 Takasaki M. Blood concentrations of lidocaine, mepivacaine and bupivacaine during caudal anaesthesia in children. *Acta Anaes Scand* 1984, **28**, 211.

33 Eyres R.L., Brown T.C.K., Hastings C. Plasma level of bupivacaine during convulsions. *Anaes Intens Care* 1983, **11**, 385.

34 Campbell R.J., Ilett K.F., Dusci L. Plasma bupivacaine concentrations after axillary block in children. *Anaes Intens Care* 1986, **14**, 343.

35 Rothstein P., Arthur G.R., Feldman H.S., Kopf G.S., Covino B.G. Bupivacaine for intercostal nerve blocks in children: blood concentrations and pharmacokinetics. *Anesth Analg* 1986, **65**, 625.

36 Eyres R.L., Bishop W., Oppenheim R.C., Brown T.C.K. Plasma bupivacaine concentrations in children during caudal epidural anaesthesia. *Anaes Intens Care* 1983, **11**, 20.

37 Ecoffey C., Desparmets J., Maurey M., Bordeaux A., Guidicelli J.F. Bupivacaine in children: pharmacokinetics following caudal anaesthesia. *Anesthesiology* 1985, **63**, 447.

38 Eyres R.L., Hastings C., Brown T.C.K., Oppenheim R.C. Plasma bupivacaine concentrations following lumbar epidural anaesthesia in children. *Anaes Intens Care* 1986, **14**, 131.

39 Eyres R.L., Kidd J., Oppenheim R.C., Brown T.C.K. Local anaesthetic plasma levels in children. *Anaes Intens Care* 1978, **6**, 243.

40 Ecoffey C., Desparmets J., Bordeaux A., Maurey M., Guidicelli J.F., St Maurice C. Pharmacokinetics of lignocaine in children following caudal anaesthesia. *Br J Anaes* 1984, **56**, 1399.

41 Eyres R.L., Bishop W., Oppenheim R.C., Brown T.C.K. Plasma lignocaine concentrations following topical laryngeal application. *Anaes Intens Care* 1985, **11**, 23.

42 Pelton D.A., Daly M., Cooper P.D., Conn A.W. Plasma lidocaine concentrations following topical aerosol application to the trachea and bronchi. *Canad Anaes Soc J* 1970, **15**, 628.

43 Martelete M., Ferriera F.C., Bau M.I., Bainy R.J., Santos J.C. *Rev Braz Anest* 1970, **20**, 512.

44 Eather K.F. Regional anaesthesia for infants and children. *Int Anaesthesiol Clin* 1975, **13**, 19.

45 Zsigmond E.K., Downs J.R. Plasma cholinesterase activity in newborns and infants. *Canad Anaes Soc J* 1971, **18**, 278.

46 Gianelly R., Van der Groeben J.O., Spivack A.P., Harrison D.C. Effect of lidocaine on ventricular arrhythmias in patients with coronary heart disease. *New Engl J Med* 1967, **277**, 1215.

47 Lutsch E.F., Morris R.W. Circadian periodicity in susceptibility to lidocaine hydrochloride. *Science* 1967, **156**, 100.

23: Induced Hypotension

PHYSIOLOGICAL PRINCIPLES

The aim, when inducing hypotension during surgery, is to reduce bleeding, so that the need for blood transfusion is avoided or reduced, allowing the surgeon a clearer view of the operating field. This results from reduced blood flow through the area being dissected, or from decreased filling of the veins due to vasodilatation and pooling of blood elsewhere in the body. It is important when blood pressure is lowered that tissue perfusion, particularly to vital organs such as the brain and the heart, is not impaired. As blood pressure depends on cardiac output and peripheral resistance, pressure may be reduced by decreasing either or both of these.

Vasodilatation increases the capacitance of the circulation so that blood volume is relatively decreased. This reduces venous return and central venous pressure, which can easily be further reduced by raising the mean intra-thoracic pressure with intermittent positive pressure ventilation (IPPV). Healthy infants and children are much less likely than adults to have catastrophic falls in blood pressure if large doses of vasodilators are used. If blood pressure does drop more than desired, the administration of intravenous fluids increases blood volume and also reduces viscosity, which aids tissue perfusion. When vasodilators are used, it is usually desirable to give extra sodium-containing intravenous fluids, so that they remain in the circulation and help to prevent the difference in capacitance of the vessels and the blood volume becoming such that venous return is inadequate.

Compensatory tachycardia mediated by a baroreceptor reflex may occur. If, despite the administration of fluids, tachycardia develops and bleeding increases, beta-adrenergic blockade may be used to depress the response. Drugs which increase heart rate, such as atropine, should be avoided. Hypercarbia stimulates catecholamine secretion and causes tachycardia. If the vasodilating drug does not dilate the cerebral vessels directly, a low Pa_{CO_2} will cause vasoconstriction, which may be dangerous if cerebral perfusion pressure is low. It is desirable to keep the Pa_{CO_2} above 30 mmHg.

Blood pressure may be reduced by decreasing myocardial contractility. Beta-adrenergic blocking drugs have this effect due to their negative inotropic action. Inhalation agents, such as halothane, and to a lesser extent isoflurane, which do not stimulate catecholamine release, also do this as the concentration is raised. Isoflurane has a potent hypotensive action, by peripheral vascular dilatation.

The blood pressure at any site in the body depends on posture and the pressure difference between that site and the heart. If, for example, the point is about 13 cm above the heart the pressure will be 10 mmHg (1.3 kPa) lower. When the patient is vasodilated the effect is relatively greater, because 10 mmHg (1.3 kPa) will be a greater proportion of left-ventricular systolic pressure and more pooling of blood will occur in dependent areas. Reflex vasoconstriction, which normally maintains arterial pressure, may be impaired by anaesthesia and prevented by the vasodilating drug. The two conclusions are that posture is a useful adjunct to the use of drugs to reduce blood pressure at the operative site if it can be elevated and, if head-up tilt is employed, the perfusion pressure of the brain must be considered. If intra-arterial monitoring is being used, the transducer should be set at head level so that cerebral arterial pressure is measured. Although cerebral blood flow is well maintained and may be increased during nitroprusside hypotension, mean cerebral arterial pressures below 50 mmHg (6.6 kPa) should be avoided. When the operation is prolonged and head-up tilt is used, the degree of elevation should be limited and the head can be lowered periodically as an extra precaution.

INDICATIONS FOR INDUCED HYPOTENSION

Reduction in blood loss

Hypotension reduces blood loss and hence the need for blood transfusion. This is particularly important when transmission of infections such as human immunodeficiency syndrome (AIDS) or hepatitis virus is of concern. It is also useful in the management of patients who refuse blood transfusion or children whose parents wish transfusion to be avoided, such as Jehovah's Witnesses.

A significant reduction in blood loss has been achieved with hypotensive anaesthesia in major surgery such as the correction of scoliosis.

Control of acute haemorrhage

Bleeding occurs from a site that the surgeon cannot pinpoint because the flow of blood obliterates his view, and can lead to massive haemorrhage and transfusion, endangering the patient's life and causing extreme stress to the surgeon and anaesthetist. The short-term use of hypotension may solve the problem. The surgeon should control the bleeding with pressure, the blood volume should be restored adequately and extra fluid given, and then sodium nitroprusside can be infused slowly until the blood pressure falls sufficiently to allow the pack compressing the bleeding area to be removed. The bleeding points can then easily be controlled and the blood pressure can be allowed to return to normal.

It is desirable to have experience with sodium nitro-prusside before using it in this situation and it is essential that blood volume is adequately restored before it is used.

It is not essential to have direct arterial pressure measurement for this very short period provided one monitors pulse pressure and blood pressure carefully with a cuff, and infuses the sodium nitroprusside (50 mg in 500 ml solution) very slowly.

Operating field

Reduced bleeding in the operating field, especially during microsurgery, provides the surgeon with a clear operating field, lessens the chance of damage to important structures, and usually shortens the duration of surgery.

Management of hypertension

When the blood pressure rises acutely to high levels, as sometimes happens when the aorta is cross-clamped prior to resection of a coarctation of the aorta, it is advisable to lower it with a vasodilator.

Phaeochromocytoma

In patients with phaeochromocytoma, it is important to be able to control blood pressure and increase the capacitance before and during angiography and operations for removal of the tumour. Preoperative alpha-blockade with phenoxybenzamine and intravenous fluids, for some days before operation, will overcome the vasoconstriction caused by high levels of circulating catecholamines and increase the blood volume to normal. If this is achieved, hypotension is unlikely to follow the removal of the tumour and the postoperative problems will be reduced. If the blood pressure still rises when the tumour is manipulated during surgery, it can be controlled promptly with sodium nitroprusside. Lowering the blood pressure with the latter will also abolish dysrhythmia during removal of phaeochromocytoma.

Beta-blockade may also be useful for additional control of hypertension or tachycardia.

Other surgical uses

Vasodilators can be used in other situations to reduce the hazards of surgery. For instance, during extensive dissection of tumours around tense, partially obstructed major blood vessels, a temporary reduction in pressure will make these less likely to tear during dissection.

Reduction of afterload

Vasodilatation is beneficial when peripheral vaso-constriction leads to excessive afterload, left-ventricular strain and eventually heart failure. Such situations may follow open heart surgery, and can be prevented or treated by reduction in afterload with a vasodilator — phenoxybenzamine is useful for this purpose because of its long action. Another advantage of reducing peripheral resistance is that myocardial work and oxygen requirement is reduced.

Vasodilatation, preferably with phenoxybenzamine which does not dilate the cerebral vessels, may be beneficial in selected cases of neurogenic pulmonary oedema. In this condition, acute hypertension is followed by left-ventricular failure, a fall in blood pressure and pulmonary oedema. If the head injury is not accompanied by severe cerebral oedema, then phenoxybenzamine may be used to reduce afterload and increase capacitance, allowing fluid redistribution away from the lungs. If cerebral oedema is present, lowering the arterial blood pressure may result in inadequate cerebral perfusion. If raised intracranial pressure is due to increased intracranial blood volume rather than oedema (CT scan can be used to differentiate these), vasodilatation may reduce intra-cranial pressure by redistribution of blood away from the head.

METHODS AND DRUGS USED

Vasodilators

SODIUM NITROPRUSSIDE

Sodium nitroprusside is a vascular smooth-muscle relaxant which causes vasodilatation, particularly of resistance vessels, and a fall in blood pressure. This action is due to a nitroso ($-NO$) group in the molecule. It interferes with sulphydryl groups or blocks intracellular calcium activation. It may also increase cyclic GMP. It has a rapid onset, a fairly consistent effect and a short half-life. The effect of a single dose lasts only a few minutes and its action is only slightly longer with a larger dose. In infants, the systolic blood pressure rarely falls below 50 mmHg (6.6 kPa), whereas in adults similar doses can have a much greater hypotensive effect. This feature plus the lack of atherosclerosis in children makes hypotensive anaesthesia relatively safer in than in adults.

Sodium nitroprusside is usually given by infusion, in concentrations varying from 0.01 to 0.1 mg/ml. It is often diluted to 50 mg in 500 ml, but in paediatric anaesthesia the addition of 1 mg/kg body weight to 100 ml in a burette ensures that a safe dose is not exceeded with 100 ml, and allows a direct reading of the dose/kg which has been used. Its administration can be controlled by a simple flow control device or by an infusion pump, which can be controlled by a microprocessor computer with arterial pressure feedback if such facilities are available.

Nitroprusside is rapidly metabolized to cyanide, hence its short duration of action. Most of this cyanide is taken up in red blood cells leaving a small amount of free active cyanide which is converted to thiocyanate by an enzyme, rhodanase, in the liver and kidneys. Thiosulphate is needed for this action. The thiocyanate is then slowly excreted via the kidneys. Excess thiocyanate can cause hypothyroidism, so infusions of nitroprusside lasting days should be avoided.

The occasional patient requires an increased dose of sodium nitroprusside to achieve the desired hypotensive response. If the dose requirement increases and is approaching 10 µg/kg/min, sodium nitroprusside should be discontinued, and other means of lowering blood pressure should be introduced. If the sodium nitroprusside is not stopped, these patients may develop severe metabolic acidosis due to poisoning of the cytochrome oxidase system by cyanide. A few patients have died as a result. These had all received more than 4 mg/kg within a 4–6-hour period. Toxicity and severe metabolic acidosis is unlikely if the dose is kept below 3 mg/kg over a 5-hour period or 10 µg/kg/min.

The treatment of cyanide toxicity involves:

1 Treatment of the metabolic acidosis.

2 Intravenous infusion of sodium thiosulphate (150 mg/kg in 50 ml water over 15 minutes). This combines with cyanide to form thiocyanate.

3 Hydroxycobalamine (Neo-Cytamen) 0.1 mg/kg (which acts as vitamin B_{12}). The hydroxy group is replaced by cyanide and it is converted to cyanocobalamine, which is commonly known as vitamin B_{12}. It is preferred for patients with renal impairment because thiocyanate excretion may be reduced.

4 An intravenous infusion of sodium nitrate (5 mg/kg) in 20 ml of water given over 3–4 minutes. This produces methaemoglobin, which has a much higher affinity for cyanide than does cytochrome oxidase.

The contraindications to the use of sodium nitroprusside are renal and liver failure, malnutrition, vitamin B_{12} deficiency unless hydroxycobalamine is given concurrently, and Leber's optic atrophy. Previous resistance to the hypotensive effect of sodium nitroprusside suggests that another agent should be used.

Sodium nitroprusside is relatively unstable in solution in light. The powder is therefore dissolved just prior to use. Stability is improved by covering the infusion bottle and line with foil when longer-term infusions are used, but during surgery this does not seem to be a practical necessity.

The main advantage of this drug for inducing hypotension or vasodilatation is its rapid transient action which makes it easy to control. If the blood pressure falls too low, it will recover within 2–5 minutes if the infusion is stopped or the rate is reduced. Cerebral blood flow is well maintained with sodium nitroprusside, but in neurosurgery the vasodilatation of cerebral vessels resulting from its direct action on vascular smooth muscle produces rather congested vessels and less ideal operating conditions than an alpha-adrenergic blocking drug.

Sodium nitroprusside is useful in determining whether vasodilatation is beneficial, before using a long-acting vasodilator such as phenoxybenzamine.

Rebound systemic or pulmonary hypertension can occur after abrupt cessation of its use.

NITROGLYCERINE

Nitroglycerine or glyceryl trinitrate (GTN) is a direct smooth-muscle relaxant which has a predominant effect on venous capacitance vessels, resulting in decreased preload. Its effect on arterioles and afterload is less than sodium nitroprusside. It is short-acting even though its dinitro metabolites have some vasodilator activity. It is infused in concentrations two to three times those used for sodium nitroprusside, and the infusion rate is titrated to produce the required effect (about $5\,\mu g/kg/min$). It dilates cerebral blood vessels, which can be a disadvantage in neurosurgery. It is a better drug than sodium nitroprusside in the treatment of myocardial ischaemia. In babies with pulmonary hypertension, nitroglycerine is the most effective pulmonary vasodilator currently available. A major advantage is the absence of toxic metabolites, so that dosage can be increased until the desired effect is produced. Significant amounts are absorbed into the PVC plastic in the infusion set, so that the dose given is not really known unless special tubing is used.

TRIMETAPHAN

A rapid, short-acting ganglion blocking agent which is best administered as an infusion (1 mg/ml), the rate being adjusted to maintain the desired blood pressure. It causes histamine release, which may contribute to its hypotensive action and can cause bronchospasm. It is preferred by some anaesthetists for neurosurgery because of its sympathetic blocking rather than direct smooth-muscle relaxing effects.

PHENOXYBENZAMINE

Phenoxybenzamine is an alpha-blocker with a long action (24 hours +) due to covalent bonding. It is used as a vasodilator in paediatric cardiac surgery to reduce vascular resistance and afterload (see Chapter 13) and it can be used for hypotension during anaesthesia.

In phaeochromocytoma it is often used orally to gradually expand the vascular volume, but it can be given intravenously (1 mg/kg) with the concurrent administration of blood or plasma volume expanders.

Phenoxybenzamine can be used in lower doses (0.3–0.5 mg/kg) to provide background vasodilation for long operations. This has advantages in the surgical management of intracranial arteriovenous malformations and aneurysms, where 0.3–0.5 mg/kg will reduce the blood pressure by 20–25%. It causes peripheral vasodilatation, which does not affect the cerebral vessels because they lack a sympathetic nerve supply and hence do not dilate unless hypercarbia develops. The other advantage is that the blood pressure recovers slowly and rebound hypertension is avoided. If the pressure needs to be lowered further during the critical phases of the operation, this can easily be achieved with very small doses of sodium nitroprusside or the use of isoflurane.

PHENTOLAMINE (REGITINE) AND TOLAZOLINE

These drugs have alpha-adrenergic blocking effects and a direct action on vascular smooth muscle, leading to vasodilatation. They are short-acting and are not often used for hypotensive anaesthesia. Phentolamine has been used to determine whether sympathetic block might be useful in patients with suspected reflex sympathetic dystrophy, and tolazoline has been advocated for treating pulmonary hypertension.

HYDRALLAZINE

Hydrallazine is an arteriolar dilator with a slower onset and longer duration of action than sodium nitroprusside. An initial bolus is usually needed to initiate the hypotensive effect. One should then wait 10–15 minutes to assess the response, as the dose varies between individuals. Further doses can be given according to response, or an infusion can be used. The offset of effect may be slow. It is partially metabolized by acetylation, and in up to 50% of the population this reaction may be slow, leading to a prolonged action. Reflex tachycardia may occur.

LABETALOL

This is a relatively new drug which combines alpha-$_1$ and beta-blockade; it will lower blood pressure with less compensatory tachycardia than occurs with alpha-blockade alone. Its hypotensive action is less than some of the other drugs and thus the desired level of blood pressure may be more difficult to attain. It has been used in the management of phaeochromocytoma.

Inhalation anaesthetic agents

Isoflurane is being used increasingly to lower blood pressure, because its predominant cardiovascular effect is on systemic vascular resistance rather than on cardiac output. Its hypotensive effect increases as the inspired, and hence the alveolar and plasma, concentrations increase. Reflex tachycardia may occur.

Halothane, which dilates certain peripheral vascular beds, causes hypotension more through myocardial depression. It can be used as an adjunct to the use of other vasodilators, but deep halothane anaesthesia is not used much to produce hypotension. It tends to cause bradycardia, particularly in children, rather than tachycardia, in deeper levels of anaesthesia.

Epidural and spinal anaesthesia

Epidural and spinal blocks affect sympathetic outflow and in adults cause some hypotension, depending on the level of block. In children the influence on blood pressure is much less marked, especially below 8–10 years of age. The clinical impression is that bleeding is less, even in younger patients, probably as a result of the more effective afferent blockade.

Posture

Posture, by elevating the operative site relative to the rest of the body, can be a useful adjunct to hypotensive anaesthesia, especially for operations on the head, which can be easily elevated.

MONITORING

It is important to observe the clinical signs of pulse, colour and skin perfusion as well as more complex methods of monitoring. The pulse becomes softer and less easily palpable. Skin perfusion is usually improved. A delay in capillary refill indicates excessive hypotension and, usually, an inadequate circulating blood volume. The amount of bleeding from the wound can also be a useful guide to the efficacy of the hypotension.

Although intra-arterial pressure monitoring is desirable during hypotensive anaesthesia, and has the advantage of continuous readout, it is possible to monitor satisfactorily with non-invasive blood pressure measurement and careful observation of pulse pressure, especially in children. The blood pressure does not tend to fall as dramatically as it can in older patients. When intra-arterial pressure is monitored during intracranial or head and neck surgery, the transducer should be set at brain level so that cerebral arterial pressure is measured.

Pulse oximetry is important in assessing tissue oxygenation and peripheral perfusion.

The measurement of central venous pressure is helpful in assessing fluid requirements, particularly when the blood pressure is being allowed to return to normal.

Temperature should be monitored, because peripheral vasodilatation will increase heat loss unless steps are taken to prevent it.

ECG and EEG may be useful in detecting myocardial and cerebral ischaemia, but these are less likely in children than in older patients.

An adequate urine output is a good indicator of adequate renal perfusion.

Monitoring during hypotensive anaesthesia must be continuous and thorough if accidents due to excessive hypotension and inadequate cerebral perfusion are to be avoided.

COMPLICATIONS

The main hazard of hypotensive anaesthesia is uncontrolled hypotension, leading to an inadequate cardiac output. The early administration of intravenous fluids, to maintain an adequate blood volume and care in assessing the patient's response to the hypotensive drug, will reduce this complication. The second serious problem results from inadequate cerebral perfusion pressure, leading to neurological complications which may include permanent brain damage or even death. It is very important to measure or estimate the blood pressure at brain level rather than heart level when the head is elevated.

Rebound hypertension can occur, although it is uncommon, after induced hypotension. It is more likely to follow the use of short-acting drugs than the longer-acting agents where the blood pressure returns to normal slowly.

During induced hypotension, very low levels of blood pressure are less common in children than adults, and it is unusual for the systolic arterial pressure to drop below 50 mmHg (6.6 kPa) in a small child, even with substantial doses of vasodilators. This, and the absence of atherosclerosis, reduces the risk of induced hypotension in children. When hypothermia is used as well, the risk of problems associated with low blood pressure is reduced. Vigilance and good monitoring are of paramount importance. Tragedies can still follow the use of induced hypotension, and the anaesthetist must be satisfied that its use offers a justifiable benefit to the child.

24: Induced Hypothermia

RATIONALE

Induced hypothermia is used to reduce metabolic rate and hence oxygen consumption, thereby increasing the duration of hypoxia that tissues will tolerate without developing irreversible damage.

USES

Cardiac surgery

Deep hypothermia (below 20°C) is used for the surgical correction of congenital heart defects in infants. It allows long periods of cardiac standstill while the operation is performed [1].

Hypothermia during cardiopulmonary bypass is achieved with a heat exchanger in the bypass circuit. This allows the interruption of bypass for short periods if problems with perfusion occur during the operation, or periods of low-flow perfusion to reduce intracardiac bleeding. It limits myocardial ischaemic damage during periods of aortic cross-clamping.

Neurosurgery

Hypothermia (surface cooling) is now less commonly used in neurosurgery but is still occasionally employed for operations on intracranial aneurysms, arteriovenous malformations or vascular tumours such as choroid plexus papilloma, especially when access is difficult or major bleeding is possible. It protects the brain if periods of reduced tissue perfusion occur, and allows temporary occlusion of the vessels. Hypothermia also causes some reduction in intracranial pressure.

Hepatic surgery

Moderate hypothermia (30–34°C) is used during the resection of liver tumours. Liver metabolism, and therefore oxygen consumption, are reduced while clamps are applied, the liver is divided and the tumour is removed. More importantly, it provides cerebral protection in the event of reduced cardiac output during haemorrhage, or while the inferior vena cava is occluded to control bleeding (see Chapter 11) [2].

It may also have a place in the management of the ruptured liver (see Chapter 11).

Intensive care

Hypothermia to reduce brain damage following head injuries or cardiac arrest is now rarely employed.

SUMMARY OF PHYSIOLOGICAL CHANGES

Metabolic rate and oxygen consumption are reduced by hypothermia, and hence longer periods of ischaemia are tolerated. Hypothermia also reduces damage to tissues when perfusion is recommenced [3]. The early recommendations for periods of safe circulatory arrest were

330

from 8 minutes at 30°C to 60 minutes at 15°C [4], although the apparent safety of 60 minutes' arrest at 20°C has been repeatedly confirmed [5]. These figures refer to obvious organic changes. Studies on piglets showed histological evidence of neuronal damage after 1 hour's arrest at 20°C [6]. More recent studies using psychological testing suggest the safe period to be less than 60 minutes [7]. These differences may be due to subtle variations in oxygen supply to the brain before circulatory arrest (see below).

When temperature falls cardiac output declines as a result of decreasing heart rate, whereas stroke volume and contractility are maintained along with blood pressure down to approximately 27°C; at lower temperatures all of these fall. At any point below 30°C, usually below 26°C, ventricular fibrillation may occur [8]. This depends on the state of the myocardium. In babies the heart may not arrest in asystole until the temperature is below 20°C.

Blood pressure is sustained partly by the maintenance of vascular tone and partly by an increase in the viscosity of the blood. The latter is due to the physical tendency of fluids to become more viscous with cooling, and partly due to an apparent decrease in plasma volume and an increase in haematocrit. There is a decrease in platelets and leucocytes, apparently due to sequestration, which becomes marked below 30°C.

In unanaesthetized individuals, ventilation decreases as oxygen requirements and CO_2 production fall. Ventilation is reduced during induced hypothermia by drugs (central nervous system depressants, muscle relaxants, etc). Recent debate on the management of hypothermia has evolved around what the optimum ventilation and CO_2 levels should be. Formerly, a corrected pH was maintained at 7.4 by the addition of CO_2, which compensated for the changes in $Paco_2$ resulting from the increased solubility of gases (including CO_2) as temperature decreased. This is now referred to as the 'pH stat' concept of acid–base control during hypothermia, in contrast to the 'alpha stat' concept which has evolved from the work of Rahn and Howell [9] and Reeves [10]. The pH of water is temperature-dependent, neutrality being pH 7.0 at 24°C. The dissociation of water decreases as temperature falls, resulting in a higher pH, and vice versa. Likewise the pH of poikilothermic animals such as reptiles changes with temperature in parallel with the pH changes of water, so that at 37°C acid–base measurements approximate those of man. Other support for the alpha stat regimen is that pH measurements in man in cold

peripheral tissues and in hot exercising muscle follow the changes expected with temperature. There is also biochemical evidence relating to optimal enzyme function, which suggests that cooling should follow the alpha stat regimen, allowing blood to become alkaline during hypothermia [11]. In contrast a pH stat regimen where hypothermia is induced, maintaining a corrected pH at 7.4 by adding CO_2 to the anaesthetic gases or oxygenator, results in a pH which is acid relative to the alpha stat regimen (Fig. 24.1) when ventilation is maintained at normal or near normal levels. To assess acid–base status at any temperature a correction factor (the Rosenthal factor) is applied [12]. This is done automatically by most acid–base measuring systems as the pH and Pco_2 electrodes are held at 37–38°C and samples are measured at these temperatures. For a corrected pH, the Rosenthal factor (pH rises 0.0147 per °C fall in temperature) may be applied automatically by the measuring apparatus to give a correct pH as if the electrode had measured at that given temperature (pH at T°C = pH at 37°C + 0.0147 × 37 − T). Using the alpha stat philosophy, if the pH measured at 37°C is within normal limits (i.e. 7.4, $Paco_2$ 40 mmHg) then the pH status of the patient at the temperature at which the sample was obtained is

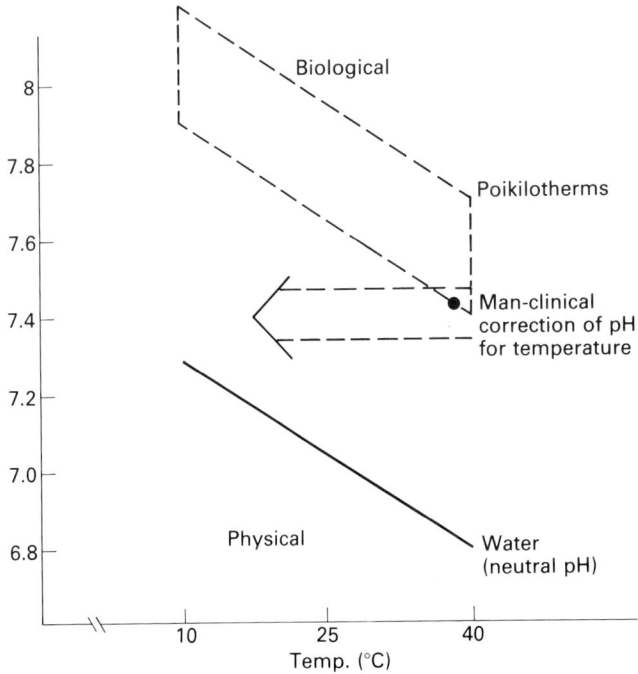

Fig. 24.1 pH changes with temperature, showing how the biological pH changes (alpha stat) run parallel to the changes in neutral pH of water, whereas the 'pH stat' line with correction for temperature runs horizontally.

appropriate. No correction factor should be applied. The main biochemical differences between the two philosophies are shown in Table 24.1.

During hypothermia O_2 requirements are decreased, but so is O_2 delivery due to the following changes:

1 there is a shift to the left of the oxygen dissociation curve (Fig. 24.2);

2 as chemical reactions are slowed, oxyhaemoglobin dissociation is slowed;

3 diffusion is slower.

This may be only partly offset by the increase of oxygen in solution (plasma) and an increase in the time the red blood cells spend in the capillary bed. Cerebral blood flow is normally autoregulated, but CO_2 can act as a cerebral vasodilator, altering this autoregulation. Studies during cooling with computer-controlled $FECO_2$ have shown that temperature differentials within the brain were less when the $FECO_2$ level was normal or slightly elevated than when it was reduced to 3% [13]. On the other hand, measurement of total and regional blood flow with microspheres demonstrated better maintenance of both cardiac output and autoregulation in the brain with an alpha stat regimen [14]. At present the alpha stat regimen is generally favoured during hypothermia in cardiac surgery. It is unusual to add CO_2 during hypo-

Table 24.1 Changes in acid—base measurements under alpha stat and pH stat regulation when body temperature is lowered

	Normothermic values	Alpha stat regulation	pH stat regulation
pH	7.4	↑	0
P_{CO_2}	40 mmHg	↓	0
OH^-/H^+ ratio	16	0	↓
CO_2 stores		0	↑
$[HCO_3^-]$	24 mmol/l	0	↑

thermia in other types of surgery. The possible advantage of adding CO_2 would be to increase oxygen release from haemoglobin by shifting the dissociation curve to the right just before circulatory arrest.

In infants undergoing surface cooling with $Paco_2$ (corrected for temperature) being maintained at about 40 mmHg (5.3 kPa), there is a decrease in plasma potassium and a parallel decrease in plasma insulin (Fig. 24.3) [15]. The changes in plasma sodium and magnesium are insignificant, while alterations in plasma calcium vary. The tendency to develop dysrhythmia at lower temperatures (25–27°C) is related to the decrease in plasma potassium, which is about 2 mmol/l by 27°C (Fig. 24.3). The administration of potassium chloride will restore sinus rhythm (Fig. 24.4). The resulting rise in plasma potassium is accompanied by a concurrent rise in plasma insulin. Blood glucose is usually raised during hypothermia and may reach very high levels if glucose is infused intravenously. This may be due to reduced utilization, depressed enzyme activity in the liver, reduced insulin levels and failure of glucose to cross cell membranes. When insulin levels rise following the injection of potassium during cooling, blood glucose levels decline [15].

Central nervous system activity decreases during hypothermia. This is demonstrated by EEG activity decreasing until it flattens out, and at the same time the pupils dilate as cold narcosis supervenes between 26° and 24°C.

Renal plasma flow, glomerular filtration and tubular function all decrease with temperature. Urine flow continues until about 20°C, below which it almost ceases.

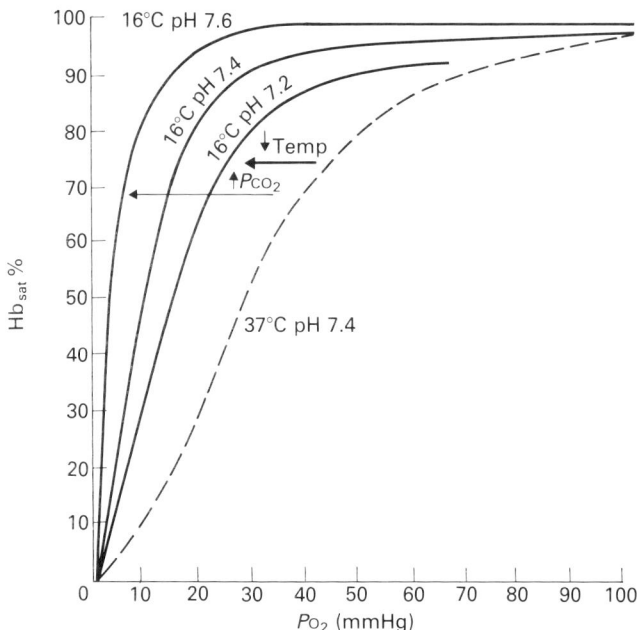

Fig. 24.2 The effect of hypothermia on the oxygen haemoglobin dissociation curve. pH changes with temperature are largely associated with changes in P_{CO_2} due to increased solubility of gases at low temperature.

ANAESTHETIC MANAGEMENT

The anaesthetic management of patients undergoing hypothermia usually includes the use of a muscle relaxant and controlled ventilation, to prevent shivering and en-

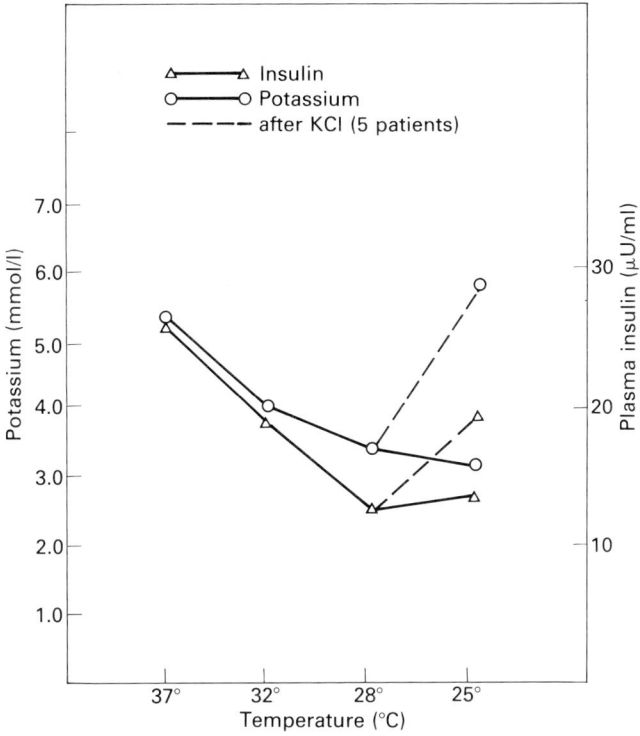

Fig. 24.3 Relationship of plasma potassium and insulin during hypothermia. The dotted line indicates changes which occur when KCl is given to stop dysrhythmias [15].

sure adequation ventilation. Vasodilatation aids cooling. A specific vasodilator such as sodium nitroprusside may be infused, or halothane or isoflurane can be used as they have a peripheral vasodilator action.

Thiopentone, a non-depolarizing relaxant, with halothane or isoflurane and possibly fentanyl are frequently used. If a pH stat regimen is used, gradually increasing concentrations of oxygen and carbon dioxide are given to compensate for the increased solubility of gases at lower temperatures. For an alpha stat regimen the above technique is used with normal ventilation without the addition of carbon dioxide.

METHODS OF COOLING

1 Surface cooling using a cold-water circulating blanket supplemented by ice packs placed around the patient, especially over major superficial vessels. It is important to ensure that the fingers, toes and ears are protected with cotton-wool to prevent ischaemic damage, and that the ice packs do not come into direct contact with the skin. When surface cooling is used alone, the cooling should be stopped one or two degrees above the desired minimum temperature, as there is a tendency for continued cooling to occur before the temperature stabilizes.

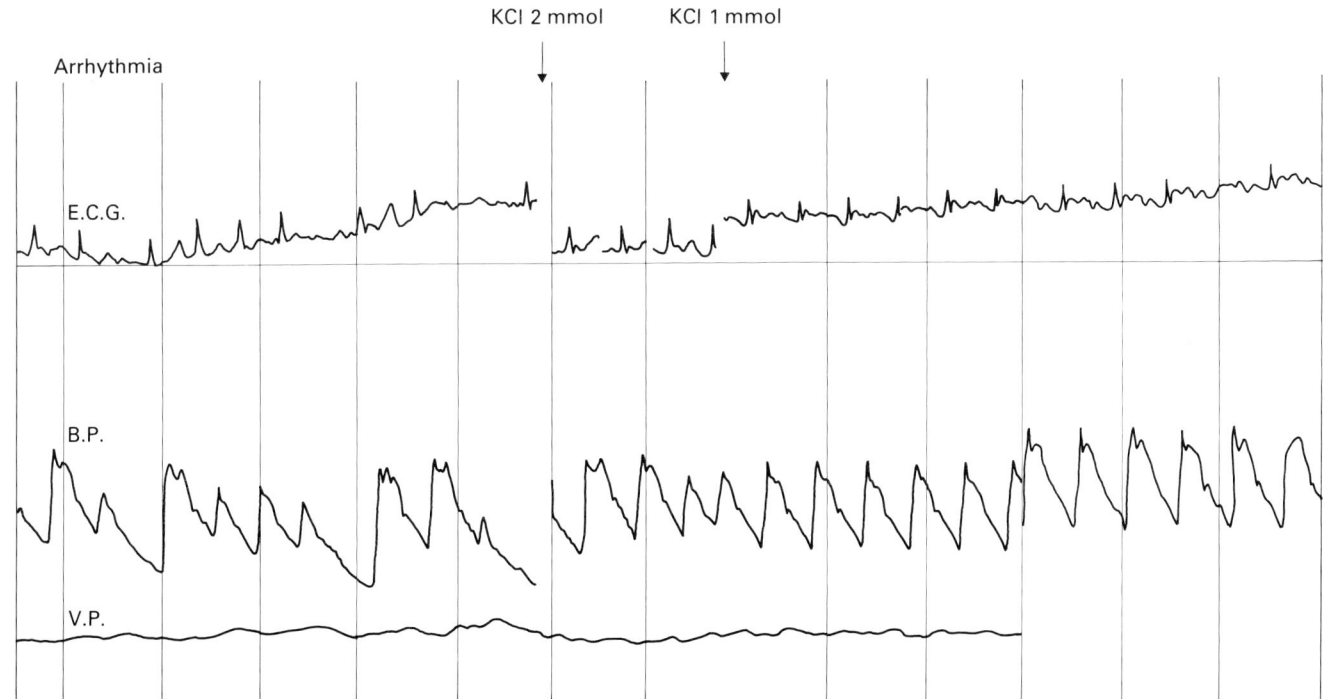

Fig. 24.4 Dysrhythmia occurring during cooling and the response to the administration of intravenous potassium chloride in an 8.7 kg patient aged 14 months [15].

2 Surface cooling in a water bath. This involves transferring the patient to and from the bath, attached to the anaesthetic and monitoring equipment, and although it produces satisfactory cooling it is an inconvenient method.

3 Bypass cooling using a heart–lung machine with a heat exchanger in the circuit is commonly employed during cardiac surgery. It has the advantage that the rate of cooling can be easily controlled and is quicker. It is also a more rapid means of rewarming the patient. It is important that the maximum temperature differential between the blood leaving and that returning to the patient should not exceed 10°C, otherwise large temperature gradients develop in the body; with the decrease in solubility of gases as temperature rises, bubbles may form, which can cause neurological complications. It is safer if cooling is conducted over a longer period, with a smaller difference in temperature.

4 Local tissue cooling is occasionally used; for example, in operations such as partial nephrectomy or removal of stones from the renal pelvis, the kidney can be cooled locally before cross-clamping the renal artery and vein for the duration of the operation. Local cooling of the heart with cardioplegia is now routine (see Chapter 13).

ADJUNCTS TO COOLING

Vasodilators

Vasodilators such as sodium nitroprusside or phenoxybenzamine will significantly increase the rate of cooling and rewarming by increasing peripheral perfusion (see Chapter 23). Sodium nitroprusside can be used either by infusion during surface cooling, taking care not to exceed a dose of 1.5 mg/kg to avoid toxicity, or by addition to the blood in the heart–lung machine. The exact change in nitroprusside pharmacokinetics and its toxicity in hypothermia is unknown. Rewarming time can also be reduced. If the patient is vasodilated when bypass is discontinued and the pressures are normal, the blood volume will have been adequately replaced.

Carbon dioxide

The addition of carbon dioxide has several effects, including the shift of the haemoglobin dissociation curve to the right, allowing greater oxygen release in the tissues, and more even brain cooling [13]. In infants, the blood pressure declines more slowly when higher levels of $Paco_2$ are maintained. It also has a peripheral vasodilating effect. The amount required to maintain a normal corrected $Paco_2$ will depend on ventilation and the rate of cooling, but the addition of 5% at 32°C and 8–10% at 25°C and lower will usually maintain a $Paco_2$ (corrected for temperature) around 40–45 mmHg (5.4–6.0 kPa) [1].

Alcohol

Ten per cent alcohol has been used at a rate of 5 ml/kg in the first hour, reducing to 4 ml/kg in the second hour to increase the rate of cooling by 20–30%, presumably by causing peripheral vasodilatation [8]. Animal studies have shown that mice treated with alcohol had a lower arrest temperature than untreated controls, and had a higher rate of recovery during rewarming.

TEMPERATURE MONITORING

Tissues cool at different rates, which depend on the method of cooling. Surface cooling reduces peripheral temperature more rapidly than core temperature, whereas on bypass the core, especially the vessel-rich organs, is cooled more rapidly. The evenness of cooling is related to the rate of cooling. Temperatures vary according to the site where they are measured depending on their perfusion at that time. The problem is which temperatures are most useful in deciding when to stop cooling and rewarming.

1 Oesophageal temperature probably most closely reflects heart and therefore central blood temperature. It is easily monitored in the lower one-third of the oesophagus. The distance of insertion of the probes should be measured. It is useful to monitor oesophageal temperature when coronary flow is to be stopped by aortic cross-clamping.

2 Nasopharyngeal or tympanic membrane temperature reflects brain temperature more closely, and one of them should be monitored when circulatory arrest is employed, because the temperature of the brain determines how long hypoxia will be tolerated. Accurate placement of nasopharyngeal temperature probes is more difficult than an oesophageal probe, and tympanic membrane probes can be traumatic in very young patients.

3 Rectal temperature is a useful guide during rewarming to ensure that an adequate body temperature is reached. During rapid changes in temperature, as in cooling or rewarming on bypass, rectal temperature often lags behind oesophageal temperature. It may reflect the average temperature of the less well-perfused tissues, and if bypass is discontinued before the rectal temperature reaches 33–34°C, there is often a drift of oesophageal or nasopharyngeal temperature as the body equilibrates. This differential is used to assess adequacy of total body rewarming. In slow surface cooling and rewarming, rectal temperature is more representative of true body temperature.

4 A temperature probe placed on the skin at a peripheral site such as the big toe identifies the gradient between the core and the periphery. Like rectal temperature, it can be used as an indication of total body change when cooling and rewarming, but its main advantage is in assessing the adequacy of perfusion in cardiac surgery.

Thus at least two sites should be monitored, one as a guide to the temperature of the organ most critically affected, and the other as a guide to rewarming. In addition, it is important to monitor the temperature of the warming blanket, the temperature of arterial blood returning from the heart–lung machine, and the inspired gas temperature when warmed, humidified inspired gases are used to aid rewarming.

ACTION OF DRUGS

Although anaesthesia is usually induced and concluded at normothermia, it is relevant to understand the general principles of drug action at lowered temperatures, so that overdosage is avoided.

At temperatures around 24–26°C, cold narcosis occurs and EEG activity ceases. This depression of cerebral function means that lower concentrations of inhalation anaesthetics are needed at lower body temperatures.

Non-depolarizing muscle relaxant requirements are reduced and recovery is slower during hypothermia (Fig. 24.5) [16].

Drugs which are inactivated by the liver or excreted by the kidney will have a longer action at low temperature, due to depression of hepatic and renal function.

CONCLUSION

Although hypothermia is not widely used except in open heart surgery, it is still useful in dealing with difficult and potentially dangerous situations. The safety margin provided enables the patient to survive such operations neurologically intact makes the extra time spent cooling and rewarming worthwhile.

REFERENCES

1 Brown T.C.K., Clarke C.P., Shanahan E.A., McKie B.D., Wood H.M., Thorp E.A. Management of infants for cardiac surgery under deep hypothermia. *Anaes Intens Care* 1972, **1**, 137.

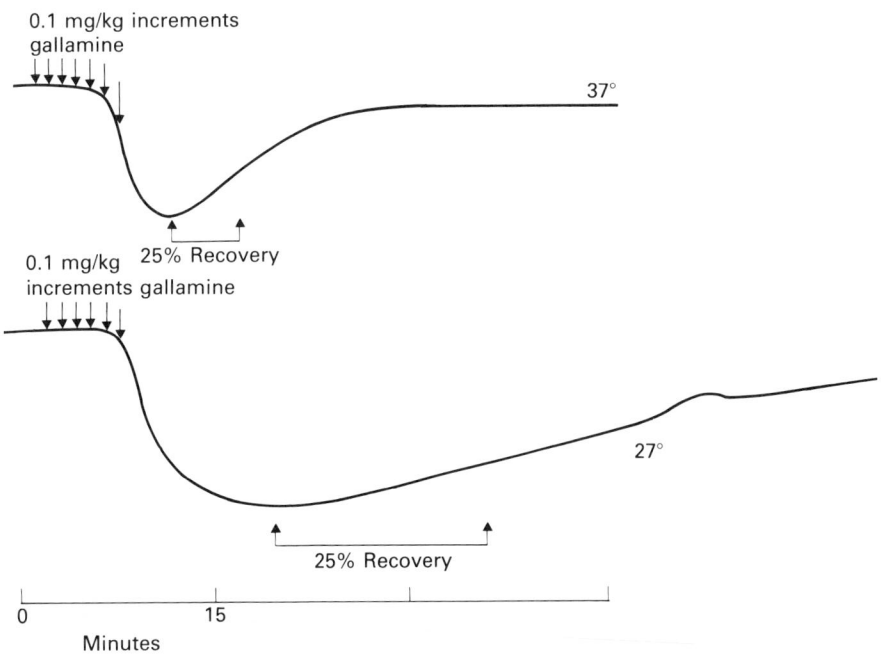

Fig. 24.5 The effect of temperature on the onset and recovery from gallamine at 37°C and 27°C.

2 Brown T.C.K., Davidson P.D., Auldist A.W. Anaesthetic considerations in liver tumour resection in children. *Pediatr Surg* 1988, **4**, 11.

3 Hickey P.R. Deep hypothermic circulatory arrest: current status and future directions. *Mount Sinai J Med* 1985, **52**, 541–549.

4 Bjork V.O., Hultquist G. Contraindications to profound hypothermia in open heart surgery. *J Thorac Cardiovasc Surg* 1962, **44**, 1.

5 Barratt-Boyes B.G., Neutze J.M., Seelye E.R., Simpson M. Complete correction of cardiovascular malformations in the first year of life. *Prog Cardiovasc Dis* 1972, **15**, 229.

6 Fisk G.C., Wright J.S., *et al*. Cerebral effects of circulatory arrest at 20°C in the infant pig. *Anaes Intens Care* 1974, **2**, 33.

7 Wells F.C., *et al*. Duration of circulatory arrest does influence the psychological development of children after cardiac operations in early life. *J Thorac Cardiovasc Surg* 1983, **86**, 823–831.

8 Hewer A.J.H. Hypothermia for neurosurgery. *Int Anesth Clin* 1964, **2**, 919.

9 Rahn H., Howell B.J. The OH−/H+ concept of acid–base balance: historical development. *Resp Physiol* 1978, **33**, 91–97.

10 Reeves R.B. An imidazole alphastat hypothesis for vertebrate acid–base regulation: tissue CO_2 content and body temperature in bullfrogs. *Resp Phsyiol* 1972, **14**, 219–236.

11 White F.N. A comparative approach to hypothermia. *J Thor Cardiovasc Surg* 1981, **82**, 821.

12 Rosenthal T.B. The effect of temperature on pH of blood and plasma *in vitro*. *J Biol Chem* 1948, **173**, 25.

13 Brown T.C.K., Lampard D.G., Brown W.A., Coles J.R. Computer-controlled studies in surface-cooling hypothermia — the effect of CO_2 on brain temperatures. *Anaes Intens Care* 1976, **4**, 36.

14 Becker H., Vinten-Johansen J., Buckberg G.D., *et al*. Myocardial damage caused by keeping pH 7.40 during systemic deep hypothermia. *J Thor Cardiovasc Surg* 1981, **82**, 810.

15 Brown T.C.K., Dunlop M.E., Stevens B.J., Clarke C.P., Shanahan E.A. Biochemical changes during surface cooling for deep hypothermic open heart surgery. *J Thor Cardiovasc Surg* 1973, **65**, 402.

16 Lam H.S., Brown T.C.K., Lampard D.G. D-tubocurarine requirement during hypothermia. *Anaes Intens Care* 1979, **7**, 222.

FURTHER READING

Blair E. *Clinical Hypothermia*. McGraw-Hill, New York, (1964).

Hunter A.R. (Ed.) *Hypothermia*. International Anesthesiology Clinics, Vol 2. Little, Brown & Co, Boston, (1964) pp. 801–1014.

25: Medical Diseases and Anaesthesia

INTRODUCTION

It is important for anaesthetists to appreciate the salient features of medical conditions that patients may have when they present for anaesthesia and surgery.

In this chapter, an attempt has been made to present concisely some of the commoner conditions that are not dealt with in the specialty chapters elsewhere in the book. A number of conditions that are less common are also included; some of these are rare, but they may have anaesthetic implications or, occasionally, require anaesthesia for their management. Because some of them may cause problems during anaesthesia, brief comments are included to provide a ready source of information. It is obviously impossible to include every paediatric disease or syndrome in an anaesthetic textbook.

CARDIOVASCULAR DISEASES

The management of special problems relating to anaesthesia in specific types of heart disease is considered in Chapter 13. The unrecognized heart murmur and myocardial disease will be considered here.

Heart murmurs

As many as 3 out of 4 children may have a transient murmur (e.g. with exercise), whilst 1 in 4 may have a murmur persisting over months. The anaesthetist must make a series of decisions when a murmur is detected at a preoperative examination:
1 Is this an innocent murmur?
2 What needs to be done perioperatively if the murmur is not definitely innocent?
3 What medical follow-up is needed?

Is this an innocent murmur? This may be a difficult diagnosis to make with certainty, especially with the rapid heart rate and limited co-operation of the small child. An isolated innocent murmur is associated with an otherwise normal cardiorespiratory history and examination.

Venous hums are common. A continuous whining or surging, varying with posture, is best heard at the upper sternal edge and lower neck. They disappear in the supine position or with pressure on the jugular vein above the site of auscultation.

All other innocent murmurs are systolic. Timing of the murmur with the carotid pulse is important, any diastolic murmur being pathological. There are two main types of innocent murmur. The first is the 'musical' or 'vibratory' murmur, with a characteristic rasping or honking quality, usually best heard at the lower left sternal edge. It may be loud and confused with the murmur of a ventricular septal defect. There may be an associated soft short aortic ejection murmur, or a venous hum. The second is a systolic ejection (crescendo–decrescendo) murmur best heard at the upper left sternal edge ('pulmonary area') exaggerated by increases in cardiac output (e.g. with exercise, fever, anaemia or anxiety). This murmur is caused by turbulence in the pulmonary artery. The distinction from an atrial septal defect (ASD) causing increased pulmonary flow may be subtle, an ASD classically causing fixed splitting of the second heart sound and a hyperdynamic parasternal impulse, the latter being mimicked by any situation with increased cardiac output.

What needs to be done perioperatively if the murmur is not definitely innocent? A well child with no gross signs, even if the murmur is of structural origin, is likely to tolerate routine anaesthesia and surgery well. If the child is asymptomatic, feeding well, not breathless, normally active without episodic syncope or 'funny turns', and has no signs of cardiac failure, cyanosis or a palpable precordial thrill or heave, then it is reasonable to proceed with surgery under appropriate antibiotic cover as long as investigation and follow-up is initiated. Detection of a severe stenotic lesion (e.g. aortic ejection murmur with a slow rise in the carotid pulse, or depressed femoral pulses in a coarctation) is of particular importance, as cardiovascular collapse at induction may occur in these patients. The opportunity to examine the child carefully when anaesthetized should not be missed, while in some centres echocardiography in theatre or the recovery room could save a small child the need for sedation for echocardiography on another occasion.

The management of children with significant impairment due to specific congenital anomalies is discussed in Chapter 13.

What medical follow-up is needed? Children who have a murmur that the anaesthetist believes may not be innocent, even if asymptomatic, must have follow-up arranged. Having the child survive the present operation is of little credit to the anaesthetist if the child presents years later with severe pulmonary hypertension or life-threatening valve stenosis, which could have been avoided by appropriate diagnosis, follow-up and well-timed corrective surgery.

If any doubt exists about the innocence of a murmur, elective referral to a suitable physician is appropriate, whose expertise in cardiac examination of children cannot be expected from anaesthetists; investigations will clarify the diagnosis. An electrocardiogram may show hypertrophy or strain of one or both ventricles, atrial hypertrophy, or conduction defects. The chest X-ray may show pulmonary plethora or oligaemia, enlargement of specific cardiac chambers, or calcification, especially of valves. The echocardiogram has revolutionized the diagnosis of congenital heart disease, giving detailed diagnoses non-invasively and dramatically reducing the need for cardiac catheterization.

Bacterial endocarditis

There is a risk of bacterial endocarditis after surgery in patients with structural cardiac abnormalities such as valvular disease, septal defects and patent ductus arteriosus. This may follow bacteraemia associated with operations in the mouth and nose, tracheal intubation and surgery of the bowel and urinary tract. The appropriate antibiotic cover for procedures around the mouth or tracheal intubation is penicillin (or erythromycin), and for bowel and urinary surgery a broad-spectrum antibiotic is used.

Myocardial diseases

ENDOCARDIAL FIBROELASTOSIS

The cause is unknown but it may be due to intrauterine mumps or Coxsackie B viral infection. The disease is endocardial but may also involve the myocardium. The affected muscle fibres are fibrotic and disorganized, and may have increased vascularity. Most patients develop symptoms of heart failure within the first year of life. Treatment is with digoxin and diuretics, but most eventually die of intractable heart failure unless heart transplant is undertaken.

As this vessel arises from the pulmonary artery, myo-cardial ischaemia may develop initially from the desatu-rated blood supplying the left ventricle. During the first 2 months, ischaemia worsens as pulmonary artery pressure falls and flow decreases. If the infant survives, collateral channels from the right coronary artery may supply the left coronary territory. The left coronary then acts as a fistula into the pulmonary artery, producing low coronary diastolic pressures, which jeopardize left-ventricular per-fusion. Death usually results from 'ischaemic cardio-myopathy' causing dilatation of the heart and congestive failure unless the left coronary artery is anastomosed to the aorta.

KAWASAKI DISEASE

This is a systemic angitis affecting the coronary arteries, as well as bowel and biliary vessels. It is also called mucocutaneous lymph node syndrome. It is an acute exanthematous disease, affecting mainly infants and chil-dren under 4 years of age. The most serious complications are myocardial involvement with dilatation and aneurysm formation in the coronary arteries (17–30% of patients), which tend to regress within 6 months, but may remain abnormal for longer periods. Occasionally, coronary artery stenosis follows. Myocardial ischaemic damage may result in mitral incompetence. Aspirin has been widely used in treatment.

Patients may present for surgery for complications of the disease, but more often for other operations. It is desirable to postpone these until at least 6 months after the acute phase, when the vessels will usually have returned towards their normal state. Preoperative ECG and echocardiography are, and liver function tests may be, indicated. Salicylates should be discontinued a few days before operation, to allow platelet function to re-cover. During anaesthesia, the ECG (leads II and V5 or CM5) should be monitored for myocardial ischaemia [1, 2].

In all patients with myocardial disease, anaesthesia carries an increased risk. Careful anaesthesia, minimizing myocardial depression, hypotension or hypertension and ensuring an adequate oxygen supply, is important (see Chapter 13).

HYPERTENSION

Hypertension is relatively uncommon in childhood, although there are many possible causes. Among them are coarctation of the aorta affecting the upper half of the body, and renal hypertension resulting from acute nephritis, chronic renal disease and renal artery stenosis. Catecholamine-secreting tumours such as phaeo-chromocytoma and, occasionally, neuroblastoma cause intermittent hypertension.

Antihypertensive treatment should be continued. The danger of complications, due to the disease and associ-ated with anaesthesia, is greater if treatment is ceased.

RESPIRATORY DISEASES

Assessment of the respiratory system

The preoperative history and examination should alert the paediatric anaesthetist to potential respiratory prob-lems. The presentation and spectrum of these disorders is different from that in adults.

HISTORY

Extreme prematurity requiring prolonged ventilation may be associated with relatively asymptomatic chronic lung disease, which is only apparent when a high FiO_2 is required for normal saturations perioperatively, even at several years of age. This group of patients is also at increased risk of perioperative apnoea in the first months of life.

Specific enquiry about nocturnal cough, snoring and associated sleep disruption may suggest unsuspected asthma or sleep apnoea respectively.

Breathlessness may have to be assessed indirectly, in terms of 'keeping up with other children,' or in infants difficulty feeding. Observant parents will sometimes describe tachypnoea, compared to other children.

Recurrent acute respiratory problems, even if the child is currently well, may be the only clue to underlying aspiration, subglottic narrowing, asthma or lung disease.

EXAMINATION

Note should be made of the child's weight and general condition, as failure to thrive may have respiratory ori-gins, but also, whatever the cause, a child who is not thriving or is neurologically abnormal is likely to have less respiratory reserve, especially postoperatively.

Observation of quiet respiration, noting the pattern, rate and associated chest, abdominal and neck movements, coordination or retractions, is the single most important step in the preoperative respiratory examination of the small child. The crying child is difficult to assess, although the deep inspiration associated with crying will exaggerate the retraction associated with obstructive lesions. Auscultation may localize pathology, or demonstrate crepitations, rhonchi or prolonged expiration, but should serve as a supplement to the history and observation, rather than being the primary respiratory diagnostic tool.

INVESTIGATIONS

A chest X-ray is only occasionally indicated, usually to assess a child with respiratory symptoms not adequately diagnosed on history and examination.

Pulse oximetry can non-invasively demonstrate abnormalities that may not be clinically apparent, and is useful if significant respiratory disease is suspected. Pulse oximetry also has a special role in the assessment of patients who may have sleep apnoea syndrome.

Blood gas estimation may be indicated in children with marked chronic lung disease. If a child is upset by the sample being taken, the result may be inaccurate because of breath-holding, causing hypoxia, or hyperventilation, lowering CO_2. Despite this, chronic CO_2 retention can usually be detected by the relationship between pH, $Paco_2$ and estimates of base excess, whilst with atraumatic samples Pao_2 may be helpful. Abnormalities in either of these factors may change perioperative management.

Spirometry has several roles but requires good patient co-operation.

Bronchial obstruction will reduce the rate at which air can be exhaled, decreasing the forced expiratory volume in 1 second (FEV_1) (compared to expected value for height) and the FEV_1/FVC (forced vital capacity) ratio (normally >70%), the FVC also being decreased by airway closure at higher lung volumes, with alveolar gas trapping and hyperinflation. Pre- and post-bronchodilator measurements may show acutely reversible bronchospasm, whilst further improvement may be shown by repeat measurements after chronic therapy. Provocative tests may be used in respiratory laboratories for diagnosis. Children with chronic or frequent episodic asthma may use home peak expiratory flow rate (PEFR)

measurements and their preoperative state can be easily compared to their 'usual' or 'best'. These simple portable devices with appropriate charts of the normal ranges may be very useful, as full spirometry is often impractical in the anaesthetic setting.

Patients with significant lung or chest-wall disease will often have a 'restrictive' pattern on spirometry, a markedly decreased FVC, with a relatively normal FEV_1/FVC ratio. These measurements are useful in patients with neuromuscular disorders. This latter group may also be assessed by the maximum inspiratory and expiratory pressures they can develop against an obstruction. In adults, the minimum vital capacity required to cough effectively is about 15 ml/kg. Abdominal or thoracic surgery may decrease vital capacity by about 50%, although this may be improved with optimal analgesia. Patients with an FVC less than 50% of predicted normal prior to major thoracic or abdominal surgery are at substantial risk of respiratory failure, and facilities for postoperative mechanical ventilation should be available.

Other tests such as diagnostic bronchoscopy, flow−volume loops for large airway obstruction, measurement of residual volume, or the diffusing capacity of carbon monoxide may be indicated occasionally in centres with the appropriate facilities and expertise.

Upper respiratory tract infection

An URTI or cold is the most common respiratory complaint confronting the anaesthetist. The dilemma of whether to proceed with the operation or not is discussed in Chapter 6.

Asthma

Bronchial asthma is a syndrome with varied presentation affecting as many as 20−30% of children. As the basic abnormality has not been defined and the clinical patterns are so protean, the best definition at present would be 'episodic cough or wheeze when asthma is likely and other rarer conditions have been excluded.' The symptoms are due to mucosal oedema, bronchial muscle constriction and increased secretions. It is important to consider asthma as a likely diagnosis in any child with recurrent cough or wheeze, so that appropriate preventive medication can be given preoperatively. Attacks of asthma may be precipitated by infection, allergens, mechanical factors such as over-inflation, laughing, coughing, local irritation and changes in temperature. As no cure is currently known, treatment is aimed at avoiding precipitating factors, using drugs such as bronchodilators, cromoglycate, anticholinergics and steroids. The basic pathological process is considered to be inflammatory so that prophylactic anti-inflammatory agents are used long-term in those with frequent symptoms. Bronchodilators are used for the treatment of acute attacks.

The primary bronchodilator therapy for asthma is with aerosol beta-adrenergic stimulants. Salbutamol, terbutaline and fenoterol are relatively specific beta-2 stimulants, with a more specific action on the bronchial mucosa than adrenaline or isoprenaline. They may exert their effect by stimulation of adenyl cyclase. They are most effective when given as an aerosol and should be administered by this route whenever possible. A metered aerosol should be delivered as the patient inspires. A spacer is a device placed between the spray and the patient, which holds the aerosol until the patient breathes in. These are now used to enable young children to use a metered aerosol. If this is not possible, a nebulizer can be used. Xanthines such as theophylline or aminophylline are used as adjuncts in the long-term treatment or acute management of severe asthma. Disodium cromoglycate has proved to be an effective prophylactic administered as an aerosol. Its precise mechanisms of action have not been clearly defined, but it can be shown experimentally to prevent release of bronchoactive mediators from mast cells. Steroids given by aerosol are important prophylactic agents, now used in relatively high doses. Oral or intravenous steroids are used for the management of acute, severe asthma. Steroids have a variety of mechanisms of action, including modification of the inflammatory process and potentiation of the effect of sympathomimetic agents on adenyl cyclase.

It is important to recognize the various presentations of asthma before surgery is undertaken. Those with recurrent wheezing are usually diagnosed appropriately, but those with recurrent cough or recurrent 'pneumonia' due to mucus plugs and atelectasis may be incorrectly diagnosed as having primary infection. When a child has an acute asthma attack, surgery should be deferred until the airway obstruction is controlled. This can usually be achieved fairly readily with aggressive bronchodilator and steroid therapy.

Patients receiving long-term therapy should not have their treatment stopped before surgery, although drugs usually taken by mouth may be given by another route if possible. Most can be given by aerosol or intravenously. If patients have had prolonged steroid therapy, including high-dose aerosol steroids, additional hydrocortisone must be given intravenously at induction, or intramuscularly beforehand. For those with episodic treatment regimens, the necessity for preoperative bronchodilators should be assessed individually. An antihistamine tranquillizer such as promethazine may be used for premedication, often with pethidine, if an analgesic is needed preoperatively. Drugs with a propensity to release histamine, such as morphine and D-tubocurarine, should be avoided in asthmatics. Pancuronium and vecuronium are the muscle relaxants of choice. Unless specially indicated, anti-sialagogues should be avoided. Bronchospasm may develop when the airway is stimulated during light anaesthesia.

The treatment of wheeze during anaesthesia should include a check that the endotracheal tube is patent and not irritating the carina, and increasing the inspired oxygen and inspiratory pressure. Deepening anaesthesia with a bronchodilator agent such as halothane may help. If bronchospasm still persists, aminophylline (5 mg/kg) can be given slowly intravenously over 10−20 minutes, unless the patient is on long-term theophylline therapy. Salbutamol can be introduced into the breathing system, using a spacer and a metered aerosol, or be given intravenously by injection (5−7.5 μg/kg) over 4−5 minutes. Hydrocortisone (approximately 4−5 mg/kg) can also be used.

Diethyl ether is a potent bronchodilator that has been used successfully to terminate status asthmaticus and bronchospasm during anaesthesia. It also stimulates the production of secretions in the respiratory tract, if atropine or hyoscine have not been given in adequate dosage. This may facilitate the removal by suction of thick mucus and plugs.

Halothane and isoflurane are also bronchodilators. Of the intravenous anaesthetics, ketamine has sympathomimetic properties and has been used successfully in the treatment of asthma.

Cystic fibrosis

Cystic fibrosis is an inherited condition affecting 1 in every 2500 children of European background. It is an autosomal recessively inherited condition, caused by an abnormality on the long arm of chromosome 7. The primary abnormality is dysfunction of the chloride channels affecting fluid and electrolyte transport across cell membranes. It is now recognized very early in life, and with aggressive therapy most children reach adulthood in reasonable health. The median age of survival is now well into the 30s.

Cystic fibrosis is characterized by dysfunction of all exocrine glands. The major features are chronic obstructive airway disease with secondary infection, pancreatic insufficiency leading to malabsorption and malnutrition, and excessive salt loss in the sweat. The loss in sweat and from the bowel may lead to hyponatraemia when the patient is febrile or during hot weather. Hypokalaemic alkalosis may also occur in an ill child. Electrolytes and acid-base status should be checked preoperatively.

These children are liable to sinusitis, otitis media, nasal polyps and oedema of the nasal mucosa causing airway obstruction. In older patients, abnormal glucose tolerance and even insulin-dependent diabetes may develop. Cirrhosis and portal hypertension are seen in up to 15% of patients after adolescence.

Patients present for surgery in infancy, with meconium ileus and bowel obstruction. About 25% of neonatal small bowel obstructions are caused by cystic fibrosis. Bowel obstruction due to meconium plugs can be relieved in many patients with a gastrografin enema, avoiding the need for surgery. This procedure is only performed when the diagnosis is made early, the baby is fit and complications have not developed. Bowel obstruction may be associated with perforation and peritonitis. Surgery is indicated in infants with complications or those who fail to respond to a gastrografin enema. Although the postoperative mortality is still significant, the results in recent years have improved due to better preoperative preparation, control of respiratory infection, attention to fluid, electrolyte and acid−base disturbances, and adequate postoperative parenteral nutrition.

Biliary obstruction may occur in the neonatal period, leading to prolonged jaundice, which eventually resolves spontaneously. Infants may be at an increased risk of bleeding from vitamin K deficiency and should be given vitamin K prior to surgery.

Older children may present for removal of nasal polyps, laparotomy for abdominal pain, portocaval shunting for portal hypertension, or lung surgery for haemoptysis or pneumothorax. They may also need anaesthesia for other surgical conditions, such as injuries. Any surgery is potentially lethal for a child with cystic fibrosis; it is essential that it be carried out in a centre where appropriate preoperative evaluation and operative and postoperative care can be undertaken. These patients should be well prepared for operation with physiother-

apy and antibiotics, which will need to be continued postoperatively.

The anaesthetist should ensure that the child is adequately hydrated during surgery, by giving intravenous fluids and humidifying inspired gases. On theoretical grounds, atropine and hyoscine are better avoided because they dry secretions, but, if necessary, atropine may be given intravenously in modest doses.

Inhalation induction may be slow, due to chronic lung disease with ventilation/perfusion disturbances. Anaesthesia can be induced intravenously. Anaesthesia, especially when the patient is intubated, provides an excellent opportunity to improve the patient's condition by bronchial toilet. Instillation of a few ml of normal saline may make this more effective.

Postoperative respiratory depression is undesirable, but postoperative pain relief is essential to enable to the patient to cough adequately. In these patients the use of regional anaesthetic methods such as intercostal blocks is useful, where applicable, to provide analgesia without respiratory depression and minimize pulmonary complications. In some cases, mechanical ventilation for a short period may be justified. Aggressive antibiotic therapy, physiotherapy and attention to appropriate nutrition are vital in the postoperative period.

Recurrent croup

Any child with a history of recurrent croup may have a narrow subglottic region. Care must be taken during intubation to ensure that the correct tube size is used, allowing a slight leak, otherwise laryngeal obstruction may develop postoperatively. If such precautions are not taken and obstruction does occur, nebulized adrenaline may be useful (see Chapter 27).

Respiratory distress syndrome

Premature infants with respiratory distress syndrome may present for operations such as closure of a perforation or resection of dead gut, in necrotizing enterocolitis, or closure of a patent ductus. These babies also have a high incidence of inguinal herniae, which are often repaired at a few weeks of age, usually after they have recovered from RDS. The principles of anaesthesia for these babies is discussed in Chapter 9 (neonatal anaesthesia).

Bronchopulmonary dysplasia

A significant number of small, pre-term infants requiring aggressive ventilator and oxygen therapy will go on to develop a chronic lung disease of infancy known as bronchopulmonary dysplasia. This is considered to be present when a child remains oxygen-dependent after 1 month of age. These children are prone to recurrent lower respiratory illness during their early years of life. They may also need surgery for the usual surgical problems of infancy. Inguinal herniae are common and present for repair in the early months of life. Treatment for bronchopulmonary dysplasia usually consists of added oxygen, diuretics, bronchodilators and steroids. More aggressive therapy may be required before and after operation, to prevent deterioration. They should be monitored with oximetry postoperatively (see Chapter 9).

BLOOD DISORDERS

Assessment of bleeding tendencies

Any child presenting for operation with a history of unusual bleeding following trauma, surgery or dental extraction, a tendency to bruise easily or a family history of a bleeding disorder should be investigated before surgery.

A history should be taken to determine the site, onset, duration and severity of bleeding, the presence of other diseases and current drug therapy.

Laboratory studies are necessary to identify defects of haemostatic mechanisms (Table 25.1).

Table 25.1 Tests for haemostatic defects

Test	Coagulation factors measured
Platelet count	
Prothrombin time (PT)	VII (extrinsic system) V and X (extrinsic and intrinsic)
Partial thromboplastin time (PTT)	VIII IX XI XII (intrinsic system) V X (intrinsic and extrinsic system) fibrinogen, fibrin
Ivy skin bleeding time (standard skin incision with increased venous pressure)	Haemostatic capacity of platelet–vessel wall interaction
Platelet function studies	

Disorders of coagulation

These usually result from abnormal synthesis of the clotting factors. Disorders due to increased utilization (disseminated intravascular coagulation) or inhibition of clotting factors (circulating anticoagulants) are rare.

Hereditary clotting defects usually involve only one factor, and the defect persists at a constant level throughout life. This level may differ between individuals, but tends to be similar within an affected family.

HAEMOPHILIA

Haemophilia A is an X-linked recessive hereditary deficiency of Factor VIII (antihaemophilic globulin — AHG) affecting males. Carrier females are not usually clinically affected. About 20% of cases are due to spontaneous mutation. The severity of the disease depends on the Factor VIII level. Severe haemophilia occurs when the level is less than 1% of normal; these children have a history of bleeding from infancy and suffer from haemarthroses. Moderate cases have Factor VIII levels of 1–5% and have occasional haemarthroses, while mild cases (5–10%) may not be recognized until adolescence.

Patients with haemophilia have a normal prothrombin time and platelet count but a prolonged PTT (Table 25.1). Specific diagnosis requires the measurement of Factor VIII (AHG) levels.

Replacement therapy is essential to prevent the crippling effects of the disease and to enable surgery to be performed. Cryoprecipitate is no longer used because of the risk of blood-borne virus transmission (hepatitis B and C, HIV). High-purity concentrates containing 200–300 units of Factor VIII, heated to 80°C to prevent blood-borne virus infection, are the treatment of choice. Factor VIII concentrate is presented as a powder, which is dissolved in sterile water. The amount required to achieve the therapeutic levels in Table 25.2 is calculated from the formula:

$$\frac{\text{Body weight} \times \text{desired rise in Factor VIII}}{1.5} = \text{no. of units required.}$$

This can be injected intravenously immediately before surgery, using a plastic syringe. It may be desirable, especially after head injury, to maintain these levels by giving replacement therapy 12-hourly or as indicated by Factor VIII levels. The half-life of Factor VIII is 8–12 hours.

Antibodies to Factor VIII develop in about 5–10% of

Table 25.2 AHG levels recommended for various operations

Condition or operation	AHG level recommended
Haemarthrosis	30–50%
Dental	50%
Major surgery	60–80%
Intracranial surgery	100%
Normal	1 u/ml (range 0.5–1.5)

patients with haemophilia. This generally precludes further treatment, and conservative management must be relied upon. Prothrombin concentrates have been shown to reduce bleeding in haemophilic patients with antibodies, and their role is being assessed. Steroid and immunosuppressive drugs have not proved helpful.

Some patients will be HIV-antibody positive and appropriate precautions will be necessary to protect the staff involved.

CHRISTMAS DISEASE

Christmas disease is an X-linked hereditary deficiency of Factor IX. Clinically, it is indistinguishable from classic haemophilia. Diagnosis is established by specific assay of Factor IX levels.

The principles of replacement therapy are similar to Factor VIII deficiency except that prothrombinex (Factors II, VII, X and 300 u of Factor IX per vial) is used.

VON WILLEBRAND'S DISEASE

This is a familial bleeding disorder that occurs in both sexes. Mucosal bleeding, petechiae and epistaxis are common features; haemarthrosis is rare. Symptoms appear early in childhood and may decrease with age. Diagnosis is established by prolonged skin bleeding time, decreased Factor VIII levels, normal platelet count and abnormal platelet function in response to ristocetin.

Patients with Type I von Willebrand's disease may be treated with desmopressin (DDAVP or 1-deamino-8-D-arginine vasopressin) for most episodes of bleeding and all except major surgical procedures. Type II von Willebrand's and Type I requiring major surgery should be treated with Factor VIII concentrate. Laboratory differentiation of the two types is useful in determining appropriate treatment.

When patients with any of these coagulation disorders have mouth bleeding or need dental treatment, the antifibrinolytic agent epsilon amino caproic acid (EACA, Amicar) or tranexamic acid (Cyklokapron) will reduce the amount of replacement therapy needed and prevent secondary haemorrhage 7–10 days later.

Platelet disorders

Haemostasis depends on the adhesion and aggregation of platelets, followed by fibrin formation and clot retraction. Platelets are also responsible for maintaining vascular integrity. Platelet disorders are due to either decreased numbers or impaired function.

THROMBOCYTOPENIA

This may be due to:

1 marrow damage by drugs or irradiation;

2 marrow replacement by neoplasm such as leukaemia;

3 ineffective formation due to Vitamin B_{12} or folate deficiency;

4 familial thrombocytopenia;

5 idiopathic thrombocytopenic purpura (ITP) — increased destruction by an immune mechanism;

6 increased consumption, as in disseminated intravascular coagulation (DIC);

7 splenomegaly — platelets pool in the spleen, decreasing the circulating levels. It is uncommon in children but can occur in thalassaemia with hypersplenism.

8 in the operating theatre, the commonest cause of acute thrombocytopenia is dilution by large volumes of crystalloid or colloid solutions or bank blood.

Idiopathic thrombocytopenic purpura is the most common cause of thrombocytopenia in childhood. A small number of these patients (10%), who do not recover spontaneously with steroids or with i.v. gammaglobulin, will require splenectomy. They are usually taking steroids and will require extra cover for operation. Platelet transfusion is not usually necessary, because the count rises rapidly after the spleen is removed. If surgery is necessary to control haemorrhage or for any other reason, a platelet transfusion in a dose of 4–6 units/m² may be required. This should be given together with steroids or gamma-globulin, which for some unexplained reason increases platelet count in this condition. Repeated transfusion can lead to sensitization and further transfusion is then ineffective.

FUNCTIONAL DISORDERS

Functional disorders of platelets are uncommon. The

cause most significant to anaesthetists is the ingestion of aspirin within 7–10 days of surgery or for postoperative analgesia. Aspirin prevents ADP-mediated aggregation, which normally follows adhesion of platelets. Its unwitting use preoperatively has caused postoperative bleeding following operations such as tonsillectomy. This can be controlled by platelet transfusion. A history of any aspirin ingestion should be sought.

Other causes of platelet dysfunction include dipyridamole, inhibitory substances such as dextrans and macroglobulins, uraemia and cardiopulmonary bypass.

Anaemia

OXYGEN TRANSPORT

Anaemia, with a haemoglobin below 10 g/100 ml, used to be taken by many as a contraindication to elective surgery. Certainly it is desirable to have more than adequate oxygen carriage during anaesthesia, but rigid adherence to such a limit does not allow consideration of many relevant factors in individual patients [3].

Using adult figures and assuming complete oxygen extraction and no change in resting cardiac output (5 l/min) 4 g/100 ml haemoglobin could carry more than the basal oxygen requirements of 250 ml/min – (4 × 1.34 + 0.3 ml in solution) × 5000/100 = 280 ml.

Several other factors must also be considered:
1 Cardiac output increases when the haemoglobin decreases to 7–8 g/100 ml, thus increasing transport.
2 Oxygen consumption usually decreases during anaesthesia.
3 Inspired oxygen concentration is usually increased, providing a small increase in oxygen carried in solution.
4 In chronic anaemia, 2-3-DPG levels are increased, shifting the haemoglobin dissociation curve to the right, thereby increasing oxygen release in the tissues. There is thus a lower venous saturation for a given $P\text{vo}_2$.
5 Anaemic patients' blood has a lower viscosity, thereby reducing that component of peripheral resistance (Pouiseuille's equation).
6 Neonates have a dissociation curve moved to the left due to haemoglobin F, and have a greater oxygen requirement per kg. This is compensated by higher haemoglobin levels, as well as greater blood volume and cardiac output relative to body weight.
Sometimes it may be justified to proceed with anaesthesia even with low levels of haemoglobin, particularly in chronically anaemic patients, provided blood loss is likely to be minimal, or the operation is urgent and the patient's heart is not likely to decompensate. In such cases any blood loss should be promptly replaced, preferably with packed cells, remembering that oxygen-carrying capacity is reduced in stored blood. If oxygen-carrying capacity is critically important, fresh blood may be needed. Additional packed cells may be given slowly to raise the haemoglobin. The inspired oxygen concentration should be increased and oxygen should be continued in the recovery room and even longer, if anaemia is severe.

BLOOD LOSS

Anaemia in surgical patients is often the result of recent blood loss, which may be the reason for surgery. If the patient is hypovolaemic, preoperative resuscitation, possibly including blood transfusion, is needed.

PHYSIOLOGICAL ANAEMIA

In infants aged about 2–3 months, the haemoglobin levels may fall to 10–11 g/100 ml. It may decrease to much lower levels in those who were born prematurely. The anaemia is associated with the change to adult haemoglobin, lack of erythropoietin and an immature bone marrow. It may be aggravated if the infant has had blood sampled frequently.

HEREDITARY SPHEROCYTOSIS

This is an autosomal dominant condition in which the abnormal red cells are prematurely removed by the spleen, leading to a haemolytic anaemia. Splenectomy will prevent further haemolysis although it does not correct the basic red-cell defect. Splenectomy should be deferred until at least 5 years of age or later, because of the increased risk of overwhelming infection after splenectomy in young children. Preoperative transfusion is usually unnecessary.

THALASSAEMIA MAJOR

This is an autosomal recessive condition with shortened red-cell survival time, ineffective erythropoiesis and severe anaemia. It is due to a quantitative deficiency in beta chains in adult haemoglobin. These patients are transfusion-dependent. Anaesthetists, because of their expertise at venepuncture, occasionally become involved in their care. Application of EMLA cream 1–2 hours beforehand reduces the child's distress from repeated venepuncture. Haemosiderosis and hypersplenism can occur if an adequate chelation programme is not followed. The former may lead to cardiac failure and the latter is an indication for splenectomy.

Preoperative transfusion is necessary if the patient is very anaemic. Extra blood can be autotransfused from the spleen by clamping the splenic artery first, or injecting adrenaline into the spleen (if halothane is not being used). Preoperative assessment of cardiac function is important, especially if the patient has haemosiderosis.

AUTOIMMUNE HAEMOLYTIC ANAEMIA

Splenectomy is occasionally needed for patients who do not respond to conservative treatment (including steroids). Preoperative transfusion is indicated only if anaemia is severe. Steroid cover may be needed.

SICKLE-CELL DISEASE

This is an autosomal recessive disease most commonly occurring in people of African descent. It is due to the presence of haemoglobin S, in which a valine molecule is substituted for glutamic acid in the beta chain. This causes the haemoglobin S molecule to form polymers at low oxygen tension, leading to sickling, increased rigidity of red cells and increased viscosity. This may cause infarcts, which are characteristic of the disease. The severity of the anaemia depends on the amount of HbS present.

In homozygous sickle-cell disease the HbS content is 80−100%, the remainder being HbF. Sickle-cell thalassaemia (SF) has 67−82% HbS and is less severe, but should be managed as sickle-cell disease when the patient is undergoing anaesthesia. The homozygous sickle-cell disease is less severe in the newborn because of the presence of a greater amount of HbF.

Sickling crises are precipitated by hypoxia, acidaemia, stasis and cooling, and it is of the utmost importance to avoid these during anaesthesia. Prophylaxis may include treatment with sodium bicarbonate and low-molecular-weight dextran. Additional oxygen, mild hyperventilation and an intravenous infusion are desirable during anaesthesia; steps should be taken to prevent cooling. Postoperatively, care must be taken to ensure that hypoventilation and hypoxia do not occur. Continued bicarbonate and oxygen therapy are helpful prophylaxis. The haemoglobin is usually 7−8 g/100 ml, but transfusion is not absolutely necessary unless the haemoglobin is below 5 g/100 ml. Ideally surgery is undertaken when the haemoglobin is 8 g/100 ml, or more [4].

OTHER CAUSES OF ANAEMIA

These are listed in medical and paediatric textbooks. In some countries, chronic anaemia may result from worm infestation or malaria. The same principles apply to the anaesthetic management of these patients.

OVERVIEW

When a child's haemoglobin is less than 11 g/100 ml the reason should be sought. It may be in the normal physiological range in babies 3−6 months old. Recent blood loss from haemorrhage or burns are obvious causes. It is desirable to have haemoglobin levels over 10 mg/100 ml in otherwise normal patients before anaesthesia for elective surgery. Anaemic patients should be considered individually, and lower haemoglobin levels may reasonably be accepted. Below 7 g/100 ml, at which level cardiac output increases to compensate for the anaemia and decompensation becomes more likely, the risks of anaesthesia and the possibility of tissue hypoxia will increase as the haemoglobin level drops.

MUSCLE DISEASES

General considerations

Muscle disease can be broadly divided into three categories:
1 Muscular dystrophy
2 Myotonia
3 Other myopathies.

Most of these are genetically determined. Although most anaesthetists do not encounter them very often, they are a cause for concern because of some unusual responses to drugs, and because these patients are prone to respiratory and cardiac complications as the diseases progress. Lack of respiratory reserve may not be obvious because the patient may not exercise and heart disease may be subtle and not easily recognized. The patient may die suddenly, during or after the operation, sometimes several hours after apparently adequate recovery from anaesthesia. This has happened following halothane, ketamine, and nitrous oxide relaxant anaesthesia. The cause of death cannot always be explained, although the effects of hypoxia and hypercarbia must often be suspected. Although the deaths were usually in severely debilitated children, this was not always the case.

The other cause for concern among anaesthetists is the possibility of malignant hyperpyrexia. This condition is discussed elsewhere (see Chapters 2 and 27) but is associated in many cases with a myopathy, which may not be clinically obvious. An elevated creatinine phosphokinase (CPK) level is usual, but this can also be elevated in some patients with muscular dystrophy such as Duchenne's, who do not often develop malignant hyperpyrexia.

Preoperative assessment is important, especially when the disease is advanced. It is helpful to know the diagnosis because some of these conditions are associated with abnormal responses to drugs, particularly muscle relaxants. The extent of the muscle disease and its effect on respiratory function should, where possible, be defined by spirometry (vital capacity, tidal volume, FEV_1, etc.) and other respiratory function tests. Clinical assessment of cardiovascular function should be supplemented, when indicated, by chest X-ray, ECG and, if necessary, echocardiography. Respiratory and myocardial depressant drugs should be used with care, or avoided altogether, if there is any suspicion that function may be impaired. Local anaesthetic blocks may be useful for analgesia.

Some of these diseases, such as dystrophia myotonica, involve other organ systems; there may be endocrine dysfunction such as diabetes mellitus and hypothyroidism.

The effective dose of muscle relaxants may be significantly reduced in patients with severe muscle disease. Atracurium, due to its rapid breakdown, is the muscle relaxant of choice. When muscle relaxants are used, neuromuscular monitoring should be used. The anaesthetist should aim to avoid postoperative respiratory depression by ensuring adequate antagonism of the muscle relaxants at the end of the operation. Analgesia must be provided, but opioids should be titrated carefully to avoid respiratory depression.

Specific diseases

DYSTROPHIES

Duchenne

Duchenne pseudohypertrophic muscular dystrophy is an X-linked recessive disease that usually presents between 2 and 6 years of age. Clumsiness, easy tiring when walking, and a tendency to fall are early symptoms. The muscles are infiltrated with fibrous fatty tissue that increases muscle bulk. There is ECG evidence of cardiac involvement in up to 70% of children [5]. Impaired contractility or dysrhythmia may contribute to anaesthetic mortality [5, 6]. Seventy-five per cent of these children die before the age of 20, frequently succumbing to pneumonia.

A wide variety of anaesthetic agents has been used successfully. Although suxamethonium and halothane have been used on many children with Duchenne dystrophy who suffered no untoward effects, these have been associated on occasion with serious perioperative complications. While some of these appear to be typical malignant hyperpyrexia (MH) reactions, others only manifest some of the features of MH, such as temperature elevation, hypokalaemia or rhabdomyolysis [5, 7, 8]. Creatine phosphokinase (CPK) levels are usually high in these patients and cannot be used to indicate propensity to MH [9].

Sensitivity to non-depolarizing relaxants depends on how far the disease has progressed. Some children may even show a slight resistance. When muscle relaxants are used, neuromuscular monitoring is needed.

Weakness, inadequate cough and restrictive lung disease (kyphoscoliosis) make inadequate ventilation a major perioperative problem. Heavy sedation should be avoided. IPPV may be required; it may also be needed after operation, if vital capacity is less than 50% of the predicted value [10]. Acute gastric dilatation is an occasional postoperative complication, with increased risk of aspiration.

Children with Duchenne muscular dystrophy undergoing spinal surgery have an increased bleeding tendency, even if induced hypotension is used. A vessel abnormality associated with the myopathy may be the cause.

Anaesthetic problems can be reduced by avoiding potent inhalational agents, using non-depolarizing muscle relaxants instead of suxamethonium, careful assessment of respiratory function, and monitoring for malignant hyperpyrexia.

Becker's

Becker's muscular dystrophy is similar to Duchenne but usually has a later onset and slower progression. Muscle enzymes may not be as elevated.

Limb girdle

In limb girdle dystrophy (Leyden–Mobius and Erb's juvenile types), the pelvic girdle and then usually the shoulder girdle become involved. The disease gradually progresses over 15–20 years.

Facio-scapulohumeral

Facio-scapulohumeral muscular dystrophy (Landouzy–Dejerine) usually develops in late childhood, up to the early twenties. It is a static, or only slowly progressive, disease.

MYOTONIA

Myotonia is delayed relaxation after muscle contraction, which may be aggravated by cold or emotional stress. It cannot be prevented during anaesthesia by the use of muscle relaxants or spinal or epidural anaesthesia, as the defect is in the muscle itself. It is improved by procainamide, steroids or quinine [11, 12].

Myotonia congenita

Myotonia congenita (Thomsen's) presents at any time during childhood and causes only mild disability. Myotonia is exacerbated by cold and is often accompanied by muscle hypertrophy. One case has been reported of generalized spasms precipitated by suxamethonium, which made ventilation almost impossible [13]. This was in an adult patient. Hypothermia and anaesthetic agents that cause shivering, such as halothane, should be avoided.

Myotonic dystrophy

Juvenile and adult-onset myotonic dystrophy are inherited autosomal dominant myopathies. Children presenting before 5 years of age are nearly always the offspring of affected mothers [14]. Neonates with this condition present as 'floppy babies' due to generalized hypotonia. Respiratory distress is common. The cry is weak; swallowing and sucking mechanisms are impaired. Facial diplegia with a 'tent-shaped' mouth and arthrogryposis are common. Over the first years of life, tone and muscle power improve, but mental retardation and delayed speech development become apparent. Progression to the adult multi-system disease — cataracts, gonadal atrophy, frontal baldness, thyroid dysfunction, diabetes mellitus, cardiac conduction defects and impaired pulmonary function — is inevitable. By the age of 10 years, 75% of these children have clinical myotonia.

Surgery is usually for correction of talipes equinovarus (present in 50%), myringotomy (disordered swallowing and palatal muscle function) and inguinal hernia repair (disordered skeletal muscle).

Anaesthetic problems depend on the progression of the disease. Hypotonic neonates require greatly reduced doses of non-depolarizing muscle relaxants [15], but older children respond normally [16]. Dystrophic changes in the adult indicate a reduced dose [17]. Depolarizing relaxants can induce generalized contracture and ventilatory embarrassment, even in those patients whose myotonia is not obvious [18].

Despite previous teachings, thiopentone can be safely used in these patients, provided care is taken with dose and rate of injection when there is myocardial involvement or borderline respiratory function. Papaveretum and hyoscine have been used without adverse effect [16].

Aspiration is a major contributor to mortality in all age groups, and precautions should be taken against this. Muscle relaxation should be monitored and full recovery achieved before the patient leaves the operating room. There is a risk of silent aspiration when spontaneous ventilation with a mask is used. Agents causing a significant decrease in postoperative conscious state should be avoided. Prophylactic antacids or H_2 receptor antagonists should be considered.

Myocardial involvement, characterized both by defects in the conduction system and by abnormalities of the contractile mechanism, is present even in neonates [19]. The myocardial depressant effects of potent inhalational agents must be considered. Cardiac decompensation from enflurane has been reported in a patient with myotonia dystrophica [20].

The response to reversal of the non-depolarizing block in the adult form of the disease may be normal, neuromuscular blockade can increase, or a tonic response may ensue [20]. Mechanical ventilation to treat residual paralysis has been advocated as the safest course of action [21], although in one series there were no ill effects in six children reversed with neostigmine [16]. A logical approach if relaxation is required is to use atracurium because it is rapidly metabolized. If reversal is necessary, neostigmine can be titrated in small doses.

Local or regional anaesthesia is often an alternative to general anaesthesia. Caudal anaesthesia has been advocated in those children undergoing lower-extremity surgery [22].

Anaesthesia must be tailored to the individual patient. The degree of muscle weakness, the risk of aspiration, cardiomyopathy, the response to muscle relaxants and the occurrence of myotonic contractures must all be considered. ECG and neuromuscular blockade monitoring are advisable. Facilities should be available for postoperative ventilation.

OTHER MYOPATHIES

Oculocraniosomatic syndrome

This usually presents at about 10 years of age with ptosis and limitation of eye movements. It may be accompanied by neurological disorders and cardiac conduction defects.

Congenital myopathies

These often present in infancy with hypotonia.

Familial periodic paralysis

Hypokalaemic type. This presents with severe, episodic asymmetric weakness or paralysis of limb and trunk muscles, which may last 12–48 hours. It can be precipitated by cold, exercise, a large carbohydrate meal, insulin or adrenaline. It may be associated with cardiac dysrhythmia and respiratory insufficiency, which should be treated with potassium chloride.

If these patients present for anaesthesia it is important to check the potassium level preoperatively, to monitor the electrocardiogram and electrolytes if the procedure is prolonged, and to avoid cold and stimuli that may increase catecholamine secretion. Beta-blockade may be useful. Postoperative weakness or dysrhythmia should be treated with potassium chloride if potassium is low [23, 24].

Hyperkalaemic type. These patients may have more frequent attacks of paralysis which last 2 or 3 hours. The attack may be precipitated by suxamethonium, potassium chloride, cold and fasting. During anaesthesia, ECG should be monitored and plasma potassium kept within normal limits. If potassium rises, diuretics, glucagon, adrenaline or salbutamol may help to reduce it [25].

Dermatomyositis (polymyositis)

The main clinical features of this disease are:
1 pathognomonic skin rash involving the upper eyelids and extensor surfaces of knuckles, elbows and knees;
2 weakness of the proximal muscles, and sometimes the pharyngeal and laryngeal muscles;
3 vasculitis, with intimal proliferation and thrombosis.
Anaesthetic problems include muscle weakness, particularly involving the muscles of respiration and deglutition. Occasionally there are contractures that make intubation difficult. Patients may be taking steroids and need cover for surgery (see Chapter 6).

In one patient studied, the effect of suxamethonium was to produce a contracture (upward EMG baseline drift) at the same time as relaxation began. The degree of paralysis and duration of action were normal after 1 mg/kg. As there is a lack of studies with nondepolarizing relaxants these drugs should be used cautiously [26].

Myositis ossificans progressiva

This is a rare disease with bony infiltration of the tendons, fascia, aponeuroses and muscles. It develops at any time from birth to late childhood. The patients usually die from respiratory failure in early adult life, due to thoracic involvement, which leads to decreased compliance, aspiration and asphyxia.

If anaesthesia is required, intubation may be difficult because of ankylosis of the neck and involvement of the masseter and the temporomandibular joints.

Central core disease

These patients have a diffuse weakness and are slender, without any focal muscle wasting. They may have congenital dislocation of the hip, lordosis or kyphoscoliosis. The site of the abnormality is in the central core of the muscle fibre.

There are several families with the disease who are malignant-hyperpyrexia susceptible, some with normal CPK. If this is suspected, muscle biopsy is advisable [27] (see Chapter 27).

Muscle biopsy

This is probably the most common reason for anaesthesia in children with muscle disease or muscle wasting from neurological disease. General anaesthesia is usually preferred, especially for small children, but the procedure should be performed quickly and the patient monitored carefully, especially for temperature changes.

When there has been no family history of malignant hyperpyrexia, nitrous oxide, oxygen and halothane, with or without thiopentone, has often been used.

Sedation and local or regional anaesthesia can be used, but local infiltration of the biopsy site is undesirable because the biopsy tissue may be distorted by the injection.

NEUROMUSCULAR AND NEUROLOGICAL DISEASES

Myasthenia gravis [28, 29]

This is a condition where there is interference of normal transmission at the neuromuscular junction, resulting in weakness. About 10% of myasthenics are under 16 years of age. These children fall into three groups:

1 Neonatal transient myasthenia gravis is uncommon and affects the newborn of 10–15% of mothers with the disease. It is due to passive transfer of acetylcholine (ACh) receptor antibody or to immune cell transfer to the fetus. The condition usually resolves after 5 weeks and responds to anticholinesterase.

2 Congenital myasthenic syndromes: these include several rare conditions which differ from the neonatal and autoimmune forms. Acetylcholine receptor antibodies are not present [30].

3 Juvenile myasthenia gravis occurs in children over the age of 1 year (mean onset 13 years), predominantly in females. It has similar features to the adult disease in which there is a reduction in acetylcholine receptors at the neuromuscular junction, due to the sustained release of acetylcholine receptor antibodies. It may be limited to the extrinsic eye muscles (about 25%) or affect all voluntary muscles. Thymectomy is usually performed in the more severe cases. This initially improves the remission rate and is more successful within a year of presentation [31].

The usual diagnostic tests for myasthenia gravis are:

1 Edrophonium (Tensilon) 20–200 µg/kg will improve muscle power.

2 Repetitive supramaximal nerve stimulation at 2 Hz results in a decremental response (fade) and post-tetanic facilitation, followed, after about 30 seconds, by post-tetanic exhaustion.

3 D-tubocurarine (0.05 mg/kg) can be used as a provocative test. This normally insignificant dose will cause a marked increase in weakness.

Facilities for assisted ventilation must be available when these tests are performed.

Myasthenia is treated with an anticholinesterase such as neostigmine or pyridostigmine. In the neonatal transient type, dosage can be gradually reduced as the weakness decreases. If secretions are troublesome, the dose is reduced and a small dose of atropine can be given.

Treatment of the disease may include thymectomy. Preoperatively, anticholinesterase treatment is continued until the night before or, in severe cases, up to the time of operation. If the patient is being treated with steroids, extra cover may be needed. The choice of anaesthesia will depend on the degree of weakness at induction. Because anticholinesterase treatment has been stopped, there is some muscle weakness which may make intubation possible without the aid of muscle relaxants. An inhalation anaesthetic can be used and local anaesthetic can be applied to the larynx. Thiopentone, sometimes followed by a muscle relaxant, nitrous oxide and an inhalation or opioid supplement, may be used. Neuromuscular monitoring is desirable with such an anaesthetic. Myasthenic patients are resistant to suxamethonium and sensitive to non-depolarizing relaxants (Figs 25.1, 25.2). The latter can be used, but in increments of one-tenth the usual dose. The short action of atracurium is advantageous (Fig. 25.3).

Postoperative problems may include respiratory muscle weakness and retention of secretions due to the inability to cough adequately. Myasthenic crisis may result from lack of treatment, or cholinergic crisis from over-treatment with anticholinesterases. In the latter case, management is complicated by excessive bronchial secretions. All these complications can be controlled by intubation or tracheostomy and mechanical ventilation. When a cholinergic crisis occurs, atropine with a small dose of non-depolarizing relaxant is given, to rest the neuromuscular junction while the patient is ventilated. Infection should be prevented or treated and adequate nutrition must be maintained.

Epilepsy

Children with epilepsy, particularly those requiring continuous medication, should be effectively controlled preoperatively and their anti-epileptic treatment continued. Some of these children are mentally retarded.

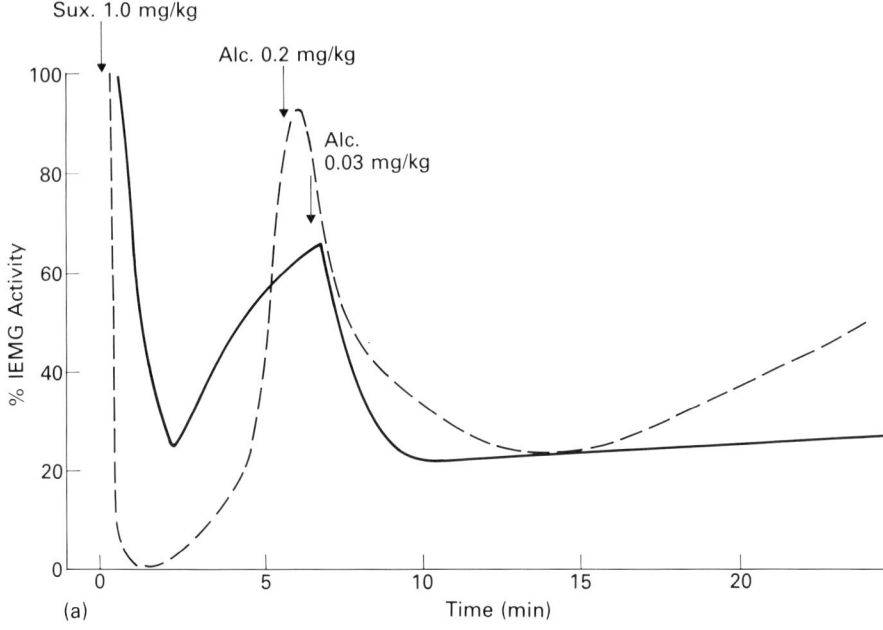

(a)

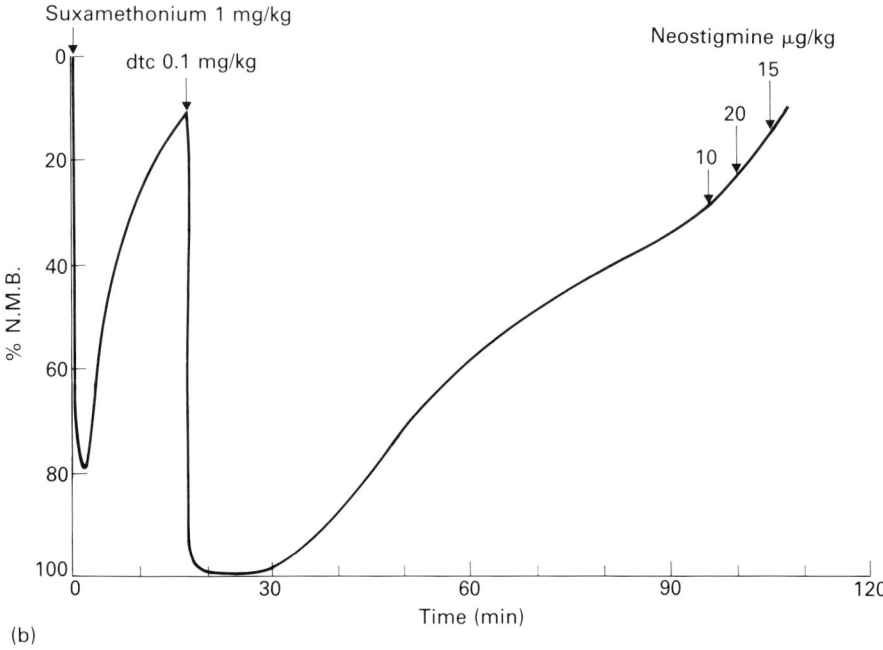

(b)

Fig. 25.1 Electromyographic recordings of patients with myasthenia gravis showing resistance to suxamethonium, and marked sensitivity to small doses of (a) alcuronium and (b) D-tubocurarine.

The anticonvulsant drugs are often involved in drug interactions. Enzyme induction by barbiturates and the closely related hydantoins will increase the metabolism of many drugs, including volatile anaesthetics such as halothane. The dose of thiopentone needed may be unpredictable. Phenytoin makes patients resistant to pancuronium, vecuronium and alcuronium, but not atracurium [32]. Increased phenytoin toxicity in the postoperative period may follow enzyme inhibition by drugs sharing a common metabolic pathway, or depression of liver function during general anaesthesia.

Anaesthetic agents that increase EEG activity, such as enflurane, ketamine and methohexitone, and factors that may precipitate convulsions, such as hypoxia or hypocarbia, should be avoided.

Long-term treatment with phenytoin (Dilantin) causes hyperplasia of the gums, but this does not usually cause any anaesthetic problem.

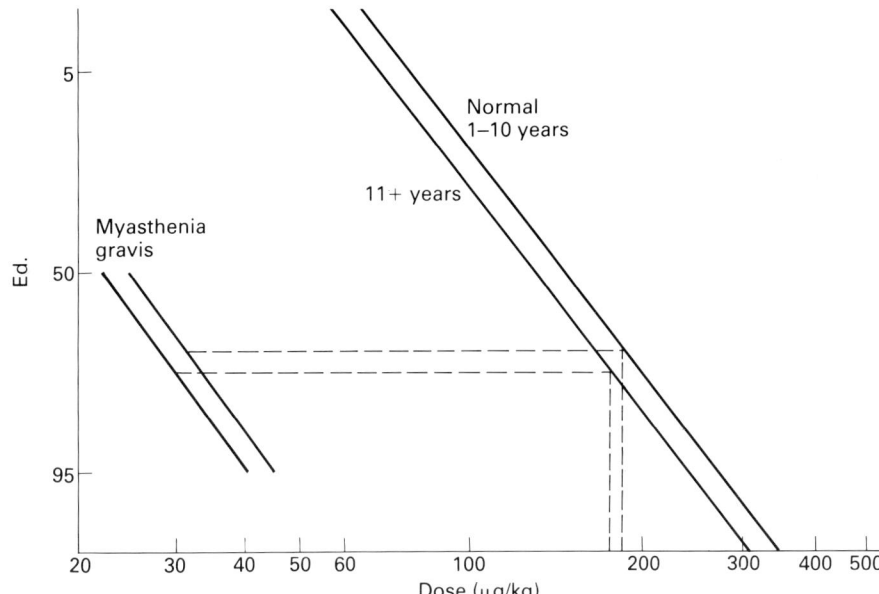

Fig. 25.2 Comparison of the alcuronium dose responses of normal children with two myasthenic children.

Cerebral palsy

This term covers disorders of motor function resulting from pre- and perinatal damage to the CNS. They are non-progressive, with various causes and prognoses. They are divided into:

1 spastic (75%), involving from one to all four limbs;
2 choreoathetosis (20%);
3 ataxia (1–2%).

Associated defects include seizures (60%), mental retardation in many, particularly spastic tetraplegics, and impaired speech and sensory functions. It may be difficult or impossible to communicate with these children. Sometimes it is helpful to the anaesthetist to have the person who cares for the child to accompany the patient to the operating theatre.

The cause may be obscure. Among those known are intrauterine bleeding, infections, toxins, congenital malformations, birth trauma and hypoxia, neonatal infections, hypoglycaemia and kernicterus.

The anaesthetic problems are predominantly due to drug therapy, e.g. anticonvulsants may alter the

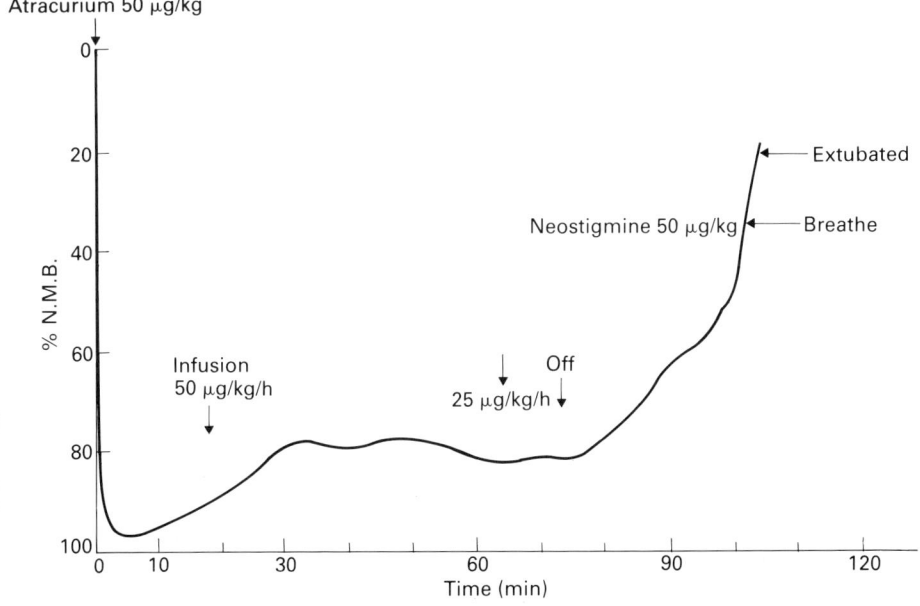

Fig. 25.3 Electromyographic recording of the effect of very small doses of atracurium in a myasthenia gravis patient, demonstrating extreme sensitivity. It also shows the value of monitoring neuromuscular block in these patients when muscle relaxants are used.

metabolism of anaesthetic agents such as thiopentone. Deformities may make posturing on the operating table difficult and special care is then necessary to prevent pressure necrosis.

Spinal cord injury

QUADRIPLEGIA

This usually follows neck trauma and these patients have several problems that affect anaesthesia [33]:

1 A recent quadriplegic may have an unstable cervical spine leading to intubation difficulties, particularly if neck movement may destroy any further chance of recovery from recent trauma. Muscle atrophy makes these patients susceptible to severe hyperkalaemia when suxamethonium is used, leading to dysrhythmia and cardiac arrest. This may occur from a few days up to 6 months after injury. Suxamethonium should be avoided in this period [34, 35].

2 Quadriplegics may develop muscle spasms and autonomic hyperreflexia and they may need anaesthesia to control spasms during surgery, even though there is no sensation at the operative site. Acute hypertension may occur.

3 Respiratory failure is common because they have lost their intercostal muscle function and may have partial diaphragmatic palsy, resulting in ineffective cough with a tendency to respiratory infection. They are usually treated lying supine because of the instability of the cervical spine. Vital capacity is often considerably reduced.

4 These patients are also prone to gastric dilatation, inhalation of gastric content and paralytic ileus leading to a distended abdomen. Pulmonary emboli can occur due to immobility. Extra fluids may be needed if induction causes vasodilatation. Care must be taken to avoid overloading with fluids, leading to pulmonary oedema or, alternatively, a vasoconstrictor may be indicated.

Respiratory reserve may be so tenuous that anaesthesia may depress respiration sufficiently to require postoperative controlled or intermittent mandatory ventilation. If respiratory assistance is needed for prolonged periods, a tracheostomy may be helpful for removal of secretions. In some patients, continuing ventilatory support which can eventually be carried out at home will be necessary. Insertion of a diaphragmatic pacemaker is another alternative.

5 Temperature regulation is disturbed by transection above C7. As the sympathetic outflow is below this level the ability to sweat and to vasoconstrict in response to cooling is abolished.

6 The cardiovascular compensatory mechanisms may be impaired, with difficulty in compensating for postural changes, IPPV and fluid loads. These patients may be particularly susceptible to central depressant drugs, such as thiopentone, which may lead to vasodilatation and hypotension. If this occurs, intravenous fluid loading or a vasopressor drug may be needed.

7 Antidiuretic hormone is often increased, increasing the risk of cerebral oedema, if too much water is administered. Plasma sodium levels should be monitored.

8 Nutritional deficiency may develop and anaemia is common.

9 Urinary tract infection leading to renal impairment is common in these patients. It is of utmost importance that, if the bladder is catheterized, this should be undertaken under strict sterile conditions. Neomycin bladder washouts may also help to reduce the incidence of urinary infection.

10 Acid−base and electrolyte imbalance and respiratory acidosis from alveolar hypoventilation are common. Metabolic alkalosis may be compensatory or due to vomiting and gastric suction, in which case there may be hypokalaemia as well.

11 These patients are prone to pressure sores and pressure areas must be well padded, especially during anaesthesia.

12 The need for non-depolarizing muscle relaxants is minimal, as these patients are already paralysed and their muscles atrophied.

13 Other occasional problems include perforated ulcers, which may be silent, and myositis ossificans.

PARAPLEGIA

Paraplegia may be a consequence of trauma, tumour or spinal haemorrhage, and occasionally follows operations for spinal abnormalities.

Many of the problems of quadriplegics may exist in paraplegics, although some to a lesser extent depending on the level of the block [36].

The mentally retarded child

Mentally retarded or intellectually handicapped children present for a variety of procedures under anaesthesia, especially dental conservation and extraction. It appears that intellectual impairment does not increase the risk of anaesthesia, but the cause of the impairment may do so.

The difficulty the anaesthetist faces is in determining how much the child can communicate and respond to people. It is sometimes helpful to have a parent or person who knows the child well to accompany him or her to the induction room, especially if the child becomes agitated on separation. Similarly their presence may be helpful in the recovery room.

Neurofibromatosis (von Recklinghausen's disease)

This condition is characterized by cafe-au-lait spots and tumours of the nerve trunks and sometimes the central nervous system. There is a wide variety of manifestations, including an increased incidence of phaeochromocytoma and kyphoscoliosis; about 10% may be mentally retarded. Some of the problems arise from compression of surrounding structures by the tumour. Tumours growing in the laryngeal region, for instance, can cause stridor or difficulty with intubation and access for surgical removal. In some cases the abdominal aorta is abnormal, often with renal artery stenosis, causing hypertension.

Werdnig—Hoffman disease (spinal muscular atrophy)

This is an infantile, progressive spinal muscular atrophy presenting as a floppy infant. Onset may be *in utero* or during the early months of life. These infants may have intercostal paralysis and be dependent on diaphragmatic respiration. Bulbar involvement will further embarrass respiration. Pneumonia, commonly following aspiration, is the most common complication. Most infants die by the age of 2—3 years. Less severe forms are referred to as the chronic spinal muscular atrophies.

Muscle biopsy is the most likely reason for anaesthesia. This shows a denervation pattern, with large bundles of atrophied fibres interspersed with bundles of normal or hypertrophied fibres.

Careful preoperative assessment of respiratory reserve is essential. A light halothane anaesthetic can be used for muscle biopsy, but care must be taken to ensure adequate oxygenation and ventilation. Local anaesthetics can be used.

Friedreich's ataxia

This is the most common of the hereditary ataxias and the most variable in its manifestations. Onset is in late childhood, and the findings include a typical foot deformity (pes cavus), kyphoscoliosis, ataxia and a variety of clinical features relating to cerebellar disease. Cardiac disease is present in most patients on presentation, and eventually all patients develop cardiomyopathy. When heart disease is present dysrhythmia may occur.

During anaesthesia, care must be taken with cardiac depressant drugs. Muscle relaxants may be used, and although normal responses have been recorded with atracurium, vecuronium and tubocurarine [37, 38], a patient who exhibited extreme sensitivity to tubocurarine has been reported [39]. Atracurium with neuromuscular monitoring is probably the best approach. Careful monitoring, especially of the ECG, is needed, as myocardial degeneration and fibrosis may be present. Epidural morphine has been used successfully as part of the anaesthetic for major abdominal surgery [37].

Leigh's syndrome (sub-acute necrotizing encephalomyelopathy)

This occurs in the first 2 years of life with respiratory symptoms, cranial nerve dysfunction, abnormal movements and incoordination; it may present with nonspecific problems such as feeding difficulties, hypotonia or pyramidal tract signs. The CT and MRI scans are characteristic; serum and CSF lactate and pyruvate levels are elevated. In some patients with respiratory symptoms, respiratory failure has been precipitated by general anaesthesia [40a].

Dystonia musculorem deformans

This condition is characterized by involuntary dystonic movements of the limbs, trunk or both. These patients have a normal response to muscle relaxants and the spasms relax with anaesthesia [40].

Familial dysautonomia (Riley—Day syndrome) [41, 42]

Familial dysautonomia is a rare autosomal recessive disease associated with autonomic dysfunction. The clinical features in the newborn include episodes of vasomotor instability, pallor, unresponsiveness, impaired response to pain, hypotonia, inability to suckle and gastric reflux. The latter leads to a high incidence of aspiration pneumonia in infants, who sometimes present for fundoplication. In older children, retarded growth, emotional lability, periodic vomiting, abdominal pain, lack of tears and unstable temperature control may be presenting symptoms. Episodic crises of vasomotor instability with hypotension, nausea and vomiting, can be controlled with diazepam. Patients may be indifferent to pain, being able to identify it but unaware of discomfort. This results in some patients developing corneal ulceration, aggravated by lack of tears. A smooth tongue, with absent taste buds, and postural hypotension are common features. A swallowing defect contributes to secondary respiratory disease, a common cause of death. The clinical features appear to be associated with insufficient acetylcholine and abnormal catecholamine metabolism. The latter leads to hypersensitivity to infused noradrenaline. Changes in the hypothalamus, brain stem and autonomic ganglia have been observed; there is a marked decrease in unmyelinated nerve fibres.

The most common anaesthetic problems are cardiovascular instability, postoperative vomiting, aspiration and recurrent chest infection. Defective respiratory response to CO_2 and hypoxia and unstable temperature control may add to the difficulties of anaesthetic management.

Premedication with chlorpromazine has been suggested and diazepam has been used. In most instances these patients appear to respond normally to atropine. They have been induced with intravenous and inhalation techniques, but doses of thiopentone and inhalation agents should be minimal, to avoid cardiovascular instability. Halothane, for example, causes cardiovascular depression and blood pressure instability when normal doses are used. The response to D-tubocurarine appears normal, although it is wise to titrate the dose, as a smaller than usual dose may provide satisfactory relaxation [43]. A combination of nitrous oxide, oxygen, nondepolarizing relaxant and fentanyl in small doses, with controlled ventilation, appears to be the safest anaesthetic for these patients.

Postoperatively, diazepam may settle a restless child with this condition better than an analgesic. Monitoring needs to be continued.

Moebius anomalad

This condition is due to agenesis of, usually, the VIth and VIIth cranial nerve nuclei, leading to mask-like facies. Micrognathia is a common feature that may make intubation difficult. Aspiration may cause lung complications and failure to thrive.

RENAL DISEASE

Introduction

It is unusual to have to anaesthetize children with acute renal disease such as glomerulonephritis. Anaesthesia for urological problems is discussed in Chapter 11. Chronic renal disease may progress to renal failure.

Assessment of renal function

In normal, healthy children routine urine testing is not always essential, but dipstick testing for glucose and protein can easily be done.

In patients with suspected renal disease the urine should be examined for protein and, if present, for casts and cells. The specific gravity of a first morning specimen gives some indication of concentrating ability, and usually exceeds 1.020.

Blood urea elevation above normal may be due to decreased glomerular filtration from impaired renal function or dehydration. It can be moderately elevated when protein intake is high, as urea is the principal nitrogenous breakdown product of protein metabolism (normal range 2.5–6.7 mmol/l)

Creatinine is normally below 0.06 mmol/l under 4 years of age, 0.08 mmol/l under 10 years and 0.1 mmol/l thereafter. It rises when glomerular filtration rate falls and 75% of function is lost. It is independent of protein intake. Creatinine clearance, which requires a 24-hour urine collection, is a sensitive test of glomerular function.

These are the most commonly performed; for more elaborate tests reference should be made to an appropriate textbook.

Renal failure

The features of renal failure in patients with renal disease will depend on its severity and may be modified by dialysis.

ACID–BASE DISTURBANCES

The kidney is responsible for excretion of excess acid; in renal failure severe metabolic acidosis may develop. This is usually compensated by hyperventilation and a decrease in Pa_{CO_2}. This compensation can be disturbed by respiratory depression during anaesthesia.

ELECTROLYTES

Alterations in electrolytes are common during renal failure. The main dangers are associated with hyperkalaemia and hypocalcaemia, which may cause increased myocardial irritability.

Hypertension is common in patients with chronic renal disease, but can usually be controlled by drugs. When anaesthesia is required, these should be continued, as untreated hypertensives may become hypo- or hypertensive during anaesthesia. Patients taking adrenergic blocking drugs should be given atropine intravenously before induction, to overcome relative parasympathetic overactivity. Alpha-methyldopa, reserpine and propranolol lower the minimum alveolar concentration (MAC).

ANAEMIA

Anaemia is present in patients with chronic renal failure unless they are treated with erythropoietin. Haemoglobin levels may be as low as 4 g/100 ml, but the increase in 2-3-DPG levels and cardiac output allows adequate oxygen transport to the tissues to be maintained. Depression of cardiac output by anaesthetic drugs may decrease the oxygen supply to critical levels in very anaemic patients.

FLUID BALANCE

Patients in renal failure who are anaemic and hypertensive have little cardiac reserve and, if also hypoalbuminaemic, may easily develop congestive cardiac failure and pulmonary oedema. If there is some renal function, larger than usual doses of diuretics may be needed to increase urine output.

Anaesthetic considerations

Most drugs used in general anaesthesia may be employed in patients with renal disease and renal failure. The exceptions are enflurane and methoxyflurane, which are nephrotoxic when used in high dosage, for prolonged periods or in association with other nephrotoxic drugs such as gentamicin. The older muscle relaxants, gallamine and decamethonium, are excreted unchanged by the kidney. D-tubocurarine, alcuronium and pancuronium have an alternative means of elimination via the liver and bile. Vecuronium is 85% excreted by this route and can be used, but atracurium is considered the drug of choice in renal failure because it is totally metabolized. Suxamethonium, which causes a small rise in potassium in normal patients, should be used with caution in patients who have uraemia and a high plasma potassium. Sleep time may be prolonged after thiopentone. Plasma albumin and thus plasma protein binding are reduced in uraemia. The potential for bleeding caused by platelet dysfunction makes regional blocks more hazardous, although brachial plexus blocks are used for the insertion of shunts in the forearm.

Patients with chronic disease or renal failure may be receiving a number of drugs, including antihypertensives and steroids. End-stage renal failure requires renal transplantation. The anaesthetic problems are similar to those in chronic renal failure. These patients are more prone to infection.

LIVER DISEASE

When there is extensive disease of the liver, interference with the biotransformation of drugs might be expected. Drug action may be prolonged in severe liver disease, but there is usually sufficient reserve function for biotransformation to continue, unless liver failure is imminent. There is no substantial evidence that the use of analgesics, sedatives or tranquillizers is contraindicated in the presence of hepatic disease, provided the patient does not have encephalopathy due to liver failure. These drugs should be used carefully, in smaller and less frequent doses, until the patient's response is determined. Central nervous system depressants and local anaesthetics should be used cautiously if hepatic damage is severe.

All anaesthetic agents and techniques may reduce liver blood flow by lowering cardiac output and mean arterial blood pressure, or by altering splanchnic resistance. Maintenance of normal Pa_{CO_2} and avoidance of hypotension and myocardial depression will help to limit these changes in patients with liver disease.

Patients with severe liver disease may develop a coagulopathy.

Patients with acute viral hepatitis should not undergo elective surgery, as there is often further deterioration in liver function postoperatively. Hepatitis A and B are the usual forms of viral hepatitis; a marker for posttransfusion hepatitis or hepatitis C has recently been isolated and its presence can be detected serologically. Cytomegalovirus, Epstein−Barr and herpes simplex viruses may also cause hepatitis.

Liver transplantation for end-stage liver disease is now performed in many specialist centres, with 1-year survival rates in children between 65% and 85%. The anaesthetist has to cope not only with the problems of advanced liver disease, but also those of a prolonged surgical procedure, massive blood loss, profound circulatory changes, rapid and complex electrolyte disturbances, renal hypoperfusion and hypothermia (see Chapter 11).

GASTROINTESTINAL DISEASES

Malabsorption and protein loss from the gut result in poor general health, and cause some specific problems that require consideration and, if possible, treatment before surgery.

Malabsorption of fat may be accompanied by deficiency of fat-soluble vitamins (A, D, E, K). The latter may result in hypoprothrombinaemia, which should be treated with vitamin K injection preoperatively.

Iron and folate deficiency anaemias may occur. Malnutrition may be severe enough to cause hypoproteinaemia.

There are many causes of protein-losing enteropathy. The two main mechanisms are blockage of lymphatics, and increased mucosal permeability to protein. Protein loss may occur in coeliac disease, tropical sprue, gastrointestinal infections and infestations, ulcerative colitis, radiation enteritis, and in association with polyps.

Low plasma protein results in alterations in fluid distribution, with oedema formation, and in changes in the protein binding of drugs.

Protein deficiency may also result from inadequate intake in the diet, as in kwashiorkor. The resulting hypoalbuminaemia has been shown to reduce protein binding of thiopentone by 10−15% in these patients.

Specific disorders

CHRONIC INFLAMMATORY BOWEL DISEASE

These include ulcerative colitis and Crohn's disease, both of which are likely to be accompanied by mild-to-moderate anaemia. Protein-losing enteropathy may be present. These patients will usually have been under prolonged medical care and are usually sick if they require surgery for their disease.

COELIAC DISEASE

Hypoprothrombinaemia due to vitamin K deficiency may be present in untreated or poorly controlled coeliac disease. Other problems include anaemia due to folate

or iron deficiency, oedema as a result of hypoproteinaemia, and rickets secondary to vitamin D malabsorption. In well-controlled coeliac disease, none of these should be present.

INTESTINAL LYMPHANGIECTASIA

Rupture of dilated lymphatics results in the loss of lymphocytes, immunoglobulins and fat, resulting in steatorrhoea. Hypoproteinaemia is common and gamma-globulins especially are likely to be low. Thus both cellular and humoral immunity may be depressed. Consideration should be given to the administration of gammaglobulin while the child is anaesthetized.

PANCREATIC ACHYLIA

In childhood this is usually associated with cyclical or constant neutropenia, making the child more prone to infection.

SHORT GUT SYNDROME

Loss of the terminal ileum may limit vitamin B_{12} and bile salt absorption. Colectomy results in a reduced ability to reabsorb water, and sodium and salt depletion occur very rapidly from an ileostomy. Ex-premature babies who have long segments of gut resected for necrotizing enterocolitis may suffer from under-nutrition and need parenteral nutrition for survival — 50 cm of gut is estimated to be necessary for independent survival.

ENDOCRINE DISEASES

Introduction

Apart from patients with diabetes mellitus, children with endocrine diseases do not often present for anaesthesia. If they do, they have usually been diagnosed and well prepared. The major problems for the anaesthetist are deficiency or over-secretion of the relevant hormone. Surgery may be undertaken to correct the latter, in which case decreased secretion after operation may require replacement until the patient is stabilized. The endocrinologist or physician who has been caring for the patient will usually supervise this. In this section, therefore, the management of the patient with diabetes mellitus will be highlighted; some of the other paediatric endocrine problems that may confront the anaesthetist will be outlined. Phaeochromocytoma is considered in Chapter 11.

Diabetes mellitus

A diabetic child who needs anaesthesia may present a number of problems. In acute surgical illness or trauma, loss of diabetic control with hyperglycaemia and possibly ketosis is likely. In the perioperative period, maintaining appropriate blood glucose levels may not be a problem in an otherwise healthy diabetic child undergoing elective surgery, but in unstable patients careful diabetic control is essential to prevent hypoglycaemia or hyperglycaemia. Persistent hyperglycaemia may lead to increased risk of wound infection, dehydration and ketosis.

Children with diabetes are usually insulin-dependent and prone to ketosis. This occurs clinically as a result of the progressive destruction of beta cells by an auto-immune process which may start months or years before presentation. At that time about 70% of tissue may have been lost, but with resuscitation and stabilization some return of beta-cell function will occur, particularly in older children. During the resulting period of remission they may be unstable and have wide variation of plasma glucose concentrations during the day. In this stage, they may be well controlled on small doses of insulin, but children are very insulin-sensitive and prone to hypoglycaemia. A diabetic child's clinical state depends on many factors, including the degree of persisting beta-cell function, the type of insulin used, diet, compliance with treatment and emotional state. The family background and their comprehension of the disease are also significant. Thus, at the time of presentation for anaesthesia, a child's diabetes may be stable or unstable and well or poorly controlled. Occasionally, diabetic ketoacidosis mimics an acute abdominal condition, with vomiting, abdominal pain and tenderness, maximal on the right side. Recognition of this may save an unnecessary laparotomy.

PREPARATION FOR ANAESTHESIA

The state of hydration, ketonuria and blood glucose concentration should be assessed to exclude hypoglycaemia and severe hyperglycaemia. If dehydration or ketonuria is present, estimation of electrolyte concentrations and acid−base status is necessary.

Dehydration is usually best corrected with 0.9% (isotonic) or 0.45% solutions of saline, and as de-hydration is usually associated with hyperglycaemia, intravenous glucose is best avoided. If ketoacidosis is present, partial correction of dehydration and acidosis can usually be achieved safely within 6 hours, at which time it should be safe to embark on emergency surgery. If surgery is not urgent, full correction should be carried out over 24 hours.

It is essential to correct hypoglycaemia before the child is anaesthetized. Before elective surgery, food may be given up to 6 hours before operation and glucose fluids up to 2−3 hours before, with appropriate insulin. If hypoglycaemia is present or likely to occur during preoperative fasting, intravenous glucose will be necessary. Fifty per cent dextrose will quickly restore low blood glucose concentrations to an adequate level, but 10% dextrose over some hours may be more appropriate if there are no symptoms of hypoglycaemia.

Neither moderate hyperglycaemia in the absence of dehydration, nor ketonuria, which can be caused by apprehension, in the absence of ketoacidosis are contra-indications to emergency anaesthesia and surgery.

For all but short surgical procedures it is wise to set up an intravenous infusion preoperatively, usually during induction of anaesthesia. If there is some insulin present, 4% dextrose and $\frac{1}{5}$ isotonic saline may be adequate to prevent hypoglycaemia.

It is difficult to give specific guidelines for insulin administration, as each child will present a unique clinical situation. The management will depend on the child's current clinical state, the last dose of long-acting insulin, the type of insulin given, and the stress produced by the illness, trauma or operation.

The stress of anaesthesia and surgery normally causes a rise in blood glucose. The aim of management of the diabetic is to provide enough insulin to prevent hyperglycaemia and ketosis and enough glucose to prevent hypoglycaemia. When a diabetic is having a lengthy operation, an infusion of insulin (0.5 u/kg/h) in saline with a concurrent 5% or 10% glucose infusion running throughout the operative period, is desirable. If the patient is hyperglycaemic or ketotic, less or no glucose is necessary. Blood glucose should be monitored with strip tests such as dextrostix to ensure that hypoglycaemia or severe hyperglycaemia do not occur.

As an alternative approach, if there is severe hyperglycaemia, subcutaneous unmodified insulin in a dose of approximately 10% of the usual daily dose may be given, and may be followed by intravenous infusion of 5% dextrose solution. In the absence of hyperglycaemia, insulin may be withheld preoperatively, provided the child is still within the time of action of the usual dose of long-acting insulin and the anaesthetic will be brief. A more appropriate procedure is to give one-sixth of the usual total insulin dose as unmodified insulin subcutaneously at the usual injection time. This dose is to suppress ketosis and hyperglycaemia.

MANAGEMENT DURING AND AFTER ANAESTHESIA

Whereas prevention of hypoglycaemia is a major concern during anaesthesia, hyperglycaemia and ketosis are additional risks in the postoperative period, when the stress of operation and physical inactivity will together lead to substantially increased insulin requirements. A child should have intravenous glucose (usually 5% concentration) in the postoperative period. If a prolonged blood transfusion is required, blood glucose estimates should be performed at least hourly to determine the need for intermittent or simultaneous glucose infusions, because the amount of glucose in blood, even with ACD or CPD, may be inadequate.

If the child is unable to tolerate oral fluids or food postoperatively, it is usually best to give unmodified insulin by intravenous infusion or, where facilities to control infusions are not available, in 6-hourly subcutaneous injections, rather than continue the child's usual long-acting insulin. The dose is based on the child's usual dose requirements and his weight. In general, from one-eighth to one-quarter of the child's usual daily dose requirements can be given 6-hourly or, if the child is fully insulin-dependent, 0.25 u/kg body weight may be given each 6 hours. The dose may be adjusted according to the response to previous doses, judged by blood glucose estimates. Blood glucose levels are maintained by intravenous dextrose infusion. This regimen is continued until the child is able to tolerate oral feeding. After that the child's normal insulin, in appropriately adjusted dosage, should be given.

KETOACIDOSIS

The diabetic with ketoacidosis is dehydrated and sodium-depleted. There will be glycosuria and ketonuria and, if severe, hyperventilation with depressed consciousness. Vomiting and abdominal pain are common. If ketoacidosis is suspected, laboratory assessment of blood glucose, electrolyte concentrations and acid−base status is essential.

Severe dehydration accompanying ketoacidosis requires initial rapid resuscitation with isotonic saline and insulin (0.1 u/kg/h). As the circulation improves, the rate of infusion should be slowed as there is a danger of developing cerebral oedema. As potassium re-enters the cells when insulin is given, the plasma levels must be monitored and intravenous potassium chloride administered as required. Potassium is not usually infused at a rate exceeding 0.3 mmol/kg/h. It is important to have urine output when administering potassium. Even in the presence of severe acidosis, it is seldom necessary or desirable to give sodium bicarbonate.

The response is monitored by blood glucose, acid−base and electrolyte estimation, frequently at first and then 3−6-hourly.

In such cases anaesthesia and surgery should be delayed, if possible, until circulation is restored, with at least partial correction of dehydration and acidosis, and the potassium level normal. If the operation is not urgent, time should be taken to correct the disturbance before commencing anaesthesia.

HYPOGLYCAEMIA

During prolonged anaesthesia, regular monitoring of blood glucose levels is needed to detect hypoglycaemia. After operation, the patient must be watched for signs and symptoms of hypoglycaemia. These are of two types: those due to rapidly falling concentration of blood glucose, and those due to a level of blood glucose below that needed for normal cerebral function. This level varies from one child to another, but cerebral function may be depressed if the blood glucose falls below 2 mmol/l.

The symptoms and signs of rapidly falling blood glucose concentration are due to adrenaline. If the child is conscious, he may feel tremulous, hungry and sweaty, complaining of headache or feeling odd. Signs include pallor, tachycardia and sweating.

Children with a very low level of blood glucose are often unable to recognize hypoglycaemia. There may be behaviour changes, and they may become truculent or quiet, tearful or ataxic. They may develop a headache, convulse, have muscular spasms or lapse into coma. It is quite possible for a diabetic child to develop hypoglycaemia within hours of having recorded a high blood glucose level.

If the child is conscious and able to drink, 15–30 g of glucose or other sugars may be given orally. Most commercial soft drinks contain 10% sugar. If not, intravenous glucose should be given either as 0.3–0.5 ml/kg of 50% dextrose if there is cerebral depression, or as 10% dextrose infusion if the child is asymptomatic. If hypoglycaemia has been prolonged, cerebral swelling may occur and full recovery of cerebration may be delayed.

INSULIN REGIMEN

Most children are managed on a mixture of short-acting (unmodified) and intermediate-acting insulins given once or, more usually, twice a day. Some children, especially in the teenage years, are managed on four injections a day, giving short-acting insulin before meals and intermediate or long-acting insulin before bed. They will use one of the pen systems for this regimen. In most countries, insulin is produced by genetically engineered bacteria and is identical with human insulin. A few children may be using pork- or beef-derived insulin. It is important not to change the species of insulin in the pre- or postoperative state without careful consideration.

BLOOD GLUCOSE MONITORING

Most, if not all, children or their parents will monitor diabetes control by blood glucose tests at home using a reflectance meter. Unless the hospital ward has a reliable meter and experienced staff, it is often wise to ask the child or parent to bring their meter and test strips to hospital for bedside monitoring. Nursing staff may need to rehearse the technique. Test strips must be fresh in order to obtain reasonably accurate results.

Insulinoma

This is a rare tumour of the beta cells of the pancreas, which produces excessive insulin, leading to hypoglycaemia. The presenting features depend on the degree to which hypoglycaemia disturbs cerebral function. There may be swings of mood, inconsistency of temperament and loss of concentration. In the more severe, subconvulsive levels of hypoglycaemia, episodes resembling deep sleep, delirium or temper tantrums occur. Eventually, there may be epileptiform convulsions that do not respond to normal anticonvulsant therapy. About 40% of reported cases occur in children less than 2 years old.

The tumours are often small (1.5 cm) and are most often found in the tail of the pancreas.

If there is difficulty in locating a tumour, partial pancreatectomy is performed, because there may be beta-cell hyperplasia causing hypoglycaemia.

These patients should have a 10% dextrose infusion running before induction, and preoperative blood sugar levels should be measured and be within normal limits. Operation may be prolonged by difficulty in locating the tumour. In 14% of patients there are multiple tumours. Blood sugar should be measured at intervals during the operation. Once the tumour and thus the source of excess insulin has been removed, the blood sugar should rise spontaneously. Continued monitoring of blood sugar is essential, so that the amount of dextrose infused is appropriate to the patient's need. This will usually decline as the patient readjusts to the normal level of insulin release.

Beckwith–Wiedemann syndrome

Macroglossia, most prominent in infancy (Fig. 25.4), exomphalos, hypoglycaemia, visceromegaly and hemihypertrophy are the commonest features, although not all of them are always present [44]. The hypoglycaemia is probably due to hyperinsulinism, but lack of glucagon has been suggested. In some patients, hypoglycaemia is severe.

It is postulated, but not proven, that this is a genetically determined, autosomal recessive disease. It has been suggested that it may be non-progressive, hypothalamic dysfunction mainly affecting the hormone-releasing factors. It is a rare disease.

Because severe hypoglycaemia can occur, an intravenous infusion of glucose should be running during the operation and postoperatively. The large tongue may make intubation difficult and can cause airway obstruction.

These patients may present in infancy for repair of omphalocoele (see Chapter 11). Partial glossectomy is sometimes required to reduce the bulk of the tongue and occasionally to relieve airway obstruction. A central wedge is usually excised. It can be a bloody procedure and steps should be taken to reduce blood loss, such as hypotensive anaesthesia, injection of a vasoconstrictor (ornithine vasopressin — POR8) into the tongue or both. Liver or kidney tumours develop in 10–15% of these patients. They occur most commonly in patients with hemihypertrophy [44].

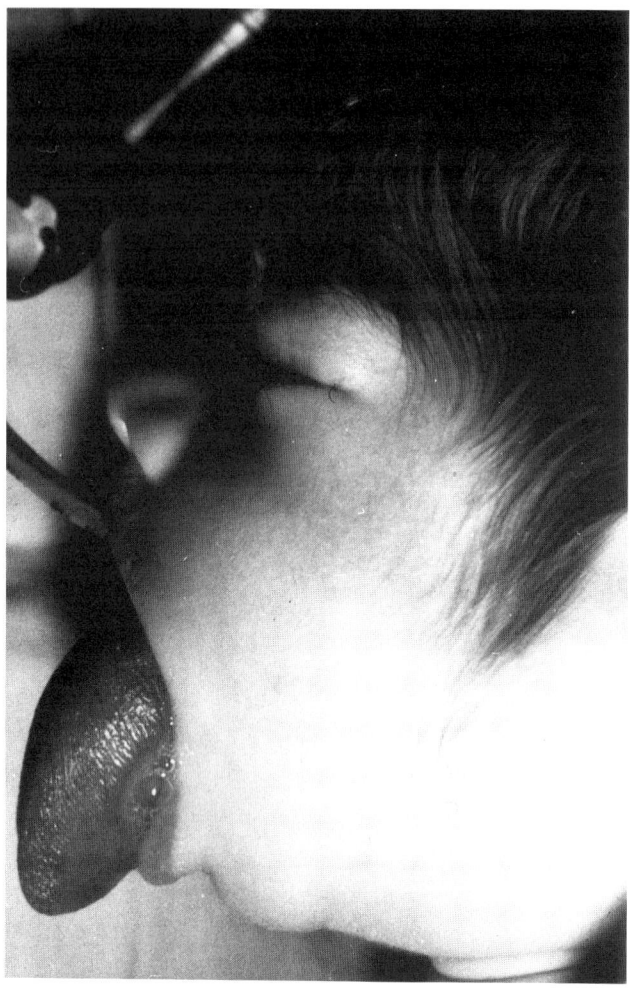

Fig. 25.4 Beckwith–Wiedemann syndrome: an example of the grossly enlarged, protruding tongue.

Prader–Willi syndrome

These children are short and mentally retarded. They are hypotonic infants, who initially fail to thrive, but between 1 and 3 years of age become obese. A diabetic type of glucose tolerance curve is often found, especially in very obese patients. They occasionally develop diabetes mellitus.

The anaesthetic problems result from the obesity — difficult venepuncture, altered drug responses, increased uptake into fat during long anaesthetics with fat-soluble inhalation anaesthetics, and a tendency to respiratory complications. It is more appropriate to administer induction agents and muscle relaxants according to lean body mass.

Adrenal cortex

TUMOURS AND HYPERFUNCTION (Cushing's syndrome)

Tumours of the adrenal cortex are rare. The resulting hypersecretion produces clinical features dependent on the predominant hormone involved. Virilization occurs when androgenic steroids are secreted in excess, producing either sexual precocity in males or masculinization in girls.

Cushing's syndrome with obesity, hypertension and stunted growth occurs when the secretion is chiefly cortisol. A mixed syndrome of virilization with some Cushingoid features, due to hypersecretion of both androgens and cortisol, is one of the most common consequences of corticocarcinoma or adenoma. Feminization of males, due to excess secretion of oestrogens, is rare.

The treatment of these tumours is by excision through a thoracoabdominal approach. Blood pressure tends to be labile during surgery.

CONGENITAL ADRENAL HYPERPLASIA

This is a congenital familial disorder resulting from deficiency of an adrenal cortical enzyme. Various types are recognized, depending on which enzyme is deficient. Some features of Addison's disease may be present. Hyperkalaemia may arouse suspicion of the disorder in the newborn. Insufficient cortisol production results in excessive adrenocorticotrophic hormone (ACTH) secretion, leading to congenital hyperplasia of the cortex with consequent increased production of androgens. Administration of cortisone acetate will suppress ACTH secretion.

Girls with congenital adrenal hyperplasia are virilized at birth due to excess androgen production. They almost always require corrective genital surgery. They may also require mineralocorticoid therapy. Steroid cover is essential for operation and postoperatively. Hypoglycaemia may occur and is sometimes severe.

ADDISON'S DISEASE

Addison's disease is an autoimmune disease that causes adrenal cortical insufficiency. The main features are weakness, fatigue, vomiting, diarrhoea and hypotension accompanied by hyponatraemia and hyperkalaemia.

Replacement therapy includes hydrocortisone or cortisone acetate and a mineralocorticoid such as fludrocortisone.

Preoperative fasting may result in severe hypoglycaemia. Hypotension may be unresponsive to treatment unless steroids are given.

Thyroid

HYPERTHYROIDISM

In children, the initial treatment is medical, with carbimazole or propylthiouracil. Potassium iodide may be used for short-term and preoperative preparation. Tachycardia and dysrhythmia are due to increased sensitivity to catecholamines and should be treated with beta-adrenergic blocking drugs. Surgical treatment may be indicated, but is rare in children.

Thyroid function must be assessed preoperatively. Surgery should be postponed if thyrotoxicosis is not adequately controlled. If the gland is enlarged, tracheal obstruction may lead to difficult intubation. This can usually be overcome by employing a smaller tube. Long-standing tracheal compression may cause tracheomalacia and a tendency to tracheal collapse when the tube is removed at the end of thyroid surgery. Special care must be taken to protect the eyes if the patient is exophthalmic.

HYPOTHYROIDISM

This may present as congenital cretinism or as an acquired juvenile form. There is growth retardation, dry skin, thick hair, diminished physical activity, constipation, thick tongue, poor muscle tone, hoarseness and intellectual retardation. Treatment consists of replacement therapy with thyroxine.

An unrecognized cretin or hypothyroid patient may present for emergency surgery. These patients are at risk from enhanced effects of depressant drugs, including thiopentone. Hypotension and cardiovascular collapse may occur and should be treated initially with hydrocortisone, because these patients have a considerably reduced response to stress. Triiodothyronine or thyroxine, which have a slower onset of action, should then be started.

Recovery from anaesthesia may be delayed in hypothyroid patients unless doses of depressant drugs are significantly reduced, to as little as one-third of the usual doses.

Hypothyroidism may be secondary to hypopituitarism, in which case thyroid stimulating hormone levels will not be elevated.

GOITRE

An enlarged thyroid may result from inflammation, infiltrative processes or neoplasm, but in most instances is due to either autoimmune thyroiditis or to deficiency of a thyroid enzyme.

The enlarged gland may vary greatly in size, shape, consistency and functional activity. Thyroid function should be assessed preoperatively and the patient made euthyroid before surgery if possible. Patients with goitre may present for surgical resection and the problems of tracheal compression may occur. A lateral X-ray of the neck may demonstrate this.

CARCINOMA

Carcinoma of the thyroid is uncommon in childhood but there is an increasing incidence, which appears to be related in a significant number of patients to irradiation of the neck or chest.

Diabetes insipidus

See Chapter 14.

SKIN DISORDERS

Eczema

This is an allergic skin disease frequently affecting the flexures at the elbows or knees, although in some severe cases it may be more widespread. These children are atopic and thus more likely to have adverse responses to histamine-releasing drugs such as morphine and D-tubocurarine.

Epidermolysis bullosa [45]

Epidermolysis bullosa is an uncommon hereditary disease of the squamous epithelium, in which there is deficiency of collagen in the dermis. Physical contact, especially of a shearing nature, results in separation of the epidermis and the formation of bullae. The lesions may be relatively mild in the simplest type of the disease, but in the dystrophic forms of epidermolysis bullosa the lesions are severe; continued formation of bullae throughout the child's life results in considerable scarring, particularly of the face and hands. Several genetic variations are recognized, the dominant dystrophic forms being less severe than the recessive ones. The lesions are most severe in early infancy and tend to diminish with the passage of time. The teeth are abnormal; lesions occur in the mouth, pharynx, oesophagus and anus, resulting in strictures. Anaesthesia may be needed for intercurrent disease, dental treatment, plastic surgery on scarred fingers and dilatation of oesophageal and anal strictures.

Various methods of managing anaesthesia for these children have been described, including the use of ketamine, which has the advantage that the airway can be maintained without handling the face. In the largest series in which general anaesthesia was used [45], intubation was complicated in some by microstomia (6 of 131 cases) caused by previous scarring, and in a few others by loose carious teeth (4 of 131). Very occasionally the laryngoscope damaged the tongue, but oral damage was more often due to other manipulations. The nasal route was used on 18 occasions. There were no postoperative complications due to intubation, contrary to the widely held view that intubation is dangerous in these patients. A ruptured bulla, bleeding in the mouth during anaesthesia, has been reported and subglottic stenosis has followed difficult emergency intubation. It is important to lubricate the laryngosope well before use and not to apply suction directly to the mucosa. Regional anaesthesia has been successfully used, either alone or as an adjunct to general anaesthesia [46].

When a face mask is used it should be cushioned; and vaseline gauze should be applied to the face for protection. With these precautions, less than 6% developed bullae [45]. In infants, general anaesthesia can be induced with inhalation agents, using a simple head box, into which the anaesthetic agents are introduced.

Adhesive tape should be avoided and alternative atraumatic methods for fixing endotracheal tubes and intravenous cannulae should be used. A weighted, monitoring stethoscope avoids the need for strapping. A clip-on pulse oximeter probe should be applied gently. The application of a tourniquet may damage the skin, unless it is protected by, for instance, vaseline gauze.

These children are sometimes given steroids and may require extra operative cover.

The essence of anaesthesia for these patients is extreme gentleness and avoidance of any abrading injury — this includes during transfer on and off the operating table.

Stevens–Johnson syndrome

This, the most serious form of erythema multiforme, is an acute eruptive disorder of the skin and mucous membranes, which is more common in children. There is a mortality of up to 12%, usually from pulmonary complications or infection. Recurrence may follow apparent resolution. The cutaneous lesions progress from erythematous areas to macules, papules, vesicles and bullae, followed by scaling and sloughing of epithelium, with large areas being left denuded. These areas weep fluid and protein until they are re-epithelialized. Mucous membranes, especially those of the respiratory tract, may be similarly involved.

There are widespread systemic manifestations, of variable severity. These include pyrexia, infection, mucosal ulceration, anaemia, oedema, pneumonitis, myocarditis and acute inflammatory renal disease. Rupture of pleural blebs has also been described, with pleural effusion and pneumothoraces.

The anaesthetic management [47] includes preoperative assessment of the extent of skin loss and fluid and electrolyte deficiencies. The mouth and pharynx should be inspected if intubation is contemplated. It is important to avoid trauma. Ketamine offers many advantages if controlled ventilation and muscle relaxation are not necessary. Induction with intramuscular ketamine can be followed by percutaneous venous cannulation, if possible, for the administration of increments of ketamine or other drugs, fluids and blood. It is preferable to avoid intubation in severe cases.

Monitoring may be a problem. A weighted stethoscope, which does not require strapping, is useful and a clip-on pulse oximeter probe should be used. A blood pressure cuff should be placed over an unaffected area. The axilla may be the least traumatic site for temperature monitoring. A blanket that will allow warming or cooling may be used to maintain normal body temperature.

Antibiotics are necessary for severe infection. Steroids and antihistamines have been used, with variable results.

Diffuse cutaneous scleroderma

This is a rare, chronic, self-limiting disease that progresses from an oedematous phase to one of an atrophic, immobile dermis involving some or all of the skin. It is refractory to all drugs. Plastic surgery is sometimes indicated to relieve contractures and constrictions.

Venepuncture is difficult. Scarring of the face and

mouth causes problems with the airway and intubation. Limitation of movement interferes with positioning of the patient for surgery. Careful preoperative assessment of cardiopulmonary function is important, because changes include pulmonary and myocardial fibrosis.

The patient may be taking steroids and need extra cover [48].

Congenital anhydrotic ectodermal dysplasia

This is a very rare condition, predominantly of males, in which there is diffuse ectodermal malformation and atrophy. The skin is atrophic, dry, translucent and smooth. There are no sweat glands and hair follicles and sebaceous glands are almost completely absent.

Water is lost insensibly through the skin, but the important heat-dissipating mechanism of sweating is abolished, making these children prone to hyperthermia in hot weather. Temperature must be monitored during anaesthesia, the operating theatre should be kept moderately cool and equipment such as a cold-water circulating blanket should be available. As lacrimation is also depressed, the eyes should be moistened, protected and kept closed throughout the operation.

Patients usually lack mucous glands in the tracheobronchial tree, making them prone to respiratory complications. Inspired gases should be humidified during anaesthesia.

Impetigo

This is a staphylococcal or streptococcal infectious disease of the skin, presenting with crusted scabs on the affected areas. It should be treated by removing the infected scabs, cleansing the underlying skin and applying antibiotic cream.

Its significance in anaesthesia is the danger of contamination of equipment and the possible spread of infection to the wound and to staff. If the skin anywhere near the operative site is involved, the procedure should be postponed, if possible, until the infection is treated.

CONNECTIVE TISSUE DISORDERS

Marfan's syndrome

These patients tend to be tall, with long, thin extremities and redundant ligaments and joint capsules. They often have a high arched palate and spinal and chest deformities. Lens subluxation and dilatation of the aorta, with secondary aortic regurgitation, are commonly seen. Dissection of the aorta may result.

It is an autosomally dominant inherited condition, affecting mainly the skeletal and cardiovascular systems and eyes. The primary problem is degeneration of the elastic lamellae, but it is uncertain whether the basic defect is in elastic or, more likely, collagen tissue. With the exception of patients with severe cardiovascular lesions, these patients generally tolerate anaesthesia well during childhood. Careful assessment of the cardiovascular status is important because serious complications, such as aortic rupture, can occur at any age. It is therefore important to know beforehand if the aorta is dilated.

Ehlers–Danlos syndrome

This disease is characterized by hyperextensible joints, which are liable to dislocate, and velvety, easily stretched skin, which is fragile and heals poorly. The patients bruise easily and have very friable veins, which make the insertion of an intravenous infusion and control of bleeding difficult. They may appear normal in infancy and only after 6 months of age do the loose skin and friable tissue become noticeable. Visceral manifestations include rupture of the great vessels, diaphragmatic and other herniae, gastrointestinal diverticula and a tendency for bowel and lung rupture.

These patients usually need surgery for inguinal herniae, which often recur, or for orthopaedic procedures.

Osteogenesis imperfecta

This is a generalized disorder of the connective tissue. The bones, which tend to be fragile, are especially affected. It is discussed more fully in Chapter 19.

Homocystinuria

This condition is due to cystathionine synthetase deficiency. Arterial lesions, such as thrombosis and partial luminal obstruction, are common features. The tunica media becomes thin, with arterial dilatation. Other features are ectopia lentis, skeletal changes and brain involvement, leading to mental deficiency. Thrombosis may be a problem after venepuncture. Surgery should be avoided where possible. The condition has some similarities to Marfan's syndrome.

Pseudoxanthoma elasticum

These patients have thickened, yellowish skin in the flexures. It appears to be due to degeneration in the collagenous elastic tissue, with accumulation of elastic fibres, many of which are fragmented.

The tunica media of the arteries is affected and the endocardium, including valve cusps, is thickened. There is a tendency to bleed, often into the gut.

Cutis laxa

This connective tissue disorder is characterized by laxity of the skin and abnormalities of the arteries and lungs, which may be emphysematous. There may be herniae and diverticula of the bladder or gut; redundant ureters and prolapsed rectum may occur.

The significant features for the anaesthetist are that upper airway obstruction may result in cor pulmonale, and that there may be redundant mucosa around the larynx. Careful preoperative assessment of the cardio-vascular and respiratory systems is needed.

STORAGE DISORDERS

Lysosomes contain specific hydrolases to break down complex macromolecules. When, as a result of genetic alteration, one of these is inactive, the substrate of the enzyme accumulates in the lysosomes of the tissues, producing the characteristic clinical picture. Several defects exist and they are classified as mucopolysaccharidoses and lipidoses, depending on the material that accumulates.

Mucopolysaccharidoses [49—52]

Mental retardation, corneal clouding, coarse facies and skeletal changes are present in this group. Difficulties with the airway and intubation occur in many, but not all, of these syndromes.

HURLER'S SYNDROME

These children have coarse facies, hypertrophied alveolar ridge and gums, stiff joints and mental retardation; they develop cloudy corneae by 2 years of age (Fig. 25.5). They have macroglossia and nasopharyngeal obstruction and are prone to frequent respiratory infections. Cardiac

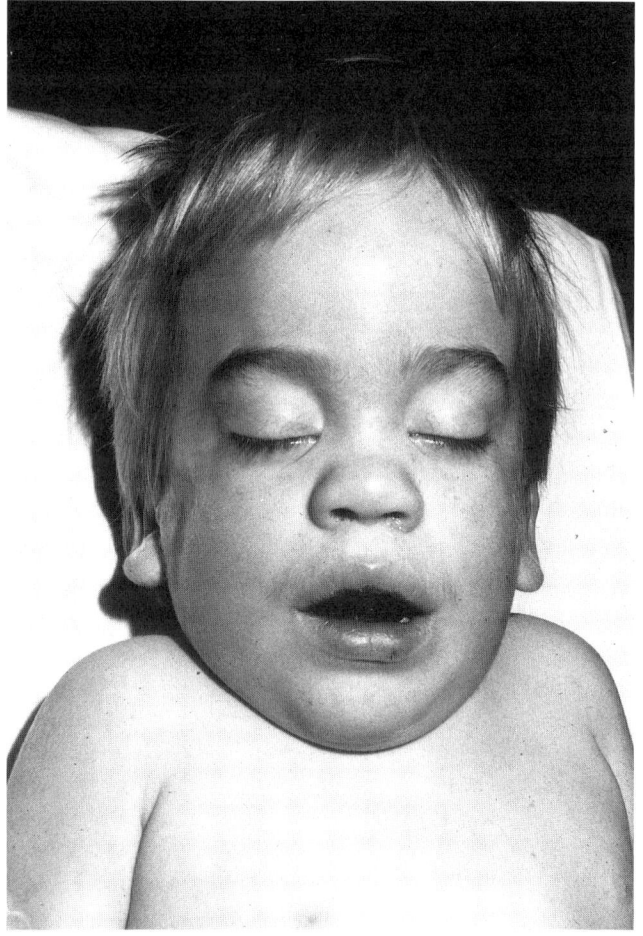

Fig. 25.5 A boy with Hurler's syndrome, demonstrating the typical facies and the short neck.

failure, due to intimal thickening of the coronary vessels and cardiac valves, may contribute to their demise. They usually die young, before the age of 10 years.

They most often need surgery for umbilical or inguinal herniae, adenoidectomy (to clear the airway and improve the quality of life) and myringotomy. Occasionally, ventriculoperitoneal shunts are needed for raised intra-cranial pressure. They present some of the most difficult problems encountered by paediatric anaesthetists, because of the difficulty in maintaining the airway and with intubation. The upper cervical vertebrae may include an underdeveloped odontoid and an unfused anterior arch of the atlas (C1) [51]. These abnormalities shorten the neck, and the larynx is consequently relatively high (opposite C2 or C3). An oral airway tends to push the epiglottis over the laryngeal inlet, worsening the

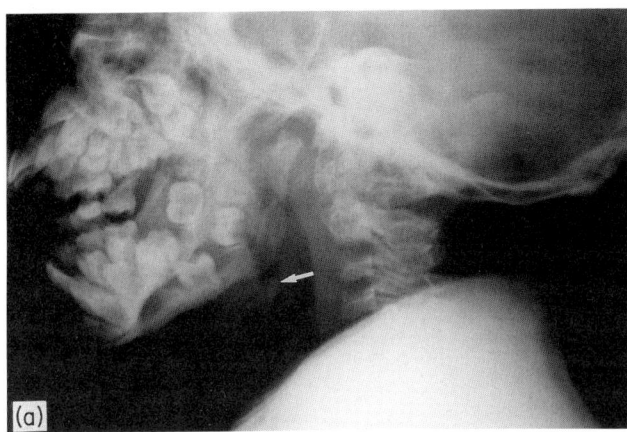

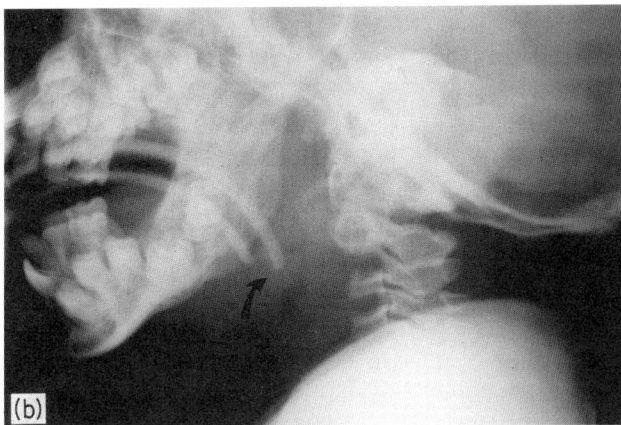

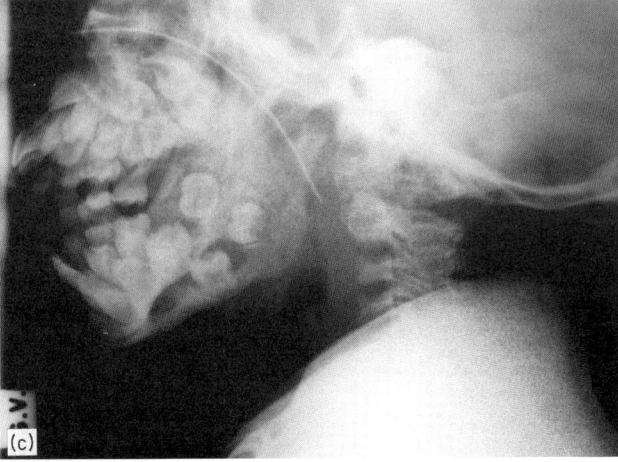

Fig. 25.6 Lateral X-ray of the neck, showing the abnormal upper cervical vertebrae. (a) The arrow points to the epiglottis. (b) An oropharyngeal airway can cause obstruction in these patients by pushing the epiglottis over the glottic opening. (c) The insertion of a nasopharyngeal tube overcomes this problem.

obstruction (Fig. 25.6) [53]. A nasopharyngeal airway will usually provide a good airway, if it can be inserted through the swollen nasopharyngeal tissues; a small tube may be necessary [49]. The high larynx makes intubation difficult. This can usually be overcome by using the techniques described in Chapter 7 for difficult intubation, such as one anaesthetist handling the laryngoscope and manipulating the larynx while an assistant inserts the tube. It is always wise to take a lateral X-ray of the neck preoperatively, so that the position of the larynx can be determined.

The other hazard is that these children sometimes have mucopolysaccharide deposits in their coronary arteries [54], which may compromise the myocardium, especially if hypoxia develops as a result of difficulty with ventilation [49] (Fig. 25.7).

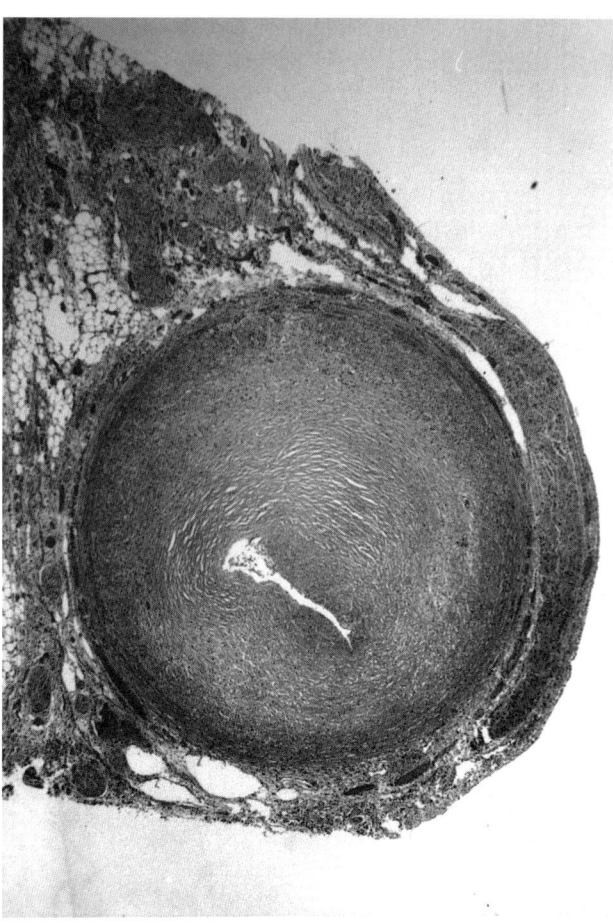

Fig. 25.7 Cross-section of a coronary artery, showing the mucopolysaccharide deposit almost occluding it from a patient with Hurler's syndrome.

SCHEIE SYNDROME (IS)

This condition has the same enzyme deficiency as Hurler's syndrome, but is less severe. The patients have normal intelligence; they may have aortic regurgitation.

HUNTER'S SYNDROME (II)

These children are similar to those with Hurler's, but have no clouding of the cornea; the course is milder, but death may still occur by 15 years of age in severe cases. They are mentally retarded, have a large tongue and are very difficult and often impossible to intubate, for the same reasons as described above. They may also have heart murmurs. The mild form has a longer life-span and less mental impairment, but may have heart disease.

SANFILIPPO SYNDROME (III)

These children present with progressive mental deterio-

ration, aggressive behaviour and sometimes seizures. Intubation may become difficult as they grow older, but is not usually so in young patients. They may present for CSF drainage shunts or liver biopsy [49].

MORQUIO'S SYNDROME (IV)

These children have bone changes, including flat vertebrae, a short unstable neck and kyphoscoliosis. The odontoid process may be fractured or absent, making the occipitoatlantoaxial region unstable [55, 56] (Fig. 25.8). Spinal cord compression is a hazard (Fig. 25.9) which can be aggravated by hyperextension or flexion. The anaesthetist should therefore be careful to avoid excessive neck movement during intubation, and a preoperative lateral neck X-ray is advisable. Cloudy corneae and aortic regurgitation are also seen. These patients sometimes present for upper cervical fusion.

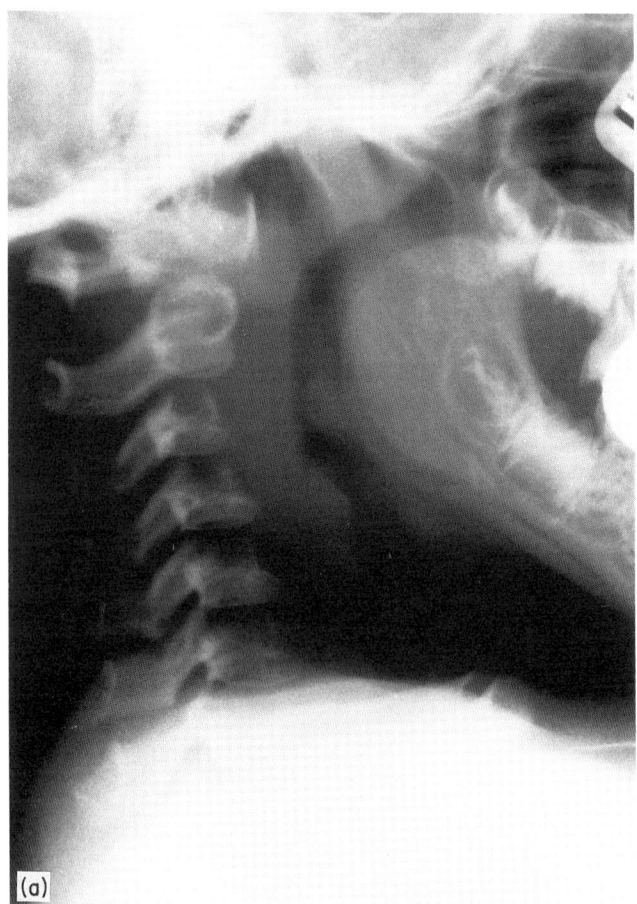
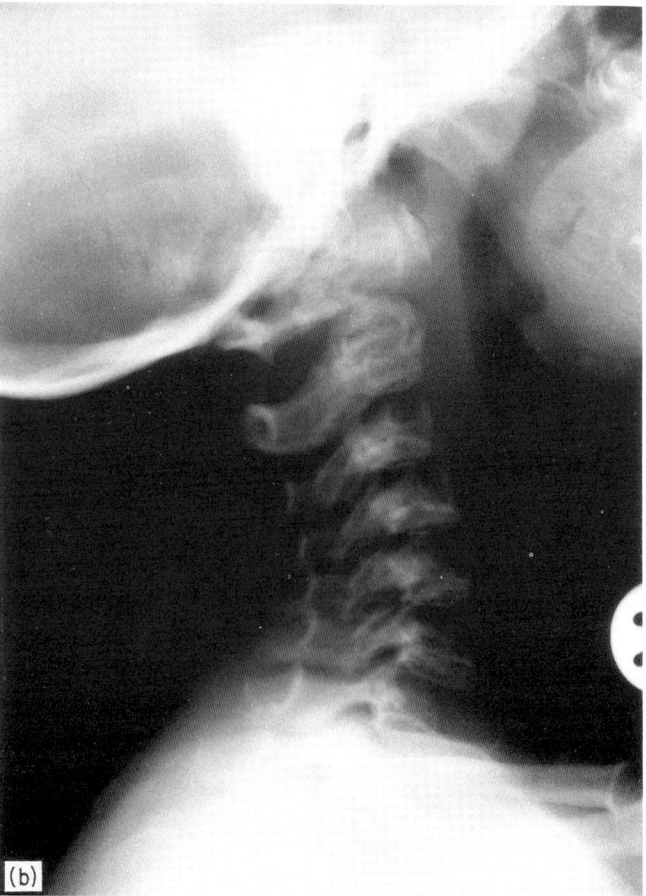

Fig. 25.8 Lateral neck X-ray in flexion (a) and extension (b) in a patient with Morquio's syndrome, showing atlantoaxial instability.

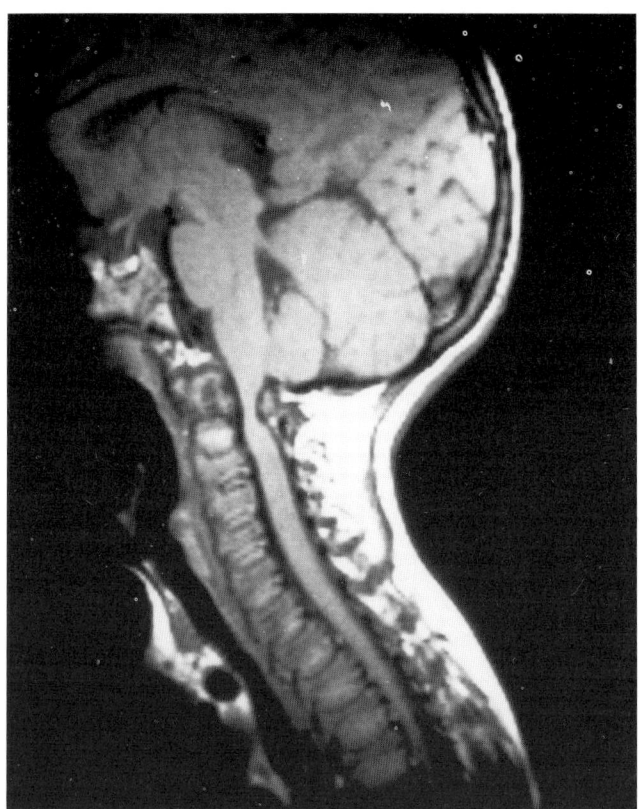

Fig. 25.9 An MRI film of the same patient with Morquio's syndrome, showing spinal cord compression.

MAROTEAUX—LAMY SYNDROME (VI)

The features are similar to Hurler's syndrome, but the children are not mentally retarded. They can have severe airway obstruction and the anaesthetist can have difficulty maintaining the airway and with intubation [51].

Bone marrow transplantation has been beneficial to some of these patients [57].

Lipidoses

These disorders are associated with the accumulation of specific lipids in the brain lysosomes. They include Gauchers, Tay—Sachs, Niemann—Pick, Krabbe's and other diseases. They generally have a poor prognosis, a short life-span, and only very rarely present for anaesthesia.

Glycogen storage diseases

These are a group of enzymatic abnormalities that inter-fere with the normal breakdown or synthesis of glycogen [58].

VON GIERKE'S DISEASE

This is the commonest glycogen storage disease to pre-sent for anaesthesia, most often for liver biopsy. These infants have impaired renal and hepatic function, lactic acidosis, severe attacks of hypoglycaemia, thrombocyto-penia and convulsions. During anaesthesia, a 5% dextrose infusion should be running. The acid—base status should be checked if the procedure is prolonged. Increasing metabolic acidosis has been reported and it should be treated with sodium bicarbonate. Hartmann's solution is inappropriate in these patients because the lactate may not be metabolized.

POMPE'S DISEASE

These infants are extremely hypotonic, have a large tongue, which can cause airway obstruction, and develop massive cardiomegaly with heart failure. They usually die before the age of 2 years.

FORBES' DISEASE

This is a similar, though milder, form of von Gierke's disease. No special anaesthetic problems should occur.

ANDERSEN'S DISEASE

This is a rare disease with early onset of cirrhosis and portal hypertension. Oedema, ascites, oesophageal varices and hypoprothrombinaemia with bleeding may occur.

MCARDLE'S DISEASE

This is a muscular disorder characterized by rapid exhaus-tion of otherwise normal muscle. It is rare.

HER'S DISEASE

A hepatophosphorylase deficiency that causes mild forms of von Gierke's disease.

GLYCOGEN SYNTHETASE DEFICIENCY

The deficient synthesis of glycogen is characterized by

hypoglycaemia and starvation in infancy. A high glucose intake is necessary.

OTHER DISORDERS OF METABOLISM

Pyruvate dehydrogenase deficiency

An increasing number of metabolic enzyme disturbances are being described, and patients with some of these will present from time to time for anaesthesia. Reports of such cases are rare. One of these is pyruvate dehydrogenase deficiency, which results in failure to metabolize pyruvate, with the resultant accumulation of pyruvate and lactate. To avoid lactic acidosis it is recommended that lactate-containing solutions be avoided, as well as hypocarbia, which can increase lactate levels, and halothane, which can inhibit gluconeogenesis [59].

DISEASES WITH SKELETAL INVOLVEMENT

Klippel−Feil syndrome

In this anomaly, the cervical vertebrae are usually fused, although hemivertebrae and other vertebral defects may be found. There may also be a secondary web neck, torticollis and/or facial asymmetry.

There may be associated anomalies, including deafness, congenital heart disease, mental deficiency, cleft palate, rib defects and scoliosis.

These patients may present problems with intubation due to the short neck and restricted movement of the cervical spine, but this is not always the case (Fig. 25.10).

Juvenile rheumatoid arthritis

This disease may present in several forms. The first is an acute febrile illness that usually occurs before the age of 4 years, and in which remission usually occurs within a year. The second, polyarticular, pattern resembles the adult disease, with chronic pain and swelling in many joints. The third affects only a few joints; up to 30% of these may develop iridocyclitis, which may lead to blindness.

The essential features of the disease are non-migratory arthropathy, with a tendency to involve large joints or proximal interphalangeal joints, and systemic manifestations. These include fever, erythematous rashes, rheumatoid nodules and leucocytosis; occasionally, there may be iridocyclitis, pleurisy, pericarditis, hepatitis and nephritis.

If this disease is rapidly progressive in childhood, there may be involvement of the temporomandibular or laryngeal joints, which could affect intubation; the anaesthetist should be aware of possible lung and pericardial manifestations of rheumatoid disease.

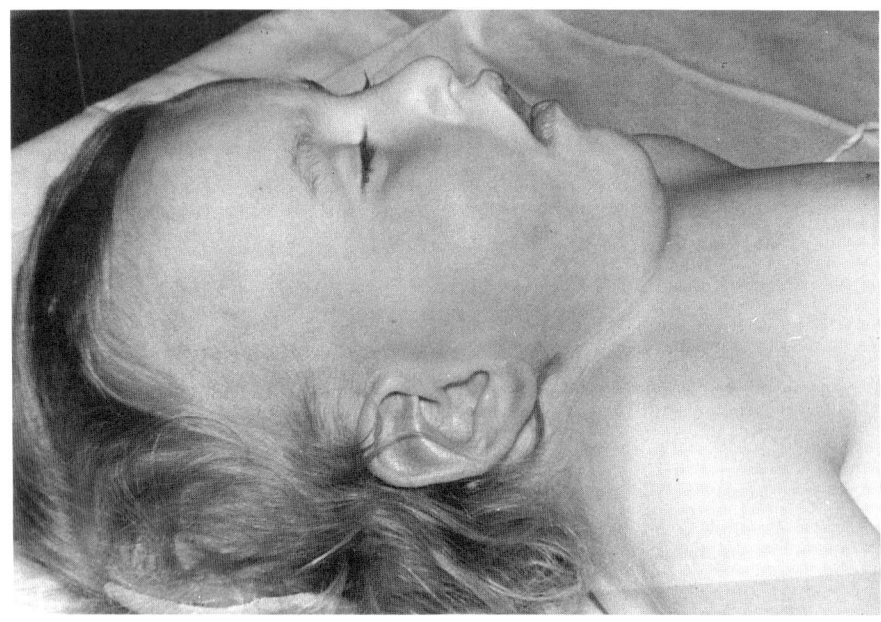

Fig. 25.10 Klippel−Feil syndrome, showing the short neck, which may make intubation more difficult.

Spondyloepiphyseal dysplasia congenita

This rare condition presents a hazard if intubation is attempted in a child with odontoid hypoplasia and instability of the atlantoaxial joint. Other features are short stature, myopia, susceptibility to retinal degeneration and detachment, cleft palate and scoliosis.

ASPECTS OF IMMUNOLOGY RELEVANT TO ANAESTHESIA

The immunodeficient patient

There is an obvious need for increased vigilance with regard to infection in patients with immune deficiency. These include conditions such as rare thymic aplasia, agammaglobulinaemia, diGeorge syndrome (cardiac anomaly, no thymus and a tendency to hypocalcaemia) and acquired immunodeficiency associated with organ transplantation, chemotherapy, HIV infection and, to a lesser extent, splenectomy. These patients are particularly prone to infection from cytomegalo virus from infected blood; if blood transfusion is necessary the blood should be irradiated or leukocyte-filtered. Splenectomized patients are particularly sensitive to encapsulated organisms such as pneumococcus. Care must be taken to avoid introducing infection when cannulae and tubes are inserted. Gammaglobulin may be administered intravenously during anaesthesia to provide some protection to patients with hypogammaglobulinaemia.

HIV infection

When immunodeficiency is due to HIV infection, particular care is needed to avoid infection of staff. This involves wearing gown and gloves and following strict procedures for handling all contaminated equipment and linen. Disposable anaesthetic equipment such as tubes and breathing system should be used where possible. Needles and sharp objects should be disposed of promptly in appropriate containers. The operating theatre and any remaining equipment must be thoroughly cleaned afterwards. The patient should be nursed in isolation in the recovery room.

A particular problem for paediatric anaesthetists is the hazard of unknowingly anaesthetizing a baby of an HIV-positive mother. Routine practices to minimize staff risk should be followed and care taken to avoid cross-infection.

Procedures carried out on immunodeficient patients

Immunodeficient patients may need anaesthesia for diagnostic or therapeutic procedures. They may undergo lung biopsy, usually percutaneous, to diagnose *Pneumocystis carinii* pneumonia, or lymph node biopsy. Often the lymph nodes are small and difficult to find, and the operation may take much longer than expected. Biopsy may be needed after organ transplantation, particularly of heart or lung, to check for possible rejection.

Effect of anaesthesia on immunity

After operation, there is a state of relative immune deficiency, probably due to the secretion of steroids in response to the stress of anaesthesia and surgery.

There have been studies that suggest diminished response to infection, and the suppression of immune mechanisms during halothane anaesthesia. Prolonged nitrous oxide administration causes bone marrow suppression.

CHROMOSOME ABNORMALITIES

Many patients with chromosome abnormality syndromes are intellectually handicapped.

Down's syndrome (Trisomy 21)

These children are mentally subnormal, with a high incidence of congenital heart disease, a large tongue and poor muscle tone. An abnormality of the atlantoaxial joint, which could be unstable, occurs in 10−22% of these children, although only about 3% develop symptoms [60]. Clinical features that suggest instability include alteration of gait, bowel or bladder function or neck posture, neck pain or limitation of movement and weakness of the extremities. If there are any such clinical signs, preoperative lateral neck X-rays should be taken in flexion and extension. If the distance between the anterior arch of the atlas and the adjacent odontoid process exceeds 5 mm the diagnosis of atlantoaxial instability can be made with reasonable certainty [60]. The anaesthetist must be aware of this potential problem and take care to avoid excessive movement of the neck during intubation, especially extreme flexion. Many children with Down's syndrome have been anaesthetized without any difficulty and reports of atlantoaxial complications with anaesthesia are rare.

Children with Down's syndrome have an increased incidence of subglottic stenosis [61]; about 20% need a smaller tube than expected for their age. In some cases this is because they are small for their age [62].

The large tongue may make intubation more difficult. Poor muscle tone combined with the large tongue may be associated with obstructive sleep problems. Opioid premedication should be used only cautiously in such patients.

These children have also been reported to be sensitive to atropine [63], but this has been refuted in recent studies with the usual clinical doses [62]. The mydriatic response may be exaggerated. As there is evidence of decreased sympathetic function, vagal blockade is advised when bradycardia may be a problem [64]. Blood pressure is significantly lower than in normal children.

Although thyroid antibodies are found, thyroid function is normal in these children, but about half of them become hypothyroid in adulthood [65].

Turner's syndrome

Girls affected by Turner's syndrome have short stature, webbing of the neck and ovarian dysgenesis. Coarctation of the aorta occurs in about 15%. The relatively small mandible, narrow maxilla and short neck can, but rarely do, cause difficulty during intubation. Bronchial intubation, due to a very short trachea, has been reported [66].

Noonan's syndrome

This occurs in males and has some similarities to Turner's syndrome. The patients have a small penis with cryptorchidism. They may have pulmonary stenosis, septal defects and pectus excavatum. Micrognathia can make intubation difficult.

Trisomies 18 and 22

These children may have micrognathia.

'Cri du chat' syndrome

This is a syndrome of mental deficiency, microencephaly and hypotonia associated with an unusual cry. The larynx appears anatomically normal.

OTHER CONDITIONS

Conjoined twins

The birth of conjoined twins is rare — estimates vary between 1:50000 and 1:200000 births. Between 75 and 90% are stillborn or die within 24 hours. Only about 6% survive separation.

Most conjoined twins are joined anteriorly (73%) at the thorax (thoracopagus), upper abdomen (xiphopagus) and lower abdomen (omphalopagus). Other connecting sites include the skull (craniopagus) and pelvis (ischiopagus). Ischiopagus twins are further classified according to how many lower limbs they have, bi-, tri- or tetrapus.

Thorough preoperative assessment of conjoined twins is essential before separation. A variety of diagnostic studies is necessary to define organ sharing, and to demonstrate coexisting congenital abnormalities. It is equally important to organize the separation teams. Discussions should include surgeons, anaesthetists, operating theatre nurses and technicians. The position of the operating tables, monitoring equipment, lighting and personnel needs must be planned meticulously. Special attention needs to be paid to the transfer of one twin at separation to a second operating table, so that it is accomplished quickly and safely. A rehearsal is valuable to plan the arrangement of the equipment and co-ordinate the activities of all those involved. Prior arrangement with the blood bank and biochemistry staff is essential. The requirements for blood and blood products may be high in major cases.

It should be assumed that there will be significant cross-circulation. If difficulties are envisaged it may be safer to intubate them awake, but the use of muscle relaxants is preferable if the airways are accessible — one baby is ventilated by mask while the other is intubated, followed by intubation of the second one.

Anaesthesia can be provided by high-dose opioids or inhalation agents.

Each twin should be monitored and ventilated individually, so that unpredictable drug responses from cross-circulation, extraordinary intravascular volume shifts and thermal instability can be detected and quickly rectified.

Monitoring should include individual direct blood pressure, central venous pressure, oximetry, capnography, ECG, urine output and temperature. Ventilation tubing and monitoring lines should be colour-coded to prevent confusion. Blood loss should be measured accurately and replaced appropriately. Large volumes of replacement fluid and blood may be required during separation. Maintenance of an adequate circulation is one of the most important aspects of the operation.

Measurements of arterial blood gases, glucose, electrolytes, ionized calcium, haemoglobin, platelets, prothrombin and partial thromboplastin times should be frequent when there is major blood loss.

The transfer of the second twin to the other table is a critical time during the operation, but it can be accomplished quickly and safely, especially if the preoperative preparation was thorough.

Specific problems arise that are related to the point of fusion and skin or organ deficiencies in one or both twins. If there are significant deficiencies, an attempt is usually made to ensure, if possible, that one baby is left with enough of the essential organs to survive.

Postoperatively, separated twins are usually transferred to the intensive care unit for respiratory and pharmacological support and monitoring.

The results of separation depend on the anatomical attachment and components of the babies, on carefully planned anaesthesia and surgery and on adequate resuscitation when necessary.

Infant effects of maternal drug use

Maternal drug consumption may be teratogenic, or result in significant withdrawal or pharmacological effects in the neonate. For example, if the mother is treated with beta-blockade the baby may have bradycardia and hypoglycaemia. Cocaine is a vasoconstrictor and causes maternal hypertension and vasoconstriction of the placental vessels, with secondary developmental effects. Cocaine blocks re-uptake of noradrenaline and dopamine at the postsynaptic junctions, and it may act directly on the fetus, increasing neurotransmission, central nervous system irritability and causing direct toxicity to the developing brain, leading to brain damage. Stopping the mother from taking cocaine during pregnancy may still be too late to prevent damage [67].

The babies of opioid-dependent women usually develop the neonatal abstinence syndrome. The commonest signs are central nervous system irritability (70%), respiratory and gastrointestinal problems (50%) and autonomic dysfunction. Hyperpyrexia and convulsions are rare. Excessive sweating in premature infants may provide a clue to opioid withdrawal [68].

In cases of maternal drug addiction, both mother and newborn infant may have HIV infection (see immunology section). The patient may be growth-retarded and premature. In the early neonatal period, the residual drug effects may increase the opioid and anaesthetic drug requirements; sedation may be needed to suppress irritability. The neonatal abstinence syndrome may need to be treated. Methadone 1−2 mg b.d. or diazepam 1−2 mg b.d. initially, reducing by 20% a day, can be used for opioid withdrawal.

Bardet−Biedl syndrome

The Bardet−Biedl syndrome is a rare disorder with autosomal recessive inheritance. It is characterized by obesity (85%) (Fig. 25.11), mental retardation (80%), polydactyly (75%), retinitis pigmentosa (68%) and hypogenitalism (60%). Males are more commonly affected. Renal abnormalities are frequent (90%), making

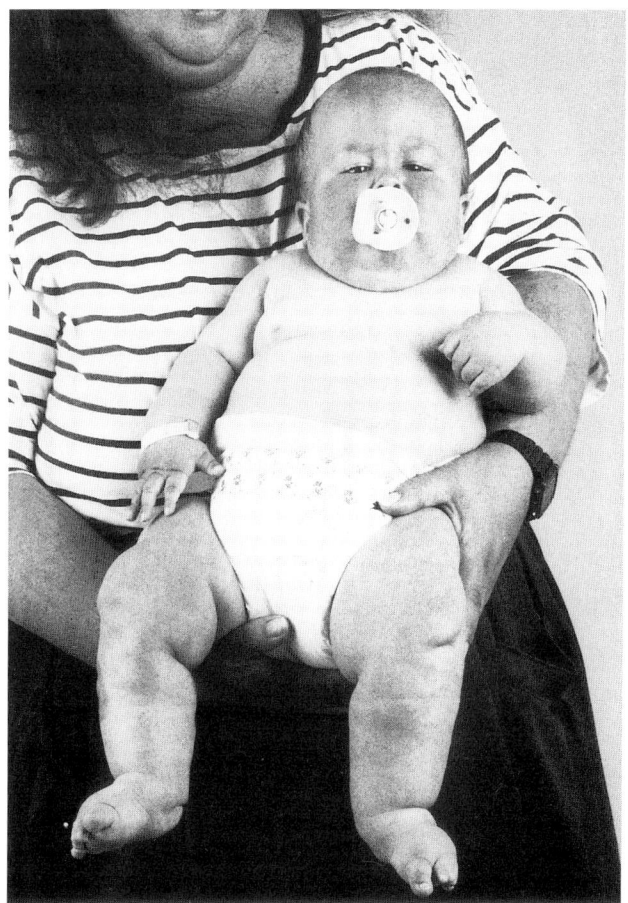

Fig. 25.11 Bardet−Biedl syndrome showing gross obesity in a 10-month-old infant.

preoperative assessment of renal function important. There are often other associated abnormalities. The main anaesthetic problems relate to obesity. Venepuncture can be difficult; altered pulmonary mechanics render the patients prone to hypoxia. The assessment of drug dosage is complicated by the obesity. It may be more difficult to determine the depth for injection, when performing regional or nerve blocks.

Laurence and Moon originally described patients in a family with retinitis pigmentosa who were not obese. The condition with obesity was described by Bardet and Biedl so that the syndrome is sometimes referred to as the Laurence−Moon − Bardet−Biedl syndrome.

Sotos syndrome

This disorder of unknown cause is characterized by the prenatal onset of excessive growth, acromegalic features and a varying degree of mental deficiency, despite normal growth hormone levels. There is a high incidence of tumours and cardiac abnormalities and some patients present for scoliosis surgery. They are poorly coordinated and seem weak, although this may be partly due to insufficient strength for support and control of their large head and limbs. Although difficult intubation and abnormal response to muscle relaxants might be anticipated, neither problem arose in the patient reported [69].

Other syndromes

There are many other syndromes, some of which may have anaesthetic implications, but they are rare. Reference texts should be consulted to find out what the syndrome involves. Some general principles are that patients with micrognathia or short necks may be difficult to intubate, cervical spine instability should be handled with care and excessive flexion or extension should be avoided, and, in those syndromes with associated heart disease, careful preoperative assessment and full monitoring should be undertaken.

Conditions described in other chapters

Acute intermittent porphyria (Chapter 2)
G6PD deficiency (Chapter 2)
Osteogenesis imperfecta (Chapter 19)
Arthrogryposis multiplex congenita (Chapter 19)
Moyamoya disease (Chapter 14)
Apert's and Crouzon's syndromes (Chapter 17)
Pierre Robin and Treacher−Collins syndromes (Chapter 17)
Goldenhar syndrome (Chapter 17)

REFERENCES

1 Kojima Y., Kitahara Y., Nozaki F. Anesthetic management of the patient with a history of Kawasaki disease. *J Anesth (Japan)* 1990, **4**, 162.

2 McNiece W.L., Krishna G. Kawasaki disease — a disease with anesthetic implications. *Anesthesiology* 1983, **58**, 269.

3 Rawstrom R.E. Preoperative haemoglobin levels. *Anaes Intens Care* 1975, **4**, 175.

4 Gilbertson A.A. Anaesthesia in West African patients with sickle-cell anaemia, haemoglobin SC disease and sickle-cell trait. *Br J Anaes* 1965, **37**, 614.

5 Sethna N.F., Rockoff M.A., Worthen H.M., Rosnow J. Anesthesia-related complications in children with Duchenne muscular dystrophy. *Anesthesiology* 1988, **6**, 462.

6 Sanyal S.K., Tierney R.C., Rao P.S., *et al.* Systolic time interval characteristics in children with Duchenne's progressive muscular dystrophy. *Pediatrics* 1982, **71**, 958.

7 Wang J.M., Stanley T.H. Duchenne muscular dystrophy and malignant hyperthermia: two case reports. *Can Anaes Soc J* 1986, **33**, 492.

8 Kefler H.M., Singer W.D., Reynolds R.N. Malignant hyperthermia in a child with Duchenne muscular dystrophy. *Pediatrics* 1983, **71**, 118.

9 Richards W.C. Anaesthesia and serum CPK levels in patients with Duchenne muscular dystrophy. *Anaes Intens Care* 1972, **1**, 150.

10 Milne B., Rosales J.K. Anesthetic considerations in patients with muscular dystrophy undergoing spinal fusion and Harrington rod insertion. *Can Anaes Soc J* 1982, **29**, 250.

11 Kaufman L. Anaesthesia in dystrophia myotonica. *Proc Roy Soc Med* 1960, **53**, 183.

12 Thiel R.C. The myotonic response to suxamethonium. *Br J Anaes* 1967, **39**, 815.

13 Paterson I.S. Generalized myotonia following suxamethonium. *Br J Anaes* 1962, **34**, 340.

14 Harper P.S., Dyken P.R. Early onset dystrophia myotonica. *Lancet* 1972, **2**, 53.

15 Bray R.J., Inkster J. Anaesthesia in babies with congenital dystrophia myotonica. *Anaesthesia* 1984, **39**, 1007.

16 Anderson B.J., Brown T.C.K. Congenital myotonic dystrophy in children — a review of 10 years' experience. *Anaes Intens Care* 1989, **17**, 320.

17 Azar I. The response of patients with neuromuscular disorders to muscle relaxants: a review. *Anesthesiology* 1984, **61**, 173.

18 Anderson B.J., Brown T.C.K. Anaesthesia for a child with congenital myotonic dystrophy. *Anaes Intens Care* 1989, **17**, 351.

19 Sarnat H.B., O'Connor T., Byrne P.A. Clinical effects of myotonic dystrophy on pregnancy and the neonate. *Arch Neurol* 1977, **33**, 459.

20 Meyers M.B., Barash P.G. Cardiac decompensation during enflurance anesthesia in patient with myotonia atrophia. *Anesth Analg* 1976, **55**, 433.

21 Buzello W., Krieg N., Schuckewei I. Hazards of neostigmine in patients with neuromuscular disorders. *Br J Anaes* 1982, **54**, 529.

22 Alexander C., Wolf S., Chia J.N. Caudal anaesthesia for early onset myotonic dystrophy. *Anesthesiology* 1984, **39**, 1007.

23 Siler J.N., Discavage W.J. Anaesthetic management of hypokalemic periodic paralysis. *Anesthesiology* 1975, **43**, 489.

24 Melnick B., Chang J.L., Larson C.E., *et al*. Hypokalemic familial periodic paralysis. *Anesthesiology* 1983, **5**, 263.

25 Egan T.J., Klein R. Hyperkalemic familial periodic paralysis. *Pediatrics* 1959, **24**, 761.

26 Johns R.A., Finhold D.A., Stirt J.A. Anaesthetic management of a child with dermatomyositis. *Can Anaes Soc J* 1986, **33**, 71.

27 Eng G.D., Epstein B.S., Engel W.K., McKay D.W., McKay R. Malignant hyperthermia and central core disease in a child with congenital dislocating hips. *Arch Neurol* 1978, **35**, 189.

28 Brown T.C.K., Gebert R., Meretoja O.A., Shield L.K. Myasthenia gravis in children and its anaesthetic implications. *Anaes Intens Care* 1990, **18**, 466.

29 Davies D.W., Steward D.J. Myasthenia gravis in children and anaesthetic management for thymectomy. *Can Anaes Soc J* 1973, **20**, 253.

30 Engel A. Congenital myasthenic syndromes. *J Child Neurol* 1988, **3**, 233.

31 Rodriguiz M., Gomez M.R., Howard F.M., Taylor W.F. Myasthenia gravis in children: a long-term follow-up. *Annals Neurol* 1983, **13**, 504.

32 Meretoja O.A., McHutchison G., Brown T.C.K. Alcuronium requirement in patients receiving phenytoin. *Anaes Intens Care* 1990, **8**, 483.

33 Quimby G.W., Williams R.N., Greifenstein F.E. Anaesthetic problems of the acute quadriplegic patient. *Anesth Analg* 1973, **52**, 533.

34 Stone W.A., Beach T.P., Hamelberg W. Succinylcholine — danger for spinal cord injured patient. *Anesthesiology* 1970, **32**, 168.

35 Smith R.B. Hyperkalaemia following succinylcholine administration in neurological disorders. *Can Anaes Soc J* 1971, **18**, 199.

36 Rocco A.G., Vandam L.D. Problems in anaesthesia for paraplegics. *Anesthesiology* 1959, **20**, 348.

37 Campbell A.M., Finley G.A. Anaesthesia for a patient with Friedreich's ataxia and cardiomyopathy. *Can Anaes Soc J* 1989, **36**, 89.

38 Bell C.F., Kelly J.M., Jones R.S. Anaesthesia for Friedreich's ataxia. *Anaesthesia* 1986, **41**, 296.

39 Kume M., Zin T., Oyama T. Anaesthetic experience with a patient with Friedreich's ataxia. *Jap J Anesth* 1976, **25**, 877.

40 Davis N.L., Davis R. Anesthetic management of the patient with dystonia musculoram deformans. *Anesthesiology* 1975, **42**, 630.

40aGrattan Smith P., Hopkins I.J., Shield L., Collins K. Acute respiratory failure precipitated anaesthesia in Leigh's syndrome. *J Child Neurology* 1990, **5**, 137.

41 Meridy H.W., Creighton R.C. General anaesthesia in eight patients with dysautonomia. *Can Anaes Soc J* 1971, **10**, 583.

42 Crichman N.N., Schwartz H., Papper E.M. Experiences with general anesthesia in patients with familial dysautonomia. *JAMA* 1959, **170**, 529.

43 Cox R.G., Sumner E. Familial dysautonomia. *Anaesthesia* 1984, **38**, 293.

44 McManamny D.S., Barnett J.S. Macroglossia as a presentation of the Beckwith−Wiedemann Syndrome. *Plas Reconst Surg* 1985, **75**, 170.

45 James I., Wark H. Airway management during anaesthesia in patients with epidermolysis bullosa dystrophica. *Anesthesiology* 1982, **56**, 323.

46 Boughton R., Crawford R.W., Vonwiller J.B. Epidermolysis bullosa: a review of 15 years' experience, including experience with combined general and regional anaesthetic techniques. *Anaes Intens Care* 1988, **16**, 260.

47 Cucchiara R.F., Dawson B. Anesthesia in Stevens−Johnson syndrome — a report of a case. *Anesthesiology* 1971, **35**, 537.

48 Birkham J., Heifetz M., Hairn S. Diffuse cutaneous scleroderma: an anaesthetic problem. *Anaesthesia* 1972, **27**, 89.

49 Kempthorne P.M., Brown T.C.K. Anaesthesia and the mucopolysaccharidoses: a survey of techniques and problems. *Anaes Intens Care* 1983, **11**, 203.

50 Baines D., Keneally J. Anaesthetic implications of the mucopolysaccharidoses. *Anaes Intens Care* 1983, **11**, 198.

51 Belani K., Floyd T., Liao J., Whitley C., Krivit W., Day D., Buckley J. Anesthetic considerations in patients with mucopolysaccharidoses. *9th World Congress of Anesthesiology*, 1988.

52 Herrick I.A., Rhine E.J. The mucopolysaccharidoses and anaesthesia: a report of clinical experience. *Can Anaes Soc J* 1988, **35**, 67.

53 Brown T.C.K. The airway in mucopolsaccharidoses. *Anaes Intens Care* 1984, **12**, 178.

54 Brosius F.C., Roberts W.C. Coronary artery disease in the Hurler syndrome. *Am J Cardiol* 1981, **47**, 649.

55 Beighton P., Craig J. Atlantoaxial subluxation in the Morquio syndrome: report of a case. *J Bone Joint Surg* 1973, **55B**, 478.

56 Birkinshaw K.J. Anaesthesia in a patient with an unstable neck: Morquio's syndrome. *Anaesthesia* 1975, **30**, 46.

57 Hobbs J.R. Bone marrow transplantation for inborn errors. *Lancet* 1981, **2**, 735.

58 Cox J.M. Anesthesia and glycogen storage disease. *Anesthesiology* 1968, **29**, 1221.

59 Dierdorf S.F., McNiece W.L. Anaesthesia and pyruvate dehydrogenase deficiency. *Can Anaes Soc J* 1983, **30**, 413.

60 Williams J.P., Sommerville G.M., Miner M.E., Reilly D. Atlantoaxial subluxation and Trisomy 21: another perioperative complication. *Anesthesiology* 1987, **67**, 253.

61 Steward D.J. Congenital abnormalities as a possible factor in the aetiology of post-intubation subglottic stenosis. *Can Anaes Soc J* 1970, **17**, 388.

62 Kobel M., Creighton R.E., Steward D.J. Anaesthetic considerations in Down's syndrome. *Can Anaes Soc J* 1982, **29**, 593.

63 Harris W.S., Goodman R.M. Hypersensitivity to atropine in Down's syndrome. *New Engl J Med* 1968, **279**, 407.

64 Keele D.K., Richards C., Brown J., Marshall J. Catecholamine metabolism in Down's syndrome. *Am J Mental Def* 1969, **74**, 125.

65 Baxter R.G., Larkins R.G., Martin F.I.R., Heyma P., Myles K. Down's syndrome and thyroid function in adults. *Lancet* 1975, **2**, 794.

66 Divekar V.M., Kothari M.D., Kamdar B.M. Anaesthesia in

Turner's syndrome. *Can Anaes Soc J* 1983, **30**, 417.
67 Chasnoff I.J. Cocaine and pregnancy: clinical and methodologic issues. *Clin Perinatol* 1991, **18**, 113.
68 Hoegerman G, Schnoll S. Narcotic use in pregnancy. *Clin Perinatol* 1991, **18**, 51.
69 Jones R.D.M. Anaesthesia in Sotos syndrome (in press).

FURTHER READING

Smith D.V. *Recognizable patterns of human malformation*. W.B. Saunders Co., Philadelphia & Toronto (1976).
McKusick V.A. *Heritable disorders of connective tissue* (4th edn.). C.V. Mosby Company, St. Louis (1972).

26: Anaesthesia for Surgical and Other Emergencies, Including Major Trauma

INTRODUCTION

When a child suffers a severe injury or develops an illness requiring emergency surgery, the problems involved in assessment and management can differ quite markedly from those of elective surgery. A number of these psychological and physical problems are dealt with in other chapters: neurosurgical (Chapter 14), thoracic (Chapter 12), cardiac (Chapter 13), orthopaedic (Chapter 19), burns (Chapter 20). There are a number of problems common to many of these conditions which can be considered together. They include the psycho-logical implications of the emergency situation, the assessment of the patient and the problem of food and other materials in the stomach. When a child has suffered multiple injuries, the order of assessment and resuscitation must be determined by allocation of priority to each problem; these need frequent reassessment so that the special skills of the several disciplines involved may be coordinated in the best interests of the patient.

PSYCHOLOGICAL EFFECTS

When a child sustains a minor injury, such as a greenstick fracture of the radius, the injury and its treatment may be seen by both the child and parents to be straight-forward. On the other hand, a number of factors can influence the effects of both the acute problem and its management. The injury or acute illness is almost always unexpected. This will restrict any time available for preparation of the child for the experience of admission to hospital, anaesthesia and surgery. The circumstances of the injury or illness may have a marked effect on the child's reaction. Thus a severe injury, perhaps an automobile accident or exposure to fire, may so frighten the child as to make further communication with him extremely difficult. Other members of the family may have been injured or even killed in the same accident. The sudden onset of acute abdominal pain or severe airway obstruction can be terrifying.

The injury or acute surgical condition can also be seen by the child and by the parents as a threat for the future, possibly leading eventually to disability, disfigurement or even death. It is important to remember that these fears may appear illogical to the medical and nursing staff, but can have a marked effect on the behaviour of the child and his parents and on their ability to communicate sensibly. Consciously or subconsciously, the child and the parents may be influenced by feelings of guilt. The child may feel punished for some wrongdoing, particularly if the injury has occurred during an activity forbidden by the parents. Similarly, the parents may feel that they might have prevented the injury or that they should have sought advice earlier. These reactions can influence the interpersonal relations between all those involved, i.e. the child, the parents and the medical and nursing attendants who may or may not be aware of the problem. It is important therefore that the child be treated with understanding and that unguarded remarks be avoided.

The feeling of abandonment which may follow the admission of young children to hospital, and the pain associated with the injury or illness, combine with the other problems to form a psychological management problem which may be quite complex. The management itself depends on the particular patient, but is largely a matter of common sense and of appreciating that these problems may exist.

As far as possible the principles of preoperative preparation set out in Chapter 6 should be applied. The events of anaesthesia and recovery, including the use of intravenous infusions, catheters and so on, should be explained to both the child and the parents so that the parents can supplement these descriptions and the reassurance needed with them. The positive results of surgery, such as relief of pain and repair of deformity, need to be emphasized. The child's fear of unconsciousness should be recognized and, where possible, mitigated. Unnecessary separation from parents during preparation for operation should be avoided. Premedication with sedative and analgesic drugs is indicated as part of the management, but the use of heavy sedation purely to avoid recognition of these problems is an inferior method of treatment, as the difficulties may only be deferred. The choice of premedication will depend on the anaesthetist and the particular problems affecting the patient. However, if he is in pain and distressed then premedication with papaveretum and hyoscine is often useful.

PREOPERATIVE ASSESSMENT

As well as considering the psychological effects discussed above, the preoperative assessment of a child who requires urgent surgery must include an assessment of general physical status, other medical conditions (outlined in Chapter 7), the extent of the injury or acute surgical condition, and the possibility of a full stomach. Acute gastric dilatation may also be present following trauma. As this may cause circulatory and respiratory embarrassment, the stomach may need to be decompressed immediately. Enquiry about past health and previous

anaesthetics and the importance of the physical examination should not be forgotten in an emergency. There may be effects on other systems, requiring modification of preoperative, intraoperative or postoperative management. The effect of drugs and anaesthesia on intracranial pressure must be considered in head injuries or neurosurgical emergencies. Resuscitation is frequently necessary before emergency operations. Deficits of blood and extracellular fluid volume, and electrolyte and acid–base imbalance must be recognized.

MAJOR TRAUMA

Epidemiology

Trauma is the most common cause of mortality in children over 1 year of age. Behavioural, environmental and social factors place a child at risk from trauma. Children exist in an environment created by adults, primarily for adults. They often require adult supervision, which may be inadequate. They have poor perceptions of speed and distance and are unpredictable and impulsive in behaviour. Children are unable to defend themselves and may be subject to deliberate trauma and abuse. A history of trauma that is inconsistent with examination findings, or the frequent attendance of a child sustaining trauma, in particular several injuries sustained at different times, should raise the suspicion of child abuse.

Blunt trauma and immersion injuries are most common, penetrating injuries being less common, although the relative incidence varies in different communities. Minor trauma is common in children, particularly from falls and tripping over objects. The main causes of traumatic death in children are injuries of pedestrians (42%), vehicle passengers (17%) and cyclists (13%) [1]. Immersion injuries (20%) are more common in children under the age of 4 years.

The tragedy is that in many cases, trauma and fatal injuries are avoidable and up to 50% of fatalities are preventable by wearing safety devices and children being supervised while negotiating traffic [1]. While the introduction of seat belts, bicycle helmets and swimming pool fences has helped reduce the incidence of accidental deaths, compliance with such safety measures is often poor.

Retrospective studies of paediatric trauma deaths has provided valuable information enabling improvement in initial patient care, and transport with a co-ordinated approach towards trauma management. Most errors of management occur between the time of injury and the arrival of the medical or paramedical assistance, but errors also occur at the site, during retrieval, and in hospital. Three main areas where errors occur are:

1 in airway management, such as delayed intubation or inadequate airway protection;

2 inadequate or inappropriate fluid and blood volume replacement;

3 in diagnosis resulting in inappropriate investigations or the failure to perceive progressive deterioration, particularly when there are complex interacting injuries. Avoiding such errors is important as they may significantly affect the patient's outcome.

Central nervous system injury is common after major trauma. A review of intensive care trauma admissions at the Royal Children's Hospital in Melbourne, Australia, over a 5-year period, showed that 66% of all trauma admissions were associated with CNS injury. If immersion injuries are added to this group the incidence increases to 80%. Isolated CNS trauma is more common than that associated with multi-system trauma. The important point is that the presence of serious central nervous system injury is the major factor determining mortality and underlines the importance of early intervention and aggressive management in these cases.

General assessment

When a child is admitted to hospital with multiple severe injuries, the anaesthetist is often asked to assist in assessment and resuscitation at an early stage so that his special skills in the management of respiratory and circulatory problems may be used, and so that he may take part in the assignment of priorities in resuscitation and surgical treatment. As in so many examples of clinical assessment and decision making, the procedure and order will depend on the clinical circumstances, and are the same whether the patient is a child or an adult. Important principles must not be forgotten just because the patient is an infant. In the following discussion, the order is that in which problems are usually assessed, but this order may need to be altered and must be frequently reviewed in any individual patient.

The first step must be to stop and look at the child as a whole. At this stage an assessment is made. This should always include the obvious sites of trauma, whether the child is breathing or not, appears to have an obstructed airway, is conscious, cyanosed or in acute distress, has grunting respiration, active bleeding, shocked and so on.

Obvious abnormalities may indicate the need for closer immediate assessment and treatment. For example, if the child is not breathing, the airway must be established and ventilation controlled before further assessment. Bleeding requires immediate control and the shocked patient *urgently* needs intravenous fluid.

Systematic assessment

A more careful assessment may now follow. If possible, a history of the injury and previous health should be obtained. Frequent reassessment is needed so that changes in the patient's condition are noted, and if necessary, the order of assessment altered. Resuscitation may be started by one or more members of the team during assessment, with particular attention to maintenance of airway, ventilation and restoration of blood volume and circulation. The important steps are as follows:

AIRWAY

The airway may be obstructed, because the patient is unconscious and hypotonic, or by foreign material. Careful inspection of the pharynx is essential to make sure that teeth and foreign material are not present. Severe continued bleeding into the airway may be an indication for early tracheal intubation. Maxillary injury may make intubation difficult and application of a face mask for inflation of the lungs almost impossible. When there is much laceration of the pharynx, inflation using a mask can cause extensive surgical emphysema. The presence of cerebrospinal fluid draining into the pharynx warns of the possibility of producing intracranial emphysema and the risk of meningitis. Marked surgical emphysema of the neck and face may suggest rupture of the trachea (Figs 26.1a,b, 26.2), in which case there is a danger that an endotracheal tube may pass outside the trachea. A blow to the front of the neck can cause rupture of the posterior part of the trachea in children, in the absence of other obvious injuries.

BREATHING

If the child is apnoeic or hypoventilating there is an obvious need to assist his breathing. The compliant chest wall, the increased dependence on the diaphragm for ventilation, and gastric or abdominal distension if present, make infants more prone to respiratory failure.

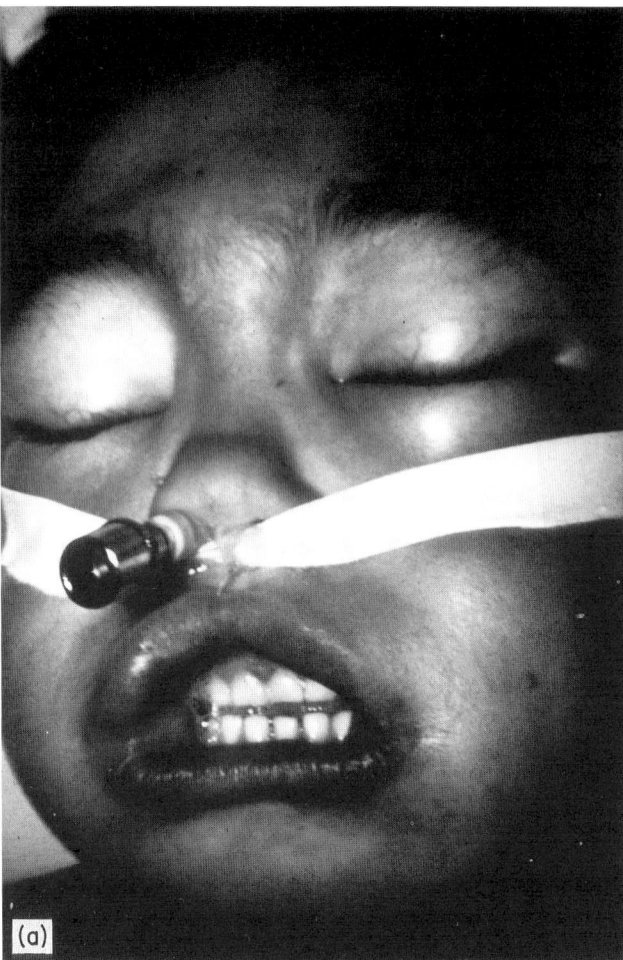

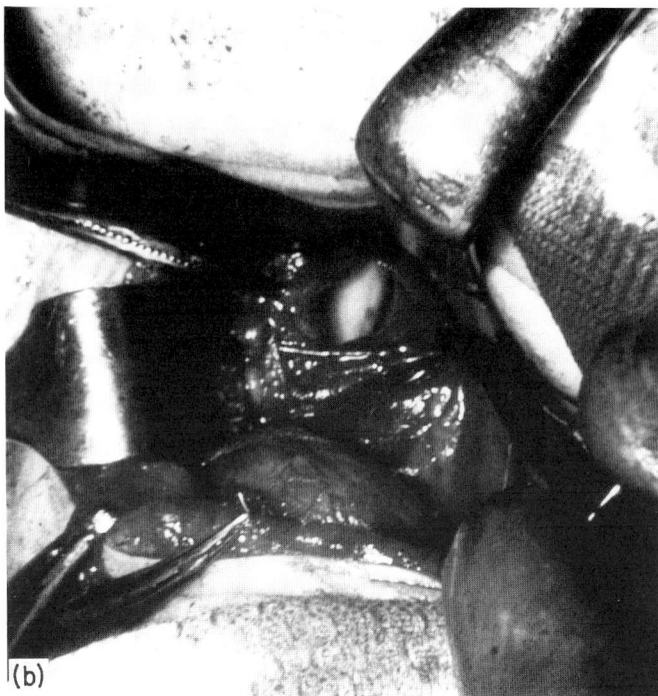

Fig. 26.1 Tracheal rupture. (a) Subcutaneous emphysema of the face of a child with a ruptured trachea. (b) Surgical exposure of a posterolateral hole in the patient's trachea.

Their high oxygen consumption and diminished oxygen reserve from an increased closing volume make them more likely to become hypoxaemic. Apnoea may be due to severe head injury, may follow hypoxia or cardiac arrest, or result from high spinal cord injury. In the latter case, if the child is conscious, movement of the accessory muscles of respiration, particularly sternomastoid or alae nasi, may be noted in the absence of other respiratory movements. When injuries to the lung or the chest have occurred, breathing movements may be ineffective and the patient may become hypoxic. A check should be made for tension pneumothorax. A chest X-ray, preferably in the upright position or, failing this a lateral film using a horizontal beam with the patient supine must be taken to rule out pneumothorax and massive haemothorax. Widening of the mediastinum will suggest damage to the aorta or pulmonary artery. Haemopericardium may cause tamponade with a large cardiac shadow. In

young children, crush injuries of the lower chest may result in a ruptured diaphragm, especially on the left.

CIRCULATION

In the early stages after injury in children, hypotension, tachycardia and other signs of low cardiac output are almost always the result of blood loss. This is an indication for starting intravenous resuscitation at once. If external bleeding is continuing, this should be stopped by application of pressure. Failure to respond to resuscitation suggests further internal bleeding; if this is not apparent on the chest X-ray then it is most likely within the abdomen.

CONSCIOUSNESS

Provided the patient is ventilating adequately and the airway is secured, unconsciousness by itself is not an

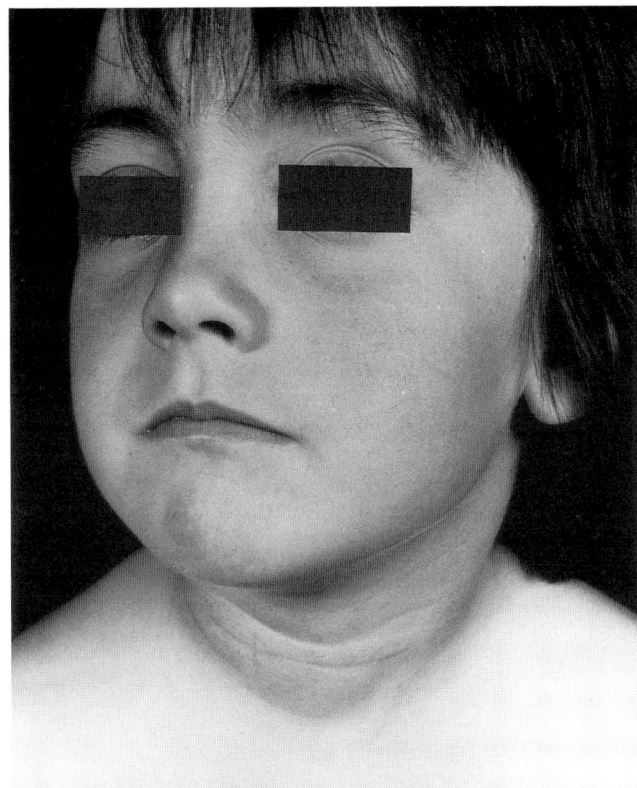

Fig. 26.2 The same patient as shown in Fig. 26.1, 2 months later.

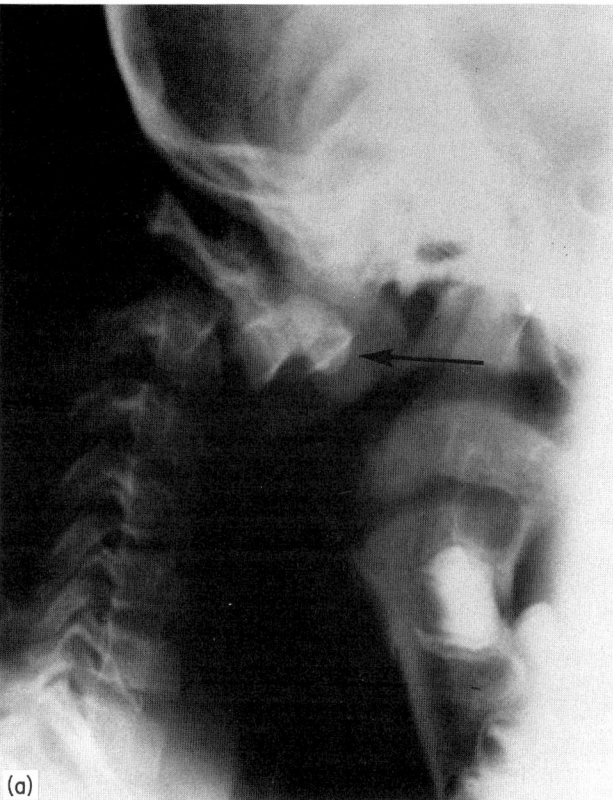

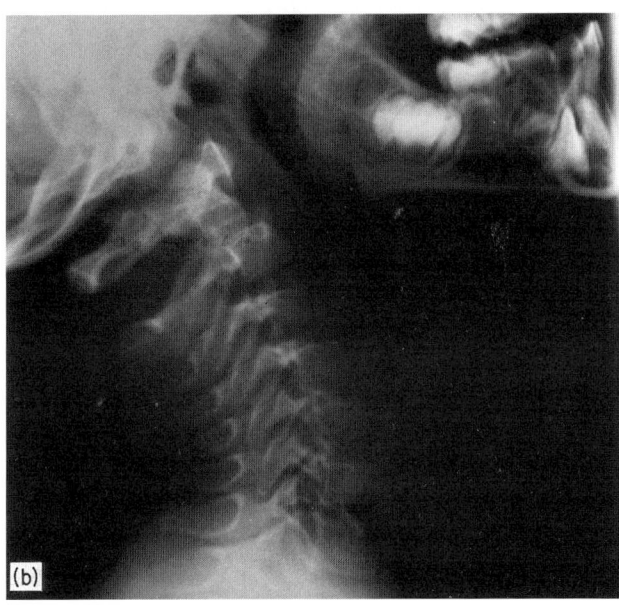

Fig. 26.3 Lateral neck X-rays showing subluxation of the atlantoaxial joint on (a) flexion, which was not obvious in (b) extension.

indication for urgent neurosurgical intervention. However, rapid deterioration in consciousness and the development of a unilateral fixed dilated pupil suggest continuing intracranial bleeding requiring urgent decompression by burr holes or, in infants, subdural tap (see Chapter 14).

THE NECK

The possibility of cervical spine injuries must always be considered, because injudicious movement of the neck may produce quadriplegia if not already present. A lateral X-ray of the neck is essential in all patients after multiple trauma (Fig. 26.3).

Spinal cord injury without radiological abnormality on plain films is a significant problem in children. While spinal cord injury is rare, it must be suspected in all patients with head injury. Up to 50% of spinal-cord injured patients will have no X-ray abnormality on presentation [2]. This relates to the flexible vertebral column yet relatively inelastic spinal cord. While vertebral fractures or displacement may not be seen on X-ray, prevertebral swelling may indicate a possible cord injury. If neck injury is suspected, the neck must be immobilized in a neutral position and injudicious movement avoided.

The other problem arising from neck trauma is rupture of the trachea, leading to the rapid development of subcutaneous emphysema. Urgent tracheal intubation may be needed to prevent airway obstruction. If this is not possible, immediate surgical exploration may be required.

ABDOMINAL INJURIES

Major abdominal trauma in children commonly involves solid viscera. This is due to a relative visceromegaly with an increased proportion of liver and spleen below the costal margin, associated with poor abdominal musculature and a flexible costal margin. Isolated abdominal trauma is rarely fatal in children, unless a major vessel or the liver is torn. Abdominal distension is common, but this is often due to gastric distension rather than intraperitoneal bleeding. Percussion of the abdomen may help to differentiate these. Abdominocentesis is not performed routinely, but is indicated in patients who are unstable despite aggressive volume replacement and in patients who have other injuries, particularly central nervous system injuries in which an unstable circulation is to be avoided. If continued bleeding occurs, as for example from a ruptured liver, early surgical intervention may be indicated (see Chapter 11). Guarding or rebound tenderness may be due to intraperitoneal blood or soiling from rupture of the bowel. Haematuria suggests renal injury, which may be defined by intravenous pyelography.

After initial resuscitation and stabilization, an abdominal CT scan with contrast can be performed to determine the extent of injury and to assist subsequent assessment.

THORACIC INJURIES

Major thoracic trauma in children may cause fractured ribs with associated pain and hypoventilation, but can often occur with relatively few external signs of injury, because the chest wall is very compliant in children. Significant lung injury, such as contusion, haemothorax or pneumothorax, and cardiac injury such as contusion, tamponade, septal and cusp rupture, may occur with few external signs of injury, rib fractures or flail segments. Examination of the chest wall, auscultation and chest X-ray are necessary in assessing chest injuries. Rate and depth of ventilation and adequacy of oxygenation must be determined.

OTHER INJURIES

The child should be examined for fractures of the spine, pelvis and limbs and for superficial injuries.

Fractures, lacerations, abrasions and dog bites are common injuries in children. They may be isolated injuries that do not require urgent or immediate surgery. However, it is important to appreciate that these injuries are often painful and distressing to the patient. Significant blood loss may also occur from both fractures and lacerations.

Trauma scoring systems

The development of scoring systems for patients following trauma has been advocated to improve field triage, planning, allocating and evaluating medical resources, and assessing the effectiveness of medical care in reducing morbidity and mortality. Such scoring systems also provide an indication of patient prognosis and the need for early transfer to appropriate centres.

The Paediatric Trauma Score incorporates physiological and anatomical measures in the assessment of injury severity, and has been found to be a useful guide to severity and outcome. The Paediatric Trauma Score is calculated by adding the numerical scores of its six components (see Table 26.1). The score ranges from +12, indicating no injury, to −6, indicating fatal injury. The Paediatric Trauma Score is accurate, reliable and predictable, enabling appropriate triage and transfer [3].

Resuscitation

As indicated in the previous section, resuscitation following multiple injuries must often start during the initial assessment and continue throughout. The first priorities are to establish the airway and ventilation, prevent soiling of the airway by blood and other materials, and deal with the problems of air leak into the pleural cavity and into the tissues.

AIRWAY

The establishment of a clear and protected airway is important after trauma but requires careful consider-

Table 26.1 Paediatric trauma score

	Severity category		
Component	+2	+1	−1
Size	>20 kg	10−20 kg	<10 kg
Airway	Normal	Maintainable	Unmaintainable
CNS	Awake	Obtunded	Comatose
Systolic BP	>90 mmHg	90−50 mmHg	<50 mmHg
Open wounds	None	Minor	Major or penetrating
Skeletal	None	Closed fracture	Open/multiple fractures

If a proper sized BP cuff is not available BP can be assessed by assigning:
+2 Pulse palpable at wrist;
+1 Pulse palpable at groin;
−1 No pulse palpable.

ation, particularly if associated with faciomaxillary trauma or possible spinal cord injury.

Careful inspection of the pharynx is essential to exclude foreign material and possible dislodged teeth. Maintaining the head in a neutral position with the mouth open and using jaw thrust may help maintain the airway. In other situations an oral airway may be necessary. However, severe faciomaxillary trauma, continued bleeding into the airway, or associated pharyngeal and laryngeal trauma may be an indication for early tracheal intubation. Significant swelling and haematoma around the neck, or surgical emphysema of the neck and face may suggest rupture of the trachea, in which case there is danger that an endotracheal tube may not enter the trachea but form a false passage into the tissues. If upper airway obstruction is severe and tracheal intubation is difficult, then urgent tracheostomy may be required.

In an unconscious patient, early airway control and, if necessary, ventilation is essential to prevent secondary cerebral injury from hypoxia and hypercapnia. If the child is not comatose and protective airway reflexes are intact then observation of the airway, supplementary oxygen and frequent reassessment of the level of consciousness may be all that is required. Patients who are comatose and have obtunded airway reflexes, particularly if transport is required, need airway control and protection with tracheal intubation.

Oral intubation is used for patients when difficulty with nasotracheal intubation is foreseen, including patients with severe faciomaxillary trauma. Nasal intubation may be preferred for transport and if prolonged airway support and ventilation are expected.

An appropriately sized endotracheal tube must be used, so that there is only a small leak when positive pressure is applied to the breathing system. Fixation is important so that accidental bronchial intubation or extubation is avoided (see Fig. 7.14).

Ideally, the tip of the endotracheal tube should be at the level of the clavicles on X-ray. It is important to note that small endotracheal tubes may be easily obstructed by secretions but intermittent suction will reduce the likelihood of this complication.

In patients with severe faciomaxillary trauma or subcutaneous emphysema, endotracheal intubation may be difficult. Consultation with surgical colleagues regarding the possible need for tracheostomy or cricothyroidotomy is important in such situations.

Intubation in the patient with a concomitant cervical spine injury may be difficult and may exacerbate underlying cervical cord trauma. Maintaining the head in a neutral position, as well as axial traction will often assist oral intubation in these patients.

VENTILATION

If ventilation is inadequate, assisted ventilation with a bag and mask may be required. Care must be taken to avoid gastric distension, which will splint the diaphragm. If ventilatory failure ensues, intubation and controlled ventilation is required.

CIRCULATION

Assessment of the circulation is primarily clinical. Hypovolaemia must be corrected. Depending on the extent of blood loss and the severity of shock, a crystalloid solution, such as Hartmann's, or a colloid plasma volume expander may be administered. In severe shock, as much as 30 ml/kg of colloid may be required initially, followed by blood when available. Blood loss may be readily concealed within the chest, abdomen and pelvis. Significant blood loss may occur from lacerations, particularly in smaller children and infants whose total blood volume is small.

Establishing venous access in shocked children may be very difficult. Peripheral sites in the limbs and scalp need to be looked for initially. Femoral and external jugular veins are useful alternatives. If no peripheral veins are apparent, a venous cut-down on the cephalic vein on the medial side of the wrist or in the deltapectoral groove or on the median cubital vein at the elbow is an alternative, although this may consume valuable time. If the necessary skill is available, central venous access via an internal jugular or subclavian vein is ideal as it also allows central venous pressure measurement. A direct intraosseous infusion is a good alternative if intravenous access has not been obtained and urgent volume replacement is necessary. The bone marrow is part of the vascular compartment and intramedullary veins are held open by the bone. Interosseous bone needles are available, or alternatively a 22 G spinal needle may be inserted. In children less than 1 year old, the needle may be inserted at the junction of the upper and middle thirds of the tibia; between 1–5 years the needle may be inserted just above the medial malleolus of the tibia and in children over 5 years the iliac crest may be used. The sternum should not be used because of the risk of potential insertion of the needle through the sternum into mediastinal structures. Once inserted, fluid may be readily injected with a syringe into the interosseous space and hence into the vascular compartment.

A warming device should be used when large volumes of fluid and blood are likely to be infused (see Chapter 3). Warming blood during rapid transfusion avoids cooling of the myocardium and the development of dysrhythmia, which sometimes lead to cardiac arrest. It minimizes general cooling with its complications such as decreased metabolism of citrate. When citrated blood is infused rapidly, the body may not be able to metabolize or store the citrate ion, and the resulting low plasma-ionized calcium may result in myocardial depression. This can be prevented by the administration of calcium chloride or calcium gluconate solution. The infusion of large volumes of stored blood may lead to pulmonary insufficiency if platelet aggregates accumulate in the pulmonary capillaries. Several blood filters are available to remove these aggregates, but they may slow infusion due to increasing resistance to flow through them, particularly when aggregates collect in them.

The bladder should be catheterized to monitor urine output in response to resuscitation.

HEAD INJURIES

The management of head injuries is discussed in Chapter 36, but it is important to emphasize aspects of initial management. Factors affecting cerebral perfusion press-

ure and intracranial pressure must be considered. Hypovolaemia must be corrected early; it is important to remember that significant blood loss may occur from scalp lacerations or be concealed in scalp or intracerebral haematomata. Prevention of airway obstruction and early intubation with controlled ventilation may be required to prevent secondary cerebral insults from hypoxaemia or hypercapnia.

Timing of surgery

In some quite severe cases of multiple injury, anaesthesia and surgery may not be the needed at all during the acute phase. If respiration and circulation are adequate, and blood volume is restored without further bleeding, the indications for surgery may be the need to explore the abdomen for visceral injury, the debridement and suturing of open wounds, especially with compound fractures, and the splinting and fixation of such fractures. Continuing bleeding, whether this is into the head, thorax or abdomen is the most urgent indication for surgery. If bleeding is rapid and severe it may not be possible to restore the blood volume until surgery has started and the bleeding points are controlled. Opening a body cavity or a large wound where there is a significant bleeding point may result in further massive bleeding and a sudden drop in blood pressure. It is essential that resuscitation continue, and that adequate supplies of cross-matched blood be obtained as soon as possible and administered through a blood warmer. On occasions, uncross-matched blood, preferably of the patient's own blood group, may need to be used initially. Attention to blood pressure, pulse rate, peripheral perfusion, central venous pressure and urinary output is essential. Direct arterial pressure monitoring can be most useful in the severely injured patient. The timing and nature of surgical intervention is a decision to be made by assessing the urgency of the problems. The priorities must be continually reviewed so that they are appropriate to the patient's interest. Antibiotics will be needed when surgery is deferred, if there are open wounds or peritonitis.

THE PROBLEM OF A FULL STOMACH

When emergency anaesthesia is necessary, the problem of a full stomach and gastric distension must be considered. There are a number of aspects to consider:
1 Gastric distension readily occurs after major trauma

and may be enhanced by unsuspected airway obstruction or assisted ventilation. This will limit diaphragmatic movement and increase the risk of regurgitation and aspiration.

2 The autonomic response to injury or acute illness can delay normal gastric emptying in children for many hours. Injuries may occur a short time following a meal, or in other circumstances drinks or sweets may have been given after an injury in an attempt to comfort the child.

3 The administration of opioids delays gastric emptying [4].

4 In abdominal emergencies, obstruction of the gastro-intestinal tract, whether mechanical or functional, will further prevent gastric emptying. Except in the case of pyloric obstruction, reverse peristalsis can rapidly refill the stomach, even though it may have been decompressed by aspiration of a nasogastric tube.

5 Intragastric bleeding or trauma to the upper airway, particularly the nose, mouth or pharynx, may result in gastric distension with blood and blood clot.

The patient with a full stomach and gastric distension is at greatest risk when this problem is not recognized or suspected. Following minor trauma, surgical procedures may be delayed for some hours to allow gastric emptying. In emergency situations such a delay is generally not possible; the anaesthetist, in consultation with the surgeon, must weigh up the potential risks of aspiration against the surgical indications to proceed with the operation.

Attempts can be made to empty the stomach prior to urgent surgery. The intravenous injection of metoclopramide (100 μg/kg) has been advocated to hasten gastric emptying in patients awaiting surgery after injuries. The reduction of psychological stress may allow more rapid gastric emptying.

Induction of vomiting or the passage of a large-bore (19–20 Fr gauge) tube passed through the mouth into the stomach may be considered, although there are few benefits to be obtained with such an unpleasant assault on the child and it may be dangerous in critically injured children. For similar reasons, the intravenous administration of apomorphine is unacceptable.

Blood and solid matter in the stomach present a particular problem because even though fluid can be removed by the nasogastric tube, clots and solid food may remain.

Anaesthetic management

The important points in the anaesthetic management of a child for emergency surgery are adequate resuscitation and avoidance of aspiration from a 'full' stomach.

If the patient is inadequately resuscitated, cardiac output is decreased and blood is distributed preferentially to the brain and the heart. The usual doses of depressant drugs such as thiopentone and opioids will have an enhanced depressant effect on these organs, sometimes with dangerous consequences. Drugs given intramuscularly will be poorly absorbed due to decreased muscle blood flow.

Aspiration is avoided by preventing regurgitation into the pharynx when the patient is anaesthetized. Evenly distributed pressure on the cricoid cartilage should compress and occlude the oesophagus (see Fig. 7.5) until the endotracheal tube is passed.

When general anaesthesia is used in the presence of a full stomach, an endotracheal tube should be inserted. If not the anaesthetist must always be prepared to deal with copious vomiting. Most anaesthetists prefer to pass an endotracheal tube after inducing the patient with thiopentone and a muscle relaxant. The use of cricoid pressure has made tracheal intubation and general anaesthesia in the presence of a full stomach relatively safe. Cricoid pressure should be applied as soon as anaesthesia is induced and maintained until the endotracheal tube is in place. Excessive pressure may cause airway obstruction and make it difficult to pass the tube. Many children, particularly older ones, can be given oxygen to breathe for a minute or two before induction, thus allowing the endotracheal tube to be passed without inflation of the lungs. In less co-operative children it may be safer to apply firm cricoid pressure and gently inflate the lungs with oxygen after induction and before intubation. The choice of muscle relaxant depends on the individual anaesthetist. A rapid onset is desirable. Suxamethonium is still preferred by many because the onset of profound relaxation is rapid. This is partly because the doses commonly used are three to four times ED95. If a large dose of atracurium (e.g. 0.6–0.8 mg/kg) is used, the onset of action will also be more rapid (see Chapter 2). This usually allows intubation of the pre-oxygenated patient without further ventilation of the lungs. Patients can be ventilated and intubated using newer short-acting agents provided cricoid pressure is properly applied. If a nasogastric tube is left in place, the cardio-oesophageal junction may become incompetent and there is a danger of leakage around it. Suxamethonium in large doses has been shown to increase intragastric pressure during the muscle fasciculation but as the rise in pressure in the lower oesophagus exceeds the rise in intragastric pressure, the suggested prior administration of a very small dose of a non-depolarizing relaxant (one-tenth of the usual dose) to reduce the rise in intragastric pressure is probably unnecessary.

An alternative approach which allows non-depolarizing relaxants to be used in infants and small children is to pass a Foley catheter into the stomach, blow up the balloon (having previously checked that it balloons evenly around the catheter), and pull it up against the cardio-oesophageal junction to form a seal. The balloon must be kept in position by taping the catheter securely, under slight tension, to the face. The catheter then acts as a vent to the outside and prevents soiling of the airways (Fig. 26.4). If properly placed it requires very high intragastric pressures to make this incompetent, a situation which does not occur if the catheter is open.

An endotracheal tube may be passed following an inhalation induction, but the patient should be placed on his left side, for two reasons: if vomiting or regurgitation occurs the vomitus will tend to drain out of the mouth, and secondly, during laryngoscopy the tongue will tend to fall to the left, allowing an unobstructed view with the laryngoscopes most commonly used.

At the end of the procedure the endotracheal tube should be left in place until the child has recovered muscle tone and reflexes and is virtually awake.

The management of the child with a full stomach must be made as safe as possible in the circumstances. Recognition of the risk and the appropriate management are the two most important considerations.

The use of regional anaesthesia, such as axillary brachial plexus block or intravenous regional anaesthesia for injuries to the upper limb, can solve some of the problems but care must be taken not to exchange the hazards of general anaesthesia in a child with a full stomach for the complications of regional anaesthesia, which may be more hazardous in this situation. Depending on age and psychological make-up, the child may cooperate sufficiently for the anaesthetist to perform a regional block.

SPECIAL CASES

Throughout this book, surgical emergencies which may

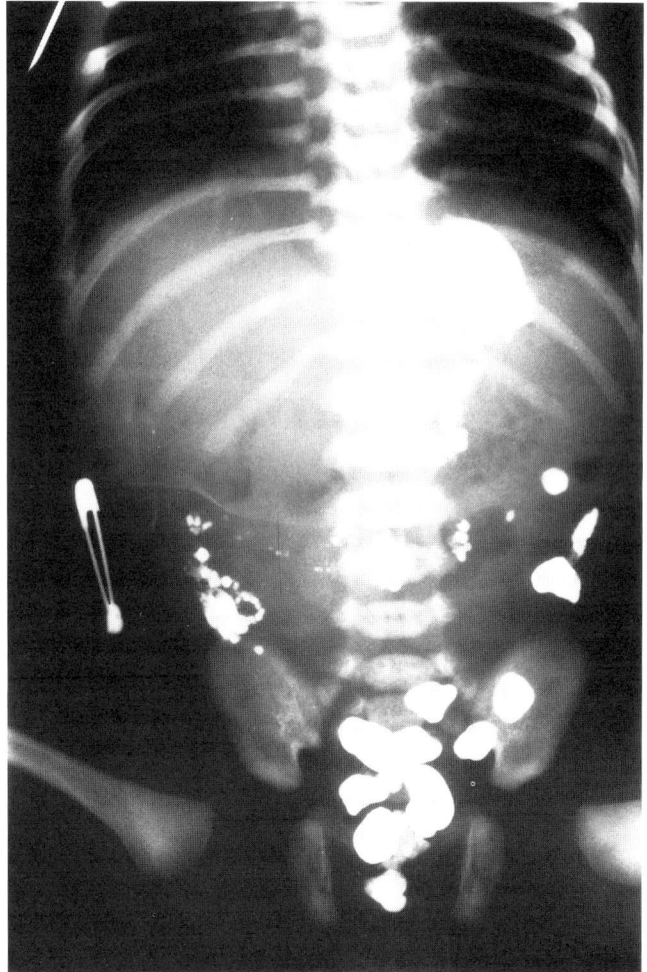

Fig. 26.4 Infant with bowel obstruction who had had a gastrografin enema (incompletely expelled). A Foley catheter with the balloon inflated and pulled up against the cardio-oesophageal junction used to prevent regurgitation.

require anaesthesia urgently are discussed in the context of the various sub-specialties of paediatric anaesthesia. A few further conditions that may not be fully covered in the other chapters are mentioned here.

The obstructed airway

Airway obstruction is a severe life-threatening emergency. It may occur in association with trauma, when teeth, blood or other foreign matter may be the cause, from inhalation of foreign bodies such as peanuts (see Chapter 15), or may be a result of tumours, cysts or infection. In the management of severe obstruction it is important to assess as rapidly as possible the site of the obstruction. When this has been done, the obstruction must be overcome. Tracheal intubation will usually overcome airway obstruction in children. In the severely obstructed child this may be accomplished without anaesthesia, although if possible, inflation of the child's lungs with 100% oxygen before intubation is desirable. In other patients some form of anaesthesia, with or without muscle relaxation, may be necessary. When the obstruction is above the glottis, and in many cases when it is below, inhalation induction (e.g. halothane) with a high concentration of oxygen may be safer. Ventilation should be assisted because the obstruction, if severe, usually reduces tidal volume. Induction of anaesthesia is usually slower if there is significant airway obstruction. If the anaesthetist is confident that he can inflate the lungs with oxygen and pass an endotracheal tube a muscle relaxant may be used, but one must always be aware of the danger that sudden paralysis may relax the tone of the muscles which are maintaining the airway and result in sudden complete obstruction. An alternative is to continue with inhalation anaesthesia and assisted ventilation; if necessary, spray the larynx with lignocaine before intubation. When the airway has been secured with an endotracheal tube, management of the cause can be undertaken. After intubation, acute swellings such as retropharyngeal abscess or a cyst can be incised and drained. When more prolonged treatment is necessary, a nasotracheal tube may be substituted; the oral tube should not be removed until the patient is well-oxygenated and the nasal tube is ready to pass into the larynx.

In some patients, often infants, with a narrow larynx, subglottic stenosis or papillomata the airway may be so narrow that intubation is either impossible or provides an inadequate airway, and tracheostomy is needed. When the obstruction is less severe but is a long-term problem, tracheostomy may again be indicated. A more extensive discussion of the causes of obstruction and their management can be found in the section on Respiratory Failure (see Chapters 32 and 33).

In a crisis, when ventilation is impossible, the insertion of a large needle or cannula through the cricothyroid membrane into the trachea may be life-saving. Oxygen can be insufflated, but care must be taken to ensure that the rate of gas escape is not exceeded by the inflow, otherwise the pressure in the lungs will rise, resulting in the risk of pneumothorax.

The battered child

These children may present with numerous and bizarre injuries. The most common conditions requiring anaesthesia and surgical intervention are intracranial bleeding resulting from head injury, fractures, abdominal injuries and even burns. The psychological problems discussed earlier in this chapter are very much to the fore and can affect not only the parents and relatives but also the medical and nursing staff, who can be distressed by the problems with which they are faced. Once again the need is for careful team work and an attempt by all concerned to understand the problems. Only one of the medical team should closely question the parents and child about the circumstances of the injury. All other staff should avoid a threatening attitude. They should be supportive and friendly and must not be seen to be suspicious or angry. At the time of tracheal intubation, the anaesthetist should examine the mouth and pharynx, recording the presence or absence of lacerations, bruising, and loose or recently removed teeth.

Facial injuries from dog bite

This is a common acute injury occurring in young children. German shepherds or Alsatians are the most common offenders. The psychological problems can be quite severe, particularly where the injury follows a sudden unexpected bite from a well-loved family pet; the parents may have conscious or unconscious feelings of guilt compounded with their fear of permanent disfigurement. A sympathetic team approach is needed with preoperative reassurance, comforting and sedation. The same general principles apply to these emergencies.

Other lacerations, injuries and fractures

The psychological effects, the need for preoperative preparation and the management of the full stomach have been outlined earlier in this chapter. No matter how minor the injury may appear, these factors can complicate the anaesthetic management.

REFERENCES

1 Wheatley J., Cass D.T. Traumatic deaths in children: the importance of prevention. *Med J Aust* 1989, **150**, 72.

2 Pang D., Pollack I.F. Spinal cord injury without radiographic abnormality in children: the SCIWORA syndrome. *J Trauma* 1989, **29**, 654.

3 Ramenofsky M.L. The predictive validity of Pediatric Trauma Score. *J Trauma* 1988, **28**, 1038.

4 Nimmo W.S., Heading R.C., Wilson J., Tothill P., Prescott L.F. Inhibition of gastric emptying and drug absorption by narcotic analgesics. *Br J Clin Pharmacol* 1975, **2**, 509.

27: Important Emergencies During Paediatric Anaesthesia

INTRODUCTION

A life-threatening emergency may occur during induction, maintenance or recovery from anaesthesia. Unexpected developments or some hitherto unsuspected abnormality in the patient may cause such problems. In most cases, failure to detect the early signs of abnormality in the patient or the equipment sets the stage for disaster. Careful monitoring of the patient and the equipment, together with appropriate responses to the information this provides, will prevent many potential problems from becoming emergencies. Pulse oximetry has been a major advance in monitoring, as it warns the anaesthetist very rapidly if peripheral oxygen supply decreases, and thus allows prompt assessment and management of the cause.

Cyanosis develops as the oxygen saturation falls to critical levels and more than 5 g/100 ml haemoglobin is desaturated. It is an important sign that all is not well with the patient, whether it be peripheral or central in origin. Peripheral pooling of blood causes peripheral cyanosis, especially in association with hypothermia, hypovolaemia, dehydration, acidosis and polycythaemia. It is essential that the cause be rapidly established and appropriate management undertaken. When a surgeon says that the blood 'looks dark' the comment must never be ignored. A careful inspection of the patient's ventilation and circulation and of the equipment and oxygen supply should be made. A particularly dangerous situation occurs when central cyanosis is mistakenly interpreted as peripheral cyanosis, with consequent inappropriate management. The appearance of central cyanosis indicates that respiratory problems need correction, the most common cause being failure to ventilate the patient's lungs with the appropriate gas mixture. Inexperienced anaesthetists using the T-piece with an open-tailed bag for controlled ventilation, may fail to adjust the leak from the bag to provide adequate ventilation.

Other aspects of monitoring, as outlined in Chapter 4, are also important in detecting the incipient emergency, and particular attention should be paid to unexplained tachycardia, bradycardia, dysrhythmia or inappropriately low or high blood pressure. Any such abnormality may warn of an impending problem, some common examples of which are discussed.

CARDIAC ARREST DURING ANAESTHESIA

The underlying principle in the management of this emergency at any stage is that oxygenated blood must be supplied to the brain as soon as possible. All other considerations are secondary to this in the early management of cardiac arrest. A detailed discussion on the management of cardiac arrest is presented in Chapter 35.

Recognition and management of cardiac arrest during anaesthesia is similar to that in other circumstances. However, there are several notable differences in the aetiology.

Predisposing factors

ANAESTHETIC AGENTS

All agents depress vital functions. The margin between good surgical conditions (unconsciousness, obtunded reflexes and lack of movement) and excessive depression of vital function — particularly ventilation and cardiac output — may be quite narrow. This is especially so if vital functions are already compromised by illness or accident. All the halogenated inhalation agents depress ventilation and cardiac output, although there are some differences in depression potency at equivalent MAC values. Halothane, for example, depresses myocardial contractility more than isoflurane. The intravenous induction agents (e.g. thiopentone) cause hypotension if injected too quickly or in excessive dose. Bradycardia, and hence diminished cardiac output, may be caused by excessive halothane or repeated doses of suxamethonium. In neonates and small infants, bradycardia is particularly significant because alternations in cardiac output are almost entirely dependent on changes in heart rate, not stroke volume. Tachycardia may be caused by some agents such as pancuronium, that release catecholamines. The cause of tachycardia may be difficult to discern, as it may also be due to other causes such as hypovolaemia, surgical stimulation or hypoxaemia.

If cardiac arrest does occur during anaesthesia, all agents should be immediately discontinued and the patient ventilated with 100% oxygen.

EQUIPMENT AND MONITORING

The safe conduct of anaesthesia — particularly general anaesthesia — is dependent upon reliable function and correct use of equipment. Equipment function should be checked periodically and the anaesthetic machine and breathing system should be checked before commencing anaesthesia.

Any equipment can malfunction unexpectedly, at any time. Fortunately, most of the equipment used by an anaesthetist is reliable, and adequate monitoring of the function of the equipment (see Chapter 5) can detect problems early and prevent the development of a life-threatening emergency. An emergency may arise most frequently from failure of the gas supply to provide the appropriate mixture to the breathing circuit, from obstruction to the flow of gases, or from leaks in the system. When such abnormalities are detected, it is important to remember that care of the patient and especially ventilation of the lungs with an adequate supply of oxygen is more urgent than fixing the apparatus. In the case of major failure, expired air ventilation or, if readily available, a self-inflating bag can be used while the apparatus is either replaced or repaired.

Unfortunately not all failures of equipment can be anticipated, so that constant vigilance is essential. Sometimes observation of the patient's colour, feeling the pulse and hearing the heart sounds with a stethoscope are essential to differentiate between the patient's physiological dysfunction and equipment failure with presentation of abnormal information.

The anaesthetist should always be able to monitor aspects of vital function such as blood pressure, heart rate and rhythm, ventilation and tissue oxygenation. If the surgical procedure makes access to the patient difficult it is particularly important that all monitors are properly attached and working reliably.

SURGERY

Although the ultimate aim of surgery is to correct some lesion, defect or illness, surgery, like anaesthesia, may temporarily compromise the patient's vital functions. Such problems as blood loss, obstructed venous return, compressed lung and bradycardia caused, for example by extra-ocular muscle retraction, can all diminish oxygen transport.

PRE-EXISTING DISEASE

Pre-existing illness adds to the risk of anaesthesia and surgery, especially if it is not possible to correct the underlying abnormality preoperatively. Cardiac failure, septicaemia or chronic lung disease, for example, add significantly to the hazard of anaesthesia.

Mishaps during anaesthesia and surgery

Despite the utmost care taken by anaesthetists and surgeons in their interference with the patient's homeostatic mechanisms, mishaps do occur. Errors of judgement, failure to notice significant physiological changes, mistakes and unanticipated events may lead to cardiac arrest. Examples are unrecognized oesophageal intubation, anaphylactic reaction to a drug, mistaken drug dosage or lacerated major vessel.

DYSRHYTHMIA

In small children, bradycardia is a common response to hypoxia and overdosage with drugs such as halothane or suxamethonium; it may occur reflexly, particularly during retraction of eye muscles, laryngoscopy, tonsillectomy and intrathoracic manipulation of mediastinal vessels. While it is sometimes necessary to administer atropine to prevent severe bradycardia, it is equally important to search for the cause of the bradycardia, to ensure that it is not hypoxia or obstruction of some major blood vessel. If it is, it is better to treat the cause rather than mask the symptom with atropine.

Sinus tachycardia is common in anaesthetized children, particularly in infants; it may be difficult to distinguish tachycardia caused by surgical stimulation during light anaesthesia from other causes.

A wandering atrial pacemaker with nodal rhythm is the most common dysrhythmia occurring during anaesthesia in children. Ventricular ectopic contractions and other forms of dysrhythmia are not common in the absence of cardiac disease.

Dysrhythmia may be detected by feeling the pulse, listening to the heart sounds and by ECG. One of the commonest causes is the association of hypercarbia with certain inhalation agents such as halothane. Such dysrhythmia respond to increasing ventilation.

LARYNGOSPASM

Laryngospasm is continuous adduction of the vocal cords, usually alone but maybe simultaneously with tonic contraction of the abdominal and thoracic muscles during light planes of anaesthesia. It is more common with certain agents such as halothane and enflurane. It is usually precipitated by the presence of secretions or by stimulation during attempted intubation or insertion of an oral airway when the patient is inadequately anaesthetized, or it may follow extubation. The incidence of laryngospasm is increased more than five times in patients with upper respiratory tract infections [1]. Rigidity of the trunk muscles in association with laryngeal spasm is rare, but is most likely to occur in unpremedicated children induced with halothane if airway instrumentation is begun before an adequate depth of anaesthesia is achieved (i.e. when the pupils are still divergent).

Muscle relaxants prevent laryngeal spasm and a rapidly acting one such as suxamethonium will relieve it. Local anaesthesia on the larynx decreases the responsiveness to tactile stimuli, making spasm unlikely. If intubation or endoscopy is carried out under inhalation anaesthesia alone, an adequate depth of anaesthesia must be reached first. Usually 3.5–4% halothane breathed spontaneously for 5 minutes will achieve this unless there is partial airway obstruction, which will slow uptake. Laryngeal spasm can follow extubation. Some anaesthetists extubate while the patient is still deeply anaesthetized but these children are more likely to develop stridor in the recovery room. Others turn the inhalation anaesthetic off early so that anaesthesia is light enough for spasm not to occur after extubation. Inhalation anaesthetic supplementation, particularly with halothane and enflurane, during a relaxant anaesthetic increases the incidence of laryngeal spasm and stridor following extubation if it is not turned off soon enough.

Stridor associated with anaesthesia may be due to incomplete spasm caused by laryngeal irritability. It may also occur with partial airway obstruction, or occasionally with laryngomalacia, which has less serious connotations than the former causes. In many cases this is relieved by applying CPAP.

The management of laryngospasm is based on the need to supply oxygen. In situations where it is likely to occur, such as after removal of an endotracheal tube, the administration of high inspired concentrations of oxygen before extubation can help the patient to tolerate a period of obstruction without significant hypoxia.

When laryngospasm does occur it is important to maintain a clear pharyngeal airway, and administer 100% oxygen so that whatever gas does enter the lung may be of the greatest value in relieving hypoxia.

In severe laryngospasm, gentle positive pressure should be continuously applied by a face mask, so that whenever spasm relaxes, even to the slightest degree, some oxygen will enter the trachea. Unless there is some obvious anatomical problem preventing achievement of a clear pharyngeal airway, attempts at laryngoscopy and forcible tracheal intubation waste time that should be used to introduce oxygen into the trachea. The use of muscle relaxants to overcome laryngospasm is appropriate where this can be done without interfering with the efforts of the most skilled person present to oxygenate the child. It should be remembered that the administration of suxamethonium to a severely hypoxic patient may worsen bradycardia and lead to cardiac arrest. In the unlikely event that all other methods fail, the passage of a relatively large-bore needle through the cricothyroid membrane will allow some oxygen to be introduced. When laryngospasm is recurrent or continues, muscle paralysis and the passage of an endotracheal tube to secure the airway is appropriate; the tube can then be left in place until the patient is conscious.

OTHER CAUSES OF AIRWAY OBSTRUCTION

Babies and children may present with conditions associated with airway obstruction (see Chapter 31). An operation may be needed to relieve the obstruction, for example tonsil and adenoidectomy (see Chapter 15), but often the tendency to obstruct adds to the difficulty of maintaining the airway during anaesthesia. Intubation may bypass the obstruction and solve the problem, but in some conditions with micrognathia (e.g. Pierre Robin and Treacher−Collins syndromes — Chapter 17), with tissues swollen by infiltrates (e.g. Hurler's or Hunter's syndromes — Chapter 25), or with infection (e.g. quinsy), obstruction and difficult intubation may co-exist. Sometimes opening the mouth before placing the mask on the face and then pulling the jaw forward will provide a clear airway, but it may be difficult to maintain this for prolonged periods (see Chapter 7). The insertion of an oropharyngeal airway or laryngeal mask may help in some circumstances or a nasopharyngeal airway may be a more effective way to bypass the obstruction.

If airway obstruction develops during anaesthesia, oxygen saturation will decline and inflation pressures will rise; rapid action needs to be taken, including increasing the inspired oxygen concentration. Any of the above steps which seem appropriate can be taken. If the patient is already intubated the tube may be kinked, compressed, obstructed by blood, sputum or adenoid tissue, misplaced

or disconnected. The passage of a catheter through the length of the tube will ensure at least some patency. If in doubt, laryngoscopy may be necessary to check the tube placement or to insert a new tube. The differential diagnosis of bronchospasm must be kept in mind.

If another form of artificial airway is in use, airway obstruction suggests that it is not fulfilling its function and that another approach, possibly endotracheal intubation, is needed.

If intubation is not possible, ventilation is inadequate and the situation is becoming desperate, the insertion of a large-bore cannula through the cricothyroid membrane and insufflation with oxygen may be life-saving. Once the situation is under control, intubation may again be attempted, if necessary using one of the techniques described in Chapter 7.

Postoperatively, the cause of the airway obstruction may still be present. To avoid problems it is important that recovery from anaesthesia is prompt and that analgesia is provided with minimal respiratory depression. It is wise to wait until the patient's airway reflexes have returned before extubation or removal of the artificial airway.

If there is likelihood of airway problems and hypoxaemia in the recovery room the patient should be observed carefully, monitored with oximetry if available and given supplemental oxygen. Resuscitation equipment must be readily available.

On occasions when hypoxaemia progressively worsens despite oxygenation, inspection of the airway by laryngoscopy may elucidate the cause — possibilities include vomited food, blood clot and even a swab not removed at the end of the operation.

Laryngeal obstruction after extubation may occur from the use of too large an endotracheal tube, or a tube which may be irritant, whether from the materials of which it is made or from contamination with substances used in cleaning or disinfection. Since the recognition of both these problems such damage is now rare. However, stridor after extubation can still occur, despite the use of a non-irritant tube of appropriate size. This may occur in a child who has a history of recurrent attacks of subglottic oedema (croup), perhaps associated with a congenitally narrow subglottic airway, or in a child who has a viral upper airway infection. Supraglottic or laryngeal injury may result from bronchoscopy, especially if the bronchoscope is inserted several times, or rarely from unduly forceful or clumsy attempts at laryngoscopy or intubation. Postoperative stridor due to laryngeal oedema following intubation is usually apparent in the first hour; it is very rare for it to develop after 2 hours.

If the obstruction is severe and life-threatening, oxygen under gentle positive pressure, as recommended for the management of laryngospasm, should be administered, and if necessary this can be followed by reintubation. Less severe episodes of stridor can often be relieved by inhalation of racemic adrenaline (2.25% solution, 0.05 ml/kg up to a maximum of 1.5 ml) as a mist nebulized with an oxygen flow of 8 l/min. If the stridor recurs, the treatment can be repeated. The merits of systemic corticosteroid drugs for extubation stridor are debated. They may be more useful if given before extubation, but some anaesthetists will give 0.1–0.25 mg/kg of dexamethasone (or equivalent) intravenously with the object of reducing oedema. Most cases of extubation stridor are amenable to conservative management in this way and subside in an hour or two. Occasionally, reintubation, sometimes for up to a few days, may be necessary, in which case the possibility of some abnormality should be considered and looked for.

ASPIRATION OF GASTRIC CONTENTS

Inhalation of gastric contents during anaesthesia in patients who have been formally prepared is uncommon, but is most frequent between 0 and 9 years [2]. The preoperative use of antacids such as sodium citrate and H_2 antagonists (e.g. ranitidine) has been shown to reduce the acidity of gastric contents in some, but not all, children [3]. This practice has not yet been widely adopted in children. If aspiration of gastric contents does occur following an episode of regurgitation or vomiting, the principles of providing a clear airway, adequate oxygenation and aspirating foreign material from the trachea through an endotracheal tube, should first be applied. Clinical examination, chest X-ray and monitoring of oxygen saturation should determine whether any lung changes have occurred. In some cases of more severe aspiration, intubation and mechanical ventilation may be necessary.

Despite care taken to the contrary, the possibility that children awaiting elective surgery have inadvertently obtained food and drink is always present. Children who have been subjected to stress such as trauma or have had morphine for analgesia may have considerable delay in gastric emptying. The time from feeding until trauma is the most relevant in assessing increased risk (see Chapters 7 and 26). Severe pain may also slow gastric emptying; boys with torsion of the testis are a special risk group. Infants who are fed excessive volumes, particularly of cows' milk — over 25 ml/kg — less than 3 hours before anaesthesia are at increased risk, as are babies with undiagnosed pyloric stenosis.

Other foreign materials may obstruct the airway. Deciduous teeth or faulty pieces of equipment are high on the list of suspects.

BRONCHOSPASM

Bronchospasm during anaesthesia may be due to histamine release by drugs such as some of the muscle relaxants, especially D-tubocurarine, or morphine in susceptible individuals, and is a feature of anaphylaxis. It may also result from mechanical stimulation of the airway, aspiration, or in atopic individuals such as asthmatics. Although not commonly used in children, non-specific beta-blocking drugs can cause bronchospasm.

Treatment is to administer bronchodilating drugs. Halothane is commonly recommended, although ether and methoxyflurane, which are now rarely used, were more potent. Ketamine has sympathomimetic bronchodilating properties and has been used successfully. Other more conventional drugs such as aminophylline (5 mg/kg by very slow intravenous injection) and β-adrenergic stimulants including adrenaline and nebulized salbutamol can be used, but care must be taken to avoid interactions with drugs such as halothane, which might cause dysrhythmia.

ANAPHYLAXIS

Minor allergic phenomena such as hyperaemia, or wheals at an injection site, are common during anaesthesia. Rarely, a severe reaction occurs with bronchospasm and/or severe hypotension with cardiovascular collapse. Urgent treatment is required. Adrenaline, preferably by slow intravenous injection, is the usual initial treatment. As little as 10 μg/kg (0.01 ml/kg of 1:10 000) adrenaline intravenously may relieve bronchospasm and produce myocardial stimulation, although more can be given cautiously when necessary. Hypotension, due to vasodilatation and capillary leakage, should be treated by raising the legs and administering intravenous fluids including a plasma volume expander (e.g. albumin, stable plasma protein solution, or Haemaccel). Hydrocortisone (8 mg/kg) may also be used. Antihistamines are too slow-acting in the acute situation.

Patients who exhibit hypersensitivity responses should be skin-tested with the drugs given. Usually 0.1 ml of a 1:1000 dilution is injected intradermally on the forearm and compared with controls. In small children a more dilute solution may be used initially. A wheal of 1.5 cm persisting for 30 minutes is positive [4].

A full range of resuscitation equipment must be available when these tests are carried out.

PNEUMOTHORAX

Abnormalities of the lung, in which there is over-distension of the alveoli or lung cysts, may give rise to spontaneous pneumothorax during anaesthesia. Contributory factors may be severe coughing or straining associated with tracheal intubation or over-distension of the lung with mechanical ventilation. Over-distension can be aggravated in lung segments where air trapping occurs when nitrous oxide is used, because it can rapidly diffuse into these areas. On the other hand, even when the lungs are normal, the use of high-flow breathing systems, such as the T-piece, or jet ventilation during bronchoscopy, can set the scene for accidental over-inflation of the lungs, resulting in pneumothorax and surgical emphysema. If the expiratory limb of a T-piece is occluded, by kinking or from the accidental obstruction of the tail of a reservoir bag, hyperinflation can occur very rapidly. The use of pressure-limiting devices on anaesthetic machines may reduce this hazard (Chapter 3). Pneumothorax may also follow insertion of a central venous catheter.

When over-distension of alveoli from abnormalities of the lung is present or accidental hyperinflation has occurred, the anaesthetist must be on the look-out for the presence of pneumothorax. The physical signs of pneumothorax may be difficult to detect in a small baby during mechanical ventilation when the body is covered with surgical drapes. Difficulty in inflating the lungs, particularly in the presence of cyanosis and bradycardia, can indicate a tension pneumothorax. Breath sounds may be diminished on the side of the pneumothorax, but if it is difficult to detect this, the marked shift in the precordial heart sounds may indicate that the mediastinum is being pushed either to the left or to the right. If the thorax is easily accessible, transillumination of the chest, especially in infants, may be diagnostic. When tension pneumothorax is present and life-threatening, there is unlikely to be time for X-ray confirmation of the diagnosis, and insertion of an appropriate needle into the area of tension is essential. This is most simply done by using a standard 16-gauge plastic intravenous cannula to which, after the sharp introducing needle has been removed, a three-way stopcock may be attached. Air should escape with a pronounced hiss when the needle is inserted, and further air may be aspirated using a syringe attached to the stopcock. If air continues to leak from the lung, an appropriate intercostal drain should then be inserted and connected to an underwater seal (see Chapter 12).

HAEMORRHAGE

One of the most important hazards of surgery is the possibility of severe haemorrhage, especially if this is unexpected. Sudden, exsanguinating haemorrhage can be an unwelcome complication of many surgical operations.

Severe surgical haemorrhage arises when bleeding from relatively large arteries or veins is uncontrolled, or when an operation involves areas of highly vascular or infected tissue. It is usually possible to anticipate the situations where such haemorrhage may occur and to be prepared for their occurrence. Such preparation includes a well-running intravenous infusion through which is administered an appropriate amount of balanced salt solution, so that blood volume is well maintained despite lesser degrees of haemorrhage and other loss of extra-cellular fluid earlier in the surgery. A blood pump or three-way tap and syringe to facilitate rapid transfusion can be included in the intravenous line. Adequate supplies of plasma volume expanders and cross-matched blood should be available, as well as the apparatus to warm blood before transfusion (Chapter 3). Calcium may be needed when relatively large volumes of blood are transfused.

The situation can arise in which severe haemorrhage occurs when an intravenous infusion is not available, or has for some technical reason become ineffective. In this case the commencement of an effective infusion is urgent. While this can usually be fairly rapidly achieved using peripheral veins, these may be difficult to find, particularly in the presence of vasoconstriction from haemorrhage. Rapid central venous cannulation may be necessary. When all else fails it may be possible for one member of the surgical team to cannulate a large vessel, either vein or artery, within the wound, through which fluid can be rapidly administered for resuscitation until a satisfactory infusion has been started in another site.

During laparotomy or thoracotomy in babies, an 18-gauge needle can be inserted by the surgeon into a central vein or the abdominal or thoracic aorta.

Vasoconstrictors or induced hypotension may be used in operations in which haemorrhage from vascular tissues is expected to be a hazard (see Chapter 23). In some instances, when the anaesthetist is familiar with the use of vasodilators and induced hypotension, the surgeon can control the bleeding with pressure while the anaesthetist catches up with the blood loss, gives extra intravenous fluids and then gives very small incremental doses of a vasodilator such as sodium nitroprusside. When the blood pressure has decreased the surgeon can release his pressure, look for and control the bleeding points.

Abnormal haemostasis can also be responsible for severe and unexpected haemorrhage during surgery; a number of important medical conditions which cause 'uncontrollable' haemorrhage are outlined in Chapter 25. In most cases the abnormality will be suspected and investigated before operation, and the appropriate management undertaken in consultation with a haematologist. When abnormal bleeding which has not been anticipated occurs, the patient may have a bleeding diathesis or depletion of platelets and other coagulation factors due to disseminated intravascular coagulation (DIC). The latter is often associated with severe infection or prolonged hypovolaemic shock. When such a situation occurs the appropriate management is to obtain direct consultation with a haematologist, who can have the appropriate diagnostic tests carried out as an emergency and advise immediate and further management of the condition. While such investigation is under way, it is essential that the anaesthetist ensures that blood volume and red-cell mass are appropriately maintained by infusion of warmed blood or packed cells and other appropriate fluids, and that the surgeon makes every effort to control the haemorrhage until the haemostatic mechanisms are improved. This may or may not involve using packs and pressure rather than further surgical exploration until the situation is controlled. Until such time as the abnormality of haemostasis is identified, it may be appropriate to administer fresh frozen plasma as part of the overall resuscitation fluid management. It is important that blood samples for diagnosis of the bleeding disorder are taken before fresh frozen plasma is given. In some places fresh blood may be more readily available.

When disseminated intravascular coagulation occurs, there is a deficiency of most of the factors involved in haemostasis. In particular there is prolongation of plasma thromboplastin and prothrombin time with thrombocytopenia. The most important aspect of the management of disseminated intravascular coagulation is the correction of the underlying cause, whether it be septicaemia or circulatory depression. Fresh frozen plasma and platelet transfusions should be used as advised by the haematologist. In some conditions, heparin administration may arrest the process of intravascular coagulation for a period and enable the vicious cycle of thrombosis and fibrinolysis to be broken. Such treatment is best undertaken only in consultation with a haematologist.

Assessment of blood loss can be difficult. Measurement of pulse, arterial and central venous pressure are all useful in assessing blood loss and its replacement. To the trained ear, diminution of heart sounds is also a sensitive indicator of decreasing cardiac output. The anaesthetist should also watch the wound and the swabs to see how much bleeding is occurring. Attention should be paid when the surgeon says that bleeding is increasing.

Sometimes babies are undertransfused because of a widespread belief that they tolerate overtransfusion poorly. If they have normal hearts, hypovolaemia is more likely to cause adverse effects than mild overtransfusion. The aim should be to return cardiovascular function to normal.

MALIGNANT HYPERPYREXIA

This uncommon condition in which the patient becomes overheated worries anaesthetists because it can occur without warning, unless there is a family history, and lead to cardiac arrest and death. It can occur at any age, although clearly identified cases are very rare under the age of 3 years. There are patients with other conditions such as osteogenesis imperfecta and arthrogryposis multiplex congenita who sometimes develop fever during anaesthesia, but these are not life-threatening (see Chapter 19).

The metabolic derangement

This is due to an excess of calcium ions in the cytosol released from the sarcoplasmic reticulum on exposure to caffeine, succinylcholine and inhalation agents such as halothane. In susceptible individuals there is an abnormal calcium-induced calcium release mechanism in the sarcoplasmic reticulum membrane [5]. The excess calcium stimulates and maintains muscle contraction, sometimes causing severe muscle rigidity.

Normally sarcoplasmic reticulum and mitochondria pump calcium inwards, helping in the regulation of cytosolic calcium concentration (10^{-7}M). The physiological actions of calcium are (a) binding to troponin C, initiating muscle contraction, (b) activation of phosphorylase kinase and phosphorylase B, initiating glycogen breakdown, and (c) activation of pyruvate dehydrogenase complex. In this pathological situation calcium uncouples mitochondria, leading to uncontrolled respiration [6]. Immediate consequences of this are increased oxygen consumption, generation of heat and a decrease in ATP/ADP ratio. The latter in turn stimulates phosphofructokinase and pyruvate dehydrogenase, enhancing glucose metabolism [7, 8]. In these circumstances glucose is metabolized to lactic acid, leading to metabolic acidosis.

Malignant-hyperpyrexia (MH) susceptible people develop intracellular acidosis in muscle more quickly than normal individuals during light exercise [9].

Precipitating factors

Malignant hyperpyrexia is triggered by exposure to many inhalation anaesthetic agents, especially halothane and halogenated ethers. It is safe to use nitrous oxide. Suxamethonium has often been implicated as it causes a myotonic type of contracture with failure to relax in susceptible patients. Masseter spasm is a common feature but not all patients with this response develop malignant hyperpyrexia [10]. When this spasm occurs, the anaesthetist should watch for the development of further clinical features of MH and treat the patient if they develop, but frequently this does not happen.

Clinical features

At varying periods after exposure to the above agents, the patient develops tachycardia, dysrhythmia, hyperpnoea, a rapidly rising body temperature (at a rate of 1°C in 15 minutes or less) and sweating. The hypermetabolic state is reflected in an enormous increase in output of carbon dioxide which can render soda-lime absorbers too hot to touch. Hypoxia, severe nonrespiratory acidosis, cardiac dysrhythmia, hypertension and disseminated intravascular coagulation follow. Hyperkalaemia and myoglobinuria may occur.

Preoperative recognition of risk

Several groups of patients appear to be susceptible to malignant hyperpyrexia. One group has a clinical or subclinical myopathy associated with strabismus or undescended testis, and a tendency to develop rigidity when exposed to triggering agents. Susceptibility to malignant hyperpyrexia is inherited as an autosomal dominant with incomplete penetrance; a family history is very important in alerting anaesthetists to the possibility. High creatinine phosphokinase (CPK) levels in a patient with a suspicious family history suggests that the patient may be susceptible, although this test is now regarded as diagnostically unreliable because there have been false positives and negatives, and there are other situations such as following exercise or trauma where CPK can be elevated. The responses in patients with myopathies such as Duchenne are confusing. Some who had high CPK levels developed pyrexia during halothane anaesthesia [11], or others have developed masseter spasm and had a positive muscle caffeine contracture test but no temperature [12]. Patients with Duchenne muscular dystrophy have had cardiac arrest on exposure to halothane or suxamethonium, possibly due to myocardial involvement or hyperkalaemia [13, 14], but many others with this condition have not developed features suggestive of malignant hyperpyrexia [10, 11].

Apart from exposing the patient to triggering agents such as halothane, MH susceptibility is currently most reliably diagnosed by contracture of a muscle biopsy on exposure to caffeine or halothane in a tissue bath.

Clinical reports of patients developing malignant hyperpyrexia fall into two categories, those with pronounced muscle rigidity (rigid variety) and those without (non-rigid or sporadic variety). It is possible that the latter is a separate entity or that the rigidity is masked by the use of non-depolarizing muscle relaxants. It is now thought that the MH gene is on the long arm of chromosome 19 and its position is close to the ryanodine receptor [15, 16]. Maybe a specific blood test for MH susceptibility will become available which will make muscle studies unnecessary [17].

Recognition during anaesthesia

Malignant hyperpyrexia carries a high mortality if inadequately treated. Early detection of the onset of the condition followed by prompt termination of anaesthesia, the intravenous administration of dantrolene and vigorous symptomatic treatment appear to be useful in reducing this mortality. A high index of suspicion must be combined with careful monitoring. Monitoring of body temperature in all cases of general anaesthesia has been recommended, especially for children. This has by no means been widely accepted, although temperature monitoring for other reasons is frequently used in infants and young children undergoing prolonged operations. Any patient who feels hot to touch should have his temperature measured. It has been suggested that an unexplained tachycardia not due to light anaesthesia, infection or other obvious causes should alert the anaesthetist to the possibility of malignant hyperpyrexia. A careful watch should then be kept for signs of a hyperkinetic state, that is, a temperature rising rapidly towards 40°C, increased oxygen consumption and carbon dioxide production, and unexplained acidosis. Capnography and pulse oximetry may help early detection of the hypermetabolic state. The time taken in many hospitals to obtain the results of blood gas analysis, if this cannot be done in the operating theatre area, means that the detection of acidosis would only be useful as a confirmation of other signs of developing malignant hyperpyrexia.

Treatment

If the patient's temperature rises during anaesthesia and malignant hyperpyrexia is seriously suspected, surgery should be terminated, help sought and the following treatment instituted:

1 All inhalation anaesthetics should be discontinued. The breathing system and preferably the whole machine should be changed as soon as convenient to one free of inhalation agents.

2 Hyperventilation with 100% oxygen (high flows).

3 Establish an intravenous infusion if one is not already running. Infuse solutions (not containing lactate) at ambient temperature.

4 Administer i.v. dantrolene — 2.5 mg/kg followed by 1 mg/kg increments until the signs reverse, up to a maximum of 10 mg/kg (vials contain 20 mg dantrolene, 1 g mannitol to be diluted in 60 ml warm sterile water). It has been used successfully in children, in whom the elimination half-life is about 10 hours [18]. It has also been shown to be synergistic with calcium-channel blocking agents (diltiazem and verapamil) [19]. Because it is very expensive, several hospitals in an area may stock a starter dose and have an arrangement with neighbouring hospitals to obtain additional emergency supplies when necessary.

5 Cooling — all heating devices should be turned off. Ice packs or cold-water circulating blankets should be placed around the body and head.

Gastric lavage with iced water.

If a body cavity is open it can be lavaged with cold solutions.

A vasodilator infusion such as sodium nitroprusside will facilitate heat exchange by allowing warm blood to reach the periphery.

6 Measure blood gas and electrolyte levels. Treat metabolic acidosis — usually sodium bicarbonate is used but trihydroxymethylaminomethane (THAM), if available, has theoretical advantages because it lowers Pa_{CO_2} and plasma potassium and does not contain sodium. Its disadvantages are that it is slow to dissolve and may cause hypoglycaemia and thrombosis.

7 Additional monitoring such as capnography, ECG and direct arterial pressure, should be set up if not already in use.

8 If hyperkalaemic, give insulin 0.25 u/kg and glucose.

9 Insert a urinary catheter to measure output — it should be maintained at about 2 ml/kg/h using mannitol (0.5 g/kg). Urine colour may indicate haemo- and myoglobinuria, but a sample should be taken for confirmation.

10 After control of the initial episode, dantrolene 1.5 mg/kg should be given intravenously as necessary for 48–72 hours. Up to 10% of patients may relapse with a rise in temperature up to 36 hours after the initial episode.

11 Because late complications may include acute renal failure, disseminated intravascular coagulopathy and heart failure, these patients should be managed postoperatively in an intensive care unit.

Management of a recognized susceptible patient

Children susceptible to malignant hyperpyrexia sometimes present for anaesthesia. These patients may have survived a previous episode or have a family history of malignant hyperpyrexia. Where possible, confirmation of the diagnosis by muscle biopsy and *in vitro* testing by exposure to halothane is desirable. This has been done in children as young as 2 years [20].

It is a worthwhile precaution to ensure that all tubing and reservoir bags as well as plastic containers and soda lime are new and have not been previously exposed to agents such as halothane, in case the gases leach some remaining agent out of these and deliver them to the patient. A machine from which the vaporizers have been removed can be cleared of halothane in 6 minutes with a 12 l/min oxygen flow [21]. When a malignant-hyperpyrexia susceptible patient is being anaesthetized, special arrangements should be made to have the necessary equipment and drugs, outlined above, available for treatment should reaction occur. Blood-gas analysis should be promptly available. Capnography should be used if available.

Adequate sedation should be given the night before the operation, as these patients are sometimes very apprehensive. Oral dantrolene does not provide adequate prophylaxis. Intravenous dantrolene (2.5 mg/kg i.v.) administered 1–2 hours before induction has been suggested, but it is expensive and unreliable. It should not be given before muscle biopsy.

All drugs known to precipitate malignant hyperpyrexia should be avoided, especially potent inhalation agents, suxamethonium, and anti-histaminic and neuroleptic drugs. Nitrous oxide was once incriminated as a precipitating agent, but there are numerous reports of its uneventful use with non-depolarizing muscle relaxants and opioids. Clinically, thiopentone, and experimentally in susceptible animals, propofol [22, 23], etomidate and ketamine [24] are safe. Local anaesthetics are safe to use [25].

The choice of anaesthesia lies between local or regional anaesthesia in conjunction with a benzodiazepine, or general anaesthesia. Pre-oxygenation followed by thiopentone, non-depolarizing muscle relaxant, nitrous oxide and fentanyl seems to provide satifactory anaesthesia without triggering the hyperpyrexic response.

As the mortality is greater when the rate of rise of temperature and the peak temperature are higher, cooling to 34–35°C at induction of anaesthesia may be worthwhile [26].

Reduction of mortality from malignant hyperpyrexia depends on the early detection and prompt treatment of susceptible patients.

In the recovery room, vital signs should be monitored more frequently than usual and temperature monitoring should be continued. In the ward, frequent observations including temperature should continue at least every 2 hours.

OVERDOSAGE OF LOCAL ANAESTHETIC AGENTS

When local anaesthetic agents are used for topical application, local infiltration or regional blocks, excessive uptake, overdose and accidental intravascular injection cause high plasma levels which result in convulsions, depression of consciousness and respiration, or cardiovascular depression. When large doses of these agents are being used, a vein should be cannulated for administration of fluids or drugs, in case of hypotension due to sympathetic blockade from major blocks, or total spinal anaesthesia or accidental overdosage.

Convulsions should be treated immediately. The first priority is to administer oxygen so that hypoxia does not occur. The airway must be cleared as soon as the major fit has passed. Diazepam, in an initial dose of 0.1–0.2 mg/kg intravenously, is probably the most effective way of terminating the fit, although thiopentone which is often readily available may also be used. Fitting may be transient; it will cease as the plasma level falls during redistribution of the local anaesthetic. Whatever means are used to control the fitting, it is probable that respiration will be depressed. Controlled ventilation and tracheal intubation may be needed for a time.

If the convulsive phase is brief, oxygenation may be all that is needed.

Bradycardia and circulatory depression may need to be treated by judicious use of inotropic agents, with appropriate monitoring and administration of intravenous fluids as indicated. Such treatment should only be used after pulmonary ventilation and oxygenation have been established. Further details regarding toxic plasma levels and overdosage are discussed in Chapter 22.

ACCIDENTAL INTRA-ARTERIAL INJECTION

Thiopentone, when injected intra-arterially, can cause vasospasm and thrombosis leading to ischaemia and sometimes necrosis of distal tissue. It is more likely to cause damage if injected as a 5% than the more commonly used 2.5% solution. This accident is recognized by acute pain and blanching of the skin. The needle should be left in the artery.

Treatment includes:

1 Dilution of the drug by flushing the artery with saline.
2 Injection of a small dose of dilute heparin into the artery, followed if necessary, by a full heparinizing dose intravenously to prevent thrombosis.
3 Relief of spasm with a vasodilator such as sodium nitroprusside (0.01 mg/kg) and/or the injection of

papaverine (0.5 mg/kg in 5–20 ml saline) into the artery.

4 Relief of pain by the intra-arterial injection of procaine (0.2 ml/kg 0.5% solution) or performance of an appropriate regional block (before full heparinization), which may also dilate the vessels.

5 Keeping the limb warm.

MISCELLANEOUS CONDITIONS

It would be possible to produce a lengthy list of possible emergencies which may arise during paediatric anaesthesia, but those outlined above are probably the most important. A number of emergencies, for example air embolism during neurosurgical operations in the sitting position, are dealt with in the appropriate chapters. In all of these cases the development of an emergency can often be prevented by meticulous attention to the details of technique and monitoring, and by being aware of significant indicators that an emergency may arise.

REFERENCES

1 Olsson G.L. Complications of paediatric anaesthesia. *Curr Opin Anaesthesiol* 1990, **3**, 385.

2 Olsson G.L., Hallen B., Hambraeus-Jonzon K. Aspiration during anaesthesia: a computer-aided study of 185 358 anaesthetics. *Acta Anaes Scand* 1986, **30**, 84.

3 Sandhar B.K., Goresky G.V., Maltby J.R., Shaffer E.A. Effect of oral liquids and ranitidine on gastric fluid volume and pH in children undergoing outpatient surgery. *Anesthesiology* 1989, **71**, 327.

4 Fisher M. Intradermal testing after severe histamine reaction to intravenous drugs used in anaesthesia. *Anaes Intens Care* 1976, **4**, 97.

5 Endo M. Mechanisms and their pharmacology of mobilization of calcium ion in muscle cells. *Nippon Yakurigaku zasshi* 1989, **94**, 329.

6 Cheah K.S., Cheah A.M., Fletcher J.E., Rosenberg H. Skeletal muscle mitochondrial respiration of malignant-hyperthermia susceptible patients. Ca^{2+}-induced uncoupling and free fatty acids. *Int J Biochem* 1989, **21**, 913.

7 Cohen R.M., McNamara P.D., Herman R.H. *Principles of metabolic control in mammalian systems.* Plenum Press, New York, (1980).

8 Lehninger A.L. *Principles of biochemistry.* Worth Publishers Inc., (1984), pp. 452, 732.

9 Webster D.W., Thompson R.T., Gravelle D.R., Laschuk M.J., Driedger A.A. Metabolic response to exercise in malignant hyperthermia sensitive patients. *Mag Reson Med* 1990, **15**, 81.

10 Richards W.C. Anaesthesia and serum CPK levels in patients with Duchenne pseudohypertrophic muscular dystrophy. *Anaes Intens Care* 1972, **1**, 150.

11 Sethna N.F., Rockoff M.A., Worthen H.M., Rosnan J.M. Anaesthesia-related complications in children with Duchenne muscular dystrophy. *Anesthesiology* 1988, **68**, 462.

12 Brownell A.K.W., Paasuke R.T., Elash A., Fowlow S.B., et al. Malignant hyperthermia in a child with Duchenne muscular dystrophy. *Anesthesiology* 1988, **68**, 462.

13 Genever E.E. Suxamethonium-induced cardiac arrest in unsuspected pseudohypertrophic muscular dystrophy. *Br J Anaes* 1971, **43**, 984.

14 Seay A.R., Ziter F.A., Thompson J.A. Cardiac arrest during induction of anaesthesia in Duchenne muscular dystrophy. *J Paediatr* 1978, **93**, 88.

15 McCarthy T.V., Healy J.M., Heffron J.J., Lehane M., Deufel T., Lehmann-Horn F., Farrall M., Johnson K. Localization of the malignant hyperthermia susceptibility locus to human chromosome 19q12–13.2. *Nature* 1990, **343**, 562.

16 MaLennan D.H., Duff C., Zorzato F., et al. Ryanodine receptor gene is a candidate for predisposition to malignant hyperthermia. *Nature* 1990, **343**, 559.

17 Ellis F.R. Predicting malignant hyperthermia. *Br J Anaes* 1990, **64**, 411.

18 Lerman J., McLeod M.E., Strong H.A. Pharmacokinetics of intravenous dantrolene in children. *Anesthesiology* 1989, **70**, 625.

19 Foster P.S., Hopkinson K.C., Denborough M.A. Effect of diltiazem, verapamil, and dantrolene on the contractility of isolated malignant-hyperpyrexia susceptible human skeletal muscle. *Clin Exp Pharmacol Physiol* 1989, **16**, 799.

20 Krivosic-Horber R., Adnet P., Krisovic I., Reyford H. Diagnosis of susceptibility to malignant hyperthermia in children. *Arch Fr Pediatr* 1990, **47**, 421.

21 McGraw T.T., Keon T.P. Malignant hyperthermia and the clean machine. *Can Anaes Soc J* 1989, **36**, 530.

22 Krivosic-Horber R., Reyfort H., Becq M.C., Adnet P. Effect of propofol on the malignant-hyperthermia susceptible pig model. *Br J Anaes* 1989, **62**, 691.

23 Raff M., Harrison G.G. The screening of propofol in MHS swine. *Anesth Analg* 1989, **68**, 750.

24 Dershwitz M., Sreter F.A., Ryan J.F. Ketamine does not trigger malignant hyperthermia in susceptible swine. *Anesth Analg* 1989, **69**, 501.

25 Dershwitz M., Ryan J.F., Guralnick W. Safety of amide local anaesthetics in patients susceptible to malignant hyperthermia. *J Am Dent Assoc* 1989, **118**, 276.

26 Nelson T.E. Porcine malignant hyperthermia: critical temperatures for *in vivo* and *in vitro* responses. *Anesthesiology* 1990, **73**, 449.

28: Day-Care Surgery

INTRODUCTION

Day-care surgery, in which the patients are admitted, usually to special units which may include their own operating room, and discharged on the same day, is being used increasingly in paediatric surgery. The short stay means that separation from the parents is minimized and the child will not have to be away from home overnight. As well as the psychological advantages, day-care surgery is more economical; it helps to alleviate nursing shortages, because night and weekend shifts are not needed.

SITUATION AND COMPONENTS OF A DAY-SURGICAL UNIT

Day-surgical units can be in a separate building, which many prefer because they can be set up as a place where well children go for relatively minor operations, thereby avoiding the stigma of going to hospital where everyone is sick. If the unit is in a hospital, it should preferably have a separate ward. The organization of surgery and postoperative care is easier if the operating theatre(s) is in the same unit, or at least close by, as it reduces transfer time to and from the theatre and makes pre- and postoperative visiting by the medical staff easier.

A day-surgical unit requires a separate area for the patients to be admitted to and cared for before and after surgery. There should be a play area with toys, books and other occupations for the children while they wait. In some centres, preoperative assessment clinics are held on the ward, so that the child has an opportunity to become familiar with the ward and staff. Additional space is required for this.

When planning a day-surgical unit, the expected patient throughput per day must be assessed and appropriate spaces should be set aside for reception, waiting, changing and play areas. If the operating theatres are included, adequate space will be required for them and for induction rooms, set-up, storage, sterilization areas and recovery room. Administrative areas for admission clerks and the nursing staff are also needed. An interviewing room for the doctors to examine the patients and speak to the parents is useful. There should be adequate parking with access to the unit clearly signposted.

STAFF

The day-care ward should have its own nursing staff who are familiar with the routine of the area. It is important that they are good at handling children and relate to parents well. Most parents willingly accept responsibility for the care of their children before surgery and when they return from the recovery room. This reduces the load on the nursing staff and therefore the numbers needed.

A day-surgical unit should have its own clerical staff to handle bookings, admission and discharge procedures and medical records. It is possible to handle 20 patients a day in a ward staffed by 3–5 nurses, a clerk and a cleaner. Additional staff will be needed if there is a theatre and recovery room.

SELECTION OF PATIENTS

Operation

There are many procedures which can be undertaken satisfactorily in children. In general they are short (an hour at the most and preferably less than 30 minutes) and are not likely to be associated with considerable pain, postoperative bleeding or excessive vomiting. Non-operative procedures such as examination under anaesthesia, endoscopy, organ-imaging and manipulation and plastering of joints and bones are suitable for day care. Commonly performed operations include myringotomy and the insertion of tubes, herniotomy, circumcision, minor superficial operations, probing of lacrimal ducts, squint correction and dental restoration and extraction. In some units the range of procedures may include orchidopexy, adenoidectomy and tonsillectomy; on the other hand where there is a risk of postoperative bleeding it may be better to have the patient in hospital overnight. Children having squint surgery can have a high incidence of postoperative vomiting unless antiemetics are used. It may be advisable to keep these patients longer before discharge.

Patient

The health of the child is important when considering a child for day admission. Usually ASA Class 1 and 2 patients are suitable but, in specialist paediatric units, children with other conditions may be included, particularly for investigations. Patients with bleeding or metabolic disorders, or with potential airway obstruction (e.g. obstructive sleep apnoea, severe micrognathia, Hurler's or Hunter's syndromes), are preferably managed as inpatients because more preoperative preparation and a longer period of postoperative observation are needed.

Babies who have been born prematurely and are still at the age when postoperative apnoea may be a problem, should be admitted to hospital where their respiration can be monitored. Opinions vary as to how long this problem exists, but most agree that premature infants up to at least 44 weeks and some consider that up to 52 weeks' post-conceptual age are at risk.

Social circumstances

The social background and location of the child's home should be considered. If there is any uncertainty regarding the parents' ability to look after the child in the early postoperative phase, day care should be avoided.

There are a few very anxious parents who are unwilling and unable to accept responsibility for the postoperative care. This should be recognized and inpatient care arranged without making the parents feel inadequate or incompetent. This may apply especially in families that have lost a child from sudden infant death syndrome (SIDS). In addition, there may be a few disturbed parents who regard surgery and hospitalization as a punishment the child should endure. If this severe and rare parental disturbance can be detected, the operation should be recommended as an inpatient procedure, so that the child will receive adequate care, sympathy and attention.

Children who live considerable distances from the hospital are at a disadvantage due to the travelling time, and lack of close accessibility to help should postoperative bleeding occur. This problem can be overcome if the family can stay near the hospital for the nights before and after surgery.

Language difficulties may lead to inadequate understanding of the procedure and precautions, so that it may be better to admit the child overnight.

It is important that the surgeon who selects the patients for day-care surgery should be aware of conditions which may cause difficulties during anaesthesia and postoperatively, so that such patients are not included.

PREADMISSION INSTRUCTIONS TO PARENTS

Appropriate written instructions should be given to the parents before they come to the hospital. This should usually be done by the surgeon when surgery is organized. The information sheet should include the patient's name, doctor's name and the proposed operation. It should give instructions for time, date and place of admission, and preoperative examination if these are to be held before the day of admission.

A map of the unit showing parking and public transport access is useful for the parents.

Information for the nursing staff or anaesthetist should be included, including a brief history of previous operations, complications, adverse responses to hospitalization or serious illnesses. A medical history questionnaire ensures that the important points are covered.

Arrangements should be made to investigate any family history of bleeding or sickle-cell disease before admission is contemplated for day care.

If a consent form can be signed and witnessed by the surgeon when the admission is arranged, time will be saved on the day of surgery.

Fasting

Instructions for preoperative fasting must be clearly stated and repeated to the parents when they are given the sheet, indicating when the last food or fluid intake may be given. Usually solid foods are avoided for at least 5 hours before the expected time of surgery. Opinions vary about the interval between last fluid intake and operation. Some studies have shown greater volumes with lower pH in children given fluids less than 4 hours before anaesthesia, and yet clinical experience with clear fluids given up to 2 hours beforehand (maximum 5 ml/kg) has not been associated with an increased incidence of vomiting or regurgitation. Breast-feeding of infants is permissible up to 3 hours before, but a longer interval is desirable with cows' milk because it is less easily digested.

The information sheet should include general information about the routine for going home and arrangements for postoperative follow-up. It should indicate whom the parents should contact in case of difficulties.

If these instructions are carefully explained, the parents will usually ensure that they are carried out because they are concerned for the well-being of their child.

Preadmission visit

In some units, particularly when the surgical consultation takes place nearby, the parents are encouraged to visit the day-care unit to make their booking, and at the same time to familiarize themselves with the surroundings.

Admission time

Admission time will depend on the expected time of surgery. The advantage of a unit which has its own operating theatre(s) is that admission can be staggered, so that patient waiting is minimized and the unit work flow is spread throughout the day. When the day-care patients are integrated into normal operating lists and the theatre is separated from the ward, it may be necessary for the patients to attend before the operating list

begins so that the anaesthetist can see the patients beforehand without disrupting the operating schedule.

The last admission for the day should be timed to allow the patient to recover before the unit's closing time.

PREOPERATIVE MANAGEMENT

Timing of assessment

This may be undertaken 1–3 days before admission, or time should be left between arrival in hospital and the beginning of the anaesthetic for adequate assessment and preoperative examination.

History and examination

The history, which may be a questionnaire, should indicate whether the child has had croup, stridor, asthma, pulmonary infection or abnormal bleeding. Information regarding any drugs being taken, allergies or anaesthetic complications should also be sought.

The anaesthetist's assessment should be the same as described in Chapter 6 (Preoperative Preparation). Particular attention should be paid to the presence of fever or upper respiratory infection. Patients exhibiting these should usually be postponed. An exception might be the child who is recovering from an upper respiratory infection who has had to travel a long distance and whose operation is short and does not require intubation. There is a slight but usually acceptable added risk, which should be discussed with the parents.

The anaesthetist's preoperative visit is important as it provides an opportunity to gain rapport with the patient and to reassure the parents, as well as to assess the child and decide whether premedication is necessary.

If the preoperative assessment is performed by a person other than the actual anaesthetist, accurate history and examination notes are essential, but the anaesthetist still has the responsibility for examining the patient before inducing anaesthesia.

Premedication

Many anaesthetists feel that premedication is unnecessary for day patients, as it may delay recovery. It helps if a parent accompanies the child to theatre or, especially in larger units, there is a kindly person available to look after children while they wait. Adequate reassurance by the anaesthetist at the preoperative visit is important.

On the other hand some anaesthetists prefer their patients to have premedication, in which case an oral sedative or tranquillizer is preferable. In children under 4 years chloral hydrate (40 mg/kg) is useful, although some children may become restless before they become sedated. In older children a benzodiazepine such as diazepam (0.3 ml/kg) or flunitrazapam are satisfactory. Nasal midazolam (0.2 mg/kg) has been tried. Plasma levels rise rapidly when it is given by this route. Opioid premedication requires an injection and tends to increase the incidence of postoperative vomiting, both of which are undesirable. It is preferable to give a short-acting drug such as fentanyl intravenously at induction if an analgesic is needed.

Oral paracetamol (10–20 mg/kg) can be added to provide some postoperative analgesia. This can be sufficient to relieve the discomfort of less painful procedures such as myringotomy. Alternatively, a suppository can be inserted after induction.

ANAESTHETIC MANAGEMENT

The anaesthetic technique should allow early awakening and minimal postoperative drowsiness. Induction may be intravenous or inhalational, depending on age and preference, which can be established at the preoperative visit. Halothane provides a smooth, fairly rapid induction but an agent such as seuoflurane, which has an even lower blood–gas solubility coefficient has a very rapid onset and may become particularly useful for paediatric day surgical anaesthesia (see Chapter 2). Intravenous induction agents which are rapidly metabolized or eliminated have advantages for short stay surgery. Propofol has these advantages but commonly causes pain on injection, which can be offset by the addition of a small dose of lignocaine (50 mg in 20 ml). It has a very variable dose requirement and it is relatively expensive. Thiopentone or methohexitone are still widely used. Methohexitone has the advantage over thiopentone of more rapid recovery, but it also causes some pain on injection and involuntary movements. As redistribution is more rapid in children, awakening following thiopentone and methohexitone is more rapid than in adults.

If a muscle relaxant is used, atracurium is the drug of choice. If the procedure is very short suxamethonium may still be used but sometimes muscle pains can occur especially in older children.

If the child is intubated, care must be taken to select the correct size of tube so that there is a gas leak around it when pressure is applied to the anaesthetic bag. Patients who have been intubated should be observed for at least 2 hours after extubation. Laryngeal oedema is uncommon when the correct size of non-irritant tube is used, but when it occurs it usually develops within an hour of extubation.

Local anaesthetic technique such as penile block or caudal anaesthesia for circumcision and ilioinguinal block for hernia repair are useful for both surgery and postoperative analgesia. Infiltration of the incision site or instillation into the wound can also provide analgesia. Bupivacaine can provide good prolonged analgesia. When used for caudal anaesthesia its action can be extended by the addition of adrenaline, but it can also, unless diluted to 0.25% or less, cause prolonged weakness of the legs, which may delay discharge.

POSTOPERATIVE MANAGEMENT

Patients should remain in the recovery room until conscious and stable. They can then be returned to the care of their parents. This can occur sooner if the theatre, recovery room and postoperative holding area are adjacent to each other. Lemonade and ice blocks can be offered to the children after recovery. Local anaesthesia or paracetamol often provide adequate analgesia.

Opioid analgesics should be given if required, but patients will then usually need to remain longer in the recovery/postoperative area. Opioids may triple the incidence of postoperative nausea and vomiting, and this may be aggravated by motion so that vomiting may occur on the way home. There may be less nausea and vomiting with codeine phosphate 1 mg/kg. The incidence of vomiting is less in infants than in older children. If several doses of parenteral analgesic are needed for postoperative pain the surgery is not suitable for a day-care programme.

Each child should be checked before discharge to ensure that there are no airway problems, bleeding, or other complications. The surgeon usually checks the patient and speaks to the parents postoperatively.

The parents should be given the name and telephone number of the person to be contacted should problems arise after discharge.

Although a minimal recovery time is not necessary for simple procedures, the children being allowed to go when they are safe, based on clinical observation and common sense, they often remain in the unit for an hour at least after the anaesthetic. A longer minimum postoperative stay of at least 2 hours is appropriate when there may be blood loss (e.g. adenoidectomy), after topical laryngeal analgesia.

COMPLICATIONS

The main complications are delayed recovery from anaesthesia, nausea and vomiting (especially in older children), and surgical complications such as bleeding. Rarely, postoperative stridor may develop, but it is unlikely if due care is taken with intubation. In well-organized units the number of patients requiring admission overnight for any reason is usually less than 2%. If large numbers of children are requiring overnight admission, the arrangements should be reviewed to ensure that the operations being performed are suitable for day care and that the timing of surgery is appropriate.

Complications occasionally reported following discharge are sore throat (especially if an airway has been used), headache, muscle pains (if suxamethonium has been used), restlessness, irritability and sleep disturbances. Psychological complications are less common after day surgery because the period of separation from the parents is short.

CONCLUSION

Day care has become an important part of paediatric surgery. The selection of patients is important. They should be having operations for which day care offers advantages to the child and parents. Time spent by the surgeon and anaesthetist explaining to the parents and child what is going to happen is invaluable in making the hospital visit easier. Most of the discussion in Chapter 5, on the child in hospital, is as relevant to these patients as it is to children who are hospitalized for longer periods.

29: The Management of Fluid, Electrolyte and Acid—Base Abnormalities

NORMAL DISTRIBUTION AND REQUIREMENTS

Distribution of body water

During fetal life the body is about 90% water. Total body water decreases to 75−80% at full term and gradu-ally decreases during the first 2 years towards the adult proportion of 60−65%. The main change occurs in extra-cellular water, which exceeds intracellular volume until about 4 months of age when extracellular and intra-cellular water are both about 35% of body weight (Fig. 29.1) [1, 2].

Infants born prematurely have a greater water content, most of which is extracellular, and this acts as a buffer against dehydration. The larger total body water in proportion to body weight must be taken into account when calculating electrolyte replacement following losses in pre-term babies. The larger extracellular volume also affects drug distribution.

The increased extracellular volume in the infant is interstitial water rather than plasma. The latter is about the same volume per kg as in older children.

Daily water requirement

Daily water turnover is greater in the newborn than the older child or adult when related to body weight, but the differences are less when related to surface area or metabolic rate. Insensible loss from the skin depends on the permeability of the skin and its area relative to weight, which are greater in the newborn. Respiratory losses are about one-third of insensible loss, being greater when ambient humidity is low than when it is high (about 10−25 ml/kg/day in newborn infants) [3]. Total insen-sible water loss in the newborn averages 30−50 ml/kg/day, depending on relative humidity.

Fluid requirements are influenced by many factors. Tables 29.1 and 29.2 show normal maintenance intra-venous fluid requirements, and some of the factors that affect the need for water.

In newborn babies, the kidney cannot concentrate as effectively as in the older child. Maximum urinary con-centration is only about 700 mmol/l compared with about 1300 mmol/l in adults. Thus the immature kidney cannot conserve water as effectively, making the infant more prone to dehydration than older children.

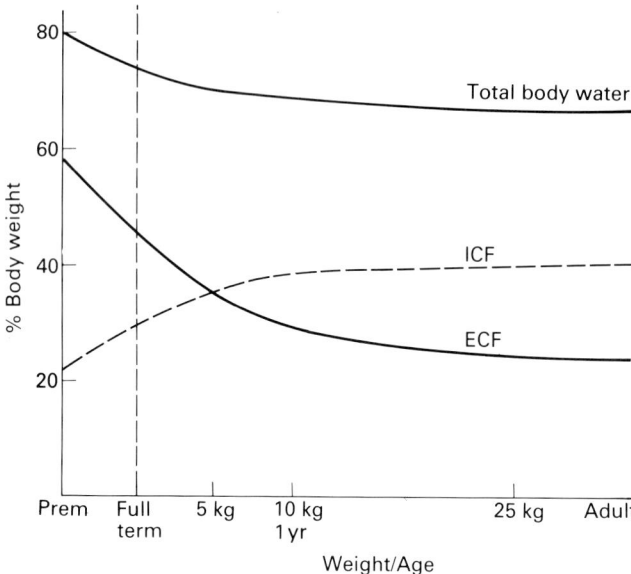

Fig. 29.1 Distribution of body water between intra- and extracellular compartments during early life. (Derived from Friis Hansen, and Cheek D.B.)

Normal electrolyte distribution

Sodium is the major extracellular cation (140 mmol/l) with small amounts of potassium (3–5 mmol/l), calcium (2.25–2.75 mmol/l) and magnesium (0.7–1.0 mmol/l). Chloride is the main extracellular anion (98–107 mmol/l) with the remainder of the total 154 mmol being made up of bicarbonate (24 mmol/l), protein, phosphate, sulphate and organic acid radicals.

In contrast, the main intracellular cations are potassium (140–150 mmol/l) and magnesium (30–40 mmol/l), with only a small amount of sodium (10 mmol/l). The intracellular anions are mainly inorganic phosphates and protein with a small amount of bicarbonate. It should be noted that intracellular fluid has a higher ionic concentration than extracellular fluid.

Table 29.1 Maintenance intravenous fluid and calorie requirements (one calorie is needed for each ml fluid)

0–10 kg	100 ml/kg
10–20 kg	1000 ml + (50 ml/kg for each kg over 10 kg)
>20 kg	1500 ml + (20 ml/kg for each kg over 20 kg)

e.g. a 14 kg child needs 1000 + [(14 − 10) × 50] = 1200 ml/day

Table 29.2 Maintenance intravenous fluid requirements

Newborn:	Day 1 of life : 2 ml/kg/h
	Day 2 of life : 3 ml/kg/h
	Day 3 of life : 4 ml/kg/h

Weight (kg)	ml/h	Weight (kg)	ml/h
4	16	18	60
6	24	20	65
8	32	30	70
10	40	40	80
12	45	50	90
14	50	60	95
16	55	70	100

Decrease	*Adjustment*
Humidified inspired air	× 0.75
Basal state (e.g. paralysed)	× 0.7
High ADH (IPPV, brain injury)	× 0.7
Hypothermia	− 12% per °C
High room humidity	× 0.7
Renal failure	0.3 + urine output
Increase	
Full activity + oral feeds	× 1.5
Hyperventilation	× 1.2
Neonate 1–1.5 kg.	× 1.2
Radiant heater	× 1.5
Phototherapy	× 1.5
Fever	+ 12% per °C
Room temperature >31°C	+ 30% per °C
Burns, first day	+ 4% per 1% area burnt
Burns, subsequently	+ 2% per 1% area burnt

Daily electrolyte requirements

The newborn baby needs 1–1.5 mmol/kg/day sodium during the first 14 days, increasing to 2–3.0 mmol/kg/day at about 2 weeks as renal function improves. If more than 10 mmol/kg are given per day it accumulates in the body because the kidneys cannot excrete large amounts [4]. The total body sodium of a full-term infant is about 80 mmol/kg and, as the baby grows, total body sodium increases proportionately.

Potassium requirements are about 2 mmol/kg/day in the neonate, decreasing slightly in older children. Total body potassium is about 40–45 mmol/kg in full-term infants. The gain during the first 20 weeks is about 0.2 mmol/kg/day. Chloride requirements are about 2 mmol/kg/day and total body chloride is about 50 mmol/kg at birth.

Table 29.3 summarizes body content, average gain per day and requirements. The content of human and cows' milk is also shown.

Table 29.3 Electrolytes — body content and requirements/kg in newborns

Electrolyte	Na	K	Cl	Ca	Mg	PO$_4$	Fe
Total body content of full term newborn/kg	70 mmol	43 mmol	46 mmol	8 g	217 mg	4.6 g	90 mg
Gain/kg/day (1st 20 weeks)	0.33 mmol	0.20 mmol	0.22 mmol	38 mg	1.03 mg	15 mg	2.3 mg
Daily requirement (mmol/kg)	1.3	2	2	0.75−1.5	0.25	1−1.5	
per 100 ml	mmol	mmol	mmol	mg	mg	mg	mg
Content human milk	0.65	1.33	1.80	33	3	15	0.04
Content cows' milk	2.16	4.10	2.75	125	14	96	0.09

Figures derived from Widdowson [9].

For maintenance, a fluid which contains an appropriate amount of sodium is selected. Potassium is added as required, but it should not normally be infused more rapidly than 0.5 mmol/kg/h or exceed 3 mmol/kg/day.

The electrolyte content of various commonly used solutions is summarized in Table 29.4. Isotonic solutions contain about 290−310 mmol/l. In some solutions glucose is added to make them isotonic, but in others the glucose content makes them hypertonic. Five per cent glucose is about 270 mmol/l, but as glucose is metabolized the osmolality declines. Glucose 5% provides only 20 cal/100 ml.

Rapid infusion of a concentrated glucose solution (10% or more) may raise plasma glucose so that the renal tubular maximum for reabsorption is exceeded, leading to osmotic diuresis.

FLUID DEPLETION

Clinical features of dehydration

A recent study of 102 children [5] found that some of the traditional signs of dehydration are unreliable, and that doctors overestimate the degree of dehydration. It was

Table 29.4 Content of intraenous fluids (mmol/l)

Solution	Na$^+$	Cl$^-$	K$^+$	Mg^{++}	Ca^{++}	HCO$_3$	Lactate	kJ/l*	Approx pH
Isotonic, 0.9% (Normal)	154	154	—	—	—	—	—		5.4
0.45% saline + 2.5% dextrose	77	77	—	—	—	—	—		—
0.45% saline	77	77	—	—	—	—	—		5.9
0.45% saline plus 5% dextrose	77	77	—	—	—	—	—	794	4.4
0.18% saline plus 4% dextrose	30	30	—	—	—	—	—	638	4.3
Hartmann's	131	112	5	—	2	—	30		6.3
Hartmann's with 5% dextrose	131	112	5	—	2	—	30	794	4.9
5% dextrose	—	—	—	—	—	—	—	794	4.5
10% dextrose	—	—	—	—	—	—	—	1588	4.2
SPPS	140	102	5	2.3	1.5	28			

* 1 kJ = 0.24 cal.

not associated with a history of oliguria, or the presence of restlessness or lethargy, sunken eyes, dry mouth, a sunken fontanelle, or the absence of tears.

Mild-to-moderate dehydration was predicted by the presence of poor peripheral perfusion (pallor or reduced capillary return), deep breathing, decreased skin turgor, high urea, low pH, and a large base deficit; a history of increased thirst just failed to reach statistical significance. Clinical signs of dehydration became apparent at 3–4% rather than 5% dehydration [5].

The signs of dehydration are mainly due to extracellular fluid depletion. It should be noted that these may be less obvious in hypertonic dehydration, where extracellular fluid volume is maintained at the expense of intracellular fluid.

Urine volume and osmolality reflect renal function. In a normally hydrated patient, a urine flow of at least 0.5 ml/kg/h would be expected. The specific gravity of urine increases as the kidneys attempt to conserve water. Because the concentrating ability of the infant kidney is limited to about 700 mmol/l, urine osmolality and maximum specific gravity will be lower (about 1.020–1.025) than in older patients.

Abnormal urinary losses of sodium, potassium and chloride can be measured. Blood urea rises in dehydration, in association with impaired renal function, and if insufficient carbohydrate is given to exert a protein-sparing effect.

Assessment of type of dehydration (Table 29.5)

Isotonic dehydration — the decrease in ECF volume is proportional to water loss: plasma sodium is 130–150 mmol/l and osmolality is normal. The clinical features will depend on the degree of dehydration.

Hypotonic dehydration — the plasma sodium is low (below 130 mmol/l) and the reduced osmolality is accompanied by shifts of water into the cells and a marked decrease in ECF volume. The clinical features of dehydration are therefore exaggerated.

Hypertonic dehydration — the plasma sodium is raised (above 150 mmol/kg) and water loss exceeds electrolyte loss. ECF osmolality is increased; there is a shift of fluid out of the cells and the degree of ECF depletion is relatively less, so that the clinical features may suggest that the patient's condition is better than it really is.

Assessment of degree of dehydration

The clinical features are related to ECF depletion, which is relatively greater in hypotonic dehydration (see Table 29.5).

3–4% Poor peripheral perfusion (pallor, reduced capillary return), deep (acidotic) breathing, decreased skin turgor, urea >6.5 mmol/l, pH <7.35, base deficit >7.0.

10% Accentuation of the above signs, with sunken eyes, tachycardia and low central venous pressure.

15% Clinical signs of shock.

PRINCIPLES OF MANAGEMENT OF FLUID AND ELECTROLYTE ABNORMALITIES

Water

The volume required is calculated from the body weight × percentage dehydration. Additional fluid must be added for maintenance requirements and adjustments

Table 29.5 Features of various types of dehydration

Type of dehydration	Plasma sodium (mmol/l)	Relative electrolyte water loss	ECF volume	ICF volume	ECF osmolality	Treatment
Isotonic	130–150	E $\propto$ H$_2$O	↓ $\propto$ loss	=	=	Water + some electrolytes
Hypotonic	↓ 130	E > W	↓↓	↑	↓	Water + ↑ electrolytes
Hypertonic	↑ 150	E < W	↓ or normal	↓	↑	Water + ↓ electrolytes

made for pyrexia, environmental temperature and humidity (see Table 29.1). As a rule, dehydration of acute onset and short duration may be corrected more rapidly than longer-standing dehydration of more gradual onset. Rapid changes of osmolality should be avoided.

Sodium

Changes in plasma sodium usually reflect changes in total body water, rather than changes in body sodium. Hyponatraemia caused by water excess should be corrected by fluid restriction; hypernatraemia caused by water deficit should be corrected by giving water.

It is most important that abnormalities be corrected slowly, particularly if they are long-standing. The rate of change in plasma sodium should not exceed 0.5 mmol/l/h [6].

Although sodium is predominantly an extracellular cation, when fluid depletion occurs there may be some leakage into cells. The amount required to restore the sodium content of the body fluids will be related to the extracellular fluid volume, which is greater in newborns and infants (30–40% of body weight). After excess water loss an extra amount equivalent to 10–20% of body weight is commonly added, to compensate for loss of weight due to dehydration and electrolyte measurements being made on relatively concentrated plasma. The amount required, for example, in a dehydrated 5 kg infant with a plasma sodium of 120 mmol/l will be:

Body weight		deficit		ECF: body weight ratio		extra amount (see above)		
5	×	(140 − 120)	×	(0.4	+	0.2)	=	60 mmol

This is contained in 385 ml normal saline (60/156 × 1000 ml). To this should be added basal daily requirements (2 mmol/kg × 5 kg = 10 mmol), and any continuing losses should be replaced.

In hypernatraemic dehydration, the sodium loss is proportionately less than water loss. The correction of the fluid and electrolyte deficit should be carried out gradually with solutions containing adequate sodium but less than normal saline. Osmotic equilibrium exists between the ECF and ICF compartments. If solutions with little or no sodium are used the ECF will become hypotonic relative to ICF and, because water equilibrates more rapidly than solute, water may enter cells and produce cerebral oedema. The rate of correction of the water deficit is much more important than sodium content; rehydration should take *at least* 48 hours [7].

Potassium

Deficiency in potassium is difficult to assess, because most potassium is in the ICF and only the extracellular component can be measured. If ECF potassium concentration is low it is likely that total body potassium is low, but if it is normal it does not necessarily mean that intracellular potassium is normal. Acid–base status also influences plasma potassium concentration — it is reduced in alkalosis by increased excretion and by increased movement into the cells. Thus the administration of sodium bicarbonate results in a prompt reduction in plasma potassium. Acidosis has the opposite effect.

A dehydrated patient has often lost potassium as well as water (e.g. in gastroenteritis). Low concentrations of potassium (e.g. 20 mmol/l) can be included in the rehydration solution without waiting for the patient to pass urine, providing he does not have chronic renal disease. In severe hypokalaemia, potassium should not usually be given faster than 0.25 mmol/kg/h, and never faster than 0.5 mmol/kg/h. Hypokalaemia may be associated with a metabolic alkalosis, but this is probably caused by a deficit of chloride rather than potassium. In such circumstances the kidney retains hydrogen at the expense of potassium and thus potassium chloride will be required for correction of the metabolic alkalosis.

Hyperkalaemia (over 5.5 mmol/l) may be dangerous. Extreme hyperkalaemia should be treated by hyperventilation (which lowers pH and shifts potassium into the cells), 50% glucose (2 ml/kg) and insulin 0.1 u/kg intravenously (which also shifts potassium into cells), 10% calcium gluconate (0.5 ml/kg) given slowly i.v. (to counteract the effects of potassium on the myocardium and neurones) and sodium polystyrone sulphonate (Resonium) 1 g/kg rectally. Consideration should also be given to starting dialysis or haemofiltration.

Anion requirements — chloride and bicarbonate

The amount of anion required is equivalent to the cation. Usually sodium chloride and potassium chloride are used in replacement therapy, but in the presence of a metabolic acidosis sodium bicarbonate may be needed to provide base.

Calcium

Calcium is present mainly in bone, which provides a large body pool, but the small amount in plasma (2.25–

2.75 mmol/l) affects the function of myocardial muscle, skeletal muscle and neurones. It is the concentration of ionized calcium (normal concentration 1.0–1.3 mmol/l in plasma) that is important, not the total plasma calcium.

Calcium loss has been shown to be significant in infants following ileostomy. As much as 4 mmol/kg/day has been measured from ileostomy drainage at 2 months, gradually decreasing with age [8]. Calcium may be more than half the cation in the ileostomy fluid.

Magnesium

This is an important intracellular cation (about 40 mmol/l), but the plasma concentration is low (0.7–1.0 mmol/l). Magnesium deficiency may be caused by prolonged diuretic therapy, nasogastric suction, diarrhoea, losses from biliary or intestinal fistula and major gut resection. Deficits can be replaced by 0.5–1 mmol/kg/day but care should be taken not to give too much, as hypermagnesaemia may cause muscle weakness.

Protein

Loss of protein can be significant in patients who have increased capillary permeability, as in inflamed bowel, peritonitis or severe burns. This may lead to hypovolaemia due to decreased intravascular colloid osmotic pressure. If the patient is hypovolaemic and shocked, protein solutions (albumin or stabilized plasma protein solution, SPPS) will be required during resuscitation; they are often given as 25–50% of the replacement solution.

ACID–BASE DISTURBANCES

Acidosis

Acidaemia is present when the pH is less than 7.35. The pH (or hydrogen ion concentration) is determined by a respiratory and a metabolic component.

Acidosis, if uncorrected, leads to acidaemia.

Respiratory acidosis develops when there is retention of carbon dioxide (rise in $Pa\text{co}_2$). This is an indication of inadequate gas exchange.

A *metabolic* or *non-respiratory acidosis* can be caused by the addition of an acid load (e.g. administration of ammonium chloride) or the excessive accumulation of the acid products of metabolism. This can result from increased acid production (e.g. lactic acidosis in hypoxia, or ketoacidosis due to the incomplete combustion of fat in diabetes or starvation) or from failure of the kidney to excrete the acids normally removed by this route. A non-respiratory acidosis can also result from bicarbonate loss from the gut (e.g. in diarrhoea) or from the kidneys (renal tubular acidosis).

Alkalosis

Alkalaemia is present when the plasma pH is greater than 7.45.

Alkalosis, if uncorrected, leads to alkalaemia.

Respiratory alkalosis results from hyperventilation and a decrease in $Pa\text{co}_2$.

Metabolic or *non-respiratory alkalosis* results from the loss of hydrogen ion. This loss may be from vomiting, as in pyloric stenosis, or from the kidney due to diuretic therapy, chloride depletion or as compensation for respiratory acidosis. Metabolic or non-respiratory alkalosis may also result from the ingestion or infusion of bicarbonate, or from the metabolism of ingested or infused lactate, citrate or acetate. Diuretic therapy may cause alkalosis by increasing the hydrogen ion excreted in the urine.

The compensatory changes for these acid–base disturbances are indicated in Fig. 29.2. Respiratory changes are compensated by renal mechanisms which may take 2–3 days to develop fully, while metabolic or non-respiratory changes are compensated by changes in ventilation. Respiratory compensation occurs rapidly, especially when the acid stress is severe, as in salicylate poisoning or diabetic ketoacidosis. Because the respiratory centre responds to CSF pH, it may take 6–12 hours for equilibrium to be reached. Figure 29.3 illustrates the changes in the Siggaard Andersen nomogram.

Correction of the disturbance differs from compensation and requires correction of the primary abnormality.

EXAMPLES OF ACID–BASE AND ELECTROLYTE DISTURBANCES

Metabolic acidosis

Metabolic acidosis commonly results from poor tissue perfusion caused by hypovolaemia or poor myocardial contractility. Treatment should include restoration of blood volume, infusion of inotropic agents such as

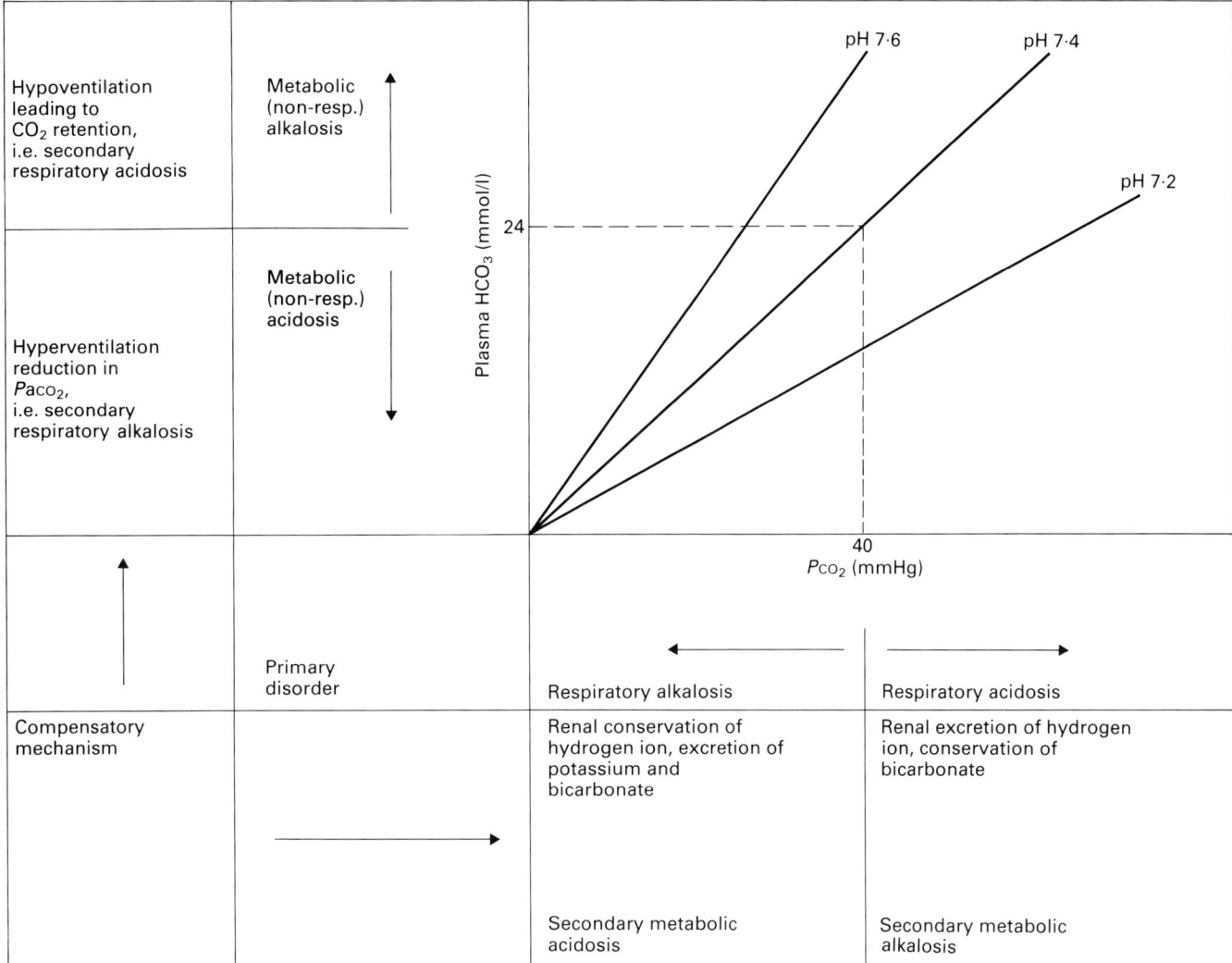

Fig. 29.2 Acid—base disturbances and their compensation.

dopamine, and the administration of sodium bicarbonate. Paralysis and ventilation assist the failing myocardium by removing the work of breathing.

Severe hypoxic metabolic acidosis occurs in infants with respiratory distress syndrome, and in some conditions such as congenital diaphragmatic hernia or severe cyanotic congenital heart disease (e.g. transposition of the great vessels) which can be treated surgically.

Respiratory acidosis

Respiratory acidosis is an accompaniment of respiratory insufficiency, unless it is compensating a non-respiratory alkalosis. This subject is dealt with in Chapters 32 and

33. The most common significant causes associated with anaesthesia are overdosage with depressant drugs (inhalation anaesthetics, narcotics, etc.), and incomplete reversal of muscle relaxants. The patient may need to be ventilated. Naloxone will reverse narcotic depression but also decreases analgesia. Residual non-depolarizing block can be treated with further doses of neostigmine or, occasionally, when due to antibiotic potentiation, with calcium.

Mixed respiratory and metabolic acidosis

This combination can occur, for example, in status asthmaticus. The situation is very grave if the pH is

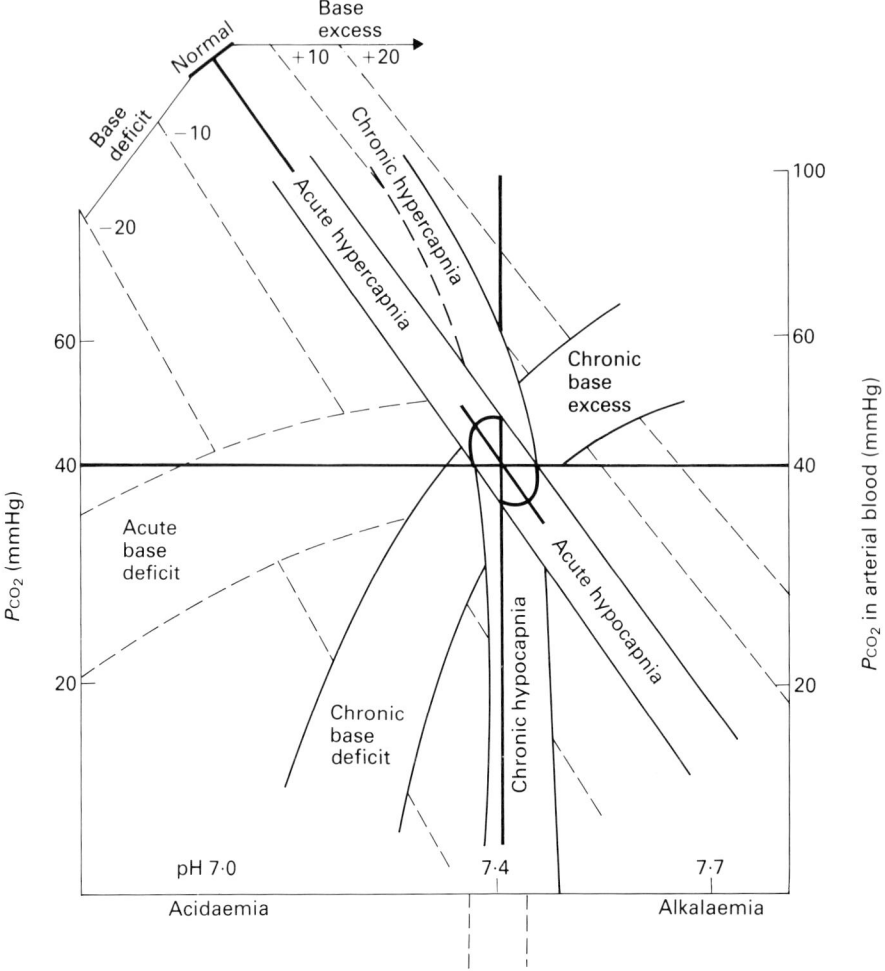

Fig. 29.3 Acid–base disturbances as represented on the Siggaard Andersen chart.

below 7.0 (100 nmol/l H⁺) and survival is unlikely if the pH remains below 6.90. At these levels myocardial contractility and the response to catecholamines are severely impaired.

Alkalosis — respiratory and non-respiratory

A primary alkalosis usually has less serious clinical consequences than a severe acidosis, but it may cause hypokalaemia and cardiac dysrhythmia. Primary respiratory alkalosis is due to hyperventilation; it causes decreased cerebral blood flow, and may result in cerebral ischaemia if the Pa_{CO_2} is lowered too far. Primary metabolic alkalosis is commonly seen in infantile pyloric stenosis where hydrochloric acid and potassium have been lost during prolonged vomiting. The treatment is to replace the deficit of water, chloride, sodium and potassium over 24–28 hours.

Small intestinal losses

Fluid loss from the small intestine is usually alkaline and isotonic, with 10–15 mmol/l of potassium and about 40 mmol/l of bicarbonate. If there is an obstruction just beyond the ampulla of Vater, the bicarbonate concentration may be higher due to pancreatic secretions.

Diarrhoea

In developed countries, severe diarrhoea is usually caused by rotavirus; the stool contains about 30 mmol/l of sodium, potassium, chloride and bicarbonate. In cholera, sodium losses are much greater because the copious stools contain 100 mmol/l of sodium.

Although water absorption is impaired in severe diarrhoea, the glucose transport mechanism still functions in the small bowel. Each molecule of glucose transported takes water and sodium with it into the body. This is the basis of oral rehydration therapy; absorption of water can be achieved by drinking a 1−2% solution of glucose, even with very severe diarrhoea. Higher concentrations of glucose cause osmotic diarrhoea. Breast-feeding and solids should be continued because they activate amino acid transport mechanisms that promote the absorption of water. For mild diarrhoea caused by rotavirus, salt should not be added, but a solution containing sodium (e.g. Gastrolyte) is desirable for severe rotavirus diarrhoea or cholera.

MANAGEMENT OF SURGICAL PATIENTS

Preoperative

Patients should be rehydrated and acid−base and electrolyte abnormalities corrected before surgery, if possible. The duration of the illness, the amount of vomiting, diarrhoea or other losses and the length of the period of starvation are all factors determining the severity of the disturbance. Clinical assessment of the child, and estimations of acid−base and electrolyte status are needed to guide therapy; assessment should be repeated periodically to assess the progress of treatment and guide further management.

The solution required to return the patient to normal will depend on the fluid deficit and the electrolytes needed to replace losses. Usually a sodium chloride solution (154 (isotonic saline), 77 or 38 mmol/l) is used with appropriate glucose for tonicity, the strength depending on the type of dehydration. To this are added sodium bicarbonate to correct metabolic acidosis, potassium chloride and other appropriate electrolyte solutions, as indicated by the biochemical findings.

If the patient is hypovolaemic with poor tissue perfusion, initial resuscitation may need to be rapid and a plasma protein solution may also be needed, especially if protein loss has occurred. Hypo- or hypernatraemia should be corrected gradually over 24−48 hours, once the circulating blood volume has been restored.

The progress of therapy should be monitored with repeated clinical and biochemical reassessment; careful records of fluid and electrolyte intake and output should be kept. Reversal of the clinical signs of dehydration, such as poor skin turgor, depressed fontanelle and sunken eyes, indicates improvement. The child becomes more alert, with improved cardiovascular status (slowing pulse,

improved perfusion, rising central venous and arterial pressures, increased output of less concentrated urine, and decreasing blood urea.

Over-infusion of fluids is recognized by a rise in central venous pressure to greater than 10−12 mmHg (1.2−1.6 kPa) and the development of peripheral and pulmonary oedema.

It should be noted that sodium bicarbonate solutions are usually hypertonic (8.4% has 1 mmol of sodium and bicarbonate per ml). This is nearly seven times the osmolality of plasma, and should therefore not be given too rapidly as rapid fluid shifts from the cells may result.

Replacement of blood loss is discussed elsewhere (Chapter 26).

Very prolonged periods of preoperative starvation should be avoided, especially in young children who generally have a lower fasting blood sugar level than older children. This is particularly important in sick or premature neonates, who have fewer glycogen reserves. Another situation where prolonged starvation can occur is when a child has an investigation under anaesthesia and it is decided to proceed to operation before the child has had time to recover from the first anaesthetic and have a meal. The operation should then either be postponed, so that the child can be fed, or intravenous fluids containing glucose should be given.

Glucose intake should be calculated in mg/kg/min: a neonate requires about 4 mg/kg/min on day 1, increasing over 2 or 3 days to 8 mg/kg/min (with 12 mg/kg/min needed in some children).

Operative

Normal children, apart from small infants, sleep for 8−10 hours without food or fluid intake and should therefore be able to tolerate a comparable period of fasting from before surgery until postoperative fluids can be taken. If the period of starvation is likely to be longer, if major surgery with associated fluid loss is undertaken, or if the weather is hot so that insensible water loss is increased, intravenous fluids which contain glucose and some electrolyte (e.g. sodium chloride 30−40 mmol/l) may be given preoperatively. Intraoperative fluids should be given if there is prolonged fluid deprivation.

Although hypoglycaemia is uncommon following a 6−8 hour fast, it occasionally occurs, especially in infants. The stress response to anaesthesia and surgery usually causes a rise in blood sugar, so that intraoperative hypoglycaemia is unlikely unless the patient has inadequate glycogen stores. Usually glucose solutions are now given during operation only to babies aged up to 3 months and to patients receiving parenteral nutrition. Blood glucose should be measured in such patients if there is a possibility of hypoglycaemia.

Extra water may be lost by evaporation from open cavities or wounds (increased if gut is brought out of the abdomen and not covered), and by redistribution from the intravascular to interstitial spaces. The latter is more significant in major surgery.

How much fluid should be given during surgery? Several factors have to be considered:

1 maintenance fluid requirements, which are about 4 ml/kg/h in the neonate after the first week of life, to 2.5 ml/kg/h in 8–12 year olds;

2 the duration of preoperative starvation;

3 the likely additional losses from cavities and redistribution of fluids;

4 the use of dry anaesthetic gases, which increases water loss;

5 the degree of metabolic response to anaesthesia and surgery — antidiuretic hormone secretion increases, leading to fluid retention, and increased adrenal corticoid secretion may lead to sodium retention.

It is difficult to provide concise rules for intraoperative fluid therapy because of the variability of the above factors in different circumstances. The following comments provide guidelines for intravenous fluids during surgery.

(a) Replacement of insensible and other losses (excluding blood). This can amount to about 10 ml/kg/h but because the sequestration of fluids into the tissues decreases with time, the volume should be reduced in the later stages of operations lasting more than 2 or 3 hours unless large wounds, body cavities or bowel are exposed for long periods allowing greater evaporation of fluid.

(b) Maintenance requirements for intravenous fluids are summarized in Tables 29.1 and 29.2. A 1–2-year-old requires about 90 ml/kg/day so that if the pre-operative and operative period of starvation is 8 hours, then $8/24 \times 90 = 30$ ml/kg can reasonably be given if the child has not been receiving intravenous fluids preoperatively. To avoid too rapid a rate of infusion and fluid overload, this volume should be given over 1.5–2 hours. When the operation is of shorter duration, fluids can be continued postoperatively if necessary. Shorter operations may disturb the physiology less and intraoperative fluid may not be needed.

(c) The types of fluid most commonly employed in children are Hartmann's solution or isotonic saline, and 0.18% or 0.44% saline with 4% and 2.5% dextrose respectively, if it is felt that additional calories are necessary to prevent hypoglycaemia, which may occasionally occur when infants are fasted for prolonged periods.

(d) Blood loss is replaced initially with electrolyte or colloid solutions; blood is needed only when 15–20 ml/kg have been lost and continuing losses are expected, or the patient is anaemic preoperatively.

Postoperative

The need for postoperative intravenous fluid therapy will depend on the nature of the operation and the state of hydration of the patient. For example, following abdominal surgery where the bowel has been handled, ileus is likely and postoperative intravenous therapy is desirable although children often tolerate oral fluids and food sooner after surgery than adults. Any continuing losses, such as nasogastric drainage, should be replaced.

The metabolic response to surgery is largely caused by increased adrenal corticoid activity, with increased protein breakdown and glycolysis for 3–7 days after operation. This catabolic phase is one of negative nitrogen, potassium and energy balance, with sodium and water retention. It can be modified by the administration of glucose, which is needed for its protein-sparing effect, and by the infusion of intravenous amino acids (see Chapter 37). However, care must be taken with hyperosmolar fluids if undesirable fluid shifts between compartments and osmotic diuresis are to be avoided. Fluid retention is caused by increased antidiuretic hormone secretion.

Inappropriate ADH secretion is discussed in Chapter 14.

Prolonged parenteral nutrition is discussed fully in Chapter 37.

CONCLUSION

Intravenous fluid therapy should supply basic daily requirements of water and electrolytes, taking into consideration the factors such as temperature and humidity which modify insensible losses, and should replace any added losses. Infusion of at least 20% of energy requirements (5% dextrose) reduces protein breakdown.

The routes of administration of intravenous fluid are considered in Chapter 7 and the equipment in Chapter 3.

REFERENCES

1 Friis Hansen B. Body composition during growth. *Pediatrics* 1971, **47**, 264.
2 Cheek D.B. Extracellular volume: structure and measurement and the influence of age and disease. *J. Pediatr* 1961, **58**, 103.
3 Hey E.N., Katz G. Evaporative water loss in the newborn baby. *J Physiol* 1969, **200**, 605.
4 Gamble J.L., Wallace W.M., Eliel L., *et al*. Effects of large loads of electrolytes. *Pediatrics* 1951, **7**, 305.
5 Mackenzie A., Barnes G., Shann F. Clinical signs of dehydration in children. *Lancet* 1989, **2**, 605–607.
6 Correspondence: Ellis J.; Farfel Z., *et al*; Illowsky B.P., Laurens R.; Sterns R.H.; Ayus J.C., *et al*. Correction of hyponatremia and its relation to brain damage. *New Engl J Med* 1988, **20**, 1335–1337.
7 Banister A., Matin-Siddiqi S.A., Hatcher G.W. Treatment of hypernatraemic dehydration in infancy. *Arch Dis Child* 1975, **50**, 179–180.
8 Winters R.W. *The body fluids in pediatrics*. Little, Brown & Co., Boston, (1973) p. 617.
9 Widdowson E.M. Nutrition. In: *Scientific foundations of paediatrics* (Davis J.A., Dobbin J., eds). Heinemann, London (1974).

FURTHER READING

Arnold W.C., Kallen R.J. (Eds). Fluid and electrolyte therapy. *Pediatr Clin N Amer* 1990, **37**, 241–512.
Finberg L., Kravath R.E., Fleischman A.R. *Water and electrolytes in pediatrics*. WB Saunders, Philadelphia, (1982).

30: The Evolution of Intensive Care For Children

Intensive care for children evolved from the need to relieve airway obstruction and to maintain ventilation in respiratory failure. In 1885, O'Dwyer reported the use of special tubes to relieve airway obstruction from diphtheria [1, 2] (Fig. 30.1). In 1927 Scholes, at Fairfield Hospital in Melbourne, reported 1175 patients treated with these tubes [3].

The worldwide poliomyelitis epidemic from 1948 to 1952 was a major stimulus to the establishment of respiratory care units and, hence, intensive care. Although Crafoord had developed a positive pressure ventilator at the Karolinska Thoracic Clinic, Stockholm, in 1937, many patients were treated in tank respirators and some remained in them for years afterwards.

In 1962, Bernard Brandstater introduced prolonged nasotracheal intubation in Beirut [4]. Tom Allen and Ian Steven in Adelaide (Fig. 30.2), John Stocks and Ian McDonald (Fig. 30.3) in Melbourne and Alan Conn and his colleagues in Toronto first used prolonged intubation in about 1963; their reports began to appear in 1965 [5, 6, 7]. The introduction of polyvinyl chloride (PVC)

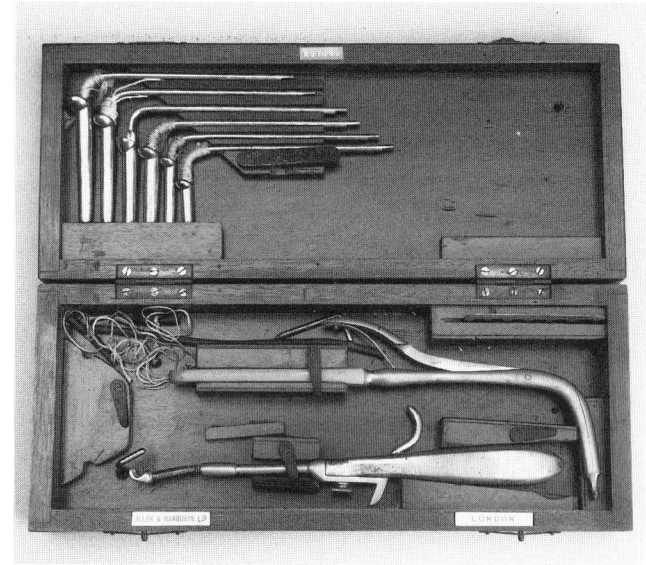

Fig. 30.1 A set of O'Dwyer tubes (Geoffrey Kaye Museum).

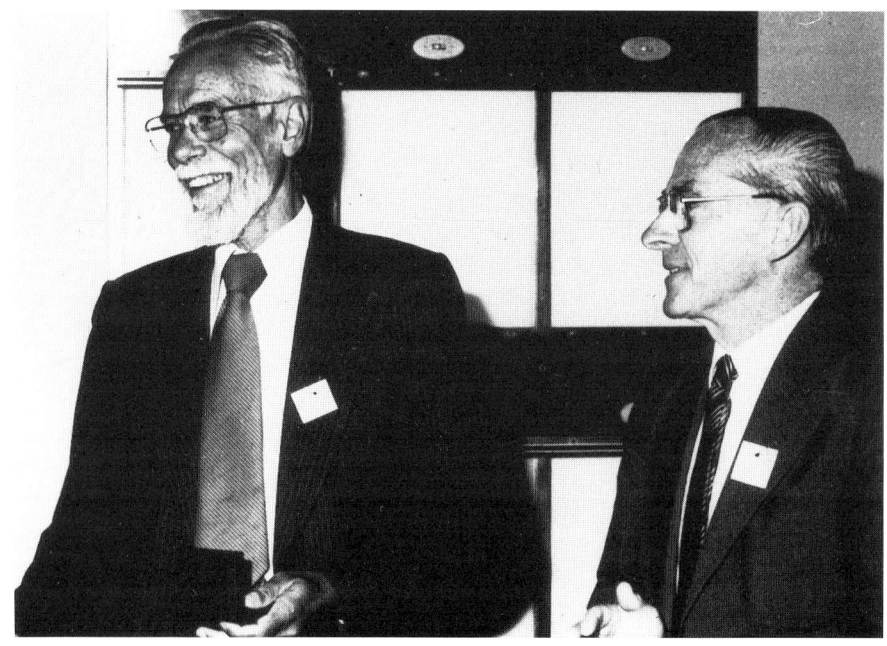

Fig. 30.2 Drs Tom Allen and Ian Steven of Adelaide.

416

tubes contributed to the success of the technique because they were less irritant than red rubber ones.

Subglottic stenosis was an occasional complication — 3 out of 60 cases in McDonald and Stocks' series [6]. Implantation testing of PVC was introduced to ensure that the tissue reaction was not due to toxic material in the tubes. After this, it became apparent that subglottic stenosis was more likely to occur if the tube fitted the larynx tightly. When care was taken to ensure that there was a slight leak around the tube, the problem was overcome and Stocks subsequently reported that there were no stenoses in their next 300 cases [8].

Accidental extubation was another potentially lethal problem and some ingenious methods were used to avoid it. Jackson Rees designed a complex tube that was attached around the head to overcome the problem (Fig. 30.4). Tunstall, in Aberdeen, developed a clip attached to the forehead to hold the tube [9]. In most centres, strapping on the face such as shown in Fig. 7.14 was used. Prolonged tracheal intubation became commonplace during the late 1960s and early 70s. This needed skilful nursing and medical care. The longest recorded intubation with ultimate recovery was 3 years [10]. One unusual consequence was that one of these infants, who had had a tube in for 3 months, could not sleep for a long time afterwards unless she had a pencil stuck in her nose!

Tube blockage focused attention on humidification

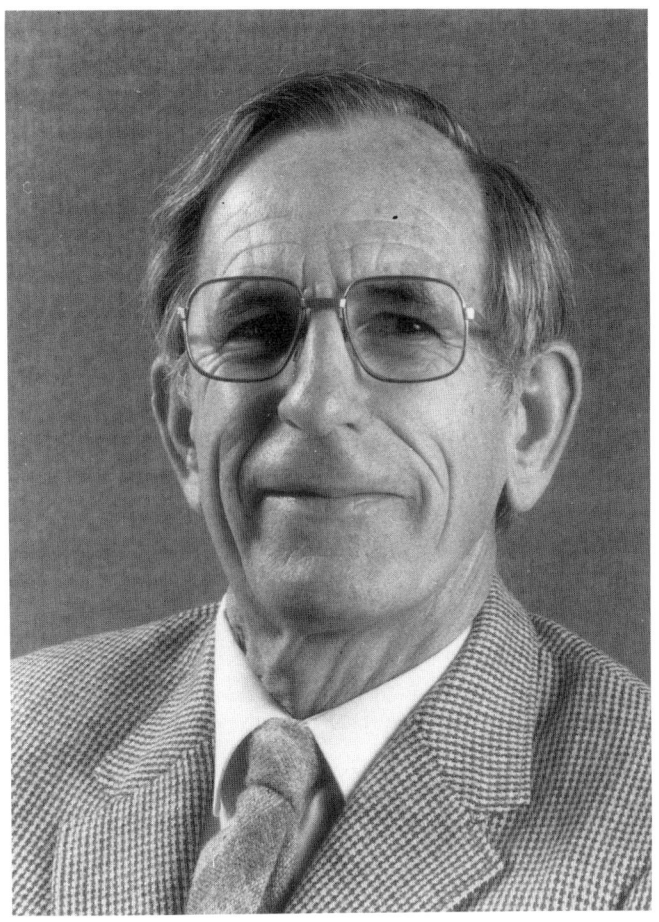

Fig. 30.3 Dr Ian McDonald of Melbourne.

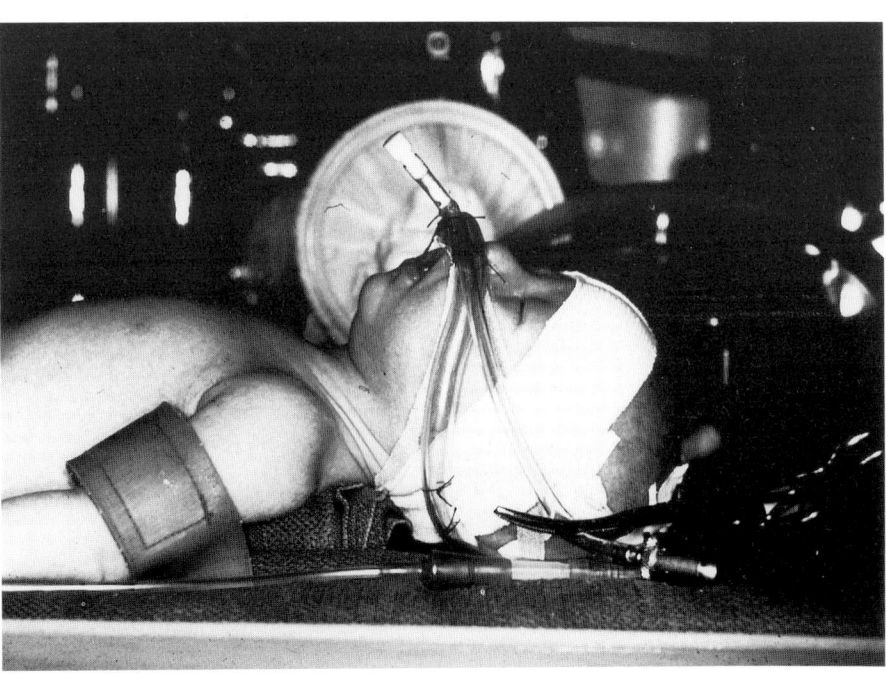

Fig. 30.4 A baby being ventilated with a Jackson Rees nasotracheal tube. Note the inspiratory and expiratory limbs attached around the head and the suction port opposite the tube.

and suction. Simple humidifiers in which the inhaled gas passed through thermostatically controlled hot water tanks, such as the Donnelly−Wilson [11] (Fig. 30.6), were used effectively for some years; others approached the problem by developing ultrasonic nebulizers. The potential hazard of these was that too much water could be delivered. Jet nebulizers such as the Puritan, which could be heated and could deliver air or varying concentrations of oxygen (40%−100%), were also popular (Fig. 30.7). An ingenious nebulizer, the Winliz, developed by the respiratory technicians at the Hospital for Sick Children in Toronto, used a gas jet to bombard water droplets on to a semicircular bar, creating small water particles. Its unique attribute was that the film of water over the gas jet was kept constant by floating the whole assembly in the water tank (Fig. 30.5). The depth

of the layer of water over the jet was thereby kept constant even though the water level in the tank dropped.

More recent humidifiers such as the Fisher−Paykel (see Fig. 33.3) and Nicholas use a heating element through the full length of the delivery tube. The water temperature is controlled to produce sufficient vapour for full saturation at body temperature. The heater in the tube keeps it above dew point until it reaches the end connected to the endotracheal tube (see Chapter 33). This system prevents droplet precipitation in the tube, but because the water in the tank is at a temperature at which bacterial growth can occur, there is a risk of contamination that was avoided in the older hot-water tank systems by the pasteurizing effect.

Infection has sometimes caused serious complications. In the late 1960s, *Pseudomonas* was the dominant organ-

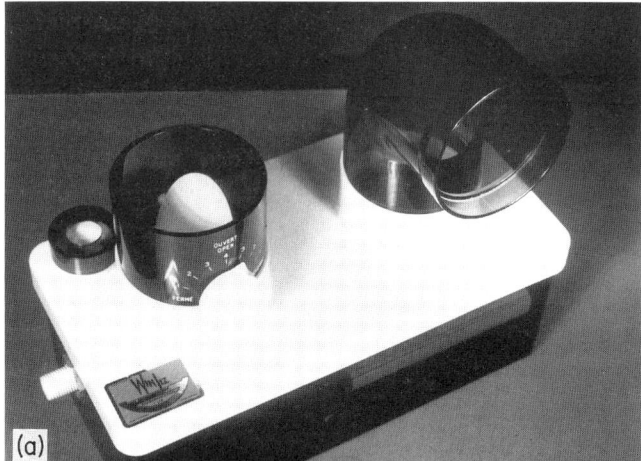
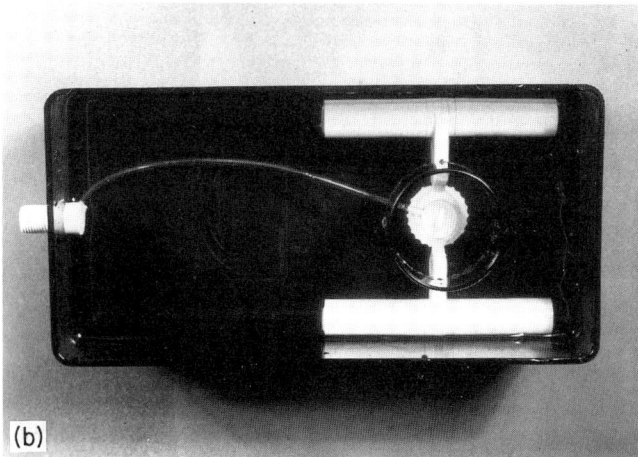
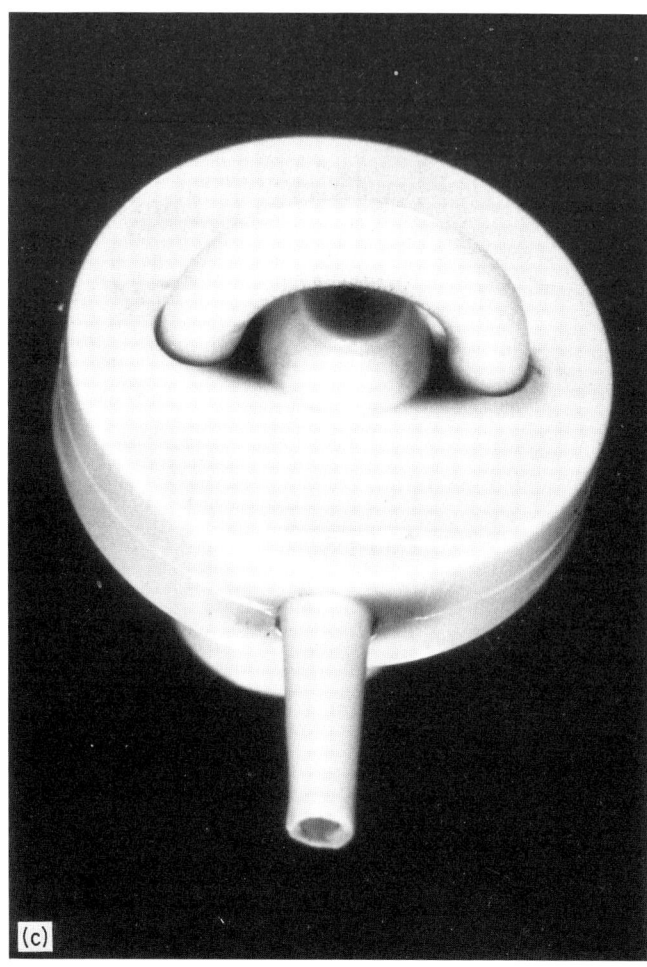

Fig. 30.5 The Winliz Humidifier. (a) The gas inlet on the left; variable inlet which allowed variable air dilution; exit port on right. (b) The tank showing the tubular floats, the gas line leading to nebulizer. (c) The nebulizer with the gas inlet; the gas lifts a film of water and bombards it on to the semicircular bridge, where it shatters into fine water particles.

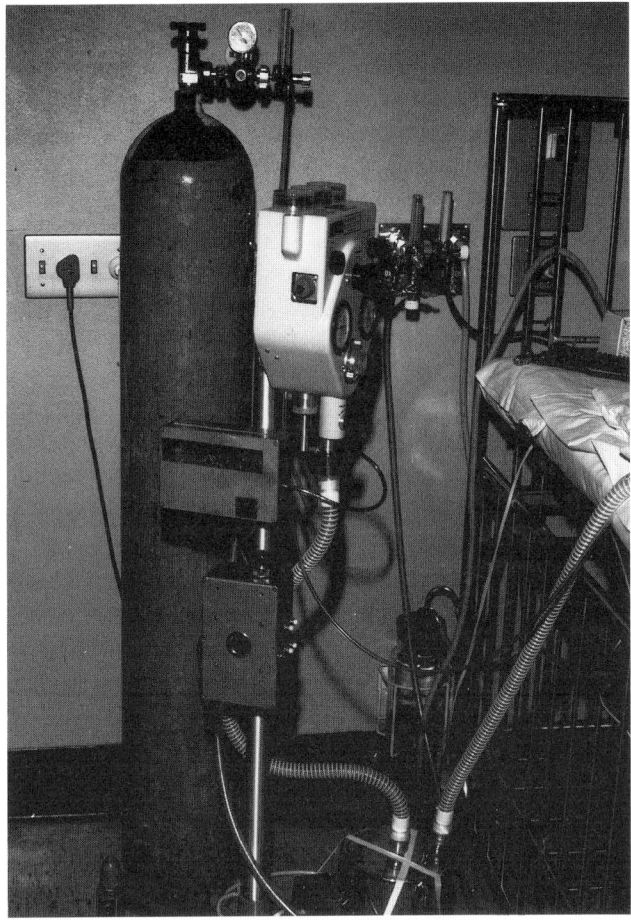

Fig. 30.6 A Bennett PR2 ventilator with a Donnelly–Wilson humidifier.

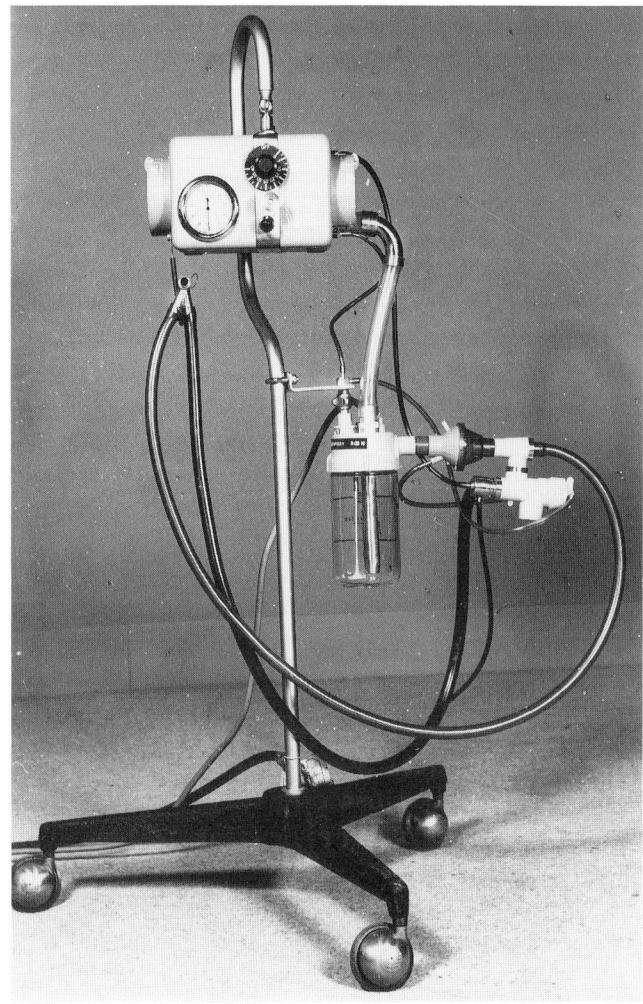

Fig. 30.7 A Bird ventilator with a Puritan nebulizer, a nebulizer for administering drugs and the paediatric circuit.

ism until effective broad-spectrum antibiotics were introduced. More recently, multiply resistant *Staphylococcus aureus* (MRSA) has been a challenging problem. Manufacturers need to keep developing new and effective drugs to overcome the resistant organisms. Clinicians must improve standards of cleanliness by regular hand washing when moving from one patient to another, and wearing gloves during procedures such as suctioning.

Suction is necessary to clear secretions, but atelectasis and hypoxaemia can result if excessive or prolonged negative pressure is used [12]. The application of positive pressure to the airways before and after suctioning helped to counteract this, but the introduction of the Stocks 'bullet' (see Fig. 33.4) allowed suctioning while IPPR was continued. This prevented the hypoxaemia and atelectasis that otherwise occurred during suctioning [13].

Tracheostomy, which is the alternative artificial airway, has been used for over 2000 years. Asclepiades

described it in 100 BC, followed by many others, such as Celsus (AD 14), Paul of Aegina (7th C), Rhazes, an Arab physician (9th C) and Pedro Virgili of Cadiz (18th C) [14]. Its use in paediatrics was established early this century by Chevalier Jackson [15]. It had similar complications to prolonged intubation, but in addition, pneumothorax occasionally resulted and subglottic stenosis was a major problem that occurred when a segment of tracheal cartilage was excised. Intubation replaced tracheostomy because there were more people, mainly anaesthetists, available with the skills for intubation than for tracheostomy. On the other hand, the prolonged use of strapping on the face inhibited the development of the muscles of facial expression. Intubated patients needed to be nursed in intensive care units, whereas patients with a tracheostomy could eventually go home. Now, when an artificial airway is needed for a long time a tracheostomy is usual. Severe laryngeal and subglottic stenosis have always been indications for tracheostomy.

At first there were no specific ventilators for infants, and ventilators such as the Engstrom and the then popular Bird (Fig. 30.7) and Bennett PR2 (Fig. 30.6) were used with modified breathing systems, until the advent of ventilators for infants, such as the Loosco flow generator. Now, there are a number of ventilators specifically designed to provide a full range of positive pressure therapy for infants and children, including continuous positive airway pressure (CPAP) and intermittent mandatory ventilation (IMV). In the early days, postoperative ventilation was only used for actual respiratory failure. The concept of prophylactic postoperative ventilation, particularly after paediatric cardiac surgery and some major neonatal and neurosurgical operations, developed in the mid 1960s [16]. Before that, postoperative ventilation was unusual.

Relatively rapid assessment of acid—base status, using small volumes of arterial or capillary blood, became available in the mid 1960s, when the Astrup triple pH method was developed [17]. Methods of measuring Po_2 soon followed. The diagnosis of respiratory failure no longer depended on clinical assessment and difficult, tedious laboratory measurements that were not suitable for infants.

The next significant advance was the introduction of continuous positive airways pressure (CPAP) and positive end-expiratory pressure (PEEP) in about 1970 [18]. Before then, babies with respiratory distress syndrome who had a Pao_2 below 60 mmHg when breathing 100% oxygen usually died. The introduction of positive airway pressure therapy, PEEP, with mechanical ventilation, and CPAP with spontaneous breathing, dramatically changed the prognosis, but this led to other problems associated with the survival of very premature babies, such as intraventricular haemorrhage and necrotizing enterocolitis. The rapid improvement in oxygenation with positive airway pressure therapy was not always appreciated when it was first used, and inspired oxygen concentration was sometimes left too high for too long. Some babies who died then had pathological signs of pulmonary oxygen toxicity. The risk of retrolental fibroplasia (retinopathy of prematurity) was also inadvertently increased.

Babies lose heat more readily than older patients (see

Chapter 1). Increased metabolism is needed to compensate for this when the baby is exposed to cold. The resulting increased respiratory gas exchange requires increased ventilation and cardiac output, placing significant stress on a sick infant. Premature infants also have smaller glycogen reserves. The use of servo-controlled overhead radiant heaters to control the temperature of the babies' environment within the thermoneutral zone has been a major advance in dealing with the above problems.

The development of drugs such as the sympathetic agonists and antagonists, prostaglandins, new antibiotics and a host of others have increased the potential for the successful treatment of very sick patients.

Survival following complex neonatal surgery, such as repair of oesophageal atresia and fistula, improved significantly with better respiratory care, intravenous fluid therapy and, later, parenteral nutrition. More recently, intensive preoperative care has enabled seriously ill babies to come to operation in better condition. Now that many more doctors skilled in neonatal and paediatric intensive care are available, better results and further advances are possible.

Transport of the critically ill child, and the management of many problems cared for in modern intensive care units are dealt with in the next few chapters.

REFERENCES

1 O'Dwyer J. Two cases of croup treated by tubage of the glottis. *NY Med J* 1885, **42**, 605.

2 Gifford R.R.M. The O'Dwyer tube: development and use in laryngeal diphtheria. *Clin Pediat* 1970, **9**, 179.

3 Scholes F.V.G. *Diphtheria, measles, scarlatina*, 2nd. edn. Ramsay, Melbourne, (1927).

4 Brandstater B. Prolonged intubation: an alternative to tracheostomy. *Proc 1st European Congress Anaesth* (1962) p. 106.

5 Allen T.H., Steven I.M. Prolonged endotracheal intubation in infants and children. *Br J Anaes* 1965, **37**, 566.

6 McDonald I.H., Stocks J.G. Prolonged nasotracheal intubation. *Br J Anaes* 1965, **37**, 161.

7 Markham W.G., Blackwood M.J.A., Conn A.W. Prolonged nasotracheal intubation in infants and children. *Canad Anaes Soc J* 1967, **14**, 11.

8 Stocks J.G. Management of respiratory insufficiency (types of tube). *Proc. 5th World Congress Anesth* 1972, Exerpta Medica, Amsterdam, p. 365.

9 Tunstall M.E., Cater J.I., Thomson J.S., Mitchell R.G. Ventilating the lungs of newborn infants for prolonged periods. *Arch Dis Child* 1968, **43**, 486.

10 Zelt B.A., LoSasso A.M. Prolonged nasotracheal intubation and mechanical ventilation in the management of asphyxiating thoracic dystrophy. *Anesth Analg* 1972, **51**, 342.

11 Donnelly G.L., Wilson A. A new respiratory gas humidifier. *Med J Aust* 1966, **1**, 720.

12 Brandstater B., Muallem M. Atelectasis following tracheal suction in infants. *Anesthesiology* 1969, **31**, 468.

13 Kerr D.R., Vonwiller J.B., Abrahams N. The Stocks suction bullet. *Anaes Intens Care* 1978, **6**, 185.

14 Watts J.McK. Tracheostomy in modern practice. *Br J Surg* 1963, **50**, 954.

15 Jackson C. Tracheostomy. *Trans Am Laryngo Rhinol Otol Soc* 1909, **19**, 285.

16 Brown K., Johnston A.E., Conn A.W. Respiratory insufficiency and its treatment following paediatric cardiovascular surgery. *Canad Anaes Soc J* 1966, **13**, 342.

17 Astrup P., Jorgensen K., Siggaard-Anderson O., Engel K. The acid−base metabolism: a new approach. *Lancet* 1960, **1**, 1035.

18 Gregory G.A., Kitterman J.A., Phibbs R.H., Tooley W.H., Hamilton W.K. Treatment of the idiopathic respiratory distress syndrome with continuous positive airway pressure. *New Engl J Med* 1971, **284**, 1333.

31: Transport of the Critically Ill Patient

INTRODUCTION

Transfer of a critically ill or injured patient to a centre with more facilities and expert care is desirable if the patient's survival and outcome are likely to be improved.

Apart from a lack of local expertise in management, other factors which need to be considered before transporting the patient include the patient's condition, the distance, mode of transport and its rapidity and, most importantly, whether adequate care can be provided during transport. The important question is whether the patient can be better managed where he is or whether the optimal location can be reached without further deterioration during transport.

A regular transport service for critically ill children should be appropriately equipped and staffed and be capable of operating at any time at short notice [1, 2]. The team should be able to give advice to attending staff before arrival, be capable of treating and stabilizing the patient at the point of embarkation, whether this be at the home, roadside, doctor's surgery or referring institution, and be able to provide optimum care during transport, so that survival is improved and morbidity is reduced. Long-distance transport, even intercontinental, is quite feasible with adequate organization [3].

Most work of paediatric emergency transport services is with patients with respiratory illness and trauma, particularly head trauma [4−7]. It is important that the service director is capable of assigning priorities to requests for transport. For less critically ill patients, advice to attending personnel may render transport safe in the hands of referring personnel [8]. Alternatively, transport may be safe without a doctor in attendance [9].

ESSENTIAL MEDICAL CAPABILITIES OF A PATIENT TRANSPORT SERVICE

The capabilities of the transport service and the personnel undertaking the transport of a critically ill patient are essentially those of an intensive care unit or emergency department operating with limited resources for a defined interval. Essentials are:

1 *Airway management*: the facilities for tracheal intubation (oral and nasal), tracheostomy and cricothyrotomy.

2 *Mechanical ventilation*: bag−mask ventilation and a simple portable ventilator with oxygen therapy and CPAP capability.

3 *Oxygen therapy*: a supply of oxygen sufficient to ensure uninterrupted supply for the duration of transport.

4 *Suction*: a portable suction generator and appropriate plastic catheters and pharyngeal suckers to maintain airway patency.

5 *Thoracentesis*: chest-drain tubes for drainage of air or fluid from the pleural cavity, and a one-way valve to prevent entry of air.

6 *Intravenous access and blood volume expansion*: percutaneous intravenous cannulation and an alternate technique such as bone-marrow puncture or surgical venous cut-down. Appropriate intravenous infusions sets and fluids.

7 *Drug therapy*: anticonvulsant, antidysrhythmic, antibiotics, bronchodilator, diuretic, inotropic, anaesthetic, muscle relaxant and analgesic. Inotropic drugs should be given by constant infusion.

8 *Anaesthesia*: local anaesthesia by nerve or regional block, or local infiltration. General anaesthesia by an intravenous technique and the use of an anaesthetic machine at the referring hospital.

9 *Defibrillation*: a defibrillator with paediatric-sized paddles (4.5 cm diameter) able to deliver low energy (5 J).

10 *Patient monitoring*: pulse oximeter, non-invasive blood pressure, electrocardiograph and temperature monitor.

11 *Body temperature conservation*.

EQUIPMENT

A list of essential equipment and medications is given in Tables 31.1 and 31.2. The complement of equipment should be kept to the minimum, but adequate to ensure patient safety. Electronic devices should be easily portable and be capable of continuous battery-powered operation for the anticipated duration of the transport.

MEMBERS OF THE TRANSPORT SERVICE

The service may use an existing ambulance service or have its own vehicles. The team members may consist of personnel from the retrieving hospital or a combination of these with members of the ambulance service. A team should always have at least two members. The medical member should be adequately trained and experienced in managing the patient's anticipated condition, and be capable of coping with likely problems during transport. It is not a task to be assigned to junior staff. The second member of the team should be a qualified critical care nurse or ambulance officer.

STABILIZATION OF THE PATIENT

In many cases, resuscitation and stabilization may commence before the arrival of the transport team. Arrangements can be made by telephone for special treatment to be started. Equipment such as an anaesthetic

Table 31.1 Essential equipment for a patient transport service

Airway, oxygen and ventilation equipment

Endotracheal tubes cuffed 6.5, 7 mm	Laryngoscope handle, batteries and bulbs
Endotracheal tubes uncuffed 2.5–6 mm	Magill forceps — small
Endotracheal tube introducer — small, medium, large	Heat and moisture exchanger (HME) (1)
Endotracheal tube suction catheters — 6, 7, 8, 10, 12 Fr (2 each)	Oxygen catheters — 6, 10 Fr Oxygen tubing (2 m)
Guedel airways, sizes 0, 1, 2, 3	Portable ventilator (with infant adaptation kit) e.g. Oxylog
Hudson oxygen masks — small, medium, large	
Humidivent (1)	HME (1)
Resuscitator — child size (1000 ml)	T-piece breathing system with small, medium and large bags
Masks, sizes 00–5 (6 masks)	
Laryngoscope blades (adult — McIntosh, baby — e.g. Robertshaw)	Yankauer sucker — large

Intravenous

Cannulae: Short 14 G (2)	Syringe pump
Cannulae: Short 20, 22, 24 G (2)	Intraosseous needle 14, 18 G
Cannulae: Long 22 G (2)	Needles 19, 21 G (2)
Cannulae: Seldinger guide wire and catheter (2)	Syringes 1, 5, 20 ml (2), 2 ml (4),
Extension set, long (2)	10 ml Luer lock (4), 50 ml (1)
Extension set, min. volume (2)	Three-way tap (2)

Miscellaneous

Artery forceps (1)	Multifunction monitor (invasive pressure, non-invasive pressure temperature, ECG oximeter)
Chest drains 10, 16 G (2)	
Dextrostix (1 pack)	Scalpel blade #11 (1), #23 (1)
Drug additives labels (4)	Scissors
Drug dose book	Silk ties (1 packet)
ECG electrodes	'Space' blanket
Gloves, size 6.5, 7, 7.5, 8	Sutures 30 (2)
	Tape: waterproof 1″ (1) Elastoplast 1″ (1) Elastoplast 3″ (1)
Heimlich valves (2)	
Defibrillator–Monitor	Tincture of Benzoin 10 ml
Nasogastric tubes 8, 10, 12, 14 Fr (1)	Torch

Table 31.2 Essential drugs for a patient transport service

Adrenaline 1:1000 1 ml (2)	Methylprednisolone 500 mg (1)
Adrenaline 1:10 000 10 ml (2)	Midazolam 15 mg (2)
Aminophylline 250 mg (2)	Naloxone 0.8 mg (1)
Atropine 0.6 mg (2)	Neostigmine 2.5 mg (2)
Benzylpenicillin 600 mg (2)	Noradrenaline 1:1000 (4)
Calcium chloride 10% 5 ml (1)	Pancuronium 4 mg (3)
Cefotaxime 1 g (1)	Phenobarbitone 200 mg (2)
Chloramphenicol 1.2 g (1)	Phenytoin 250 mg (2)
Clonazepam and diluent (2)	Propranolol 1 mg (2)
Dobutamine 250 mg (1)	Racemic adrenaline (1)
Dopamine 200 mg (2)	Sodium bicarbonate 8.4% 10 ml (1)
Dextrose 50% 10 ml (1)	Sodium bicarbonate 8.4% 100 ml (1)
Diazepam 10 mg (2)	Salbutamol resp soln 0.5% (1)
Frusemide 20 mg (2)	Salbutamol i.v. 5 mg (2)
Heparin 1000 u/ml 5 ml (1)	Saline 10 ml (2)
Ketamine 500 mg (1)	Suxamethonium 100 mg (3)
Lignocaine 1% 5 ml (2)	Thiopentone 500 mg + diluent (1)
Mannitol 12.5% 100 ml (1)	

Miscellaneous
Alcohol swabs (6)

machine, special supplies and cross-matched blood, if necessary, can be prepared. This forward planning can expedite stabilization, save valuable time and allow earlier transport.

Upper airway obstruction

Laryngotracheobronchitis (croup) and epiglottitis are common indications for transport to a paediatric centre. Croup may occasionally necessitate tracheal intubation, but epiglottitis almost always. Septicaemic shock and pulmonary oedema may occur if epiglottitis is recognized late in the course of illness. Croup may respond transiently to an inhalation of nebulized adrenaline (2−5 ml of 1:1000 solution) or racemic adrenaline (0.05 ml/kg of 2.25% solution). If the duration of transport is short (less than 1 hour) and the severity of obstruction not

great, administration of nebulized adrenaline before and during transport may minimize deterioration and obviate intubation. Epiglottitis, on the other hand, is not alleviated by inhalation of adrenaline; these patients should be intubated before transport unless there is no obstruction, the duration of transport is short and antibiotic therapy has already been started. In these circumstances, the patient should be transported in a sitting position. It is very dangerous to embark on a journey without determining the aetiology of upper airway obstruction, especially in the case of epiglottitis, in which complete obstruction may develop in a few hours or less.

When the patient is intubated it is desirable to check the position of the tube on X-ray before leaving. The distal tip of the tube should lie opposite the sternoclavicular joints on a supine film. The lengths of tube inserted by oral and nasal routes is given in Chapter 33. The tube should be firmly secured to the face to prevent both accidental extubation and endobronchial intubation [7]. Reliable fixation is more easily achieved with nasal intubation. Adequate humidification and airway aspiration are essential in intubated patients. This applies especially to croup or epiglottitis, in which airway secretions have usually been retained and are viscid. The use of sedation is optional, but the arms should be splinted to prevent the child pulling the tube out en route.

Neurological trauma

In the case of head or spinal cord injury, it is essential that all efforts are made to minimize secondary insults. Spinal injuries can easily be missed. Burr holes may be needed urgently prior to transportation, or immediately on arrival at the referral centre. The priorities are to ensure an adequate cerebral perfusion pressure and transport of oxygen to the damaged neural tissue. Blood pressure must be maintained and factors which influence intracranial pressure controlled, including $Paco_2$ (30−35 mmHg). Although monitoring of $Paco_2$ is not possible during transport, a reasonable appreciation of the required ventilation may be obtained during pre-embarkation stabilization. Hypotension, hypoxaemia or hypoventilation must be avoided. Head-injured unconscious patients require both airway protection and artificial ventilation to control intracranial pressure. Unfortunately, head-injured comatose patients are often transported, even to neurosurgical units, without adequate airway protection, mechanical ventilation or correction of hypoxaemia or hypotension [10]. Muscle relaxants, mannitol and diuretics may be useful. Fitting and hyperthermia must also be controlled.

Peripheral circulatory failure (shock)

This may be associated with a variety of pathological conditions, the most common being trauma, septicaemia, dehydration and myocardial failure. Reliable venous access is essential before transportation. The transport personnel should be skilled at circulatory access in adverse circumstances. Central venous cannulation, peripheral venous cut-down or intraosseous infusion (usually into the tibia) are essential. Adequate volumes of resuscitative fluids should be available for the journey. A means of administering fluids rapidly and a device for constant infusion of vasopressor/inotropic drugs should be available. Small volume-controlled infusion pumps with prepared drug infusion tables facilitate the preparation of infusates and obviate errors [11]. Monitoring is essential.

The management of respiratory failure (Chapter 33), circulatory insufficiency (Chapter 34) and neurological problems (Chapter 36) can be initiated before transportation. The airway must be secured and ventilation and the circulation maintained with other specific treatment.

Meningitis

Bacterial meningitis may present with many problems, including unconsciousness with raised intracranial pressure, shock, electrolyte abnormalities (hyponatraemia) and fitting. The most common causative organisms are *Haemophilus influenzae*, *Streptococcus pneumoniae* and *Neisseria meningitidis*. In advanced illness, intubation with mechanical ventilation and inotropic support are often necessary. It is hazardous, although necessary, to administer an anticonvulsant (CNS depressant) to a fitting patient with meningitis. Apnoea is a common consequence. Lumbar puncture in advanced meningitis may cause severe cardiovascular decompensation and even brain-stem coning. Antibiotics (ceftriaxone alone or chloramphenicol and penicillin) should be administered after urine and blood have been taken for culture and examination for bacterial antigen. Only when intracranial hypertension has been excluded and cardio-vascular support established should lumbar puncture be undertaken. If *Haemophilus influenzae* antigen has been detected in a body fluid and if the patient's condition is responding to antibiotics, a lumbar puncture is not necessary for identification.

Asthma

Effective oxygen therapy is essential. Inhalation salbutamol may be safely administered continuously in a concentration of 0.2−0.5%. Provided that a theophylline preparation has not been administered already, a loading dose of aminophylline (10 mg/kg over 1 hour) may be given followed by a continuous infusion of 1.0 mg/kg/h. Serum theophylline levels should be used to guide therapy once the patient is in hospital. A steroid, such as hydrocortisone 2−4 mg/kg 3−6-hourly, may also be beneficial. Failure to respond to conventional therapy may necessitate intravenous infusion of salbutamol (1−20 µg/kg/min). Poor gas exchange, loss of consciousness or metabolic acidosis necessitate mechanical ventilation with 100% oxygen. Air leak from the lung is a possible cause of therapy failure.

MODE OF TRANSPORT

Transport usually involves an ambulance, fixed-wing aircraft or helicopter. The retrieval team may travel to the patient in the vehicle intended for patient transport, but, if necessary, any means of transport to the referring hospital may be used to save time. The time taken for the transport team to arrive at the child's bedside is more critical than the time taken for the return journey [6]. The degree of urgency and the destination must also be considered when organizing the outward trip. As a general rule, road vehicles are suitable for use within a radius of 50 km from the referral hospital, helicopter within 50−150 km and fixed-wing aircraft beyond 150 km.

If the same vehicle is available for both the outward and return journeys, it should remain at the referral hospital, even if prolonged stabilization is needed before transfer; it will be out of service while waiting.

Patient-transfer vehicles should be equipped with an oxygen supply, suction, heating and lighting and be spacious enough to permit adequate access to the patient. Other equipment necessary to ensure adequate patient management must be standard in the vehicle, or be supplied by the transport team.

PROBLEMS AND DIFFICULTIES DURING TRANSPORT

Some difficulties can be anticipated and therefore reduced by forward planning, whilst others arise *de novo* and test the skills and ingenuity of the transport personnel.

Physiological problems

The behaviour of gases at increasing altitude are predictable from Dalton's Law of Partial Pressures and Boyle's Law ($P \propto 1/V$ at constant T). The important consequences are related to hypoxia and changes in pressure during transport by aircraft.

HYPOXIA

The percentage of oxygen in the atmosphere remains constant whatever the altitude. At 1800 m (6000 ft) the partial pressure of oxygen is 21% of 609 mmHg, so that the inspired Po_2 is 128 mmHg compared with 160 mmHg at sea level (where it is 21% of 760 mmHg). At high altitude, the cabin pressure is usually maintained at a pressure equivalent to that at 1800–2000 m. This predisposes all occupants to hypoxaemia and, in the case of a critically ill patient, may by itself or in association with other factors, such as lung disease, hypovolaemia or poor myocardial contractility, lead to poor oxygen transport to tissues. The treatment of hypoxaemia at high altitude is to administer oxygen. If the patient is already dependent on increased inspired oxygen (FiO_2) at sea level, the new amount of inspired oxygen needed to compensate for altitude can be calculated from the following equation [12]:

$FiO_2 = FiO_2$ (sea level) $\times$ 760/altitude pressure (mmHg)

FiO_2 at sea level breathing air is 21 $\times$ 76 mmHg. Altitude pressure drops about 1/3 for each 10 000 ft and 350 mmHg at 20 000 ft.

PRESSURE EFFECTS

With increasing altitude, gases contained in natural cavities, in pathological locations and within equipment expand and may severely compromise the patient's condition. At an altitude of 1800 m (the cabin pressure of high-flying commercial aircraft and low-flying un-pressurized craft), the volume of gas is 25% more than that at sea level. If the gas is confined in a cavity, the pressure within it will rise with ascent of the aircraft and fall with descent. The problems of gas expansion may be alleviated by limiting the altitude of flight, if practical, and by ensuring that confined gas cavities are free to decompress. Some gas-containing cavities have natural mechanisms to relieve pressure. Examples of this are the middle ear and nasal sinuses, relieved by swallowing or yawning, which allows the Eustachian tube to open. In the comatose patient in whom swallowing or yawning does not occur, severe middle ear pain and damage to the tympanic membrane may occur (barotitis media). The same problem arises if the Eustachian tube is blocked by oedema associated with trauma or inflammation of the upper airway. Likewise, severe pain may be experienced in the nasal sinuses if pressure equalization is not possible (barosinusitus).

Air-containing organs which expand on ascent may compromise the function of the organ or nearby organs. Expansion of bowel gas may lead to perforation, bowel-wall ischaemia, surgical anastomosis breakdown or impairment of diaphragmatic excursion. In the case of a diaphragmatic hernia, in which gas-containing bowel may be located within the thoracic cavity, expansion of bowel gas may lead to further deterioration of lung function. A pneumothorax or pneumoperitoneum should be drained before leaving and the drainage tube connected to a one-way valve (Heimlich valve) to prevent entry of air.

Air introduced into plastic-walled cavities, such as an endotracheal tube cuff or Swan–Ganz catheter balloon, may expand and exert pressure on surrounding tissues. The volume of air in an endotracheal cuff should be checked on ascent and reduced to the minimum volume necessary to obtain an airtight seal of the trachea. Conversely on descent, reduction in cuff volume may necessitate introduction of more air to maintain a seal. This problem can be overcome by filling the cuff with water or saline.

Intravenous fluids, particularly those used to deliver potent drugs, should be administered by volume-regulated devices rather than by drip-rate regulation. Changes of pressure within the fluid containers with changes in altitude might change the infusion rate. Glass bottles containing air should not be used because of the potential for breakage with ascent, and of air embolism if uncontrolled flow occurs.

HEAT LOSS

Critically ill patients, because of their illness and exposure during treatment, may lose heat. Infants, whose large body surface area in relation to small mass and poor insulation, are especially prone to cooling. For a patient who is comatose or purposely paralysed, generation of heat by shivering is impossible. During transport, additional factors such as suboptimal humidification of inspired gas and exposure to poorly controlled environmental temperatures may lead to hypothermia.

At an altitude of 1800 m (6000 ft), the environmental temperature is 12°C less than the temperature at sea level. Although the temperature of aircraft cabins is usually regulated, the adjustment of the ambient temperature may be slow, due to rapid fall in outside temperature during ascent.

Every effort should be made to conserve body heat by utilizing adequate protective body covering, such as reflective blankets or mylar foil. Exposure of the body should be minimized. It is rarely possible to utilize fully warmed and humidified gases for mechanical ventilation, but an in-line heat and moisture exchanger should be incorporated in the ventilator circuit. Infants should be transported in a temperature-controlled humidicrib. All patients should have their temperature monitored.

DESICCATION

Several factors predispose patients to the problem of airway desiccation during transport. Artificial airways bypass the natural humidifying function of the upper airway. When mechanical ventilation is provided with compressed gas, the respiratory tract receives no moisture at all. At high altitude, when air is used to ventilate a patient or the patient spontaneously breathes air, there is still a risk of mucosal desiccation because the moisture content decreases with increasing altitude. In unpressured, low-flying aircraft, the humidity in the cabin falls steadily with time and increasing altitude. In high-flying pressurized aircraft, the humidity is usually regulated to 60–70%. Encrusted secretions may threaten the patency of endotracheal tubes and is the most common preventable problem during air transport [8]. The use of a heat and moisture exchanger (HME) in the airway, regular instillation of small amounts of normal saline into the endotracheal tube or tracheostomy and regular aspiration, are necessary to ensure patency.

FLUID SHIFTS

Autonomic regulation of vessel tone may be lost in the critically ill patient. During take-off and landing, gravitational forces may alter the venous return, with undesirable effects. If a head-injured patient is positioned head-aft, the intracranial pressure during take-off may rise due to impeded venous return. On the other hand, if such a patient is positioned head-forward, decreased venous return may compromise cardiac output and cerebral perfusion. Similar effects occur during landing. Acceleration and deceleration manoeuvres should be undertaken gently.

Practical problems

Motion, vibration, noise and turbulence render patient monitoring and treatment less than ideal during transport. The measurement of blood pressure using a stethoscope and chest auscultation are unreliable. Palpation of the pulse is also difficult; poor lighting often further frustrates accurate assessment of skin and mucosal colour. Continuous pulse oximetry, non-invasive blood pressure monitoring and an electrocardiograph are invaluable.

Transfer of the patient in and out of ambulances, often several times, may pose the greatest threat to stability. These are the times when vital pieces of apparatus become disconnected or dislodged. Good communication between members of the transport team and careful patient movement are important in preventing such problems as accidental dislodgement of endotracheal tubes or intravenous cannulae. These should be well secured. If the patient is conscious, his arms should be splinted to prevent dislodgement of these devices. Sedatives may be needed to ensure compliance.

Working conditions for the transport team are often less than ideal. Space is often restricted and the seating made awkward for the sake of better patient surveillance. Motion sickness, the anxiety associated with departure at short notice, possibly dangerous travel and being expected to deal competently with a hitherto unseen clinical problem in an unfamiliar setting, often aided by strangers, are additional stresses.

ADMINISTRATION AND ORGANIZATION

A patient transport service for critically ill patients is

frequently the responsibility of a parent service such as an intensive care unit, anaesthetic or emergency department. Careful organization and allocation of resources is required to operate a transport service while conserving the capability of the parent service.

New team members should have an adequate period of orientation and training and be accompanied on initial patient retrievals by a more experienced member.

Ideally, a roster should be organized so that both the transport service and the parent unit are not short-staffed. Patient retrieval trips may occupy many hours, especially if the travelling time is long and the patient's condition requires prolonged stabilization before transportation.

Adequate lines of communication are needed to organize the mode of transport, staffing, optimal patient management before arrival of the transport team at the referring hospital and during transfer. Special procedures may need to be undertaken immediately upon arrival at the destination. In these circumstances, appropriate personnel and facilities must be organized.

Auditing and review of the service are necessary to identify problems, improve efficiency and effectiveness, and ensure safety and optimal patient care.

The physical and mental well-being of the transport personnel should not be overlooked. The conditions, duration and safety of travel need to be considered. Comfortable accommodation should be organized if the retrieval entails overnight delay at the referring hospital. Adequate insurance should be established for all transport team members.

CONCLUSION

Safe transport of critically ill patients is made possible by a prepared and experienced transport team. The crucial factors which ensure success are careful assessment and stabilization before embarkation, securing devices attached to the patient, an adequate supply of therapeutic and monitoring equipment and awareness of potential problems. Consultation by the transport team before arrival at the pick-up site and communication with the referral hospital before returning often expedite and improve management.

REFERENCES

1 Dobrin R.S., Block B., Gilman J.I., Massaro T.A. The development of a pediatric emergency transport system. *Pediatr Clin North Am* 1980, **27**, 633–646.
2 Harris B.H., Orr R.E., Boles E.T. Aeromedical transportation for infants and children. *J Pediatr Surg* 1975, **10**, 719–924.
3 Merlone S., Hackel A. Care of patients during long-distance transport. *Int Anesthesiol Clin* 1987, **25**, 105–116.
4 Kissoon N., Frewen T.C., Kronick J.B., Mohammed A. The child requiring transport: lessons and implications for the pediatric emergency physician. *Pediatr Intens Care* 1988, **4**, 1–4.
5 Owen H., Duncan A.W. Towards safer transport of sick and injured children. *Anaes Intens Care* 1983, **11**, 113–117.
6 Black R.E., Mayer T., Walker M.L., *et al*. Air transport of pediatric emergency cases. *New Engl J Med* 1982, **307**, 1465–1468.
7 Sweeney D.B., Turtle M.J. Paediatric retrievals in South Australia. *Anaes Intens Care* 1985, **15**, 410–414.
8 Kanter R.K., Tompkins J.M. Adverse events during inter-hospital transport: physiologic deterioration with pre-transport severity of illness. *Pediatrics* 1989, **84**, 43–48.
9 McClaskey K.A., King W.D., Byron L. Pediatric critical care transport: is a physician always needed on the team? *Ann Emerg Med* 1989, **18**, 247–249.
10 Gentleman D., Jennett B. Audit of transfer of unconscious head-injured patients to a neurosurgical unit. *Lancet* 1990, **335**, 330–334.
11 Shann F. Continous drug infusions in children: a table for simplifying calculations. *Crit Care Med* 1983, **11**, 462–463.
12 Lachenmyer J. Physiological aspects of transport. *Int Anesthesiol Clin* 1987, **25**, 15–41.

32: Acute Respiratory Failure in Infancy and Childhood

INTRODUCTION

Respiratory illness is common in children. It is estimated that 75% of the problems seen in neonates, 25% of all admissions to paediatric hospitals and 50% of the chronic diseases of childhood are related to respiratory disease. Acute respiratory failure exists when ventilation and/or oxygenation are impaired sufficiently to prove an immediate threat to life. Established or imminent respiratory failure is the commonest reason for admission to neonatal and paediatric intensive care units. Respiratory failure is frequently the result of pathology primarily affecting other organ systems, e.g. congenital heart disease or central nervous system disturbances. A number of predisposing factors render the infant vulnerable to respiratory failure. The principles of management of respiratory failure are common to all aetiologies and are discussed in Chapter 33. Management of individual conditions is discussed below.

PREDISPOSING FACTORS

There are many respiratory, anatomical and physiological differences between infants, children and adults that help to explain the high incidence of acute respiratory failure, particularly in the first year of life [1]. Detailed discussion of these differences can be found in Chapter 1.

To maintain homeostasis, respiratory function must be coupled to metabolic demands. Oxygen consumption in the neonate is approximately 7 ml/kg/min compared with 3−4 ml/kg/min in the older child and adult. Fever, illness and restlessness may dramatically increase metabolic demands. In the apnoeic infant, Pa_{CO_2} rises at approximately twice the adult rate and an oxygen debt, accompanied by severe metabolic acidosis, develops rapidly. The low respiratory reserve in infants and neonates is due to a number of factors:

1 *Structural immaturity of the thoracic cage*. The ribs are short and horizontal, and the bucket-handle motion that increases the anteroposterior and lateral dimensions of the thorax is minimal. The infant is therefore more dependent on diaphragmatic displacement of the abdominal contents to increase the length and volume of the thoracic cavity. Any impairment of diaphragmatic function, such as abdominal distension or phrenic nerve palsy, may precipitate respiratory failure. Structure and function of the rib cage alter between 12 and 18 months of age, possibly related to assumption of the upright posture.

The infant's chest wall is very compliant and is a poor basis for increased respiratory effort. Retraction of both the bony structures and the soft tissues of the chest wall occurs with any marked reduction in lung compliance or increase in airway resistance. Resting intrapleural pressure in the infant is −1 to −2 cmH$_2$O (−0.1 to −0.2 kPa) compared with −5 to −10 cmH$_2$O (−0.5 to −1 kPa) in the adult. This is due to the compliant nature of the chest wall (which tends to collapse in) and a lower elastic recoil of the lung itself. The result is an increased tendency to airway closure, atelectasis and intrapulmonary shunting.

In the neonate, the diaphragm and intercostal muscles have relatively fewer Type 1 (slow twitch, high oxidative) muscle fibres that fatigue more readily [2]. Respiratory fatigue may lead to sudden apnoea, particularly in the premature infant. Although gas exchange has been shown to be efficient under normal circumstances, these factors make it difficult for the infant to meet increased demands in the presence of increased respiratory work.

2 *Narrow airway diameter*. Relative to body size the infant's airways are large compared with the adult, but in absolute terms the airways of the infant are small. Developmental anomalies, acute inflammatory conditions and other acquired lesions can reduce the diameter, with dramatic results. In the newborn infant, it is estimated that a 50% reduction in airway diameter demands an increase in pressure (and therefore work) required to maintain breathing by 32 times. Airway obstruction accounts for 15−20% of admissions to a general paediatric intensive care unit.

3 *Immature development of the respiratory system*. Surfactant deficiency in the premature infant may lead to alveolar instability, atelectasis, intrapulmonary shunting and reduced lung compliance (see Chapter 1).

4 *Immaturity of respiratory control*. Inadequate respiratory drive due to immaturity of the respiratory centre is one of the factors leading to apnoeic spells, particularly in the premature (see Chapter 9).

5 *Congenital abnormalities*. Defects of the respiratory system or associated organs, such as the heart, often present with respiratory failure in the neonatal period. Examples include reduced lung development in diaphragmatic hernia, anatomical narrowing, compression or collapse of the major airways and congestion of the lungs due to a large cardiac shunt, such as in ventricular septal defect.

6 *Perinatal asphyxia or injuries*. Injuries or asphyxia associated with the birth process may result in respiratory failure, due to either central nervous system or respiratory complications.

7 *Increased susceptibility to infection*. The immaturity and inexperience of the immune system results in a markedly increased susceptibility to infection in the first 6 months of life. Both cell-mediated (T-cell) and humoral (B-cell) systems may be impaired.

CLINICAL FEATURES

Respiratory distress is manifested by tachypnoea, distortion of the chest wall (sternal and rib retraction, recession of intercostal, subcostal and suprasternal spaces), and the use of accessory muscles (flaring of the alae nasae and contraction of neck muscles). The early recognition of respiratory failure in small infants depends on careful observation of the effort of breathing and a high index of suspicion. Non-specific signs, such as lethargy and pallor in an infant or child who has severe respiratory distress, are an indication for blood gas analysis and close monitoring.

Neonates respond differently to hypoxia, compared with older children and adults. In the older child and adult acute hypoxia results in cyanosis, tachypnoea, tachycardia, hypertension, confusion, increased psycho-motor activity and vomiting, followed by cardiovascular and central nervous system depression with bradycardia, hypotension, coma and death.

In the neonate (especially the premature infant) sympathomimetic responses are less pronounced; lethargy, pallor, apnoea, bradycardia and hypotension are often the first signs of hypoxia. The physiological anaemia of infancy may delay the recognition of cyanosis. Sweating, a feature of carbon dioxide retention in older children, is not seen in the newborn period.

In neonates hypoxia may have additional effects not seen in older children. Massive pulmonary or intracranial haemorrhage may occur. Hypoxia and acidosis may be associated with the development of pulmonary hypertension and persistent fetal circulation, with right-to-left shunting through a patent ductus arteriosus and foramen ovale. If untreated, increasing hypoxaemia, progressive acidosis and death may follow.

Routine clinical examination of the child's chest should be performed to detect clinical features pointing to the diagnosis. In the neonate, however, chest examination is of more limited value as breath sounds may be transmitted uniformly throughout the chest, even in the presence of tension pneumothorax, lobar collapse or bronchial intubation. Chest radiology is an essential part of the assessment. The clinical features of specific disease processes are discussed below.

AETIOLOGY (Table 32.1)

The causes of respiratory insufficiency in infancy and childhood are classified according to age and the site of the underlying problem. All may culminate in respiratory failure. Acute respiratory failure in the newborn period is usually the result of asphyxia or other injury associated with birth, developmental anomalies including congenital heart disease, immaturity of development associated with prematurity or increased susceptibility to infection.

In the older infant and child, acute respiratory failure most commonly results from airway obstruction (upper and lower), congenital heart disease, central nervous system disorders or childhood accidents.

CAUSES IN THE NEONATE

Upper airway obstruction

CHOANAL ATRESIA

Nasal obstruction from choanal atresia may be unilateral, bilateral, bony or membranous. It is important if it is bilateral because in the first month of life many babies cannot breathe through the mouth except when crying. It presents shortly after birth with respiratory obstruction, retraction and cyanosis; the signs disappear on crying. The diagnosis is confirmed by inability to pass a catheter through the nostrils. Insertion of a carefully positioned and secured oral airway or the passage of a wide-bore orogastric tube acting as a splint should relieve obstruction in the short term; only rarely will intubation be required before operative relief of the nasal obstruction.

PIERRE ROBIN SYNDROME

This consists of a posterior cleft palate, mandibular hypoplasia and a relatively large, posteriorly fixed tongue that may become impacted in the cleft, obstructing the airway. The severity of the deformity varies, but it may present as a neonatal emergency. Airway obstruction is most marked in the supine position. Nursing the infant in the prone position or passage of a nasopharyngeal tube may relieve the obstruction. The optimal length of nasopharyngeal tube can be estimated from the crown-to-heel length [3] (Fig. 32.1). Occasionally, in the most severe deformities, tracheostomy may be needed for the first year of life.

CYSTIC HYGROMA

Cystic hygroma is a relatively rare cause of upper airway obstruction in young infants. The tumours consist of masses of dilated lymphatic channels. They usually occur in the neck and may involve the tissues of the tongue and larynx. Occasionally extension into the mediastinum

Table 32.1 Causes of respiratory insufficiency in infancy and childhood

Cause	Neonate	Older infant and child
Upper airway obstruction		
Nasal	Choanal atresia	
Pharyngeal	Pierre Robin syndrome	Macroglossia
	Cystic hygroma	Tonsillar and adenoidal hypertrophy
		Retropharyngeal abscess
		Obstructive sleep apnoea syndrome
Laryngeal	Infantile larynx	Croup
	Vocal cord palsy	Epiglottitis
		Diphtheria
	Subglottic stenosis	Post-intubation oedema and stenosis
	Subglottic haemangioma	Foreign body
	Webs and cysts	Papillomata
Lower airway obstruction		
Tracheal	Tracheomalacia	Foreign body
	Vascular anomalies	
	Tracheal stenosis	Mediastinal tumour
Bronchial	Bronchomalacia	Foreign body
Bronchiolar	Meconium aspiration	Status asthmaticus
	Lobar emphysema	Bronchiolitis
Disorders of lung function		
	Aspiration syndromes	Pneumonia
		Cystic fibrosis
	Hyaline membrane disease	
	Bronchopulmonary dysplasia	Aspiration syndromes
	Perinatal pneumonia	Pulmonary oedema
	Massive pulmonary haemorrhage	Congenital heart disease
	Pulmonary oedema	Near drowning
	Pulmonary hypoplasia	Trauma
	Diaphragmatic hernia	Burns
		Adult respiratory distress syndrome
Pulmonary compression		
	Diaphragmatic hernia	Pneumothorax
	Pneumothorax	Pleural effusion
	Repaired exomphalos	Empyema and gastroschisis
	Gastroschisis	

Neurological and muscular disorders

Diaphragmatic palsy	Poisoning
Birth asphyxia	Meningitis
Convulsions	Encephalitis
Apnoea of prematurity	Status epilepticus
	Guillain–Barré syndrome
	Envenomation

occurs. Sudden airway obstruction may be due to infection or haemorrhage into the lesion. Surgical excision is currently the treatment of choice, but it is difficult to remove the whole mass and recurrence is common. Successful treatment using sclerosing therapy with a bleomycin emulsion has been reported [4]. In severe cases, long-term tracheostomy may be required.

LARYNGOMALACIA

This is the commonest congenital cause of stridor. The supporting tissues of the larynx are lax and, on inspiration, the epiglottis, which is large and omega-shaped, and the arytenoids prolapse into the laryngeal vestibule. It usually

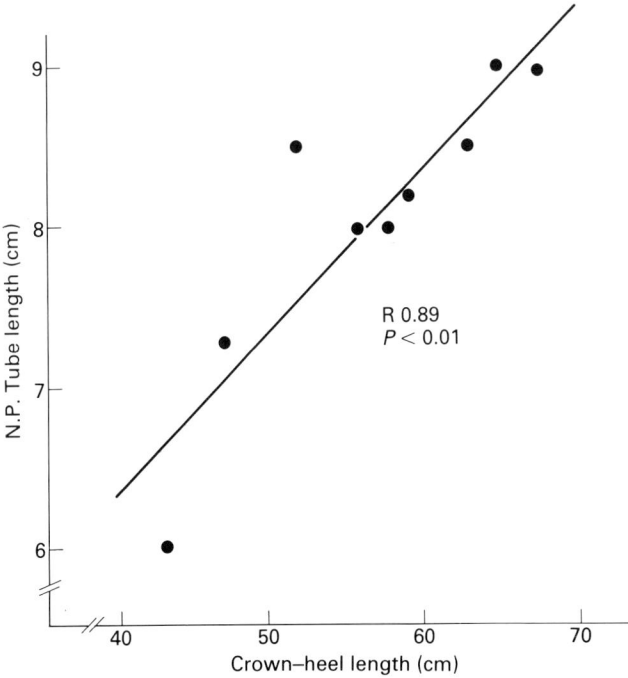

Fig. 32.1 Relationship between crown–heel length and length of nasopharyngeal tube (reproduced with permission from Heaf *et al.*, *J Pediatr* 1982, **100**, 698–703).

presents in the first days of life. The stridor is predominantly inspiratory, characteristically intermittent and affected by posture; it is not usually associated with significant obstructive episodes. Obstruction and failure to thrive, severe enough to require an artificial airway, are very rare. The stridor usually begins to resolve at 4–5 months of age and nearly always disappears by 12 months. Direct laryngoscopy should be performed to confirm the diagnosis and exclude more serious causes of stridor (see Chapter 15).

VOCAL CORD PALSY

This may be unilateral or bilateral. Presentation may vary from mild stridor with hoarseness of the voice or a weak cry to severe stridor with obstruction requiring urgent relief. The cause is not usually apparent. It may also be associated with meningomyelocoele, especially if the Arnold–Chiari malformation and hydrocephalus are present, with herniation through the foramen magnum and cervical cord compression. A recurrent laryngeal nerve may be injured by birth trauma or during left thoracotomy. The diagnosis is confirmed by direct laryngoscopy. In unilateral vocal cord palsy, a flaccid, often bowed vocal cord is seen on the affected side. Bilateral vocal cord palsy is evidenced by apposition of the vocal cords during inspiration. Intubation may be required, especially in neonates, but usually only if both cords are paralysed. Recently, laryngeal electromyography has been used to determine whether or not the muscles are functional (see Chapter 15). Stridor usually disappears over several months and most patients become asymptomatic by 12 months of age.

SUBGLOTTIC STENOSIS

Subglottic stenosis may be congenital or acquired. The congenital form may be due to soft-tissue narrowing of the subglottic region. Rarely, the cricoid cartilage is abnormal. The symptoms are recurrent croup or persisting stridor, exacerbated by intercurrent infection. Subglottic stenosis may also follow prolonged intubation with secondary pressure necrosis; its occurrence is then related to the size of the tube, duration of intubation and the number of reintubations.

Several operations have been devised for the surgical relief of subglottic stenosis, but prolonged tracheostomy may be required (see Chapter 15).

SUBGLOTTIC HAEMANGIOMA

These lesions characteristically cause variable inspiratory and expiratory obstruction, with inspiratory and expiratory stridor and a croupy or brassy cough. Unless the larynx is involved, the cry is normal. Symptoms are usually absent at birth and develop in the second or third months of life. Obstruction is typically exacerbated by crying or struggling, and by upper respiratory tract infection. It may also result in failure to thrive. The diagnosis is confirmed by endoscopy. Acute obstruction is readily relieved by an endotracheal tube, although tracheostomy is usually required for long-term care. The lesions usually regress spontaneously over a period of 1−2 years. Laser surgery has been beneficial.

LARYNGEAL WEB

This may be supraglottic, glottic or subglottic. The symptoms consist of stridor and respiratory distress. If the vocal cords are affected, the infant will also be hoarse or completely aphonic. Diagnosis is made by direct laryngoscopy. The web can usually be easily divided.

LARYNGEAL CYST

This may be in the epiglottis, the aryepiglottic folds, the arytenoids and down to and including the ventricles. Cysts also occur above the larynx and may arise from the dorsal surface of the tongue, in which case they may be found by direct palpation. Simple aspiration may reduce their bulk, but marsupialization may be necessary to prevent recurrence.

Lower airway obstruction

TRACHEOMALACIA, TRACHEAL STENOSIS AND VASCULAR COMPRESSION

Instability of the tracheal wall is most commonly seen in association with oesophageal atresia, tracheo-oesophageal fistula and various vascular anomalies. It may also follow tracheostomy, especially in infants, if cartilage has been excised. Rarely, tracheomalacia may occur without associated anomalies. The most common causes of vascular compression are a double aortic arch and the complex of a right-sided aortic arch, left ductus arteriosus and an aberrant left subclavian artery. These produce a true vascular ring, with encirclement of the trachea and oesophagus. Anterior tracheal compression may also be due to an anomalous innominate artery. Lower tracheomalacia or tracheal stenosis may occur in association with an anomalous left pulmonary artery (pulmonary artery sling).

Division of the vascular ring and ligation or repositioning of the aberrant vessel, while removing the cause of obstruction, do not immediately re-establish normal airway dimensions or function. Although the severity of symptoms may be alleviated by surgery, problems may persist for a number of years. Tracheomalacia may sometimes be stabilized by a prolonged period of nasotracheal intubation or tracheostomy with continuous positive airway pressure (CPAP).

BRONCHOMALACIA

Bronchomalacia, congenital cartilage deficiency, may occur as an isolated lesion or in association with other abnormalities. It may also be secondary to bacterial or severe adenoviral infection. It is characterized by persistent cough, wheezing and copious production of mucopus. Intercurrent respiratory infection may make matters worse.

MECONIUM ASPIRATION SYNDROME

Meconium aspiration is seen in approximately 0.3% of live births and is most common in term or post-term infants. There is usually a history of fetal distress in labour or prolonged and complicated delivery. Asphyxia during labour results in the expulsion of meconium. With the first few breaths the bulk of the material in the upper airway consisting of amniotic fluid, meconium, vernix and squames is inhaled, obstructing small airways and producing areas of atelectasis and obstructive emphysema. The irritant nature of meconium causes a chemical pneumonitis. With recovery, the aspirated material is absorbed and phagocytosed.

Clinical signs include tachypnoea, retraction and cyanosis. The chest may become hyperexpanded and pneumomediastinum or pneumothorax are frequent complications. Pulmonary hypertension and persistent fetal circulation are common.

The chest X-ray confirms the diagnosis, with coarse mottling and streakiness radiating from the hila. The lungs are over-expanded, with flattened diaphragms and an increase in the A-P diameter of the chest (Fig. 32.2). The condition is largely preventable if the airway can be aspirated rapidly and completely following the delivery of the head, before the first breath.

Most of these infants will require controlled oxygen therapy. The most severely affected require mechanical ventilation, which may be extremely difficult because of the high pressures required, uneven ventilation and the danger of pneumothorax. Extracorporeal membrane oxygenation has been shown to be effective in some infants [5]. The cerebral effects of severe intrapartum asphyxia contribute to some of the deaths that occur in babies with this condition.

LOBAR EMPHYSEMA

Seventy per cent of cases present in the first month of life, with tachypnoea, wheezing, grunting and cough. Signs include hyperresonance, decreased air entry and deviation of the trachea and heart away from the affected lobe. There may be asymmetry of the chest due to bulging of the affected hemithorax. Cyanosis may be associated with periods of increased respiratory distress. Once symptoms and signs develop, they may progress rapidly.

Radiologically, the affected lobe is over-distended with compression and deviation of the surrounding structures (Fig. 32.3). The left upper lobe, right middle lobe and right upper lobe are the most frequently affected sites, in that order.

The pathogenesis is unknown in over 50% of cases. Twenty-five per cent have localized bronchial cartilaginous dysplasia. The remainder have obstruction of a lobar bronchus from a mucous plug, redundant mucosa,

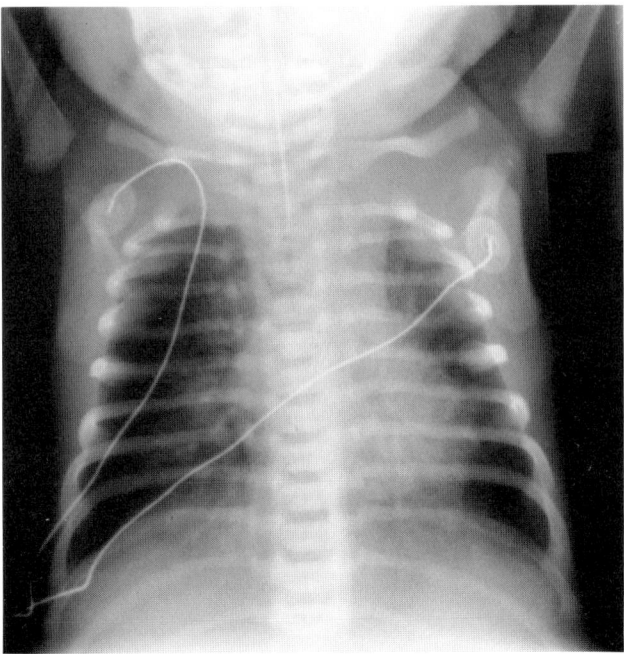

Fig. 32.2 Meconium aspiration syndrome. A-P chest radiograph demonstrating coarse mottling and streakiness radiating from the hila, and hyperinflation of the lungs.

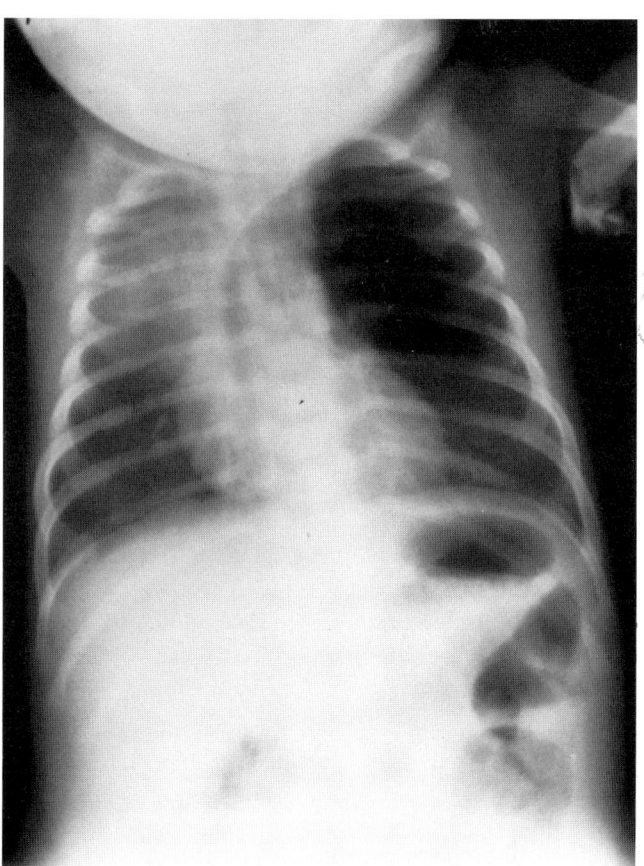

Fig. 32.3 Lobar emphysema involving left upper lobe, with displacement of the mediastinum.

aberrant vessels, bronchial stenosis or enlarged hilar lymph glands.

Lobar emphysema may be managed conservatively, but if there is progressive deterioration lobectomy is indicated.

Disorders of lung function

ASPIRATION

This may occur if there is incoordination of the swallowing mechanism, or impairment of upper respiratory tract reflexes, as may be seen in prematurity, brain damage or drug depression. Inhalation is frequently associated with abnormalities of the upper alimentary tract, such as cleft palate, oesophageal atresia with spillover from the upper oesophageal pouch, tracheo-oesphageal fistula and hiatus hernia with reflux.

Inhalation of gastrointestinal contents may produce both large and small airway obstruction and inflammatory oedema of the airways and lung parenchyma. The severity of the inflammatory reaction is related to the nature of the fluid aspirated. Gastric contents with a pH less than 5 are more likely to cause pneumonitis. The sudden onset of tachypnoea, rib retraction, grunting and cyanosis in a newborn, especially after a feed, suggests inhalation.

HYALINE MEMBRANE DISEASE (neonatal respiratory distress syndrome)

This condition occurs in 1% of all live births and approximately 10% of premature births. The main predisposing factor is prematurity. It also occurs more frequently in infants of diabetic mothers, in the second of twins and following caesarean section. The cause of the disease is deficiency of lung surfactant at birth. Surfactant production is also inhibited by postnatal hypoxia and acidosis. Lack of surfactant leads to alveolar instability, atelectasis, intrapulmonary shunting and increased work of breathing (see Chapter 1).

Clinical signs appear shortly after birth and consist of tachypnoea, chest-wall retraction, expiratory grunting and a progressive increase in oxygen requirements. Chest X-rays show a characteristic reticulogranular pattern (ground-glass appearance), with air bronchograms extending beyond the heart border (Fig. 32.4). The natural history is of progressive deterioration in the first 24–48 hours. In uncomplicated cases, where Pao_2 is

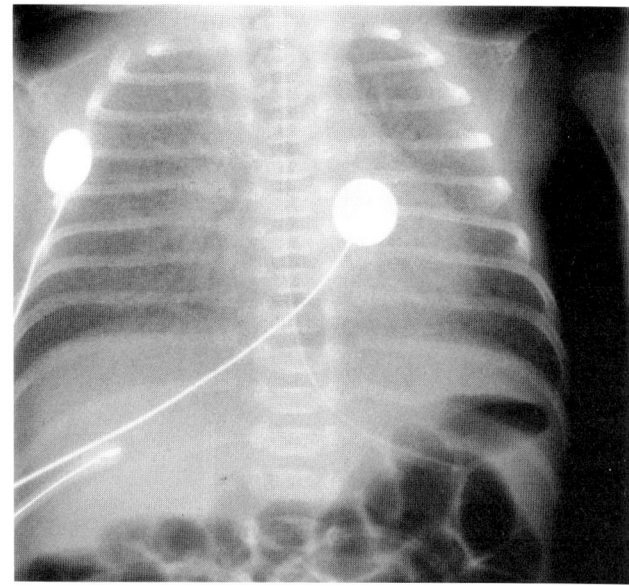

Fig. 32.4 Hyaline membrane disease. A-P chest radiograph demonstrating air bronchograms and reticulogranular pattern in the lung fields.

maintained over 60 mmHg (8.0 kPa) the disease is self-limiting and resolves in 4–5 days. Ninety per cent of deaths occur within the first 3 days. Respiratory failure may require increasing oxygen concentrations, CPAP, intermittent mandatory ventilation (IMV) or continuous mechanical ventilation (CMV). CPAP prevents alveolar collapse until surfactant is formed, and thereby improves oxygenation; the pattern and regularity of respiration improve, the progression of the disease slows and morbidity is reduced.

Arterial Po_2 should be maintained in the range of 50–80 mmHg (6.6–10.6 kPa) to avoid tissue hypoxia and the development of retrolental fibroplasia (due to hyperoxia, particularly in premature infants).

BRONCHOPULMONARY DYSPLASIA

This chronic lung disease may occur in the survivors of respiratory therapy. Its development correlates with lung immaturity, high airway pressures and the occurrence of air leak leading to pneumothorax, pneumomediastinum and pulmonary interstitial emphysema. Bronchopulmonary dysplasia is a cause of chronic respiratory failure in infancy, and occasionally progresses to cor pulmonale and death in the first 2 years of life.

Intrauterine pneumonia may occur as a result of transplacental spread of a maternal infection. It may also follow passage through an infected birth canal after prolonged rupture of the membranes, or as a result of cross-infection in the nursery. The immunoparetic state of the newborn and the need for invasive procedures such as intubation and vascular cannulation increase the risk of infection.

Clinical and radiological features may be indistinguishable from hyaline membrane disease. Antibiotics, such as penicillin and gentamicin, should be given until negative cultures exclude the diagnosis. The most common organisms include group B haemolytic streptococcus, *Escherichia coli*, *Pseudomonas aeruginosa*, *Klebsiella pneumoniae* and *Staphylococcus aureus*. Group B haemolytic streptococcal infection is frequently associated with septic shock and persistent fetal circulation. Failure to suspect group B haemolytic streptococcal infections and treat them promptly with penicillin will result in a poor outcome. Multi-resistant staphylococcal and Gram-negative bacillary infections must be suspected in longer-stay patients in neonatal intensive care units.

MASSIVE PULMONARY HAEMORRHAGE

This usually presents as acute cardiorespiratory collapse, accompanied by outpouring of blood-stained fluid from the trachea, mouth and nose. It is seen in association with severe birth asphyxia, hyaline membrane disease, congenital heart disease, erythroblastosis fetalis, coagulopathy and sepsis. Hypoxia is often a precipitating factor. The condition is believed to be the result of haemorrhagic pulmonary oedema due to acute left-ventricular failure.

Treatment is that of the underlying condition with oxygenation, mechanical ventilation and correction of any coagulation disturbance.

PULMONARY OEDEMA

Pulmonary oedema in the newborn period is due most often to congenital heart disease, especially coarctation of the aorta, patent ductus arteriosus, critical aortic stenosis and, rarely, total anomalous pulmonary venous drainage. Pulmonary oedema due to circulatory overload may also occur in erythroblastosis fetalis, the placental

transfusion syndrome or as a result of inappropriate fluid therapy.

The clinical features are those of respiratory distress in the newborn period, but specific clinical features of congenital heart lesions may be evident. There is a spectrum of severity, from tachypnoea with a widened alveolar−arterial oxygen gradient to life-threatening respiratory failure requiring urgent support. Chest X-ray usually shows an enlarged heart (except in total anomalous pulmonary venous drainage) and a ground-glass appearance fanning out from the hilar regions.

Details of management of congenital heart defects can be found in Chapter 13.

PULMONARY HYPOPLASIA

This is seen most often in association with congenital diaphragmatic hernia, but bilateral pulmonary hypoplasia may also occur in association with renal agenesis or dysgenesis (Potter's syndrome), in babies with severe rhesus isoimmunization and in the presence of chronic amniotic fluid leak. It may also present as an isolated malformation. Unilateral hypoplasia can occur as an isolated anomaly or in association with cardiovascular defects.

Pulmonary compression

DIAPHRAGMATIC HERNIA

Congenital diaphragmatic hernia presenting in the neonatal period results in respiratory failure, partly due to lung compression but more to the associated lung hypoplasia. Commonly, the hypoplasia is extreme on the affected side, with a variable degree of hypoplasia on the contralateral side.

The disturbance of pulmonary function ranges from mild to severe. In severe cases, life-threatening respiratory distress is present from birth, with cyanosis, intercostal retraction, mediastinal displacement and poor or absent breath sounds on the affected side. The abdomen is usually scaphoid, due to much of its usual contents being in the chest.

Chest X-ray shows loops of bowel in the affected hemithorax, with pulmonary compression and mediastinal displacement to the contralateral side (Fig. 32.5).

Perioperative care is dealt with in Chapter 9. Surgical correction should occur once the infant's condition has been stabilized, but there may not be an immediate

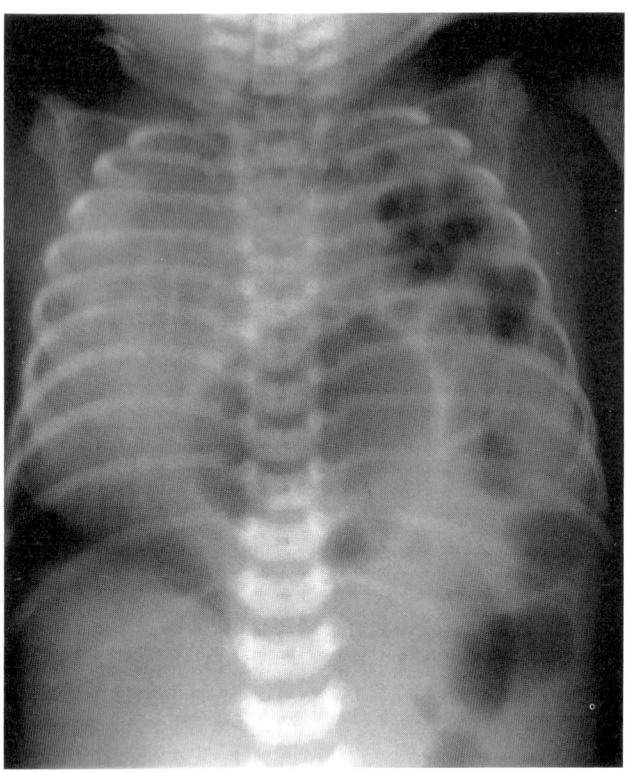

Fig. 32.5 Left-sided diaphragmatic hernia. A-P radiograph demonstrating gas-filled stomach, loops of bowel in the left chest and mediastinal displacement.

improvement in pulmonary compliance and gas exchange.

The major problems are pulmonary hypertension, with persistent fetal circulation and difficulties with mechanical ventilation and air leak.

Cyanosed neonates presenting in the first 4 hours of life have major lung hypoplasia, and continue to have a mortality of approximately 50%, despite maximal supportive therapy. Those presenting after 4 hours of age should all survive. Prolonged support of ventilation is often required, but the overall outlook for survivors is excellent. Some centres have shown improved survival in poor-risk cases using extracorporeal membrane oxygenation. Intrauterine diagnosis and repair has been described, but the indications for this are still unclear.

PNEUMOTHORAX

Spontaneous pneumothorax may appear at birth in otherwise normal babies. It may also occur secondary to hyaline membrane disease or meconium aspiration. Tension pneumothorax is particularly likely to occur when mechanical ventilation is required in the presence of immaturity, hypoplasia and non-uniform disease of the lungs, as well as diseases characterized by air trapping, such as meconium aspiration and bronchiolitis.

Whenever the condition of an infant being mechanically ventilated suddenly deteriorates, tension pneumothorax must be suspected. In older children, the classic signs of pulmonary collapse with hyperresonance and mediastinal shift are evident, but these are of limited value in neonates. Unilateral chest hyperexpansion and abdominal protuberance due to depression of the diaphragm and congestion of the liver are prominent signs. Transillumination of the thorax is a simple and rapid diagnostic technique in pre-term infants. A chest X-ray should be taken urgently, but must be preceded by needling or drainage if the infant's condition is critical. Unilateral pulmonary interstitial emphysema, evident on a previous chest X-ray, may also provide a clue to the side of the pneumothorax.

REPAIRED EXOMPHALOS OR GASTROSCHISIS

Complete repair of abdominal wall defects may cause marked elevation of intra-abdominal pressure when the intestines are enclosed in a poorly developed peritoneal cavity. The diaphragm is elevated, compressing the lungs. In addition, compression of the inferior vena cava may lead to peripheral oedema, reduced cardiac output and oliguria. The associated paralytic ileus may further increase intra-abdominal pressure.

Disturbed lung function with inadequate gas exchange may require postoperative mechanical ventilation for several days. In the case of large defects it may be necessary to house the abdominal contents in a prosthesis in order to allow gradual reduction into the abdominal cavity (see Chapter 11).

Neurological disorders

DIAPHRAGMATIC PALSY

Phrenic nerve palsy is a relatively common complication of cardiothoracic surgery. It occasionally occurs as a congenital abnormality or it may result from birth trauma. Paralysis and paradoxical movement of the affected diaphragm lead to reduced lung volume and tidal volume, hypoxaemia and increased work of breathing. A chest X-ray taken without positive airway pressure confirms the elevation of the hemidiaphragm (Fig. 32.6).

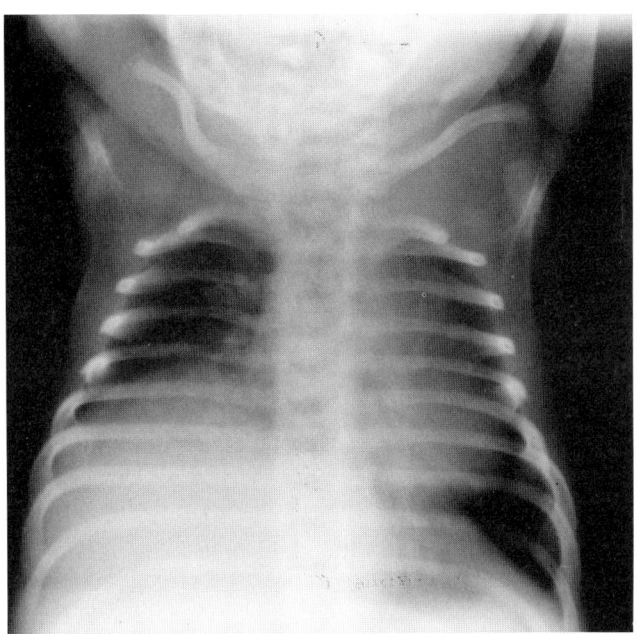

Fig. 32.6 Congenital right diaphragmatic palsy. A-P radiograph demonstrating elevated right hemidiaphragm.

Paralysis of the hemidiaphragm may cause protracted respiratory failure in infants, particularly if associated with another disorder affecting lung function. The problems are greatest in children under 3 years of age, due to the poor stability of the chest wall. CPAP may be an effective method of increasing lung volume, stabilizing the rib cage and reducing paradoxical movement. Surgical plication of the diaphragm is necessary in some cases that fail to resolve with conservative management [6].

BIRTH ASPHYXIA

Birth asphyxia may result from placental failure, obstetric difficulties or maternal sedation. The resulting central respiratory depression, convulsions, intracerebral haemorrhage, meconium aspiration and persistence of fetal circulation can all play a part in causing respiratory failure.

The Apgar score at 1 minute is an objective means of evaluating the newborn's degree of asphyxia, and the score at 5 minutes is a guide to prognosis. Delayed onset of spontaneous respiration (longer than 5 minutes) is also a poor prognostic sign. It is important to avoid further postnatal hypoxaemia, hypercapnia and brain ischaemia [7]. Severely asphyxiated infants need mechanical ventilation after delivery, with correction of acidosis and hypovolaemia; inotropic drugs may be needed to maintain cerebral blood flow. It is important to avoid hypoglycaemia and to control convulsions.

CONVULSIONS

Convulsions in the newborn are most frequent during the first 3 days of life. They are commonly due to birth asphyxia, trauma, intracranial haemorrhage, metabolic abnormalities such as hypoglycaemia or hypocalcaemia and meningitis.

Generalized convulsions may cause central respiratory depression, loss of protective upper airway reflexes and upper respiratory tract obstruction; this can lead to aspiration of stomach contents. Initial management consists of ensuring a clear airway, adequate oxygenation and ventilation, and controlling the seizures with anticonvulsants. The underlying cause must then be determined and treated (see Chapter 36).

APNOEA OF PREMATURITY

Recurrent apnoeic episodes are common in premature infants, occurring in 25% of infants less than 2500 g and in 84% of infants under 1000 g. Central apnoea unrelated to an underlying disease has been attributed to hypoxia, immaturity of the nervous system, altered chemoreceptor responsiveness, diaphragmatic fatigue and the active (REM) sleep state. Apnoea may also occur in association with aspiration of mucus or feed, hypoglycaemia, hyperbilirubinaemia, infection, dehydration, intracranial haemorrhage and raised intracranial pressure.

It is now recognized that many premature infants also suffer obstructive apnoea or mixed apnoea (central and obstructive), both being disorders of control of respiratory and airway musculature. The infant airway is easy to collapse, and this is aggravated by neck flexion.

Apnoeic attacks often respond to simple tactile stimulation. Low dose theophylline, 2–3 mg/kg 12-hourly, is used in premature infants as a respiratory stimulant to reduce the frequency of attacks. CPAP delivered by nasal 'prongs' or endotracheal tube will also decrease the incidence of apnoeic attacks and make breathing more regular. There is evidence to suggest that CPAP alters the reflex control of respiration, possibly by elimination of the Hering–Breuer deflation reflex. If apnoeic attacks persist, intermittent mandatory ventilation may be required (see Chapter 33).

CAUSES IN THE INFANT AND CHILD

Upper airway obstruction

MACROGLOSSIA

A large tongue is a feature of congenital syndromes such as Beckwith's and Down's and, occasionally, cystic hygroma. It may be sufficiently large to obstruct the oral airway and sometimes, particularly in Beckwith's syndrome (see Chapter 25), backward protrusion will obstruct the pharyngeal airway. Macroglossia may also be acquired in angioneurotic oedema or as a result of haemorrhage due to blood dyscrasia. Massive swelling of the tongue may follow partial glossectomy for any of the above conditions.

A carefully placed, patent nasopharyngeal airway will usually relieve respiratory obstruction. It may be preferable to leave a nasotracheal tube in place after glossectomy, because progressive swelling of the tongue may obstruct the airway.

TONSILLAR AND ADENOIDAL HYPERTROPHY;
RETROPHARYNGEAL ABSCESS

Upper airway obstruction can be caused by enlarged adenoids and tonsils, which may be associated with obstructive sleep apnoea (see Chapter 15). This obstruction can lead to hypoxia, hypercarbia and eventually to pulmonary hypertension and cor pulmonale. The conservative approach to tonsillectomy and adenoidectomy has led to an increased incidence of chronic upper airway obstruction due to hypertrophy.

Acute infective tonsillitis occasionally causes airway obstruction, dysphagia and drooling, mimicking epiglottitis. Other infections such as peritonsillar abscess, retropharyngeal abscess, Ludwig's angina and infectious mononucleosis, if it involves the tonsils, may produce similar features. Antibiotics should be given. If airway obstruction is marked, a nasopharyngeal or nasotracheal tube may be needed. The anaesthetic and surgical aspects of these conditions are considered in Chapter 15.

OBSTRUCTIVE SLEEP APNOEA SYNDROME

Obstructive sleep apnoea syndrome (OSA) is characterized by intermittent upper airway obstruction during sleep, with heavy snoring, and an abnormal, irregular respiratory pattern. These episodes are most frequent during rapid eye movement (REM) sleep and are accompanied by variable degrees of oxygen desaturation. OSA may be associated with enlarged tonsils and adenoids, a large uvula or long soft palate, macroglossia and retrognathia. Obesity is common. Daytime somnolence, learning difficulties and failure to thrive may result.

If OSA is severe and protracted, chronic hypoxia and hypercarbia may lead to pulmonary hypertension and cor pulmonale. In extreme cases, there may be evidence of left-ventricular failure and pulmonary oedema. The urgency of treatment is dictated by the mode of presentation. Critically ill children require immediate relief of the airway obstruction with a nasopharyngeal or nasotracheal tube, oxygen and diuretic therapy. Tonsillectomy and adenoidectomy are necessary after stabilization and are often dramatically beneficial. As an expendable part of the airway, these are best removed even when not grossly enlarged. Sometimes a degree of obstruction, due to such factors as a lax palate and tissue swelling, persists after the operation (see Chapter 15).

CROUP

Croup (acute laryngotracheobronchitis) is the commonest cause of laryngeal obstruction in childhood. It is due to inflammation and oedema of the glottic and subglottic regions. The narrowest part of the upper airway of the child is the subglottic region, and this is the point at which critical narrowing occurs (Fig. 32.7). Three subgroups are recognized: viral croup, spasmodic croup and bacterial tracheitis.

Viral croup, due to parainfluenza viruses, respiratory syncytial virus (RSV), rhinovirus and, rarely, measles, is characterized by nasal catarrh, low-grade fever, harsh barking cough and hoarse voice. The peak incidence is in the second year of life. In many cases the condition is mild and self-limiting, but in about 5% obstruction progresses until inspiratory stridor is constant and associated with retraction of the ribs, indrawing of the suprasternal tissues, tracheal tug and dilatation of the alae nasae. Desaturation detected by continuous pulse oximetry may be an early warning sign of deterioration.

If obstruction becomes marked, the child may no longer be able to compensate; signs of carbon dioxide retention and hypoxia are added to those of obstruction — stridor is severe, the child is restless and sweating and pulse rate and blood pressure rise. Finally, such children become exhausted and no longer attempt to

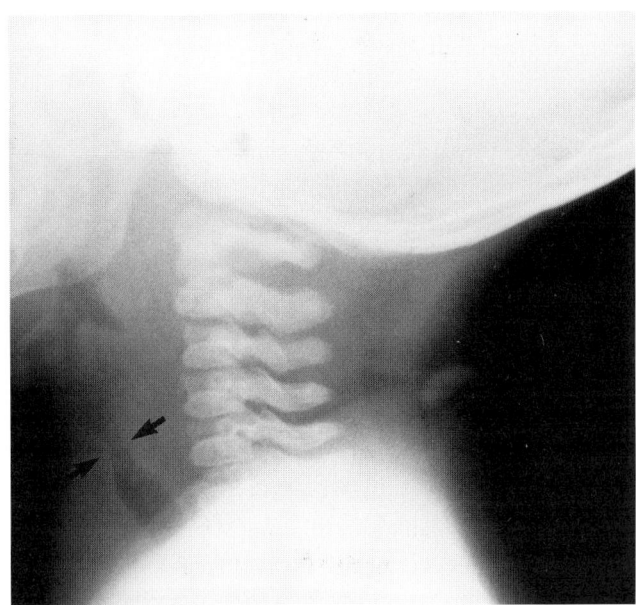

Fig. 32.7 Lateral neck radiograph of a child with severe croup. Arrows indicate subglottic narrowing due to mucosal oedema.

compensate. Respiration becomes shallow and stridor may be minimal.

Spasmodic or recurrent croup usually develops suddenly and without prodromal symptoms. There is often an allergic predisposition and the condition may represent part of the asthma spectrum.

Bacterial tracheitis is uncommon but should be suspected when croup is associated with high fever, marked leucocytosis and copious purulent secretions. The course of the disease is more rapid. Sudden, complete airway obstruction from oedema and purulent secretions may occur. *Staphylococcus aureus* is usually identified as the causative organism, although *Haemophilus influenzae* and group A streptococci are sometimes responsible.

Croup is uncommon under 6 months of age and its appearance at this age may suggest an underlying structural lesion, such as subglottic stenosis or haemangioma, with superimposed infection. Endoscopy should be considered in the convalescent phase if there is a prior history of stridor or if symptoms persist.

The management of croup requires minimal handling and repeated observation of pulse rate, respiratory rate, colour and retraction of the chest wall and soft tissues. Oxygen therapy may mask the signs of respiratory failure, but is needed to prevent hypoxia. Its use can be guided by pulse oximetry. In general, the need for oxygen therapy often predicts the need for an artificial airway.

The role of corticosteroids in uncomplicated croup has not been defined, mostly because of methodological difficulties. Recent studies have shown benefit in both spasmodic croup and viral laryngotracheobronchitis [8, 9].

Nebulized adrenaline will often provide at least temporary relief of acute obstruction. In viral croup, relief usually lasts 1−2 hours. It is debatable whether the course of the disease is altered. Its use is dramatically effective in spasmodic croup. It is particularly valuable when the child needs to be transferred to a specialized centre. The empirical dose is 0.05 ml/kg of 1% (i.e. 1:100) adrenaline diluted to 2 ml with saline and nebulized with oxygen. If only 0.1% (1:1000) adrenaline is available, it is recommended that the dose be limited to 5 ml at a time. Antibiotics are indicated only for bacterial tracheitis, in which case, antistaphylococcal cover is recommended.

Relief of airway obstruction by intubation is required in 2−5% of admissions for croup. The need for intubation is indicated by increasing tachycardia, tachypnoea, restlessness and oxygen saturation persistently less than 90%. One should not wait for signs of exhaustion and respiratory failure. Blood gas estimation is not helpful in the assessment.

Nasotracheal intubation is the preferred method of relieving airway obstruction. It is best performed under inhalation anaesthesia using halothane in oxygen. An endotracheal tube smaller than one normally predicted for age should be chosen. Infants less than 6 months of age require a 3.0 mm ID tube and from 6 months to 1 year, 3.5 mm. Beyond 1 year of age, the tube is predicted by the formula: (age divided by 4) + 3 = the internal diameter in mm.

Extubation can be performed when the child is afebrile, secretions are diminished and a leak is audible around the tube with coughing or positive pressure (25 cmH$_2$O, 2.5 kPa). The average duration of intubation is 5 days. Children less than 1 year of age generally need to be intubated more often than older patients and the tube is usually needed for longer. Steroids have been shown to shorten the duration of intubation and increase the success of extubation [10].

EPIGLOTTITIS

Epiglottitis is a life-threatening cause of supraglottic obstruction due almost exclusively to infection with *Haemophilus influenzae* type B. Streptococci, staphylococci and pneumococci are very occasionally responsible. Airway obstruction results from acute inflammatory hyperaemia and gross oedema of the epiglottis and aryepiglottic folds (Fig. 32.8). In about 30% of cases there is radiological evidence of subglottic swelling. Epiglottitis has been reported from the neonatal period through to adult life, although the peak incidence is between 2 and 3 years of age.

The diagnosis is usually obvious from the history and clinical features. There is acute onset of high fever and noisy breathing. The child adopts a characteristic posture, preferring to sit, usually breathing through an open mouth and drooling saliva. Cough is typically absent but its presence does not exclude epiglottitis. These features are due to an intensely painful pharynx, with difficulty in swallowing. The general appearance of the

child and severity of illness often appear out of proportion to the degree of airway obstruction. This is a reflection of the septicaemia that is almost always present. The stridor is characteristic; a low-pitched inspiratory stridor is accompanied by an expiratory snore.

Sudden complete obstruction is not infrequent and may be precipitated by examination of the pharynx, the supine position or stressful procedures such as intravenous cannulation. The spectrum of the illness is wide. About 10% of children with epiglottitis present with a milder form where the diagnosis may be in doubt. In these cases, a lateral X-ray of the neck should be taken in the sitting position, in the intensive care unit (Fig. 32.9). Examination of the pharynx must not be undertaken unless both personnel and facilities are available for immediate intubation.

Eighty-five per cent of children with epiglottitis require nasotracheal intubation for the relief of airway obstruction [11]. Milder cases may be treated with antibiotics

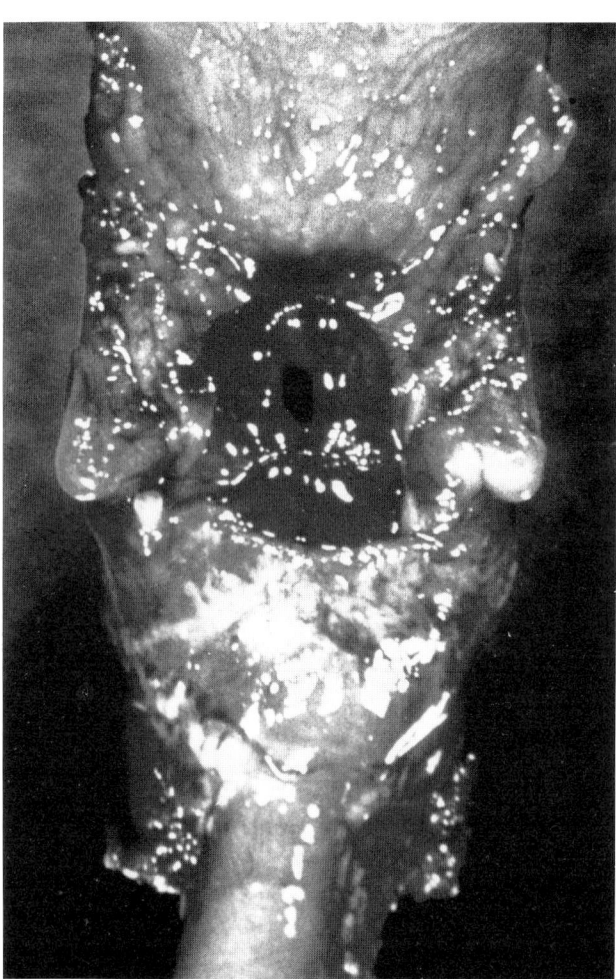

Fig. 32.8 Acute epiglottitis. Postmortem specimen demonstrating gross hyperaemia and oedema of epiglottis, aryepiglottic folds and arytenoids.

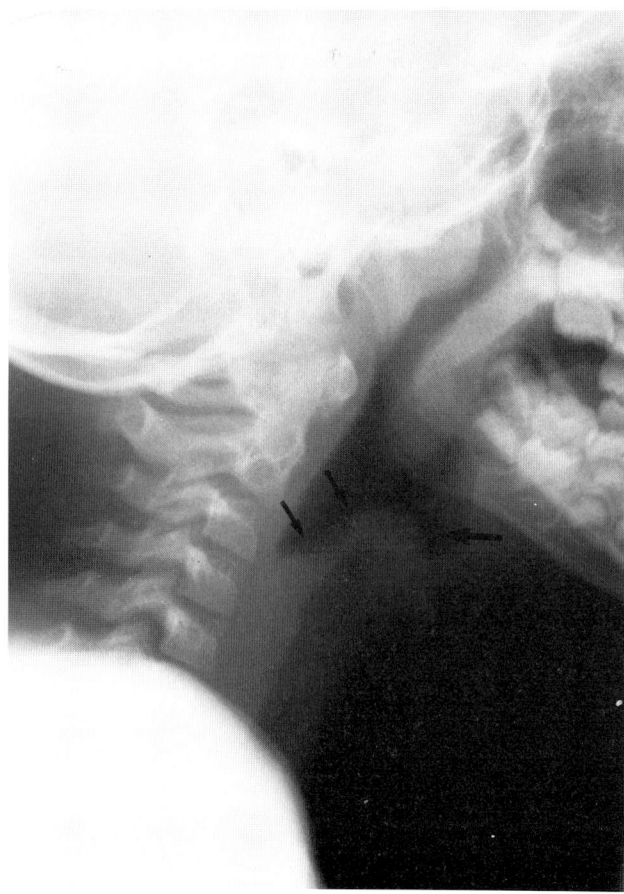

Fig. 32.9 Lateral neck radiograph showing swelling of epiglottis, aryepiglottic folds and arytenoids in a child with epiglottitis.

alone, provided staff who can intubate are immediately available. Until recently ampicillin (200 mg/kg/day) or chloramphenicol (100 mg/kg/day) have been the antibiotics of choice. The emergence of resistant strains of *Haemophilus* has led to the increased use of cefotaxime (200 mg/kg/day). Nebulized adrenaline is of no benefit in this condition, and may be harmful [12].

Inhalation anaesthesia using halothane in oxygen with CPAP provides adequate and safe conditions for intubation. Extubation can be undertaken when the temperature falls and the child no longer appears toxic. Most can be extubated in less than 18 hours [11]. Only cases complicated by pulmonary oedema, pneumonia or cerebral hypoxia will require intubation for longer than 24 hours. It is not necessary to examine the larynx again before extubation.

DIPHTHERIA

This was a common cause of laryngeal obstruction before the immunization of children. As immunization is no longer compulsory, the possibility of diphtheria as a cause of acute infective upper airway obstruction should be borne in mind.

POST-INTUBATION OEDEMA AND STENOSIS

Subglottic stenosis may follow tracheal intubation, whether for general anaesthesia or for prolonged management. It is usually due to the passage of too large an endotracheal tube. Children with congenital narrowing of the upper airway (e.g. subglottic stenosis, Down's syndrome) are at particular risk. Compression of the subglottic mucous membrane causes oedema and if obstruction follows, stridor usually develops within 1–2 hours of extubation.

Management involves minimal handling and supplemental humidification. Nebulized adrenaline is often dramatically effective (see above), but in some patients the benefit is transient and symptoms recur within 2 hours. If persistent obstruction occurs, reintubation with a smaller size endotracheal tube may be required. An alternative approach is to use nasal CPAP, a technique that is tolerated in some infants, and which avoids the need for further damage to the airway.

Subglottic stenosis develops when mucosal compression is so severe that ischaemia destroys the basement membrane, and normal mucosal cells are replaced by granulation and fibrous tissue. Obstruction may take several days to develop. The initial management is as for subglottic oedema, but if obstruction is severe or prolonged, a tracheostomy may be required. Severe permanent subglottic stenosis can be treated by surgical laryngotracheoplasty (see Chapter 15).

LARYNGEAL PAPILLOMATA

Multiple laryngeal papillomata are among the less common causes of laryngeal obstruction in infancy and childhood. They are usually confined to the larynx but can seed down the trachea. They are usually benign histologically, but tend to recur and require periodic surgical removal. In more extensive cases tracheostomy is necessary. They may resolve spontaneously after a year or two, but sometimes continue recurring. Their anaesthetic and surgical management is discussed in Chapter 15. They are usually removed with laser.

Hoarseness is the usual presenting symptom, although some children may have stridor and signs of airway obstruction.

FOREIGN BODY

A foreign body lodged in the region of the larynx of an infant or young child may cause acute respiratory distress that may progress to cardiorespiratory arrest if the airway is occluded. Thin foreign bodies with sharp points which stick in the larynx may only cause stridor or aphonia (see Chapter 15). Urgent laryngoscopy will be required if acute respiratory distress is present.

Lower airway obstruction

MEDIASTINAL TUMOUR

Mediastinal tumours may press on the trachea or bronchi, causing symptoms such as dry cough, stridor or wheeze. A brassy cough and hoarseness may be due to pressure on the recurrent laryngeal nerve. Occasionally, airway compression may result in hyperinflation or atelectasis, with respiratory distress. A concurrent pleural effusion is not uncommon and may add to respiratory embarrassment.

Increased difficulty with breathing can occur if the surrounding vessels become engorged. Biopsy is usually necessary to determine the nature of the tumour, so that the most appropriate chemotherapy can be given. Respiratory difficulties can occur during anaesthesia, especially in the supine position (see Chapter 12). It is safer to leave an endotracheal tube in postoperatively, until chemotherapy reduces the size of the tumour.

FOREIGN BODY

An inhaled foreign body that passes the larynx usually enters a main bronchus and may result in obstructive emphysema or atelectasis. Respiratory failure is rare unless there is obstruction of the trachea or both main bronchi. Inspiratory and expiratory chest X-rays or fluoroscopy are usually diagnostic. The clinical features and management by bronchoscopy are discussed in detail in Chapter 15. In an emergency, some relief of respiratory distress can be obtained by pushing a tracheal foreign body distally into one or other bronchus.

STATUS ASTHMATICUS

Asthma is the commonest reason for admission to most paediatric hospitals. Airway obstruction in asthma is due to mucosal oedema, mucous plugging, and bronchial muscle spasm. Under 2 years of age, bronchial and bronchiolar muscle is poorly developed and muscle spasm is probably of less importance and there is less response to bronchodilator therapy.

The clinical picture consists of loud wheezing, tachypnoea and a marked increase in the work of breathing. Cyanosis in room air is common. The chest is hyperinflated and there are widespread rhonchi, especially on expiration. The child is distressed, with tachycardia and hypertension.

Blood gas estimation is indicated for any child with the clinical features of acute severe asthma, if pulsus paradoxus greater than 20 mmHg (2.6 kPa) is present or if the child fails to respond to optimal drug therapy.

Hypoxaemia is the usual finding, and is the main cause of morbidity and mortality. High inspired oxygen therapy is therefore important. Hypocarbia in response to hypoxic drive is the rule; normocarbia or a rising $Paco_2$ are signs of worsening asthma or fatigue, and require increased medical therapy or mechanical ventilation.

Nebulized beta-2 sympathomimetic amines, intravenous methylxanthines and corticosteroids form the mainstay of drug therapy; maximal therapy should be introduced early. Salbutamol is nebulized as 0.05 mg/kg of 0.5% solution diluted to 2 ml with sterile water, given 2–4-hourly initially, or more frequently in severe cases. A greater and more sustained response may be achieved by more frequent or continuous salbutamol nebulization.

Children under 9 years of age have increased metabolism and require higher doses of theophylline (0.85 mg/kg/h equivalent to an aminophylline infusion rate of 1.1 mg/kg/h). Serum levels should be measured to ensure that they are in the therapeutic range (60–110 μmol/l). Continuous intravenous infusion of salbutamol has been shown to reduce the need for mechanical ventilation; it should be added to the regimen when $Paco_2$ is rising or is greater than 60 mmHg. An infusion is started at 1 μg/kg/min and increased every 20 minutes until $Paco_2$ decreases by about 10%, or a maximum dose of 14 μg/kg/min is reached.

Metabolic acidosis may occur as a result of hypoxaemia and increased work of breathing. Intravenous bicarbonate therapy may be used to restore pH and responsiveness to drug therapy, although it may cause an increase in carbon dioxide.

With aggressive medical therapy, mechanical ventilation should not often be needed. Its use should be based predominantly on clinical features rather than solely on blood gas analysis. It should not, however, be withheld out of fear of the difficulties. Mechanical ventilation may worsen air trapping and lead to hypotension or pneumothorax. Controlled hypoventilation with a long expiratory time is advocated to minimize airway pressures and air trapping. A trial of positive end-expiratory pressure may be justified.

BRONCHIOLITIS

Acute viral bronchiolitis is the most common serious acute lower respiratory tract infection in infants. Respiratory syncytial virus (RSV) is the cause in approximately 80% of cases. Parainfluenza type 3, rhinovirus and influenza type A2 may produce a similar illness. In 15–20% of cases, no pathogen can be identified.

Bronchiolitis usually occurs between 1 and 6 months of age, and is rare beyond 12 months. The illness typically begins with coryzal symptoms followed by wheeze and tachypnoea. There is evidence of chest hyperinflation and fine crepitations are heard towards the end of inspiration. Progression of the disease leads to exhaustion and respiratory failure in 1–2% of cases. Recurrent apnoea may be a problem, especially in infants who were born prematurely.

Management consists of minimal handling and oxygen

therapy. If respiratory distress is marked, feeds should be withheld and fluids administered intravenously. Continuous positive airway pressure [13] and/or aminophylline therapy are reported to reduce the work of breathing, lower $Paco_2$ and eliminate recurrent apnoea. Mechanical ventilation is required in some cases, particularly when the disease occurs in association with other problems, such as congenital heart disease. High airway pressures may be required, increasing the risk of pneumothorax.

Disorders of lung function

CYSTIC FIBROSIS

This is the most common cause of chronic suppurative lung disease in children. The lungs are affected in more than 95% of patients with cystic fibrosis.

The pathological changes in the lungs are suppurative bronchitis and bronchiolitis. *Staphylococcus aureus* and *Pseudomonas aeruginosa* are the most common causative organisms in young children. Permanent damage to the airway eventually results in bronchiectasis, fibrosis, atelectasis, pulmonary hyperinflation, localized areas of pneumonia and abscess formation.

Acute rapid deterioration in the later stages of the disease may result from pneumothorax, pneumomediastinum or massive haemoptysis. Occasionally children will require intensive care after thoracotomy for control of a bronchopleural fistula.

The prompt treatment of all lower respiratory infections with antibiotics and physiotherapy are probably the most important factors in minimizing permanent lung damage. With aggressive therapy, the prognosis for survival has improved greatly with most patients now reaching adolescence. The mode of death is progressive respiratory failure with pulmonary hypertension and cor pulmonale.

PNEUMONIA

Most pneumonia in infants and young children is of viral origin. The viruses commonly implicated are respiratory syncytial virus (RSV), influenza A1, A2, and B, and parainfluenza types 1 and 3. Adenovirus and rhinovirus are less common causes. The spectrum of illness is wide. Many infants and children have cough, fever and tachypnoea, with X-ray evidence of patchy consolidation, all of which resolve rapidly. Occasionally, infants develop life-threatening respiratory illness with extensive pneumonic changes and marked tissue necrosis. Permanent lung damage with bronchiolitis obliterans and pulmonary fibrosis may occasionally complicate severe adenoviral pneumonia.

Bacterial pneumonia is also seen. Pneumococcal pneumonia is common and usually responds dramatically to appropriate antibiotic therapy. Staphylococcal pneumonia is relatively uncommon, but is important because it may result in life-threatening respiratory failure and is often associated with complications such as empyema, pneumatocoele, tension pneumothorax and suppuration in other organs (Fig. 32.10). Aspiration of an effusion may be useful for diagnostic purposes. Tube thoracotomy or rib resection may be necessary in the treatment of empyema, and is believed to hasten resolution of the disease. In severe cases with bronchopleural fistula, surgical resection of the necrotic area offers the best chance of survival (see Chapter 12).

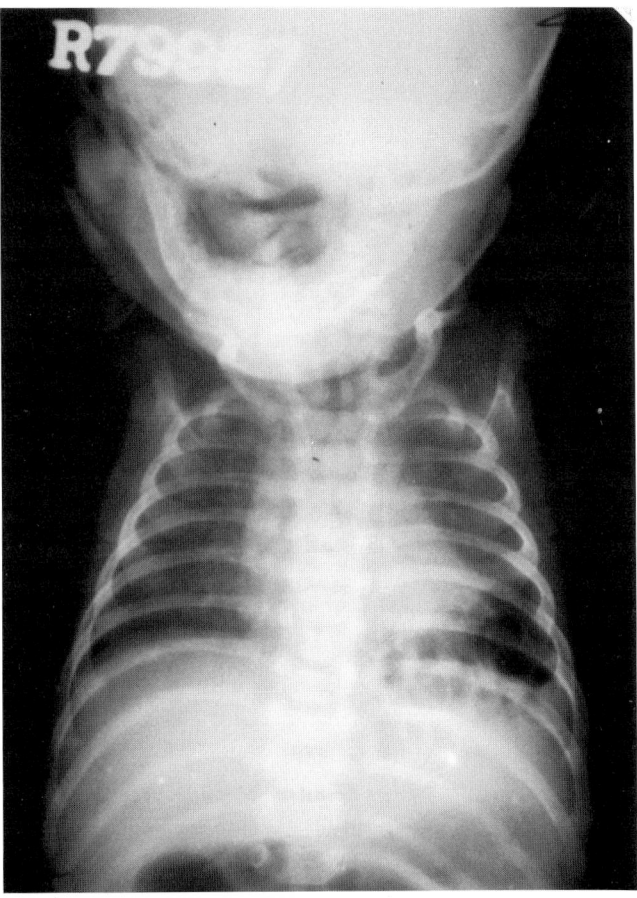

Fig. 32.10 Staphylococcal pneumonia. A-P chest radiograph demonstrating empyema and pneumatocoele formation.

Pneumonia due to *Haemophilus influenzae* may also occur and be associated with epiglottitis, meningitis, pericarditis or middle ear disease.

Gram-negative pneumonia is seen mostly in infants with debilitating conditions who are hospitalized for prolonged periods. It is a particular risk for patients in intensive care units with endotracheal or tracheostomy tubes. Other opportunistic infections, such as *Pneumocystis carinii*, *Candida albicans*, *Aspergillus* and cytomegalovirus, may occur in immune deficiency states, e.g. malignancy and chemotherapy, AIDS and subacute combined immune deficiency.

CONGENITAL HEART DISEASE

Infants with congenital heart disease may develop respiratory failure for a number of reasons, depending on the nature of the cardiac lesion, the presence of intercurrent infection and postoperative complications.

Congenital heart lesions resulting in acute respiratory failure fall into 5 main groups:

1 *Left heart obstruction*, such as critical aortic stenosis, interrupted aortic arch and coarctation of the aorta, may lead to left-ventricular failure, pulmonary oedema and respiratory failure.

2 *Large left-to-right shunts*, such as ventricular septal defect and patent ductus arteriosus. Respiratory failure in this group with excessive pulmonary blood flow results from overloading of the left ventricle and pulmonary oedema, small airways obstruction (due to peribronchial oedema), bronchial compression by enlarged pulmonary arteries or left atrium, or intercurrent infection.

3 *Hypoxaemic lesions with reduced pulmonary blood flow*, such as tetralogy of Fallot and pulmonary atresia. With these lesions, lung compliance is high. Excessive use of positive pressure ventilation may further impede pulmonary flow, leading to increased hypoxaemia and, occasionally, carbon dioxide retention.

4 *Hypoxaemic lesions with increased pulmonary blood flow*, such as truncus arteriosus and transposition with ventricular septal defect. These lesions have problems of reduced lung compliance and air trapping from small airways disease (due to peribronchial oedema) and bronchial compression, in addition to hypoxaemia from mixing of systemic and pulmonary venous blood.

5 *Vascular lesions* associated with compression or stenosis of the large airways, such as vascular rings and pulmonary artery slings. These were discussed earlier in this chapter.

Recurrent pneumonia and bronchiolitis are common in infants with congenital heart disease, especially those with high pulmonary blood flow.

Respiratory failure may follow repair of cardiac lesions; it may be due to low cardiac output with pulmonary oedema, adult respiratory distress syndrome, lobar collapse, pneumonia, respiratory depressant drugs, abdominal distension and ascites.

NEAR DROWNING

Respiratory failure after near drowning may be the result of aspiration pneumonitis, or may be from central nervous system depression as a result of the hypoxic—ischaemic encephalopathy. Acute gastric dilatation associated with the immersion itself or with resuscitation is common and may be a contributing factor.

Pulmonary oedema may be secondary to water and particulate matter inhaled, or to chemical pneumonitis from aspiration of gastric contents. Secondary infection occasionally leads to necrotizing pneumonia.

Prophylactic antibiotics are not of proven benefit and may lead to infection with resistant organisms. Antibiotic therapy, when given, should be guided by culture of tracheal aspirate. Steroids are of no benefit and may impair lung healing.

Respiratory failure in hypoxic—ischaemic encephalopathy may be due to the comatose state or associated seizures. Immersion hypothermia may protect the brain but may also contribute to central nervous system depression. Resuscitation and rewarming should be performed before deciding the prognosis (see Chapter 36).

TRAUMA

Respiratory failure may follow trauma to the brain, spinal cord, chest or abdomen. Most trauma in children results from pedestrian or bicycle accidents; isolated head injuries are common. Respiratory failure may be due to altered conscious state with airway obstruction or pulmonary aspiration, or to brain-stem injury or compression (see Chapter 36).

Because the child's chest wall is so compliant, impact injuries can severely damage intrathoracic structures without obvious external evidence of trauma. Respiratory failure may be due to pulmonary contusion, haemopneumothorax or flail chest.

Acute gastric dilatation almost invariably accompanies severe trauma and may exacerbate respiratory failure. Emergency decompression of the stomach with a wide-bore nasogastric tube will often improve cardiorespiratory function and reduce the risk of aspiration.

High spinal cord injuries may be difficult to detect in the presence of severe brain injury, and should be suspected in any patient with flaccidity, apnoea or paradoxical respiration (see Chapter 36).

BURNS

With more effective control of burn wound sepsis, respiratory complications are now the major cause of mortality in children who are burnt. Respiratory failure may be due to a number of factors. Local burns cause upper airway obstruction. Small airway obstruction may result from oedema and the inhaled products of combustion. Other causes include chemical pneumonitis, carbon monoxide poisoning, fluid overload with pulmonary oedema, and secondary infection.

Adult respiratory distress syndrome

Despite the name, adult respiratory distress syndrome (ARDS) may occur in children of all ages in response to a variety of lung insults. ARDS is characterized by respiratory distress or failure, diffuse pulmonary infiltrates, reduced pulmonary compliance and hypoxaemia, in the presence of a known precipitating cause. In children, the common causes include shock from any cause, pneumonia with septicaemia, near drowning, aspiration and pulmonary contusion.

The underlying pathology consists of 'non-cardiogenic pulmonary oedema' and an inflammatory response in the lung. Complement activation and leucocyte sequestration in the lung with mediator release are believed to be central to the pathogenesis.

Pulmonary compression

Pneumothorax, pleural effusions and empyema compress the lungs and require drainage to allow the lungs to expand. The principles are similar to those described in the neonatal section.

Neuromuscular disease — neurological causes (see Chapters 25 and 36)

POISONING

Poisoning resulting in respiratory insufficiency in children may be caused by accidental ingestion of drugs that depress respiration or decrease the activity of respiratory muscles. In older children, suicidal overdoses are sometimes taken. Tricyclic antidepressants, antihistamines, anticonvulsants and benzodiazepines are the commonest central nervous system depressant drugs ingested. Iatrogenic overdosage, particularly with opiates, occasionally occurs in hospital.

Convulsions and the therapy required for their control may enhance the central depression.

MENINGITIS AND ENCEPHALITIS

Meningitis is common in the early years of life. After the neonatal period, the usual causative organisms are *Haemophilus influenzae*, *Neisseria meningitidis*, and *Streptococcus pneumoniae*. Rapid diagnosis and appropriate antibiotic therapy form the cornerstone of treatment. Respiratory failure is mainly associated with uncontrolled convulsions or raised intracranial pressure.

Encephalitis may cause unconsciousness and raised intracranial pressure. Associated problems are upper airway obstruction, pulmonary aspiration and central respiratory depression. Encephalitis is usually viral in origin and may be complicated by hyperpyrexia, convulsions and cerebral oedema. Herpes encephalitis is uncommon, but important in that effective antiviral therapy is available. Acyclovir should be administered early if viral encephalitis is considered likely (see Chapter 36).

GUILLAIN−BARRÉ SYNDROME

Guillain−Barré syndrome is the most common cause of acute polyneuritis in infancy and childhood. The duration of onset is variable but may be rapid, with respiratory failure occurring within 48 hours. Respiratory failure may be due to weakness of the respiratory muscles or bulbar palsy with impaired cough reflex and aspiration of saliva, food or gastric contents.

The need for assisted ventilation is based on clinical assessment that the cough reflex and bulbar function are depressed, measured vital capacity of less than 15 ml/kg and evidence of hypoxaemia (oxygen saturation less than 90%). Elevated $Paco_2$ is a late feature, when the vital capacity is in the tidal range, i.e. less than 5−7 ml/kg. The condition may be improved by the early use of plasmapheresis (see Chapter 38) or intravenous immunoglobulin therapy [14, 15]. A tracheostomy is advised if the use of mechanical ventilation or an artificial airway is likely to be prolonged (see Chapter 36).

STATUS EPILEPTICUS

Seizures in children commonly occur with fever, idiopathic epilepsy, central nervous system infection, poisoning, trauma and other metabolic disturbances, such as hypoglycaemia and hypocalcaemia. Respiratory failure with generalized seizures may be due to airway obstruction, aspiration, apnoea or respiratory depression. During grand mal seizures, ventilation may be inadequate and oxygen consumption and carbon dioxide production may be increased by the associated muscle activity. It must be remembered that anticonvulsant drugs used to control seizures may further depress respiration.

Oxygen should be administered during seizures because cerebral and total body oxygen consumption are increased and it is difficult to assess the ventilation. If there is any doubt about the adequacy of ventilation and oxygenation during status epilepticus, the child can be paralysed and ventilated, as well as being given anticonvulsant drugs (see Chapter 36).

ENVENOMATION

Some animal venoms, such as those of some snakes, ticks and the blue ringed octopus, are neurotoxic and may cause muscle weakness and respiratory insufficiency.

The Sydney funnel-web spider causes widespread acetylcholine release and symptoms similar to poisoning with the anticholinesterases, malathion and parathion. These symptoms include intense salivation, lacrimation, sweating, laryngeal and muscle spasm and pulmonary oedema.

Paralysis due to tetrodotoxin may rapidly follow puffer-fish ingestion.

In Australia and many other countries, specific anti-venom therapy is available for most potentially lethal envenomations. Supportive therapy is required until anti-venom is administered and recovery occurs [16].

REFERENCES

1 Stocks J.G. The management of respiratory failure in infancy. *Anaes Intens Care* 1973, **1**, 486–506.
2 Keens T.G., Bryan A.C., Levison H., Ianuzzo C.D. Developmental pattern of muscle fibre types in human ventilatory muscles. *J Appl Physiol: Respirat Environ Exercise Physiol* 1978, **44**, 909–913.
3 Heaf D.P., Helms P.J., Dinwiddie M.B., Mathew D.J. Nasopharyngeal airways in Pierre Robin syndrome. *J Pediatr* 1982, **100**, 698–703.
4 Tanaka K., Inomata Y., Utsunomiya H., Uemoto S., Asonuma K., Katayama T., Ozawa K., Hasida M. Sclerosing therapy with bleomycin emulsion for lymphangioma in children. *Pediatr Surg Int* 1990, **5**, 270–273.
5 O'Rourke P.P., Crone R.K., Vacanti J.P., Ware J.H., Lillehei C.W., Parad R.B., Epstein M.F. Extracorporeal membrane oxygenation and conventional medical therapy in neonates with persistent pulmonary hypertension of the newborn: a prospective randomized study. *Pediatrics* 1989, 84, 957–963.
6 Lynn A.M., Jenkins J.G., Edmonds J.F., Burns J.E. Diaphragmatic paralysis after pediatric cardiac surgery: a retrospective analysis of 34 cases. *Crit Care Med* 1982, **11**, 280–282.
7 Fletcher J., Shann F., Duncan A. The dangers of premature extubation after severe birth asphyxia. *Aust Paediatr J* 1987, **23**, 27–29.
8 Koren G., Frand M., Barzilay Z., Maclean S.M. Corticosteroid treatment of laryngotracheitis vs. spasmodic croup in children. *Am J Dis Child* 1983, **137**, 941–944.
9 Super D.M., Cartelli N.A., Brooks L.J., Lembo R.M., Kumar M.L. A prospective randomized double-blind study to evaluate the effect of dexamethasone in acute laryngotracheitis. *J Pediatr* 1989, **115**, 323–329.
10 Freezer N., Butt W., Phelan P. Steroids in croup: do they increase the incidence of successful extubation. *Anaes Intens Care* 1990, **18**, 224–228.
11 Butt W., Shann F., Walker C., Williams J., Duncan A., Phelan P. Acute epiglottitis: a different approach to management. *Crit Care Med* 1988, **16**, 43–47.
12 Kissoon N., Mitchell I. Adverse effects of racemic epinephrine in epiglottitis. *Pediatr Emerg Care* 1985, **1**, 143–144.
13 Beasley J.M., Jones S.E.F. Continuous positive airway pressure in bronchiolitis. *Br Med J* 1981, **283**, 1506–1508.
14 Yoshioka M., Kuroki S., Mizue H. Plasmapheresis in the treatment of the Guillain–Barré syndrome in childhood. *Pediatr Neurol* 1985, **1**, 329–334.
15 Shahar E., Murphy E.G., Roifman C.M. Benefit of intravenously administered serum globulin in patients with Guillain–Barré syndrome. *J Pediatr* 1990, **116**, 141–144.
16 Sutherland S.K. *Australian animal toxins.* Oxford University Press, Melbourne, (1983).

FURTHER READING

Rogers M.C. *Textbook of pediatric intensive care*, vol. 1. Williams and Wilkins, Baltimore, (1987) Chapters 4–10.
Gregory G.A. *Respiratory failure in the child.* Clinics in Critical Care Medicine, Churchill Livingstone, New York, (1981).
Phelan P., Landau L.I., Olinsky A. *Respiratory illness in children* (3rd edn). Blackwell Scientific Publications, Oxford, (1990).

33: Management of Acute Respiratory Failure

INTRODUCTION

The object in the management of acute respiratory failure is to provide support that allows the time needed for specific therapy to take effect or for the underlying disease to resolve. The general principles are common to all conditions, and involve the provision of an adequate airway and maintainance of oxygenation and ventilation. Specific therapies for individual conditions are outlined in Chapter 32.

Children with acute respiratory failure are best managed in an intensive care unit. Apart from brief, treatable episodes they should be transferred, where possible, to a specialized paediatric intensive care unit that is designed to cope with the special physical, psychological and equipment requirements of the child and the needs of the family. Prolonged care of children in adult intensive care units is undesirable.

Emergency transport services have been developed in many paediatric centres. These extend the facilities of a children's intensive care unit to general hospitals and remote locations and enable the safe retrieval of critically ill patients [1]. The effectiveness of such services depends on the skill and experience of the medical and nursing staff. Up to 40% of transfers may involve upper airway obstruction; most others involve actual or potential respiratory failure. Retrieval staff must be skilled in handling paediatric emergencies and be able to provide safe anaesthesia. Special equipment for advanced paediatric life support must be carried.

GENERAL MANAGEMENT

Oxygen therapy

METHODS

The flow rates provided by conventional oxygen delivery systems approximate or exceed the peak inspiratory flow rates of most infants and small children. Thus it is possible to attain high inspired oxygen concentration (FiO_2). Despite this advantage it is difficult to apply continuous oxygen therapy to the restless, hypoxic and mobile young child.

In the newborn period and during infancy, it is possible to nurse the whole body or the head and neck in a high oxygen concentration. Incubators are used as a means of delivering oxygen and providing a neutral thermal environment. Although it is possible to obtain inspired oxygen concentrations as high as 85%, the need for this is usually an indication for other methods of oxygen delivery, or techniques such as continuous positive airway pressure (CPAP) and mechanical ventilation. The major problems are the high oxygen flow rates, difficult access to the patient and the long time taken for the concentration to build up again after opening the incubator.

Oxygen is often administered to the newborn and infants by a head box which encases the patient's head and neck (Fig. 33.1). It is common practice to use such a box within an incubator when high FiO_2 is required. The oxygen concentration delivered depends on the flow rate, the volume of the box, the size of the leak around the neck, the position of the head in the box and frequency of opening. An oxygen concentration of 100% can be achieved, but the concentration falls rapidly on removal of the lid. The time taken for the concentration to be restored after opening depends on the oxygen flow rate and the volume of the head box. Rebreathing may occur with low flow rates and a close seal around the neck. Mixtures of air and oxygen should be added to the box at high flows to flush CO_2 from the system and to shorten the recovery time after opening. It is essential to monitor oxygen concentration at a point close to the face.

Nasal catheters will deliver continuous oxygen therapy

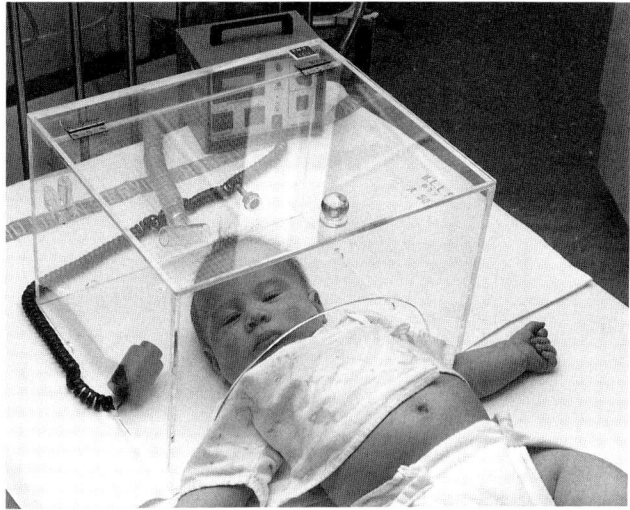

Fig. 33.1 Infant in an oxygen headbox; the oxygen sensor is close to the face.

to infants and small children, and allow them to feed at the same time. A single catheter in the postnasal space, taped to the side of the face, is often well tolerated (Fig. 33.2). When a nasogastric tube is in place, the oxygen catheter should be placed in the same nostril, to avoid complete nasal blockage and increased airway resistance. The nasopharynx acts as an oxygen reservoir and is loaded with oxygen for the next breath during the expiratory pause. Oxygen enrichment is provided with both nose and mouth breathing. The inspired oxygen concentration varies both during and between breaths, depending on the rate and depth of breathing, the length of the expiratory pause, body size and metabolic rate. A flow rate of 150 ml/kg/min provides an inspired oxygen concentration of about 50% in children under 2 years of age [2]. High oxygen flow rates may lead to discomfort and drying of the nasal mucosa. For prolonged therapy, heated humidification should be added.

Older children will tolerate face masks. Face masks, however, make the control of oxygen concentration and its measurement difficult; they are often dislodged, leading to intermittent therapy.

Larger children can be nursed in oxygen tents or cots, although it is difficult to achieve an oxygen concentration above 40%. The concentration falls rapidly when the tent is opened and rises slowly when closed. As access and observation are very restricted and the environment may be frightening to children, tents are now not often used.

Oxygen therapy can be accurately controlled and

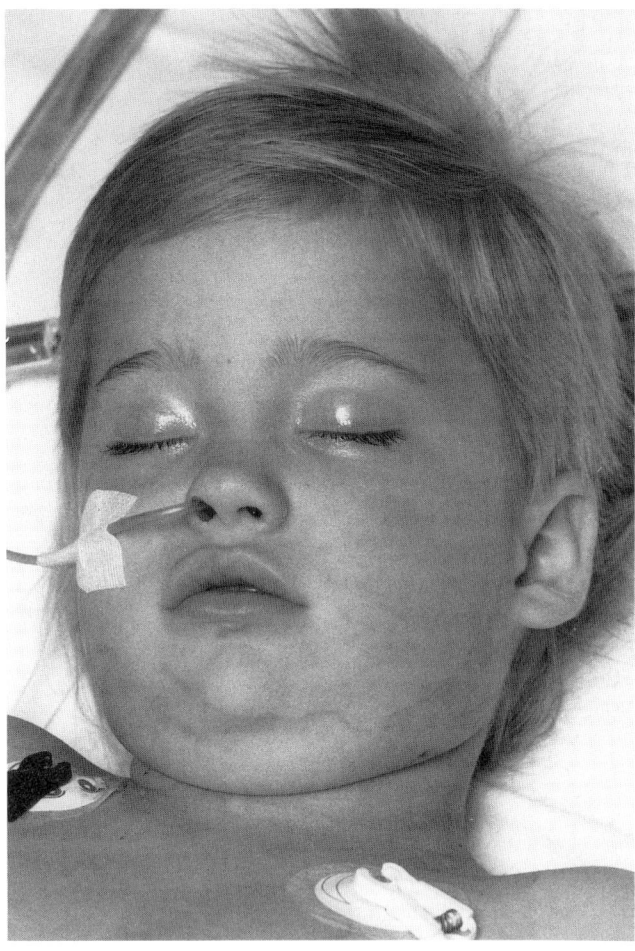

Fig. 33.2 Intranasal oxygen therapy with a single nasal catheter in the postnasal space.

monitored when delivered via an endotracheal or a tracheostomy tube.

The concentration of oxygen required must be carefully titrated, depending on the underlying disease. All patients having prolonged oxygen therapy require measurement of blood oxygen saturation or tension. Any handling of the patient, during transport, diagnostic imaging, insertion of vascular cannulae and other procedures, can cause hypoxia; the inspired oxygen concentration may need to be increased during these procedures.

COMPLICATIONS

Retinopathy of prematurity

This condition, also called retrolental fibroplasia, is mostly seen in premature infants exposed to increased arterial oxygen tension before 36 weeks' gestational age, when retinal vessels are susceptible to vasoconstriction.

Visual impairment is due to fibroproliferative changes in the retina, or to the subsequent retinal detachment. Neither the safe level nor the duration of increased retinal artery Po_2 associated with the retinopathy have been identified.

Retinopathy has been reported in premature infants who have not been given oxygen therapy. Pao_2 should be maintained between 50 and 80 mmHg (6.6–10.6 kPa), by careful adjustment of the inspired oxygen concentration.

Pulmonary oxygen toxicity

Prolonged exposure to high oxygen concentration (greater than 40%) causes pulmonary damage. Oxygen toxicity is characterized by hypertrophy of the pulmonary vasculature and fibroproliferative changes in the lung parenchyma. These changes are not specific to oxygen toxicity but are also seen in circumstances that lead to adult respiratory distress syndrome. Exposure of normal lungs for many days to concentrations below 40% does not appear to cause harm, but diseased lungs may be more susceptible.

Bronchopulmonary dysplasia

This condition complicates severe hyaline membrane disease in the premature infant. It is characterized by focal air trapping, cyst formation and fibrosis, and is accompanied by hypoxaemia and carbon dioxide retention. Lung immaturity and barotrauma from mechanical ventilation are thought to be the major aetiological factors; pulmonary oxygen toxicity is believed to contribute. Some infants remain in chronic respiratory failure, requiring home oxygen therapy; rarely, there is progression to cor pulmonale and death in the first 2 years of life.

Similar pathology may develop in very low-birthweight premature infants given oxygen therapy without mechanical ventilation. The condition, known as Mikity–Wilson syndrome, progresses over the first few weeks of life before undergoing gradual resolution.

It is important to remember that hypoxia is common, and its effects on the brain, heart and kidneys may be serious and permanent. Pulmonary oxygen toxicity is relatively uncommon, its development takes days or even weeks and its effects are often reversible. Fear of oxygen toxicity must never be allowed to militate against the need to treat hypoxaemia.

Fluid therapy

Oral feeding should be suspended when dyspnoea is severe, as absorption is impaired and there is a danger of vomiting, regurgitation and aspiration. In infants, feeding may also result in abdominal distension, interfering with descent of the diaphragm and further impairing respiratory function. Even uncomplicated feeding may be associated with increased hypoxia.

An intravenous infusion must be established, to enable fluid, electrolytes and calories to be given, dehydration, metabolic acidosis or hypoglycaemia to be corrected and essential drug therapy to be administered, with minimal disturbance of the child.

Lung disease is often associated with increased secretion of antidiuretic hormone (ADH), leading to fluid retention. Increased airway pressure (continuous positive airway pressure, mechanical ventilation) may also increase ADH secretion. The efficient use of humidification with an endotracheal or tracheostomy tube prevents insensible loss from the airway and diminishes fluid requirements. Most patients with acute lung disease benefit from some degree of fluid restriction. Fluid balance and biochemical status must be monitored carefully. In prolonged respiratory failure, it is essential to minimize wasting of the respiratory muscles and to provide energy for increased work of breathing. High calorie oral or nasogastric feeding may be employed. In some cases, parenteral nutrition is indicated, especially when fluids need to be restricted.

General nursing care

Skilled one-to-one nursing is vital in the care of the infant or child with acute respiratory failure. Such care may minimize respiratory distress, ensure safety of the therapy used, warn of further deterioration and provide support for the child and family. The importance of this aspect of management cannot be over-stressed. It is a major difference between general and paediatric intensive care units.

THE NURSING ENVIRONMENT

Maintenance of body temperature is of major importance in the seriously ill neonate. The immature newborn is particularly vulnerable to cold stress, which increases metabolism, rapidly depletes carbohydrate stores and may result in cardiorespiratory deterioration. In a normal newborn, oxygen consumption may rise three-fold on exposure to moderate environmental temperatures of 20–25°C, which are below the thermoneutral range (see Chapter 1). Conditions are optimal when the abdominal skin temperature is 36–36.5°C.

The most satisfactory appliances to maintain temperature homeostasis are servo-controlled infrared-heated open cots. These devices allow excellent conditions for observation of and access to the exposed infant, without the danger of cold stress. Insensible loss is increased under radiant heaters, especially in the premature infant; this must be taken into account when determining fluid requirements.

In an incubator, the environmental temperature is less stable, especially when procedures must be performed on the infant. Access to the patient is difficult. Double-glazed incubators reduce radiant heat loss.

Older infants and children can be nursed in standard cots and beds. It is important that the room is air-conditioned and free from draughts, so that oxygen consumption is not increased by shivering.

POSTURE

Neonates are best nursed prone with the hips and knees flexed and the head turned regularly. This posture may reduce or even abolish apnoeic episodes in premature infants. It also decreases gastric emptying time and makes aspiration of vomitus less likely. However, if the clinical state is unstable and especially if bag and mask ventilation or other intervention is likely, the supine position is preferred.

Older infants and young children are usually nursed in the position they find most comfortable. Provided cardiovascular function is stable, the semi-upright posture is encouraged, because of improved respiratory function and less interference with diaphragmatic excursion when compared with the supine position.

Physiotherapy

In infants, gentle pharyngeal suction performed at intervals (e.g. half-hourly) not only removes secretions that tend to pool in the pharynx, but also stimulates coughing and the expulsion of tracheobronchial secretions. This is also useful in patients with altered conscious state and impairment of bulbar function. Pharyngeal suction may avert the necessity for intubation to remove retained secretions.

The role of conventional physiotherapy with posturing, percussion and vibration in older infants and children in the paediatric intensive care setting, is unproven. It is most likely to be of value with suppurative lung and airway disease. Physiotherapy may cause a significant fall in Pao_2; inspired oxygen concentration should be increased beforehand. Physiotherapy must be used with caution in patients with cardiovascular instability or raised intracranial pressure.

Procedures

Handling should be gentle and procedures performed as rapidly as possible, with a minimum of disturbance. Appropriate analgesic and sedative techniques should be used to minimize stress. Physical upsets may induce bouts of crying or restlessness that lead to increased oxygen consumption and possible deterioration. Intra-cardiac right-to-left shunting may be precipitated. Particular care is necessary to ensure that oxygen therapy is maintained or even increased during such interference.

ASSESSMENT

Clinical

Once the patient has been stabilized, the most important part of continuing management is usually skilled observation and assessment by experienced medical and nursing staff. A very seriously ill child may require one-to-one medical and nursing attention for some hours.

Observation is particularly directed to the presence, degree and progression of the following signs:

1 Evidence of hypoxia, such as central cyanosis and restlessness.
2 Increased work of breathing appearing as tachypnoea and intercostal, suprasternal or subcostal retraction.
3 Inadequate tidal exchange with a weak cough or cry, inability to speak, reduced air entry on auscultation and laboured inspiration.
4 Circulatory embarrassment with tachycardia or bradycardia, hypotension, pallor and poor peripheral perfusion.

Progression of the illness may lead to fatigue, with slowing of the respiratory rate, apnoeic episodes and general lethargy. Any evidence of deterioration must be recorded, reported and acted upon. It may be due to progress of the disease or to an intercurrent complication. Common complications include pneumothorax, lobar collapse, vomiting with aspiration, and accidental reduction in inspired oxygen concentration.

Monitoring

PULSE OXIMETRY

Pulse oximetry represents a major advance in monitoring. It provides continuous non-invasive measurement of arteriolar oxygen saturation and rapidly indicates hypoxaemia. Useful information is given even in adverse clinical situations such as:

1 when the oxyhaemoglobin dissociation curve is shifted to the left (fetal haemoglobin or alkalosis) or to the right (sickle haemoglobin or acidosis);
2 in the presence of carboxyhaemoglobin where the functional saturation of haemoglobin is accurate;
3 with severe desaturation, as in cyanotic heart disease;
4 with anaemia (down to a haemoglobin of approximately 5 g/dl);
5 with skin pigmentation.

Errors occur with extreme hypoperfusion, excessive movement and with rapidly changing ambient light. Movement artefact is reduced with pulse oximeters that incorporate ECG tracking. A range of sensors is now available for monitoring children of all ages.

TRANSCUTANEOUS Po_2 AND Pco_2 MONITORING

Oxygen and carbon dioxide diffuse through well-perfused skin from the superficial capillary network, and can be measured using modified polarographic and glass electrodes respectively. The electrodes are heated to $43-45°C$ to increase capillary flow and 'arterialize' the capillary blood. Under optimal conditions, there is good correlation between arterial and transcutaneous gas tensions. Continuous monitoring of blood gas tensions is therefore possible, using this non-invasive technique. The transcutaneous-to-arterial tension gradient is widened when peripheral perfusion is poor. These devices are not reliable outside the neonatal period. Unlike pulse oximetry, the electrodes need frequent recalibration. Skin burns can occur and electrodes should therefore be moved every few hours.

OTHER CARDIORESPIRATORY MONITORS

Electronic monitors should be used to warn of alterations in heart rate, blood pressure, respiratory rate and apnoeic spells in all patients with respiratory failure, but they are no substitute for close and skilled nursing observation. Their major virtue lies in the immediate indication of alarm when unexpected complications occur, so that appropriate action may be taken.

Measurement of blood gases and acid—base status is an essential part of cardiorespiratory assessment in the critically ill.

Arterial blood may be obtained either from an indwelling arterial cannula or by direct puncture of peripheral arteries. The latter may be distressing to the child and time-consuming; the results from difficult collections may not accurately reflect the blood gas status in the stable state. Topical anaesthesia using EMLA cream should be considered for non-urgent percutaneous sampling.

Peripheral arterial cannulation is routine practice in paediatric intensive care, even in infants weighing less than 1 kg. It allows continuous blood pressure monitoring and reduces sampling errors.

Umbilical arterial catheters may be used in the newborn period, but are best avoided because of vaso-occlusive complications such as lower limb ischaemia, renal artery thrombosis, necrotizing enterocolitis and paraplegia.

The radial, ulnar, brachial, femoral, posterior tibial and dorsalis pedis arteries are suitable for cannulation. Radial and ulnar or posterior tibial and dorsalis pedis vessels must not be cannulated in the same limb, even at different times, because of the danger of distal limb ischaemia if blood flow through both is reduced. The safety of brachial and femoral cannulation lies in the collateral vessels around the elbow and hip joints. The complications of arterial cannulation include distal ischaemia, infection, haemorrhage and retrograde embolization when the cannula is flushed.

The patency of arterial cannulae is maintained by continuous flushing with heparinized saline or dextrose solutions. Cannulation by cut-down should be considered when the percutaneous method fails. In the neonate with acute respiratory failure, a preductal vessel, such as the right radial artery, should be used. Preductal sampling is important, because it indicates the Pa_{O_2} of blood perfusing the retina.

Knowledge of the inspired oxygen concentration is essential for interpretation of information from all forms of oxygen monitoring.

The measurement of end-tidal CO_2 in the intubated patient provides a continuous guide to the adequacy of alveolar ventilation. In the presence of severe lung disease, the absolute value fails to reflect arterial P_{CO_2} due to the wide alveolar—arterial gradient. The instrument may still provide valuable trend information and is useful to detect sudden reductions in cardiac output.

Serial chest X-rays are an important part of continuing assessment of infants and children with respiratory failure. Supine anteroposterior X-rays usually provide the necessary information; lateral or lateral decubitus (A-P, lying on the side) views may be useful to localize pathology in the lungs, or to confirm the presence of air or fluid collections. Particular attention should be paid to the presence of focal or general lung disease, signs of air leak, the size and shape of the cardiac contour, and the position of the endotracheal tube and vascular catheters.

Multiple chest X-rays may be required in rapidly changing clinical situations. To aid interpretation, an attempt should be made to standardize the technique of chest X-ray examination in a given patient.

EMERGENCY MANAGEMENT

A proportion of patients will present with severe asphyxia or with respiratory or cardiac arrest due to rapid progress of the illness, the occurrence of complications or late referral. Management should be directed towards restoration of adequate pulmonary ventilation and oxygenation, restoration of the circulation and treatment of the cause and complications.

Restoration of ventilation

The airway should be cleared by posture and suction if necessary. Oxygen is initially administered by bag and mask, but this method of ventilating infants may be difficult for inexperienced hands. The head should not be hyperextended as this may cause airway obstruction. The mask should be held carefully on the face. When the mandible is drawn forward to maintain the airway, care must be taken to avoid pressure on the tongue, forcing it back into the pharynx (see Fig. 7.9). Once oxygenation has been achieved, the trachea may be intubated. In acute situations, it is preferable to pass an oral tube first, to oxygenate the child. When conditions are more stable, one can change to a nasotracheal tube. Ventilation is then assisted or controlled as necessary.

Special measures may be appropriate for some forms of supraglottic obstruction. In choanal atresia, an oral airway or wide-bore orogastric tube may be fixed in position until surgery relieves the nasal obstruction. The passage of a nasopharyngeal tube will relieve the obstruction in Pierre Robin syndrome and other lesions such as adenotonsillar hypertrophy.

In some children, inflation of the lungs with a mask may be impossible and intubation is the first step, possibly without the use of drugs. If time permits and upper airway tone is present, the patient should be anaesthetized before intubation. Inhalation anaesthesia is preferred for most cases of upper airway obstruction. In other situations, emergency rapid-sequence induction and intubation can be used.

Treatment of complications

METABOLIC ACIDOSIS

In the presence of severe tissue hypoxia, metabolic acidosis develops rapidly and should be presumed to be present in the absence of blood gas determination. Sodium bicarbonate (2 mmol/kg) may be given empirically and additional doses can be based on acid–base analysis. It should be given slowly, especially in neonates, because of the high osmolality of the solutions (8.4% = 1 mmol/ml). Additional carbon dioxide is produced by the buffering action of sodium bicarbonate.

CARDIAC ARREST — see Chapter 35

ACTIVE MANAGEMENT

Depending on the underlying cause, ventilation may be improved by the provision of an artificial airway alone, application of CPAP, or intermittent positive pressure ventilation (IPPV) and its variants. Definitive therapy, such as tube thoracostomy for pneumothorax, reversal of muscle relaxant effect or reversal of narcotic overdosage, may occasionally avert the need for assistance.

The use of IPPV increases the complexity of management and the need for nursing surveillance and monitoring.

Indications

Mechanical ventilation may be used in acute and chronic respiratory failure and for other reasons listed in Table 33.1 [3]. The decision to ventilate a patient with respiratory failure is based on a knowledge of the natural history of the disease and an assessment of the severity of the disturbance in each patient. Clinical estimation of the degree of respiratory insufficiency is based on the following factors: colour, respiratory rate, nasal flaring, expiratory grunting, use of accessory muscles, intercostal, suprasternal and subcostal retraction, air entry, cardiovascular stability, mental alertness, arterial blood gas tensions and acid–base balance.

It is generally agreed that a Pao_2 of 60 mmHg (8.0 kPa) with the patient breathing 100% oxygen or a $Paco_2$ of 60 mmHg (8.0 kPa) and rising, combined with clinical signs of respiratory failure, require close observation, if not immediate intervention.

The rate of change in a child's condition will also influence the decision to intervene. Concurrent disease such as congenital heart disease, and technical difficulties anticipated with some conditions, such as asthma and bronchiolitis, may alter the threshold for intervention.

Table 33.1 Indications for mechanical ventilation [3]

1 To maintain gas exchange in acute and chronic respiratory failure

2 During general anaesthesia:
  (a) to ventilate when muscle relaxants are used
    (i) when muscle relaxation is needed
    (ii) to permit light, balanced anaesthesia
  (b) when ventilation is needed for thoracotomy, craniotomy, etc.

3 To increase CO_2 excretion:
  (a) to reduce $Paco_2$ in order
    (i) to achieve normal ECF [H^+] in metabolic acidosis
    (ii) to cause cerebral vasoconstriction
    (iii) to restore cerebrovascular autoregulation
    (iv) to reduce pulmonary vascular resistance
  (b) when CO_2 production is increased

4 To reduce work of breathing in cardiorespiratory failure

5 To reduce afterload on a failing left ventricle, by increasing intrathoracic pressure and so reducing end-diastolic wall tension

6 Prophylactically (with or without PEEP), to avoid complications after major surgery

7 To splint a flail chest internally

Some children require ventilation when signs of fatigue appear, regardless of results of blood gas analysis.

Some general principles can be stated, depending on the cause of the respiratory failure.

UPPER AIRWAY OBSTRUCTION

Such patients usually present with increasing respiratory distress without blood gas abnormalities. At the stage where an artificial airway is considered, the child is restless, anxious, pale, often sweating and has tachycardia. The blood gases may be almost normal. This is not true of neonates and young infants, who often have falling Pao_2 and rising $Paco_2$; restlessness may not be seen. Pulse oximetry is useful in monitoring these children.

In the neonate, blood gas determination may be of value in deciding when to intervene, but in older infants and children such determinations are not only misleading but potentially dangerous if the sampling technique distresses the child, increasing oxygen consumption.

Children with lesions above the larynx often present with intermittent obstruction and cyanotic attacks. If these attacks cannot otherwise be prevented, an artificial airway is needed.

LOWER AIRWAY OBSTRUCTION

The indications for mechanical assistance are mainly clinical. If the clinical state is deteriorating despite maximal oxygen and drug therapy, intervention is necessary. Warning signs include disturbed conscious state, cyanosis with high inspired oxygen concentration, increasing tachycardia, tachypnoea, falling respiratory rate or ineffective respiratory effort, indicated by decreased intensity of wheezing and decreased breath sounds.

Arterial blood gas estimation should complement clinical observation. There is no absolute level of $Paco_2$ that indicates the need for mechanical ventilation. Hypocapnia is a common finding in the early phase of an asthmatic attack; an increase to the normal range may be evidence of fatigue and cause for concern. $Paco_2$ more than 90 mmHg (12.0 kPa) for short periods may be associated with recovery without the need for mechanical ventilation, but a progressively rising $Paco_2$ with deteriorating clinical status is an indication to intervene.

PULMONARY DISEASE

The indications for assistance depend on clinical observation and/or trends in arterial blood gas tensions.

Survival without assistance is unlikely if, when breathing 100% oxygen, there is considerable respiratory distress associated with central cyanosis or Pao_2 less than 60 mmHg (8.0 kPa) and persistent respiratory acidosis resulting in a pH of less than 7.25; these are therefore logical indications for assistance. In neonates and infants, intervention is necessary if severe respiratory distress is associated with more than one or two apnoeic episodes that do not respond rapidly to bag and mask inflation.

The use of CPAP in the management of hyaline membrane disease reduces oxygen requirements, shortens the duration of oxygen therapy, hastens resolution of the disease and reduces morbidity and mortality. Early introduction of CPAP is now recommended. A Pao_2 less than 60 mmHg (8.0 kPa) in 60% oxygen is used in many centres as the indication for CPAP. In extremely low-birth-weight infants with rapid disease progression, earlier intervention is advised; many of these infants will need intermittent mandatory ventilation (IMV) at this stage.

NEUROLOGICAL DISEASE

Premature infants who develop apnoeic episodes that do not respond rapidly to tactile stimulation should be ventilated by bag and mask, with the same concentration of oxygen as the atmosphere in which the infant is nursed between episodes. If these episodes persist, theophylline therapy may be tried (see Chapter 32). If they are severe or recurrent, CPAP or IMV should be used.

Children with meningitis, encephalitis and head injuries should be ventilated if there is evidence of hypoventilation or clinical signs of raised intracranial pressure. A rising $Paco_2$ will increase cerebral blood volume and intracranial pressure making permanent damage or death more likely. Raised intracranial pressure should be suspected with any or all of the following signs: deep coma, inability to protect the airway, head retraction or other abnormal posturing, unilateral or bilateral pupillary dilatation, loss of light reflex, respiratory embarrassment, bradycardia and hypertension. Other indications for mechanical ventilation in head injury include persistent seizures, severe extensor rigidity and extreme hyperventilation.

In peripheral neuromuscular disease, weak or absent cough and gag reflex, difficulty swallowing saliva, oxygen desaturation and hypoventilation, are all indications for intervention. Vital capacity <15 ml/kg, peak expiratory flow <25% predicted and maximum subatmospheric inspiratory force <25 cmH$_2$O (2.5 kPa) usually indicate the need for an artificial airway, if not mechanical ventilation.

Postoperative assistance

A number of factors must be taken into account after major operations. These include the effects of surgery itself, blood loss and adequacy of replacement, acidosis, accidental hypothermia, residual effects of anaesthetic agents, especially muscle relaxants, and the impact of postoperative pain. After major cardiac and thoracic surgery, acute respiratory failure may be avoided by a period of mechanical ventilation until the child's condition is stable. Controlled ventilation removes the work of breathing and is important for myocardial support after open heart surgery.

INTUBATION

A correctly placed endotracheal tube with an adequate internal diameter will overcome upper respiratory tract obstruction, protect the airway, allow direct access for tracheal suction and enable modification of airway pressure. It does this at the cost of considerable narrowing of the airway, bypassing of the humidifying, heating and filtering mechanisms of the upper respiratory tract and, because closure of the glottis is impossible, preventing effective coughing and grunting. Impaired cough renders the patient more dependent on regular suction, whilst grunting is a protective mechanism which minimizes alveolar collapse.

Technique

Ideally, an oral endotracheal tube is used at first. Insertion is easier and quicker than nasotracheal intubation and allows ready assessment of the airway and the size of nasotracheal tube to be used. Once adequate oxygenation, ventilation and removal of secretions have been achieved, the oral tube is replaced by a nasal one.

The tube may be inserted without the use of drugs in very ill neonates and in other dire emergency situations. Sedation or anaesthesia, however, can prevent rises in anterior fontanelle pressure that may be associated with intracranial haemorrhage in low-birth-weight infants. Unless they are comatose or profoundly ill, older infants and children usually require general anaesthesia for intubation.

In the presence of upper airway obstruction, inhalation anaesthesia, such as halothane in oxygen with CPAP or assisted ventilation, is usually preferred to the use of muscle relaxants. A high Pao_2 is easier to achieve and maintain, and there is less danger of being unable to ventilate the patient if intubation is difficult. Short-acting muscle relaxants may be used when the ability to intubate and ventilate can be relied upon, as when changing to a nasal tube after oral intubation.

Suxamethonium increases the risk of dysrhythmia, bradycardia and cardiac arrest, especially in the presence of hypoxia or hypercarbia; atropine should be used to prevent these.

The choice of endotracheal tube is important; guidelines for selection and positioning of endotracheal tubes are included in Table 33.2 [4]. The tube selected must be large enough to provide an adequate airway, but not so large that the subglottic mucous membrane is compressed, leading to oedema or stenosis. The normal criterion for selection of a tube is that it should allow a small leak of gas from the larynx when the lungs are inflated with a pressure of 25 cmH$_2$O (2.5 kPa).

There are exceptions to this rule. In neonates a gas-tight tube may be used, provided that it passes easily, since, for reasons not understood, subglottic complications are rare at this age. Subglottic stenosis in the neonate correlates mainly with the number of re-intubations and the duration of intubation; its incidence can be reduced by skilful insertion, good fixation technique and careful nursing care.

A 3.0 mm tube may be used in almost all neonates weighing more than 1000 g. It may be important not to have a large air leak around the tube during mechanical ventilation in order to maintain mean airway pressure and oxygenation, especially when lung compliance is low.

In older children, extremely stiff lungs or high airway resistance, as occurs in severe asthma, may need a leak-free tube to ensure adequate ventilation. In cases of respiratory obstruction such as laryngotracheobronchitis, a leak-free tube may be used provided it is the smallest tube that will provide an adequate airway.

It is essential that the tube be positioned correctly with

Table 33.2 Choice and positioning of endotracheal tube [4]

Age	Wt (kg)	Int dia (mm)	Ext dia (mm)*	At lip (cm)†	At nose (cm)†	Sucker (FG)
Newborn	<1	2.5	3.4	5.5	7	6
Newborn	1.0	3.0	4.2	6	7.5	7
Newborn	2.0	3.0	4.2	7	9	7
Newborn	3.0	3.0	4.2	8.5	10.5	7
Newborn	3.5	3.5	4.8	9	11	8
3 months	6.0	3.5	4.8	10	12	8
1 year	10	4.0	5.4	11	14	8
2 years	12	4.5	6.2	12	15	8
3 years	14	4.5	6.2	13	16	8
4 years	16	5.0	6.8	14	17	10
6 years	20	5.5	7.4	15	19	10
8 years	24	6.0	8.2	16	20	10
10 years	30	6.5	8.8	17	21	12
12 years	38	7.0	9.6	18	22	12
14 years	50	7.5	10.2	19	23	12
Adult	60	8.0	11.0	20	24	12
Adult	70	9.0	12.2	21	25	12

* External diameter of Portex tubes.
† Average length to mid-trachea.

the end in mid-trachea. If the end is too low, bronchial intubation may occur, while if too high, accidental extubation is more likely. In the term neonate, the change from extension to flexion of the neck may advance the tube by 2 cm. Head position should be noted when interpreting endotracheal tube position on the chest X-ray.

It is useful to note that from 1–8 years of age, the length of a nasal tube can be estimated by the formula: age in years plus 13 cm. A guide to the length of oral and nasal endotracheal tubes is provided in Table 33.2 [4].

Clinical assessment of the tube position must be checked radiologically. Once in position, the tube must be securely fixed. Many methods of fixation have evolved. Some incorporate a circumferential head band over the forehead, to which is fixed a wire frame with an attachment for the tube. Another technique is to strap the tube to the upper lip and nose with adhesive tape. The skin may be protected and adhesion increased by applying compound tincture of benzoin to the skin (see Fig. 7.14).

Cuffed tubes are not usually needed until puberty. Up to this age the cricoid ring is the narrowest part of the airway and is circular in cross-section. Children over 9 years of age may require tubes with low-pressure, large-volume cuffs when high airway pressures are necessary for adequate ventilation, as in status asthmaticus.

The tube should be thin-walled and made of a material proven by implantation testing to be chemically inert. PVC tubes are most often used.

Management

HUMIDIFICATION

Whenever the upper respiratory tract is bypassed, it is essential to provide artificial humidification. Inadequate humidification results in drying of secretions, alteration in the characteristics of mucus and suppression of ciliary function. This is especially significant in the very young, as inspissated mucus is more likely to block the branches of the bronchial tree or the lumen of a narrow endotracheal tube. Fever, dehydration and increased ventilation associated with respiratory distress are contributing factors.

Humidified oxygen–air mixtures are best delivered to the airway by a system directly connected to a heated water-bath humidifier. The most suitable devices incorporate heating along the delivery tubing and temperature monitoring at the patient's end. A servo-controlled mechanism maintains the inspired gases at 37°C and 100% relative humidity, independent of gas flow. The problem of condensation in the expiratory limb can be overcome by the insertion of water traps or, better, by controlled heating of the expiratory limb. (Fig. 33.3).

Adequate humidification is more difficult in the active, intubated child with croup or epiglottitis. Light-weight condenser–humidifiers such as the Humidivent (Portex) and Thermovent (Gibeck) have proved very useful for this [5]. The humidifier should be changed every 24 hours to reduce contamination and resistance. Oxygen enrichment can be provided if needed.

Condenser–humidifiers are also suitable for in-line humidification during positive pressure ventilation for short periods such as during anaesthesia or medical evacuation.

In the presence of very viscid secretions, humidification may have to be supplemented by the instillation of 0.5 ml of normal saline before endotracheal suction.

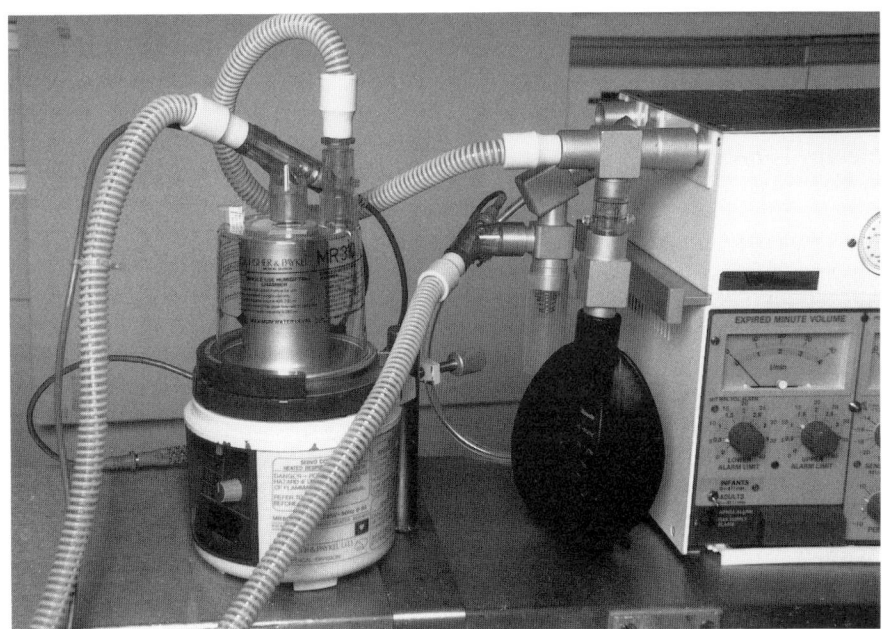

Fig. 33.3 Fisher–Paykel humidifier and ventilator system, demonstrating heated inspiratory and expiratory limbs.

SUCTION

Endotracheal suction is necessary to remove secretions. Intubation prevents apposition of the vocal cords and impairs coughing, which may also be obtunded by muscle weakness, neurological disturbance, sedation and muscle relaxants. Clearance of airway secretions then depends entirely on posture, physiotherapy, hand ventilation and good suction technique. Endotracheal suction is usually performed at hourly intervals, but may be required more frequently.

Endotracheal suction may be associated with hypoxia, atelectasis, a fall in lung compliance and the introduction of infection. It may also cause airway trauma and bleeding, especially in the presence of coagulopathy. Vagal reflexes may lead to bradycardia and dysrhythmia. Hypoxia and cardiac reflex effects are particularly dangerous in children with congenital heart disease, because shunt reversal and increased hypoxaemia may lead to sudden deterioration.

These effects of suction must be minimized; it is essential to use sterile technique. The external diameter of the catheter should be less than half that of the endotracheal tube, the endotracheal tube connection should be as large as possible and the catheter should be introduced rapidly. The catheter should be withdrawn slowly over the first 3–4 cm and then removed quickly.

The suction regulator should limit subatmospheric pressures to 200 mmHg (26.2 kPa), and the lungs should be inflated with oxygen both before and after suction, to prevent hypoxaemia and atelectasis.

The late John Stocks designed a 'bullet' device which is inserted into the ventilator circuit. It has a central lumen that allows the continuation of gas flow, positive pressure ventilation and constant positive airway pressure whilst suction is performed. This reduces the fall in Pao_2 and minimizes atelectasis (Fig. 33.4) [6]. A 'bullet' with a central lumen, appropriate to the size of catheter, is placed in the E-piece attached to the endotracheal tube

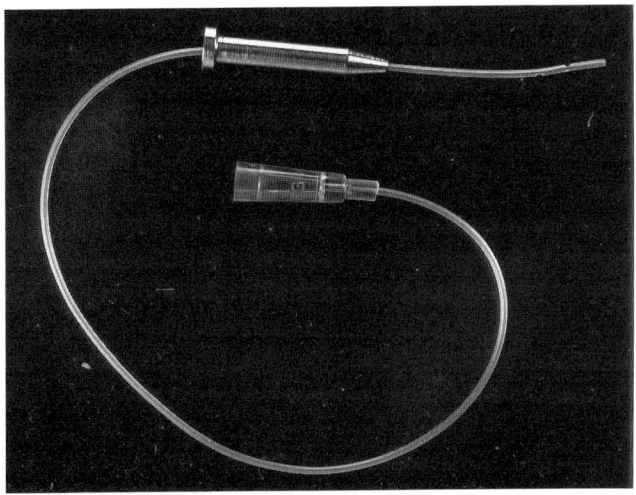

Fig. 33.4 Stocks 'Bullet' and suction catheter.

connector covered by a gas-tight cap. For endotracheal suction, the cap is removed and a catheter introduced into the lumen of the 'bullet', giving an almost gas-tight fit. The fall in the system pressure during positive pressure therapy is minimal.

PREVENTION OF CROSS-INFECTION

This is of great importance, because the airway provides direct access to the trachea. The risks are greatest in premature and in chronically ill, debilitated patients with impaired host resistance. In the past, the Gram-negative organisms such as *Pseudomonas* and *Klebsiella* have been the major organisms involved in cross-infection in intensive care units, but contamination with any organism is possible.

Spread from one patient to another is usually by the hands of medical and nursing staff. Respiratory apparatus, especially humidifiers and ventilator systems, may be a reservoir for organisms; the equipment must be sterilized regularly and always before use on a new patient. While in use, samples should be obtained regularly from the apparatus for bacteriological culture.

Cross-infection can only be prevented by strict aseptic technique during endotracheal suction, by hand-washing and gloving before carrying out procedures, and by maintaining a one-to-one nurse/patient ratio in those particularly at risk.

Complications

Blockage of the endotracheal tube and accidental extubation are potentially the most serious complications. Adequate humidification, effective endotracheal suction and secure fixation of the endotracheal tube are fundamental to the success of the technique. Nursing staff must be taught to recognize either complication and manage until medical assistance arrives. This usually entails removing the endotracheal tube, administering oxygen by mask and, if appropriate, assisting ventilation.

Subglottic oedema and stenosis are due to the pressure effects of the tube. Oedema results from minor degrees of trauma. Stenosis occurs if the lamina propria is destroyed and heals by granulation. Airway obstruction due to subglottic oedema is often relieved by the inhalation of nebulized adrenaline.

Laryngeal granulomata and thickening of the vocal cords may result from abrasions, especially with the use of large tubes, but rarely require operative treatment.

Ulceration and scarring of the nostril may occur with prolonged intubation, especially in premature infants. It can be avoided by good fixation technique and by angling the protruding part of the tube downwards and forwards.

The complications of tracheal intubation are mostly avoidable and provide an indicator of the quality of respiratory care in an intensive care unit. There should be no reason for the duration of intubation to be limited for fear of complications.

TRACHEOSTOMY

In most paediatric centres, tracheostomy has been replaced by prolonged nasotracheal intubation for acute care. Tracheostomy, however, remains a life-saving procedure and must be undertaken if endotracheal intubation is impossible, or if equipment or personnel are unavailable.

For chronic airway problems, tracheostomy is more comfortable. It allows better nasopharyngeal toilet and may permit the child to leave the intensive care unit and eventually go home. The airway is shorter and wider than that provided by intubation, but a surgical operation is needed, which has more immediate complications. The morbidity and the mortality with the two techniques are similar.

Technique

Attention to detail is important. Whenever possible, respiratory failure should be managed at first by tracheal intubation. Tracheostomy is best performed using endotracheal anaesthesia, with the neck extended. A longitudinal slit is made through the second and third tracheal rings without excision of cartilage. Stay sutures in the tracheal wall, lateral to the incision, aid recannulation should accidental dislodgement occur before a track is formed (after 4 days).

Commonly available paediatric tracheostomy tubes and their dimensions are listed in Table 33.3 [4]. The choice of tube depends on availability, the patient's needs and the preference of the operator. After insertion, the tube should be fixed securely by tapes, tied whilst the head is flexed.

Management

The principles of humidification, suction and prevention of cross-infection for tracheostomy are similar to those

Table 33.3 Tracheostomy tube sizes [3]

	Portex			Shiley				Gt. Ormond St.		
Age	ID (mm)	OD (mm)	Lth[a] (mm)	No.	ID (mm)	OD (mm)	Lth[a] (mm)	ID (mm)	OD (mm)	Lth[a] (mm)
Term	3.0	4.2	26	00	3.1	4.5	30/39	3.0	4.5	38[b]
<6 mo	3.5	4.9	28	0	3.4	5.0	32/40	3.5	5.0	41[c]
1 yr	4.0	5.5	29	1	3.7	5.5	34/41	—	—	—
2–3 yr	4.5	6.2	31	2	4.1	6.0	42	4.0	6.0	41[c]
4–5 yr	5.0	6.9	33	3	4.8	7.0	44	4.5	7.0	47[c]
6 yr	—	—	—	—	—	—	—	5.0	7.5	49[c]
8 yr	6.0	8.3	38	4	5.5	8.0	46	5.5	8.0	51[c]
12 yr	7.0	9.7	45	6	7.0	10.0	68	6.0	9.0	52[c]
14 yr	7.5	10.4	49	—	—	—	—	—	—	—
Adult	8.0	11.0	53	—	—	—	—	7.0	11.0	53[c]
Adult	9.0	12.4	60	8	8.5	12.0	71	—	—	—
Adult	10.0	13.7	68	10	9.0	13.0	71	—	—	—

[a] Horizontal length from mid-stoma to tip of tube.
[b] Portex Infant Tracheostomy Tube.
[c] Franklin GOS Paediatric Tracheostomy Tube.

for intubation. Infants should be nursed with the head extended for the first 12–24 hours after tracheostomy, to reduce the risk of accidental decannulation.

Complications

The major complications are related to surgical technique and early postoperative care. They can usually be prevented. Pneumothorax is likely if the tracheostomy is too low or the dissection strays from the midline. Respiratory obstruction may cause air to track into the mediastinum, from where it may rupture into a pleural cavity. A chest X-ray should be obtained immediately after tracheostomy, to check the position of the tip of the tube and to exclude pneumothorax. If the neck is extended too much during the operation, the stoma may be too low and the tube may enter a bronchus.

Blocked tube and accidental decannulation may occur, especially in the first 24 hours, when there is a risk of blood clot in the airway. The danger of accidental decannulation is greatest in the first few days, before a track is formed. Replacement of the tracheostomy tube may be very difficult, especially with a low tracheostomy;

tracheal intubation may be required in an emergency.

Rigid tracheostomy tubes can erode the trachea and may even perforate a major vessel, causing massive haemorrhage. This complication is rarely seen with the plastic tubes now commonly used.

The percutaneous tracheostomy techniques used in adults should probably be avoided in children until their safety is established.

'Retained tracheostomy tube' occurs when the underlying airway abnormality persists or tracheomalacia develops at the site of the tracheostomy, most likely if cartilage is excised. Bronchoscopic inspection may reveal a surgically treatable cause, such as a granuloma. Otherwise, a period of tracheal intubation may be needed to allow decannulation. If this fails, surgery may be necessary, to enlarge and stabilize the trachea.

CONSTANT POSITIVE AIRWAY PRESSURE (CPAP)

CPAP is a technique by which a constant positive pressure is applied to the airway of a spontaneously breathing patient.

Clinical applications

CPAP was intially used for the management of hyaline membrane disease in premature infants. Subsequently, it has been useful in a wide variety of conditions, particularly those characterized by hypoxaemia, atelectasis, alveolar instability and intrapulmonary shunting. The indications for CPAP are listed in Table 33.4 [7].

CPAP prevents airway closure and its effect is to re-expand atelectatic areas, decrease intrapulmonary shunting and increase Pa_{O_2}. Functional residual capacity and compliance are increased towards normal. If suitably designed equipment is used correctly, the work of breathing is reduced.

Premature infants with irregular breathing and periods of apnoea breathe more regularly when CPAP is applied, because the airways are kept open and the work of breathing is reduced. CPAP is also useful in weaning patients from mechanical ventilation.

CPAP systems

A CPAP system requires a high gas flow, an expiratory resistance in the breathing system and a method of interfacing the breathing system with the patient. A flow rate exceeding peak inspiratory flow is needed to maintain positive pressure throughout the breathing cycle. In neonates, infants and small children this can be accomplished using standard flow meters. In larger children, a reservoir bag is necessary. Continuous flow systems are generally preferable to demand systems, because the work of breathing is reduced (Fig. 33.5).

The CPAP system may be applied to the child by an

Table 33.4 Indications for continuous positive airway pressure (CPAP) [7]

Prophylactic:
Intubated patients
Adult respiratory distress syndrome
Surfactant conservation
Adult respiratory distress syndrome
Hyaline membrane disease
Left-ventricular failure and pulmonary oedema
Postoperative respiratory support
Pneumonia
Inhalation burn injury
Bronchiolitis
Meconium aspiration syndrome
Apnoea of prematurity
Diaphragmatic paralysis
Flail chest
Obstructive sleep apnoea
Bronchomalacia and tracheomalacia

endotracheal tube, nasal 'prongs' or mask, face mask or body chamber. Nasotracheal intubation is often the safest and most efficient method of applying CPAP. A single nasopharyngeal tube is effective in neonates and young infants, who are obligatory nose-breathers.

Expiratory resistance may be provided by such devices as a spring-loaded valve, a weighted valve, an underwater column, a venturi device, an electronically controlled constriction (e.g. scissor valve) or a pressure-actuated solenoid valve (Fig. 33.6).

Devices may be classified as either flow resistors or threshold resistors. With threshold resistors, the pressure generated is virtually independent of flow rate. Expiratory retard may be provided either deliberately or in-

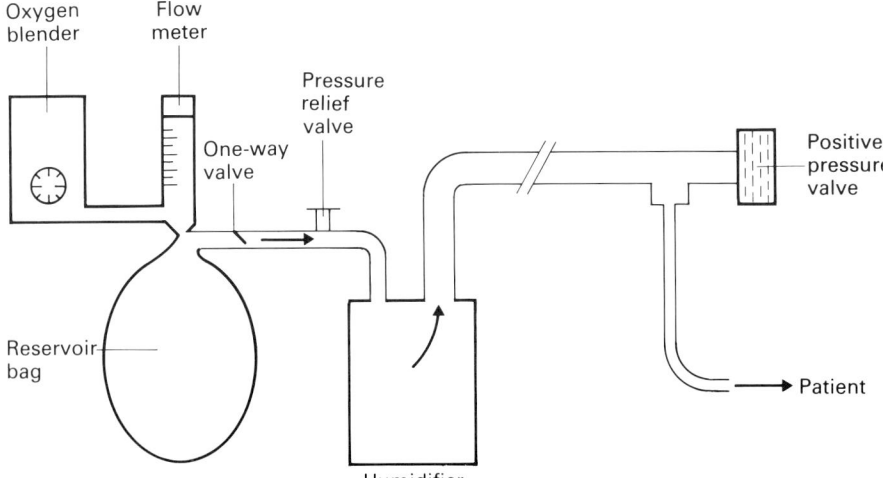

Fig. 33.5 A continuous flow CPAP circuit incorporating a reservoir bag.

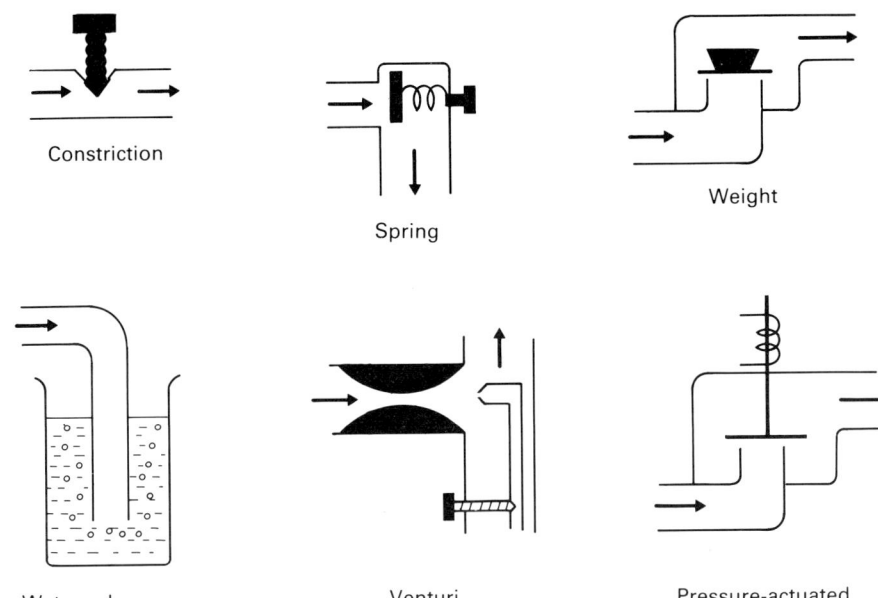

Fig. 33.6 Various forms of PEEP valves. (From Oh T.E. (ed) *Intensive care manual*, Butterworth (1990), with permission.)

Constriction

Spring

Weight

Water column

Venturi

Pressure-actuated solenoid

advertently by the use of small-calibre tubing in the expiratory circuit.

With nasal CPAP, positive pressure is lost during crying or mouth breathing, and abdominal distension may occur. Blood gas sampling during mouth breathing may lead to errors in oxygen therapy. The stomach should be decompressed continuously with a nasogastric tube.

The CPAP level is chosen to improve oxygenation and minimize side-effects. Small amounts of CPAP (2–5 cmH₂O, 0.2–0.5 kPa) should be applied, if practicable, to all intubated children to prevent airway closure. In infants with hyaline membrane disease or with pulmonary congestion, oedema or haemorrhage, CPAP levels of 5–10 cmH₂O (0.5–1.0 kPa) may substantially improve oxygenation and allow inspired oxygen concentration to be reduced. If no improvement occurs, the CPAP level can be increased in increments to 15 cmH₂O (1.5 kPa), or more.

Complications

Complications of CPAP therapy are more likely at high levels, especially in non-uniform lung disease. The application of CPAP in any patient may cause barotrauma, such as pneumothorax, pulmonary interstitial emphysema, pneumomediastinum, pneumoperitoneum and subcutaneous emphysema.

CPAP increases mean intrathoracic pressure and in-

hibits venous return. This is compensated by an increase in venous pressure, which may cause peripheral oedema (puffy eyes). High levels of CPAP may depress cardiac output and, hence, oxygen delivery, especially with normally compliant lungs or when the patient is hypovolaemic. CPAP may increase pulmonary vascular resistance and right-ventricular afterload by a Starling resistor effect. This effect may be balanced by the beneficial effect of CPAP in preventing atelectasis, thereby reducing pulmonary vascular resistance.

Increased antidiuretic hormone (ADH) secretion and fluid retention are also seen, although the exact mechanism for this is disputed.

INTERMITTENT POSITIVE PRESSURE VENTILATION (IPPV)

A ventilator is used to inflate the patient's lungs with humidified air, oxygen or mixtures of both (IPPV). Positive end-expiratory pressure is often added (PEEP). If the breathing system is arranged so that the patient can breathe spontaneously without generating sub-atmospheric airway pressure, the ventilator can be used to provide background ventilation at a slower rate. This is called intermittent mandatory ventilation (IMV) (Fig. 33.7). A constant positive pressure can be, and usually is, provided, adding the advantages of PEEP and CPAP. IMV is useful for patients who have apnoeic

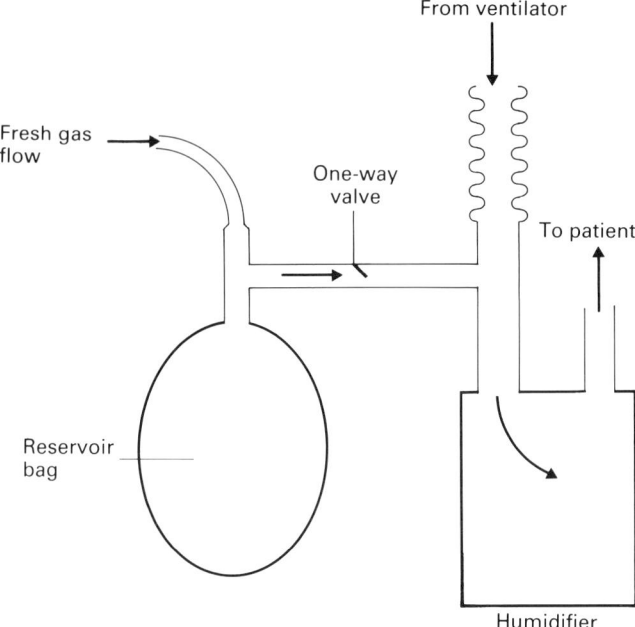

Fig. 33.7 An IMV attachment for incorporation into a ventilator circuit.

spells or tend to hypoventilate. It is valuable during weaning from mechanical ventilation.

Physiological principles

Intrapleural pressure is normally subatmospheric during inspiration. This not only draws air into the lungs but aids venous return to the heart. IPPV creates positive intrathoracic pressure as air is blown into the lungs, so that venous return may be impeded. The pattern of ventilation is important in determining the effectiveness of gas exchange and the effects on venous return and cardiac output. Very rapid and short inspiration results in uneven ventilation, while more prolonged inspiration, particularly with an end-inspiratory plateau, will allow time for areas of higher airway resistance to be ventilated. The longer inspiratory time, unless compensated by prolonged expiration, will cause higher mean intrathoracic pressure and hence greater impedance to venous return. This is compensated by an increase in venous pressure, unless the patient is hypovolaemic. In infants with rapid respiratory rates, the inspiratory and expiratory times are shorter, but the ratio of inspiratory to expiratory time is still important in determining mean airway and intrathoracic pressures.

Ventilators

Numerous ventilators that are designed for, or can be adapted for, neonates and infants are available. The principles of some of these are discussed in Chapter 3. In addition to the general requirement for mechanical ventilators, the ideal paediatric ventilator should incorporate the following features:

1 It must be capable of delivering small tidal volumes (as low as 10 ml) over a suitable period of time (0.3–1 second).

2 It should be able to ventilate at rates up to 60 per minute (up to 150 per minute for neonatal applications). Specifically designed ventilators are required for high frequency ventilation and oscillation.

3 Inspiratory and expiratory times should be independently adjustable.

4 The compressible volume and resistance of the ventilator and breathing system should be minimal.

5 The gas flow should be variable, up to 3 l/kg/min.

6 Gas flow should be immediately available for spontaneous respiratory effort (IMV).

7 The breathing system should be lightweight, with minimal dead space.

Both volume-preset and pressure-preset ventilators are used for infants and children. Volume-preset ventilators are valuable in conditions in which lung compliance and airway resistance are changing, but they do not compensate for leaks from the system. Air leak around the endotracheal tube often varies; this may lead to alveolar hypoventilation in neonates and infants with small tidal volumes. Moreover, the compressible volume of the circuit may be greater than the tidal volume and small tidal volumes are difficult to set and maintain. Barotrauma remains a threat when volume-preset ventilators are used with immature lungs.

Most neonatal intensive care units employ ventilators that are constant flow and time-cycled, but with a pressure limit. Examples of these are the Bourne's BP 200, Bear Cub BP 2001, Sechrist V-100B and Newport E100i. This form of ventilation has some characteristics of both volume- and pressure-preset systems. It achieves adequate gas exchange in newborn infants with minimal barotrauma. Provided the flow rate is adequate, there is some compensation for leaks from the system, but there is no compensation for changes in lung compliance.

Inadequate flow rate or a large leak (e.g. bronchopleural fistula) prevent the development of an inspiratory plateau. This means lower mean airway pressure and impaired oxygenation. The value of the plateau at the end of inspiration is that inspired gas is redistributed to poorly ventilated areas (slow compartments). The effect is similar to that of a sigh; it prevents atelectasis.

Ventilator settings

The risks of barotrauma and oxygen toxicity, especially in premature infants, demand that precise ventilator settings be prescribed. These should include rate, peak inspiratory pressure (pressure-preset and pressure-limited ventilators), positive end-expiratory pressure (PEEP) or CPAP, flow rate (IMV and constant flow ventilators), inspiratory time, minute volume (volume-preset ventilators) and inspired oxygen concentration. When pulmonary function deteriorates, it may be useful to increase each component of the prescription in steps. The alternative with the least potential for harm should be altered; increasing FiO_2 is probably safer than increasing PEEP. Increased PEEP demands an equivalent increase in peak inspiratory pressure if the same tidal volume is to be maintained, unless the effect is to move the lung volume to a more favourable part of the compliance curve.

The pattern of ventilation has many effects, but mean airway pressure is the main determinant of oxygenation. It is dependent on rate, peak inspiratory pressure, flow rate, inspiratory time and PEEP. Monitoring of airway pressure and wave-form is particularly useful with constant-flow time-cycled ventilators. The aim is to optimize gas exchange with minimal barotrauma.

Patient-triggered systems for ventilation, CPAP and IMV are generally unsuitable for use in infants less than 10 kg. The negative pressure generated by an inspiratory effort is dissipated within the relatively large volume of the ventilator and breathing system. With current equipment, the response time is too slow to synchronize with the rapid respiratory rates in young infants with lung disease.

IMV is important in infants and children for minimizing barotrauma and weaning from mechanical ventilation. Continuous-flow systems are preferred.

Unless there is some contraindication, low levels of PEEP (2−5 cmH₂O, 0.2−0.5 kPa) are applied routinely during mechanical ventilation of infants.

Sedation

When children are mechanically ventilated, sedation should be used whenever necessary to reduce restlessness and discomfort and to minimize energy wasted 'fighting the ventilator'. It may be required to prevent coughing, straining, unwanted autonomic responses and elevation of intracranial pressure in brain injury. Heavy sedation may be needed, with or without muscle relaxants. This can be applied safely, provided adequate medical and nursing supervision is available, with suitable monitoring devices. A continuous infusion of morphine, 10−50 µg/kg/h, will prevent awareness and discomfort in most children. The addition of midazolam, 0.1 mg/kg/h, induces a tranquil state and compliance with the ventilator, which may avoid the need for muscle relaxants.

Complications

Mechanical failure may occur with any ventilator; many have characteristic types of malfunction, which should be known to the operator. Constant vigilance is needed to detect accidental disconnection and other complications. Ventilators must have alarms for disconnection and high pressure. Mechanical ventilation increases the demands on both medical and nursing staff; it should not be undertaken lightly. Whenever muscle relaxants or heavy sedation are used, particular care must be provided.

Any form of increased airway pressure raises mean intrathoracic pressure and may reduce venous return and cardiac output, especially in volume-depleted patients. Volume expansion, with 10−20 ml/kg of colloid solution, may be required at the commencement of mechanical ventilation. Depression of cardiac output by mechanical ventilation is less of a problem in infants and children than in adults.

Barotrauma may result in pulmonary interstitial emphysema, pneumothorax, pneumomediastinum and pneumopericardium; it is likely with immature lungs, non-uniform lung disease or when very high airway pressures are needed. Facilities for decompressing a pneumothorax must be immediately available whenever mechanical ventilation is applied. Pulmonary barotrauma also contributes to the development of pulmonary oxygen toxicity and bronchopulmonary dysplasia.

Fluid retention and oedema may occur, especially with high intrapulmonary pressures. Fluid therapy must be adjusted according to needs and state of hydration. Allowance should be made for the lack of water loss from the airway and the effects of positive pressure ventilation on ADH secretion.

Weaning from ventilatory support

The decision to wean from respiratory support is based on improved clinical signs, radiological examination and blood gas status. Weaning can start when the condition needing mechanical ventilation has resolved sufficiently, the cardiovascular system is stable and the child is awake and active.

It is unlikely to be successful if oxygen concentration exceeding 50%, or peak airway pressure more than 25 cmH$_2$O (2.5 kPa) are needed. PEEP or CPAP should be reduced to 5 cmH$_2$O (0.5 kPa) or less before extubation. The rate of weaning depends on the nature of the underlying pathology and the anticipated and actual response to weaning. Progression through IMV and CPAP is advised, other than when weaning from a short period of ventilation.

Meticulous attention to the function of all organ systems is needed for successful weaning. Some degree of fluid restriction is usually indicated. Cardiovascular support with inotropic and vasodilating agents should be maintained during the weaning period, if these are needed. The increased work of breathing associated with weaning places additional demands on the cardiovascular system, and may divert blood flow from other vital organ systems. The patient should be fasted and the abdomen decompressed before extubation. Fasting for 24 hours after extubation is recommended in the newborn and some other children, when they have had a long period of intubation, to allow for return of laryngeal competence.

High-frequency ventilation

The term high-frequency ventilation (HFV) now generally refers to ventilation at respiratory rates greater than 4 Hz, with tidal volumes close to or less than anatomical dead space. Methods of HFV most commonly used are: high-frequency jet ventilation, high-frequency flow interruption, and high-frequency oscillation. All three, when combined with PEEP, can produce adequate oxygenation and CO$_2$ removal in infants, children and adults with restrictive lung disease, often using lower peak and mean airway pressures than in conventional ventilation.

Studies in pre-term infants have not shown any improvement in mortality, morbidity or long-term lung function with HFV compared with conventional venti-lation. Similarly, studies in adults with ARDS did not show improvement in mortality, hospital stay or intensive-care stay.

Necrotizing tracheitis is much more common with the use of high-frequency jet ventilation and high-frequency flow interruption than with conventional ventilation or high-frequency oscillation, even when improved methods of humidification are used. The eventual role of HFV in patients of all ages is not yet settled, but there have been many favourable case reports of its use, especially in severe pulmonary air leak.

CONCLUSION

The complex techniques involved in the treatment of acute respiratory failure in infants and children require a paediatric intensive care unit with high standards of nursing and medical care, specially designed facilities and 24-hour biochemistry and radiological services.

Such services are very expensive and should not be duplicated in every hospital. Regional centres, with facilities for safe and effective transport to such centres, are needed for all but very short-term respiratory support.

REFERENCES

1 Owen H., Duncan A.W. Towards safer transport of sick and injured children. *Anaes Intens Care* 1983, **11**, 113−117.
2 Shann F., Gatchalian S., Hutchinson R. Nasopharyngeal oxygen in children. *Lancet* 1988, **1**, 1238−1240.
3 Henning R. Clinical applications of mechanical ventilation. *Anaes Intens Care* 1986, **14**, 267−280.
4 Shann F., Duncan A.W. (Eds) *Drug doses in paediatric intensive care*. 5th edn, Melbourne, Royal Children's Hospital, (1989).
5 Duncan A.W. Use of disposable condenser humidifiers in children. *Anaes Intens Care* 1985, **13**, 330.
6 Kerr D.R., Vonwiller J.B., Abrahams N. The Stocks suction bullet. *Anaes Intens Care* 1978, **6**, 185−199.
7 Duncan A.W., Oh T.E., Hillman D.R. PEEP and CPAP. *Anaes Intens Care* 1986, **14**, 236−250.

FURTHER READING

Rogers M.C. *Textbook of paediatric intensive care*, Vol. 1. Williams and Wilkins, Baltimore, (1987) Chapters 4−10.
Gregory G.A. *Respiratory failure in the child*. Clinics in Critical Care Medicine, Churchill Livingstone, New York, (1981).
Stocks J.G. The management of respiratory failure in infancy. *Anaes Intens Care* 1973, **1**, 486−506.
Bohn D. High-frequency ventilation. *Br J Anaes* 1989, **63**, 16S.

34: Intensive Care of Children With Shock and Cardiac Failure

In circulatory failure, the cardiovascular system is unable to supply the metabolic needs of the tissues. Shock is acute circulatory failure. Cardiac failure is a more chronic process due to abnormality of heart function, and includes states in which tissue needs are only met by the development of abnormally high filling pressures.

PHYSIOLOGY

The nutrition of a tissue depends on blood flow through the capillaries supplying that tissue and on the number of perfused capillaries per unit cross-sectional area of the tissue. Blood flow through a tissue depends on mean arterial blood pressure (BP) and on the resistance of the arteriolar/capillary network of that tissue. Mean arterial blood pressure is proportional to cardiac output and total peripheral resistance (Fig. 34.1). Total resistance is the sum of the resistances of individual tissue capillary beds. If the vessels in one bed dilate, redistribution of cardiac output diverts blood away from other areas, which may include vital organs.

Cardiac output is proportional to heart rate and stroke volume. Stroke volume depends on (i) ventricular end diastolic volume, and (ii) the velocity and extent of shortening of the ventricular muscle.

Figure 34.2 shows the effect of ventricular filling on ventricular contractility. In a failing heart, ventricular stroke volume is lower for a given preload or filling

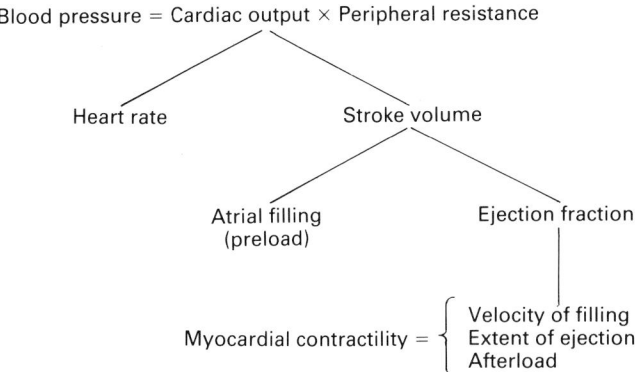

Fig. 34.1 Factors relating to cardiac output.

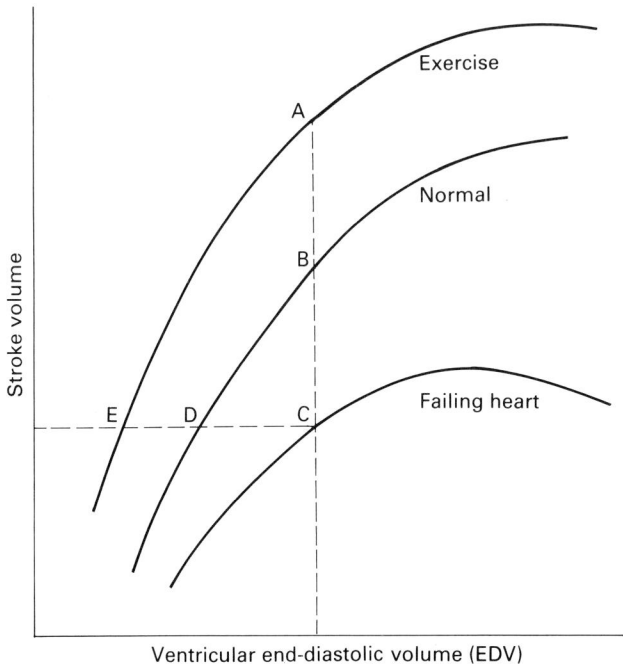

Fig. 34.2 The relation between ventricular filling and stroke volume in normal and failing hearts. In the failing heart EDV increases (D−C) and stroke volume decreases (B−C). The opposite occurs in exercise (D−E and B−A).

467

volume, and for a given stroke volume a higher preload is necessary.

Myocardial contractility depends on the extent and velocity of ventricular contraction and after load (Fig. 34.1) [1]. Thus, for a fixed level of contractility, the greater the afterload the smaller the velocity and extent of shortening. Afterload is the ventricular wall tension (T) during systole and is related to ventricular radius (R) and transventricular pressure thus:

$$T = \frac{(P_1 - P_2) \times R}{2\,H}$$

where P_1 is pressure within the ventricle, P_2 is intrathoracic pressure and H is ventricular wall thickness. Therefore the greater the intraventricular pressure or ventricular radius, the greater is the afterload.

Ventricular end-diastolic volume (or preload) depends on venous return to the ventricle in question, and on ventricular compliance, where compliance equals

$$\frac{\text{ventricular end-diastolic volume}}{\text{ventricular end-diastolic pressure}}$$

Ventricular compliance is low in a hypertrophied heart and in infiltrative cardiomyopathy; it is reduced by ischaemia and by inotropic drugs [2]. Ventricular compliance is high in dilated cardiomyopathy and in conditions such as atrial septal defect, in which ventricular dilatation rather than hypertrophy occurs. It has been observed that vasodilator drugs increase ventricular compliance.

Increased dilatation of the atria causes release of atrial natriuretic hormones (which have natriuretic and vasodilator actions) and sends afferent nerve impulses which inhibit central sympathetic outflow. This causes dilatation in the skin, splanchnic circulation and kidneys, and inhibits renin release from the juxtaglomerular apparatus [3].

Afferent impulses from arterial and atrial stretch receptors inhibit the output of vasopressin. In heart failure and shock, the effect of osmoreceptors on vasopressin release is unimportant compared with that of arterial pressure receptors. Arterial stretch also inhibits sympathetic outflow. In heart failure, arterial pressure is low and atrial volume is high, so that contradictory messages are sent to the medulla from the arterial and atrial stretch receptors, but the effect of low arterial pressure predominates.

Phylogenetically the cardiovascular reflexes evolved to defend arterial blood pressure (the major determinant of tissue perfusion) in exercise and trauma, when peripheral resistance and circulating blood volume respectively are low. In cardiac failure these reflexes have deleterious effects, such as vasoconstriction and sodium and water retention, causing pulmonary and peripheral oedema [4].

CARDIAC FAILURE

A child may have a cardiac abnormality for years without overt heart failure, but intercurrent infection with its associated increased metabolic demands, anaemia or dysrhythmia may cause decompensation [5]. Therefore in heart failure, both the underlying cause and the precipitating cause should be sought and treated. When one of the underlying causes of heart failure is present the body compensates by the following means:

1 Hypertrophy: reduces afterload by ventricular wall thickness but also reduces diastolic compliance (i.e. raises LVEDP for the same LVEDV).

2 Expansion of the central blood volume due to sodium and water retention by the kidney which increases cardiac output (Starlings Law).

3 Neuroendocrine responses associated with the actions of renin−angiotensin−aldosterone, noradrenaline, vasopressin, atrial natriuretic hormone and various vasoactive peptides increase blood volume and peripheral resistance [4].

4 Raising systemic vascular resistance redistributes the cardiac output to the heart and brain and away from the skin, splanchnic circulation and kidneys.

In congestive heart failure from any cause, there is evidence of abnormal excitation−contraction coupling, impairing calcium delivery to contractile sites. The mechanism has not been defined [6]. Energy demand is increased by tachycardia and increased ventricular-wall tension. Energy supply is reduced due to the presence of fewer capillaries and fewer mitochondria per unit area of tissue. Diastolic relaxation is impaired, reducing diastolic compliance and slowing diastolic ventricular filling. This is especially important at high heart rates and in the hypertrophic heart [7].

In the failing myocardium, the density of beta 1 (but not of beta 2) receptors and the noradrenaline stores are reduced, while circulating noradrenaline concentration increases and the sensitivity of beta 1 receptors to catecholamines declines [8]. In chronic heart failure, pump failure may be due to fibrosis and less efficient ventricular size and shape.

An infant's heart has less contractile tissue per unit mass, so that there are fewer mitochondria and less myosin ATP-ase than in the adult. The heart depends on increase in rate rather than in contractility to adapt to stresses such as hypovolaemia, anaemia, hypoxia and acidosis (see Chapter 1). Inefficient calcium transport and storage in T-tubules and sarcoplasmic reticulum mean that excitation−contraction coupling in the infant's heart is more dependent on trans-sarcolemmal calcium flux and on plasma-ionized calcium concentration than in the adult [9].

Sympathetic innervation is less developed than parasympathetic in neonates and infants. The infant's response to increasing hypovolaemia, hypoxia, trauma and acidosis proceeds from tachycardia to bradycardia more rapidly than in adults.

Dopamine has both direct and indirect sympathomimetic actions. Infants require relatively higher doses of dopamine than adults because they have smaller myocardial noradrenaline stores and have less sensitive beta-receptors.

Signs and symptoms

Feeding is slow, and often associated with sweating and dyspnoea. The child may fail to gain weight. Examination reveals tachycardia, tachypnoea, low-volume pulses, cardiomegaly and hepatomegaly. There may be a gallop rhythm. There may be clinical and chest X-ray signs of lung congestion, oedema and air trapping (due to bronchial mucosal oedema in the presence of large left-to-right shunts). In addition there may be signs of the underlying causative lesion (Table 34.1).

Management

The methods of managing failure are:

1 Maintain the systemic circulation and reduce venous congestion.

(a) Reduce preload with a diuretic and by salt and water restriction, head elevation and possibly venodilator infusion (e.g. nitroglycerine (GTN)).

(b) Reduce afterload with infusion of a short-acting vasodilator such as sodium nitroprusside or GTN. If necessary and if there is no contraindication, such as hypotension or obstructive valvular lesion, a longer-acting vasodilator such as phenoxybenzamine or captopril can be used.

(c) Increase contractility with digoxin and, if necess-

Table 34.1 Causes of heart failure in childhood

Volume load
PDA in pre-term babies
VSD after age 6 weeks
Common atrioventricular canal
Truncus arteriosus
Transposition of the great arteries with VSD
Arteriovenous fistula (in heart, brain, liver, kidney)
Regurgitation of atrioventricular or semilunar valves

Pressure load
Coarctation of the aorta
Aortic stenosis
Mitral stenosis
Cor triatriatum
Total anomalous pulmonary venous drainage
Persistent pulmonary hypertension of the newborn (of any cause)

Myocardial dysfunction
Cardiomyopathy (drugs, inborn error of metabolism)
Myocarditis
Myocardial ischaemia (Kawasaki disease, anomalous origin of the left coronary artery) mucopolysaccharidoses I & II
Asphyxia (peripartum, near drowning, etc.)

ary, infusion of dopamine or dobutamine. The latter is preferred if the patient does not have a central venous catheter or if vasoconstriction is not desirable.

2 Mechanical ventilation using muscle relaxants and positive end-expiratory pressure. This helps to control cardiac failure by improving gas exchange, correcting acidaemia and reducing the demand by respiratory muscles for blood flow.

3 Correct the precipitating cause, such as intercurrent infection with fever, lung collapse, dysrhythmia, endocarditis or anaemia.

4 Identify and correct the underlying cause. For example, repair of a coarctation or large VSD, or replacement of a regurgitant valve.

SHOCK

Pathophysiology

Shock is acute circulatory failure resulting in inadequate supply and use of oxygenated metabolic substrates, leading to multiple organ dysfunction. The commonest types of shock in childhood are hypovolaemic, cardiogenic, septic and distributive (neurogenic, drug-induced and anaphylactic).

Depletion of the ATP stores in hypoxic cells results in

failure of sodium/potassium pumping, calcium accumulation in the cytoplasm and finally in cell death. Increased cytosol calcium concentration increases phospholipase A_2 activity, releasing arachidonic acid from membrane phospholipids to be transformed into the vasoactive prostaglandins, prostacyclin and thromboxane A_2, and leukotrienes C_4 and D_4. Free oxygen radicals released in this process cause cell membrane lipid peroxidation, resulting in damage and cell death [10].

Circulating antigen−antibody complexes, bacterial toxins and the breakdown products of tissue destruction are taken up by macrophages, causing the release of monokines such as interleukin-1 (IL-1) and tumour necrosis factor (TNF). IL-1 stimulates neutrophil release and increases amino-acid oxidation, causing muscle proteolysis, while TNF appears to be responsible for most of the injurious effects of bacterial endotoxin. Infusion of TNF into animals causes peripheral circulatory changes, lactic acidosis, fever, disseminated intravascular coagulation (DIC) and increases the permeability of systemic and lung capillaries [11]. The circulating level of TNF correlates closely with mortality and with the extent of purpura fulminans in meningococcal septicaemia in children [12]; high TNF levels are also found in Gram-negative septic shock.

Complement activation by antigen−antibody complexes and tissue debris releases peptide fragments such as C_5A which activate neutrophils and cause them to accumulate in lung capillaries, releasing lysosomal enzymes and free oxygen radicals with subsequent damage to lung capillary endothelium and lung parenchyma. This and other mechanisms may cause adult respiratory distress syndrome 12−36 hours after the onset of shock [13].

Ischaemia of the intestinal wall due to splanchnic vasoconstriction in shock states allows the absorption of gut bacterial toxins into systemic blood, perpetuating the complement activation and monokine release described above [11].

Activation of platelets and the coagulation, fibrinolytic and kinin cascades with the release of histamine contribute to the small-vessel obstruction, loss of microvascular control and the DIC seen in children with shock from any cause [14].

In shock myocardial performance is depressed by several factors, including relative myocardial ischaemia, reduced responsiveness to catecholamines, myocardial metabolic derangements and circulating cardiotoxic substances.

Types of shock

HYPOVOLAEMIA

Hypovolaemia due to blood loss or dehydration is the commonest cause of shock in childhood. Early signs include those of external or internal bleeding, or of water loss in severe dehydration caused by intestinal losses (including diarrhoea and vomiting), polyuria and burns. The patient will usually be shocked when more than 30 ml/kg of blood is lost. At this stage, tachycardia, hypotension, narrowed pulse pressure and oliguria (less than 0.5 ml/kg/h) are associated with pale, mottled or cyanosed skin, slow capillary refill, tachypnoea and stupor or coma.

CARDIOGENIC SHOCK

Cardiogenic shock is due primarily to 'pump' failure. In the first few days of life it is most commonly caused by obstructive lesions of the left heart (coarctation of the aorta with or without VSD, critical aortic stenosis, interrupted aortic arch or hypoplastic left-heart syndrome), supraventricular tachycardia or congenital heart block.

In an older child it may be due to progressive deterioration of congenital or acquired heart disease.

Cardiogenic shock may also present in a previously well child, due to myocarditis or toxic cardiomyopathy. In addition to signs of a specific heart lesion, there are usually tachycardia and hypotension. Pulse pressure is narrow and pulses may be difficult to feel. There are usually cardiomegaly, hepatomegaly and widespread chest rales. The heart sounds are often faint and there may be a gallop rhythm.

SEPTIC SHOCK

The organisms which commonly cause septic shock in the newborn are Gram-negative bacilli, group B beta-haemolytic streptococci, *Staphylococcus aureus*, *Listeria monocytogenes* and echo and coxsackie viruses. After the first 6 weeks of life, *Haemophilus influenzae*, *Meningococcus*, *Pneumococcus*, *Staphylococcus aureus* and Gram-negative bacilli cause most cases of septic shock.

Tachycardia, hypotension, oliguria and depressed conscious state are present from the start. In early septic shock, the skin of the extremities is warm, with low pulse pressure and dilated veins. In late septic shock the extremities are cool and cyanosed. Pulse pressure is narrow and there is tachypnoea and coma. This clinical course is seen with Gram-positive, Gram-negative, fungal and viral pathogens. Meningococcal septic shock, however, follows the course of cardiogenic or hypovolaemic shock [15]. In small infants the signs of sepsis are subtle and non-specific, for example, lethargy, vomiting, irregular breathing or apnoea. They may not be febrile. Neonates and infants less than 6–12 months old present with a hypodynamic rather than a hyperdynamic state, and appear pale and floppy with cool cyanosed extremities from the start.

DISTRIBUTIVE SHOCK

This is an abnormal distribution of cardiac output resulting in hypotension and reduced blood flow to the vital organs. Neurogenic, anaphylactic and drug-induced shock are examples. The clinical picture is dominated by profound hypotension with tachycardia. In neurogenic shock, there is wide pulse pressure and warm, pink extremities, but in anaphylactic shock the fluid loss from capillaries causes hypovolaemia, with reduced pulses.

The late signs of shock are similar whatever the cause; they include disseminated intravascular coagulation, bloody diarrhoea, renal failure, increasing jaundice, fitting and coma.

Patient assessment

A rapid examination of the child will establish whether shock is present. Depressed conscious state, tachypnoea and mottled skin can be seen from the end of the bed; palpation reveals a rapid, low-volume pulse (in hypovolaemic or cardiogenic shock) or a bounding pulse in septic or distributive shock.

To reduce the mortality of shock, one must be aware of predisposing conditions and intervene early when signs of cellular injury or circulatory deterioration occur (e.g. metabolic acidosis, hyponatraemia, thrombocytopenia, falling fibrinogen concentration and increasing clotting time and catecholamine output with tachycardia and glucose intolerance).

MANAGEMENT OF THE SHOCKED CHILD

The child's airway, breathing and circulation should be secured during the initial assessment. The information which must be obtained by history, examination and investigation during this assessment is:
1 is this child shocked?
2 what is the cause of the shock?
3 how advanced is the shock state?
4 what complications of shock are present?
Investigations which are performed immediately in any shocked patient should include: arterial pH, Po_2 and Pco_2; urea; creatinine; electrolytes and glucose; haemoglobin; platelet count; total and differential white-cell count; prothrombin ratio; blood group and cross-match; chest X-ray.

If the cause of shock is unknown, hypovolaemia is usually revealed by history and examination. If necessary, chest X-ray (small heart shadow) and measurement of right atrial pressure by central venous catheter may assist in diagnosis.

Although cardiogenic shock can usually be excluded on clinical grounds (see above), investigations such as electrocardiogram, echocardiography and cardiac catheterization may be needed for diagnosis and management. When pulmonary oedema is associated with shock, measurement of pulmonary capillary wedge pressure (PCWP) can distinguish cardiogenic pulmonary oedema (high PCWP) from non-cardiogenic (adult respiratory distress syndrome in which PCWP is normal or low).

In the newborn, dysrhythmia can be excluded by an electrocardiogram, and systemic arteriovenous fistula diagnosed by collapsing pulses and a murmur over the head, liver, kidneys or limbs. Obstructive left-heart lesions are suspected if the pulses are absent or unequal, and can be confirmed by echocardiography.

If septic shock is suspected on clinical grounds, several blood cultures should be taken, as well as samples of pus for culture and Gram staining. Tracheal or pharyngeal aspirate, urine, CSF and drain fluid should also be cultured. Urine should be assayed for bacterial antigens (especially *Haemophilus influenzae* and *Pneumococcus*). Samples of urine, faeces and nasopharyngeal aspirate should be collected for viral culture, as well as blood for viral serology. Differential white-cell count and C-reactive protein assay are useful to differentiate infective from non-infective causes of shock. The primary infective focus must be found.

Drug screening of urine, gastric aspirate and blood, and urine metabolic screening for amino and organic acids may elucidate a toxic or metabolic cause.

Complications of shock to be looked for include acute renal failure, coagulopathy (especially disseminated intravascular coagulation), liver impairment with hypoglycaemia and jaundice, upper gastrointestinal bleeding, bloody diarrhoea with mucosal sloughing, and encephalopathy with fits.

Variables which should be monitored in a shocked child include heart and respiratory rates, core and toe temperatures, blood pressure by intra-arterial catheter, central venous pressure and/or pulmonary capillary wedge pressure, and cardiac output by physical signs, Doppler or bio-impedance, or invasively by dye dilution. Urine output, pulse oximetry and Glasgow coma score (motor response only) [16] should also be recorded.

Shocked children compensate well for most insults; decompensation is late and catastrophic. A well-resuscitated child can recover without sequelae from insults that would kill most adults. Therefore one should be more aggressive in resuscitating children than one would be with an adult: it is better to intubate and ventilate or give inotropic drugs unnecessarily than not to be aggressive enough.

The steps in management of a shocked child are:

1 *Airway*: should be secured immediately by turning on the side, with jaw support.

2 *Breathing*: every shocked child should receive oxygen by mask at a flow which will avoid CO_2 retention (at least 4 l/min). Tracheal intubation and mechanical ventilation using muscle relaxants reduces the work of breathing, diverts the limited cardiac output away from the respiratory muscles; it should be performed urgently if there is clinical or biochemical evidence of poor gas exchange, or if the shock cannot be reversed in less than 30 minutes. The disadvantages are that muscle relaxants prevent neurological assessment and that high intrathoracic pressure during IPPV can reduce cardiac output by impeding venous return. The advantages of muscle relaxants must outweigh the disadvantages if they are to be used.

3 *Circulation*: in severe shock with hypotension, the primary aim is adequate perfusion of the heart and brain, which requires systolic and diastolic pressures at least 80% of normal for age.

When this has been achieved (usually by colloid infusion and inotropic drugs including, if necessary, vasoconstrictors such as high-dose dopamine and/or noradrenal-

ine), the kidney and gut vessels are dilated and perfusion is improved by low-dose infusion of dopamine (2.5 μg/kg/min) and reduction of vasoconstrictors. Later, blood flow to muscle and skin may be improved by the use of vasodilators such as sodium nitroprusside.

Preload is improved by rapid infusion of 10 ml/kg aliquots of blood or colloid; the effect of each aliquot is assessed by heart rate, skin perfusion, blood pressure, urine output and liver size. If more than 20 ml/kg is needed, central venous pressure, cardiac output and occasionally PCWP should be monitored so that fluid overload is avoided. If a fluid challenge improves cardiac output with a small increase in atrial pressure, then another bolus may be given. Larger increases in atrial pressure for small increases in cardiac output means that the top of the volume–contractility curve (Starling, Sarnoff) (Fig. 34.1) is close and that further improvement in output will require improved contractility or afterload reduced.

Contractility may be increased by infusing an inotropic drug at high dose (e.g. dopamine or dobutamine 10 μg/kg/min) initially and reducing the dose as soon as possible. Children often need a higher dose of inotropic drug per kg than adults. In the initial resuscitation dobutamine may be given through a peripheral i.v. infusion while a central catheter is being inserted through which to infuse dopamine, adrenaline or noradrenaline (all of which cause skin necrosis if infused into peripheral veins). The choice of inotropic drug depends on the amount of vasoconstriction present, and on the previous response to inotropes. In septic or other distributive shock, a vasoconstrictor such as noradrenaline (0.1–5.0 μg/kg/min) or dopamine (10–20 μg/kg/min) may be needed to achieve an adequate blood pressure. Dopamine depletes myocardial noradrenaline stores; dopamine and dobutamine reduce the sensitivity (down-regulation) of beta-1 receptors. If the cardiac output is low after 48 hours of either drug, then a trial of (i) calcium gluconate (10%) infusion (0.2–0.5 ml/h vasoconstricts and improves myocardial contractility), or (ii) either noradrenaline + sodium nitroprusside (this combination stimulates myocardial alpha-receptors while reducing afterload) or salbutamol (which stimulates myocardial beta-2 receptors) may improve the circulation.

Afterload should be reduced to improve myocardial performance, provided diastolic blood pressure is over about 80% of normal. Infusion of short-acting drugs such as sodium nitroprusside and nitroglycerine is safer than that of long-acting drugs.

Metabolic acidosis (base deficit >10 mmol/l) may be corrected with sodium bicarbonate. This increases intracellular pH in the newborn animal with lactic acidosis, though not in the adult [17].

Neither high-dose steroids nor naloxone improve survival in septic shock, and their use is not justified [18, 19].

Granulocyte transfusion and exchange transfusion may be useful in neonates with sepsis and neutropenia, although their value is not proven in older children.

Supportive measures for the shocked child include the prevention of gastric ulceration with sucralfate or H_2 receptor antagonists, transfusion of platelets and fresh-frozen plasma for consumption coagulopathy, and peritoneal dialysis or veno-venous haemofiltration (see Chapter 38) for renal impairment.

REFERENCES

1 Sonnenblick E.H., Strobert J.E. Derived indexes of ventricular and myocardial function. *New Engl J Med* 1977, **296**, 978.

2 Calvin J.E., Sibbald W.J. Applied cardiovascular physiology in the critically ill, with special reference to diastole and ventricular interaction. In: Shoemaker W.L., Ayres S., Grenvik A., Holbrook P.R., Thompson W.L. (Eds) *Textbook of critical care*. WB Saunders, Philadelphia, (1989) p. 312.

3 Covell J.W. Neurohumoral control of the circulation. In: West J.B. (Ed) *Best and Taylor's physiological basis of medical practice*, 12th edn. Williams & Wilkins, Baltimore, (1991) p. 76.

4 Harris P. Congestive cardiac failure: central role of the arterial blood pressure. *Br Heart J* 1987, **58**, 190.

5 Braunwald E. Heart failure. In: Braunwald E., Issellbacher K.J., Pelerodorf R.G., Wilson J.D., Martin J.B., Fauci A.S. (Eds) *Harrison's principles of internal medicine*, 11th edn. McGraw Hill, New York, (1987), p. 905.

6 Braunwald E. Normal and abnormal myocardial function. In: *Harrisons principles of internal medicine*, 11th edn. McGraw Hill, New York, (1987), p. 904. *op. cit.*

7 Katz A.M. Cellular mechanisms in congestive heart failure. *Am J Cardiol* 1988, **62**, 3A.

8 Poole-Wilson P.A. Current therapeutic principles in the acute management of severe congestive heart failure. *Am J Cardiol* 1988, **62**, 4C.

9 Maylie J.G. Excitation–contraction coupling in neonatal myocardium of cat. *Am J Physiol* 1982, **242**, H834.

10 Zimmerman J.J. Oxyradical species and their relationship to pathophysiology in pediatric critical care illness. *Crit Care Clin* 1988, **4**, 645.

11 DeCamp M.M., Demling R.H. Post-traumatic multisystem organ failure. *JAMA* 1988, **260**, 530.

12 Girardin E., Graw G.E., Dayer J.M., Roux-Lombard P. The J5 Study Group, Lambert PH. Tumor necrosis factor and interleukin-1 in the serum of children with severe infectious purpura. *New Engl J Med* 1988, **319**, 397.

13 Vercellotti G.M. Role of neutrophils in endothelial injury. In: Bihari D.J., Cerra F.B. (Eds) *New horizons: multiple organ failure*. Fullerton Society of Critical Care Medicine (1989), p. 77.

14 Wetzel R.C. Shock. In: Rogers M.C. (Ed) *Textbook of pediatric intensive care*. Williams & Wilkins, Baltimore, (1987), p. 483.

15 Mercier J.C., Beaufils F., Hartmann J.F., Azema D. Hemodynamic patterns of meningococcal shock in children. *Crit Care Med* 1988, **16**, 27.

16 Jagger J., Jane J.A., Rimel R. The Glasgow Coma Scale: to sum or not to sum? *Lancet* 1983, **2**, 97.

17 Sessler D., Mills P., Gregory G., Litt L., James T. Effects of bicarbonate on arterial and brain intracellular pH in neonatal rabbits recovering from hypoxic lactic acidosis. *J Pediatr* 1987, **111**, 817.

18 Bone R.C., Fisher C.J., Clemmer T.P., *et al*. A controlled clinical trial of high-dose methyl prednisolone in the treatment of severe sepsis and septic shock. *New Engl J Med* 1987, **317**, 653.

19 De Maria A., Heffernan J.J., Grindlinger G.A., *et al*. Naloxone versus placebo in treatment of septic shock. *Lancet* 1985, **1**, 1363.

35: Cardiopulmonary Resuscitation

INTRODUCTION

Cardiac arrest in infants and children usually follows hypoxia. Respiratory arrest often precedes circulatory arrest. Diseases and abnormalities of the upper airway that cause obstruction and lung diseases are the common causes of hypoxia. Occasionally, cardiac dysrhythmia occurs in patients with abnormalities of the conduction system, after poisoning with cardioactive drugs such as tricyclic antidepressants and carbamazepine, after cardiac surgery or as a consequence of myocarditis, hypotension or ischaemia.

Normal brain function after cardiopulmonary resuscitation of children has been variously reported in between 5% and 40% of patients [1], depending on whether the arrest was respiratory alone or both cardiac and respiratory. Whatever the circumstance, the neurological outcome is mostly determined by the time taken to start resuscitation and the effectiveness of the resuscitation.

It is important to realize that bradycardia, rather than tachycardia, is the cardiac response to hypoxaemia or ischaemia in infants and children, especially the newborn. Spontaneous tachydysrhythmia is uncommon.

MANAGEMENT

The immediate goal of cardiopulmonary resuscitation (CPR) is to restore circulation and oxygenate the blood.

The outcome, in particular the survival of the brain, depends mostly on the time taken to achieve adequate, oxygenated cerebral blood flow. Recovery of sinus rhythm and spontaneous cardiac output is determined by the delay before effective cardiopulmonary resuscitation is started and, during resuscitation, by adequate coronary perfusion pressure, i.e. the difference between pressure at the aortic root and left atrial pressure when compression is released [2]. Basic life support (basic CPR) is the establishment of a patent airway, artificial ventilation and external cardiac compression. Basic life support can be started immediately without special equipment.

Advanced life support includes all further measures to restore and maintain function. Advanced life support can be started when appropriate equipment is available.

Airway and ventilation

When there is sudden loss of consciousness, apnoea or absent pulses, patency of the airway and the presence or absence of ventilation should be checked immediately. Any movement of the chest or abdomen during attempted inspiration indicates that the respiratory centre in the brain stem is still capable of generating respiratory drive. Paradoxical respiration, indrawing rather than expansion of the chest wall during inspiratory effort, immediately signifies airway obstruction. Likewise, noisy breathing suggests partial obstruction. Both airway and ventilation should be checked simultaneously. The quickest way to do this is to lift the chin upwards with the fingers of one hand while checking for expired gas impinging on the palm. At the same time, observation of chest movement allows a rapid decision as to whether respiration is adequate. The well-known first aid techniques to improve the upper airway in the supine position (backward head tilt, jaw thrust and chin lift) may be all that are necessary to avert respiratory arrest in early obstruction. All of these manoeuvres extend the atlanto-occipital joint and flex the neck slightly to attain the so-called 'sniffing position'. It is not necessary, particularly in small infants whose heads are relatively large, to place an object beneath the head, neck or shoulder to achieve this position. Hyperextension of the head and extension of the neck may compromise the airway and should be avoided. If respiratory effort is present, but obstructed, and not improved by the above first-aid measures, the pharynx should be inspected and any obstructing material removed, by turning the patient on the side or by sweeping the pharynx with a finger. If available, a laryngoscope and suction should be used. Expired air resuscitation by a mouth-to-mouth technique for children or a mouth to mouth-and-nose technique for infants should be given until resuscitation equipment is available. Care should be taken to protect the operator whenever possible, for example, by the use of latex rubber gloves and eye glasses.

In hospital areas where resuscitation equipment should be close at hand, such as in the operating or procedural theatres, anaesthetic induction rooms, emergency departments and wards, the patient should be ventilated with oxygen using a resuscitation bag (Laerdal, Ambu, Air Viva), mask and oropharyngeal airway. Early tracheal intubation is desirable, unless rapid recovery occurs. Intubation not only maintains and secures the airway, but also allows tracheal and bronchial suction and protects from further contamination. The lungs can be ventilated with oxygen without risk of gastric dilatation, and some resuscitation drugs can be instilled into the trachea.

Bag and mask ventilation, the use of an oropharyngeal airway and intubation are described in Chapter 7. Equipment appropriate to the size and age of infants and children is described in Chapter 3. It is essential that appropriate equipment of all the different sizes that may be needed is readily available. All personnel who work in areas where there are children who are sick or at risk of cardiorespiratory arrest must be thoroughly trained in the use of such resuscitation equipment.

The first few breaths of ventilation for resuscitation should have a prolonged inspiratory phase, to ensure that the lungs are as near to normally inflated as possible.

If tracheal intubation is difficult, it is better to ventilate the patient with oxygen, using bag and mask, than to allow hypoxia during repeated, unsuccessful attempts at intubation. In the hurried and sometimes flustered circumstances of cardiopulmonary resuscitation, care must be taken to ensure that the tube enters the trachea rather than the oesophagus and does not subsequently slip out of the larynx or enter a bronchus. The endotracheal tube should be tied securely in place to prevent both accidental extubation and bronchial intubation. Table 35.1 gives the appropriate size and length of insertion of endotracheal tubes [3]. The correct size of tube is one that enters the trachea without much resistance, and allows adequate ventilation of the lungs with unobstructed expiration. There should be a small audible leak of gas around the endotracheal tube when the lungs are inflated using moderate pressure ($20-25$ cmH$_2$O). If the tube is too large, ischaemic or traumatic damage to the tracheal mucosa may occur. High ventilation pressure (>30 cmH$_2$O) may be needed during simultaneous external cardiac compression, or when there is severe lung disease.

If cardiorespiratory arrest is the result of airway obstruction at or above the vocal cords (supraglottic), which cannot be relieved by posture or intubation, emergency cricothyrotomy or tracheostomy may be needed. Special cricothyrotomy apparatus is available for near-adult size children, but a relatively large-bore ($14-12$ SWG) intravenous cannula can be used.

Circulation

The pulse should be assessed by palpation of the carotid artery in children, or the brachial or femoral artery in small infants. Inaudible or faint heart sounds indicate absent or poor cardiac output. In the absence of pulse or heart sounds, or if there is severe hypotension or bradycardia, external cardiac compression should be started at once. If two persons are resuscitating, ventilation and

Table 35.1 Guide to oral endotracheal tube size and length (lips to mid-trachea) according to weight and/or age

Body weight/age	Size (internal diameter) (mm)	Length (mm)
1000 g/27 weeks' gestation	2.5	6.5
2000 g/34 weeks' gestation	3.0	8.0
3500 g/40 weeks' gestation	3.0	9.5
1–6 months	3.5	11.0
6–12 months	4.0	12.0
1–2 years	4.5	13.0
3–4 years	5.0	13.5–14.0
5–6 years	5.5	14.5–15.0
6–7 years	6.0	15.0–15.5
8–9 years	6.5	16.0–16.5
9–10 years	7.0	16.5–17.0
11–12 years	7.5	17.5–18.0
12–15 years	8.0	18.0–19.5

cardiac compression should be in a ratio of 1:5. With single-person resuscitation, the ratio of ventilation and external cardiac compression should be 2:15. These ratios apply at all ages [4]. The first breaths should have a prolonged inspiratory phase, to ensure initial inflation of the lungs. Thereafter, ventilation should be interposed in the external cardiac compression sequence so that both ventilation and compression are effective. This is important because during simultaneous ventilation and compression, it is difficult to judge whether ventilation is expanding the chest. The recommended rates of external cardiac compression and ventilation per minute for the different age groups are given in Table 35.2. The recommended depths of compression are: newborn 2−3 cm, infants and small children 2.5−4 cm, and for large children and teenagers 3−5 cm.

Strictly coordinated compression and ventilation is not essential when using an endotracheal or tracheostomy tube, because movement of the chest and compliance are easier to estimate than during expired air resuscitation or bag and mask ventilation. It is possible to ventilate an intubated patient with simultaneous external cardiac compression. As blood flow is generated by external cardiac compression or by positive pressure ventilation, which raises intrathoracic pressure, there may be more flow when they are simultaneous [5]. The heart functions as a conduit rather than as a valved pump during cardiopulmonary resuscitation [6]. The direction of blood flow is determined not by the cardiac valves, but by the different resistances of the great vessels entering and leaving the heart. The aorta and pulmonary artery offer less resistance to flow than the collapsed great veins, so that blood flows in the desired direction. The direction of flow also depends on the valves of major veins entering the thorax, which prevent backflow. Nevertheless, until there is clinical evidence to support changes in the routine of CPR it is best to use the ratios of external cardiac compression and ventilation recommended in Table 35.2.

External cardiac compression should be confined to the lower sternum to prevent rib fractures, pneumothorax and damage to abdominal organs. Compression should be of a squeezing nature, not a sharp blow. Each compression should occupy half of the compression–relaxation cycle. The technique of external cardiac compression varies with the age of the patient, but compression should always be applied only to the lower half of the sternum [4]. Good compression technique can achieve 30−40% of the patient's basal cardiac output, with a systolic arterial pressure near normal. In newborns, the index and middle fingers of one hand are used (Fig. 35.1), pressing vertically on the lower sternum. Alternatively, in a two-handed technique, both thumbs compress the sternum (Fig. 35.2). Higher blood pressure is obtained with the latter method [7], but care is needed to avoid restriction of chest expansion during ventilation. Obviously, this technique is only applicable to newborns

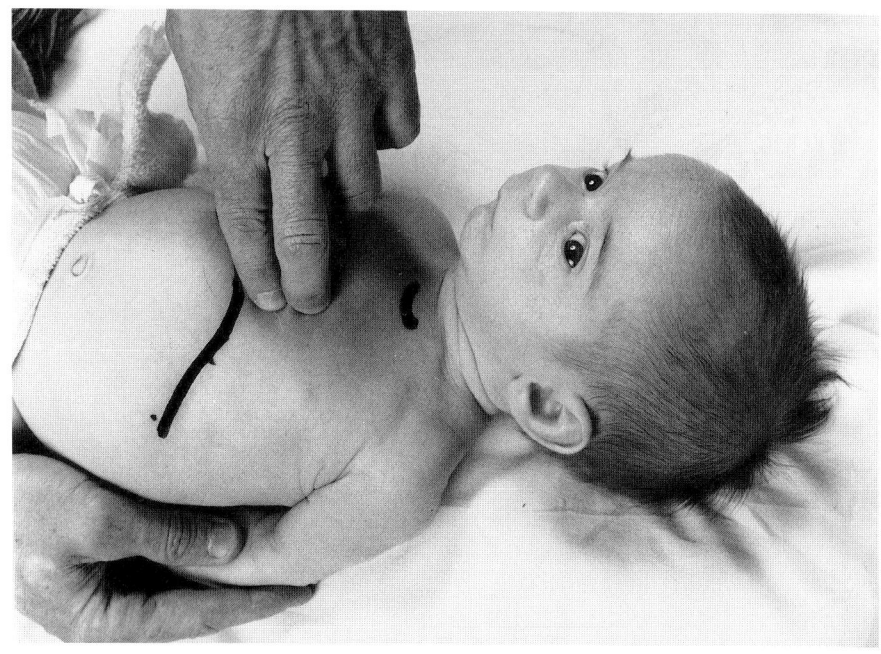

Fig. 35.1 External cardiac compression in a newborn with two fingers compressing the lower half of the sternum.

Table 35.2 Guide to ventilation—compression rates per minute in basic life support for a large child/teenager, small child/infant and newborn

	Large child/ teenager	Small child/ infant	Newborn
Two-person resuscitation			
Ventilation	16	20	24—30
Compression	80—100	100	120—150
(ratio 1:5)			
One-person resuscitation			
Ventilation	8—12	12	16
Compression	60—90	90	120
(ratio 2:15)			

and smaller infants. In infants up to the age of 12 months, the sternum may be compressed with all four fingers aligned over the lower sternum (Fig. 35.3). For small children over 1 year old, the heel (thenar and hypothenar eminences) of one hand is used (Fig. 35.4). In larger children and teenagers, the technique is the usual bimanual method applied to adults. In all patients, the compression should be applied vertically to the lower sternum, with the patient supine on a firm surface.

The effectiveness of external cardiac compression should be assessed regularly by feeling a pulse. It should be remembered that the pulse is a pressure wave and does not necessarily mean adequate blood flow. The latter is shown by normal colour and perfusion of skin and mucous membranes. External cardiac compression should be continued until adequate pulse rate, blood pressure and perfusion are restored. The perfusion may be restored spontaneously or need support by injections or infusions of drugs. Both effective cardiac output and ventilation are essential; one without the other is useless. Direct cardiac compression via thoracotomy may be appropriate in special circumstances, such as following cardiac surgery, when the chest can be easily re-opened.

Treatment of dysrhythmia

A routine precordial thump is not recommended for paediatric cardiopulmonary resuscitation, because ventricular fibrillation is rare as a primary dysrhythmia. The electrocardiogram is essential to determine the cardiac rhythm before drugs are used. The size (weight) of the child determines the dose of all drugs and of DC shock. Life-threatening dysrhythmia requiring immediate treatment may be severe bradycardia/asystole, ventricular fibrillation or electromechanical dissociation. The management of these is discussed below and presented in Table 35.3.

BRADYCARDIA/ASYSTOLE

This is the usual finding in cardiac arrest in children. The drugs of choice are catecholamines with predominant

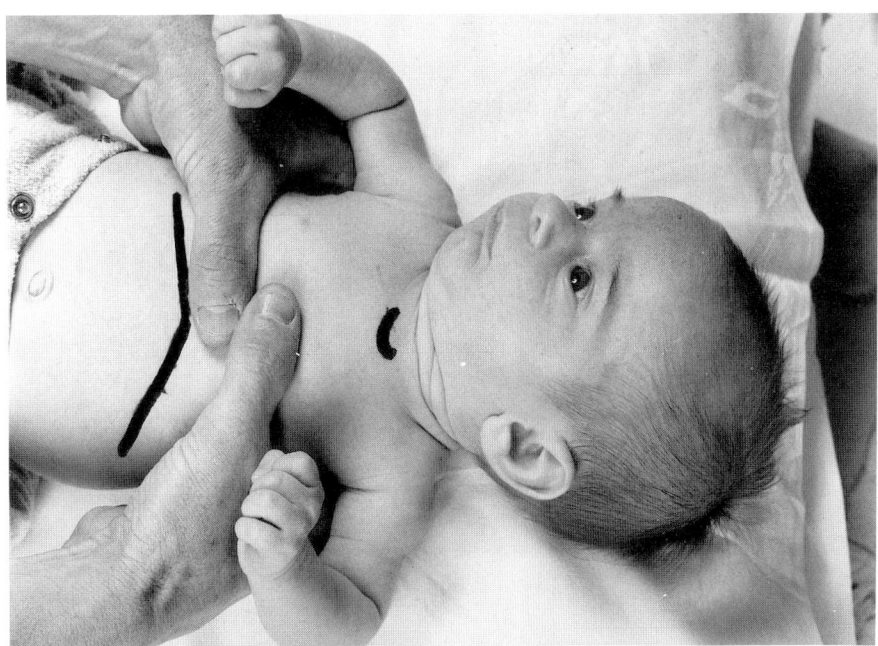

Fig. 35.2 External cardiac compression in a newborn supporting the back with the fingers and compressing the lower half of the sternum with the thumbs.

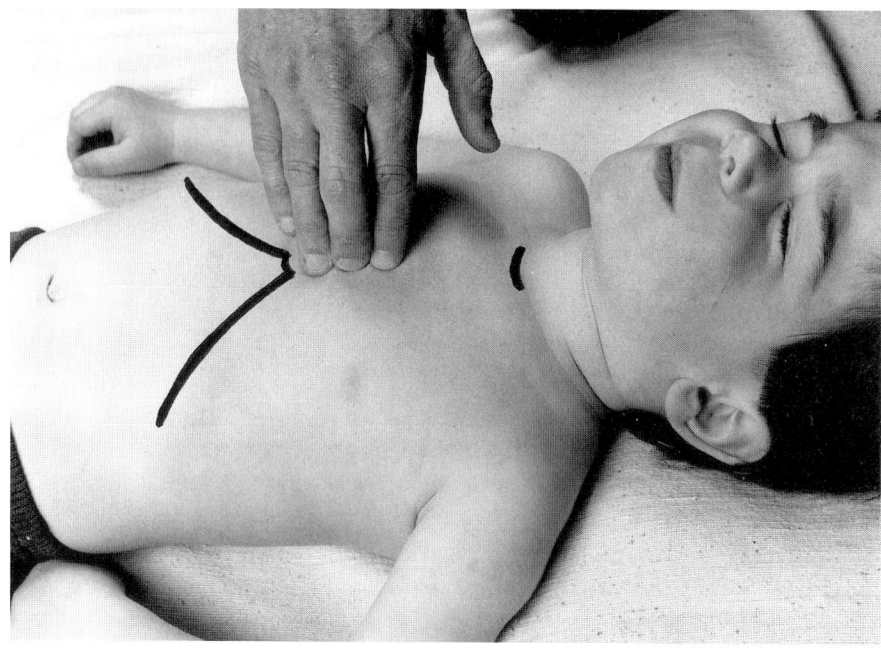

Fig. 35.3 External cardiac compression in infants up to 12 months is achieved by compressing the lower half of the sternum with three or four fingers.

alpha-agonistic activity, because the vasoconstriction and rise in diastolic pressure improve coronary and cerebral perfusion. Adrenaline is most often used. The initial dose is 0.01 mg/kg intravenously, although much higher doses (up to 0.2 mg/kg) [8], repeatedly, may be needed, or an infusion of 0.1–1.0 µg/kg/min. Similar drugs, such as methoxamine, dopamine and noradrenaline, may be

useful. Isoprenaline, a beta-agonist without substantial alpha effects, should not be used because its peripheral vasodilation shunts bloods away from vital organs, although it may be a second choice (after atropine) to treat normotensive, mild-to-moderate bradycardia. If asystole, confirmed by ECG, does not respond to external cardiac compression, ventilation with oxygen and re-

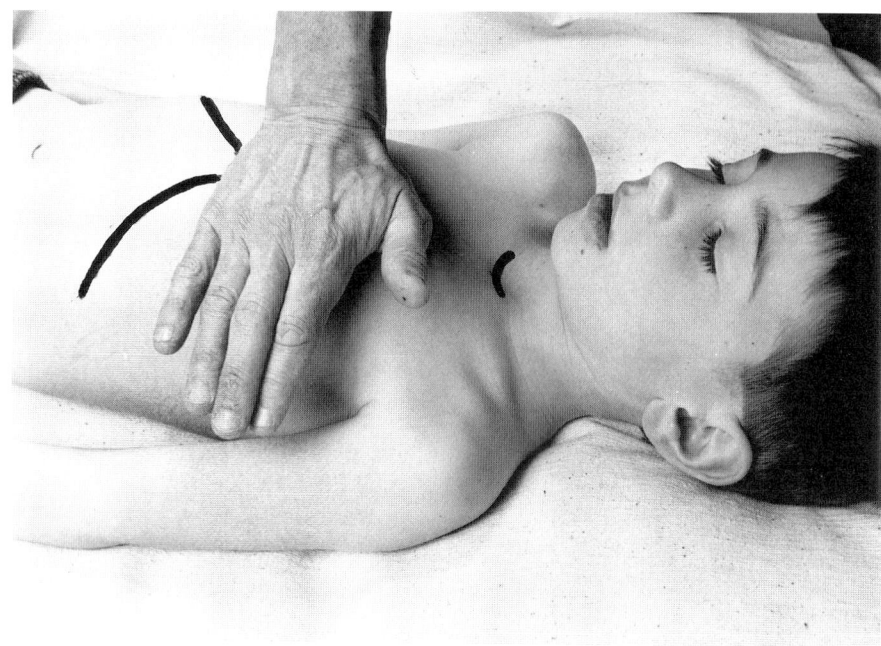

Fig. 35.4 External cardiac compression in a child compressing the lower sternum with the heel (thenar and hypothenar eminences) of the hand.

Table 35.3 Management of life-threatening dysrhythmia

Asystole	Ventricular fibrillation	Electromechanical dissociation
Basic CPR ↓ Intubate, ventilate O$_2$, i.v. access ↓ Adrenaline i.v. or tracheal 0.02−0.2 mg/kg × 3 ↓ Sodium bicarbonate i.v. 0.5−1 mmol/kg ↓ Adrenaline i.v. or tracheal repeated/larger dose ↓ Atropine i.v. or tracheal 20 μg/kg ↓ Defibrillate 2−4 J/kg ↓ Consider stopping	Basic CPR ↓ Defibrillate 2−4 J/kg × 3 ↓ Intubate, ventilate with O$_2$, i.v. access ↓ Defibrillate 2−4 J/kg ↓ Adrenaline i.v. or tracheal 0.01−0.2 mg/ 0.01−0.2 mg/kg ↓ Defibrillate 2−4 J/kg ↓ Sodium bicarbonate i.v. 0.5−1 mmol/kg ↓ Defibrillate 2−4 J/kg ↓ Consider lignocaine, or bretylium, adrenaline and sodium bicarbonate before repeated defibrillation	Basic CPR ↓ Intubate, O$_2$ ventilate with O$_2$ i.v. access ↓ Adrenaline i.v. or tracheal 0.02−0.2 mg/kg ↓ Sodium bicarbonate i.v. 0.5−1 mmol/kg ↓ Adrenaline i.v. or tracheal repeated/larger dose ↓ Calcium chloride 0.2 ml/kg 10% ↓ Exclude hypovolaemia, pneumothorax, pericardial tamponade

peated doses of adrenaline, atropine (10−20 μg/kg) may be useful. If asystole does not respond to treatment, other factors should be considered. Fine ventricular fibrillation may simulate asystole, but DC shock should be applied [9]. Misconnection or malfunction of the electrocardiograph must be excluded. Cardiac pacing (transcutaneous, oesophageal, transvenous) may be required when other means fail [10].

VENTRICULAR FIBRILLATION

Ventricular fibrillation or ventricular tachycardia with low cardiac output should be treated by immediate countershock with 2−4 J/kg body weight although 5 J/kg are often used. The electrodes should be adequately coated with conductive gel and correctly placed: one to the right of the upper sternum below the clavicle, and the other in the left anterior axillary line at the level of the xiphoid or nipple. The defibrillator setting must be 'unsynchronized'. If defibrillation is unsuccessful, a further attempt may be made with one electrode over the left precordium and the other over the back behind the heart. If still unsuccessful, another defibrillator should be tried. Defibrillators should have paddles 8 cm in diameter for children and 4.5 cm for infants.

Several drugs may be useful in the treatment of refractory ventricular fibrillation. Adrenaline was previously considered to be helpful in the treatment of fine fibrillation because of its ability to the 'coarsen' fibrillation. However, adrenaline is beneficial in both fine and coarse fibrillation because it improves coronary perfusion pressure and so lowers the threshold for successful defibrillation. Lignocaine (1 mg/kg) has been used for refractory fibrillation because of its membrane-stabilizing property. Other drugs, such as bretylium tosylate (5 mg/kg), may also be useful, although not proven to be more effective than lignocaine.

ELECTROMECHANICAL DISSOCIATION

Regular QRS complexes without palpable pulses indicate that the heart is able to generate and conduct electrical activity but has little or no output, resulting in severe hypotension. Adrenaline or other catecholamines with vasopressor and/or inotropic action may remedy poor contractility. Repeated doses (0.01 mg/kg every few minutes) or an infusion (0.1−1.0 μg/kg/min) of adrenaline may be needed.

Poor cardiac output may be due to other causes, such as hypovolaemia, pneumothorax, pericardial tamponade or cardiac rupture. Each of these conditions requires specific correction, but temporary improvement may follow an increase in cardiac filling pressure from rapid infusion of 10 ml/kg of colloidal fluid, while preparations are made to treat the problem. Obstruction of cardiac outflow can also result in electromechanical dissociation. This may occur as a result of pulmonary embolism or acute infundibular obstruction, as in Fallot's tetralogy (see Chapter 13).

Other drugs

Sodium bicarbonate has not been used as readily in recent years as in the past to buffer metabolic acidosis in acute cardiopulmonary resuscitation. The deleterious effects of reduced extracellular hydrogen ion concentration and paradoxical increase in intracellular hydrogen ion have been recognized. Bicarbonate reacts with acid to form carbon dioxide, which enters cells more readily than bicarbonate. It follows that ventilation should be adequate before sodium bicarbonate is given. Controlled ventilation is most important in combating the combined respiratory and metabolic acidosis of cardiorespiratory arrest. Further problems derive from the use of hyperosmolar solutions of sodium bicarbonate (8.4%). Despite the disadvantages of sodium bicarbonate, there is still a place for it in severe or prolonged cardiac arrest. Marked increase in extracellular hydrogen ion concentration impairs myocardial contractility and reduces the effectiveness of defibrillation. An appropriate initial dose would be 0.5−1.0 mmol/kg. In prolonged resuscitation, further doses are given according to acid−base analysis when the dose (mmol) equals body weight (kg) multiplied by base deficit (mmol/l) multiplied by 0.2. Sodium bicarbonate should not be mixed with calcium salts because precipitation occurs, or with adrenaline because of deactivation.

Calcium salts are sometimes useful as vasopressors during hypotension, as either inotropic or vasoconstrictor agents. An appropriate bolus dose would be 5−7 mg/kg of elemental calcium (0.2 ml/kg of 10% calcium chloride or 0.7 ml/kg of 10% calcium gluconate). An infusion of 0.2 ml/kg/h of 10% calcium chloride may be necessary to maintain blood pressure. Despite frequent use, there is little or no evidence to support the efficacy of calcium salts in the management of dysrhythmia. The value of calcium salts during electromechanical dissociation is doubtful. Calcium preparations have no place in the treatment of asystole or ventricular fibrillation, but they have a definite place in the management of calcium channel blocker toxicity, hypocalcaemia and hyperkalaemia.

Drugs such as beta-adrenergic blocking agents, digoxin, amiodarone and phenytoin are rarely required urgently in the cardiopulmonary resuscitation of infants and children.

Routes of drug administration

Drugs may be administered by several routes:

INTRAVENOUS

All drugs should be administered intravenously during CPR — preferably by a central vein, since the time taken to reach the heart is much less than from a peripheral vein. It is hazardous and difficult to attempt to cannulate a central vein during initial cardiopulmonary resuscitation. On the other hand, the external jugular vein is usually quite prominent during CPR and is often the best choice, providing ready access to the central circulation and being relatively free of the complications of other central routes. For cannulation of this vein, the head should be turned to the opposite side with the neck in a neutral position.

The peripheral veins commonly used in infants and children are on the dorsum of the hand, the wrist, the cubital fossa, the ankle and the foot. In the newborn, the umbilical and scalp veins are useful and may be the preferred route for drug administration. Occasionally, the superior sagittal sinus may be used for emergency drug administration in newborns. Surgical cut-down may be useful, for example on the saphenous vein at the ankle. If access for intravenous therapy is not easily established, other routes should be used.

ENDOTRACHEAL

Adrenaline, atropine, lignocaine and naloxone may be given safely and effectively into the trachea. Maximum blood levels are reached as quickly as when a peripheral vein is used, but they are lower. The endotracheal doses should be approximately twice the intravenous. The drugs should be diluted in 0.9% sodium chloride to a volume of 1 ml for newborns, 3−5 ml for infants and small children and 5−10 ml for large children and teenagers. They should be injected into the endotracheal tube from a syringe without a needle, and dispersed throughout the respiratory tree by vigorous ventilation.

INTRAOSSEOUS

Bone marrow has a plentiful blood supply. The intramedullary vessels are patent, regardless of the state of the circulation. Before plastic catheters were available, metal cannulae were often used to infuse drugs or blood products and substitutes into the circulation via bone marrow. The intraosseous route is a valuable alternative, especially for the administration of fluids in hypovolaemia. Drugs injected into the marrow are distributed as fast and in the same concentrations as those injected intravenously [11]. Fat and bone-marrow pulmonary emboli are a frequent but minor consequence of intraosseous infusions [12].

In infants and children up to the age of 6 years, the proximal tibia over the anteromedial surface, at the junction of the upper one-third and lower two-thirds, is a suitable site. The distal tibia over the medial surface, proximal to the medial malleolus, can be used in all children and adults [13]. Both tibial sites are immediately subcutaneous, whereas the distal femur, another suitable site, is covered by muscle and fat. Special intraosseous infusion needles are manufactured. If not available, a short lumbar puncture needle (18, 20 gauge) will suffice. The needle is inserted perpendicular to the bone with a rotary action until there is loss of resistance. The required depth is usually about 1 cm.

INTRACARDIAC

If attempts at venous cannulation and tracheal intubation have both failed, the intracardiac route is an alternative. This route of drug administration may be used for the collapsed child when there is no-one skilled in tracheal intubation, especially if there is also hypovolaemia or hypothermia and the veins are collapsed. The technique is not without considerable risk of complications; these include coronary vessel laceration, pericardial tamponade, pneumothorax and myocardial damage from the needle or from injection into the muscle itself. Moreover, the technique requires that both external cardiac compression and ventilation be temporarily suspended. Pneumothorax may be avoided by injecting into the left ventricle very close to the sternum in the fourth or,

preferably, the fifth left interchondral space, where the lung is not directly behind the anterior thoracic wall (the cardiac notch). This also avoids the internal mammary artery and minimizes the risk to the anterior interventricular artery and the great cardiac vein. A narrow (22, 20 gauge) needle attached to a syringe containing the drug should be inserted vertically, and advanced with regular aspiration until blood appears in the syringe barrel. Care must be taken to prevent the injection of air, which might enter the coronary or cerebral circulation.

Further management

Resuscitation should be continued until spontaneous cardiac output and ventilation are adequate to maintain perfusion and oxygenation. Until such recovery, mechanical ventilation, oxygen therapy, inotropic support and control of cardiac rythm may be required. This may mean several, or even many, days of intensive therapy.

If, after about 45–60 minutes of resuscitation, there is no sign of response from the patient and if there are no reversible conditions, such as metabolic disturbance or hypothermia, termination of treatment can be considered.

In prolonged resuscitation, associated complications, such as abdominal and thoracic organ damage due to external cardiac compression, must be considered. Attention should be given to managing sequelae, such as cerebral oedema, fitting and renal failure. These are discussed in Chapter 36. Occasionally, the outcome of cardiopulmonary resuscitation will not be apparent for several days.

REFERENCES

1 Nichols D.G., Kettrick R.G., Swedlow D.B., Lee S., Passman R., Ludwig S. Factors influencing outcome of cardiopulmonary resuscitation in children. *Pediatr Emerg Care* 1986, **2**, 1.

2 Sanders A.B., Ewy G.A., Taft T.V. Prognostic and therapeutic importance of the aortic diastolic pressure in resuscitation from cardiac arrest. *Crit Care Med* 1984, **12**, 871.

3 Tibballs J. Practical aspects of advanced paediatric cardiopulmonary resuscitation. *Aust Paediatr J* 1988, **24**, 228.

4 Standards and guidelines for cardiopulmonary resuscitation (CPR) and emergency cardiac care (ECC). *JAMA* 1986, **255**, 2905.

5 Ewy G.A. Alternative approaches to external chest compression. *Circulation* 1986, **74**, IV–98.

6 Rudikoff M.T., Maughan W.L., Effron M., Freund P., Weisfeldt M.L. Mechanisms of blood flow during cardiopul-

monary resuscitation. *Circulation* 1980, **61**, 345.

7 David R. Closed chest cardiac massage in the newborn infant. *Pediatrics* 1988, **81**, 552.

8 Goetting M.G., Paradis N.A. High-dose epinephrine in refractory pediatric cardiac arrest. *Crit Care Med* 1989, **17**, 1258.

9 Chamberlain D.A. Advanced life support. *Br Med J* 1989, **299**, 446.

10 Dick M., Campbell R.M. Advances in the management of cardiac arrhythmias in children. *Pediatr Clin North Am* 1984, **31**, 1175–1195.

11 Orlowski J.P., Porembka D.T., Gallagher J.M., Lockrem J.D., Vanlante F. Comparison study of intraosseous, central intravenous and peripheral intravenous infusions of emergency drugs. *Am J Dis Child* 1990, **144**, 17.

12 Orlowski J.P., Julius C.J., Petros R.E., Porembka D.T., Gallagher J.M. The safety of intraosseous infusions: risks of fat and bone marrow emboli to the lungs. *Ann Emerg Med* 1989, **18**, 1062–1067.

13 Spivey W.H. Intraosseous infusions. *J Pediatr* 1987, **111**, 639.

36: Neurological Disorders Requiring Intensive Care

INTRODUCTION

The common neurological disorders of children that require intensive care are reviewed in this chapter. The physiology of the cerebral circulation, the formation of cerebrospinal fluid (CSF) and the determinants of intracranial pressure (ICP) have been dealt with in Chapter 14.

PATHOPHYSIOLOGY OF THE INJURED BRAIN

Several varieties of cerebral insult are commonly encountered in paediatric intensive care. A cerebral insult is one in which brain cells are temporarily or permanently damaged by events such as trauma, metabolic abnormality, especially hypoxia, or prolonged seizures. These have important effects on cerebral physiology.

Cerebral metabolism

When the brain is injured, the cerebral metabolic rate for oxygen is reduced roughly in proportion to the depth of coma, unless there are prolonged seizures. In some patients, cerebral blood flow is also reduced in parallel. In others, there is metabolic uncoupling and cerebral blood flow may actually increase (so-called 'luxury perfusion'), with an associated risk of cerebral oedema. Brain temperature also influences metabolic rate such that hypothermia protects against even lengthy periods of ischaemia, whereas hyperthermia may amplify cerebral damage, especially if blood flow is limited.

During hypoxia, anaerobic glycolysis produces only 5.5% of the adenosine triphosphate that is generated during aerobic conditions and is accompanied by production of lactic acid. During ischaemia, the absence of blood flow causes such toxic metabolites to accumulate. Hypoxia/ischaemia may occur locally or globally. When flow is restored after ischaemia, there may be residual perfusion abnormalities (the 'no reflow' phenomenon) which may prevent recovery.

Metabolic abnormalities may follow ischaemia. Failing membrane pumps are associated with elevated intracellular calcium, which appears to trigger a wide range of toxic metabolic reactions. Oxygen-free radicals and arachidonic acid metabolites produce further membrane damage. Hyperglycaemia may make matters worse by promoting intracerebral lactic acidosis.

Oedema

There are three types of cerebral oedema:
1 Cytotoxic oedema, which is cellular swelling secondary to local failure of sodium/potassium ATPase membrane pumps. It occurs in hypoxia—ischaemia, metabolic coma (e.g. hepatic failure) and as a result of some toxins.
2 Vasogenic oedema, which is due to disruption of the blood—brain barrier. Protein and water accumulate in the brain's extracellular spaces, especially in white matter. It occurs in trauma, prolonged ischaemia, infection and around tumours.
3 Interstitial oedema, which is an accumulation of interstitial fluid when there is obstructed drainage of CSF.

Both cytotoxic and vasogenic oedema are probably present to some degree when brain injury occurs. Oedema resolves by the restoration of cellular integrity and the blood—brain barrier, and possibly by drainage of interstitial fluid into ventricular CSF.

Intracranial hypertension

Increasing intracranial pressure is the complication most feared following cerebral insults. If detected, the accumulation of CSF (hydrocephalus) or a surface collection of blood may be readily treated. On the other hand, intracranial hypertension may be difficult to reverse if it follows vasodilatation, oedema or contusion. This may lead to global reduction of cerebral perfusion pressure, with consequent ischaemia and brain-stem compression due to cerebral herniation.

Seizures

The incidence of seizures after cerebral insults is much higher in children than in adults, especially after trauma and in meningitis and encephalitis. If seizures are not rapidly controlled, the dramatic increase in cerebral metabolic rate, coupled with the liberation of neurotoxic metabolites like glutamic acid, may considerably worsen the outcome of the primary injury.

Cerebral vasospasm

Deterioration in conscious state with focal neurological deficits, 6—7 days after an intracranial haemorrhage, is likely to be due to spasm of intracranial arteries. This spasm is caused by blood in the subarachnoid space. Deterioration due to other events, such as further bleeding, hydrocephalus, hypoxia and cerebral oedema (especially from hyponatraemia), should be excluded. Treatment consists of nimodipine infusion (15 μg/kg/h) for 2 hours then 15—45 μg/kg/h for 21 days. Normal hydration should be maintained and normal blood pressure ensured (if necessary with dopamine infusion).

MONITORING THE INJURED BRAIN

The ideal cerebral monitor would safely give continuous specific information about neuronal well-being. Such a device does not yet exist, so repeated clinical examination provides the best information at present.

Clinical signs

COMA

The level of consciousness is the most important monitor of the overall state of the brain. The Glasgow Coma Score (GCS) was described in an attempt to standardize neurological observations in head-injured patients, although it is equally useful in coma from other causes. The numerical score (see Table 36.1) allows grading of the depth of coma, and can be used for repeated assessment and for prognosis.

The scoring system is not without problems. An endotracheal tube makes verbal assessment impossible. Some patients will have spontaneous eye-opening in the ab-

Table 36.1 Modified Glasgow Coma Score

Score			
Best motor response to painful stimulus			
	>1 year	<1 year	
6	Obeys	Localizes pain	
5	Localizes pain	Withdrawal	
4	Withdrawal	Decorticate	
3	Decorticate	Decerebrate	
2	Decerebrate	Flaccid	
1	Flaccid		
Eye opening			
	>1 year	<1 year	
4	Spontaneous	Spontaneous	
3	To command	To shout	
2	To pain	To pain	
1	Nil	Nil	
Best verbal response			
	>5 years	2–5 years	0–2 years
5	Oriented/converses	Appropriate words	Appropriate smile/cry
4	Disoriented	Inappropriate words	Crying
3	Inappropriate words	Irritable cry	Irritable cry
2	Incomprehensible	Grunts	Grunts
1	Nil	Nil	Nil

Total: 3–15 points

sence of response to pain or verbal command. Alternatively, oculomotor nerve injury or periorbital swelling may prevent eye opening. In children, the GCS must be further modified; the assessment of response to command and the patient's verbal responses must be adjusted for age-dependent language skills. The best motor response to painful stimuli is the most reliable and accurate assessment of cerebral function. It should be remembered that the GCS is not a complete neurological examination. A careful history and detailed examination are also needed.

EYE SIGNS

Pupils

Although much is attributed to the size and speed of reaction to light, pupillary signs are often misleading. Constriction may be due to pontine haemorrhage or the effect of narcotics. Dilatation may be due to progressive brain-stem compression, or to local ocular trauma, mydriatic drugs or sympathetic stimulation from pain.

Retinal examination

Although papilloedema occurs with raised intracranial pressure, it is not usually seen in acute cerebral disturbances. Subhyaloid haemorrhages are seen in the presence of subarachnoid haemorrhage. Diffuse retinal haemorrhages are often seen in child abuse associated with violent shaking.

FOCAL NEUROLOGICAL SIGNS

Hemiparesis associated with increased muscle tone and upgoing plantar response is a sign of corticospinal tract injury. If accompanied by oculomotor nerve palsy, this is a warning of impending brain-stem compression needing immediate neurosurgical consultation.

Clinical signs may be difficult to interpret in the presence of sedatives, muscle relaxants or anasthetic drugs, so that additional monitoring techniques may be needed.

Investigations

BLOOD SUGAR

When the cause of coma is not clear, hypoglycaemia should be excluded and corrected, if present, by administration of 1 ml/kg of 50% dextrose i.v. The previous rate of dextrose administration should be increased and the blood sugar checked hourly for 2–4 hours. Hyperglycaemia due to excessive sugar loading should be avoided, as this may have a deleterious effect on outcome in conditions such as hypoxia/ischaemia.

OXYGEN AND CARBON DIOXIDE

Deterioration in conscious state may be due to hypoxaemia or hypercarbia, especially in the presence of cerebral oedema. Oxygen may need to be administered and the patient may need to be ventilated to ensure adequate CO_2 elimination.

COMPUTERIZED TOMOGRAPHY (CT)

CT scanning has revolutionized the diagnosis of cerebral lesions, particularly in trauma, although resolution in the posterior fossa is poor. If a CT scan is performed soon after an injury (within 1 hour), small areas of haemorrhage or early oedema may be missed. Therefore, if there is clinical deterioration, the scan should be repeated to detect evolving lesions.

The problems of this investigation include monitoring the airway, breathing and circulation inside the scanner in the supine position. These need careful management. The restless, semicomatose patient is more safely managed by general anaesthesia with positive pressure ventilation via an endotracheal tube, thus preventing airway obstruction, hypoventilation or pulmonary aspiration.

INTRACRANIAL PRESSURE (ICP)

Monitoring of ICP has not been shown to improve the outcome after neurological insults. However, as the technique allows continuous assessment, the effects of some aspects of treatment can be observed. It has an accepted place in the intensive care management of severe head trauma and Reye's syndrome. Its role in the care of hypoxic–ischaemic encephalopathy and meningitis is less clear. Several techniques are available.

Subdural

In the subdural method, a small hole is drilled through the skull and a hollow fluid-filled catheter or screw is placed below the dura. The multiple-hole subdural catheter is less prone to blockage than the screw. This is connected by a fluid column to an electronic strain-gauge transducer.

Ventricular

A soft catheter is placed directly into a lateral ventricle through a burr hole. In addition to measuring pressure, this technique allows removal of CSF as a means of lowering ICP and possibly assisting resolution of cerebral oedema (see Fig. 14.9). This method is probably the most accurate, but has a higher risk of infection, particularly ventriculitis.

Extradural

A small transducer is implanted in the extradural space, e.g. the Ladd monitor. This has the advantage of the lowest infection risk. However, the transducer cannot be recalibrated once implanted, and inaccurate readings may result from 'baseline drift'.

Measuring ICP allows calculation of the cerebral perfusion pressure (CPP) by subtracting ICP from mean arterial pressure. This can be used to evaluate the effects of management such as hyperventilation, positive endexpiratory pressure and tracheal suction. Accurate determination of CPP depends on the transducers for intracranial and arterial pressure both being referred to the same zero level (either the highest point of the skull or the external auditory meatus which is the level of the brain stem). An unexpected rise in ICP may be a sign of a space-occupying lesion, cerebral oedema, or of unrecognized seizures. Insertion of the ICP monitor itself may result in a haematoma. Persistent intracranial hypertension is associated with a poor prognosis (death or permanent disability).

The applications of ICP monitoring will be further discussed in the relevant clinical sections.

ELECTROENCEPHALOGRAPHY (EEG)

A formal 18-lead EEG may be performed to identify the nature of seizures and their origin, and for prognosis after a cerebral insult. Continuous modified EEG recordings (e.g. the frequency/amplitude cerebral function monitor and 'compressed spectral array' by Fourier analysis) may help to detect unrecognized seizures and estimate the level of consciousness of intensive-care patients paralysed by muscle relaxants.

Sensory evoked potentials are used to show the integrity of nerve pathways, and as an aid to prognosis after severe brain injury.

Global blood flow measurements can be made but may be too crude to be useful. Regional measurements provide more data but it is yet to be shown that these are clinically relevant. Thus, there has been much interest in techniques which allow some assessment of cerebral metabolism. Jugular venous oxygen tension measurement with a catheter in the jugular bulb, coupled with measurement of cerebral blood flow, permits global assessment of hemispheric oxygen delivery and extraction. Specific metabolic defects of damaged areas may be detected by positron emission tomography, or by the newer bedside tests including magnetic resonance spectroscopy and near-infrared spectroscopy. This latter technique uses infrared radiation which can pass through a child's skull to examine the tissue redox state of cytochrome C oxidase, the terminal member of the electron transport chain. It has been used to investigate the cerebral effects of hypoxia in pre-term infants. All of the above techniques will need considerable development and investigation before they find a place in routine neurointensive care.

CRANIOSPINAL TRAUMA

Trauma is the leading cause of death in children over 1 year of age. Head injuries from road trauma account for at least 50% of these deaths. Falls and child abuse are important causes of serious head trauma in the domestic environment. Many deaths are preventable by appropriate supervision and safety measures, including well-fitting car seat restraints. Bicycle crash-helmets reduce the risk of serious head injury in cyclists by at least 85%.

Pathophysiology and patterns of injury

Short stature puts the child's head level with the front of motor vehicles. The relatively large head may be hit by the car and/or strike the road. Head injuries in children are not usually accompanied by major chest and abdominal trauma. Long-bone fractures are common and easily missed.

Injuries to the cervical spine occur in approximately 5% of paediatric head injuries. However, spinal cord trauma is rare in children with head injuries who reach hospital alive. This is because most cord injuries occur above the roots of the phrenic nerve; the resulting apnoea and circulatory collapse cause death prior to reaching hospital.

About 50% of children with cervical injuries have spinal cord injury without radiographic abnormality, because of the hypermobile joints, relatively heavy head and weak neck muscles. Approximately half of these have complete and permanent neurological deficits that may need long-term ventilatory support. Unstable lower cervical spine injuries are rare.

The pathophysiology of the injured brain was discussed earlier, but some specific features of cerebral trauma are identified here:

1 The typical response to head injury is diffuse brain swelling, usually as a result of generalized hyperaemia. The vasculature may still respond to $Paco_2$, so that hyperventilation may be used to lower intracranial pressure. In more severe trauma, there is usually primary neuronal disruption secondary to shearing forces, resulting in diffuse areas of petechial haemorrhage and the development of localized or generalized vasogenic oedema.

2 Autoregulation is disturbed and cerebral perfusion becomes pressure-dependent. Therefore, sympathetic nervous system stimulation causing arterial hypertension may increase the risk of cerebral oedema. On the other hand, hypotension may cause ischaemia in areas with marginal blood flow.

3 Children are less likely than adults to have intracranial collections of blood, such as extradural or subdural haematomata, that need surgical drainage after severe head trauma. The incidence is 25% or less compared with 40–50% in adults. In babies, whose heads are relatively large, hypovolaemia may result from intracranial haemorrhage.

4 The young child's softer skull provides little protection against forceful injuries. On the other hand, before the sutures close during the second year of life, the skull can expand to a limited degree, providing a more compliant system in the presence of brain swelling. Children with multiple 'eggshell' fractures from severe injuries may show considerable decompression from head expansion.

5 Seizures often follow immediately after paediatric head trauma or occur during the next week, but these are not predictive of later seizures.

Initial management

The first priority is the rapid assessment of problems with airway, breathing or circulation, with appropriate resuscitation. At the same time, rapid but comprehensive examination should determine the level of coma and the presence of localizing neurological signs (see 'Monitoring the Injured Brain', above). Note that if there have been seizures, these may further lower the GCS. Significant injuries of the face, spine, chest, abdomen, pelvis and long bones should be identified. Hypoxia should be presumed in all trauma patients. Oxygen should be given by face mask and pulse oximetry used during this phase. Examination of oculocephalic reflexes should not be performed until cervical spine damage has been excluded.

Diagnosis of spinal cord injury may be difficult in comatose patients. Absent limb movements with are-flexia, paradoxical movement of the chest and abdomen without airway obstruction, or apnoea with rhythmic flaring of the alae nasi and sternomastoid contraction suggest a spinal lesion. Priapism is common. There may also be hypotension (see below). The neck should be immobilized during resuscitation.

Child abuse should be considered when the injuries sustained seem inconsistent with the reported history, or when presentation to hospital is delayed. Physical signs such as bruising and skin markings in unusual patterns, or injuries to the mouth or genitalia, may indicate abuse. Bilateral retinal haemorrhages from violent to-and-fro shaking may be present.

If the airway or ventilation is inadequate, oxygenation by bag and mask should be followed by tracheal intubation. As unstable cervical spine fractures in children with head injuries are very rare, the risk of further cerebral damage from untreated respiratory failure exceeds the risk of spinal cord damage from intubation. Preference must be given to establishing adequate cerebral oxygen delivery, and the trachea should be carefully intubated with the minimum necessary head and neck movement. In the initial assessment, too much time is often wasted on examination of the fundi, with neglect of diagnosis and treatment of shock or respiratory failure.

Table 36.2 Causes of shock in paediatric trauma

Hypovolaemic
25–50% blood volume loss (= 20–40 ml/kg)

Distributive
Spinal cord transection
Brain-stem injury

Refractory
Continuing blood loss
Cardiac tamponade
Tension pneumothorax
Myocardial contusion

The causes of shock in paediatric trauma are shown in Table 36.2. Hypotension is a late sign of hypovolaemia due to the child's effective compensatory mechanisms. Tachycardia, pallor and slow capillary refill are important signs of reduced cardiac output. Hypotension in trauma should be assumed to be secondary to hypovolaemia until disproven. Blood loss may be from wounds, especially of the scalp, or concealed in the chest, abdomen, pelvis, long bones or skull. A large scalp laceration and one major bone fracture may account for the loss of 30% of the circulating blood volume, causing hypovolaemic shock.

Failure of the brain stem or high spinal-cord injury abolishes control of the sympathetic nervous system. The resulting hypotension is characterized by inappropriate bradycardia and cutaneous vasodilatation, with very poor tolerance of hypovolaemia. In children, cardiogenic shock after injury is most often due to pneumothorax or haemopneumothorax. The diagnosis is suggested by distended neck veins, unilateral chest expansion, and the downward displacement of abdominal viscera creating a subcostal sulcus.

Restoration of blood volume and cardiac output are necessary if the patient is hypovolaemic (see Chapters 26 and 34). If hypotension is not controlled by rapid volume expansion, an inotropic infusion should be used to restore reasonable coronary and cerebral perfusion pressure while the cause of refractory shock is investigated. Dopamine $1-30\,\mu g/kg/min$ or adrenaline $0.1-1\,\mu g/kg/min$ may be used.

A gastric tube should be inserted, as acute gastric dilatation is common in traumatized children, causing diaphragmatic embarrassment and the risk of aspiration. An orogastric tube should be used if there are facial injuries or a possible basal skull fracture, because a nasal tube may enter the cranial cavity.

Subsequent management

After the initial assessment and resuscitation, the need for mechanical ventilation, CT scan and neurosurgery must be considered.

MECHANICAL VENTILATION

This is needed if there is:
apnoea, respiratory failure or poor airway control;
rapidly worsening coma, or GCS < 8;
evidence of increasing intracranial hypertension with bradycardia, hypertension, and localizing signs.

Orotracheal intubation must be carried out as a rapid-sequence technique using thiopentone and suxamethonium with cricoid pressure, after oxygenation with bag and mask. Thiopentone should be used with caution if the patient is shocked. Neck movement should be avoided if there is any likelihood of cervical spine injury. If the base of the skull is intact, the oral tube may be replaced later by a nasal one. Sedation (with opioids and/or benzodiazepines) and non-depolarizing muscle relaxants should be used, if necessary, to facilitate ventilation and prevent straining, but will prevent further neurological examination.

These patients should also receive mannitol 0.25 g/kg i.v., and a urethral catheter should be inserted to monitor urine output.

CT SCAN

A cranial CT scan should be performed in patients with a modified GCS less than 10, and in those with focal neurological deficits. Before anaesthesia for major surgery to treat other injuries, a CT scan should be considered even in less severe head trauma. The scan may reveal areas of focal damage, mass lesions requiring drainage, brain swelling due to hyperaemia or oedema, and skull fractures.

If there is suspected spinal column or cord injury, plain X-rays of the spine should be supplemented by a CT scan to show cord involvement by haematoma, bone fragments and foreign bodies. In cases of spinal cord injury without radiological abnormality, metrizamide myelography with CT examination may reveal cord injury with soft tissue or disc involvement and dural tears. This is usually performed 24–48 hours after injury. If there is concern about significant intra-abdominal injury, a contrast abdominal CT scan can be performed at the same time.

NEUROSURGERY

Immediate consultation with a neurosurgeon is indicated in the presence of any collection of blood around or within the brain, hydrocephalus or a depressed skull fracture.

The intracranial pressure should be monitored in all children with a modified GCS less than 8, if significant cerebral swelling is present on CT examination and in those patients requiring drainage of intracranial haematoma.

Intensive care management

The ongoing care of the patient requires constant careful observation of the general and neurological status. The aim is to prevent secondary insults to the brain by ensuring cerebral oxygen delivery, and avoiding factors such as seizures or fever that increase intracranial pressure or cerebral oxygen consumption. In addition, efforts are made to detect and treat any deterioration early, in the hope of preventing further progression.

GENERAL CARE

Careful monitoring of oxygenation, respiratory pattern, blood pressure and neurological status are essential when the patient is breathing spontaneously. Controlled ventilation may be facilitated by long-acting muscle relaxants (e.g. pancuronium 0.1 mg/kg), i.v. by bolus, when needed, or by infusion and/or sedation using intravenous drugs such as morphine 30–50 µg/kg/h with midazolam 50–100 µg/kg/h so that coughing and straining do not increase blood pressure and oxygen consumption. The ICP should be monitored when muscle relaxants are used. The Pao_2 should be over 100 mmHg (13.3 kPa) and $Paco_2$ 30–35 mmHg (4–4.7 kPa). Additional sedation may be required to prevent increased ICP during endotracheal suction, physiotherapy or painful procedures. An intra-arterial catheter is needed for continuous measurement of blood pressure and sampling arterial blood. Efficacy of ventilation is monitored by continuous pulse oximetry and, if there is no significant alveolar–arterial gradient, capnography. Blood pressure should be maintained in the range that is normal for age, i.e. systolic pressure = (80 + 2 × age in years) mmHg. Surface cooling should be used if core temperature exceeds 38°C.

PREVENTION OF INTRACRANIAL HYPERTENSION

The head should be elevated to 30° and the head and neck kept midline to prevent jugular venous obstruction. After hypovolaemia has been corrected, fluids should be restricted to 30% of maintenance water requirements for as long as mechanical ventilation is needed.

SEIZURE PROPHYLAXIS

Because at least 30% of children with severe head injury have seizures in the first week, anticonvulsants are needed. Phenytoin, 20 mg/kg i.v. over 30 minutes, is followed by 3 mg/kg 8-hourly. This drug does not interfere with neurological assessment. Seizures in the patient paralysed with muscle relaxants may present as tachycardia, with hypertension and loss of pupillary reaction to light.

TREATMENT OF INTRACRANIAL HYPERTENSION

If ICP remains persistently higher than 15–20 mmHg (2–2.7 kPa), more aggressive therapy is used.

Hyperventilation

Hyperventilation (25–30 mmHg) lowers ICP by cerebral vasoconstriction, which reduces cerebral blood volume. The effect of hyperventilation is demonstrated clearly in Fig. 36.1. Hyperventilation is only useful for short periods to control acute rises in ICP, because CSF pH returns to normal after about 4 hours and the vasoconstriction wanes. Excessive hyperventilation may cause cerebral ischaemia and pulmonary barotrauma.

Diuresis

Mannitol 0.25 gm/kg i.v., repeated if necessary 1–2-hourly to a maximum plasma osmolality of 320 mmol/kg, usually lowers ICP. If the plasma osmolality rises above 320 mmol/kg, infusions of normal saline, lactated Ringer's solution or plasma will be hypotonic to the patient's extracellular fluid and cause brain swelling. Frusemide 0.5 mg/kg i.v. lowers ICP by its diuretic effect and, possibly, by reducing CSF formation; it may act synergistically with mannitol.

CSF removal

The drainage system is shown in Fig. 14.10. It is important not to drain all the CSF, as the ventricles may collapse around the catheter and prevent further drainage.

Barbiturate therapy

Although temporary reduction of cerebral oxygen consumption, blood volume and ICP occurs with bolus

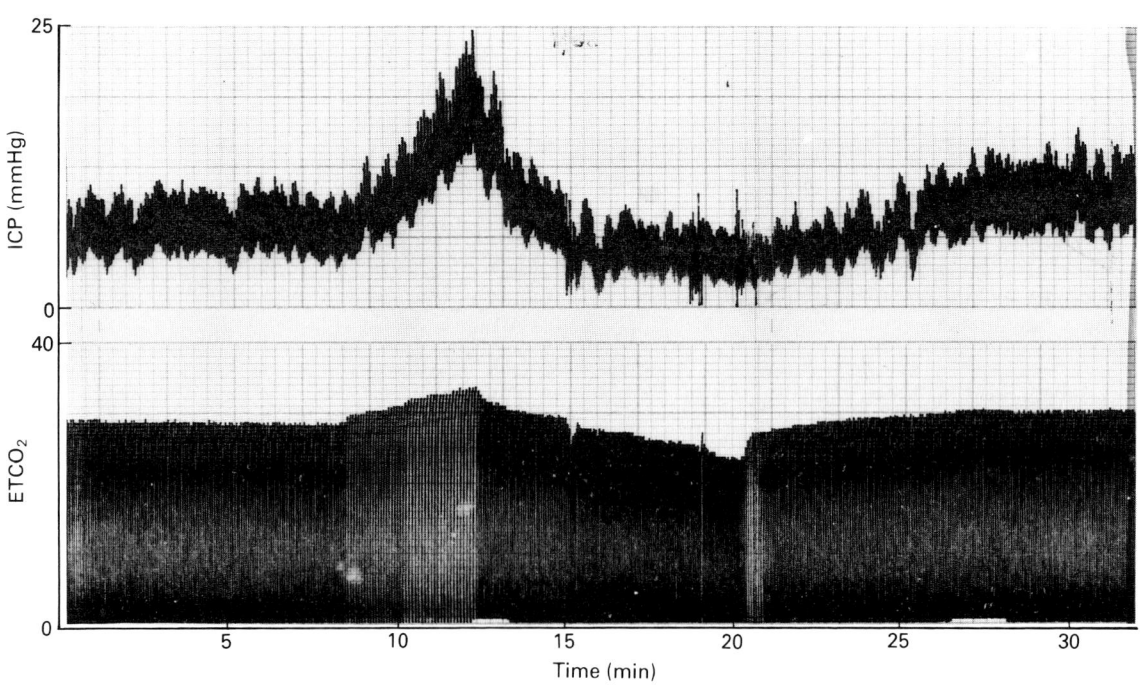

Fig. 36.1 Chart recording of intracranial pressure (ICP) and end-tidal carbon dioxide (both in mmHg) in a ventilated patient with severe head trauma. The small reduction in minute ventilation at 8 min causes the intracranial pressure to almost treble. At 12 min, ventilation is reset to the initial setting, and ICP returns to its baseline value by 15 min. Increased hyperventilation causes further reduction in ICP until 20 min, when the ventilator is again reset.

doses, there is no evidence of reduced morbidity or mortality with barbiturate infusions in severe paediatric head injury. There may be a role for barbiturates in some patients with progressive, diffuse swelling. The usual regimen is thiopentone, 1–5 mg/kg/h for 1–4 days.

Surgical decompression

Surgical decompression with bifrontal craniectomy is rarely used to treat intractable intracranial hypertension in head injury, but there have been anecdotal reports of its success. Some neurosurgeons will perform a craniectomy when a patient, whose initial neurologic and CT assessment was favourable, develops life-threatening brain swelling.

PROGNOSIS

The mortality of severe head injury in children, when the GCS is less than 8, is between 30% and 50%, little different from that in adults. However, in survivors with residual deficits, there may be progressive, sometimes remarkable, improvement over 6–12 months. The mortality in children with severe head trauma is increased as much as seven-fold if there is hypoxia, hypercarbia or hypotension on arrival at hospital. An initial GCS of 3 or 4, brain-stem reflex abnormalities and extensive cerebral bleeding or contusion are also indicators of increased mortality.

HYPOXIC–ISCHAEMIC ENCEPHALOPATHY

Aetiology

Hypoxic–ischaemic insults may be global or regional. Ischaemia causes coma in less than 10 seconds and permanent cerebral damage in as little as 2–3 minutes.

Hypoxic–ischaemic encephalopathy results when patients survive periods of inadequate ventilation or brain perfusion resulting in disruption of cerebral function. Common causes include head injury with shock or hypoxia, near drowning, asphyxia and poisoning (drugs, toxins or envenomation). Encephalopathy may follow any cardiac arrest where cardiac function is re-established after delayed or prolonged resuscitation.

The effect of active therapy on neuronal recovery after hypoxia or ischaemia has been questioned. The most important treatment is the immediate restoration of cardiac output and cerebral blood flow. At normal body temperatures, survival is unlikely after cardiac arrest if resuscitation is not started immediately, or if there is no spontaneous cardiac output on arrival at hospital. On the other hand, pre-existing hypothermia (below 30°C) or overdose with cerebral depressants lowers cerebral metabolic rate and may permit survival after cardiac arrest lasting as long as 20 minutes. It is possible that a form of the 'mammalian diving reflex' may contribute to protection of the brain in some cases of near drowning.

If the initial resuscitation is successful, subsequent therapy is directed to maintaining cerebral oxygen delivery and minimizing intracranial pressure, as discussed above. Cardiac dysfunction requiring inotropic support and hypovolaemia from bowel fluid loss ('ischaemic diarrhoea') are common after prolonged cardiac arrest. The stomach is often full of swallowed water after immersion or distended with air from attempted expired air resuscitation. It should be emptied with a gastric tube. Pulmonary dysfunction from aspiration of water or gastric contents is common, but severe damage, as seen in adult respiratory distress syndrome, is rare in children.

Children who recover consciousness soon after resuscitation have an excellent prognosis. Some patients awaken with 'cerebral irritability', needing sedation and close observation. Comatose patients with hypertonia or flaccidity and a Glasgow Coma Score of less than 8 may be best managed at first by mechanical ventilation, sedation and paralysis, although this is unproven. If the conscious level is not markedly improved in 1–2 days, a CT scan may help to diagnose cerebral oedema or areas of infarction. ICP measurement correlates poorly with outcome. Barbiturate coma and induced hypothermia are of no proven value and increase the risk of sepsis.

Prognosis

Those children who are flaccid or apnoeic after resuscitation and correction of body temperature are likely either to have serious neurological deficits or to die. Recovery is more likely in those who present comatose with flexion or extension response to pain. Patients with severe neurological deficits 1 week after hypoxia–ischaemia are much less likely to recover than those with similar lesions after head trauma.

SEIZURES

Aetiology

Inadequate anticonvulsant levels, or seizure threshold lowered by an intercurrent febrile illness in idiopathic epilepsy, are the commonest causes of childhood status epilepticus. Other children may have seizures during a febrile illness. These vary from a short, generalized seizure during a febrile illness to those who have complex seizures that last more than 10 minutes. In some patients a febrile seizure may last more than 30 minutes and be classified as status epilepticus.

Other major causes of seizures are cerebral infections (meningitis, encephalitis, abscess), trauma, hypoxia, ischaemia, and a variety of metabolic derangements, drugs and toxins.

Pathophysiology

BRAIN

Seizures increase the cerebral metabolic rate and cerebral blood flow, leading to the release of toxic metabolites. Seizures continue unabated beyond 45−60 minutes, and may cause generalized cerebral damage with diffuse swelling and neuronal loss. This is likely to be more severe if the seizures are accompanied by hypoxia, hypoventilation, hypotension or hyperthermia.

SYSTEMIC EFFECTS

Prolonged convulsions dramatically increase total body energy expenditure, oxygen consumption and carbon dioxide production. A mixed respiratory and metabolic acidosis is common. Multiple organ failure involving the kidneys and liver may result. Rhabdomyolysis has been described.

Therapy

The child presenting with status epilepticus must be treated as an emergency. Initial resuscitation is needed to restore and maintain cerebral oxygen delivery; the seizures should be controlled. Oxygen should be administered, and if convulsions persist despite anticonvulsant therapy, the patient may need to be intubated and ventilated.

The cause of seizures should be sought and treated while anticonvulsant therapy is initiated.

SEIZURE CONTROL

If hypoglycaemia is present or cannot be rapidly excluded, 1 ml/kg of 50% dextrose should be given intravenously.

Diazepam 0.1−0.2 mg/kg i.v. may be repeated up to 0.5 mg/kg. As an alternative, it may be given per rectum using a small catheter, but up to twice the intravenous dose may be required. Respiratory depression needing controlled ventilation is common when maximal doses are used. An injectable form of Lorazepam has been developed, and may have a role.

Phenytoin 20 mg/kg i.v. is given slowly over 20 minutes to avoid hypotension and arrhythmias. A common reason for failure to control seizures is inadequate dosage, e.g. 10 mg/kg. This drug should be given in 0.9% saline as it precipitates in dextrose solutions. Subsequent doses of 3 mg/kg 8-hourly should be monitored by blood levels (10−20 µg/ml).

If control is not achieved with diazepam and phenytoin, thiopentone may be used to terminate the seizures, in a dose range from 2−5 mg/kg as an i.v. bolus, followed by an infusion of 2−5 mg/kg/h. Controlled ventilation will usually be needed after oxygenation and intubation with suxamethonium and cricoid pressure. Unwanted effects include hypotension from vasodilatation and myocardial depression, and may be corrected by intravascular volume expansion and inotropic drug infusion, e.g. dopamine. Subcutaneous extravasation is a hazard.

Paraldehyde, 0.2 ml/kg (in a glass syringe) intramuscularly or rectally, is a useful alternative if intravenous access cannot be obtained. It may also be given intravenously, with caution.

Prolonged use of muscle relaxants is not indicated in status epilepticus, as it does not prevent neuronal injury but does prevent observers discovering that seizures are continuing.

The cause of seizures must be sought and treated. It should be remembered that epileptic patients may develop conditions such as meningitis or drug poisoning, which need treatment. If the core temperature is raised, surface cooling should be used to lower seizure threshold. Significant complications (see 'Pathophysiology' below) are more likely when seizures last more than 1 hour, especially if they are accompanied by hypoxaemia.

BACTERIAL MENINGITIS

Meningitis remains one of the important causes of death and permanent neurological impairment in infants and children. There has been little change in mortality since the introduction of antibiotics.

Pathophysiology

After the first 3 months of life, the common infecting organisms are *Haemophilus influenzae* type B, *Neisseria meningitidis* and *Streptococcus pneumoniae*. A child with the clinical features of meningitis but an atypical history, with slow onset and lower cranial nerve lesions, should alert one to the possibility of tuberculous meningitis, sometimes missed because it is no longer common in affluent societies. Children with meningeal or neural tube defects are at significantly greater risk for developing meningitis, as are others with CSF shunts. Neonatal meningitis is usually caused by *Escherichia coli*, group B beta haemolytic streptococci, and *Listeria monocytogenes*.

The pathological changes include pyogenic inflammation of the meninges, and, in severe cases, infective vasculitis of the superficial cortical layers. This may lead to brain swelling, small-vessel thrombosis and areas of infarction. Subdural effusion and empyema may develop.

Diagnosis

The diagnosis of meningitis requires a high index of suspicion. Older children may have fever, headache, altered conscious state, photophobia and signs of meningeal irritation with neck stiffness. Neonates and infants usually have non-specific symptoms such as lethargy, reduced muscle tone and poor feeding. The fontanelle may be tense, reflecting raised intracranial pressure. There may be signs of septic shock (see Chapter 34).

The diagnosis should be confirmed by lumbar puncture in mildly ill patients. When the patient is severely ill, with coma, shock or evidence of raised intracranial pressure, antibiotics should be given after blood for culture and urine for bacterial antigen have been collected. Lumbar puncture should be delayed until improvement occurs, because of the risk of coning. The cerebrospinal fluid should be examined for pleocytosis, elevated protein and low glucose. Rapid identification of the pathogens can be made by Gram stain and latex particle agglutination before the results of culture and sensitivity are available. CT scan will identify brain swelling in severely ill children.

Management

The first priorities should be the resuscitation of airway, breathing and circulation, and control of seizures; antibiotics are then given. Once hypovolaemia has been corrected, fluids should be restricted to one-third of normal water maintenance or less for at least 2−3 days. This is because inflammation at the base of the brain often leads to 'inappropriate' secretion of antidiuretic hormone, causing severe hyponatraemia with seizures, cerebral oedema and death.

Until antibiotic sensitivities are known, paediatric meningitis should be treated with benzylpenicillin 60 mg/ kg i.v. 4-hourly, and cefotaxime 50 mg/kg i.v. 6-hourly. The development of resistant strains of *Haemophilus* has led to these drugs superseding chloramphenicol and amoxycillin. In neonatal meningitis, amoxycillin 100−200 mg/kg and cefotaxime 150−200 mg/kg i.v. per day are used. The appropriate antibiotic, depending on clinical response and bacterial sensitivities, is continued for 14 days. There may be a role for steroids (e.g. dexamethasone 0.6 mg/kg/day for 4 days) to reduce the inflammatory response and avoid subsequent deafness.

The use of ICP monitoring in meningitis is controversial. Reduction in fontanelle tension reassures the clinician that brain swelling is improving, but invasive measurement of intracranial pressure (ICP) in older children has not been shown to improve morbidity or mortality.

The household contacts of patients with meningococcal disease, and of those patients with haemophilus infection with siblings less than 5 years old, should receive prophylactic antibiotic treatment with oral rifampicin to eradicate the carrier state. Rifampicin is potentially teratogenic; pregnant contacts can be safely treated with a single intravenous dose of ceftriaxone.

Prognosis

Persistently abnormal neurological signs, intractable generalized or focal seizures and prolonged coma all suggest structural brain damage. A CT scan may reveal cerebral oedema, infarction or subdural effusion. The need for mechanical ventilation is associated with a high mortality.

HERPES SIMPLEX ENCEPHALITIS

Aetiology and clinical features

Viral encephalitis after the newborn period is most commonly caused by herpes simplex virus type 1, but herpes encephalitis in the newborn is mostly acquired from the birth canal. In the newborn, there may be infection of the whole brain, but in infancy and childhood herpes encephalitis mostly involves the temporal and orbito-frontal areas of the brain. The encephalitis presents with fever, headache, altered consciousness and focal or generalized seizures. There may be cranial nerve palsies, hemiparesis, asymmetrical reflexes and papilloedema. Untreated herpes simplex encephalitis progresses to brain swelling, coma and death in 70% of cases.

Diagnosis

This is based on clinical suspicion. CSF may show pleocytosis (mostly lymphocytes), but may be normal at first. It should be cultured for the virus. Lumbar puncture must not be performed if there is any suggestion of brain oedema. EEG may show temporal lobe abnormality and can be useful if the diagnosis is uncertain. Brain biopsy is not justified.

Management

A child with a history suggesting herpes simplex encephalitis should be given acyclovir 10 mg/kg 8-hourly i.v., especially if there is fever or pleocytosis. Fluid intake is restricted to 30% of maintenance during any phase of acute brain swelling. If there are clinical or CT signs of brain swelling, the child should be intubated for moderate hyperventilation, sedated and nursed with a 20° head-up tilt.

GUILLAIN−BARRÉ SYNDROME

Aetiology and clinical features

Guillain−Barré Syndrome is the most common cause of acute motor paralysis in children. There is inflammation of nerves with lymphocytic infiltration and demyelination. It is believed to have an autoimmune basis, because it often follows a viral infection and antibodies to myelin can be identified in blood.

In a typical case, there is ascending symmetrical areflexic weakness, often associated with muscle pain. There may be paraesthesiae and sensory loss. There are numerous variants of the disease. There may be asymmetric or descending weakness, or cranial nerve involvement may predominate with associated ataxia (Miller−Fischer type). Autonomic nerve involvement is common. Papilloedema and encephalopathy occasionally occur.

Diagnosis

Diagnosis depends on the presence of progressive areflexic motor weakness with a low CSF cell count (<50 monocytes or 2 neutrophils) and exclusion of differential diagnoses. These include myasthenia gravis, botulism, poliomyelitis, other neuropathy, myopathy, envenomation (tick, snake) and poisoning (lead, arsenic and organophosphate insecticides). The CSF protein is usually elevated after 1 week, but may be normal before this.

Management

Many patients are managed with symptomatic treatment because of the mild nature of their disease, but the condition frequently progresses to bulbar palsy or respiratory failure needing intubation and mechanical ventilation. In young children, vital capacity is an unreliable predictor of the need for respiratory support. The decision to intubate and ventilate these children depends on clinical judgement, in which fatigue, respiratory reserve, adequacy of cough and bulbar function are assessed, assisted by pulse oximetry. In older children, intubation and mechanical ventilation are indicated when vital capacity is less than 15 ml/kg. Up to one-third of patients require ventilatory support.

Morbidity and mortality are reduced by good respiratory care, which involves carefully monitored ventilation, adequate humidification, endotracheal suction and chest physiotherapy. If, after 1 week, there is little improvement, a tracheostomy should be performed, as this is more comfortable for the patient and the reduction in anatomical dead space facilitates weaning from mechanical ventilation. Successful weaning is unlikely until vital capacity exceeds 12 ml/kg, maximum negative inspiratory force is at least 20 cmH$_2$O and there is return of bulbar function. Autonomic dysfunction has been described in children with Guillain−Barré syndrome, although serious cardiovascular disturbances (e.g. ventricular arrhythmias or hypotension) seem to be less of a problem than in adults. Great caution should be exercised when inducing anaesthesia, or using drugs known to stimulate or depress the cardiovascular system. Suxamethonium should not be used because, as in other denervating conditions, it may cause severe hyperkalaemia. Urine retention and gut dysfunction also occur.

The overall care of the patient needs a co-ordinated approach, taking the needs of a young child into account. It is as important to communicate with a young child in order to allay fear, control pain, and provide activities and mental stimulation, as it is to prevent pressure sores, maintain joint mobility etc.

Treatment of Guillain–Barré syndrome is changing. There is good evidence that plasmapheresis, if started within the first week, reduces the period of ventilation and hospitalization. However, adequate vascular access for this can be a problem and it involves a risk of infection and hypovolaemia. There is also anecdotal evidence of dramatic improvement with the use of high-dose immunoglobulin (2 g/kg i.v.). This therapy is being evaluated.

In most children, symptomatic recovery is complete after 3–12 months, although there may be permanent abnormalities of nerve conduction. If improvement does not start within 18 days from the time of maximal neurological deficit, full recovery may be less likely.

REYE'S SYNDROME

Reye's syndrome is a rare paediatric condition characterized by acute encephalopathy with brain swelling and fatty degeneration of viscera, especially the liver. Typically, it follows a viral infection (particularly influenza or varicella) and may be related to salicylate ingestion in susceptible individuals. Hepatic mitochondrial dysfunction appears to be involved in disturbed metabolism of amino acids and lipids, and accumulation of toxins including ammonia.

Clinical features

Reye's syndrome is variable in presentation and should be considered in patients with otherwise unexplained encephalopathy or seizures, particularly if preceded by persistent vomiting and personality change. Although 50% of patients have hepatomegaly, jaundice is not a feature. Cardiac failure and pancreatitis may develop. The degree of coma may be staged according to the Glasgow Coma Score, or according to the similar Lovejoy scale, which includes pupillary reflexes. Increasing coma correlates with the development of diffuse cerebral oedema.

In the absence of central nervous system infections, poisoning and other metabolic disorders, the diagnosis is confirmed by hyperammonaemia, with plasma hepatocellular enzymes at least twice the upper limit of normal, and normal bilirubin. Liver-dependent clotting factors are usually depleted. Hypoglycaemia may occur in patients under 2 years of age. Liver biopsy usually shows non-inflammatory microvesicular fat deposition, with mitochondrial disruption on electron microscopy. The coagulation defect should be corrected before performing liver biopsy.

Therapy

Patients with appropriate withdrawal responses to pain are managed symptomatically, with frequent neurological observation. The blood sugar is maintained at the upper limit of normal with intravenous dextrose infusions. Those who become decorticate or worse need intensive therapy, with monitoring of intracranial pressure, aiming to keep the cerebral perfusion pressure above 60 mmHg by measures similar to those used for head trauma. Thiopentone infusion and decompressive craniectomy have been used in those with intractable intracranial hypertension. Pancreatitis and multiple organ failure may need treatment. There is anecdotal evidence that high-dose L-carnitine, intravenously, may prevent progression of the disease.

Prognosis

The prognosis is good if cerebral perfusion is maintained, but mortality approaches 100% if the patient is decerebrate or flaccid.

FURTHER READING

Pathophysiology

Krause G.S., White B.C., Aust S.D., *et al*. Brain-cell death following ischemia and reperfusion: a proposed biochemical sequence. *Crit Care Med* 1988, **16**, 714–726.

Obrist W.D., Langfitt T.W., Jaggi J.L., *et al*. Cerebral blood flow and metabolism in comatose patients with acute head injury. *J Neurosurg* 1984, **61**, 241–253.

Monitoring the injured brain

Holbrook P.R. The child's central nervous system: assaults, monitoring and therapy. In: Vincent J.L. (Ed) *Update in intensive care emergency medicine*. Springer Verlag, Berlin, (1988) pp. 583–590.

Mendelow A.D., Rowan J.O., Murray L., Kerr A.E. A clinical comparison of subdural screw pressure measurements with ventricular pressure. *J Neurosurg* 1983, **58**, 45–50.

North B., Reilly P. Comparison among three methods of intracranial pressure recording. *Neurosurgery* 1986, **18**, 730–732.

Craniospinal trauma

Bruce D.A., Raphaely R.C., Goldberg A.L., *et al*. Pathophysiology, treatment and outcome following severe head injury in children. *Child's Brain* 1979, **5**, 174–191.

Bruce D.A., Abass A., Bilaniuk L., *et al*. Diffuse cerebral swelling following head injuries in children: the syndrome of 'malignant brain oedema'. *J Neurosurg* 1981, **54**, 170.

Thompson R.S., Rivara F.P., Thompson D.C. A case-control study of the effectiveness of bicycle safety helmets. *New Engl J Med* 1989, **320**, 1361–1367.

Mayer T.A., Walker M.L. Pediatric head injury: the critical role of the emergency physician. *Ann Emerg Med* 1985, **14**, 1178–1184.

Saul T.G., Ducker T.B. Effect of intracranial pressure monitoring and aggressive treatment on mortality in severe head injury. *J Neurosurg* 1982, **56**, 498–503.

Hypoxic–ischaemic encephalopathy

Bohn D.J., Biggar W.D., Smith C.R., Conn A.W., Barker G.A. Influence of hypothermia, barbiturate therapy, and intracranial pressure monitoring on morbidity and mortality after near-drowning. *Crit Care Med* 1986, **14**, 529–534.

Sarnaik A.P., Preston G., Lieh-Lai M., Eisenbrey A.B. Intracranial perfusion pressure in near-drowning. *Crit Care Med* 1985, **13**, 224–227.

Seizures

Menkes J.H. Paroxysmal disorders. In: Menkes J.H. (Ed) *Textbook of child neurology*. Lea and Febiger, Philadelphia, (1985), pp. 608–676.

Smith D.W., Cullity G.J., Silberstein E.P. Fatal hepatic necrosis associated with multiple anticonvulsant therapy. *ANZ J Med* 1988, **18**, 575–581.

Bacterial meningitis

Feigin R.D. Bacterial meningitis beyond the neonatal period. In: Feigin R.D., Cherry J.D. (Eds). *Textbook of pediatric infectious diseases*, 2nd edn. WB Saunders, Philadelphia, (1987), pp. 441–465.

Lebel M.H., Freij B.J., Syrogiannopoulos G.A., *et al*. Dexamethasone therapy for bacterial meningitis. *New Engl J Med* 1988, **319**, 964–971.

Guillain–Barré syndrome

The Guillain–Barré Syndrome Study Group. Plasmapheresis and acute Guillain–Barré syndrome. *Neurology* 1985, **35**, 1096–1104.

Eberle E., Brink J., Azen S., White D. Early predictors of incomplete recovery in children with Guillain–Barré polyneuritis. *J Pediatr* 1975, **86**, 356–359.

Shahar E., Murphy E.G., Rolfman C.M. Benefit of intravenously administered immune serum globulin in patients with Guillain–Barré syndrome. *J Paediatr* 1990, **116**, 141–144.

Reyes syndrome

Dean J.M., Rogers M.C. Reye's syndrome. In: Rogers M.C. (Ed) *Textbook of pediatric intensive care*. Williams and Wilkins, Baltimore, (1987), pp. 629–648.

37: Intravenous Nutrition

INTRODUCTION

Intravenous nutrition is a specialized subject. Anaesthetists are sometimes involved, especially in preparation of the route of administration. Strict asepsis in the insertion and handling of the intravenous lines is of the utmost importance. This chapter is a review of parenteral nutrition which should be a useful guide to those involved in the intensive care of children, especially neonates, and can help the anaesthetist less involved in this field to understand the general principles.

It is important that when these patients have to be anaesthetized the anaesthetic drugs are given by a separate peripheral vein rather than via the central vein, so that contamination is avoided.

Intravenous feeding of children may be of value in a number of situations:

1 Low-birth-weight babies with respiratory distress or apnoea, who often tolerate nasogastric feeds poorly. In some units nearly all such babies are fed intravenously, while others make strenuous efforts to introduce milk feeds.

2 Following major abdominal surgery, usually in the neonatal period for congenital malformations or necrotizing enterocolitis, parenteral nutrition has contributed to improved results.

3 In malabsorption, for example following an episode of severe gastroenteritis. The former practice of giving such children 0.225% saline in 5% or 10% dextrose for prolonged periods amounted to partial starvation, with adverse effects on resistance to infection, wound healing, growth and survival (Table 37.1) [1].

Although these situations can be dramatically altered by adequate parenteral nutrition [2], it must be stressed that it is a hazardous procedure that should not be attempted without adequate facilities and expertise.

REQUIREMENTS FOR INTRAVENOUS NUTRITION

Wretlind [3] has made a comprehensive review of this subject. In addition to minerals and vitamins, a patient's nutrition depends on the amount of water, protein (amino acids), carbohydrate (dextrose) and fat (Intralipid or Nutralipid) he or she receives. Average childhood requirements are set out in Table 37.2. These vary widely in disease states. Oxygen and calorie requirements are increased if the child is not in a neutral thermal environment, or if body temperature either rises above or falls below the normal range. Radiant heaters, phototherapy and fever may dramatically increase fluid and calorie requirements in small premature babies.

Calories — energy requirements

Calorie is the term used in this chapter rather than kJ because it is still in common clinical usage. Although the total calorie requirement can often be provided entirely as glucose, without the use of fat, there is a risk of hyperglycaemia, glycosuria and dehydration. The extremely

Table 37.1 Estimated survival time in days in starvation and semi-starvation [1]

	Water only	10% dextrose*
Small premature infant	4	11
Large premature infant	12	30
Full-term infant	33	80
1-year-old child	44	110
Adult	90	350

* 75 ml/kg/day for children; 3 l/day for adults.

hypertonic solution that is needed makes a central venous line desirable. There is no place for the use of fructose or Sorbitol, which may cause lactic acidosis [4]. Intralipid or Nutralipid (soyabean fat emulsion) are isotonic solutions that may be used to provide up to 30 cal/kg/day. The patient's serum must be monitored at least once daily for hyperlipaemia. Even if it is not used as a source of calories, low doses of fat emulsion (e.g. 2 g/kg twice weekly) should be given to prevent essential fatty acid deficiency.

Amino acids

Amino acid requirements in the neonatal period have not been adequately defined, but the subject has been reviewed by Vinnars [5]. Infusion of excessive amounts of amino acids is unnecessary and may cause hyper-ammonaemia, hyperaminoacidaemia, acidosis and brain damage [6, 7]. From 2.5−3 g/kg/day of L-amino acids appears to be appropriate [8, 9] with the provision of at least 30 cal/g of amino acids [5].

Of the commercial preparations presently available, Vamin appears to have the amino acid composition most

suitable for children weighing less than 5 kg [4], and Synthamin for children weighing more than 5 kg. Paedamin, a preparation designed specifically for use in children, may supersede both of these. Solutions of pure L-amino acids are preferable to mixtures of L and D forms because most of the D-amino acids cannot be utilized and are excreted in the urine. Preparations containing synthetic crystalline amino acids are preferable to hydrolysates for paediatric use. The latter have a variable composition; approximately one-third of the amino acids are in the form of small peptides which are not completely usable for protein synthesis, and they may be allergenic.

The approximate relationship between nitrogen amino acid and protein is shown in Table 37.3.

Minerals

Requirements for sodium and potassium vary widely. Premature babies may need a high sodium intake because of aldosterone resistance and high urinary sodium loss. In addition to the normal intravenous feeding regimen, losses of fluid from nasogastric and drain tubes should be measured, analysed, and replaced with intravenous fluid of similar composition. Little is known of the requirements for many trace elements and vitamins in childhood. Some information is available from balance studies and from measurements of rates of accumulation in the fetus

Table 37.3 Approximate relationship between nitrogen, amino acids and protein

1 g of N is equivalent to 7.4 g of amino acids
1 g of N is equivalent to 6.3 g of protein
1 g of amino acids is equivalent to 0.85 g of protein

Table 37.2 Average parenteral requirements for fluid, amino acids, glucose, fat and calories in childhood

Content in g/kg/day on day of treatment	Amino acids			Glucose			Fat (Intralipid)				Total calories needed per day*	Total fluid (ml/kg/day)
	1	2	3+	1	2	3+	1	2	3	4		
Neonates	1.5	2	2	10	10−15	15−20	1	2	3	3	100/kg	100[†]
Under 10 kg	1.5	2	2	10	10−15	15−20	1	2	3	3	100/kg	100
10−15 kg	1	1.5	2	5	10	15	1	2	3	3	1000 + 50/kg over 10 kg	90
15−20 kg	1	1.5	1.5−2	5	10	10−15	1	2	2	3		80
20−30 kg	1	1	1−2	5	10	10−15	1	1.5	2	2.5	1500 + 20/kg over 20 kg	70
Over 30 kg	1	1	1−2	5	5−10	10	1	1.5	1.5	2		50

* Total calories/kg/day equals g/kg/day of: (amino acids × 4) + (glucose × 4) + (Intralipid × 10).
[†] Neonates: Day 1 of life 50 ml/kg, day 2 75 ml/kg, day 3 100 ml/kg.

[3, 10]. Some trace elements (aluminium, iron, zinc, copper, manganese, selenium, calcium and magnesium) are present in significant amounts as contaminants in some intravenous solutions [11].

Although it is most important to provide adequate amounts of calcium and phosphorus [12], solubility problems make this difficult unless they are added to the amino acid solution. This arrangement is satisfactory, as the requirements for calcium and phosphorus appear to be related to protein intake [13]. Children under 5 kg are usually given 1 mmol/kg/day of calcium and phosphate (to a maximum concentration of 12 mmol/l). Children over 5 kg are normally given 7.5 mmol/day of calcium and phosphate (to a maximum of 12 mmol/l). The approximate mineral requirements of neonates are listed in Table 37.4.

Iron should not be given routinely. It may potentiate haemolytic anaemia in vitamin-E deficient premature babies [14]; in malnourished children it may further impair immune function and precipitate overwhelming infection [15].

It may be found desirable to add chromium, selenium, molybdenum and vanadium to intravenous nutrition solutions [16, 17], but this is still not common practice.

PRESCRIBING INTRAVENOUS NUTRITION

The prescribing and preparation of intravenous nutrients is fairly complex, and many formulae have been devised.

Two systems will be described. The first is a detailed prescription which is made up for individual patients by pharmacists, and the second is a simpler prescription which can be made up on the ward from available solutions.

Detailed prescription for individual patients

A prescription is written out each day in the format shown in Table 37.5. Under laminar flow, a pharmacist places all the required nutrients in a single bottle of nutrient solution, with the exception of Intralipid which remains separate. Unless otherwise specified in the electrolytes column, the nutrient solution also contains:
per day: calcium and phosphate under 5 kg 1 mmol/kg/day; over 5 kg 7.5 mmol/kg/day (to a maximum concentration of 12 mmol/l)
μmol/kg/day: manganese 0.2, zinc 3, copper 0.5, iodide 0.04, chromium 0.005.
per litre: vitamin B_{12} 20 μg, Intravite 4 ml (Vitamins B_1 20 mg, B_2 10 mg, B_6 5 mg, C 100 mg, nicotinamide 100 mg, sodium pantothenate 10 mg).
vitamin K_1 2 mg, heparin 1000 units, magnesium 4 mmol.
μg/day: folic acid 100.
The solution does not include fluoride or iron. Fat-soluble vitamins are given to patients needing intravenous nutrition for more than a week as:
under 1 kg — MVI Paediatric 1.5 ml/day,
1–3 kg — MVI Paediatric 2.5 ml/day,
3 kg–12 years — MVI Paediatric 5 ml/day,
over 12 years — MVI. 12 10 ml/bag.

The concentration of dextrose implicit in a prescription of this type can be determined from Table 37.6. This system simplifies matters for the ward in that only two bottles are needed: nutrient solution and Intralipid. It is extremely flexible, as the intake of individual nutrients can be easily adjusted within wide limits, but the greatest benefit of this system is that it expresses the intake of

Table 37.4 Approximate mineral requirements of neonates

mmol/kg/day		μmol/kg/day	
Sodium	2–4	Manganese	0.2
Potassium	3	Zinc	2–5
Calcium	0.75–1.5	Copper	0.5
Magnesium	0.25	Iodide	0.04
Phosphate	1–1.5	Chromium	0.005

Table 37.5 Sample of intravenous nutrition prescription from Royal Children's Hospital*

Weight: 3 kg

Date	Nutrient volume ml/kg/day	Amino acids g/kg/day	Glucose g/kg/day	Potassium mmol/kg/day	Sodium mmol/kg/day	Other electrolytes mmol/kg/day	Fat g/kg/day	Total calories per kg/day
	150	3.0	17.5	3	4	Ca 1.0 Phos 1.0	4	122

* This example, designed for infusion into a peripheral vein, has a larger volume than that recommended in Table 37.2 for central venous infusion.

Table 37.6 Concentration of dextrose implicit in a prescription

Fluid (ml/kg/day)	2.5	5	7.5	10	12.5	15	17.5	20	22.5	25	27.5	30
50	5%	10%	15%	20%								
60	4.2	8.3	12.5	16.7								
70	3.6	7.1	10.7	14.3	17.8%							
80	3.1	6.3	9.4	12.5	15.6	18.8%						
90	2.8	5.6	8.3	11.1	13.9	16.7	19.4%					
100	2.5	5	7.5	10	12.5	15	17.5	20%				
110	2.3	4.5	6.8	9.1	11.4	13.6	15.9	18.2				
120	2.1	4.2	6.3	8.3	10.4	12.5	14.6	16.7	18.8%			
130	1.9	3.8	5.8	7.7	9.6	11.5	13.6	15.4	17.3	19.2%		
140	1.8	3.6	5.4	7.1	8.9	10.7	12.5	14.3	16.1	17.9	19.6%	
150	1.7	3.3	5	6.7	8.3	10	11.7	13.3	15	16.7	18.3	20%
175	1.4	2.9	4.3	5.7	7.1	8.6	10	11.4	12.9	14.3	15.7	17.1
200	1.3	2.5	3.8	5	6.3	7.5	8.8	10	11.3	12.5	13.8	15

In the prescription in Table 30.5, the patient received nutrient 150 ml/kg/day, dextrose 17.5 g/kg/day, and Intralipid 4 g (20 ml)/kg/day. From the above table there would be 11.7% dextrose in the nutrient solution (or just over 10% dextrose infused overall, if allowance is made for dilution of the 150 ml of nutrient with 20 ml of Intralipid).

nutrients in amounts per kg/day, rather than just the concentration of nutrients. Previous experience with one-fifth normal saline in 5% or 10% dextrose conditioned doctors to think in terms of the composition of the solution being given to the patient, rather than the actual amount of nutrients the patient received per kg/day. This practice often resulted in gross errors of nutrition passing unnoticed.

Although this system is logical, flexible and simple for the ward, it places heavy demands on the pharmacy department, and is therefore impractical in many hospitals.

Simplified regimen (Fig. 37.1)

The pharmacy department provides a standard solution of electrolytes, in 10, 15 or 20% dextrose prepared under laminar flow. In the ward, this is mixed in the i.v. burette with amino acid solution (to which phosphorus has been added in the ward). If 3 g of amino acid, 17.5 g of glucose and 150 ml of fluid/kg/day is required, then 43 ml of 7% Vamin (containing 3 g amino acids and 1 mmol of phosphorus) is placed in the burette. 107 ml of dextrose–electrolyte mixture is then added to fill the burette to 150 ml (the volume required per kg/day). The burette would have to be refilled 3 times a day for a 3 kg baby. If the requirement of fluid/kg/day is greater than the volume of the burette (which is usually limited to 150 ml), only half the volume of both solutions is added to the burette each time but it must be filled twice as often.

It is convenient to withdraw dextrose from the bottle in a volume equal to the amount of electrolyte added (about 35 ml). Both this and the addition of amino acid solution to the burette reduce the concentration of dextrose received by the patient. Table 37.7 summarizes the composition of the solutions used.

Although this system is much simpler for the pharmacy department, it is relatively inflexible and some calculation is required to determine the quantity of nutrients infused per kg/day.

PROTEIN

Intake is determined by the volume of amino acid solutions added to the burette, e.g. with Vamin 7%: volume in burette = amount of amino acids required in g/kg/day × 100/7.

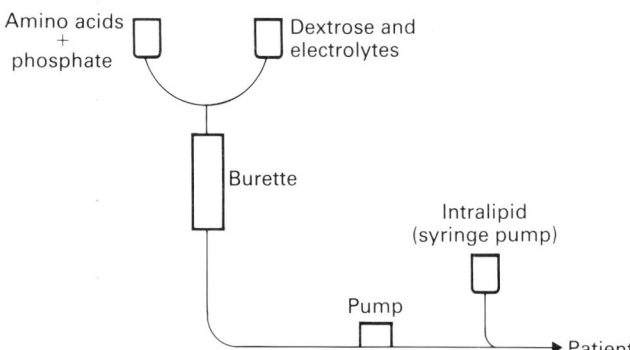

Fig. 37.1 Method suggested for preparing nutrient solution by a simplified regimen.

Table 37.7 Composition of solutions used

	Dextrose−electrolyte Content of 500 ml (Dose 107 ml/kg/day)*	Vamin 7% in 43 ml*	Total intake/kg/day*
Amino acids		3 g	3 g
Glucose	70 g (465 ml of 15%)		15 g
Na (chloride)	8 mmol	2.15 mmol	3.9 mmol
K (acetate)	2 mmol	0.86−1.72	1.2−2.1 mmol
Mg (sulphate)	1 mmol	0.065	0.28 mmol
Ca (gluconate)	4 mmol	0.11	0.9 mmol
Phosphorus	4 mmol		0.9 mmol
Copper	2.3 μmol		0.5 μmol
Zinc	14 μmol		3.0 μmol
Iodide	0.2 μmol		0.04 μmol
Manganese	1 μmol		0.2 μmol
Chromium	0.02 μmol		0.005 μmol
Heparin	500 unit		107 unit
Vitamin B_{12}	10 μg		2.1 μg
Intravite	2 ml		0.43 ml
Folic acid	1.5 mg		0.32 mg
Vitamin K1	1 mg		0.21 mg

* Calculation of total intake of 150 ml/kg/day for peripheral infusion (see Table 37.5).

GLUCOSE

Figure 37.2 is a nomogram which shows the relationship between fluid intake, composition of the solution, and intake of glucose/kg/day. The nomogram does not allow for the slight dilutional effect of adding electrolytes to the 500 ml dextrose bottle.

ELECTROLYTES

Because of the fixed concentration of electrolytes in the dextrose−electrolyte solution, the intake per kg/day is determined by the fluid intake required. On occasions, adjustment of the concentration of sodium and potassium will be required. The calculation of the amount infused is rather tedious.

FAT

Fat emulsion is infused separately to provide up to 3 g/kg/day of fat (30 cal/kg/day).

VITAMINS

Fluoride, iron and fat-soluble vitamins are not included in the nutrient. Fat-soluble vitamins should be given to children who need intravenous nutrition for more than 1 week (see above).

DELIVERY OF INTRAVENOUS NUTRITION

If a substantial proportion of the calories is given as fat, and the solution is less hypertonic, it can be delivered through peripheral cannulae that are replaced as necessary.

Alternatives are to use a silastic catheter threaded from a peripheral into a central vein [10], or a central line inserted by cut-down in an operating theatre.

Whichever route of infusion is used, meticulous care of the catheter has been clearly shown, in a number of studies, to reduce the risk of sepsis [18, 19, 20, 21]. It should be inserted by experienced staff using full sterile technique. The catheter should be used exclusively for the administration of the nutrient solutions. The administration of drugs and blood products, and the measurement of central venous pressure, should not be allowed. All flasks and intravenous tubing up to the cannula should be changed every 3 days. Using sterile technique, the skin around the catheter site is cleansed with acetone and dressed with povidone iodine (Betadine) every 2−3 days. Although this regimen has a marked effect on the incidence of sepsis, it is not clear which of the individual parts is effective. As there is evidence that candida septicaemia often follows invasion from the gut [22], oral or intragastric nystatin should be given to patients receiving intravenous nutrition.

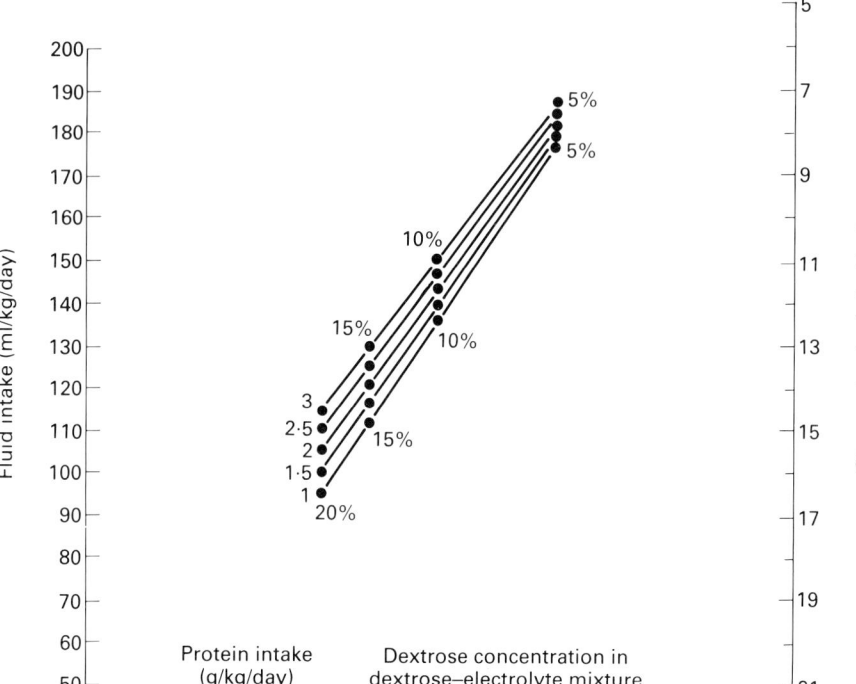

Fig. 37.2 Nomogram relating fluid and protein intake, dextrose concentration of the solution, and glucose intake/kg/day.

Solutions containing Vamin are incompatible with fat emulsion. If there is only one intravenous line available, the nutrient solution should be given for 3 of every 4 hours, and the fat solution for the other hour. This gives 18 hours of nutrient solution and 6 hours of fat infusion per day.

Solutions containing Synthamin are compatible with fat emulsion, providing the combined concentration of calcium and magnesium does not exceed 10 mmol/l, and the Synthamin and fat are mixed in the intravenous line just before it enters the patient. Synthamin solutions with more than 10 mmol/l of calcium and magnesium must be cycled in the same way as Vamin solutions.

GENERAL PRINCIPLES

Fluid losses should be replaced in addition to intravenous nutrition. The introduction and withdrawal of intravenous nutrition should be gradual (over about 3 days). A dislodged i.v. cannula should be replaced immediately in a patient on intravenous nutrition and, if the nutrient solution is not available at any time, it should be replaced with an infusion of a similar concentration of dextrose in water (e.g. 10% dextrose in 0.25 normal saline with potassium).

Care must be taken to avoid hyperglycaemia (with glycosuria and dehydration), hypoglycaemia, sepsis, extravasation of nutrient solution and fat emulsion from veins, thrombocytopenia, hypoproteinaemia, electrolyte imbalance, acidosis (possibly with hyperammonaemia), anaemia, hyperlipaemia and uraemia.

MONITORING

Patients who are being fed intravenously need to be closely monitored. Urine glucose and blood glucose (BM test or Dextrostix) should be measured every 8 hours. The rate of infusion should be reduced if there is more than a trace of glycosuria. The following should be done at least daily: inspection of the intravenous site, measurement of electrolytes and acid–base state, and screening for lipaemia (if there is more than a trace of lipaemia the rate of lipid infusion should be reduced). Haemoglobin, platelets and proteins (twice weekly), and creatinine, magnesium, calcium and phosphate (weekly) should be monitored. Once the child's intravenous nutrition has stabilized, the frequency of monitoring can be reduced.

Blood should be transfused if the child is anaemic; it may be beneficial to infuse 20 ml of stable plasma protein solution (SPPS) once a week to provide small quantities of albumin, globulin and trace elements, and other unknown nutrients that are not present in nutrient solution.

CONCLUSION

In the past, patients unable to tolerate gastrointestinal feeding were frequently subjected to semi-starvation. Intravenous nutrition has made this unnecessary but its successful use demands meticulous attention to detail. Much has still to be learnt about the requirements for intravenous nutrition, particularly in the neonatal period.

REFERENCES

1 Heird W.C., Driscoll J.M., Schullinger J.N., Grebin B., Winters R.W. Intravenous alimentation in paediatric patients. *J. Pediatr* 1972, **80**, 351.
2 Borresen H.C., Knutrud O., Vaage S. Intravenous feeding in paediatric surgery. *Progr Pediatr Surg* 1975, **8**, 49.
3 Wrethind A. Complete intravenous nutrition. *Nutr Metabol* 1972, **14**, 1-57.
4 Editorial. Intravenous feeding. *Lancet* 1973, **ii**, 1179.
5 Vinnars E. Intravenous amino acid therapy. *Acta Anaes Scand* 1974, **55**, Suppl 137.
6 Heird W.C., Winters R.W. Total parenteral nutrition. *J Pediat* 1975, **86**, 2.
7 Goldman H.I., Goldman J.S., Kaufman M.A., Liebman O.B. Late effects of early dietary protein intake on low-birth-weight infants. *J. Pediatr* 1974, **85**, 764.
8 Fomon S.J. *Infant nutrition*, 2nd edn. WB Saunders. Philadelphia, (1974) p. 141.
9 Munro H.N. Amino acid requirements and metabolism and their relevance to parenteral nutrition. In: Wilkinson A.W. (Ed) *Parenteral nutrition*. Churchill Livingstone, Edinburgh, (1972) p. 48.
10 Shaw J.C.L. Parenteral nutrition in the management of sick low birthweight infants. *Pediatr Clin N Am* 1974, **290**, 757.
11 Jetton M.M., Sullivan J.F., Burch R.E. Trace element contamination of intravenous solutions. *Arch Int Med* 1976, **136**, 782.
12 Lichtman M.A. Hypoalimentation during hyperalimentation. *New Engl J Med* 1974, **290**, 1432.
13 Ricour C., Millot M., Balsan S. Phosphorus depletion in children on long-term parenteral nutrition. *Acta Paediatr Scand* 1975, **64**, 385.
14 Dallman P.R. Iron, vitamin E, and folate in the preterm infant. *J Pediatr* 1974, **85**, 742.
15 Bothe A. Use of iron with total parenteral nutrition. *New Engl J Med* 1975, **293**, 1153.
16 WHO Technical Report Series No. 532 (1973) Geneva.
17 Greene H.L. Trace elements and vitamins. In: Bode H.H. (Ed) *Parenteral nutrition in infancy and childhood*. Plenum Press, New York, (1974) p. 131.
18 Ryan J.A., *et al.* Catheter complications in total parenteral nutrition. *New Engl J Med* 1974, 290, 757.
19 Bentley R.W., Lepper M.H. Septicaemia related to indwelling intravenous catheter. *JAMA* 1968, **206**, 1749.
20 Corso J.A., Agostinelli R., Brandiss M.W. Maintenance of polyethylene catheters to reduce risk of infection. *JAMA* 1969, **210**, 2075.
21 Bernard R.W., Stahl W.M., Chase R.M. Subclavian vein catheterizations: a prospective study. *Ann Surg* 1971, **173**, 191.
22 Stone H.H. Candida sepsis. In: Wilkinson A.W. (Ed) *Recent advances in paediatric surgery*. Churchill Livingstone, Edinburgh (1957) p. 115.

FURTHER READING

Arnold W.C. Parenteral nutrition, and fluid and electrolyte therapy. *Pediatr Clin N Am* 1990, **37**, 449-461.
Hendricks K.M. *Manual of pediatric nutrition*. B.C. Decker Inc., (1990).
Kerner J.A. (Ed) *Manual of paediatric parenteral nutrition*. John Wiley & Sons, New York, (1983).
Heird W.C. Parenteral nutrition. In: Grand R.J., Sutphen J.L., Dietz W.H. (Eds) *Paediatric nutrition; theory and practice*. Butterworths, London, (1987) p. 747.
Collier S.B. Parenteral nutrition. In: Hendricks K.M., Walker W.A. (Eds) *Paediatric nutrition*. B.C. Decker Inc., (1990) p. 110.

38: Artificial Organ Support for Children in Intensive Care

INTRODUCTION

In recent years techniques to support the heart, lung and kidneys through a period of acute failure have been developed, making recovery possible in infants and children who would probably otherwise die. The heart and lung support are extensions to developments in cardiopulmonary bypass for open heart surgery. Membrane oxygenators, which cause minimal damage to the blood, have made long periods of extracorporeal membrane oxygenation (ECMO) possible. If only lung support is needed veno-venous extracorporeal carbon dioxide removal (ECCO₂R) may suffice; ventricular assist devices (VAD) can be used when only cardiac support is required.

Chronic renal failure is managed long term by dialysis, but for acute renal failure and the removal of toxic substances which the kidney is unable to handle, various filtration methods have been developed (haemo-, ultra-, and plasma filtration).

EXTRACORPOREAL MEMBRANE OXYGENATION

Extracorporeal membrane oxygenation (ECMO) with extrathoracic cannulation is used to support patients with acute, reversible and probably fatal respiratory or cardiac failure who have not responded to conventional medical, pharmacological or surgical therapy. ECMO is a supportive, not a therapeutic, intervention [1, 2]. It provides cardiopulmonary 'rest', allowing for healing and resolution of reversible lung and heart pathology.

Currently, venoarterial ECMO is the predominant method used in newborn infants [3]: blood drains from the patient into a reservoir via a 10−14 Fr gauge cannula inserted into the right atrium through the right internal jugular vein. The blood is then pumped through a silicone membrane oxygenator, which functions as an artificial lung adding oxygen and removing carbon dioxide. After passing through a heat exchanger the warmed blood is returned to the patient's aortic arch via an 8−12 Fr gauge cannula inserted into the right common carotid artery (Fig. 38.1). Heparin is necessary to prevent clotting.

Gas exchange occurs across the membrane lung. Carbon dioxide exchange depends on fresh gas flow rate, fresh gas carbon dioxide concentration, and the membrane surface area; it is independent of blood flow rate and membrane thickness. Oxygen exchange is independent of gas flow rate, but depends on fresh gas flow oxygen concentration, blood flow rate, membrane thickness and membrane surface area.

ECMO variants

VENO-VENOUS EXTRACORPOREAL CARBON DIOXIDE REMOVAL (ECCO₂R)

This is used in adults with either one double-lumen cannula, or two single-lumen cannulae. It avoids the complications of arterial cannulation, but provides respiratory support only [4]. Therefore, in illnesses in-

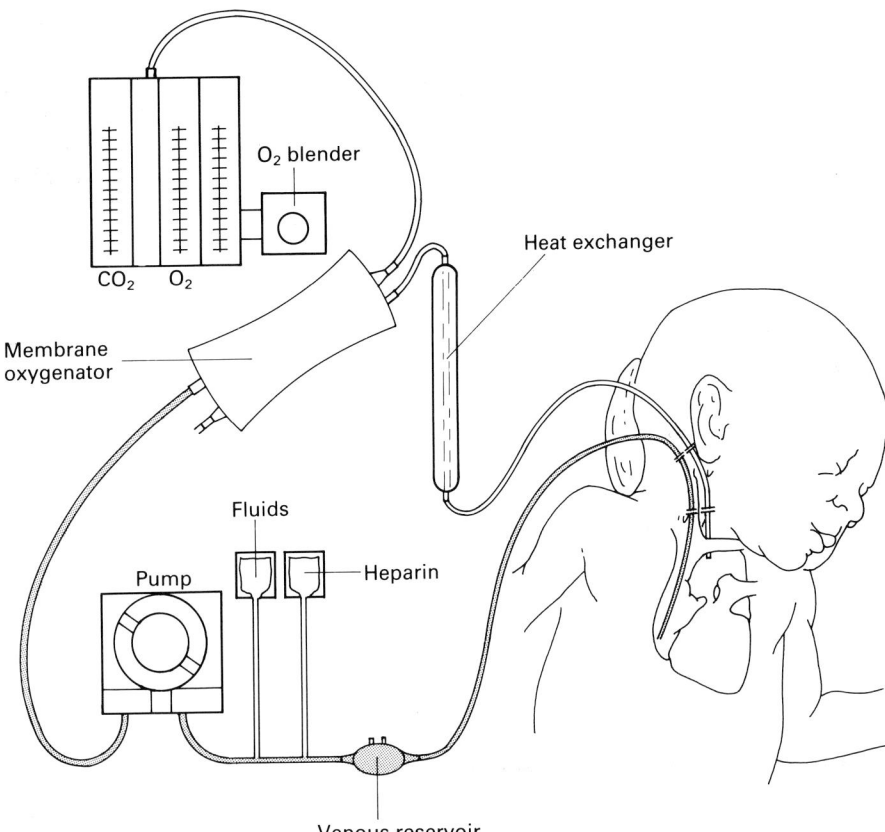

Fig. 38.1 The standard circuit for venoarterial ECMO

volving significant myocardial dysfunction, ECCO₂R is inappropriate. Veno-venous ECMO has been used as a two-cannulae, high blood flow technique in children, but it has the added problems of leg oedema and the potential need for later conversion to venoarterial ECMO [5]. Veno-venous ECMO with one single-lumen cannula and an in-and-out technique has been used successfully in a pre-term infant [6]. Veno-venous ECMO and ECCO₂R have similar respiratory indications and problems to venoarterial ECMO. Although carotid arterial cannulation is avoided, thereby reducing the risk of neurological complications, oxygenation is less efficient.

VENTRICULAR ASSIST DEVICE (VAD)

This is used to supplement cardiac output in patients with myocardial dysfunction but normal respiratory function. Blood drained by a cannula in the atrium is pumped back into a major artery, thereby providing ventricular assistance (left atrium to aorta, LVAD; right atrium to pulmonary artery, RVAD). The sternum cannot be closed until the cannulae are removed, which is usually after 1–3 days but the skin can be closed.

Great care must be taken to avoid contamination of the wound.

Patient selection for ECMO

Because ECMO is expensive, it is essential that patients are carefully selected. The aims should be to improve survival and decrease chronic lung disease, with minimal neurological handicap in survivors. The disease process must be potentially reversible within 2 weeks. Conditions that may benefit from ECMO in neonates are meconium aspiration syndrome, persistent pulmonary hypertension [7], sepsis, respiratory distress syndrome, severe lung barotrauma and congenital diaphragmatic hernia [8]; in older children, adult respiratory distress syndrome, sepsis and multiple organ failure are suitable; in children of any age it can provide perioperative myocardial support of patients with congenital heart disease and in some patients awaiting heart transplantation.

Currently, patients with these conditions are selected for ECMO if the expectation of death with conventional medical therapy exceeds 80% and there are none of the following contraindications:

1 gestation less than 34 weeks or weight less than 2000 g;

2 acute or chronic irreversible disease process;

3 underlying congenital abnormality associated with a need for long-term dependent care;

4 intracranial haemorrhage/cerebral infarct, likely to extend with anticoagulation;

5 IPPV and high FiO_2 for longer than 10 days.

There are many predictors of an 80% mortality risk in newborn infants [1]; these include:

1 $AaDO_2$ greater than 620 for 8−12 hours in 100% oxygen;

2 oxygenation index (OI) of greater than 40 on 3 of 5 consecutive blood gas measurements obtained 30−60 minutes apart. (OI = mean airway pressure (cmH$_2$O) $\times$ FiO_2/postductal Pao_2 (mmHg));

3 Pao_2 less than 50 mmHg for 4 hours.

In older children, one study developed a mortality risk predictor for children, based on oxygenation and ventilation [9]:

If OI > 0.04 and VI > 40 then there was a 77% chance of death (sensitivity 65%, specificity 74%), where OI = MAP $\times$ FiO_2/Pao_2

(OI = oxygenation index, MAP = mean arterial pressure, FiO_2 = fractional inspired oxygen concentration, Pao_2 = partial pressure of arterial oxygen, post-ductal), and where VI = RR $\times$ PIP $\times$ $Paco_2$/1000

(VI = ventilation index, RR = respiratory rate, PIP = peak inspiratory pressure, $Paco_2$ = arterial partial pressure of carbon dioxide).

Mortality rates for conditions considered for ECMO treatment vary between hospitals and may improve with new advances in treatment [10]. Thus each unit will have to develop its own criteria, based on current outcome, to decide which patients should be treated. As the complications of ECMO decrease and further technical advances occur (such as heparin-bonded circuits), ECMO will become safer and, therefore, will be used with lower predicted mortality.

It must be stressed that ECMO is an invasive, complicated and potentially dangerous therapy. It is not safe in the hands of the occasional operator. Enough patients need to be treated in a unit to develop and maintain the skills required to ensure that ECMO is performed safely — a minimum of 12 and preferably 24 patients per year is suggested. Paediatric ECMO should be performed in major centres in order to develop expertise, provide optimum care and evaluate formally the survival and long-term outcome.

Management of children on ECMO

Cannulation is usually performed in the intensive care unit, with the patient paralysed, ventilated and having been given analgesia (e.g. fentanyl 20−50 µg/kg). Once the cannulae have been inserted, heparin (1 mg/kg) has been added and the circuit attached, the flow is gradually increased to the desired setting (usually 120−150 ml/kg). Gas exchange and cardiac output usually improve rapidly [11]; $Paco_2$ decreases, blood pressure increases and heart rate decreases. The ventilator settings are then decreased to allow lung rest: a rate of 5 per minute with positive end-expiratory pressure of 10−14 cmH$_2$O, peak inspiratory pressure of the minimum amount associated with some chest-wall movement (usually 20−30 cmH$_2$O); FiO_2 is decreased to 0.21 [12]. The trachea should be regularly suctioned. All inotropic and vasodilator drugs are usually stopped.

If renal function is also compromised and is unresponsive to frusemide (0.5−1 mg/kg) or low-dose dopamine, haemofiltration may be necessary; this may be incorporated into the ECMO circuit with the use of a small arteriovenous shunt. The haemofiltration system has two pumps, which control fluid balance; one extracts the filtrate and the other replaces fluid. Fluid balance is determined by the relative flows of these two pumps. Parenteral nutrition can also be administered when haemofiltration is used. The replacement fluid volume added to the circuit must be decreased by the amount of nutrient fluid added, so that fluid balance is maintained and water overload is avoided. If replacement fluid contains colloid or platelets, care must be taken not to remove too much water and crystalloid, as there is a danger of developing hyperproteinaemia.

Haemoglobin, haematocrit, platelets, white-cell count, electrolytes and calcium are monitored every 12 hours.

Potassium loss requires replacement with 4 mmol/kg/day; sodium (2−3 mmol/kg) and calcium (50−70 mg elemental Ca^{++}/kg) are added each day. Magnesium and phosphorus levels are monitored daily. The membrane lung does not cause significant haemolysis unless clotting occurs, but platelets are damaged and sequestered, resulting in the need for frequent platelet transfusions to keep platelet counts above 60 000/mm^3 in patients without bleeding complications, and above 100 000/mm^3 if bleeding occurs from any site. Spun platelets are preferred, if available, to decrease the volume given and to avoid transfusion of degradation products present in the plasma supernatant fluid. All platelets should be transfused into the circuit distal to the membrane, to ensure they reach the patient and to minimize the adherence of platelets to the membrane, or they can be given by another intravenous line. Activated clotting times are kept at twice normal with a heparin infusion ($10-20\,u/kg/h$); all invasive procedures should be avoided.

All injection ports are cleaned with povidone iodine (Betadine) or alcohol before drawing samples from or injecting fluids into the system. One port is used for injection only and one for withdrawal only, in an attempt to reduce the risk of bacterial colonization and subsequent nosocomial infection. Blood cultures are taken daily from the circuit. Some drugs, such as vancomycin, react with heparin and should be avoided if possible.

Daily chest X-rays are obtained to follow the progression of the lung disease and to check the position of catheters. Ultrasound is done every second day to look for intracranial haemorrhage. Echocardiography is done before ECMO to exclude any structural heart disease that may need operation.

Infants are mildly sedated with opioids (morphine $10-20\,\mu g/kg/h$ or fentanyl $2-4\,\mu g/kg/h$); neuromuscular blockade is used only if movement is excessive because it interferes with clinical neurological examination; IPPR may cause peripheral oedema.

Stress ulceration is uncommon in newborn infants and in paediatric intensive care units. If prophylaxis is indicated, sucralfate is preferred to ranitidine or antacids [13].

WEANING

After an initial worsening of lung function at 24 hours there is usually gradual improvement, with increasing lung compliance and clearing of the chest X-ray. As improvement occurs, flow is decreased; eventually, after a brief period on very low flows, the pump is stopped and the patient decannulated. Blood gases are measured. Successful weaning has been accomplished with lung compliance of $0.4-0.8\,ml/cmH_2O$.

Complications

A number of complications can occur:
1 Haemorrhage (minor 25%; major 5%).
2 Technical failure (material failure, mechanical malfunction or technical error) occurred for 25% of patients in one series, although only 4% required resuscitation; the fatality rate due to technical failure was 1% [14].

3 Residual neurological deficit: abnormalities in survivors include 10–15% with residual motor deficits, 10–15% with developmental delay and 10–15% with hearing/language problems. The incidence of hemiparesis associated with carotid artery cannulation appears to be low. Seventy per cent of survivors of ECMO are normal [15]. Although carotid and internal jugular ligation have been carried out without apparent complication, the recent trend is to repair both artery and vein at decannulation.
4 Infection (5–10%).
5 Haemolysis and other cell and platelet damage, 6% [16].
6 Embolism — the incidence is unknown [17].

Results of ECMO treatment

The results of more than 4800 cases of neonatal ECMO have been reported to the Extracorporeal Life Support Organization (ELSO): 83% of these patients have survived (Table 38.1). The two controlled trials in neonates, done by Bartlett [18] and O'Rourke [7], showed improved results, but because of prior anecdotal evidence that ECMO improved survival, considerable ethical problems were encountered in conducting these trials (where death was the end-point), which prevented valid random selection being carried out.

The results of ECMO in older children are less encouraging, with about 40–50% short-term survival when it was used to treat respiratory or cardiac failure. The main reasons for the poorer outcome compared to neonatal ECMO are: (i) the wide diversity and irreversibility of illnesses leading to cardiorespiratory failure in children, and (ii) the poor clinical predictors of death in

Table 38.1 Conditions treated with ECMO and outcome (ELSO Report April 1991)

Diagnosis	Total	Survived (%)
Newborn		
Meconium aspiration syndrome	1825	93
Persistent fetal circulation	705	87
Congenital diaphragmatic hernia	877	62
Respiratory distress syndrome	705	84
Sepsis	625	77
Child		
Respiratory failure	222	44
Cardiac failure	419	47

older children, resulting in poor patient selection for ECMO. These results are similar to the results of an early controlled trial of ECMO in adults, which showed no benefit of ECMO when compared to conventional therapy [19].

Cost

ECMO is expensive (US$2000 per day) but it reduces the time spent in hospital, which balances the cost with longer-stay conventional therapy. One study showed that the cost for survivors was considerably less for ECMO-treated patients [20]. The ultimate social and economic cost of ECMO will not be determined until the consequences of long-term neurological complications is known. It is unclear whether the neurological handicap rate in survivors is related to the primary condition or to the ECMO procedure and its complications, but the handicap rate is less in ECMO survivors than in surviving patients who were not treated with ECMO.

FILTRATION IN CHILDREN

Arteriovenous filtration is now standard practice in adult intensive care, and is used to treat patients with acute renal failure, vascular congestion, haemodynamic instability and multi-organ failure or after cardiothoracic surgery [21, 22, 23]. Continuous arteriovenous haemofiltration has been used in infants in intensive care [24, 25], for children with multi-system organ failure, acute renal failure and to remove toxic substances [26, 27, 28].

Filtration variants

Continuous arteriovenous haemofiltration (CAVH) is the standard type of filtration, but a number of variations exist. These are:
1 pump-assisted continuous veno-venous filtration (CVVH);
2 pump-assisted CAVH;
3 a combination of dialysis and filtration which may increase renal solute clearance — continuous arteriovenous haemodiafiltration (CAVHD);
4 low-volume fluid and solute removal with no replacement solution — slow continuous ultrafiltration (SCUF);
5 filtration with larger, more porous filters — plasmafiltration (PF).

Principles of filtration

The ultrafiltration that occurs during CAVH is similar to ultrafiltration in the renal glomerulus. The glomerular capillary wall and the filter used in the extracorporeal circuit are each composed of semi-permeable membranes. The blood pressure of the individual provides the hydraulic force needed to produce the ultrafiltrate in both circumstances. Conversely, plasma protein oncotic pressure opposes ultrafiltrate formation in both the glomerulus and the extracorporeal circuit. The resulting ultrafiltrate in Bowman's capsule and that formed by the extracorporeal circuit are free of red cells and proteins, and have similar electrolyte composition to plasma.

Thus, filtration depends on filter blood flow and filtration fraction. Filter blood flow depends on blood pressure, the patient's total and regional cardiac output, blood viscosity and the combined circuit and filter resistance [21]. The filtration fraction (volume of filtrate flow/unit volume of blood flow) is determined by the membrane surface area, membrane permeability, transmembrane pressure (TMP) and colloid oncotic pressure (Figs 38.2, 38.3).

Technical considerations

Infants have a low blood pressure and their arteries are narrow; therefore small fine catheters and low-volume circuits with a high resistance to filter blood flow are used. This means that the volume filtered is small and solute clearance is low. In critically ill neonates, an extra stress is imposed on the infant's heart by having to pump blood through the extracorporeal circuit; diastolic hypotension may result from the large arteriovenous shunt. Veno-venous filtration with a pump (Fig. 38.4) is often used in small patients to alleviate these problems [29, 30], because a higher rate of filter blood flow decreases local stagnation and thrombus formation and allows a larger and more efficient filter to be used.

Alteration of the blood flow rate and filtration flow rate varies with the type of filtration used. For example, in the newborn:
SCUF blood flow 25 ml/min, filtrate flow 10−30 ml/h;
CVVH (low flow), blood flow 25 ml/min, filtrate flow 100 ml/h;
CVVH (high flow), blood flow 40 ml/min, filtrate flow 600 ml/h.
Since CAVH in the newborn usually has filtrate flow rates of 5−10 ml/h, CAVHD has often been used to

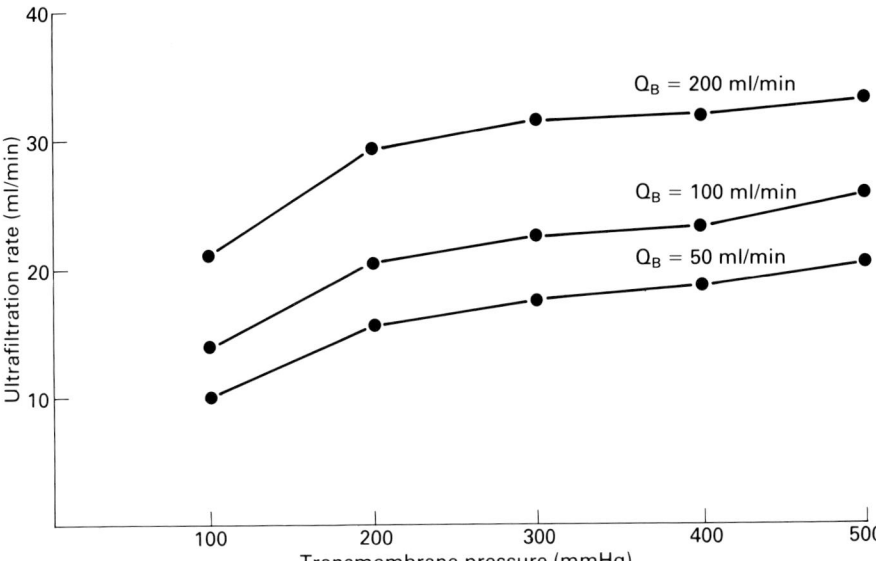

Fig. 38.2 Relationship between ultrafiltration rate, transmembrane pressure and filter blood flow (Q_B).

increase solute clearance but high-flow CVVH also produces very effective solute clearance which equals the dialysis techniques [31].

To perform veno-venous filtration, a 6.5 Fr gauge double-lumen catheter is used for blood flow rates of 25–40 ml/min. For older children with blood flow rates of 50–100 ml/min, a 11.5 Fr double-lumen catheter is used. A blood pump (e.g. Gambro MPM10) and two standard infusion pumps are used to control the rate of filtration and administration of replacement solution. Fluid balance is controlled by the flow rates of these two pumps (Fig. 38.4). If there is excess water to be removed

from the patient the filtrate flow should be greater than replacement flow. Low flow rates can be used if only water needs to be removed but higher flow rates are necessary to remove solute. Haemofiltration and plasma-filtration replacement solutions are made in the hospital pharmacy (Table 38.2).

Anticoagulation of the circuit is important; activated clotting time is maintained at 1.5 × normal. Heparin is infused pre-filter at 5–20 u/kg/h and post-filter at 1–5 u/kg/h. For plasma filtration acid–citrate–dextrose solution is also infused pre-filter (1 ml for every 50 ml blood flow).

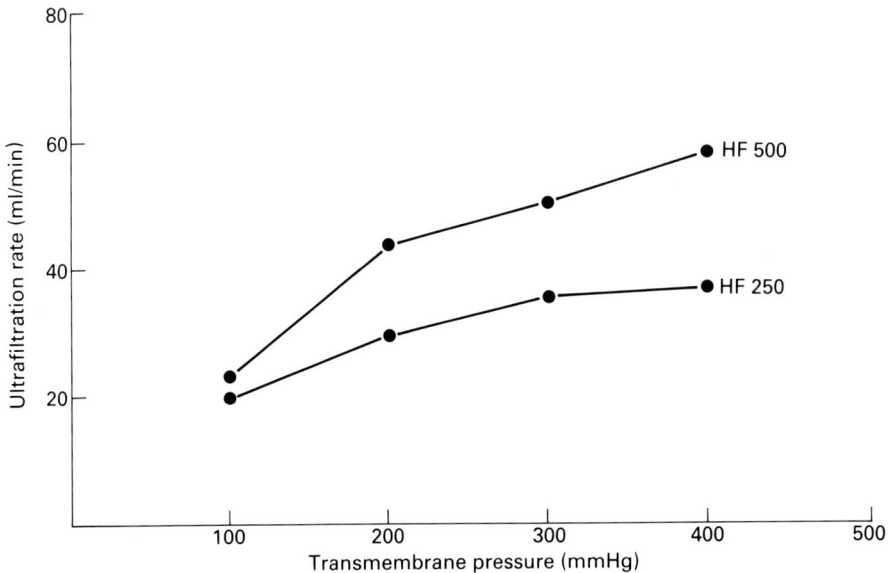

Fig. 38.3 Relationship between ultrafiltration rate, transmembrane pressures with different size filters (500 and 250 cm²) at 200 ml/min filter blood flow. TMP = (PA + PV)/2 + PN where PA = arterial pressure (prefilter), PV = venous pressure (post filter) and PN = absolute value of outlet pressure.

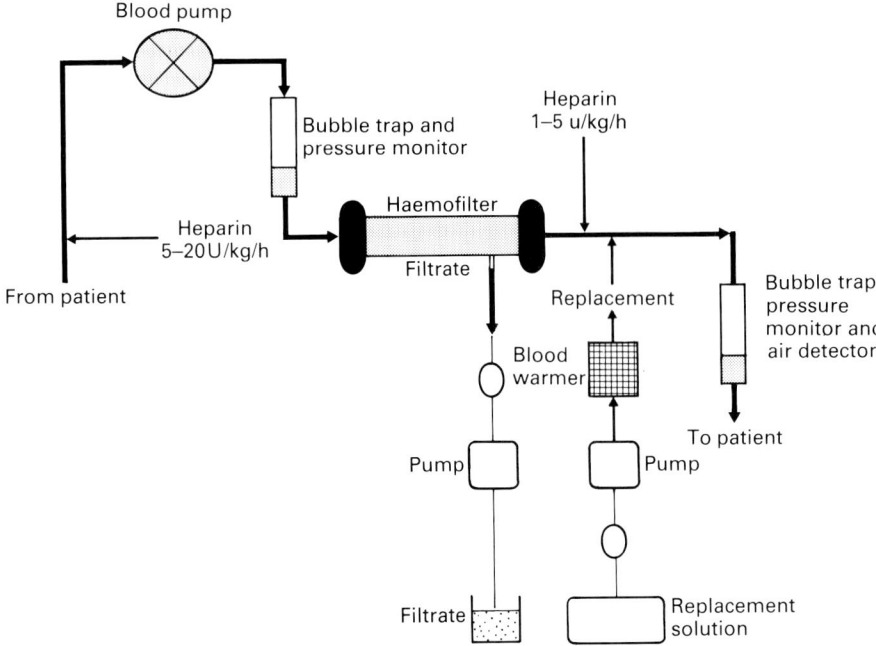

Fig. 38.4 Continuous veno-venous haemofiltration circuit. Fluid balance is determined by the relative flows of the two pumps.

Conditions treated

The conditions treated, outcome, and details of filter function are listed in Table 38.3.

Complications

Complications include infection, thromboembolism, membrane-induced haemolysis (which occurs when the filters are clotted) and electrolyte abnormalities which are corrected daily by ordering appropriate replacement filtrate solution based on biochemical and haematological monitoring. Technical problems can also occur.

Table 38.2 Composition of filtration replacement solution

Dextrose 0.3 g%
Sodium 135 mmol/l
Potassium 3.0 mmol/l
Calcium 1.5 mmol/l
Magnesium 0.7 mmol/l
Phosphate 1 mmol/l
Bicarbonate 25 mmol/l
Acetate 16.4 mmol/l
Chloride 100 mmol/l
For plasmapheresis, albumin 40 g/l is also added

Plasma filtration

This veno-venous system may be used for plasma filtration. Large volumes may be regularly exchanged to treat drug overdose [32], Guillain−Barré syndrome [33], hyperbilirubinaemia, interstitial nephritis or sepsis [34].

Table 38.3 Filtration of children at Royal Children's Hospital, Melbourne

Conditions treated	Total	Survived %
Sepsis, multi-organ failure	46	53
Guillain−Barré syndrome	13	100
Drug overdose	6	86
Metabolic disease	5	80
Interstitial nephritis	2	100
Hyperbilirubinaemia	2	100
Total	76	66%

Filter function	Arteriovenous	Veno-venous
Duration of treatment (h)	40 (14−142)	54 (3−226)
Filter life (h)	27 (4−47)	58 (3−148)
Blood flow (ml/min)	30 (15−50)	65 (25−100)
Filtration fraction (%)	17 (10−25)	13 (5−30)
Ultrafiltration rate (ml/min/m^2)	6 (2−18)	19 (5−43)

(January 1991.)

In small infants or critically ill patients, a plasma filtration replacement solution is used for the first 75% of the plasma exchange and the last 25% is replaced with fresh frozen plasma. In older, more stable patients, stable plasma protein solution (SPPS) or 5% albumin solution is used as replacement solution.

Summary

Veno-venous filtration is relatively simple and flexible: it enables a wide range of different techniques such as slow continuous ultrafiltration, haemofiltration or plasma filtration to be performed in patients of all ages from newborn infants to adults. As the same circuit and equipment is used for all patients, no extra personnel are required to supervise the procedure; this can be done by the bedside nurses as part of patient care.

Haemofiltration allows removal of large amounts of water, solutes and low-molecular-weight mediators of inflammation, and has been used to improve pulmonary gas exchange in critically ill children. Haemofiltration also allows precise control of water balance, such that adequate parenteral nutrition can usually be accomplished in critically ill patients with multi-system organ failure. Although not proven by random controlled trials to alter mortality, this therapy aids in the care of critically ill children.

REFERENCES

1 Short B.L. ECMO in management of respiratory failure in the newborn. *Clin Perinatol* 1987, **14**, 737.

2 Ortiz L. ECMO in pediatric respiratory failure. *Pediatr Clin N Am* 1987, **19**, 39.

3 Stork E. Extracorporeal membrane oxygenation in the newborn and beyond. *Clin Perinatol* 1988, **15**, 815–830.

4 Gattinoni L. ECCOR in adult respiratory failure. *Intens Care World* 1988, **5**, 42.

5 Klein M., Andrews F., Wesley J.R., *et al*. VV perfusion in ECMO for neonatal respiratory insufficiency. A clinical comparison with V-A perfusion. *Annals Surg* 1985, **20**, 520.

6 Tsuno K., Terasaki H., Tsutsumi R., Sadanaga M., Higashi K., Morioka T. To-and-fro veno-venous extracorporeal lung assist for newborns with severe respiratory distress. *Intens Care Med* 1989, **15**, 269–271.

7 O'Rourke P.P., Crone R.K., Vacanti J.P., *et al*. Extracorporeal membrane oxygenation and conventional medical therapy in neonates with persistent pulmonary hypertension of the newborn: a prospective randomized study. *Pediatrics* 1989, **84**, 957–963.

8 Heiss K., Manning P., Oldham K.T., *et al*. Reversal of mortality for congenital diaphragmatic hernia with ECMO. *Ann Surg* 1989, **209**, 225–230.

9 Rivera R., Butt W., Shann F. Predictors of mortality in children with respiratory failure: possible indications for ECMO. *Anaes Intens Care* 1990, **18**, 385.

10 Nading J.H. Historical controls for extracorporeal membrane oxygenation in neonates. *Crit Care Med* 1989, **17**, 423–425.

11 Martin G.R., Short B.L. Doppler echocardiographic evaluation of cardiac performance in infants on prolonged extracorporeal membrane oxygenation. *Am J Cardiol* 1988, **62**, 929–934.

12 Keszler M. Pulmonary management during ECMO. *Crit Care Med* 1989, **17**, 495.

13 Driks M.R., Craves D.E., Celli B.R., *et al*. Nosocomial pneumonia in intubated patients given sucralfate as compared with antacids or histamine type 2 blockers. *New Engl J Med* 1987, **317**, 1376.

14 Harais W.E., Darling E.M., Heaton J.F.G., Arensman R.M. Complications of long-term extracorporeal membrane oxygenation other than haemorrhage: an analysis of 146 cases. *Proc 5th Annual Childrens Hospital National Medical Centre*. ECMO Symposium, Colorado (1989), p. 26.

15 Data from the Extracorporeal Life Support Organisation registry. Ann Arbor, Michigan. January 1991.

16 Steinhorn J.R., Isham-Schopf B., Smith C., Green T.P. Hemolysis during long-term ECMO. *J Pediatr* 1989, **115**, 625.

17 Fink S., Bockman D., Howell C., Greer Falls D., Kanto W.P. Bypass circuits as a source of emboli during ECMO. *J Pediatr* 1989, **115**, 621.

18 Bartlett R.H., Roloff D.W., Cornell R.G., *et al*. Extracorporeal circulatory support in neonatal respiratory failure: a prospective randomized study. *Pediatrics* 1985, **76**, 479–487.

19 Zapol W.M., Swider M.T., Hill J.D., *et al*. Extracorporeal membrane oxygenation in severe acute respiratory failure. *JAMA* 1979, **242**, 2193–2195.

20 Pearson K., Short B.L. Economic analysis of infants undergoing ECMO. *J Intens Care Med* 1987, **2**, 116.

21 Kramer P., Kaufhold G., Grone H.J., *et al*. Management of anuric intensive care patients with arteriovenous haemofiltration. *Int J Artificial Organs* 1980, **3**, 225–230.

22 Mault J., Kresowik T., Dechert R., *et al*. Continuous arteriovenous hemofiltration: the answer to starvation in acute renal failure. *Trans Am Soc Artif Intern Organs* 1984, **30**, 203–206.

23 Lauer A., Saccaggi A., Ronco C., *et al*. Continuous arteriovenous hemofiltration in the critically ill patient. *Ann Intern Med* 1983, **99**, 455–460.

24 Lieberman K.V., Nardi L., Bosch J.P. Treatment of acute renal failure in an infant using continuous arteriovenous hemofiltration. *J Pediatr* 1985, **112**, 646–649.

25 Lieberman K.V. Continuous arteriovenous hemofiltration in children. *Pediatr Nephrol* 1987, **1**, 330–338.

26 DiCarlo J.V., Dudley T.E., Sherbotie J.R., Kaplan B.S., Costarino A.T. Continuous arteriovenous hemofiltration/dialysis improves pulmonary gas exchange in children with multiple organ system failure. *Crit Care Med* 1990, **18**, 822–826.

27 Leone M.R., Jenkins R.D., Golper T.A., Alexander S.T. Early experience with continuous arteriovenous hemofiltration in critically ill pediatric patients. *Crit Care Med* 1986, **14**, 1058–1063.

28 Pascual J.F., Lopez J.D., Molina M. Hemofiltration in children with renal failure. *Pediatr Clin N Am* 1987, **34**, 803–817.

29 Wendon J., Smithies M., Shepphard M., *et al*. Continuous high volume veno-venous haemofiltration in acute renal failure.

J Intens Care Med 1989, **15**, 358.

30 Bambauer R., Jutzler G., Phillipi H., *et al*. Hemofiltration and plasmapheresis in premature infants and newborns. *Artificial Organs* 1987, **12**, 20.

31 Thompson G., Butt W., Henning R., Shann F., Osborne A. Continuous veno-venous haemofiltration in management of acute decomposition in inborn errors of metabolism. *J Pediatr* 1991 (in press).

32 Laussen P., Shann F.A., Butt W., Tibballs J. The use of plasmapheresis in acute theophylline toxicity. *Crit Care Med* 1991, **19**, 288.

33 The Guillain—Barré Syndrome Study Group. Plasmapheresis and acute Guillain—Barré syndrome. *Neurology* 1985, **35**, 1096—1104.

34 Ossenkoppele G., van der Meulen J., Bronsveld W., Thijs L.G. Continuous arteriovenous hemofiltration as an adjunctive therapy for septic shock. *Crit Care Med* 1985, **13**, 102.

Appendices

1 : Electrosurgical Units

INTRODUCTION

Electrosurgery, or surgical diathermy, uses high-frequency electric currents to cut and coagulate body tissues. High-frequency currents generated inside the electrosurgical unit (ESU) are channelled to the patient via an insulated cable and a handheld active electrode. All the current is concentrated at its point of contact with the tissue, producing intense heat that can be used for either cutting or coagulation. The current leaves the patient either through another active electrode or through a large-area, dispersive electrode (often called the 'patient plate').

Because of the electrical hazards and potential for serious complications, all operating theatre staff should understand the principles of electrosurgery and follow appropriate safety procedures.

THE ELECTROSURGICAL UNIT

The electrosurgical unit is the power source that supplies and controls the high-frequency electric current used to cut and coagulate. The selected power is displayed either as a number on a control knob, or as a digital reading in watts. The displayed power is based upon the output power that would be delivered into a predetermined load impedance and is only a guide to the maximum power available at a given setting. The actual power delivered to the patient depends on the load placed on the electrosurgical unit by the total impedance between the two electrodes.

Cutting

In the cutting mode, a high-temperature electric arc is struck between the thin blade of the active electrode and the tissue. The arc is intense enough to vaporize the tissue in the immediate vicinity of the blade. With careful selection of power levels and waveform it is possible to cut so that there is very little bleeding.

The waveform commonly used for cutting is a continuous sinusoidal current with a frequency of 400–800 kHz. Coagulation is achieved by switching this waveform on and off to produce a stream of brief bursts of high-frequency energy.

Coagulation

There are two techniques for producing coagulation [1]. Desiccation occurs as a result of the intense heat produced by the current as it passes from active electrode to tissue when they are in contact.

Fulguration occurs when the active electrode is held close to but not touching the tissue and an arc is struck in the gap between electrode and tissue. It is similar to the cutting technique, except that a much larger electrode such as a ball electrode is used.

Coagulation waveforms vary with the machine, but they all have a low duty cycle. The high-frequency energy is applied to the active electrode as a train of short-duration bursts. The low duty cycle provides coagulation with very little cutting.

Blend

Nearly all ESUs have a facility for mixing cutting and coagulation waveforms to produce an output waveform that has properties of both modes. The degree of mixing can be adjusted to suit the operator's needs.

MODES

Monopolar mode

The monopolar mode of operation, in which high-frequency current enters the patient at the handheld active electrode and leaves via the large-area, dispersive electrode, is most commonly used. Very high temperatures are produced at the active electrode because the entire output of the electrosurgical unit is channelled through a very small cross-sectional area.

Bipolar mode

A bipolar technique, which is suitable for delicate procedures, has been developed in which there is no dispersive electrode. The output current, which is passed between two small electrodes such as the tips of a pair of insulated surgical forceps, is confined to the small volume of tissue between the electrodes, thereby reducing the power needed for coagulation and the risk of accidental burns. It overcomes some of the problems of the monopolar mode, including its high power requirement, substantial spacing between active and dispersive electrodes, and the consequent imprecise control over the distribution of current through the body.

Most electrosurgical units have outputs for both monopolar and bipolar electrosurgery, which are separately switched, but there are some units in which both outputs are activated by a single footswitch control.

It is safer not to use two active electrodes on electrosurgical units that can produce simultaneous activation of two or more electrodes.

ELECTRODES

Active electrode

The active electrode, for monopolar surgery, is usually a handheld pencil with the electrode protruding from the distal end. Whereas older-style pencils were unswitched and relied on footswitch control to select cut or coagulation waveforms, many modern pencils are fitted with rocker or push-button switches, one for cutting and one for coagulation. Blend is usually achieved by setting the electrosurgical unit to Blend and pressing the Cut switch. Most manufacturers follow the AAMI standard [2] with the Cut switch closest to the electrode blade. Some manufacturers are colour-coding the switches so that Cut switch is yellow and Coagulation switch is blue.

Most pencils have a blade electrode that can be exchanged for a needle or a ball. The electrodes are usually made of a material that can be bent by the operator into the desired shape.

A major problem with hand-switched pencil electrodes is the risk of burns to the patients or staff if fluid enters the switch mechanism. Most pencils are constructed to prevent this; it is important to ensure that this is so when purchasing an electrosurgical pencil.

It is imperative, particularly when more than one electrode is connected, that active electrodes should be put in a non-conductive holster (quiver) when they are not being used, so that inadvertent burns are avoided [3].

Dispersive electrode

The dispersive electrode, used with monopolar mode, is a metal plate or foil with a large surface area so that the return current can be distributed over a large area, and the heating effect at the electrode site can be minimized.

Various sizes of dispersive electrode are available, and one should be selected that is appropriate for the age and size of the patient. In general, the larger the electrode the better [3]. The complete conductive surface of the electrode should be in contact with the patient. It should be positioned as close to the operation site as possible so that the current path is as short as possible, and not across the chest. The site should be clean, shaved if necessary, and over a well-vascularized area, away from bony prominences, scar tissue and implanted prostheses.

Various dispersive electrodes are available, most of which are single-use pre-gelled disposable types. Because burns can result from whole or partial detachment of the dispersive electrode, those with adhesive over the whole surface are better [3].

Dispersive electrodes may or may not have a separate cable. Those with an attached cable are safer. The hazard of the reusable cable is that eventually strands may break, creating a fire hazard from arcing.

OUTPUT ISOLATION

Earthed patient circuits

Current standards for electrosurgical equipment recommend that all patient connections be isolated at DC and mains frequencies [1, 2, 3], to minimize the chance of electric shock and to reduce the possibility of accidental burns. Earlier electrosurgical units had a connection between the dispersive electrode and the earth which prevented the potential of the patient rising above earth potential. The disadvantage is that when the patient becomes energized with mains power, for example from a faulty medical device, mains current flows through the patient to the earthed dispersive electrode, possibly causing severe electric shock and burns.

When the connection between an earthed dispersive electrode and the electrosurgical unit deteriorates or breaks, the high-frequency current can no longer return to the electrosurgical unit. It will seek an alternative return path back to earth and the dispersive electrode terminal on the electrosurgical unit. If any earthed equipment touches the patient it will provide a return path for the high-frequency current; if the contact area is small the resultant high current density will probably cause a serious burn. For safety reasons, electrosurgical units which have earthed dispersive electrodes should be replaced.

Isolated patient connections

The isolated electrosurgical unit has no connection between the patient cables and earth; it has been developed to overcome the hazards inherent in the earthed output. Although high-frequency leakage currents cannot be completely eliminated, present design methods, standards [2, 4] and components ensure that leakage currents are very small.

The isolated electrosurgical unit is safer than earthed units, but if it is energized when the active electrode is not in contact with the patient, the dispersive electrode can rise to a substantial potential above earth, particularly if the active electrode is accidentally earthed. The entire output is then available between the dispersive electrode and the earth, and the patient is in danger of receiving a burn at any site that makes contact with earthed metal.

High-frequency earthed patient connections

To overcome the possibility of a floating dispersive electrode, some manufacturers have earthed the dispersive electrode indirectly through a capacitor which has a very high resistance to mains frequencies, but a very low resistance at electrosurgery frequencies. This configuration clamps the dispersive electrode at earth potential and overcomes the electric shock hazard of the older earthed dispersive electrode. A break in the connection between the dispersive electrode and the electrosurgical unit will still expose the patient to the possibility of burns if the patient is in contact with any earthed metal, and for this reason electrosurgical units with earth-referenced isolated outputs must be fitted with a dispersive electrode monitor.

DISPERSIVE ELECTRODE MONITORS

Cable monitor

Most new electrosurgical units are fitted with a dispersive electrode cable monitor that sounds an alarm and disconnects the output if the dispersive electrode cable breaks or becomes detached. This monitor does *not* provide the operator with any information concerning the connection between the dispersive electrode and the patient — it only monitors the condition of the cable connections.

Contact quality monitor

A more comprehensive monitor is the contact quality monitor, which measures the quality of electrical contact between the dispersive electrode and the patient. These monitors apply a test signal across the two halves of a special dual-foil dispersive electrode, and measure the electrical impedance between the two foils. If the impedance is above or below preset levels, the monitor displays an alarm indicator, sounds an alarm, and disconnects the electrosurgical unit output [3]. The contact quality monitor combines the features of a cable monitor and skin/electrode contact monitor in the one unit.

Standard single-foil electrodes can be used on electrosurgical units fitted with a contact quality monitor, but contact quality will not be measured without dual-foil electrodes. The manufacturer's instructions should be consulted if this arrangement is desired.

The level of protection offered depends on the competence of the user. The monitor is not a substitute for good training and correct use of the equipment.

ELECTROSURGERY AND PACEMAKERS

The high-frequency currents produced when an electrosurgical unit is activated near a pacemaker or pacing wires may interfere with the operation of the pacemaker and in some cases may burn the patient. The rates of internal and external pacemakers are likely to change as a result of the high-frequency interference produced; programmable pacemakers may suffer some degree of reprogramming. For these reasons it is recommended that the manufacturer of the pacemaker is consulted prior to surgery.

An isolated or high-frequency earthed electrosurgical unit should be used. An electrosurgical unit with earthed patient connections is undesirable and must not be used on a patient with an external pacemaker. If possible, the bipolar technique should be used, as it limits the high-frequency current to the region between the bipolar electrodes, and it generally produces less interference.

If the monopolar technique must be used, the dispersive electrode must be placed as close as possible to the surgical site; the dispersive electrode, active electrode and electrosurgical cables should be positioned as far away as possible from the pacemaker and pacemaker leads.

The patient's ECG must be monitored closely for signs of pacemaker interference during the use of electrosurgical units. As a precaution, an alternative pacing source should be available, particularly if the patient is highly dependent on the pacemaker. A cardiac defibrillator should be close at hand.

After the procedure, the pacemaker should be checked, to ensure that it is operating correctly and that none of the programmed functions have changed.

PROCEDURES AND PRECAUTIONS IN THE USE OF ELECTROSURGERY

1 All personnel responsible for using the electrosurgical unit must be familiar with the particular unit concerned, and have basic knowledge of its function and of the various attachments which may be used with it.

2 The manufacturer's instructions for use of the electrosurgery unit should be followed to prevent any injury to patients or staff.

3 The electrosurgical unit and accessories should be checked before use, looking for damaged, burned or broken insulation.

4 Check that the electrosurgical unit has received routine maintenance inspection and testing.

5 Make sure the audible activation tone can be heard.

6 Place the dispersive electrode (patient plate) close to the operation site, which should be dry and not over bony prominences, scar tissue or hairy areas (see above). Use the largest dispersive electrode that will make complete contact of the conductive surface with the patient.

7 Set the current at the lowest level to carry out the particular technique. When there are repeated requests for more current the machine and the attachments should be checked and, if necessary, changed. A decrease in the effectiveness of the electrosurgical unit, at otherwise normal settings, may indicate faulty application of the dispersive electrode, failure of an electrical lead, or excessive accumulation of tissue on the active electrode.

8 When the active electrode is not being used, it must be kept in an insulated sheath [3].

9 The active electrode should not be used in the vicinity of ECG electrodes. Needles should not be used as monitoring electrodes during electrosurgical procedures.

10 The use of an electrosurgical unit on a patient with a cardiac pacemaker is potentially hazardous (see above).

11 Bipolar techniques should be used for small appendages, as in circumcision or finger surgery. Monopolar electrosurgery can cause thrombosis and other unintended injury on small appendages.

12 The electrosurgical unit must not be used in the presence of flammable agents.

13 Check contact between patient and dispersive electrode if the patient is repositioned.

14 Use non-conductive eyepieces with endoscopes.

15 Operating staff must not contact ESU electrodes or cables while the unit output is energized.

REFERENCES

1 Standards Association of Australia. *Guidelines for the use of electrosurgical equipment.* Appendix F of AS 2500–1986, Guide to the safe use of electricity in patient care, (1986), pp. 51–61.
2 AAMI, American National Standard. *Electrosurgical Devices.*

Arlington, VA: Association for the Advancement of Medical Instrumentation, (1986).

3 ECRI, Update: controlling the risks of electrosurgery, and ESU return electrode contact quality monitors. *Health Devices* 1989, **18**, 433–436.

4 International Electrotechnical Commission. *High-frequency electrosurgery equipment*. IEC 601.2.2.

FURTHER READING

ECRI. Electrosurgical Units. *Health Devices* 1987, **16**, 291–342.

Gerhard G.C. Electrosurgical Unit. In: Webster J.G. (Ed) *Encyclopedia of medical devices and instrumentation*, Vol. 2, John Wiley & Sons, New York, (1988), pp. 1180–1203.

2: Cardiac Defibrillation

INTRODUCTION

Electrical defibrillation, or countershock, is the best method of terminating ventricular fibrillation. An electric current is passed through the heart to depolarize a sufficient number of myocardial cells simultaneously. This usually restores normal sinus rhythm, provided the myocardium is oxygenated and is not severely acidotic.

Only trained operators should use a defibrillator, and the safety precautions outlined here and in the operator's manual should be followed. The voltages and electrical energy required for defibrillation are hazardous. All operating theatre staff should be made aware of these dangers.

Although the treatment of ventricular fibrillation is the primary application of the electrical defibrillator, it can also be used for cardioversion of ventricular tachycardia, atrial fibrillation and atrial flutter.

DEFIBRILLATION

Energy requirements

There is a threshold below which the energy is insufficient to terminate ventricular fibrillation.

The energy required to defibrillate children successfully is usually about 2 J/kg [1, 2]. If this dose is insufficient, the energy should be increased to 4 J/kg. If this is unsuccessful twice, attention should be directed to electrode problems, such as inadequate electrode−chest-wall interface, inappropriate electrode position, excessive distance between electrodes or insufficient electrode pressure, or to other physiological problems such as acidosis, hypoxaemia and hypothermia.

For adults and older children it is recommended that an initial defibrillation of approximately 200 J (watt seconds) [3] be used. If this fails, a second shock at a similar energy level should be given immediately. If the second shock is unsuccessful the selected energy should be increased, but to no more than 360 J [4, 5].

The defibrillation energy dose should *not* be increased when the rhythm initially converts but then reverts back to ventricular fibrillation. An antidysrhythmic drug such as lignocaine should be given before further attempts at defibrillation.

Transthoracic impedance

Although defibrillators are calibrated in joules, it is the current that flows through the myocardium that actually defibrillates the heart. The magnitude of this current is determined by the selected energy and the impedance of the thorax. If the impedance is high, the defibrillator will be less effective, and defibrillation may not be possible at normal energy levels. The mean transthoracic impedance in adults is about 60 ohms and slightly less — 57 ohms — in children over 12 kg [6].

Factors that affect transthoracic impedance include energy level, electrode size, the interface between the electrode and the skin, the number and time interval of previous discharges, the phase of ventilation, the distance between electrodes, and the electrode paddle pressure. Minimizing the transthoracic impedance reduces the energy required for successful defibrillation and reduces the heat and risk of burns at paddle sites.

THE EXTERNAL CARDIAC DEFIBRILLATOR

General principles

All defibrillators employ the same basic principle. Electrical energy is stored in a high-voltage capacitor during the charge cycle and switched on to the patient electrodes when the Discharge button is pressed. The capacitor is charged slowly (usually less than 10 seconds) and discharged rapidly into the patient in less than 10 milliseconds. The most common discharge waveform is a rounded pulse in the shape of a heavily damped sinusoid. The peak current available depends upon the transthoracic impedance. The lower the impedance, the higher and more effective will be the discharge.

Most modern defibrillators will discharge the storage capacitor into an internal dummy load, if they are switched off, if the electrodes are unplugged, if the mains power fails on mains-powered units, or if not discharged within a certain preset time (normally 30–120 seconds). Operators should be aware that some older defibrillators may not have these features and the capacitor may remain charged. The operation manual should be consulted for details of the disarming conditions for such machines. A charged defibrillator must be handled with extreme care and an operator should not touch the electrodes once they are plugged into a defibrillator.

Energy indicator

The energy displayed on the energy selector and the energy level indicator on most modern defibrillators is the energy that will be delivered into a 50-ohm load but, in some older defibrillators, the display shows the energy stored in the capacitor. This is misleading, as not all stored energy is delivered to the patient — some is lost inside the machine. Present standards [4, 5] recommend that all the controls and displays indicate the delivered energy. The AAMI/ANSI standard [5] recommends that the delivered energy should be within 4 J or ± 15%,

whichever is the greater, of the selected energy indicated on the energy level indicator, when discharged into a 50-ohm resistive load.

Because the storage capacitor cannot maintain the charge indefinitely, a defibrillator should be charged just prior to discharge and not left in the charged state. Some defibrillators use an energy-refresh circuit to maintain the charge on the capacitor, but discharge may be inhibited during the refresh process.

Features

The patient circuits of defibrillators are required to be isolated from earth to ensure that current is not diverted from the patient's heart to earth, and that the patient is not burned at the site of an alternative pathway. Defibrillators are labelled with symbols indicating the degree of patient protection from leakage current.

Most defibrillators now have the discharge button on the insulated handle of the paddles. Often there is a button on each paddle and the buttons must be pressed simultaneously to effect a discharge. This arrangement ensures that there is less likelihood that the unit will be discharged prematurely. Some defibrillators are equipped with a discharge button on the main unit to enable it to be used with internal paddles which do not have their own discharge switch.

The portable battery-powered defibrillator with integral monitor has become popular in recent years [7]. These units have several advantages, and are generally to be preferred over the mains-powered units. The battery-powered units are usually more portable, can be used if the mains power fails or is unavailable, and, with the integral monitor, can provide a more rapid indication of the patient's rhythm. Most units have synchronized cardioversion and internal defibrillation ability; some are fitted with an annotating strip recorder to provide documentary evidence of the rhythm, dose, electrode impedance, time and date.

External electrodes

Most defibrillators are supplied with reusable external paddle electrodes which have insulated handles, usually with integral charge and discharge controls, and a smooth flat electrode on the opposite face. The handles are designed to have an insulated guard and a long pathway between the operator's hand and the electrode surface, to minimize the chance of electric shock due to surface leakage currents or accidental contact with the electrode.

To avoid burns, there must be low impedance between the skin and the paddle electrodes. This is achieved by using a large surface area applied with firm pressure to the paddles and by improving contact with conductive gel between the paddles and the skin. Sparks at the electrode during discharge are evidence of inadequate contact.

ELECTRODE SIZE

Most defibrillators are equipped with adult and paediatric transthoracic paddle electrodes. Small paediatric paddles, to enable adequate electrode separation and good contact on the chests of infants, have a recommended minimum contact area of 15 cm^2 (4.5 cm diameter) each; the larger paddles for older children and adults have a recommended minimum contact area of 50 cm^2 (8 cm diameter) each [8].

The largest electrode which allows good chest-wall contact over its entire surface should be used to minimize transthoracic impedance. When possible, adult paddles should be used for children [6]. The paediatric paddles should only be required for the very young, in whom the adult paddles cannot make full contact with the skin.

ELECTRODE PLACEMENT

Electrodes must be placed so that as much of the discharge current passes though the heart as possible. Usually one electrode is placed to the right of the sternum just below the clavicle, and the other just below and to the left of the left nipple in the anterior–axillary line. The other common position is to place one paddle anteriorly over the precordium and the other posteriorly behind the heart. Never place electrodes over or close to ECG electrodes or cables.

ELECTRODE GEL

There must be conductive gel between the electrode and the chest wall to minimize the transthoracic impedance and the temperature rise at the electrode skin junction. The gel must cover the entire electrode surface, but must not be allowed to create a path between the electrode surface and the handle, or between the electrodes.

If the latter bridging occurs, nearly all the current will flow between the paddles over the chest, and insufficient current will flow through the heart. If a bridge is formed, wipe excess gel completely from the chest before defibrillating.

Ultrasonic gels must not be used, as they are poor electrical conductors. Alcohol pads must never be used, as they can cause serious burns.

Alternatively, conductive pre-gelled defibrillator pads are available [7]. They reduce smearing and sliding, thereby minimizing the chance of bridging and may make cleaning after the procedure easier, but tend to dry out and lose their electrical properties fairly rapidly; they should only be opened as required and not kept beyond the expiry date.

DISPOSABLE ELECTRODES

Disposable defibrillator electrodes are now available to replace the hand-held paddle [8]. These electrodes consist of a gel-impregnated pad or solid conductive polymer covering a metal-foil electrode on one side and an insulating layer on the other. The conductive gel or polymer side is pressed against the skin and held in place by an adhesive.

Pre-gelled defibrillator pads and disposable electrodes both share the advantage that they avoid the smearing and sliding that can occur with conductive pastes and creams. Disposable electrodes eliminate the need for separate ECG electrodes.

A complete, functional set of paddles and a tube of paste or cream must remain with the defibrillator at all times, in case the disposable electrodes are found to be defective.

INTERNAL DEFIBRILLATION

During cardiac surgery, ventricular fibrillation often occurs or is induced, and when the surgical procedure is completed the heart may spontaneously defibrillate during rewarming. When defibrillation is required, the paddle electrodes are applied directly to the heart.

Because all the energy is delivered directly to the heart, internal defibrillation requires much less energy than transthoracic defibrillation. When internal paddles are attached, defibrillators limit the amount of energy that is available. The AAMI/ANSI standard [5] recommends that the energy output using internal paddles is limited to 50 J. Accidental discharge of energy over 50 J using internal paddles may lead to irreversible cardiac damage [9].

Internal electrodes

The internal electrode is usually a concave disk, which provides good electrical contact with the heart, attached to a long insulated handle. The back surface and all other exposed metal are insulated to prevent leakage of the charge to the surrounding tissue. If electrodes without insulated backs or stems are used, great care must be taken to ensure that these parts do not contact other tissue. Before use, the concave surface of internal paddles should be wet with saline.

The recommended minimum contact area for each internal electrode is 32 cm² (6.4 cm diameter) for adults and 9 cm² (3.4 cm diameter) for children [5].

Internal paddles do not usually have discharge buttons, because it is difficult to protect switches from repeated sterilization. Instead, a defibrillator with the discharge button on the front panel is used. Special care must be exercised to ensure that the defibrillator is not discharged before the paddles are correctly located.

The sterilizing process can cause the paddles' insulation to flake, peel, bubble or chip. They should be checked before use, because damage poses an electrical risk to patient and operator and the danger that flakes may be left in the body.

PROCEDURES AND PRECAUTIONS

Most defibrillators have instructions on the unit, and/or in the operator's instruction manual. All operators should familiarize themselves with these instructions before performing defibrillation.

Although the operating steps vary from one unit to another, the essential operating steps and precautions are as follows:

1 Check that other equipment connected to the patient is defibrillator-protected. If not, disconnect them from the patient.

2 Do not use a defibrillator in the presence of flammable agents, or in areas of high oxygen concentration.

3 A second trained operator should always be nearby when a defibrillator is being used or tested, just in case the operator receives a shock.

4 Check that the paddles are clean and thoroughly dry.

5 If using gel, cover the metal face of the electrodes with the gel. The paddle surfaces can be gently rubbed together to distribute the gel evenly. If using pre-gelled pads, place the pads on the chest at the intended electrode sites. Always use the correct gel, never use ultrasound gel or saline or alcohol-soaked pads.

6 Do not place paddles over or close to ECG electrodes or leads.

7 Check that the defibrillator is in the defibrillate mode and *not* in the synchronized mode.

8 Switch the defibrillator on and select the desired energy level, based on the guidelines given in this appendix.

9 Place the paddles on the patient's chest and apply firm pressure.

10 Do not touch the patient, operating table or any equipment or cables connected to the patient during defibrillation. Ensure that the patient is not touching conductive or metal objects including the table.

11 Press the Charge button. Do not leave the defibrillator whilst it is charged.

12 Warn those in the immediate area that you are about to discharge the defibrillator; check that no one is touching the patient, cables or leads.

13 Press the Discharge buttons whilst holding the paddles firmly against the patient.

14 If unsuccessful, repeat the dose, following the recommendations in this appendix. If using gel, remember to wipe surplus gel from the skin between discharges, to avoid spreading it, thereby providing a path between the electrodes.

15 Turn the unit off as soon as the procedure is complete and return to its storage location.

16 Always clean paddles thoroughly after each use. Follow the manufacturer's cleaning instructions. As a general rule, wipe all paddle surfaces with warm soapy water, but do not immerse.

17 Test the unit weekly by charging it and discharging into the internal test load. The paddles must be in their holders, not apart or shorted together.

SYNCHRONIZED CARDIOVERSION

It is possible to convert other ventricular rhythms and rapid supraventricular rhythms to sinus rhythm with a defibrillator, but for these procedures a defibrillator and a monitor are required, and the defibrillator must be fitted with a syncrhonizer circuit. Where possible, a defibrillator with an integral monitor should be used for cardioversion to ensure accurate timing and correct interconnection.

The synchronizing circuit within the defibrillator detects the patient's R-waves and synchronizes the discharge so that it only occurs on the trailing edge of an

R-wave. When the discharge button is pressed, energy will not be discharged until just after the next R-wave. A marker is usually superimposed on the ECG display to indicate the point in the cardiac cycle at which discharge will occur. If the unit is fitted with a recorder a mark is usually superimposed on the ECG tracing.

Units that have separate ECG leads are preferred for cardioversion. The electrical noise resulting from paddle movement can accidentally initiate a discharge if the external paddles are used for the ECG. Monitoring through self-adhesive defibrillator electrodes is an option that can provide a stable ECG signal. Always inspect the ECG before discharging the defibrillator to ensure that the ECG is of good quality and that the mark appears only on each R-wave. Conduct a test discharge with the paddles in their holders before placing the electrodes on the patient.

Cardioversion requires far less energy than that required for the treatment of ventricular fibrillation. The energy dose for cardioversion for children is likely to be in the range 0.2–1.0 J/kg. The recommended procedure for cardioversion [10] is to start at the lowest energy dose and increase the selected energy of each subsequent trial until the procedure is successful. Attention should be paid to correcting any hypoxaemia, acidosis, hypoglycaemia, or hypothermia. In general a maximum of 50 J is recommended for the initial dose for adults with ventricular tachycardia, 25 J for atrial flutter and 75–100 J for atrial fibrillation and paroxysmal supraventricular tachycardia [10].

Most modern defibrillators revert to the non-synchronized mode when switched off, as recommended in the AAMI/ANSI standard [5], but there are still many units in use which can be switched on in the synchronized mode. Extreme caution must be exercised with these units, as a defibrillator in the synchronized mode may not discharge during treatment of a patient with ventricular fibrillation, and valuable time can be lost.

When synchronized cardioversion is finished, always switch the defibrillator to the non-synchronized mode.

ROUTINE INSPECTIONS AND TESTS [10]

It is suggested that a defibrillator be inspected daily and after each use, to ensure that it is ready for the next emergency. Inspect the unit visually to ensure that it is clean and free from damage, and that the paddles are free from electrode cream and paste. Check the paddles for cracks in the insulation, loose components or pitting of the electrodes; check all cords, connectors, plugs and components for signs of wear or damage. Ensure that the defibrillator has received routine service. Check that all indicator lamps are on and that, if the unit has separate components, such as a separate monitor or battery charger, that they are all properly connected.

If the unit is battery-powered, check that the charger is connected, plugged in and switched on. Most chargers have some indication that the battery is charging. Consult the operator's manual for details. If the unit has a battery condition indicator, temporarily disconnect the charger, test the defibrillator, then reconnect the charger.

The defibrillator should also be tested, at least weekly, to verify that it is fully operational. Some manufacturers provide a routine test schedule in their operating manual, together with testing recommendations. Unless otherwise indicated by the manufacturer, testing should only be performed with the paddles firmly located in their holders. Do not discharge the defibrillator with the paddles shorted together or into the air. Both of these practices place enormous stress on output circuit components, and will shorten the life of the defibrillator.

Routine checks should also be made of the cart or trolley on which the defibrillator rests, to ensure that it is uncluttered, that the wheels rotate freely and that there are no obstructions to the rapid deployment of the unit. Check that there is a sufficient supply of electrode paste and/or disposable pads; if equipped with a monitor, ensure that there are appropriate and sufficient ECG electrodes.

Before leaving the unit, check that it is ready for use and that the defibrillator is *not* in the synchronize mode.

REFERENCES

1 Tacker W.A., Geddes, L.A. *Electrical defibrillation.* CRC Press, Florida, (1980).

2 Gutgesell H.P., *et al.* Energy dose for ventricular defibrillation of children. *Paediatrics* 1976, **58**, 898–901.

3 Standards and guidelines for cardiopulmonary resuscitation (CPR) and emergency cardiac care (ECC). *JAMA* 1986, **255**, 2905–2984.

4 International Electrotechnical Commission. *Particular requirements for the safety of cardiac defibrillators and cardiac defibrillator monitors.* IEC 601.2.4, 1983.

5 AAMI/ANSI, American National Standard. *Cardiac defibrillator devices.* DF2–1989, Arlington, VA: Association for the Advancement of Medical Instrumentation, (1989).

6 Atkins D.L., *et al.* pediatric defibrillation: importance of paddle size in determining transthoracic impedance. *Paediatrics* 1988, **82**, 914–918.

7 Emergency Care Research Institute. Battery-powered defibrillator monitors. *Health Devices* 1987, **16**, 183−216.

8 Emergency Care Research Institute. Disposable defibrillator pads and electrodes. *Health Devices* 1990, **19**, 33−56.

9 Emergency Care Research Institute. Line-powered defibrillators. *Health Devices* 1983, **12**, 291−314.

10 Standards Association of Australia. *Use and testing of cardiac DC defibrillators*. Appendix D of AS 2500−1986, Guide to the Safe Use of Electricity in Patient Care, (1986), pp. 43−46.

3: Cardiopulmonary Bypass

COMPONENTS

Open heart surgery requires substitution of the pumping action of the heart and the gas exchange function of the lungs. The basic components of the cardiopulmonary bypass circuit are:

1 Blood reservoir
2 Heat exchanger
3 Oxygenator
4 Pump
5 Arterial filter.

Additional pumps provide variable suction return from the chambers of the heart. The reservoir contains a large pore size polyester filter to remove large particulate matter from the blood.

Blood reservoir

This is usually integrated with the oxygenator but it may be separate. It is designed to hold a large volume of blood, and to defoam gas emboli generated by intracardiac and intrapericardial suction.

Heat exchangers

The heat exchanger is usually integrated with the oxygenator and blood reservoir in modern equipment, but can be separate. It is designed to minimize trauma to the blood components while providing an optimal surface area between the blood path and a counter-current flow of water, to maximize thermal transfer. Blood cooling and rewarming is achieved by pumping water at a controlled temperature through this device. The construction of the heat exchanger should ensure that there is no possibility of water or air leaking into the blood compartment.

Because the solubility of gases falls with rising temperature, oxygen microbubbles may form during rewarming. The heat exchanger should be placed on the venous side of the circuit to avoid this complication.

Oxygenators

Bubble oxygenators (Bentley, Harvey, Shiley, Cobe, Travenol, Rygg) achieve gas exchange in a bubble column. Oxygen (and other gases) is bubbled directly into the venous blood returning from the patient, while carbon dioxide is driven off. The blood is debubbled in a defoaming section, which has a large surface area of material, such as polyurethane foam, covered with an antifoaming agent. The blood is then collected into the arterial reservoir. The size of bubbles created by the oxygen diffuser determine the gas transfer capacity of the device. Small bubbles have an increased ratio of surface area to bubble gas volume and provide maximal oxygen transfer, but carbon dioxide removal is less efficient and the bubbles are not easily removed by the defoaming device. The opposite is true for large bubbles, so the best compromise is either medium-sized bubbles or a mixture of bubble sizes. Blood trauma and haemolysis result from excessive turbulence at the gas−blood interface. It can be minimized by improving the efficiency of the bubbling column and equalizing the flows of gases and blood.

Bubble oxygenators are still used and a number of simple, convenient, disposable units are available. The major disadvantage of these devices are the frequency and size of microemboli produced, which are very difficult to remove completely.

Membrane oxygenators (Bard, Bentley, Cobe, Medtronic, Travenol, Terumo, Sci-Med) have a gas-permeable membrane between the oxygenating gas and the blood. Gas transfer is determined by the permeability of the membrane material to the gas and the rate of diffusion, which is proportional to the difference in the pressures of the gas on either side of the membrane. It is independent of other gases which may be present. The usual pressure differential is greater for oxygen than CO_2. In order to compensate for this difference a silicone rubber membrane, which is six times as permeable to CO_2 as it is to oxygen, is often used.

The efficiency of membrane oxygenators depends on the diffusion capability of the membrane, the surface area and thickness of the blood film, and the pattern of flow of blood and gas through the oxygenator. Several efficient and reliable membrane oxygenators are currently available and widely used. The Cobe VPCML has compartmented membranes, which enables a single oxygenator with a minimal prime volume to be suitable for perfusion of small infants as well as larger patients.

Membrane oxygenators prevent direct contact between gas and blood and thereby minimize blood trauma, protein denaturation, haemolysis, platelet damage and gas emboli. Their use has been an important factor in reducing the pulmonary and cerebral complications bypass in infants.

Blood pumps

Roller pumps, which produce flow by compressing the wall of the tubing between the roller and the backing plate, are usually employed thus pushing blood out in front of the roller. Blood trauma is minimized if rollers are set so that they are slightly non-occlusive. Flow rate depends on the diameter of the tubing and the pump speed.

The *constrained vortex pump* is another device which can be used to propel blood. It is primarily used as a ventricular assist device (VAD) or for extracorporeal membrane oxygenation (ECMO). Circular motion is imparted to the blood by vaneless rotor cones which are spun by a magnetic linkage to the main drive, creating a pressure gradient from the centre to the outside of the cone. Flow is thus generated by providing an outlet on the cone periphery at a right-angle to the cone radius.

Arterial filters

Several disposable blood filters have been developed to minimize the entry of microemboli into the patient. These may result from gas bubbles or damage to blood by suction, the oxygenator, the pumps or contact with foreign surfaces. These cause platelet—leucocyte aggregation, plasma protein denaturation, and particulate microemboli. There is some argument about how effectively these filters remove air emboli or denatured proteins, but they are effective at removing fibrin material and platelet aggregates. In the extra-corporeal circuit they are placed so that the blood is filtered just before it returns to the patient. They should function at an appro-priate flow without causing undue haemolysis and should be easily primed and debubbled.

Line pressure should be monitored so that line obstruction or filter occlusion is detected.

METHOD OF OPERATION

Cardiopulmonary bypass is usually achieved either by cannulating both vena cavae via the right atrium and applying snares so that all blood returning via the vena cava drains into the bypass circuit, or by single cannulation of the right atrium. Arterialized blood is usually returned to the systemic circulation via the aorta, but sometimes the femoral artery is used, particularly in the event of re-operation.

Some blood other than that coming via the vena cava still enters the heart. The majority is coronary sinus flow, and it must be returned to the reservoir via a separate sucker.

The usual pump flow rates are 150 ml/kg for infants under 10 kg and 2.4 × surface area l/min for patients over 10 kg.

CARDIOPLEGIA

Many cardiac surgical operations have become longer and more complicated. The adequacy of myocardial protection is an important determinant of outcome. The infusion of cardioplegic solution into the coronary circulation will induce immediate cardiac arrest in diastole, with complete cessation of electromechanical activity. This enables any energy produced by anaerobic metabolism to be used in the maintenance of cell membrane integrity.

The following are the principles involved in constituting and administering cardioplegic solution:

1 Immediate arrest should be produced to reduce energy demands and avoid energy depletion by ischaemic electromechanical work. Arrest can be achieved by the use of potassium, magnesium, procaine or with a hypocalcaemic solution.

2 The solution should be administered at a temperature of 6–10°C to cool the heart, thereby reducing metabolic rate and assisting arrest.

3 A buffer such as bicarbonate, THAM or phosphate is added to provide an appropriate pH to optimize hypothermic metabolism and maintain cell membrane integrity.

4 Membrane stability (e.g. with procaine or steroids) is

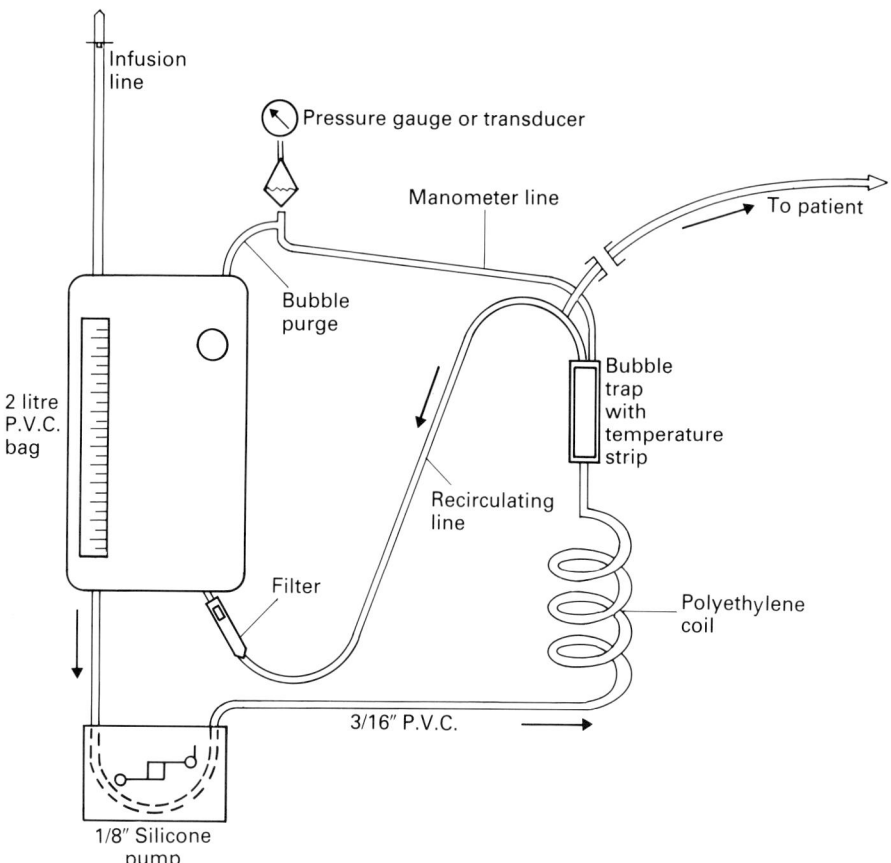

Fig. A3.1 System used for administration of cardioplegic solution. The patient line is clamped while the fluid is recirculated. When the solution is to be delivered to the patient the patient line clamp is released and the recirculating line is clamped.

important in the prevention of cell disruption. It also minimizes the potential for intracellular biochemical dysfunction. Severe hypocalcaemia must be avoided because it can damage sarcolemmal membranes.

5 The solution should be slightly hyperosmolar (about 350 mmol/l) to minimize myocardial oedema from ischaemic damage.

6 Oxygen, glucose and other substrates (e.g. aspartate, glutamate) should be provided for continued anaerobic or aerobic energy production during aortic cross-clamping.

Administration of cardioplegia

The solution is given at a rate of 110 ml/min for 4 minutes and then for 2 minutes every 20 minutes using the circuit shown in Fig. A3.1. It is usually delivered at a pressure of 30 mmHg to neonates and at 40 mmHg to patients from 4–10 kg. Pressures in larger patients are usually 40–100 mmHg, the higher pressures being used when the ventricle is hypertrophied. Pressure is monitored at all times to prevent damage from excessive pressure.

The composition of 500 ml perfusate for patients under 10 kg is one bag (385 ml) cardioplegia base solution, 100 ml 20% w/v albumin and 26 ml cardioplegia buffer solution. For children over 10 kg, to one bag of cardioplegia base solution is added 100 ml normal (0.9%) saline, 20 ml 12.5% mannitol (to provide osmolality) and 5 ml 8.4% sodium bicarbonate (1 mmol/ml) as buffer.

Reperfusion

Special formulae solutions may be used for patients with severe ventricular dysfunction who require extended ischaemic periods during cardiac surgery, resulting in impaired cell metabolism and inefficient oxygen use during reperfusion. They often have depleted energy reserves. Infusion of a warm, hyperkalaemic, hypocalcaemic, oxygenated, leucocyte-filtered blood solution can be used to resuscitate energy-depleted hearts after extended periods of aortic cross-clamping. Enrichment with amino acid precursors of Kreb's cycle intermediates improves oxygen utilization, potentially facilitating cell repair, and provides energy reserves to sustain metabolism during ischaemia.

4: Glossary of Operations for Congenital Heart Disease

Blalock—Taussig shunt Connection of subclavian artery (R or L) to pulmonary artery (R or L), either directly (classic) or via a PTFE (Gore-tex) tube (modified). Used for palliation of various cyanotic lesions with low pulmonary blood flow.

Glenn shunt End-to-side connection of SVC to RPA, with ligation of SVC at the RA end and interruption of PA between the shunt and PA bifurcation. Used for palliation in various types of univentricular hearts.

Kawashima shunt (bidirectional cavopulmonary shunt, bi-directional Glenn shunt) Connection of SVC to RPA with ligation of proximal SVC and main PA. Used for various types of univentricular hearts (or as a definitive operation if an interrupted IVC is present).

Fontan operation Routing of all systemic venous return into the pulmonary circulation, usually with part of the RA but no ventricle in the circuit. It is used as a definitive operation for various types of univentricular heart.

Jatene operation (arterial switch) Transection of the proximal aorta and PA with anastomosis of proximal PA to the distal aorta and vice versa. The coronary arteries are excised from the aortic sinus and anastomosed to the pulmonary (neo-aortic) sinuses. It is used for repair of transposition of great arteries in neonates.

Rastelli operation An intraventricular baffle is placed to route left-ventricular blood through a VSD into the aorta. The RV is connected to the PA via a valved extracardiac conduit. It is used for transposition with VSD and left-ventricular outflow tract obstruction. ('Rastelli' is often used to describe any operation involving placement of a RV-to-PA conduit.)

Senning operation (atrial switch) Flaps of atrial septum and free wall used to direct caval blood to the mitral valve and pulmonary venous blood to the tricuspid valve. It is used for infants with transposition of the great arteries.

Norwood operation (1) Connection of the proximal PA to the aorta using a homograft patch to enlarge the aortic arch, with pulmonary blood flow re-established via modified Blalock—Taussig shunt. It is used for palliation of hypoplastic left-heart syndrome in the newborn.

Takeuchi operation Connection of an anomalous left coronary artery (from PA) to the aortic root via an intra-PA baffle leading from the coronary ostium to a surgically created aortopulmonary window. It is used for ALCAPA syndrome (anomalous left coronary artery from PA).

Konno operation Enlargement of the left-ventricular outflow tract by a patch enlargement of the aortic annulus and ventricular septum, and replacement of the aortic valve with a homograft or mechanical prosthesis. It is used in the treatment of left-ventricular outflow tract obstruction with a small aortic annulus, and/or severe subaortic stenosis.

5: Standards Relating to Anaesthesia

The following represents a list, by no means exhaustive, of English-language standards relating to anaesthesia.

Australian Standards Association

AS 1169–1982	Minimizing of combustion hazards arising from the medical use of flammable anaesthetic agents
AS 1944–1987	Medical gas cylinder identification
AS 2120–1977	Rules for suction systems for medical use in hospitals
AS 2385–1980	Single-use (sterile) infusion sets for general medical use
AS 2485–1981	Single-use winged intravenous devices (sterile) for general medical use
AS 2472–1985	Valves for medical gas cylinders
AS 2473–1985	Valves for compressed gas cylinders (threaded outlet)
AS 2488–1981	Resuscitators, resuscitator containers and resuscitator kits
AS 2496–1981	Breathing attachments for anaesthetic purposes for human use
AS 2568–1987	Medical gases — Purity of compressed medical breathing air
AS 2684–1984	Medical equipment — Humidifiers, for medical use
AS 2896–1986	Medical gas systems — Installation and testing of non-flammable medical gas pipeline systems
AS 2901–1986	Medical devices — Characteristics of audible and visible alarm signals
AS 2902–1986	Medical gas systems — Low-pressure flexible connecting assemblies (hose assemblies)
AS 3655–1989	Sphygmomanometers
AS 2500–1986	Guide to the safe use of electricity in patient care
AS 3003–1985	Electrical installations — Patient treatment areas of hospitals and medical and dental practices
AS 3200–1990	Approval and test specification — Electromedical equipment — General requirements
AS 3202–1989	Approval and test specification — Electrosurgical equipment
AS 3203–1981	Approval and test specification for electrocärdiographs
AS 3204–1981	Approval and test specification for cardiac defibrillators
AS 3551–1988	Acceptance testing and in-service testing — Electromedical equipment

American National Standards Institute

ANSI Z79.2–1976	Tracheal tube connectors and adaptors
ANSI Z79.3–1983	Oropharyngeal and nasopharyngeal airways
ANSI Z79.4–1983	Anesthetic reservoir bags
ANSI Z79.8–1979	Anesthesia machines for human use, minimum performance and safety requirements for components and systems of continuous flow
ANSI Z79.9–1979	Humidifiers and nebulizers for medical use
ANSI Z79.10–1979	Oxygen analysers for monitoring patient breathing mixtures, requirements for
ANSI Z79.11–1982	Scavenging systems for excess anesthetic gases
ANSI Z79.13–1981	Oxygen concentrators for medical use
ANSI Z79.14–1983	Tracheal tubes
ANSI Z79.16–1983	Cuffed orotracheal and nasotracheal tubes for prolonged use

American Society for Testing & Materials

F927–86	Specification for pediatric tracheostomy tubes
F965–85	Specification for rigid laryngoscopes for tracheal intubation
F1054–87	Specification for conical fittings of 15 mm and 22 mm sizes

F1101−90	Specification for ventilators intended for use during anesthesia
F1161−88	Specification for minimum performance and safety requirements for components and systems for anesthesia gas machines
F1204−88	Specification for anesthesia reservoir bags
F1205−88	Specification for anesthesia breathing tubes
F1208−89	Specification for minimum performance and safety requirements for anesthesia breathing systems
F1242−89	Specification for cuffed and uncuffed tracheal tubes
F1243−89	Specification for tracheal tube connectors

British Standards Institute

DIN 13252 A1−1991	Inhalation anaesthetic apparatus: requirements for safety and testing: amendment 1
BS 3353:1987	ISO 5362−1986 Specification for anaesthetic reservoir bags
BS 3849:Part 1:1988	ISO 5356−1:1986 Conical connectors for anaesthetic and respiratory equipment. Specification for cones and sockets (excluding 8.5 mm size)
BS 3849:Part 2:1988	ISO 5356−2:1987 Conical connectors for anaesthetic and respiratory equipment. Specification for screw-threaded weight-bearing connectors
BS 3849:Part 4:1990	Conical connectors for anaesthetic and respiratory equipment. Specification for 8.5 mm cones and sockets
BS 4272:Part 3:1989	Anaesthetic and analgesic machines. Specification for continuous-flow anaesthetic machines
BS 5724:Section 2.13:1990: IEC 601−2−13:1989	Medical electrical equipment. Particular requirements for safety. Specifications for anaesthetic machines
BS 6834:1987	Specification for active anaesthetic gas scavenging systems

International Standards Organisation

ISO 5356−1−1987	Anaesthetic and respiratory equipment: Conical connectors: Part 1: Cones and sockets
ISO/DIS 5358−1990	Anaesthetic machines for use with humans (revision of ISO 5358:1980)
ISO/DIS 5367−1989	Breathing tubes intended for use with anaesthetic apparatus and ventilators
ISO/DIS 5369−1988	Breathing machines for medical use — lung ventilators
ISO/DIS 7281−1988	Anaesthetic gas scavenging systems
ISO 8185−1988	Humidifiers for medical use — Safety requirements
ISO/DIS 9360−1990	Anaesthetic and respiratory equipment: heat and moisture exchangers for use in humidifying respired gases in humans
ISO 32−1977	Gas cylinders for medical use — Marking for identification of content
ISO 407−1983	Small medical gas cylinders — Yoke type valve connections

International Electrotechnical Commission

IEC 513−1976	Basic aspects of the safety philosophy, electrical equipment used in medical practice
IEC 529−1976	Classification of degrees of protection provided by enclosures
IEC 536−1976	Classification of electrical and electronic equipment with regard to protection against electric shock
IEC 601−1988	Safety of medical electrical equipment. Part 1: General requirements. Part 2: Particular requirements for the safety of anaesthetic machines. First ed. 1977. Amendment No. 1 (1984). Part 2: Particular requirements for the safety of anaesthetic machines
IEC 825−1990	Radiation safety for laser products; equipment classification, and user's guide

Compressed Gas Association (US)

Pamphlet C9−1973	Standard color-marking of compressed gas cylinders intended for medical use in the United States
Pamphlet M1−1972	Standard for 22 mm anaesthesia breathing circuit connectors
Pamphlet V1−1977	Compressed gas cylinder valve outlet and inlet connectors
Pamphlet P2−	Characteristics and safe handling of medical gases

Canadian Standards Association

Z168.1−M83	Tracheal tubes
Z168.3−M84	Continuous-flow inhalation anaesthetic apparatus (anaesthetic machines) for medical use
Z168.5−M78	Lung ventilators

Z168.4—M83   Keyed filling devices for anaesthetic
                  vaporizers

Z168.6—M81   Oxygen analysers

Z168.8—M82   Anaesthetic gas scavenging systems

Z168.9—M86   Breathing systems for use in anaesthesia

C22.2 No
125—M1984   Electromedical equipment

6: Protocol for Checking
an Anaesthetic Machine Before Use

1 Bulk gas supply and reserve cylinders

1.1 Check bulk gas warning lights or gauges.

1.2 Check level of contents of all cylinders on the anaesthetic machine.

    1.2.1 First open and then close each cylinder valve in turn, observing the related cylinder pressure gauge.

    1.2.2 A falling pressure on the cylinder pressure gauge indicates a high pressure leak.

    1.2.3 Reopen each cylinder valve in turn and then, with the bulk gas supply disconnected, open the appropriate flowmeter to check that gas is able to pass from the cylinder through the flowmeter. Finally, close each cylinder valve after each cylinder is tested.

1.3 Replace oxygen cylinders less than one-quarter full.

1.4 Test oxygen failure warning device.

    1.4.1 With nitrous oxide flowing at 2 l/min turn off or disconnect machine oxygen supply.

    1.4.2 Press emergency oxygen button to release the oxygen pressure in the machine. The audible warning device, if present, should operate. Devices fitted which operate to interrupt the flow of nitrous oxide when the oxygen supply fails should do so within 10 seconds.

    1.4.3 Restore the oxygen supply to the machine and the warning devices should cease to operate.

1.5 'One gas' test (this eliminates the possibility of crossed pressure hoses).

    1.5.1 Check that the high-pressure gas hose for oxygen is connected to the correct wall outlet or large cylinder regulator, and to the oxygen inlet on the machine.

    1.5.2 Check that the oxygen analyser is correctly calibrated and that the low-oxygen alarm is working.

    1.5.3 With the oxygen supply 'ON', turn off or disconnect all other gas sources.

    1.5.4 After other gases have been bled from the machine, open all flowmeter controls and check that only oxygen flows as detected by the oxygen analyser.

1.6 Connect the high-pressure gas hoses for nitrous oxide to the correct wall outlet or large cylinder regulator, and to the nitrous oxide inlet on the machine.

    1.6.1 Restore nitrous oxide flow to the machine and check that nitrous oxide flows in the correct flowmeter.

1.7 If air is available, connect the high-pressure gas hose for air to the correct wall outlet or large cylinder regulator, and to the air inlet on the machine. Turn on the air flowmeter and check that the oxygen analyser detects 21% oxygen. Repeat this test for the reserve air cylinder.

2 Flowmeters

2.1 Ensure that the indicator device moves freely.

2.2 Turn off each flowmeter control and check that the position of the indicator device is at zero when no gas flows.

3 Vaporizers

3.1 Check each vaporizer in turn.

    3.1.1 That it is seated correctly and locked in place when applicable.

    3.1.2 That it *can* be turned *on*.

    3.1.3 That it *is* turned *off*.

    3.1.4 That it contains sufficient amount of the correct liquid agent.

    3.1.5 That the filling and emptying ports are closed.

3.2 If flammable agents are to be used, the appropriate safety conditions and procedures must be observed.

4 Test for leaks upstream of the common gas outlet

4.1 Turn on the oxygen rotameter to 2 l/min and occlude the common gas outlet for 10 seconds. If the rotameter bobbin does not fall, take steps to detect the sites of leakage.

4.2 Repeat this test with each vaporizer turned 'off' and 'on' in turn.

4.3 If gas flows of less than 1 l/min are to be used, more precise testing should be performed to determine the leakage flow rate.

5 Breathing system selection

5.1 Check that the gas supply is connected to the selected breathing systems.

5.2 Check that the size of the tube used to make this connection is adequate to cope with anticipated gas flows.

6 Circle absorption system

6.1 Soda lime — check that this is not exhausted. Renew if necessary, and remove dust from soda lime when refilling canister.

6.2 Breathing hoses — check that these are correctly and firmly connected.

6.3 Valve function and leaks in breathing system.

6.3.1 Close spill valve and attach a spare breathing bag to the patient connection line of the Y-piece.

6.3.2 Depress the *emergency oxygen* button to fill the breathing bag.

6.3.3 Alternatively squeeze the two bags to ensure that oxygen passes from one bag to the other and check visually that each unidirectional valve functions correctly.

6.3.4 Squeeze both bags simultaneously to raise the pressure in the circuit to approximately $30\,cmH_2O$. Maintain pressure for 5 seconds, to test for major leaks.

6.3.5 If gas flows of less than 1 l/min are to be used, more precise testing should be performed to determine the leakage flow rate.

6.3.6 Open spill valve and check that gas spills easily when both bags are squeezed.

6.4 Disconnect *spare* breathing bag and replace with a mask suitable for the patient.

7 Scavenging system

7.1 Check that the scavenging system is connected correctly to the selected breathing system.

7.2 Check that all components of the scavenging system are unencumbered and allow free gas flow.

7.3 If negative pressure is used to aid scavenging check that this does not empty the breathing system.

7.3.1 Fill the breathing system with oxygen by occluding the patient outlet and depressing the emergency oxygen button.

7.3.2 Check that the circuit does not empty when the spill valve is opened.

7.3.3 Close the spill valve again when this check has been done.

8 Apparatus mounted on the anaesthetic machine

8.1 Other apparatus to be used in the conduct of the anaesthetic should be checked according to the protocol appropriate to the device.

8.2 Special attention should be given to:

8.2.1 Equipment for intubation of the trachea.

8.2.2 Suction apparatus.

8.2.3 Gas analysis devices.

8.2.4 Monitoring apparatus.

8.2.5 Ventilators.

8.2.6 Disconnection alarm. This should be checked to ensure that the alarm functions when the breathing system is disconnected from the patient airway.

Guidelines produced by Australian and New Zealand College of Anaesthetists (T2 1990)

7: Monitoring during Anaesthesia

INTRODUCTION

Attempts to set minimal standards of monitoring have been made in several countries. An attempt is also being made to develop graded monitoring standards which can be applied in less affluent countries, but which gradually evolve to higher levels. The standards included here are those set by the Australian and New Zealand College of Anaesthetists.

The monitoring of certain fundamental physiological variables during anaesthesia is recommended. Clinical judgement will determine how long monitoring should be continued following completion of anaesthesia.

Some or all of these basic recommendations will need to be exceeded routinely, depending on the physical status of the patient, the type and complexity of the surgery to be performed, and the requirements of anaesthesia. Occasionally some of the recommended methods of monitoring may be impractical or inappropriate. Departments of anaesthesia should establish policies to deal with such circumstances.

The described monitoring methods may fail to detect unfavourable clinical developments and their use does not guarantee any specific patient outcome.

The following recommendations refer to patients undergoing general anaesthesia or major regional anaesthesia for diagnostic or therapeutic procedures, and should be interpreted in conjunction with other policy documents published by the College of Anaesthetists. All policy documents are revised from time to time as required by changing clinical practice and developments in technology.

The Health Care Facility in which the procedure is being performed is responsible for the provision of equipment for anaesthesia and monitoring on the advice of one or more designated specialist anaesthetists, and for effective maintenance of this equipment.

1 Personnel

Clinical monitoring by a vigilant anaesthetist is the basis of patient care during anaesthesia. This should be supplemented by appropriate devices to assist the anaesthetist.

A medical practitioner whose sole responsibility is the provision of anaesthetic care for that patient must be constantly present from induction of anaesthesia until safe transfer to recovery room staff or intensive care unit has been accomplished. Such medical practitioner must be appropriately trained in anaesthesia, or be a trainee anaesthetist supervised in accordance with the Faculty Guidelines for Supervision of Trainees in Anaesthesia (Faculty Policy Document E3).

In exceptional circumstances brief absences of the person primarily responsible for the anaesthetic may be unavoidable. In such circumstances that person shall delegate, temporarily, observation of the patient to an appropriately qualified person who is judged to be competent for the task.

The individual anaesthetist is responsible for monitoring the patient and should ensure that appropriate monitoring equipment is available. Where there is an environmental risk to staff, e.g. radiation, adequate facilities must exist to enable remote patient monitoring.

2 Patient monitoring

2.1 Circulation

The circulation must be monitored at frequent and clinically appropriate intervals by detection of the arterial pulse and measurement of the arterial blood pressure.

2.2 Respiration

Respiration must be monitored continuously by observation of rate and depth.

2.3 Oxygenation

The patient must be observed at frequent intervals for evidence of central cyanosis. If an oximeter is in use its displayed values should be assessed by frequent observation of the patient.

3 Equipment

3.1 Oxygen supply failure alarms

An automatically activated device to monitor oxygen supply pressure and to warn of low pressure must be fitted to the anaesthetic machine.

3.2 Oxygen analyser

A device incorporating an audible signal to warn of low oxygen concentrations, correctly fitted in the breathing system, must be in continuous operation for every patient when an anaesthetic machine is in use.

3.3 Pulse oximeter

Pulse oximetry provides evidence of the level of oxygen saturation of the haemoglobin of arterial blood and identifies arterial pulsation at the site of application. A pulse oximeter must be exclusively available for every anaesthetized patient.

3.4 Alarms for breathing system disconnection or ventilator failure

When an automatic ventilator is in use, a device capable of warning promptly of a breathing system disconnection or ventilator failure must be in continuous operation. It is desirable that this device be automatically activated.

3.5 Electrocardiograph

Equipment to monitor and continually display the electrocardiograph must be available for every anaesthetized patient.

3.6 Temperature monitor

Equipment to monitor temperature continuously must be available for every anaesthetized patient.

3.7 Carbon dioxide monitor

A carbon dioxide monitor must be exclusively available for every intubated and ventilated patient.

3.8 Neuromuscular function monitor

Equipment to monitor neuromuscular function must be available for those patients in whom neuromuscular paralysis has been induced.

3.9 Other equipment

When clinically indicated, equipment to monitor other physiological variables should be available.

ANZ College of Anaesthetists Document P 18 (1990)

Index

537